CLINICAL VIROLOGY

The Evaluation and Management
of Human Viral Infections

EDITED BY

ROBERT DEBRÉ, M.D.

and

JOSETTE CELERS, M.D.

With 58 International Authorities

W. B. SAUNDERS COMPANY

Philadelphia London Toronto 1970

W. B. Saunders Company: West Washington Square
Philadelphia, Pa. 19105

12 Dyott Street
London WCIA 1DB

1835 Yonge Street
Toronto 7, Ontario

Title of the original French Edition: DEBRÉ et CELERS *Clinique Virologique*
Editions Medicales Flammarion, Paris, 1970.

English translation published by W. B. Saunders Company.
Philadelphia, 1970.

Clinical Virology: The Evaluation and Management of Human Viral Infection   SBN 0-7216-3008-1

Print No.:   9   8   7   6   5   4   3   2   1

Contributors

DANIEL ALAGILLE, M.D.

Maître de Conférences Agrégé à la Faculté de Médecine de Paris, Médecin des Hôpitaux de Paris, Hôpital Parrot, Bicêtre

CLAUDE ATTAL, M.D.

Médecin des Hôpitaux de Paris, Hôpital des Enfants Malades, Paris

MAURICE AUBRY, M.D.

Membre de L'Académie de Médecine, Professeur de Clinique d'Oto-rhino-laryngologie, Médecin des Hôpitaux de Paris, Service d'Oto-rhino-laryngologie, Hôpital Lariboisière, Paris

BERTRANNE AUVERT, M.D.

Maître de Conférences Agrégé à la Faculté de Médecine de Paris, Ophtalmologiste de l'Hôpital Saint Louis, Paris

M. J. F. BALTAZARD, M.D.

Chef de Service, Institut Pasteur, Paris

JEAN BERNARD, M.D.

Professeur à la Faculté de Médecine de Paris, Médecin de l'Hôpital Saint Louis, Paris

ANDRÉ BOUÉ, M.D.

Maître de Recherches au Centre National de la Recherche Scientifique, Laboratoire de la Société d'Etudes et de Soins pour les Enfants Poliomyélitiques, Paris

JOËLLE G. BOUÉ, M.D.

Chargée de Recherches au Centre National de la Recherche Scientifique, Laboratoire de la Société d'Etudes et de Soins pour les Enfants Poliomyélitiques, Paris

FERNAND BRICOUT, M.D.

Professeur Agrégé à la Faculté de Médecine, Biologiste des Hôpitaux de Paris, Hôpital Trousseau, Paris

MARCEL CAPPONI, M.D.

Chef de Laboratoire, Institut Pasteur, Paris

RENÉ CARAVANO, M.D.

Maître de Recherches a l'Institut National de la Santé et de la Recherche Médicale, Centre International de l'Enfance, Paris

GENEVIÈVE CATEIGNE,
Docteur ès Sciences

Chef du Centre National de la Grippe, Institut Pasteur, Paris

JOSETTE CELERS, M.D.

Chef de Section Laboratoire National Santé Publique, Directeur Scientifique, Groupe de Recherches U73 de l'Institut National de la Santé et de la Recherche Médicale, Société d'Etudes et de Soins pour les Enfants Poliomyélitiques, Paris

ROBERT M. CHANOCK, M.D.

Chief, Laboratory of Infectious Diseases, National Institute of Allergy and Infectious Diseases, National Institutes of Health, Bethesda, Maryland, Academic Staff, Children's Hospital, Washington, D.C.

CHARLES CHANY, M.D.

Professeur Agrégé à la Faculté de Médecine de Paris, Biologiste des Hôpitaux, Groupe de Recherche sur les Virus, Institut National de la Santé et de la Recherche Médicale, Hôpital Saint Vincent de Paul, Paris

J. COLOMBANI, M.D.

Professeur Agrégé à la Faculté de Médecine de Rennes, Hôpital Saint Louis, Paris

GABRIEL COSCAS, M.D.

Chef de Clinique à la Faculté de Médecine de Paris, Assistant des Hôpitaux de Paris, Clinique Ophtalmologique, Hôtel-Dieu, Paris

JACQUES COUVREUR, M.D.

Médecin Assistant des Hôpitaux de Paris, Hôpital Trousseau, Paris

ROBERT DEBRÉ, M.D.

Membre de l'Académie des Sciences et de l'Académie de Médecine, Paris

FRITS DEKKING, M.D., Ph.D.

Professor of Virology, University of Amsterdam, Attending Bacteriologist, Emma Children's Hospital, Amsterdam

VICTORIA DROUHET, M.D.

Maître de Recherches à l'Institut National de la Santé et de la Recherche Médicale, Chef du Laboratoire de Virologie, Société d'Etudes et de Soins pour les Enfants Poliomyélitiques, Paris

PAULETTE DUC-GOIRAN, M.D.

Groupe de Recherches sur les Virus, Institut National de la Santé et de la Recherche Médicale, Paris

J. ALASTAIR DUDGEON, M.D., M.C., F.C. Path.

Consultant Microbiologist, The Hospital for Sick Children and Institute of Child Health, London

GÉRARD DUHAMEL, M.D.

Professeur Agrégé à la Faculté de Médecine de Paris, Hôpital Saint Antoine, Paris

EDITH FARKAS-BARGETON, M.D.

Maître de Recherches à l'Institut National de la Santé et de la Recherche Médicale, Attachée de Biologie, Hôpital Saint Vincent de Paul, Paris

BERTHE FERIGNAC

Unité de Recherches sur les Virus, Institut National de la Santé et de la Recherche Médicale, Hôpital Saint Vincent de Paul, Paris

SVEN GARD, M.D.

Professor of Virology, Karolinska Institutet Medical School, Stockholm

MARTHE GAUTIER, M.D.

Maître de Recherches à l'Institut National de la Santé et de la Recherche Médicale, Service de Cardiologie Infantile, Hôpital Parrot, Bicêtre

PAUL GIROUD, M.D.

Membre de l'Académie de Médecine, Chef du Service des Rickettsioses, Institut Pasteur, Paris

BERNARD GRENIER, M.D.

Professeur Agrégé à la Faculté de Tours, Assistant, Centre de Pédiatrie de Clocheville, Tours

FRANÇOISE HAGUENAU, M.D.

Directeur de Recherches à l'Institut National de Santé et de Recherche Médicale, Sous-directeur de Laboratoire, Collège de France, Paris

CLAUDE HANNOUN,
Docteur ès Sciences

Chef de Laboratoire, Institut Pasteur, Paris

JEAN HEWITT, M.D.

Professeur Agrégé de Dermatologie, Hôpital Broca, Paris

JEAN-CLAUDE JOB, M.D.

Médecin des Hôpitaux de Paris, Hôpital Saint Vincent de Paul, Paris

MICHAEL KATZ, M.D.

Associate Member, The Wistar Institute of Anatomy and Biology, Assistant Professor of Pediatrics, School of Medicine, University of Pennsylvania, Associate Physician, Children's Hospital of Philadelphia

HILARY KOPROWSKI, M.D.

Director, The Wistar Institute of Anatomy and Biology, Wistar Professor of Research Medicine, School of Medicine, University of Pennsylvania, Philadelphia

BORIS KREIS, M.D.

Professeur à la Faculté de Médecine de Paris, Médecin des Hôpitaux de Paris, Hôpital Cochin, Paris

SAUL KRUGMAN, M.D.

Professor and Chairman, Department of Pediatrics, New York University School of Medicine, Director of Pediatrics, Bellevue Hospital and University Hospital, New York

EMILE DE LAVERGNE, M.D.

Professeur à la Faculté de Médecine, Biologiste des Hôpitaux, Nancy

MARCEL LELONG, M.D.

Membre de l'Académie de Médecine, Paris

JEAN-C. LEVADITI, M.D.

Chef de Service, Institut Pasteur, Paris

RAYMOND MANDE, M.D.

Professeur Agrégé à la Faculté de Médecine de Paris, Médecin des Hôpitaux de Paris, Hôpital Bretonneau, Paris

PIERRE MOZZICONACCI, M.D.

Professeur à la Faculté de Médecine, Hôpital des Enfants Malades, Paris

ROGER NATAF, M.D.

Professeur à la Faculté de Médecine de Reims, Membre Associé de l'Institut Pasteur de Tunis, Chef de Service à l'Institut d'Ophtalmologie de Tunis

NATAN NEIMANN, M.D.

Professeur de Clinique de Pédiatrie et de Puericulture, Médecin des Hôpitaux, Nancy

ROBERT NETTER, M.D.,
Docteur ès Sciences

Directeur à la Section Virologie, Laboratoire National de la Santé Publique, Paris

JEAN NOUAILLE, M.D.

Médecin des Hôpitaux de Paris, Service de Cardiologie Infantile, Hôpital Parrot, Bicêtre

DANIÈLE OLIVE, M.D.

Chef de Clinique—Assistant, Département de Pédiatrie, Faculté de Médecine, Nancy

EVA OSETOWSKA, M.D.

Professor, Chief, Laboratory of Comparative Neuropathology, Polish Academy of Sciences, Warsaw

RENÉ PANTHIER, M.D.

Chef du Service de la Fièvre Jaune et des Arbovirus, Institut Pasteur, Paris

PAUL PIALOUX, M.D.

Professeur Agrégé à la Faculté de Médecine de Paris, Médecin des Hôpitaux de Paris, Service d'Oto-rhino-laryngologie, Hôpital Bretonneau, Paris

PIERRE RENARD, M.D.†

ALFRED ROSSIER, M.D.

Professeur à la Faculté de Médecine de Paris, Médecin des Hôpitaux de Paris, Hôpital Saint Vincent de Paul, Paris

HIROTSUGU SHIRAKI, M.D., M.Sc.

Professor of Neuropathology, Department of Neuropathology, Institute of Brain Research, School of Medicine, University of Tokyo, Tokyo

DAVID TAYLOR-ROBINSON, M.D.,
M.C.Path.

Member of Scientific Staff, Medical Research Council, Clinical Research Centre, Harvard Hospital, Salisbury, Wiltshire

STÉPHANE THIEFFRY, M.D.

Professeur à la Faculté de Médecine de Paris, Médecin des Hôpitaux de Paris, Hôpital Saint Vincent de Paul, Paris

LE TAN VINH, M.D.

Chef de Laboratoire à la Faculté de Médecine de Paris, Hôpital Saint Vincent de Paul, Paris

ROBERT WARD, M.D.

Professor and Chairman, Department of Pediatrics, University of Southern California School of Medicine, Physician-in-Chief, Children's Hospital, Los Angeles

---

†Deceased.

For the small viruses such as poliovirus, or for those with helical symmetry, whose nucleic acid is included in the capsid without a supplementary envelope, the term nucleocapsid is sometimes used to designate the virion.

In addition, certain viruses possess an *envelope* around the capsid; this is usually furnished by the host cell and is an important element in classification. The presence of this envelope can lead to the belief that the virus has a spherical form, and it is only after its rupture that the type of internal symmetry is distinguished.

Certain viruses have a structure even more complex: the vaccinia virus has several envelopes and *lateral bodies;* the envelope of the influenza virus is covered with *spicules* responsible for hemagglutination; bacteriophages have a type of binary or mixed symmetry associating the cubic symmetry of the head with the helical symmetry of the tail.

CHEMICAL CONSTITUTION

Study of the different constituents of the virion throws some light on the properties of viruses, on the mechanisms of infection and of oncogenesis,* as well as on the possibilities of action of antiviral chemotherapy.

Nucleic Acid. The nucleic acid determines the infective power of the virus; the proteins that surround it represent only a package which protects it during transport and which is removed to enable the cycle of infection to start.

The percentage of nucleic acid in the whole virion varies from 0.8 per cent for the myxoviruses, for example (p. 10), to 30 per cent for the picornaviruses, the group which includes the poliomyelitis virus (p. 11).

It is known that the nucleic acids result from the assemblage of a large number of nucleotides made up of one molecule of phosphoric acid, a sugar with five atoms of carbon, and purine (adenine, guanine) or pyrimidine (cytosine, thymine, uracil) base. (See below.)

For the ribonucleic acids the sugar is ribose and the four fundamental bases are adenine, guanine, cytosine, and uracil.

For the desoxyribonucleic acids, the sugar is desoxyribose and the four bases are

_____

*From the Greek: ογκος = tumor.

Adenine   *Guanine*   *Cystosine*   *Thymine*   *Uracil*

A fragment of ribonucleic acid can be schematized as follows:

adenine, guanine, cytosine, and thymine. In the DNA of certain bacteriophages, cytosine is replaced by 5-hydroxymethyl cytosine. If the functions of these two large groups of nucleic acids are different, their structures, on the other hand, are rather closely related. When the nucleic acid has two strands, the purine bases of one of the strands are united by hydrogen bonds to the pyrimidine bases of the other, which explains why the percentages of bases are nearly paired. When the nucleic acid has only a single strand, the percentages of each of the bases are independent.

Chemical studies of nucleic acids have not merely a speculative interest for the classification of viruses; they open onto a vaster domain, that of cancer. Attempts have been made to predict the oncogenic properties of viruses by comparing the chemical constituents of the viruses responsible in the normal state for animal tumoral diseases (rabbit papilloma, polyoma of Muridae, avian or murine leukoses) with those of the viruses that can cause, in the artificial state, tumors in the newborn hamster (SV 40, adenoviruses 12 to 18) or even the oncogenic viruses of plants (wound tumor virus).

At the present writing we can only limit ourselves to hypotheses. The nature of the nucleic acid is not decisive, since some oncogenic viruses contain less than 50 (avian leukoses) and some of DNA structure (papilloma, polyoma, adenoviruses 12 to 18). The circular characteristic of the nucleic acid of the papilloma viruses is not a good criterion either, for the adenoviruses have a linear nucleic acid. At one time it was believed that oncogenic viruses contain less than 50 per cent guanine-cytosine, but this is no longer accepted.

Proteins. The biological specificity of viral proteins (manifested by their antigenicity) is determined by the sequence of some 20 amino acids. The techniques of study are highly complex, and thus far only the protein structure of the tobacco mosaic virus has been completely elucidated.

Other Constituents. To the two essential constituents, nucleic acid and proteins, can possibly be added lipids and glucides. The presence or absence of lipids constitutes an invaluable differential factor. Thus all the grease solvents such as ether, chloroform, saponin, or desoxycholate can alter the infectious power of the viruses containing lipids. Conversely, the viruses lacking lipids are resistant to these agents. This is the basis for the ether extraction technique, long used, for example, to isolate enteroviruses from stools.

CLASSIFICATION

Principles. Earlier classifications were based on the tissue affinities of viruses, on the modifications they engendered (ectodermoses, ectoendodermoses, mesoendodermoses, neurotropic ectodermoses, neurotropic endodermoses, mesodermoses, septicemias, neoformation), or on their distribution in nature among living species: vegetable, insect, mammal, and so forth. These criteria were insufficient, for they depended in large part on the host and on various external factors and assembled very different viruses under the same heading.

Newer techniques and research have permitted establishment of new criteria for classification, perhaps still provisory but certainly more rational.

If certain viruses have not yet been studied sufficiently to be classified (the virus of lymphocytic choriomeningitis, and the viruses of avian leukoses), it has at least been possible to delimit certain large groups by taking into account the following characteristics: (1) The nature of the nucleic acid: RNA or DNA; (2) the size of the virion; (3) the type of symmetry, cubic or helical, of the capsid; (4) the number of capsomeres and even their constitution; (5) the diameter of the helix; (6) the presence or absence of an envelope; and, (7) sensitivity to ether.

On the basis of these criteria, Melnick and McCombs have proposed the classification of animal viruses into 11 groups.

Main Groups of Viruses (Tables 2 and 3)
DNA VIRUSES. *Poxviruses.* The viruses of this group are voluminous, are in brick form, and possess a common nucleoproteinic antigen. They are responsible for eruptive or tumoral diseases.

The *variola* subgroup includes the virus of smallpox (of the major and the minor types), the vaccinia viruses, cowpox virus, rabbitpox virus and ectromelia virus. Smallpox virus is essentially adapted to man; that of cowpox usually occurs in bovines but can cause small human epidemics; vaccinia is a creation by man to protect himself against smallpox. Rabbitpox or rabbit pest sometimes causes ravages in rabbit farms, while ectromelia is often latent in mouse-breeding colonies but epizootic outbreaks are not rare.

The *avian* subgroup has great economic

Table 2. *Principal Groups of Animal Viruses: DNA Viruses*

Group	Nucleic Acid	Size (mμ)	Symmetry of Capsid (H, C*)	Number and Constitution of Capsomeres (Cubic Symmetry)	Helix Diameter (Helical Symmetry)	Envelope
Poxviruses	DNA	160 × 260 to 200 × 320	H		100 Å	+
Herpex viruses		120 − 180	C	162 (150 hexamers + 12 pentamers)		+
Adenoviruses		70 − 85	C	252 (240 hexamers + 12 pentamers)		−
Papovaviruses		40 − 55	C	72 (60 hexamers + 12 pentamers)		−
Picodnaviruses		15 − 30	C	12 or 32		−

* H = helical, C = cubic.

importance because of industrial breeding. The avian variola virus can cause a pseudo-membranous form with tracheal lesions (avian diphtheria) or a pseudotumoral form (contagious epithelioma).

The next subgroup is that of *myxoma* and of *fibroma* of the rabbit, hare, or squirrel. Myxomatosis can lead to epizootics with heavy mortality.

The *orf* subgroup (orf is the name given to the contagious pustular dermatitis of sheep) is distinguished from the others by the fact that the virus is smaller and more oval; moreover, the nucleoprotein filaments visible under the electron microscope are less tangled and are disposed in parallel criss-crossed bands as in a ball of string or wool.

There is a tendency to consider that the same virus can produce milker's nodules (paravaccinia) in man, papulous stomatitis in bovines, and a contagious pustular dermatitis in sheep. The viruses of sheep pox and goatpox also doubtless belong to this subgroup.

A subgroup awaiting classification includes disparate viruses such as that of molluscum contagiosum of man, and the Yaba virus, which produces superficial tumors in the monkey.

Herpesviruses. These viruses of medium size, capable of provoking intranuclear cellular inclusions, are divided into two subgroups according to their cultural character.

Subgroup A: the virus of human herpes, or herpes simplex, is the leading member; the virus of simian herpes (B virus) can cause

Table 3. *Principal Groups of Animal Viruses: RNA Viruses*

Group	Nucleic Acid	Size (mμ)	Symmetry of Capsid (H, C*)	Number and Constitution of Capsomeres (Cubic Symmetry)	Helix Diameter (Helical Symmetry)	Envelope
Myxoviruses	RNA	80 − 120	H		90 Å	+
Paramyxo-viruses		100 − 300	H		180 Å	+
Rhabdoviruses		60 − 225	H		180 Å	+
Arbovirus		22 − 50	C	?		+
Reoviruses		70 − 75	C	92 (80 hexamers + 12 pentamers)		−
Picornaviruses		17 − 32	C	32 (20 hexamers + 12 pentamers)		−

*H = helical, C = cubic.

encephalomyelitis of extreme gravity in man. The pseudorabies virus (Aujesky's disease) attacks bovines, ovines, pigs, dogs, and cats; the disease, often fatal, is characterized by an encephalomyelitis accompanied by intense itching. An equine herpetic virus causes a rhinopneumonia or abortion; the virus of bovine infectious rhinotracheitis yields symptoms similar in bovines, as well as pustular vulvovaginal lesions.

Subgroup B: the varicella virus is now solidly associated with that of herpes zoster, with which it merges. The viruses of cytomegalic inclusions of man and animals produce inapparent salivary gland infections but often cause fatal neonatal infections with microcephaly and disseminated visceral lesions.

Adenoviruses. These viruses were formerly called APC owing to the frequent involvement of the adenoids, the pharynx, and the conjunctivia, or ARD (*a*cute *r*espiratory *d*isease).

These viruses of moderate size provoke, as do the herpesviruses, intranuclear cellular inclusions. Among the 32 types of human adenoviruses accepted at present, only certain ones are responsible for respiratory involvement or, more rarely, for eruptive or even digestive syndromes. Types 3, 7, 12, 14, 16, 18, and 31 produce tumors in the newborn hamster. The dog adenovirus causes a canine hepatitis (Rubarth's disease) and the avian adenoviruses (GAL virus: *G*allus *a*denovirus-*l*ike) have caused hepatic necrosis experimentally.

Papovaviruses. These viruses derive their name from the first syllable of the names of three of them: *pa*pilloma of the rabbit and of man (wart), *po*lyoma of Muridae, *va*cuolating agents (simian vacuolating virus: SV 40). Most of the viruses of this group are oncogenic and ether resistant (Chapter 35). Although SV 40 was present in a certain number of lots of inactivated or live antipoliomyelitis vaccine that were administered subcutaneously or orally before the danger was known, it does not seem, up to the present, that the persons vaccinated have suffered any consequences.

Numerous research works on cancer have been carried on with this group of viruses.

Picodnaviruses. This new group, whose name is still provisory, corresponds to very small DNA viruses (pico-small, plus DNA); in it are found osteolytic hamster viruses

(H virus) and different viruses associated with preparations of human and animal adenoviruses (p. 18).

RNA VIRUSES. *Myxoviruses.* This is a group of medium-sized viruses of spherical or filamentous form. They hemagglutinate the red cells of poultry or of guinea pigs, but this process can be reversed by an enzyme, neuramidase, that is packed closely between the hemagglutinating spicules of the virus. This enzyme constitutes a rare exception for viruses, which usually lack enzyme; actually, it does not intervene in metabolism. The myxoviruses are sensitive to actinomycin. The influenza viruses A, B, and C and those of porcine influenza and of avian plague belong to this group.

Paramyxoviruses. These viruses form a more heterogeneous group in which the viruses are a little more voluminous than the myxoviruses; their hemagglutinating properties are less clear cut; they sometimes hemadsorb only the red cells of certain species at the very surface of the cellular sheet, while some do not possess any hemadsorption property. The paramyxoviruses are resistant to actinomycin.

This group includes the human or animal parainfluenza viruses 1, 2, 3, and 4, the virus of mumps, and that of avian pseudopest (Newcastle virus), which is very widespread in breeding flocks and can cause conjunctivitis in man. Three viruses that are similar to one another also belong to this group: those of measles, distemper, and rinderpest. It also includes the respiratory syncytial virus, which can cause serious epidemics in young children. It has also been proposed that rubella virus be included in this group.

Rhabdoviruses. This new group (from the Greek ραβδος rhabdos = rod) has been created to include the RNA viruses shaped roughly like an artillery shell, one of the extremities being pointed and the other flattened. The rabies virus is the member of this group which interests us the most, but other viruses, such as those of bovine vesicular stomatitis and of hemorrhagic septicemia of the rainbow trout, as well as different insect viruses (including the sigma virus of the Drosophila) and plant viruses show that this new group can be extended.

Arboviruses. This is a group of more than 150 small viruses attacking man, Equidae, domestic and wild birds, bats, and serpents; its development cycle usually passes through insects (mosquitoes or ticks). There exist, however, certain exceptions as concerns size and even the necessity of arthropod vectors, a fact which emphasizes the relativity of a classification based on this criterion.

Various subgroups are based on antigenic relationships.

Subgroup A includes the viruses of Eastern, Western, and Venezuelan equine encephalitis, and the viruses Semliki, Sindbis, and Chikungunya, among others. Man can be attacked accidentally and can suffer severe sequelae. The case fatality rate due to Eastern equine encephalitis can attain 70 per cent.

Subgroup B is dominated by the yellow fever virus and by those of dengue (four types), Japanese encephalitis, and St. Louis encephalitis. The viruses of West Nile, Murray Valley, and tick-borne encephalitis and others are also included. The interest of this subgroup is obvious.

Subgroup C and various smaller subgroups include the viruses of phlebotomus fever, Bunyamwera virus, as well as the virus agents of hemorrhagic fevers.

The large number of viruses of this group and the difficulty of studying them due to their antigenic relationships render their study very complex.

Reoviruses (*Respiratory Enteric Orphan Viruses*). These viruses, of medium size, were formerly called ECHO 10. Three antigenic types are found in the feces or the respiratory tract of man and animals. They are found in the course of eruptive, digestive, or merely febrile syndromes.

Picornaviruses (pico-small and RNA). These are very small RNA viruses. The picornaviruses of human origin are divided into the enteroviruses and the rhinoviruses.

The *enteroviruses* (most often isolated from the intestine) include the poliomyelitis viruses (type I, II, and III); the Coxsackie A viruses (23 types); the Coxsackie B viruses (6 types); and the ECHO viruses (33 types) (*enteric cytopathogenic human orphan*).

The *rhinoviruses* are isolated from the respiratory tract; there are 55 types. They are responsible for the classic common cold. The multiplicity of types has so far impeded the preparation of an effective vaccine.

The picornaviruses of animal origin are also numerous (enteroviruses and rhinoviruses); they are found in monkeys, bovines, pigs (encephalomyelitis, Teschen disease), felines, and birds. The virus of bovine foot-and-mouth disease is classified among the bovine rhinoviruses.

The viruses of this human or animal group cause diseases of varied symptomatology: encephalitis, poliomyelitis, and eruptive, febrile, or digestive syndromes. These are discussed in the appropriate chapters of this book.

MECHANISM OF VIRAL INFECTION

Whereas bacteria possess the two varieties of nucleic acid and are generally capable, since they contain enzymes, of multiplying by binary fission in an artificial medium, viruses contain only a genetic material capable of orienting to their benefit the metabolism of the infected cell. This material is sometimes ribonucleic acid, sometimes desoxyribonucleic acid. Herein lies a singularity of viruses, for it was accepted previously that it was the DNA of chromosomes that, in cells, played the essential role.

The mechanism of viral infection is studied by measuring the infectiousness of cells or of the supernatant fluid at intervals spaced out in relation to the inoculation of the cells; radioactive tagging, electron microscopy, and immunofluorescence permit the research worker to follow the production of the different viral constituents in the course of their fabrication. Finally, use of antimetabolities makes it possible to cut certain chains indispensable to the formation of virions and opens certain horizons to future viral chemotherapy.

FIXATION OF THE VIRUS ON THE CELLULAR MEMBRANE

During this step the virus can be neutralized by the corresponding antibodies. From the moment that it penetrates the cell it is protected by it and is insensitive to external action, in particular to that of antibodies. Simple brownian movement cannot explain the virus's fixation on the cellular membrane, for the "fixation rate" is less than the "rate of encounter."

The first phase, adsorption, is nonspecific and reversible; presumably the forces involved are purely electrostatic and independent of temperature: a polyanionic substance such as heparin that has no action in vitro on the herpetic or vaccinial viruses exerts an inhibitory effect during the adsorption phase in tissue culture.

The second phase, attachment, is specific and irreversible; it develops well only above a certain temperature. At its surface the cell possesses mucoprotein or lipoprotein cellular receptors at the level of which certain chemical functions of the capsid of the viral envelope fix themselves. The neuramidinase of myxoviruses destroys the neuraminic acid of the cell surface, which explains why, after hemagglutination followed by elution at 37° C., the red cells cannot agglutinate again, whereas the virus is capable of causing hemagglutination if furnished with new red cells. The vaccinia virus is not very specific in its requirements and can fix itself on and develop in cells of diverse origin (even though the sensitivity is not the same). On the other hand, the complete poliomyelitis virus can be cultivated only in human or simian cells and is capable of infecting chicken fibroblasts only when it is rid of its protein matrix. The virulence of poliomyelitis strains cannot, however, be explained by a difference in adsorption, for, virulent or not, they fix themselves equally well on nerve cells.

There is thus no absolute parallel between the ability of a virus to fix itself on the cellular membrane and its infective power or its virulence. On the other hand, there is a practical application of this fixation phenomenon that is not reserved solely to the cells that permit viral multiplication; a great number of viruses can be adsorbed on red blood cells and provoke a hemagglutination phenomenon widely utilized in virological diagnosis.

PENETRATION AND ECLIPSE OF THE INFECTIOUS VIRUS

The virus penetrates, probably by phagocytosis and by *pinocytosis,* into the interior of the cell, i.e., by adsorption of the viral particle into a sort of cytoplasmic vacuole. On infection by a purified RNA, the penetration is favored by hypertonic solutions or by diethylaminoethyl dextran (DEAED). After a period of time that varies according to the virus, the virus disappears, i.e., it is no longer possible to find the viral particle or its infecting power. This is the onset of the *eclipse phase.*

The disappearance of the virus corresponds, in fact, to the liberation of the essential part of the virion: the nucleic acid. Using the nucleus of the parasitized cell as intermediary, the viral protein induces the synthesis of a cellular protein necessary to this liberation. (At this stage, puromycin, actinomycin D, or the blocking of the cellular nuclei in metaphase stops all viral development.)

For a poxvirus, the operation is laborious; a poxvirus whose capsid has been altered by moderate heating or by a mercuric derivative such as phenyl mercuric borate is no longer infectious quite simply because its protein will no longer induce the formation of the cellular protein necessary to "disrobe" the virion; if another live poxvirus brings to the first the lacking viral protein (reactivation phenomenon), liberation of the nucleic acid will be achieved.

The viral genome, be it an RNA or a DNA virus, serves as a matrix for the formation of a *viral messenger RNA* charged with transmitting the orders to the cell for the elaboration of the new viral constituents. For the viruses that contain single-stranded RNA, such as that of poliomyelitis, it is this constituent itself that will most often play the role of messenger; for the DNA viruses, elaboration of a messenger RNA occurs first, which is why the eclipse phase is slightly lengthened.

The constituents of viruses are synthesized separately, the proteins and the nucleic acids usually appearing in distinct places in the cell. Oxidative phosphorylation, a source of cellular energy, occurs at the level of the mitochondria. Other cytoplasmic organelles, the ribosomes,* sometimes assembled in "polyribosomes" or "polysomes," †play a role in the synthesis of peptides and of nucleic acids. The *RNA viruses* usually develop in the cytoplasm. Among the RNA viruses, the *Myxovirus influenzae* are exceptions to the rule, the nucleic acid seeming to be synthesized in the nucleus whereas other components such as the hemagglutinating antigen are synthesized in the cytoplasm. The *DNA viruses* are all synthe-

---

*Ribosomes are spherical or spheroid masses seeming to possess a protein envelope surrounding a nucleus of ribonucleic acid. Ribosomes are composed of two subunits. Synthesis of proteins is believed to occur at their surface.

†Polyribosomes or polysomes are complexes made up of ribosomal subunits assembled among themselves by the filaments of messenger RNA containing the genetic information.

sized in the cellular nucleus, with the exception of the poxviruses.

Inhibition or Absence of Inhibition of Regular Syntheses of the Cell. This succession of phenomena to some degree disturbs the metabolism proper to the cell. When it occurs, the blockade is more or less rapid. For the virus of poliomyelitis, it intervenes in three and a half hours. The normal cellular polysome is destroyed and replaced by a viral polysome; the polypeptide chains newly formed on contact with it are like those of the viral capsid. This blockade of the cellular syntheses is more or less intense for the myxoviruses; it is almost nil for measles virus, as well as for the reoviruses.

The synthesis of the cell's DNA is rapidly blocked after infection by a living or inactivated vaccinia virus, and in tissue culture a more or less generalized rounding of the cells by a sort of toxic effect occurs.

Synthesis of Viral Products by the Cell. We have already mentioned the messenger RNA induced when the constituent viral nucleic acid cannot itself serve as messenger.

The enzymes useful for viral nucleic acid synthesis are essentially kinases, which play a role during phosphorylation of nucleotide bases (thymidine-kinase, for example) or polymerases which serve for end-to-end association of the nucleotides. Whereas polymerases are generally specific, it is rather curious to note that the polymerase of *Escherichia coli* can be utilized for the synthesis of the RNA of the reoviruses.

The viral nucleic acids fabricated in the presence of RNA or DNA polymerase end up in the doubling of the molecule; the RNA of the poliomyelitis virus, which in general has only a single strand, acquires a second strand, a fact that for a reason not yet clarified renders it resistant to the action of ribonuclease.

The proteins of the viral capsid are synthesized by an equally complex mechanism. The messenger furnishes the model of the sequence of amino acids in accord with the sequence of its own nucleotides; the sequence of three of the nucleic acid bases suffices to determine and to localize an amino acid (code of triplets). The RNA of the cytoplasmic ribosomes fabricates them thereafter, and a transfer RNA orders them in the predetermined direction. These operations occur over three to eight hours for the vaccinia virus. It is during the construction of the capsid that the rounding of the host cell occurs in the case of poliomyelitis virus. Of course,

*repressors** of the synthesis of viral proteins limit these fabrications to the time desired, according to the models proposed by Jacob and Monod for bacteriophages.

The Assemblage of Viral Products. This stage lasts from 30 to 60 minutes for vaccinia virus, and the virus is sensitive to desoxyribonuclease during this period.

Under normal conditions, all the operations are perfectly synchronized owing to synthesis repressors, and no excessive accumulation of nucleic acid or of protein occurs. In the end, formation of the envelope completes maturation of the virus: the arboviruses mature next to the cellular membrane where they acquire a phospholipid envelope. A virus of the same group (Sindbis virus) constitutes its envelope to the detriment of the wall of certain cytoplasmic vacuoles that exist only in the infected cells. The myxoviruses, like the poxviruses, cover themselves anew with an envelope on emergence across the cellular membrane; proteins of properly viral nature communicate to them, in addition, a certain specificity.

Excretion of Virus into the Surrounding Medium. The complete virus or virion is now ready for a new cellular invasion.

Most RNA viruses (picornaviruses, myxoviruses, arboviruses) are excreted in large amounts, the reoviruses, in somewhat smaller amounts. The DNA viruses diffuse but slightly, the viruses usually passing from cell to cell. As usual in biology, nothing is absolute; it is the herpes virus that, in this group, constitutes the exception to the rule.

We have described above the multiplication mechanism of a virus under ideal conditions; certain external factors can disturb this development.

INFLUENCE OF SOME EXTERNAL FACTORS

The influence of *temperature* on the pathogenic power of bacteria has been known for a long time. At the start of the bacteriological era, did not Pasteur succeed in killing hens inoculated with anthrax bacillus simply by drenching their feet in cold water in order to lower their internal temperature and so permit the bacillus to multiply?

The same phenomenon was observed for different poxviruses inoculated into the

---

*The mechanism of repression consists in the inhibition of enzyme synthesis by the presence of the product of the enzymatic action.

chorioallantoic membrane of the embryonated egg, or even in tissue culture. The maximal temperatures permitting development of the virus vary from 38.5° C. for the smallpox virus to more than 40° C. for vaccinia virus. Similarly, Lwoff, studying poliomyelitis virus in tissue culture, found that highly virulent strains multiply as well at 40° C. as at 36° C., whereas for the attenuated strains of live antipoliomyelitis vaccine (Koprowski, Sabin) there is a considerable lowering of infectious titer at the more elevated temperature. The correlation between the results of this test and the neurovirulence for the monkey is sufficient for this test to be used during production of the attenuated strain as a "genetic marker" *(rct)* to verify the maintenance of its attenuation. It is possible that fever aids the infected organism by preventing the virus from multiplying; the disease would appear only if the virus is virulent, i.e., prepared to live under unfavorable conditions. In this case the physician would not be playing a very useful role were he to combat the fever which accompanies the viral invasion.

Another factor, no less important, is the *pH*. When the pH of the culture medium falls below 6.6, culture of poliomyelitis virus is very much slowed. Similar observations have been made with varicella virus. This slowing down no doubt reinforces the action of macrophages in the inflammatory zones, in which the pH is frequently lowered.

If we have discussed the mechanisms of infection at such length, it is because their study represents an extraordinary contribution of modern science to knowledge concerning the etiology of viral diseases and their therapy. Thus some hope concerning the future of chemotherapy may arise from our knowledge that the virus cannot multiply when a link in the complex chain that leads to the virion is lacking. The complexity of virus-cell relationships is such that it is evident that laboratories utilizing different media and cellular systems sometimes obtain diametrically opposite percentages of virus isolation. Numerous viruses unknown today will perhaps be discovered when a sensitive cellular system has been found.

DIFFERENT MODES OF INTRACELLULAR INFECTION

The mechanism of infection as it has just been set forth is a general schema. In fact,

the relationships between the virus and the host cell are highly varied.

CELLULAR DESTRUCTION; CYTOPATHOGENIC EFFECT*

If the virus manages to check or to block cell metabolism, it produces disturbances resulting more or less rapidly in cellular death; centers of destroyed cells or plaques are then observed. The progression of these centers is sometimes slow, as in the case of vaccinial virus, which transmits itself from cell to cell, and sometimes rapid, as in the case of poliomyelitis virus, which is excreted into the medium that surrounds the cells. The older authors recognized certain cytological alterations which permitted them to make, in histopathological preparations, the diagnosis of vaccinia-variola (Guarnieri-Paschen bodies), of rabies (Negri bodies), of herpes, or of cytomegalic inclusion disease.

Nucleus. The nucleus of the parasitized cells sometimes contains a characteristic inclusion body. The herpes virus dislocates the nuclear chromatin and rejects it to the periphery of the cellular membrane; the nucleus of cells infected with the varicella-herpes zoster virus undergoes a change resembling that produced by colchicine: blockade of the metaphase, and breakage and contraction of the chromosomes. The adenoviruses also create typical lesions. A good many viruses provoke chromosomal breakages, but it is not possible to attach to them a definite genetic significance, for they represent a variation in the cellular metabolism. Other chromosomal alterations (translocation) may be more significant but they are much less frequent.

The Cytoplasm. Various disturbances in the usual appearance of the cytoplasm are reflected in the denomination of the virus that has provoked them.

VACUOLES. The abbreviation papovaviruses derives from the papilloma, polyoma vacuolating viruses. The SV 40 virus, which is a possible contaminant of monkey kidney cell cultures and which possesses oncogenic properties, provokes the formation of numerous vacuoles in the cell. Cells infected with vaccinia virus fairly often contain vacuoles but in lesser quantity.

SYNCYTIUM. When syncytia that can

---

*For figures, see color plate.

reach 1 mm. in size and that contain some 100 nuclei are observed in cell culture, one immediately thinks of the respiratory syncytial virus. Smaller syncytia are also seen in the cellular sheet inoculated with *Myxovirus parainfluenzae,* varicella-herpes zoster, or vaccinia virus. During measles infection, it is not rare to observe Warthin multinucleated cells in the ganglionic or splenic tissue, the bronchial mucosa, or the alveolar secretions.

The tendency today is to think that these syncytia result from the fusion of several cells. The phenomenon appears from the moment of virus adsorption, but the cell does not die immediately and its nuclei are capable of mitosis despite the infection. Chany, discussing the herpes virus, has suggested the hypothesis that a cellular factor, "syncytine," is synthesized during the eclipse phase of the virus; Cascardo and Karson postulated the existence of a "fusion factor" of viral origin, for it can be inhibited by the antibodies corresponding to the virus responsible. There remain a certain number of unknowns, and a virus such as that of measles, which provokes the formation of vast syncytia on isolation, no longer causes, after a certain number of passages in cell culture, more than a rounding of the infected cells with a few filiform prolongations.

VIRAL INCLUSIONS. To describe these inclusions would be to pass too many viruses in review; the interested reader will refer to the various chapters of this book. We shall, however, cite the inclusion of poliomyelitis virus, which pushes back the nucleus, and that of vaccinia virus, which is either single and stuck to the nucleus or else multiple.

CELLULAR MORPHOLOGY. The cellular morphology also undergoes modifications that are manifested by a rounding effect on the cell (poliovirus, herpesvirus, adenovirus), the cell having a tendency to lose its adherence to glass; in its retraction, it sometimes leaves behind fine prolongations (vaccinia virus, varicella-herpes zoster virus).

PROLIFERATIVE BUDDINGS. Occasionally the onset of the infection is marked by a rapid cellular multiplication; proliferative buddings appear on the sheet of Hela cells infected by measles or smallpox virus. In the second case an important differential characteristic is involved, for vaccinia virus does not produce any such effect; however, there is no relation between these lesions and possible malignancy.

All these disorders, which often end with death of the cell, point up that cellular multiplication is in no wise indispensable to viral multiplication. Quite the contrary: a moderate irradiation of the cells can increase their sensitivity to viruses.

CHRONIC INFECTIONS

Certain human infections seem to indicate that the virus can persist a very long time in the organism without causing obvious disturbances. Labial or menstrual herpes which regularly reappears in the same body site is an example; the transmission of hepatitis by transfusion long after icterus in the donor is another; the occurrence of herpes zoster years after varicella is considered proof of the persistence of the virus in the human body. An infection can be latent in the animal and reveal itself by producing a disease in man; this is the case of B virus of the monkey, which causes a fatal disease in man. This is the reason for the strict precautions against the presence of this virus in the vaccines prepared in monkey cells. What becomes of the virus in the course of this silent phase? Cellular studies tend to show that in the course of chronic infection the virus multiplies without causing any modification of the cell in which it dwells; the cell has become a "healthy carrier" capable not only of surviving but also of multiplying. The detection of the virus is accomplished in this case by indirect procedures: the hemadsorption procedure described by Shelokov consists in detecting the presence of viruses by means of the adsorption that is produced when red cells are placed at the surface of infected cells; the hemadsorbing viruses of the *Myxovirus influenzae* group are thus recognized.

Various hypotheses have been proposed to explain the mechanism of chronic infections. Walker summarizes them as follows:

The slight proportion of sensitive cells in a population of resistant cells is sufficient to maintain the virus if the rate of repopulation of sensitive cells always remains greater than or equal to the rate of destruction.

The cells are sensitive to the virus, but the antibodies in the surrounding medium allow only the propagation of the infection from cell to cell. In this case there is an unstable equilibrium, which causes the balance to tip in favor of the cells at some times and in favor of the virus at others.

The cells are genetically sensitive, but the fraction that is contaminated manufactures enough interferon to protect the majority of the elements of the cellular sheet.

There remains, finally, true chronic infection, in the course of which the infected cells divide. Various authors have thus been able to maintain rubella virus, mumps virus, or measles virus at the same time as the host cells. The viruses of avian leukoses also reproduce in chicken embryo cells without hindering cellular reproduction; on the contrary, the cellular divisions increase the infectious titer of these viruses.

In conclusion, the models proposed are very different from genuine "latent" infections. In the chronic infections, the virus multiplies in the cell and only the absence of cytopathogenic power or of an indicator to uncover its presence permits the belief that the virus has momentarily disappeared. In "latent" infections we should expect the virus to be better hidden, for instance, hooked onto a chromosome of the cellular nucleus, as is the case, for example, for bacteriophages of which the prophage is fixed on the nucleic acid of the bacterium that harbors it and reproduces it at each division at the same time as its own genome. Even though the existence of a similar schema for the animal viruses is very likely, proof has so far not been furnished.

CELLULAR TRANSFORMATIONS[*]

The domain of cancer begins when the virus, instead of killing the cell, transforms it. The rate of mitoses accelerates, the metabolism is modified, and mucopolysaccharidic acid accumulates at the same time that the production of lactic acid accelerates. The fibroblastic cells grow larger and round out in form. Finally, the inhibition of contact that maintained the multiplication of the cells in only two dimensions ceases to function, and tridimensional tumoral foci develop. The change in the number and the aspect of the chromosomes indicates the passage to malignancy, confirmed in the animal by the appearance of tumors and of metastases. All these phenomena have been particularly well studied with the RNA viruses of the avian leukosarcomas and with the DNA viruses of the papova group.

The Avian Leukosarcoma Viruses. In 1910, Peyton Rous discovered the leading virus of the group, the Rous sarcoma virus

---

[*]This problem is studied in detail in Chapter 62.

(RSV). Since then, investigators have discovered that a large number of similar viruses are capable of provoking leukoses, erythroblastoses, or myeloblastoses. These viruses do not attack domestic fowl alone and can produce chromosomal anomalies in human leukocytes (Nichols, 1964) or even tumors in the monkey; it is for this reason that strict precautions are taken to assure their absence from vaccines prepared from chick embryo cells.

At high dosage, on chicken fibroblasts, the Rous virus induces rapid formation of a large number of foci of transformed cells that are productive of the virus. At low dosage, on the other hand, only a few cells are transformed, and these are not productive of virus (NP). The tumors obtained in mammals inoculated with Rous sarcoma virus also show a very high majority of nonproductive cells. This transformation certainly depends on the conditions of the medium, and a strong concentration of serum or the addition of embryo serum to the culture medium reduces the number of transformed cells. It depends above all on the viral genome, for, despite the absence of virus from the surrounding medium, it is easy to cultivate these cells for a long time and to obtain, anew, tumors in domestic fowl by inoculation of these transformed cells. Several facts demonstate that the viruses persist in the nonproductive cells in an incomplete form *(defective virus)*. Indeed, they are not neutralized by the corresponding antibodies, and the inoculation of transformed cells that are not productive of virus does not provoke antibody formation in the inoculated animal; in addition, the animal remains sensitive to a new inoculation. It is accepted today that defective Rous virus lacks the protein coat that usually communicates to viruses their specificity. Moreover, the inoculation of the RNA of Rous virus produces the same result. Defective Rous viruses are capable of acquiring an envelope protein when their development occurs contemporaneously with any one of the viruses of avian leukoses ("helper virus") such as the RAV (*R*ous *a*ssociated *v*iruses), AMV (*a*vian *m*yeloblastosis *v*irus), or erythroblastosis virus. The same cell then fabricates two complete viruses; in the nomenclature, virus that furnished the protein of the defective virus is mentioned in parentheses, e.g., RSV (RAV).

The schema shows that the infection of a fibroblast by a Rous virus transforms the cell that does not excrete virus; when a

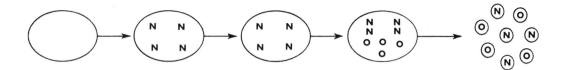

single leukosis helper virus superinfects the cell, the cell becomes capable of excreting both viruses. The rate of multiplication of the helper virus then commands that of the defective virus.

These extraordinarily interesting studies point to a few conclusions that can be applied in the study of human cancers:

A defective virus that lacks a protein envelope can provoke tumors in which the virus is not recoverable.

In the absence of a protein covering, the virus will be weakly antigenic.

The Rous virus is not fixed to the chromatin (provirus) by a process similar to that demonstrated by Lwoff and Gutman in 1950 for bacteriophages (prophage); thus the spermatozoa of the infected cock do not transmit the infection at the time of fertilization, on injection of their DNA; by analogy it is deduced that transmission of the virus from cell to cell results not from a latent infection or from heredity but from a distribution of the viral nucleic acid in the cytoplasm of two daughter cells at the moment of division.

The Viruses of the Papova Group. These are, on the other hand, DNA viruses whose action, according to the type of cells they infect, is sometimes destructive, sometimes oncogenic.

The hunters of Kansas and of Iowa are well acquainted with warty tumors of cottontail rabbits. Shope, and then Rous, toward 1933, noted that the papilloma of the wild rabbit contains many viruses concentrated in the superficial keratinized layers; the tumor is transmissible even in the absence of cells by passage of filtrates of ground-up tissue. In contrast, this ground-up papilloma inoculated into the domestic rabbit produces voluminous tumors very poor in infectious virus; the cells contain in reserve the virus in an immature noninfecting form. Extraction of the desoxyribonucleic acid of the transformed noninfecting cells revealed the existence of a papillomatous DNA capable of transmitting the infection.

The polyoma virus was discovered by Gross in 1951 and cultivated in cells in vitro

by Eddy in 1957. The destructive effect for simian or murine cells in culture varies according to the cellular species and the conditions of the surrounding medium. Each cell can produce 800 to 1000 infectious units.

In cultures of embryonic hamster cells, the percentages of transformed cells generally observed are 0.14 to 0.63 per cent; it is rather curious to learn that this rate increases to 10 per cent when the cells are incubated at 24° C.; the rest of the cellular sheet is normal in appearance. Clones of neoplastic cells that did not produce virus were established by Vogt and Dulbecco in 1960. The virus is doubtless not integrated into the genome of the cellular nucleus. The cells remain sensitive to infection with polyoma virus; it is thought, rather, that the number of infectious particles is insufficient to be detectable.

The tumors induced in the hamster lend themselves but little to multiplication of infectious virus even though the animal can acquire certain antibodies.

The polymorphism of the oncogenic power in different rodents (hamster, rat, rabbit, guinea pig) is reflected in the name of the polyoma virus: the tumors observed are epithelial or conjunctival, malignant or benign (parotid and submaxillary, renal and adrenal tumor, bone sarcomas, mammary carcinoma, mesothelioma, hemangioendothelioma).

The SV 40 virus, the importance of which for manufacturers of culture vaccines was brought to light in 1960 by Sweet and Hilleman, is a latent virus of the monkey. Rabson and Kirschstein in 1962 obtained the malignant transformation of hamster renal cells in vitro; the inoculation of these cells into the newborn hamster provoked carcinomas and sarcomas. The tumor of the hamster obtained upon inoculation of transformed cells is poor in virus, whereas that observed after inoculation of virus into nontransformed culture cells of Cercopithecus kidney contains numerous infectious units. In 1962 Koprowski, using SV 40 virus, noted the transformation of skin and buccal mucosa cells of adult subjects in two to three months.

As we see it, the problem of cancer of

viral origin is not simple, and different mechanisms are involved. The cell can thus be brought to manufacture, in greater or lesser quantity, antigens or enzymes such as arginase (cellular conversion); this phenomenon is not limited to viruses, and the strain of diphtheria bacillus is strongly toxigenic only when it is contaminated with a bacteriophage.

A very virulent virus is not generally oncogenic; moreover, the cellular transformation often results from an incomplete multiplication of the virus, which sometimes lacks its protein shell, a fact that explains the attenuation of the immunological reactions.

A vaccine that would protect only against the helper virus in the case of avian leukoses would not prevent the defective virus from provoking its neoplastic damage; the vaccine should thus also protect against the defective virus and the added protein that is furnished to it. Only in the complete infectious form does the virus accept emergence from the cell in order to pass into the surrounding medium, where the antibodies provoked by the vaccine can annihilate it.

MIXED INFECTIONS, RECOMBINATION, MUTATION, AND INTERFERENCE

Mixed Infection. In mixed infections, the two viruses multiply together without getting in each other's way.

We have seen that certain defective viruses such as the Rous virus require a helper virus in order to complete their development. This same helper virus can, on the other hand, hinder the development of Rous virus if it is inoculated before the latter. This principle is the basis for Rubin's test or RIF (*R*esistance *I*nducing *F*actor) designed to detect avian leukosis viruses contaminating egg-culture vaccines. The leukosis virus, if it exists, induces a cellular resistance to subsequent inoculation of Rous virus. Other viruses, such as adenovirus 4, which are cytopathogenic in human cells, are cytopathogenic for simian renal cells only if the latter are contaminated by a SV 40 virus, heat-inactivated or not; the mechanism here is different from that for the leukosarcomatosis viruses, for the latter contribute, precisely, to the defective viruses the protein that they lack.

Recombination. Recombination is defined as the possibility for two viruses belonging to the same species to exchange a part of their genome, an exchange manifested by a modification of genetic characteristics (virulence, aspect of plaques in cell culture, hemorrhagic character of the lesions on the chorio-allantoic membrane, and thermal stability, to name only a few). Obviously, the modification obtained is thereafter transmissible to the descendants.

The fibromatosis virus provokes in the rabbit benign tumors that progressively regress along with virus multiplication; if at the same time one inoculates a myxomatosis virus heated so as to destroy only the envelope protein, the infection rapidly becomes fatal. In this case not recombination but *reactivation* is involved, for exchange of genetic material has not occurred; the fibromatosis virus has merely furnished the myxomatosis virus with the protein it lacked. True recombination is easy between vaccinia virus and rabbitpox; it is less easy between the mouse ectromelia virus even though it belongs to the same subgroup; it is nonexistent with the fibromatosis viruses, which belong to another subgroup of poxviruses. The hypothesis has been advanced of a possible recombination in nature between cowpox and smallpox viruses having resulted in the formation of a hybrid, the vaccinial virus. Recombinations are also easy to obtain in vitro between the viruses of the influenza subgroup; however, it is more likely that the minimal changes that occur in the genetic characteristics of the influenza viruses in the course of influenza epidemics result purely and simply from mutation.

Mutation. It is by mutations induced in the laboratory under difficult living conditions (suboptimal host cell or abnormal temperature) that virulent viral strains are finally domesticated so as become vaccines (street rabies virus and fixed virus, yellow fever virus and Dakar strain or Rockefeller 17 D, wild poliomyelitis virus and attenuated strain).

Inhibitive Interference. In the phenomenon of inhibitive interference, the virus first present impedes multiplication of the second virus, especially when a certain lapse of time exists between the two infections.

The phenomenon seems very widespread; it is used to explain the rapid action of Sabin live vaccine (p. 101) in breaking epidemics of poliomyelitis; however, when certain ECHO, Coxsackie, or adenoviruses are already present in the digestive tract, the Sabin virus cannot multiply in certain cases. It is perhaps also as a result of the same mechanism that yellow fever does not propagate in Asia where dengue rages, and this despite the presence of a common vector.

The interest of the discovery of *interferons* by Isaacs and Lindenmann lies especially in the explanation that they have given of the phenomenon and the research works that they have stimulated. The word interferon is a general term that is applied to all cellular nonviral protein capable of hindering the multiplication of different viruses. The first experiment of Isaacs indicated that an inactivated influenza virus inoculated into the chorioallantoic membrane of the embryonated egg impeded the subsequent development of the same live virus. The experiment has also been reproduced in cell culture with the same success. Subsequently, it was noted that numerous live viruses or viruses inactivated by heat below 60° C., by formaldehyde, or by moderate irradiation (picornaviruses, arboviruses, myxoviruses, poxviruses) are capable of inducing a similar substance. It is somewhat curious to note that the attenuated viruses are better producers of interferon than the highly virulent viruses, which destroy cells too rapidly. Interferon production is in no way peculiar to viruses and rickettsiae; statolon (an antibiotic derived from a *Penicillium*), *Brucella*, or an endotoxin is associated with the same phenomenon.

Numerous varieties of human or animal cells, cancerous or not, can produce interferon. Almost all viruses are capable of inducing its production. Inversely, it has been possible to demonstrate varying degrees of sensitivity to interferon for all viruses except the papovaviruses and the herpes viruses. The sensitivity of the viruses to interferon is independent of the nature of the agent that has provoked its formation: for example, the interferon produced against influenza A virus is active not merely against this virus but also against Eastern equine encephalitis virus or against vaccinia.

Two facts have limited utilization of this product:

First, interferon shows cellular specificity: whatever the virus inoculated, the interferon acts only on a viral infection of cells of the same species. Fortunately an exception exists that may permit application in man; the interferon produced by simian cell cultures is active on calf renal cells, hu-man thyroid, or amniotic cells inoculated with virus.

The second problem lies in the moment of action: interferon should be administered before the infection.

Interferon is a proteinic substance of low molecular weight in the range of 20,000 to 34,000, stable at ambient temperature and inactivated only at 60° C. It also resists great variations in pH, from 2 to 11, and the action of different cellular nucleases.

How is interferon formed? Since very different viruses are capable of causing production of the same interferon by the same cell variety, in all likelihood it is not the viral genome that directly gives the order to produce. The fact that blockade of the cell DNA by actinomycin D or iodo-2-deoxyuridine arrests synthesis of interferon shows that the order to produce is registered and given by the cell nucleus. Perhaps a repressor gene that under normal conditions blocks synthesis of interferon by the cell is destroyed on introduction of the virus into the cell.

The interferon produced by the cell does not have virucidal action in vitro; it intervenes at the onset of the infection, immediately after penetration of the virus into the cell, by preventing the cell from multiplying.

GENERAL PHENOMENA OF RESISTANCE TO VIRAL INFECTION

In addition to the cellular phenomena which protect the organism at the various stages of viral penetration and multiplication, man shows general phenomena of resistance to infection by viruses.

Two systems of defense are usually distinguished: natural, nonspecific resistance, independent of earlier infection by the viral agent, and specific immunity, resulting from active immunization induced by the viral agent after vaccination or spontaneous invasion, either manifest or inapparent.

FACTORS OF NATURAL NONSPECIFIC RESISTANCE

The human organism as a whole defends itself against viral infection. The first barrier is the mucocutaneous covering, a mechanical, passive barrier, to which must be added other factors such as sweat or the sebaceous secretions, which act particularly by modifying the pH, and such factors as the ciliated epithelium and the mucous secretions.

General phenomena intervene, as we have seen, in the cell-virus system. A general rise in temperature (or a local rise in the case of an inflammatory process) inhibits viral development. A fall in pH in an inflammatory zone could have the same effect. Thus cortisone, which is known to have a harmful effect on certain viral infections, may act by reducing the inflammatory reactions and also by inhibiting the synthesis and the action of interferon.

The blood contains a certain number of substances that act in a nonspecific manner. Properdin, long considered a factor of natural resistance, seems, in fact, to owe part of its properties to minimal quantities of specific antibodies. The cellular components of blood, the lymphocytes in particular, participate in two ways, both as virus transporters and as interferon producers. The role of lymphocytes will be considered again in connection with specific defense processes and the phenomenon of delayed hypersensitivity. The reticuloendothelial system may also play a defensive role, as yet ill defined.

THE FACTORS OF SPECIFIC IMMUNITY

Immunity is linked to the production by the organism of antibodies associated essentially with three types of immunoglobulins: the G immunoglobulins (IgG), the A immunoglobulins (IgA), and the M immunoglobulins (IgM). The classification is based on their physicochemical, immunological, and biological properties.

The G immunoglobulins (IgG), formerly known as gamma globulins, are also called gamma 2, gamma 7S, or Gamma G. They have a molecular weight close to 160,000 and a sedimentation constant of 7S.* Their electrophoretic mobility is not homogeneous; it covers the gamma and beta zones.

The A immunoglobulins (IgA) correspond to a part of the beta 2 globulins. They have been called beta 2A, gamma 1A, gamma 17S, or gamma A. They have a molecular weight close to 160,000 and a sedimentation constant of 6.5 to 7S. They can yield polymers with higher sedimentation constants (9 to 13S) and are dissociable by sulfhydrylated compounds.

The M immunoglobulins (IgM) also correspond to a fraction of the beta 2M globulins. They have been called beta 2M, gamma 19S, gamma 1M, or gamma M. They have a molecular weight of 1 million and a sedimentation constant of 19S. They can be dissociated in a more or less reversible manner by sulfhydrylated compounds into monomers having a sedimentation constant of 6.5S and a molecular weight of 100,000.

The immunoglobulins are constituted of different types of polypeptide chains: two heavy chains and two light chains united by disulfide bonds. The light chains are common to all the immunoglobulins and confer on them the general properties of immunoglobulins. The heavy chains differ according to the type of immunoglobulin; they have distinct physicochemical properties, and their structure determines the biological activities peculiar to each type, in particular transplacental passage or the power to fix complement.

The G immunoglobulins, by far the most abundant, are considered, according to different authors, to represent 70 to 90 per cent of the total immunoglobulins. Their distribution is intravascular (40 to 58 per cent) and interstitial. They are also found in rhinopharyngeal secretions, but in lesser proportion. The M immunoglobulins, much less abundant, represent only about 3 to 10 per cent of the immunoglobulins. They are almost totally intravascular.

The G and M immunoglobulins appear to have different significance. After immunization, the antibodies first detected are usually IgM antibodies. Their level can increase over approximately a week before IgG antibodies appear. Appearance of IgG antibodies is accompanied by a marked reduction in synthesis of IgM antibodies, and subsequently IgG antibodies heavily predominate. A new stimulation by the same antigen is followed by almost exclusive production of IgG.

Moreover, only the G immunoglobulins are capable of traversing the placenta. This exclusive passage of the IgG in significant quantities is probably linked to a phenomenon of active transport and not simply to the lesser dimension of their molecule, which in any case differs only slightly from that of IgA. The placenta indeed appears relatively impermeable to the light polypeptide chains common to all the immunoglobulins, and it is probable that the heavy polypeptide chain peculiar to IgG carries the site (active zone)

---

*S = Svedberg units.

responsible for placental passage. This explains the intense interest attached to fractionations of globulins in the course of prenatal viral diseases. This fractionation, by showing the presence of IgM antibodies in the fetal blood, reveals the possibility of genuine immunological defense reactions during the fetal stage in the course of rubella or of cytomegalic inclusion disease (see Chapter 61).

The G and M immunoglobulins fix complement, whereas the A immunoglobulins do not.

Like the G immunoglobulins, the A immunoglobulins are found in the serum and the interstitial fluid, but it is in the secretions that they seem to play their essential role in resistance against infections. In the healthy subject, the antiviral activity of the nasal secretions is associated with the IgA, which heavily predominate, whereas the IgG are detected at this level only intermittently. Nonetheless, it has been shown that, in the course of certain respiratory viral diseases, the nasal secretions contained both A and G immunoglobulins equally endowed with antiviral activity.

Development of immunoglobulins is the result of the host's reactions to his environment. Germ-free animals live and reproduce with extremely low levels of immunoglobulins. The newborn, at birth is endowed with large reserves of G immunoglobulins of maternal origin. These are progressively catabolized, attaining their lowest level toward the second month. The subsequent synthesis of immunoglobulins depends on the number and the frequency of invasions, in particular of antigenic stimuli. The cells that produce immunoglobulins are lymphoplasmacytic or reticular cells, sometimes typical plasmacytes. Different techniques and, for example, use of fluorescent antibodies specific for the different polypeptide chains that constitute the immunoglobulins have made it possible to reveal the strict specialization of the competent cells. Although the same type of cell is capable of producing the light and the heavy chains, each cell produces individually only one type of heavy chain and one type of light chain.

It seems that immunoglobulin formation by the competent cells can be directly induced by the virus itself. It is well known that at various times after poliomyelitis or vaccinia infection, for example, virus is found in the regional lymph nodes; it has been demonstrated by in vitro experiments with actinomycin blockade that gamma globulin could be synthesized by the cellular ribosome on order from a messenger RNA or a virus playing this role.

Drescher and Jachertz recently showed, in vitro, globulins in cellular cultures obtained from peritoneal exudates of mice inoculated with influenza virus or its hemagglutinizing subunits.

It must be emphasized that antibody production—its rapidity and its intensity—depends on the quantity and quality of the antigen. In the course of natural infection, the infecting dose is generally very small and a lapse of several days is necessary to permit viral multiplication sufficient for induction of the immune response (IgM, then IgG). Considerable quantities of antibodies must be synthesized and retained in the blood before serum antibodies are detectable. It is estimated that, for a man of 60 kg., at least 10^6 molecules of antibodies must be synthesized before 0.001 mg. of antibody can be revealed in 1 ml. of serum. But this response is more rapid and much more intense in cases of reinfection by the same virus; it is even qualitatively different because G immunoglobulins are produced at the outset. The response is of *secondary* type, in contrast with the preceding one, which is a response of *primary* type. It is thanks to this secondary response that a reinfection fails to develop in the immunized subject. It is also this secondary response that occurs with booster injections after vaccination.

On the occasion of a reinfection, the antibody action can be immediate, averting recurrence. On the other hand, in the case of an initial infection this action occurs relatively later, preceded and prepared by the processes of nonspecific defense.

In addition, defensive action can exert itself on viruses only during their extracellular life, up to and including the period of fixation on the cellular membrane. After their multiplication, certain viruses such as the poliovirus are expelled from the host cell and are immediately exposed to the action of neutralizing antibodies. Thanks to this neutralization of the liberated viruses, the progress of the infection can be limited or arrested.

However, other viruses seem to escape the action of antibodies; thus, in the local lesions of recurrent herpes, the virus spreads despite high levels of antibodies in the serum and the interstitial fluid. Among the various explanations proposed, the one most commonly accepted is the direct passage of the virus from cell to cell by means of intercellular bridges that thus prevent their direct contact with the antibodies. In such infections, antibodies could hardly intervene except in passages in the intercellular spaces, the lymphatic glands, or the blood vessels. Furthermore, they would be limited in their action by the intracellular means of transport of these viruses which are contained by the macrophages.

OTHER SPECIFIC PROCESSES

The deficits or the insufficiencies of the immune phenomena dependent on immunoglobulins have created in the last few years a resurgence of interest in phenomena long known but very difficult to analyze. We shall merely cite the interaction of the components of complement with the antigen-antibody complex; its role in virology is not clearly defined. On the other hand, it seems that delayed hypersensitivity reactions represent an interesting aspect of cellular immunity.

The state of *delayed-type hypersensitivity* is recognized, in vivo, by a cutaneous lesion, complex and specific, provoked by a test injection of antigen. One of the models most currently used is the cutaneous reaction to tuberculin, which reflects both a cellular hypersensitivity and a certain degree of protection in the subject presenting it. Delayed hypersensitivity to a given antigen can be revealed in the animal at a time when only traces of specific antibodies can be discovered. It is transmissible from subject to subject by the injection of a small number of lymph cells. The prolonged duration (up to one or two years) of such a passively transmitted hypersensitivity can be due either to the particularly long life of certain lymph cells or to their capacity to "teach" the host cells this type of reaction (Lawrence's "transmissible factor").

Even though a definitive viewpoint on the relationships between delayed hypersensitivity and cellular immunity is not yet possible, the two phenomena are closely linked and the same types of cells, lymphocytes and macrophages, are implicated in the two processes. It seems more and more likely that they play a role in the fight against viral infections. Kempe in 1960 reported a case of progressive vaccinia in a child with a normal level of gamma globulins. Even though the patient responded normally to tetanus and diphtheria antigens, and even though he received massive doses of immunoglobulins, no result was obtained: the evolution of the lesions was abruptly arrested by the injection, into the neighboring skin, of leukocytes from recently vaccinated donors. At the same time, delayed sensitivity reactions to killed vaccinia virus could be demonstrated. In another connection, Rosen and Janeway noted that deaths from progressive vaccinia occur principally in children with "thymic alymphoplasia" (absence of antibody formation plus absence of delayed hypersensitivity reaction) and not in children with isolated "agammaglobulinemia."

SOME EXAMPLES OF DIFFERENT ASPECTS OF VIRAL INFECTIONS ACCORDING TO THE REACTIONAL MODALITIES OF MAN

All these defense processes confer on viral infections in man highly varied physiopathological aspects almost unique for each type of virus. Some examples can be cited.*

The clearest model—even though it is still poorly understood in many ways—seems to us to be furnished by a disease such as measles, which involves an infection that is always clinically evident, followed by an immunity that is considered definitive. This particularly solid immunity, which is manifested by the persistence of neutralizing and hemagglutination-inhibiting antibodies for a great many years, is, however, not the organism's sole defense process. Enders and his co-workers have clearly revealed the role of mechanisms of cellular defense: interferon at least in the initial rhinopharyngeal period of infection, and delayed hypersensitivity in the agammaglobulinemic subjects, who resist the disease well (whereas subjects with thymic alymphoplasia die from it).

For whatever the reason, during normally encountered measles, the virus is no longer found in the rhinopharyngeal secretions from the second day of the eruption, and it disappears from the urine a few days later, while the various antimeasles antibodies appear and develop. Acute measles infection, thus, by its clinical, virological, and immunological

---

*We shall not consider here the problem of "slow" viruses; a special chapter is devoted to them (Chapter 19).

Foreword

During the last three decades the theoretical and practical approaches of those studying animal viruses have been profoundly influenced by two events. Of these the first was the development of new techniques and the refinement and extension of older procedures which permit the recognition and measurement of the pathogenic effects of viruses *in vitro* and *in vivo*. The application of these methods soon led to the isolation from man and other warm blooded vertebrates of hundreds of agents whose existence had been wholly unsuspected or only vaguely postulated, as well as to the cultivation of agents already well known and which had proved difficult or impossible to propagate in the laboratory. Somewhat later, the concept of a science of molecular biology was formulated. By applying the principles and procedures of this discipline to problems in their own field animal virologists have succeeded within the short space of the last ten years in defining with increasing precision the nature, the properties, and the mode of replication of many of these agents. For the medical student, the clinician, the epidemiologist, and the immunologist seeking new means of prophylaxis against viral diseases one of the most helpful results to come from these investigations is a classification based upon stable physical and chemical properties of most of the known animal viruses. This accomplishment has already brought order into chaos and greatly facilitated communication among virologists themselves as well as between them and other workers in related fields. In addition, the labors of virologists during these 30 years have produced a wealth of other contributions useful to practitioners of therapeutic and preventive medicine. The more significant and valuable of these have been clearly summarized by the authors of this book.

But all this progress, as with many other sciences in our time, has not proved an unmixed blessing. Many virologists find it increasingly difficult to keep abreast of the ever expanding flood of new information except in the domain of their own particular interest. It is entirely unrealistic, therefore, to expect that the physician and others who are concerned primarily with the practical management and control of infectious diseases will find an opportunity to fish from this torrent the data relevant to their own purposes. In this predicament they are compelled to turn to the textbook or review which recapitulates our present knowledge of the animal viruses. But many of these treatises are written in large part by specialists whose eyes, quite naturally, tend to look first and longest at their major quarry, the microorganism itself. In this book, with the needs of the physician foremost in mind, the emphasis has been reversed. The patient who may be suffering from a viral infection is here the cynosure.

From this perspective the diagnosis of the disease by all available means, its management, and the protection of contacts and other members of the community become the prime objectives. An acquaintance with the techniques offered by virology forms only a part of the equipment demanded of the well-qualified physician. He must, of course, know what these techniques are and when and how they can be properly applied, but an extensive and thorough knowledge of the clinical features of viral infection is clearly his first requirement. Indeed on such knowledge he must often solely rely since virological aids are still lacking in certain instances, are impractical to invoke in others, or at best serve belatedly to confirm the clinical assessment. Moreover, as is suggested in this volume, it seems likely that through further accurate observation and description of slight differences in the response of patients to infection with different, although closely related viruses, the clinician not only will increase the chances that his initial assessment will be correct, but will also advance in his turn our understanding of the mechanisms, as yet incompletely defined, which underlie viral pathogenicity.

Writing in the spirit of this philosophy the authors of *Clinical Virology*, whose experience and accomplishment give them the right to speak with authority both as clinicians and virologists, have made a valuable addition to the didactic literature of viral infections.

In this enterprise, Professor Robert Debré has been the instigator and leader, as he has in so much else that he has contributed for so long and so brilliantly to the advancement of medical science and to medical education in France. As one of many colleagues in other lands whom he has inspired by his life and work I am happy to be able to record here my high admiration for his beneficent labors.

JOHN F. ENDERS, PH.D.
Professor Emeritus, Harvard Medical School

Editors' Note

This book is designed for clinicians. It is conceived as a practical manual available for consultation in the presence of a symptomatic picture suggestive of a viral etiology.

How does viral disease present itself, and when should viral etiology be suspected? What is the clinical and epidemiological evidence in favor of this etiology? How does one seek the help of the laboratory, which usually will be the only way to confirm the diagnosis? These are the questions that confront the practitioner, and thus is explained the scheme of presentation that has been adopted: division by physiological systems, by pathological manifestations, rather than division by viral species, as is the rule for textbooks of theoretical virology. The scheme chosen inevitably creates repetitions and also difficulties in presentation because the same pathogenic agent can (and this is frequent in virology) be the cause of various disturbances or, conversely, similar syndromes can be produced by different viruses. The practitioner also needs to know the prophylactic measures and the therapeutic actions indicated. The interest of the latter is so great that we have in some instances discussed those that are still in the experimental stage.

It was not, however, possible to approach so specific an area of human pathology without discussing the most recent data on viruses, in order to understand their mode of action and the means of defense of the organism. We have generally asked those in daily professional contact with these problems to present the most important concepts concerning pathogenic viruses and the reactions of the human host. For each group of viruses, these special chapters have been placed in the framework of the most frequent or the best-known manifestation; once again, repetitions and referrals from one chapter to the other are the inevitable result.

Although we have been rigorously critical of the facts reported, we could not limit this book to those manifestations whose viral etiology has been proved. Thus we have accorded a place to certain illnesses the pathogenic agent of which has not been isolated but which are probably of viral origin, such as infectious hepatitis or infectious mononucleosis. We have also studied, because of their close clinical kinship to the viruses, illnesses due to *Mycoplasma* or to *Rickettsia*, such as atypical pneumonia or Q fever. It appeared interesting to us, finally, to explore certain areas of special current interest, such as the relationships of viruses and tumors, diseases of the hematopoietic system, alterations of chromosomes, and the diseases provoked by the "slow" viruses.

This book has benefited from the collaboration of authors of very different nationality, culture, spirit, and notoriety. Despite an effort toward order and unity, the personality of each author appears in the manner of presenting the subject, the opinion expressed, and the interpretation given to the facts. Each author is responsible for his own concepts, but each has fullfilled his task scrupulously in order that this book might attain the double purpose of practical information and broad education that its editors assigned to it.

Contents

ENCEPHALITIDES, ENCEPHALOPATHIES, AND MENINGOENCEPHALITIDES

MENINGITIDES

VII. VIRAL INFECTIONS WITH INVOLVEMENT OF THE HEMATOPOIETIC AND LYMPHATIC SYSTEM

Introduction

By   R. DEBRÉ, J. CELERS, AND R. NETTER

Unquestionably the diseases most frequently observed in man and in mammals are caused by viruses. Medical practitioners encounter them every day. In their benign manifestations, viral infections are observed daily in the form of the common cold, herpes, and often slight discomforts to which little significance is attached. It is hardly necessary to recall that viruses are responsible for most of the infectious exanthemas so common in childhood all over the world, and for respiratory diseases related to a whole series of newly discovered viruses: rhinovirus, Myxovirus parainfluenzae, respiratory syncytial virus, reovirus, and doubtless others yet to be identified. They are perhaps also the cause of many of the gastrointestinal infections so frequently observed in early infancy. Moreover, viruses are responsible for the most severe pandemics, such as those of smallpox or influenza, which can cause thousands of deaths and which have played a major role in the history of man. Not to be forgotten are the ravages of encephalitis lethargica from 1917 through 1925, of poliomyelitis in Denmark in 1952, and, during the years 1964-1965, of German measles in the United States. Also there still persists that terrible contamination from animal to man, always fatal to man, namely, rabies. We could add many more examples; those given suffice to recall the importance of virology in the physician's everyday practice.

We must also ask ourselves what is the role of viral infections in congenital malformations, in malignant blood dyscrasias such as leukemia, in benign tumors, and finally in various cancers. We would like to examine this vast domain of human pathology under a particular light.

In which cases should the medical practitioner consider the possibility that a virus is the cause of the symptoms he observes? Which clinical manifestations suggest a disease of viral origin, and which type of virus should be suspected in a given circumstance? Which laboratory examinations are mandatory to assure a correct diagnosis? What should one ask from the biologist, whose work in this case is not simple? How should the clinician interpret the laboratory results supplied to him? How can one fight the disease when we possess but few antiviral therapeutic agents? How can a viral epidemic be limited? How, in any case, can individuals and the community be protected against the spread of viral diseases?

These are the problems we would like to help the medical practitioner to solve. He is often discouraged by the difficulties of taking specimens, by the long delay in obtaining laboratory results, and by the difficulties in interpreting them. Doubtless, in certain instances, such as eruptive fevers, mumps, or acute anterior poliomyelitis, he can make a diagnosis that is probably correct on the basis of physical examination and epidemiological background, but in other circumstances only the laboratory can assure him that his diagnosis is correct. Conversely, knowledge of well-defined clinical aspects of a disease and results of well-controlled laboratory tests should prevent the practitioner from attributing illness to a virus without the slightest proof; too often it is suggested that a disease is viral merely for want of another recognizable etiology. In this work we shall have occasion to repeat many times that the diagnosis of a viral infection requires a battery of clinical, virological, and epidemiological arguments. Thus the laboratory can suggest the role of a virus when it is isolated

1

from specimens taken early in the disease, and it can affirm the existence of viral infecion when the acquisition of specific antibodies or an increase in their level coincides with the evolution of the disease, but it does not establish a causal relation between the virus and the clinical picture.

This correlation becomes evident for the clinician only when the symptomatology is precise and when other observations, personal or otherwise, have already established the etiological role of a definite virus during identical diseases. It requires in addition a close study of the human environment, a search for similarly well established cases in the same community, and a biological study proving that no other virus can be incriminated. Today we cannot accept a vague hypothesis of a viral disease without real proof. Neither can we ask the biologist to perform a difficult and expensive task without attempting to guide him, thus sparing time, money, and the effort of laboratory workers.

Our present attempt should be to diagnose a viral disease only when it is necessary. We must apply the same standards to study of viral diseases that have been so successfully applied to those of bacterial, protozoal, and fungal origin, and the same rigorous demonstrations should be demanded. Whatever the difficulties, they engender progress.

For most viral diseases the spread of the agent in a given community is such that clinical study of a patient is inconceivable without epidemiological study of the community and even of the country or the entire continent. Since viruses cannot multiply outside a living cell, the relationships between the pathogenic agent and the human host are of particular importance. In a great number of cases, each disease represents only the visible manifestation of a virus that is widespread in the population. This spread is usually inapparent, although reactions that are extreme in their variation show the relationship between the virus and each individual host. Epidemiological study is therefore fundamental and should be pursued by the clinician, the virologist, and the statistician. Thus teamwork is necessary to help the practitioner in his difficult task.

In this field the investigation starts with the clinical manifestations. The clinician is the first to raise the problem and immediately initiates the necessary measures. The clinical work is the object of the initial and fundamental research in all the senses of this word.

The textbooks on virology are centered on the virus, and their chapters are divided according to different kinds of pathogenic viruses. Our point of view is different. We shall describe the syndrome first, presenting the results of physical examination of the patient based on the most carefully detailed observations; then we shall proceed to study the causal agent. This process should give a somewhat new form to each exposition.

Sometimes the problem seems quickly solved: the clinical picture is well defined and attributable to only one virus, as in the case of measles and chickenpox. Nevertheless, even in such circumstances virology can clarify certain clinical and epidemiological problems that confront practitioners. The relation between giant-cell pneumonia of early childhood and measles, between chickenpox and herpes zoster, or between herpes simplex and certain types of stomatitis or keratitis are examples of instances in which virology completes the knowledge established by clinical experience.

In many other clinical syndromes the etiology is difficult to ascertain. The infections of respiratory, intestinal, pharyngeal, and nasal mucosae and the involvements of the central nervous system furnish examples of these difficulties. In these syndromes a variety of viruses can be incriminated. The effect of each virus should be determined as well as is possible, for there are still a few orphan viruses in search of a disease and also a few diseases which are certainly or probably of viral origin that are still in search of an identified agent. However, it seems to us that a closer and more detailed study of the clinical symptoms and of the etiology of these diseases with apparently similar manifestations will show that they are not identical. Symptomatic study has not always been sufficiently thorough to exclude the possibility that in the future distinctions will be possible which, at present, only the virological laboratory can make. The entire history of pathology has taught us how the increasingly careful examination of the patient has led to the recognition of definite entities in the midst of a confusing picture. The task of the clinician is far from complete, and the rigorous specificity of each infectious agent no doubt is manifested by clinical reactions that it will be possible to define, although not without difficulty. Thus it may be possible to achieve a sufficiently clear description of diseases that resemble each other but are different.

The physician's concern is not only the diagnosis of a viral disease but also the fight against it. It is almost superfluous to recall here the glorious beginnings of the prevention of viral diseases before the knowledge of viruses. The discovery of Jenner and the protection against smallpox, and that of Pasteur and the vaccination against rabies, are examples known by everyone. These two discoveries marked the beginning of a series of preventive measures which, though preceding the successes of modern science, have, together with vaccinations and passive immunization, shown the way in which we are now advancing with more assured steps.

In the pages that follow we shall review the principles of vaccinations against viral diseases and of passive immunization, especially by gamma globulins. The task of the practitioner in preventive medicine becomes more and more important. He must, on the basis of valid information, select the methods of vaccination to be used, determine the dates of vaccinations, and combine them, associating them according to the geographic location, the circumstances, and the individuals, weighing in each case the advantages and the disadvantages of the schedule he will follow.

As in all medical fields, each physician's decision must not be too strictly limited by rules. In no case should the practitioner's action be automatic; it should be based upon precise and compelling indications. The application of general rules and legal obligations is not simple. In fact, new knowledge and discoveries impose frequent changes. This will be discussed in detail in connection with each disease.

The practitioner's task in preventive medicine includes, moreover, the application of a series of measures in social medicine. They will also be considered. Although the treatment of viral diseases is far from attaining the effectiveness which permitted victory over most bacteria, research in this field should not be ignored, and its principles will be discussed.

Our purpose is therefore, first, to try to provide the physician with the means to establish a correct diagnosis and, second, to supply the information that will aid him in his ever more important role as the protector of individual and public health.

The refinements of clinical examination should thus be developed first, then the team tasks based on epidemiological and etiological research, and, last, individual and collective protection. This is the work that appears desirable to us to facilitate to our utmost in the vast field of viral infections.

VIRUSES: DESCRIPTION

At this point, certain precise details concerning viruses must be given. In view of the purpose of this book, only a reminder concerning the essential and generally accepted concepts will be outlined here.

DEFINITION

The meaning of "virus" has evolved greatly in the course of time. This Latin word can be found in the writings of Cicero, Virgil, and Pliny with the general sense of venom or poison, and even then, of infection.

At the end of the nineteenth century, during the pasteurian period, the term took on a more restrictive sense. It was no longer applied except to agents of infectious diseases. Thanks to progress in the techniques of microscopy and filtration, the element of size made possible a preliminary distinction of the ultraviruses or filtrating viruses from other microbes. Ivanowski is generally considered the scientist who "found," as early as 1892, the first virus by candle filtration of the juice of tobacco plants attacked by mosaic disease. Influenced by E. Roux, he thought then that a toxin was involved, and it was Beijerinck who, in 1899, proved the viral nature of tobacco mosaic by contaminating healthy plants by use of the filtrate. The first human viruses known were those of yellow fever, the filtrating nature of which was established in 1901 by Reed, and that of rabies, the viral origin of which, suspected by Pasteur, was demonstrated by Remlinger in 1903.

The notion of parasitism began to appear, and it was considered that viruses need, in order to multiply, a cellular substrate not furnished by the media generally utilized for bacteriological cultures.

Years later, in 1916, the rickettsiae, so named in honor of Ricketts, who died of typhus in the course of his research work, were seen to constitute a group of pleomorphic agents at the limit of visibility with the microscopes of the time. The works of Charles Nicolle on typhus drew attention to the notion that arthropods were indispensable to the survival or to the transmission of these agents; this last characteristic did not, however, prove to be absolute, since certain rickettsiae such as those of Q fever do not need a vector agent, whereas most of the arboviruses are thus transmitted, from which fact derives their name of *Ar*thropod-*bo*rne viruses. The term arbovirus has replaced that of arborvirus to avoid any confusion concerning a forest origin.

Over approximately the last 20 years the discovery of numerous new viruses and the perfecting of techniques and knowledge, particularly in molecular biochemistry, have made it possible to specify accurately the physical and chemical criteria defining viruses.

Viruses are living organisms which contain (after purification to rid them of cellular constituents) only a single nucleic acid, either ribonucleic acid (RNA) or desoxyribonucleic acid (DNA), surrounded by a protein shell. The presence of nucleic acid, the bearer of heredity and the repository of the information necessary for reproduction, demonstrates that viruses are not simple proteins.

Viruses, unlike bacteria and rickettsiae, lack enzymes; to reproduce, they need living cells that furnish the enzymatic systems necessary and that carry out, under their control, the necessary syntheses. They are hence incapable of multiplying in artificial culture media.

To these two essential features characterizing viruses — the presence of a single nucleic acid and obligatory intracellular parasitism — should be added a third, namely, their insensitivity in vivo to the antibiotics known at present.

As can be seen in Table 1, bacteria and viruses represent two extremes, bacteria being independent organisms that carry two nucleic acids and are sensitive to antibiotics, while viruses are obligatory intracellular parasites, carriers of a single nucleic acid, and insensitive to antibiotics. Between the two are a series of "intermediate" agents. The mycoplasma, isolated for the first time in 1898 by Nocard and Roux from a case of bovine pleuropneumonia (hence their earlier name of PPLO — pleuropneumonia-like organism), are near in size or even smaller than certain large viruses such as those of smallpox or measles. They can be cultivated in artificial media and have two nucleic acids, features bringing them closer to bacteria.

The agents of the group psittacosis — lymphogranuloma venereum — trachoma have received various names: the term "bedsoniae" was given them by the British in memory of Bedson, who made a thorough study of psittacosis. Giroud and Jadin in 1954 proposed the term "neorickettsia" to indicate the character intermediate between rickettsia and viruses. There also appear in the literature other denominations such as "chlamydozoaceae," "chlamydiaceae" (from the Greek χλαμύς, which means coat), and "miyagawanellae." Gear suggested setting apart the *TRIC* agents (*T*rachoma *I*nclusion *C*onjunctivitis); recently, biological and chemical tests for their identification and differentiation have been described (cf. Chapter 52).

The agents of this group have close antigenic relationships. They possess the two nucleic acids, are endowed with an enzymatic system, and are sensitive to antibiotics of the tetracycline group. All these characteristics distinguish them from the viruses despite their common inability to develop in artificial media.

Nevertheless, the techniques and the methods used for both rickettsiae and the psittacosis group are so close to those employed in virology that it is most often the

Table 1. *Characteristics of Infectious Agents from Bacteria to Viruses*

	GROWTH ON ARTIFICIAL MEDIA	TWO NUCLEIC ACIDS	RESPONSE TO ANTIBIOTICS
Bacteria	+	+	+
Mycoplasma	+	+	+
Rickettsia	−	+	+
Psittacosis–lymphogranuloma venereum–trachoma group	−	+	+
Viruses	−	−	−

virologists and not the bacteriologists who study them. Moreover, most books on virology include them and thus receive titles such as "Infections Due to Viruses and Rickettsia in Man."

Since our purpose in this book is dominated by clinical considerations, we will extend our study to the agents of the psittacosis group and even to mycoplasma. Furthermore, in discussing various syndromes we will indicate the different agents that may cause them; if indicated, the therapy will also be discussed, even when the authentic viruses are not involved.

SIZE AND MORPHOLOGY

Size. As we have indicated, the size of viruses is entirely insufficient to characterize them, since certain nonviral agents as distant from them as the mycoplasma are no larger than most viruses, and a simple molecule of snail hemocyanin is even larger than a poliomyelitis virus. This small size, initially considered a criterion, was measured first by indirect procedures such as filtration and ultracentrifugation and then by means of the electron microscope, which has permitted the greatest precision.

The diameter of viruses varies from 15 mμ* for the virus of yellow fever to 260 mμ for that of vaccinia, which is at the limit of visibility with the optic microscope.

Form. Viruses have various forms. They can resemble parallelepipeds with rounded angles (vaccinia virus), spheres (myxoviruses, adenoviruses, enteroviruses), and cones (rabies virus).

Bacteriophages are viruses that are parasites of bacteria: their polygonal heads and their tails (when they exist) make them roughly resemble spermatozoa. Precise information on the ultrastructure of viruses has been obtained by such electron microscopic techniques as negative staining with phosphotungstate,† developed by Brenner and Horne, and by chemical degradation techniques. As early as 1935 Stanley obtained crystals of tobacco mosaic virus and Schaffer and Schwert obtained crystals of poliomyelitis virus; it was supposed that the extreme limit

between living matter and inanimate matter had been attained. In reality, this pseudocrystalline aspect represents a tendency common to all viruses to organize themselves according to a geometric pattern.

Structure. Lwoff applied the term *virion* to the complete viral particle capable of surviving in crystalline form and infecting a living cell: this term replaces the former denominations "elementary body" or "viral particle." Its different parts are distinguished under the electron microscope. The *nucleoid,* the viral genetic material, is a darker zone situated in the center of the virion. It appears as a biconcave disk in vaccinia virus, an eccentric rod in herpes virus, or a hexagon in adenovirus. It is constituted essentially of ribonucleic or desoxyribonucleic acid with one or two filaments (monocatenary or bicatenary strands). The RNA of the poliomyelitis virus is only a short strand; the DNA of the papilloma group, like that of bacteria, has an annular form.

The *capsid* is the shell of protein that protects the nucleic acid. Study by x-ray diffraction and under the electron microscope indicates two essential variants:

In the capsids with *helical symmetry* the protein elements constituting the capsid are bound to the nucleoid and form a sort of spiral stairway whose flight appears to be the ribbon of nucleic acid. The whole is lengthened into a tubular form (tobacco mosaic virus) or rolled up into a ball (influenza or vaccinia virus).

In the capsids with *cubic symmetry,* the nucleic acid forms a central, independent ball.

The capsid is composed of morphological units or capsomeres. The capsomeres are disposed at the surface of the nucleoid according to an icosahedral* symmetry. Each capsomere is in turn subdivided into structural units the number of which varies from two to six, so that it is possible, according to the number of these structural units, to designate the capsomeres as dimers, trimers, pentamers, hexamers (cf. Tables 2 and 3). The capsomeres of the herpes virus have, for example, the form of pentagonal or hexagonal prisms.

Certain viruses such as the adenoviruses or the reoviruses are thought to possess a double capsid, internal and external.

---

*The millimicron is the millionth part of a millimeter; one millimicron (mμ) is equal to 10 angströms (Å).

†This technique indicates the ultrafine structure of the virus on an electron-opaque film of phosphotungstate.

---

*The icosahedron is a polyhedron having 20 faces, each an equilateral triangle.

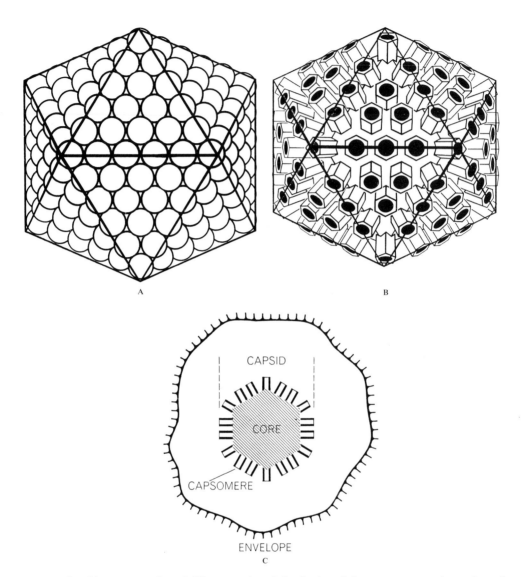

Figure 1. Graphic representation of different modes of distribution of the capsomeres at the surface of capsids with cubic symmetry. *A*, Adenovirus: 240 hexamers on the faces and the edges of the icosahedron, 12 pentamers on the apices. *B*, Herpes virus: 150 hexamers on the faces and the edges of the icosahedron, 12 pentamers on the apices. *C*, Graphic representation of a virus (herpes virus) whose capsid with cubic symmetry is surrounded by an envelope with, from the center to the periphery, the core, the capsid with the capsomers, and the envelope. (From The Structure of Viruses, by R. W. Horne. Copyright © 1963 by Scientific American, Inc. All rights reserved.)

on lymphocytic choriomeningitis (L.C.M.) virus infection in mice (32254). Proc. Soc. Exp. Biol. Med., *125*:980-983, 1967.

16a. Hotchin, J., et al.: The effects of pretreatment with X-rays on the pathogenesis of lymphocytic choriomeningitis in mice. 1. Host survival virus multiplication and leukocytosis. 2. The pathological histology. J. Immunol., *87*:675-681; 682-687, 1961.

16b. Hotchin, J., et al.: Factors affecting the induction of persistent tolerant infection of newborn mice with lymphocytic choriomeningitis. Virology, *18*: 71-78, 1962.

17. Johnsson, A. T.: Nord. Med. *55*:859, 1965; cited by Sohier.[42]

18. Komrower, G. M., et al.: Lymphocytic choriomeningitis in the newborn. Probable transplacental infection. Lancet, *268*:697-698, 1955.

19a. Kreis, B.: La maladie d' Armstrong: Chorioméningite lymphocytaire. Paris, Baillere, 1937.

19b. Kreis, B.: La maladie d'Armstrong: Chorioméningite lymphocytaire. Sem. Hop. Paris, *24*:1018, 1948.

20. Lavillaureix, J., et al.: Résultats de 18 mois d' enquête sur les maladies à virus en Alsace. Strasbourg Med., *8*:497-503, 1957.

21a. Lepine, P., et al.: Réceptivité de l'homme au virus murin de la chorioméningite lymphocytaire. Reproduction expérimentale de la méningite lymphocytaire bénigne. C. R. Acad. Sci., *204*: 1846 , 1937.

21b. Lepine, P., et al. Déviation du complément dans l' infection par le virus de la chorioméningite lymphocytaire. Ann. Inst. Pasteur (Paris), *61*:868, 869, 1938; C. R. Soc. Biol., *124*:925-927, 1938.

21c. Lepine, P., et al.: Un nouvel ultravirus: le virus de la pneumopathie des cobayes. C. R. Soc. Biol., *137*:317, 1943.

22. Levey, R. H., et al.: Lymphocytic choriomeningitis infection in neonatally thymectomized mice bearing diffusion chambers containing thymus. Science, *142*:483, 1963.

23. Lewis, J. M., et al.: Orchitis, parotidis and meningoencephalitis due to lymphocytic choriomeningitis virus. New Eng. J. Med. *265*:776-780, 1961.

24. Lippi, M., et al.: Contributo sieroimmunologico alla conoscenza delle principali virosi. Ricerca nei soggetti sani degli anticorpi devianti il complemento verso il virus della coriomeningite linfocitaria. Arch. Ital. Sci. Med. Trop., *42*:109-124, 1961.

25. McCallum, F. O., et al.: Pseudolymphocytic choriomeningitis. Brit. J. Exp. Path., *20*:260, 1939.

26. Marquezy, R. A., Chorio-méningite lymphocytaire: Maladie d' Armstrong. (1) Etude clinique, (2) Etude virologique. Sem. Hop. Paris, *36*:1211/ P211, 1216/P 216, 1960.

27. Meyer, H. M., et al.: Central nervous system syndromes of "viral" etiology. Amer. J. Med., *29*: 334-347, 1960.

28. Milzer, A.: Routine laboratory diagnosis of virus and rickettsial diseases. J.A.M.A., *143*:219-224, 1950.

29. Mollaret, P., et al.: Les bases immunologiques (dans le sang) du diagnostic actuel de la chorioméningite lymphocytaire. Paris Med., 470-478, 1939.

30. Nikolitsch, M., et al.: Immunserum und Gehirnbarriere. Arch. Hyg. Bakt., *141*:275, 1957.

31. Oker Blom, N., et al.: Nord. Med., *57*:621, 1957; cited by Sohier.[42]

32. Pfau, C. H.: Biophysical and biochemical characterization of lymphocytic choriomeningitis virus. Acta Path. Microbiol. Scand., *63*:188-197, 1965.

33. Public Health Laboratory Service: Suspected virus infections of respiratory tract and central nervous system. Lancet, *1*:85-87, 1953.

34. Reiss-Gutfreund, R. J., et al.: Etude d'un virus présentant les caractéristiques de la chorioméningite lymphocytaire (C.M.L.) isolé en Ethiopie. Ann. Inst. Pasteur (Paris), *102*:36-43, 1962.

35. Rivers, T. M., et al.: Meningitis in man caused by a filterable virus. *Science, 81*:439, 1935; *J. Exp. Med., 63*:397-414; 415-432, 1936.

36a. Roger, F., et al.: Etudes sur le pouveir pathogène expérimental du virus de la chorio-méningite lymphocytaire. II. Innoculation dans le derme du cobaye. Ann. Inst. Pasteur (Paris) *104*:274-282, 1963.

36b. Roger, F., et al.: Etudes sur le pouvoir pathogène expérimental du virus de la chorio-méningite lymphocytaire. III. Une réaction inflammatoire directement visible chez la souris, l'oedème viral du membre inférieur. Ann. Inst. Pasteur (Paris), *104*:347-360, 1963.

36c. Roger, F., et al.: Etudes sur le pouvoir pathogène expérimental du virus de la chorio-méningite lymphocytaire. VII. L'allergie dans les réactions locales chez la souris et ses conditions de demonstration. Ann. Inst. Pasteur (Paris), *107*:354-365, 1964.

37a. Scheid, W., et al.: Infektionen mit dem Virus der lymphozytären Choriomeningitis in Deutschland. Deutsch. Med. Wschr., *81*:700-703, 1956.

37b. Scheid, W., et al.: Die Bedeutung der komplementbindeuden und der neutralisieren den Antikörper für die Diagnose der Infektionen mit dem Virus der lymphozytären Choriomeningitis. Deutsch. Med. Wschr., *84*:1293-1296, 1957.

38. Schwarz, J., et al.: 1st Congr. Intern. Path. Inf. Lyon, 1956, p. 131; cited by Sohier.[42]

39. Sedallian, P., et al.: Sur un virus d'origine méningitique, apparenté au virus d'Armstrong, mais anormal par sa résistance, ses dimensions et sa répartition dans l'organisme. Ann. Inst. Pasteur (Paris), *86*:F85-F87, 1954.

40. Shvarev, A. I.: A clinical and virological study of lymphocytic choriomeningitis. (In Russian). Voprossi Virusol., pp. 323-326, 1959.

41a. Smadel, J. E., et al.: A soluble antigen of L.C. II. Characteristics of the antigen and its use in precipitin reactions. J. Exp. Med., *71*:43, 1940.

41b. Smadel, J. E., et al.: Complement fixation in choriomeningitis. Proc. Soc. Exp. Biol. Med., *40*:71, 1939.

42. Sohier, R., et al.: Meningites et méningo-encéphalites à virus observées en France. Presse Med., *62*:1248-1251, 1954.

43a. Traub, E.: A filterable virus recovered from white mice. Science, *81*:298, 1935.

43b. Traub, E.: Persistence of lymphocytic choriomeningitis in immune animals and its relation to immunity. J. Exp. Med., *63*:533-546, 1936.

44. Volkert, M., et al.: Immunological tolerance to viruses. Progr. Med. Virol., *7*:160-207, 1965.

45. Wilsnack, R. E., et al.: Immunofluorescent studies of the histopathogenesis of lymphocytic choriomeningitis virus infection. J. Exp. Med., *120*:829-840, 1964.

46. Wooley, J. G., et al.: A study of human sera antibodies capable of neutralizing the virus of lymphocytic choriomeningitis. Public Health Rep., *54*: 938, 1939.

18

Data Concerning the Different Viruses Responsible for So-Called Aseptic Meningitis

By V. DROUHET

The frequency of the lymphocytic meningitides and the percentage of cases due to the various responsible agents in different countries vary from year to year and depend, essentially, on the manner in which the virological diagnosis is carried out.

From 1950 to 1955, when the diagnosis of herpes simplex was made by inoculation into fertile eggs and onto the rabbit's cornea, that of mumps by inoculation into fertile eggs, and that of lymphocytic choriomeningitis by the use of adult mice, the percentages given for different countries were as shown in Table 18-1.

Virus-isolation, complement-fixation, or hemagglutination-inhibition tests were used by Milzer (1950)[11] for the diagnosis of 39 cases of "aseptic" meningitis and encephalitis.

Some 14 per cent of the results were positive, and of these 2.2 per cent showed western equine encephalomyelitis; 3.3 per cent choriomeningitis; and 8.8 per cent mumps meningoencephalitis. These results are abstracted from laboratory investigations carried out over a period of 18 months.

The use of tissue cultures has made considerably easier the diagnosis of infections by poliovirus, Coxsackie B, and ECHO viruses, but results obtained by this method are incomplete. Statistics from Davis and Melnick,[7] obtained by tissue culture in 219 cases of "aseptic" meningitis, yielded the figures shown in Table 18-2.

The statistics of Oker-Blom et al.[12] in 418 cases in Finland are shown in Table 18-3.

Table 18-1. *Percentages of Reported Cases of Lymphocytic Meningitis Due to Various Agents (1950-1955)*

COUNTRY	HERPES SIMPLEX	MUMPS	LYMPHOCYTIC CHORIOMENINGITIS
France[14]	0.8%	10%	3.3%
Great Britain[10]	5%	2.7%	2.2–3.7%
Sweden[2, 8]	1%	–	0%
United States[1, 6, 11]	1–5.3%	8.8% (Civilians) 9.4–17% (Army)	3.3% (Civilians) 8.1–11% (Army)
Holland	–	–	14%
Austria[4]	–	–	12%
Rumania[13]	–	–	9.4%

Table 18-2. *Viruses Recovered in Tissue Culture in 219 Cases of Meningitis**

Year	1955	1956	Total
Number of Cases	137	82	219
Recoveries of Virus in Tissue Culture	68	30	98
Poliovirus I	27	4	31
II	0	0	0
III	1	2	3
ECHO 5	1	0	1
6	22	9	31
14	2	2	4
Coxsackie A9	1	6	7
B2	5	1	6
3	2	4	6
4	7	2	9

*From Davis and Melnick.[7]

Table 18-3. *Viruses Recovered in Tissue Culture in 418 Cases of "Aseptic" Meningitis**

Etiological Agent	Cases, No.	Isolation of Virus No.	%
Poliovirus type I	85	36	42
Unidentified cytopathic agent; possibly ECHO virus	85	15	18
Mumps	79	11	14
Coxsackie	27	1	4
Herpes simplex	36	1	3
Leptospira	106	5	5
	418		86†

*From Oker-Blom et al.[12]
†The etiology was unknown in 14% of cases.

Virus isolation in cases of meningoencephalitis was carried out in a hospital in Johannesburg[3] and gave the following results: poliovirus in two of 175 cases investigated, Coxsackie A virus in 11 of 150 cases, Coxsackie B virus in 20 of 150 cases, and herpes virus in one of two cases.

Complement-fixation tests from the same laboratory gave the following diagnoses: herpes in two of 200 cases investigated, lymphocytic choriomeningitis in none of 200 cases, and mumps in 14 of 200 cases. In 25 cases, results were negative for St. Louis encephalitis, Japanese B encephalitis, eastern equine encephalitis, and western equine encephalitis.

At the Hospital for Sick Children in Toronto[5] during 1957, viruses were recovered from the stools, from the cerebrospinal fluid, and from the blood; human amnion and monkey kidney tissue cultures were used. Neutralizing antibodies against the isolated viruses were looked for and, in addition, serological tests were used for the diagnosis of mumps. In 51 cases of "aseptic" meningitis the results were as follows: ECHO 6 and ECHO 9 viruses appeared to be responsible in 48 per cent of cases and Coxsackie A9, B3, and B5 viruses in 18 per cent; 14 per cent of cases were diagnosed as being due to mumps virus. The etiology remained unknown in 20 per cent of cases of lymphocytic meningitis.

In the diagnosis of lymphocytic meningitis, some laboratories use serological examination (for mumps, herpes simplex, and some of the encephalitis viruses), combined with the virus isolation in different tissue culture systems and inoculation into animals (suckling mice, for example, to demonstrate Coxsackie virus A, and adult mice for the diagnosis of lymphocytic choriomeningitis).

Thus, for example, Lennette et al.[9] in the United States in 1958 found etiological proof in 253 of 368 cases of lymphocytic meningitis; that is, in 69 per cent of cases.* In 2 per cent polioviruses were responsible, in 2 per cent Coxsackie A, in 43 per cent Coxsackie B (Coxsackie B5 epidemic at the time of the study), in 9 per cent ECHO virus, in 9 per cent mumps virus, in 1 per cent herpes virus, and in 3 per cent miscellaneous agents. Adenovirus was implicated in one case.

---

*These figures are misleading, however, as a Coxsackie B5 virus epidemic was raging in the area at the time when the investigation was made.

BIBLIOGRAPHY

1. Adair, C. V., Gauld, R. L., and Smadel, J. E.: Aseptic meningitis, a disease of diverse etiology: clinical studies on 854 cases. Ann. Int. Med., *39*:675, 1953.
2. Alfzelius-Alm, L.: Aseptic (nonbacterial) encephalomeningitides in Gothenburg 1932-1950. Acta Med. Scand., Supplement 140, 1951.
3. Bayer, P., and Gear, J.: Virus meningo-encephalitis in South Africa of the cases admitted to the Johannesburg fever hospital. S. Afr. J. Lab. Clin. Med., *6*:22, 1955.
4. Bieling, R., and Koch, F.: Versuch einer klinischen Differentialdiagnose der abakteriellen Meningitis. Ztschr. Kinderh., *72*:85, 1952.

5. Clarke, M., et al.: Seasonal aseptic meningitis caused by Coxsackie and ECHO viruses, Toronto, 1957. Canad. Med. Assn. J., *81*:5, 1959.

6. Crawford, I. D., Meyer, H. M., Rogers, N. G., Miesse, M. L., and Banknead, A. S.: In: 4ème Réunion Europ. Stand. Biol., Bruxelles, 1957.

7. Davis, D. C., and Melnick, J. L.: Poliomyelitis and aseptic meningitis; a two year field and laboratory study in Connecticut. J. Lab. Clin. Med., *51*:97, 1958.

8. Johnsson, T.: Meningitis serosa. II. Primär och sekundär eller postinfektiös meningo-encephalit: etiologi och epidemiologi. Nord. Med., *55*:859, 1956.

9. Lennette, E. H., Magoffin, R. L., Schmidt, N. J., and Hollister, A. C.: Viral disease of the central nervous system. Influence of poliomyelitis on etiology. J.A.M.A., *128*:1456, 1959.

10. MacCallum, F. O.: Diagnosis of virus diseases. Brit. M. Bull., *7*:174, 1951.

11. Milzer, A.: Routine laboratory diagnosis of viral and rickettsial diseases. Results of an eighteen month study. J.A.M.A., *143*:219, 1950.

12. Oker-Blom, A. N., Pentinnen, K., Salminen, A., Pohjanpelto, P., Halonen, P., Haapanen, L., and Klemola, E.: Den serösa meningitens etiologi i finland virus och leptospiraunder-sökningar på 134 patienter vid aurora sjukhus i Helsingfors 1952-1955. Nord. Med., *57*:621, 1957.

13. Schwarz, J., Moscovici, O., and Samuel, J.: In: Atti 1 Congr. inst. Pathol. infettiva., Lyon, 24 mai, 1956, p. 131.

14. Sohier, R., and Buissière, J.: Méningites et méningoencephalites à virus observées en France. Presse Med., *62*:1248, 1954.

19

Diseases Caused by Slow Viruses*

By HILARY KOPROWSKI and MICHAEL KATZ

The definition of a virus as "slow" or "fast" is anthropocentric and may actually stand in the way of conceptual appreciation of the agents that are so defined. The "slow" character of certain agents is not intrinsic but refers, rather, to the host manifestation of their presence or, more correctly, to the investigator's recognition of their manifestation. The earmark of these agents is the chronic, languishing nature of the infectious process they initiate in the human or animal organism, or in an *in vitro* tissue culture system. The incubation period may extend over months or even years, and the disease that results may advance gradually (sometimes characterized by remissions and exacerbation of symptoms) but relentlessly, leading ultimately to an irreversible deterioration of the host.

In general, viruses have been identified by the influence they exert on the cell; this has been either destruction or stimulation of proliferative growth. The relatively new idea that neither may occur is based on the consideration that some viruses may coexist in some type of commensalism with the cell and ultimately—often only after a long period

of time—may cause dysfunction of the cell.† If the dysfunction is subtle, detection of the dysfunction may be long in coming. This, then, is the core of the definition of "slow" viruses (Fig. 19-1).

MECHANISMS OF PATHOGENESIS

Pathogenesis of any viral disease depends on the multiplication of the agents in the host and affection of the target tissue. For example, in poliomyelitis, the virus multiplies in the intestinal mucosa before it is carried by the blood to the central nervous system, where it causes damage by destroying anterior horn cells. Although poliomyelitis is not a "slow" virus, there is a measurable time lag between infection and development of symptoms. This delay, or incubation period, exists regardless of the pathway of spread. Similarly, in experimental scrapie in mice, the virus is present in the viscera for approximately 16 weeks, while the mice are asymptomatic, before it penetrates the central nervous system and causes symptoms. In these animals, the agent of scrapie

*This work was supported in part by Public Health Service Research Grant #1-R01-NB 06859-01 from the National Institute of Neurological Diseases and Blindness.

†An analogy may be made with the known relationship between a cell and a tumor virus. Following an abortive infection, such a cell continues to divide in a seemingly normal pattern. After many cell generations, the original virus in its infective form may still be recovered.

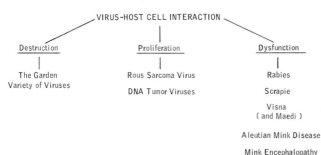

Figure 19-1. Virus-host cell interaction.

infects the lymphatic tissue long before it reaches the central nervous system.

However, this time lag for multiplication of the agent before it reaches the target tissue cannot be the only explanation for the prolonged incubation period of "slow" virus diseases. In experimental infection of mice with rabies, which classically has a prolonged incubation period, viral antigen can be detected in the spinal cord by immunofluorescence within 24 hours; yet there are no observed central nervous system symptoms for several weeks.

The consideration of rabies virus illustrates many of the problems encountered in "slow" virus infections. In man and many other homoiothermic animals, the incubation period, following exposure with the street virus, is variable, and may be several months to two years. During this interval, no clinical evidence of an infection is discernible. Moreover, when clinical symptoms ultimately develop (and even when death occurs), there are no clear pathological manifestations of the presence of this infectious agent. The only observable abnormalities are nonspecific, focal degenerative changes in the ganglia, accumulation of phagocytic cells and scattered petechial hemorrhages. Until the discovery by Negri of a specific inclusion body, no definite pathological diagnosis of rabies could be made. The presently available technique of immunofluorescence permits not only rapid identification of the rabies virus inclusion within the cell, but also tracing the pattern of its distribution.

Thus, if one did not see Negri bodies and had no fluorescent antibody technique, rabies would mimic the mysterious "slow" virus diseases. It is a progressive neuropathic disease with a long incubation period; suspensions of neural tissue from the individuals afflicted with it are infectious; the disease is

reproduced on serial passage of the infected tissues: yet there is no pathognomonic lesion.

The host-virus relationship in the animal body can be mimicked *in vitro* in tissue culture systems. Rabies virus can be present in 100 per cent of infected tissue culture cells without affecting their normal multiplication for at least 200 generations. Although these cells continue to divide and metabolize, all of them show presence of specific inclusion bodies (see also footnote, page 235).

With this concept in mind, let us summarize what is known about the several conditions that have been classified as "slow" virus infections.

SCRAPIE

Host(s)

NATURAL. Sheep, occasionally goat.

EXPERIMENTAL. Sheep, goat, mouse, hamster, rat.*

Agent. Scrapie is one of the smallest known infectious agents.

SIZE. This has been estimated by radocol (nitrocellulose) membrane filtration as 27 mμ, and by x-ray inactivation as 7 mμ.

RESISTANCE TO CHEMICAL AGENTS. It is resistant to formalin; i.e., goat brain material remains infective for goats by the intracerebral route after exposure to 8 per cent formalin. It is also resistant to ether.

RESISTANCE TO PHYSICAL AGENTS. When a crude suspension of the brain material containing virus is heated to 95.5° C., the titer drops 100-fold. After Millipore filtration, a solution containing a 10^3 to 10^4 concentration of the virus, when heated to

---

*Based on reproduction of the disease in natural host after serial passage of the agent in the experimental animal.

95.5° C., becomes noninfectious. If a pellet is produced by centrifugation at 100,000 × *g* for 45 minutes, heating to 80° C. does not kill the infectious material. No known infectious agent exhibits a similar property, although the agent of mink encephalopathy (which may be the same as the agent of scrapie) is probably also heat-resistant. The agent of scrapie has been reported also to be resistant to ultraviolet radiation.

This agent is nonantigenic for the infected animals and for a variety of laboratory animals, such as rabbits, that are not subject to infection with scrapie* (Fig. 19-2).

Tissue Culture. Mouse spleen-clot culture from affected animals will maintain the agent for as long as 28 days. Primary mouse embryo tissue culture, in a like manner, will maintain this agent for 48 days. However, it produces no cytopathic effect in primary mouse embryo tissue culture and can be detected only by infectivity for mice. There is no evidence for or against *replication* of this agent in any *in vitro* system.

Pathogenesis. Ultimate lesions are found in brain and spinal cord following an experimental infection in mice by the extracerebral route. Scrapie agent can be isolated quite early (approximately one week postinfection) in the lymph nodes and spleen and, several weeks later, also in the salivary glands, thymus, and lungs. It is recoverable from the brain at 16 weeks.

Incubation Period. Natural scrapie, in sheep, has an incubation period of two to four years. In experimental scrapie the in-

---

*Refer to footnote under Aleutian Mink Disease.

cubation period is variable and generally is longer in interspecific than in intraspecific transfer. In the latter, earlier passages take longer to produce the disease than subsequent, fixed passages (Fig. 19-3).

Clinical Symptoms

SHEEP. The animals rub their bodies and nibble on the skin of the lower extremities. They show fatigue, poor exercise tolerance, and soon begin to lose weight because of poor feeding. They exhibit a characteristically disturbed gait, walking on a broad base, with a high-stepping movement of the forelimbs. They also show involuntary tremor at rest, which is accentuated by excitement. Ultimately, they develop ataxia, which may become so severe that the animals stagger. Righting reflexes remain intact until the terminal stage of the disease. The tendon reflexes may also be unaffected or only slightly exaggerated. Occasionally the animals exhibit bizarre behavior; some may become blind; some show cardiovascular instability manifested by wide fluctuations of the heart rate; some show wide fluctuations in body temperature. The disease is progressive and invariably fatal, death following six weeks to six months after the onset of the symptoms.

GOATS. Goats exhibit a similar pattern of the disease, but also have a variant in which the animals become progressively drowsy before death.

Pathological Findings. When the central nervous system is examined, the essential lesion is a noninflammatory, diffuse degeneration of gray matter which is focal and distributed symmetrically in various parts of the brain. Perineuronal gray matter becomes

Figure 19-2. Unique properties of the scrapie agent.

Alleged Property		Factual Evidence
Size:	Smallest known infectious agent.	a. 27 mμ by Gradocol membrane. b. 7 mμ by X-ray target size. c. Irregularly dialyzable (as some larger viruses).
Effect of physical agents:	More heat-resistant than other known viruses. UV-resistant.	Resistant to > 80° C for prolonged period of time. Not confirmed.
Effect of chemical agents:	Formalin-resistant.	Resistant to 20% formalin for at lease 18 months.
Immunological response:	None.	Non-antigenic in natural and experimental hosts; also fails to produce antibodies in animals not susceptible to the disease.

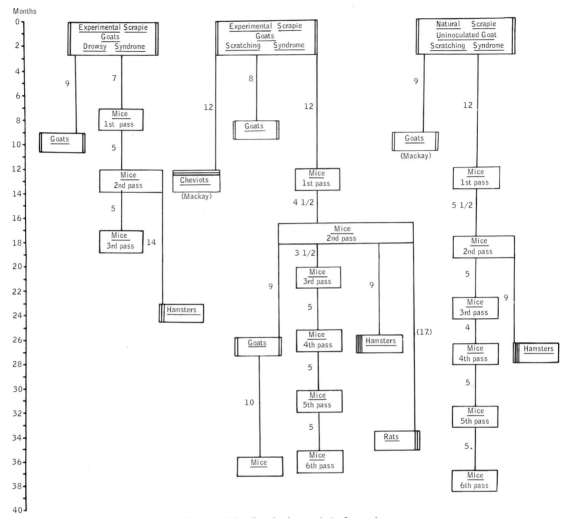

Figure 19-3.   Incubation period of scrapie.

spongy, the astrocytes hypertrophy, and there is sporadic degeneration of the myelin. Neurons become pyknotic, exhibiting necrosis and vacuolation. Eosinophilic bodies are often seen within vacuoles. Status spongiosus and edema associated with hypertrophy of astrocytes are the most common lesions of scrapie and are seen in all animals with this disease.

Experimental scrapie is characterized by similar lesions. However, in later passages in mice, the cerebral cortex, which is unaffected in the natural disease, also becomes involved. Hamsters inoculated with scrapie from mouse brain show cortical lesions in the early passages as well.

Electron Microscopy.   No particles have been seen.

VISNA

Host(s)

NATURAL.   Sheep.

EXPERIMENTAL.   Sheep.

Agent*

SIZE.   Particle size is 70 to 100 mμ, with an average of 85 mμ. There is a central core of 30 to 40 mμ.

RESISTANCE TO CHEMICAL AGENTS. The visna agent is inactivated by ether and chloroform, by exposure to acid, and by formalin. Synthesis of the virus can be stopped by actinomycin D, but infectious nucleic acid has not been isolated.

---

*All properties refer to agent obtained in tissue culture.

RESISTANCE TO PHYSICAL AGENTS. Visna virus is inactivated by heat and by ultraviolet radiation; it induces antibody production, and is also neutralized by antibodies produced against maedi (q.v.).

Tissue Culture. Visna agent has been grown in a primary diploid cell culture derived from the choroid plexus of sheep. This virus produces a cytopathic effect, preceded by a latent period of 20 hours.

Incubation Period. Incubation period is eight months to four years.

Pathogenesis. The mode of spread has not been definitely established, but the disease apparently is contagious. During the incubation period (or period of subclinical infection) the virus has been isolated from cerebrospinal fluid, blood, saliva, reticuloendothelial system, brain, and lungs.

Clinical Symptoms. The disease is insidious at onset. The earliest signs are paresis of the hind limbs. Progressively, after a few weeks to several months, the animal develops total paralysis and invariably dies.

Pathological Findings. The primary lesion is in the central nervous system. It is characterized by meningeal and subependymal infiltration and proliferation of cells of the reticuloendothelial system. Secondly, there is demyelination of white matter; gray matter is unaffected. The infected animals produce neutralizing antibodies in a high titer.

Electron Microscopy. Examination of the tissue culture material reveals particles of 70 to 100 mμ which are surrounded by an envelope covered by projections in the shape of spikes, each about 10 mμ in length. The internal structure is uncertain, but occasionally a concentric ring arrangement is discernible, suggesting a helicoid structure. The virus matures at the cell membrane and reproduces by budding.

MAEDI

The agent of maedi (hemorrhagic pneumonia of sheep) is apparently a variant of visna, and both may represent two strains of the same virus. It can be grown in the same tissue culture system and has very similar properties. This virus has a particle size of 60 to 90 mμ, with a center core identical to that of visna. It also reproduces by budding at the cell membrane, but has a somewhat longer latent period in tissue culture than visna. It produces neutralizing antibody which neutralizes maedi and visna completely. The antibody produced against visna only partially neutralizes maedi.

ALEUTIAN MINK DISEASE

Host(s)

NATURAL. Mink. The difference in the pattern of this disease in Aleutian mink and in other mink is apparently related to the difference in the mortality rate *(vide infra)*. Ferrets that have been in contact with infected mink occasionally harbor the virus. There have been reports, as yet unconfirmed, of infection in man and cattle.

EXPERIMENTAL. Mink.

Agent. The agent is very likely a virus because (1) it can be serially transferred beyond theoretical dilution endpoint, and (2) it can be transferred by cell-free filtrates.

SIZE. This agent is probably smaller than 50 mμ, but the size has not been definitely determined.

RESISTANCE TO CHEMICAL AGENTS. Formalin inactivates this agent in 12 hours. It is resistant to treatment with ether, proteases, and nucleases.

RESISTANCE TO PHYSICAL AGENTS. Purified suspension is inactivated by heating to 90° C. for 15 minutes.

Tissue Cultures. The agent has not been propagated in any tissue culture system.

Pathogenesis. The disease is contagious, but the method by which it spreads is not clearly understood. Healthy animals housed together with infected ones contract the disease. Vertical transmission from dam to kits is also probable. The manner of the disease induction by the agent is also unknown. The agent may produce an autoimmune reaction by evoking some change in the native proteins, or it may unite with native proteins and act as an antigen. Another possibility is that it may stimulate plasma cells to elaborate gamma globulins, which may be either a specific antibody or nonantibody. An unusual mechanism must operate in this disease, since the virus and gamma globulin are produced in concert. Although the antibody forms a complex with the virus, it does not neutralize its pathogenic properties.*

Incubation Period. The incubation period of Aleutian mink disease is probably 8 months to one year, but this has not been definitely established.

Clinical Symptoms. There are few symptoms or signs of the disease. Death is usually

---

*Immediate coating of the virus with gamma globulin upon its entry into the body may be the basis for failure to identify this agent serologically. Perhaps for the same reason it has been impossible to develop serological tests for identification of other agents, such as scrapie.

sudden, often by exsanguination as the result of rupture of a major blood vessel.

Pathological Findings. Liver and kidneys are most severely affected. There is capillary membrane thickening in the glomerulus of the kidney. Both organs show fibrin thrombosis and plasma cell infiltration of perivascular areas. There is amyloid and paramyloid infiltration. Ultimately, the perivascular cell infiltration characterizes all organs. Lymph nodes and spleen show plasmacytosis.

Electron Microscopy. No particles have been seen.

MINK ENCEPHALOPATHY

Host(s)
    NATURAL. Mink.
    EXPERIMENTAL. Mink.
Agent
    SIZE. Infectious particles pass through membranes of 100 mμ.
    RESISTANCE TO CHEMICAL AGENTS. Brain homogenate retains its infectivity after at least 11 months' exposure to formalin at room temperature. It is also resistant to ether.
    RESISTANCE TO PHYSICAL AGENTS. The virus is resistant to heat (analogous to scrapie).
    Tissue Culture. No successful *in vitro* system has been developed. However, explants from brains with this encephalopathy show a higher incidence of glial outgrowth than do normal brains.*
    Pathogenesis. The pathogenesis of the disease is obscure, but the naturally exposed animals apparently acquire the disease by the oral route. This route has also been utilized successfully for the experimental infection. In one epizootic, there were a few secondary cases nine months after the original disease outbreak.
    Incubation Period. The natural incubation period is eight to 11 months. This is probably inversely proportional to the infective dose. In the experimental infection, in which mink brain was inoculated by the oral route, the incubation period is eight to nine months. Serial intracerebral passage will reduce it still further to four months.

Clinical Symptoms. This progressive central nervous system disease is characterized by locomotor incoördination. The signs are insidious. As the disease advances, there may be convulsions, followed by somnolence and, ultimately, a total incapacitation and a state of semicoma. Death follows three to eight weeks after the development of the initial symptoms.

Pathological Findings. The major pathological lesions are limited to the central nervous system and consist of vacuolization of the gray matter and a reactive astrocytosis. There is also some degeneration of the neurons and, infrequently, vacuolization of cerebral neurons.

Electron Microscopy. No particles have been seen.

KURU

Host(s)
    NATURAL. Members of the Fore tribe in New Guinea.
    EXPERIMENTAL. Chimpanzee.
    Agent. The agent is unknown, but it is suspected to be a virus because a kuru-like syndrome resulted in seven of eight chimpanzees inoculated intracerebrally with the brain suspension of a human with the natural disease. A subsequent passage of brain suspension from one of the original experimentally infected chimpanzees in other chimpanzees resulted in kuru.
    Tissue Culture. None has been successful.
    Pathogenesis. The pathogenesis of kuru is unknown but is suspected to be related to cannibalism, which may be the basis for oral transmission of the infectious agent. However, cases of kuru have been known among individuals who apparently did not consume human brains. Moreover, neighboring tribes with a similar cannibalistic cultural pattern do not exhibit kuru. The possibility of a genetic predisposition to an ubiquitous agent has been suggested.†
    Incubation Period. In the natural disease the incubation period is unknown. In experimental kuru (in a single study) it was 18 to 30 months in the man-to-chimpanzee

---

*Compare these findings with similar results for scrapie mouse brain.

†This would be analogous to scrapie and Aleutian mink disease (q.v.).

passage, and 10 to 12 months in the chimpanzee-to-chimpanzee passage.*

Clinical Symptoms. Symptoms are predominantly of the type associated with cerebellar disease. Affected individuals show ataxia, disturbance of balance, tremor, and clumsy gait. Patients remain mentally alert; they have a curious awareness of their impending death, and can predict its time quite accurately. In the late stages of the disease, they show some confusion, slow thinking, and withdrawal. Death follows within one year after onset of symptoms.

In adults the disease shows a predilection for females, with a sex ratio of 2/1 in favor of women. However, no such predilection has been observed among children.

Pathological Findings. Abnormalities are limited to the central nervous system and are only microscopic. The changes are widespread, characterized by spongy degeneration of gray matter associated with hypertrophy and proliferation of the astrocytes. There is neuronal degeneration, most commonly seen in the cerebellum. Occasionally cerebellar demyelination is observed. Large neurons in the corpus striatum show vacuolization.

Electron Microscopy. No particles have been seen.

PROGRESSIVE MULTIFOCAL LEUKOENCEPHALOPATHY

Host

NATURAL. Man (?).

EXPERIMENTAL. Unknown.

Agent. The agent has not been isolated, but it can be identified morphologically under the electron microscope in lesions within the fresh and fixed tissue of the parietal subcortex in patients suffering from this disease. Since many cases of this illness exhibit arrays of numerous virus particles of identical morphology, it may be assumed that some relationship exists between the agent and the clinical syndrome.

SIZE. The particles are virus-like, ranging in size from an average diameter of 38 $m\mu$ in a fixed specimen to an average diameter of 41 $m\mu$ in a fresh specimen, with a close morphological resemblance to DNA oncogenic viruses such as SV_{40} and polyoma, as well as human wart virus.

DENSITY. The highest concentration of particles occurs in the 1.30 to 1.31 range in cesium chloride gradient.

Tissue Culture. Attempts to establish infection in various tissue culture systems, using only the preparation of progressive multifocal leukoencephalopathy (PML) brain containing virus particles and available prior to fixation, have ended in failure. A fraction containing virus particles obtained by concentration and purification of the crude suspension by gradient centrifugation (see under *Density*) was also "noninfectious" for tissue culture and animals.

Pathogenesis. Progressive multifocal leukoencephalopathy occurs mostly, but not exclusively, in patients suffering from leukemia, lymphoma, or other forms of cancer, who have been subjected to intensive therapy with immunosuppressive drugs. Isolated cases have been observed in patients suffering from tuberculosis and sarcoidosis. The possibility that leukemia or cancer patients treated with immunosuppressive drugs are predisposed to progressive multifocal leukoencephalopathy cannot be ruled out.

Incubation Period. This is impossible to determine at the present time.

Clinical Symptoms. In general, symptoms are those of a diffuse disease of the cerebral hemispheres, usually with unilateral distribution of lesions. The most frequent clinical syndrome is hemiparesis, either spastic or flaccid, accompanied by some decline in mental faculties as the disease progresses. A large proportion of patients suffer from impairment in vision and a few become completely blind. Aphasia or dysarthria were noted in the majority of cases observed. Sensory impairment, dysphagia, vertigo, and nystagmus were recorded in a few cases. None of the patients suffered from a convulsive disorder. The time from the first observation of neurological disorders until death was an average of three to four months.

Pathological Findings. Pathological changes are characterized by multiple, usually confluent, areas of demyelination, most numerous in the cerebral hemispheres, but also occurring in the cerebellum and brain stem. These lesions can be seen on gross examination. Microscopically they are characterized by the presence of eosinophilic intranuclear inclusions in oligodendrocytes. Nuclei of these oligodendrocytes are enlarged,

---

*This is also analogous to scrapie (q.v.), which shows a shortening of the incubation period in intraspecific passage compared with interspecific passage.

basophilic, and fail to show detailed structure. Hyperplasia of astrocytes leading to formation of giant astrocytes has also been observed in some, but not all, cases. Marked enlargement of nuclei of the cerebral neurons has also been seen in isolated cases. Inflammatory lesions, characterized by perivascular, lymphocytic infiltrations, were characteristically absent.

Electron Microscopy.   See under *Agent.*

SUBACUTE SCLEROSING PANENCEPHALITIS (SSPE)

(Dawson's Inclusion Body Encephalitis; van Bogaert's Sclerosing Leukoencephalitis; Panencephalitis of Pette-Döring)

Host

NATURAL. Man.

EXPERIMENTAL. A recent report describes the passage of an encephalitogenic agent from three patients to ferrets after an incubation period of five months, and its subsequent further passage in ferrets after an incubation period of three months. Disease produced in these animals was characterized by apathy and ataxia, and was associated with a burst suppression pattern on the electroencephalogram and a histological picture of meningoencephalomyelitis that consistently spared the cerebellum. The disease in ferrets was not fatal, and partial recovery with residual brain damage was noted seven months after inoculation.

Agent. The agent has not been isolated, but some patients with the disease have high titers of measles antibodies in their serum, and brain slices of some of these patients show staining with fluorescein-tagged measles antibody. Moreover, myxovirus-like particles have been seen in the electron micrographs of some of these brains.

Tissue Culture. All attempts at tissue culture isolation of an infectious agent from the brains of patients with subacute sclerosing panencephalitis have failed.

Pathogenesis. The chronic course of this disease, in the presence of an histological picture consistent with viral encephalitis, has suggested that this disease may be a slow virus infection.

Incubation Period.   Unknown.

Clinical Symptoms. This disease affects children and young adults and is characterized by an insidious onset. First symptoms are gradual intellectual deterioration, followed by motor abnormalities that evolve into myoclonic jerks, convulsions, and incoördination. Visual difficulties and ultimately blindness follow. Finally there is coma and death. Although usually the disease is relentless and terminates in death some months to one year after onset, remissions lasting several years have been recorded. The clinical diagnosis is supported by typical laboratory findings of a "first zone" colloidal gold curve of the cerebrospinal fluid with a marked increase in the IgG. The electroencephalogram is characterized by slow wave configurations and burst-suppression patterns.

Pathological Findings. Histological examination of the brain reveals astrocytosis, round cell infiltration, perivascular cuffing, and often, but not always, Cowdry type A intranuclear inclusion bodies. These are 3 to 9 μ in diameter, are eosinophilic, and are found in neuronal and glial nuclei.

Electron Microscopy.   See under *Agent.*

CONCLUSION

The nosology of slow virus diseases will undoubtedly undergo many modifications. At the present time, this classification includes only those conditions in which at least one clue to a slow viral agent has been demonstrated, such as the *in vivo* and *in vitro* cultivation of visna virus; the *in vivo* passage of the agents of scrapie and Aleutian mink disease; the experimental passage of the kuru agent from man to chimpanzee and its secondary passage into another chimpanzee, and experimental passage of SSPE from man to ferret. Progressive multifocal leukoencephalopathy, which has a slow clinical course, has been included on the basis of the morphological finding of structures resembling virions.

The etiology of other similar diseases, such as amyotrophic lateral sclerosis, and multiple sclerosis, remains to be established. However, on the basis of their slow clinical course, these diseases, as possible resultants of slow virus infection, are now the subject of intensive research.

ADDENDUM

This chapter, completed in May of 1967, does not include some of the most important recent findings in the field of slow virus diseases. The delay of its publication has occurred through no fault of the authors and extensive revision of the chapter, to bring it up to date, has not been possible.

The reader's attention is invited to the following facts:

1. A measles-like virus has been isolated from brain cells in cultures derived from patients with SSPE. It is pathogenic for ferrets (Payne, F. E., Baublis, J. V., and Itabashi, H. H.: Isolation of measles virus from cell cultures of brain from a patient with subacute sclerosing panencephalitis. New Eng. J. Med., *281*:585-589, 1963; Katz, M., Rorke, L. B., Masland, W. S., Barbanti-Brodano, G., and Koprowski, H.: Subacute sclerosing panencephalitis: Isolation of a virus encephalitogenic for ferrets. J. Infect. Dis., *121*: 188-195, 1970).

2. Kuru has now been passed serially through the chimpanzee and has also been transmitted to the spider monkey (Gajdusek, D. C., Gibbs, C. J., Jr., Asher, D. M., and David, E.: Transmission of experimental kuru to the spider monkey (*Ateles geoffreyi*). Science, *162*:633-634, 1968).

3. Spongiform encephalopathy (Creutzfeld-Jakob disease) has been passed to chimpanzee in the same manner as has kuru (Gibbs, C. J., Jr., Gajdusek, D. C., Asher, D. M., Alpers, M. P., Beck, E., Daniel, P. M., and Matthews, W. B.: Creutzfeld-Jakob disease (spongiform encephalopathy): Transmission to the chimpanzee. Science, *161*: 388-389, 1968) and therefore is now included among slow virus diseases.

BIBLIOGRAPHY

GENERAL

1. Fernandes, M. V., Wiktor, T. J., and Koprowski, H.: Endosymbiotic relationship between animal viruses and host cells. A study of rabies virus in tissue culture. J. Exp. Med., *120*:1099-1116, 1965.
2. Field, E. J.: Transmission experiments with multiple sclerosis; an interim report. Brit. Med. J., *2*:564-565, 1966.
3. Gibbs, C. J., Jr.: Search for infectious etiology in chronic and subacute degenerative diseases of the central nervous system. In: Current Topics in Microbiology and Immunology, Vol. 40: Chronic Infectious Neuropathic Agents (CHINA) and Other Slow Virus Infections. Brody, J. A., Henle, W., and Koprowski, H., eds. Berlin, Springer Verlag, 1967, pp. 44-58.
4. Sigurdsson, B.: Rida, a chronic encephalitis of sheep. With general remarks on infections which develop slowly and some of their special characteristics. Brit. Vet. J., *110*:341-354, 1954.

SCRAPIE

5. Alper, T., Haig, D. A., and Clarke, M. C.: The exceptionally small size of the scrapie agent. Biochem. Biophys. Res. Commun., *22*:278-284, 1966.
6. Beck, E., Daniel, P. M., and Parry, H. B.: Natural (Spontaneous) Scrapie in Sheep. II. The Pathology of Natural Scrapie in Sheep with Particular Reference to the Neuromuscular System. Paper No. 9. Scrapie Seminar, Washington, D.C., U.S. Dept. of Agriculture, 1964.
7. Eklund, C. M., Kennedy, R. C., and Hadlow, W. J.: Pathogenesis of scrapie virus infection in the mouse. J. Infect. Dis., *117*:15-22, 1967.
8. Pattison, I. H., and Jones, K. M.: The possible nature of the transmissible agent of scrapie. Vet. Rec., *80*:2-9, 1967.
9. Pattison, I. H., and Millson, G. C.: Scrapie produced experimentally in goats with special reference to the clinical syndrome. J. Comp. Path., *71*:101-108, 1961.
10. Zlotnik, I.: Observations on the experimental transmission of scrapie of various origins of laboratory animals. In: NINDB Monograph No. 2: Slow, Latent, and Temperate Virus Infections. Gajdusek, D. C., Gibbs, C. J. Jr., and Alpers, M., eds. U.S.P.H.S. Pub. No. 1378, Washington, D.C., U.S. Department of Health, Education, and Welfare, 1965, pp. 237-248.
11. Zlotnik, I., and Rennie, J. C.: The effect of heat on the scrapie agent in mouse brain. Brit. J. Exp. Path., *48*:171-179, 1967.

VISNA AND MAEDI

12. Gudnadòttir, M., and Kristindòttir, K.: Complement-fixing antibodies in sera of sheep affected with visna and maedi. J. Immun., *98*:663-667, 1967.
13. Thormar, H.: A comparison of visna and maedi viruses. I. Physical, chemical, and biological properties. Res. Vet. Sci., *6*:117-129, 1965.
14. Thormar, H.: Physical, chemical, and biological properties of visna virus and its relationship to other aniam viruses. In: NINDB Monograph No. 2: Slow, Latent, and Temperate Virus Infections. Gajdusek, D. C., Gibbs, C. J., Jr., and Alpers, M., eds. U.S.P.H.S. Pub. No. 1378, Washington, D.C., U.S. Department of Health, Education, and Welfare, 1965, pp. 335-340.
15. Thormar, H.: Cell-virus interactions in tissue cultures infected with visna and maedi viruses. In: Current Topics in Microbiology and Immunology, Vol. 40: Chronic Infectious Neuropathic Agents (CHINA) and Other Slow Virus Infections. Brody, J. A., Henle, W., and Koprowski, H., eds. Berlin, Springer Verlag, 1967, pp. 22-32.
16. Thormar, H., and Pálsson, P. A.: Visna and maedi, two slow infections of sheep and their etiological agents. In: Perspectives in Virology, Vol. 5, Academic Press, 1967, pp. 291-308.

ALEUTIAN MINK DISEASE

17. Gorham, J. R., Leader, R. W., Padgett, G. A., Burger, D., and Henson, J. B.: Some observations

on the natural occurrence of Aleutian disease. In: NINDB Monograph No. 2: Slow, Latent, and Temperate Virus Infections. Gajdusek, D. C., Gibbs, C. J., Jr., and Alpers, M., eds. U.S.P.H.S. Pub. No. 1378, Washington, D.C., U.S. Department of Health, Education, and Welfare, 1965, pp. 279-285.

18. Karstad, L.: Aleutian Disease. A slowly progressive viral infection of mink. In: Current Topics in Microbiology and Immunology, Vol. 40: Chronic Infectious Neuropathic Agents (CHINA) and Other Slow Virus Infections. Brody, J. A., Henle, W., and Koprowski, H., eds. Berlin, Springer Verlag, 1967, pp. 9-21.

19. Kenyon, A. J., Magnano, T., Helmboldt, R. F., and Buko, L.: Aleutian disease in the ferret. J. Amer. Vet. Med. Assoc., *149*:920-923, 1966.

20. Leader, R. W., Gorham, J. R., Benson, J. B., and Burger, D.: Pathogenesis of Aleutian disease of mink. In: NINDB Monograph No. 2: Slow, Latent, and Temperate Virus Infections. Gajdusek, D. C., Gibbs, C. J., Jr., and Alpers, M., eds U.S.P.H.S. Pub. No. 1378, Washington, D.C., U.S. Department of Health, Education, and Welfare, 1965, pp. 287-295.

MINK ENCEPHALOPATHY

21. Burger, D., and Harsough, G. R.: Transmissible encephalopathy of mink. In: NINDB Monograph No. 2: Slow, Latent, and Temperate Virus Infections. Gajdusek, D. C., Gibbs, C. J., Jr., and Alpers, M., eds. U.S.P.H.S. Pub. No. 1378, Washington, D.C., U.S. Department of Health, Education, and Welfare, 1965, pp. 297-305.

22. Marsh, R.: Studies on the Reactive Astrocyte in Mink Encephalopathy. Thesis, University of Wisconsin, 1966.

KURU

23. Gajdusek, D. C.: Kuru in New Guinea and the origin of the NINDB study of slow, latent, and temperate virus infections of the nervous system of man. In: NINDB Monograph No. 2: Slow, Latent, and Temperate Virus Infections. Gajdusek, D. C., Gibbs, C. J., Jr., and Alpers, M., eds. U.S.P.H.S. Pub. No. 1378, Washington, D.C., U.S. Department of Health, Education and Welfare, 1965, pp. 3-12.

24. Gajdusek, D. C.: Discussion on kuru, scrapie, and and the experimental kuru-like syndrome in chimpanzees. In: Current Topics in Microbiology and Immunology, Vol. 40: Chronic Infectious Neuropathic Agents (CHINA) and Other Slow Virus Infections. Brody, J. A., Henle, W., and Koprowski, H., eds. Berlin, Springer Verlag, 1967, pp. 59-63.

25. Gibbs, C. J., Jr., and Gajdusek, D. C.: Attempts to demonstrate a transmissible agent in kuru, amyotrophic lateral sclerosis, and other subacute and chronic progressive nervous system degenerations of man. In: NINDB Monograph No. 2: Slow, Latent, and Temperate Virus Infections. eds. Gajdusek, D. C., Gibbs, C. J., Jr., and Alpers, M., eds. U.S.P.H.S. Pub. No. 1378, Washington, D.C., U.S. Department of Health, Education, and Welfare, 1965, pp. 39-48.

26. Kakulas, B. A., Lecours, A. R., and Gajdusek, D. C.: Further observations on the pathology of kuru. J. Neuropath. Exp. Neurol., *26*:85-97, 1967.

27. Klatzo, I.: Neuropathological findings in kuru. In: NINDB Monograph No. 2: Slow, Latent, and Temperate Virus Infections. Gajdusek, D. C., Gibbs, C. J., Jr., and Alpers, M., eds. U.S.P.H.S. Pub. No. 1378, Washington, D.C., U.S. Department of Health, Education, and Welfare, 1965, pp. 83-84.

PROGRESSIVE MULTIFOCAL LEUKOENCEPHALOPATHY

28. Astrom, K. E., Mancall, E. L., and Richardson, E. P., Jr.: Progressive multifocal leukoencephalopathy. A hitherto unrecognized complication of chronic lymphatic leukaemia and hodgkin's disease. Brain, *81*:93-111, 1958.

29. Howatson, A. F., Nagai, M., and Zu Rhein, G. M.: Polyoma-like virions in human demyelinating brain disease. Canad. Med. Assoc. J., *93*:379-386, 1965.

30. Muller, J., and Watanabe, I.: Progressive multifocal leukoencephalopathy; a virus disease. Amer. J. Clin. Path., *47*:114-123, 1967.

31. Richardson, E. P., Jr.: Progressive multifocal leukoencephalopathy. New Eng. J. Med., *265*:815-823, 1961.

SUBACUTE SCLEROSING PANENCEPHALITIS

32. Connally, J. H., Allen, I. V., Hurwitz, L. J., and Millar, J. H. D.: Measles-virus antibody and antigen in subacute sclerosing panencephalitis. Lancet, *1*:542-544, 1967.

33. Dawson, J. R.: Cellular inclusions in cerebral lesions of lethargic encephalitis. Amer. J. Path., *9*:7-16, 1933.

34. Dayan, A. D., Gostling, J. V. T., Greaves, J. L., Stevens, D. W., and Woodhouse, M. A.: Evidence of a pseudomyxovirus in the brain in subacute sclerosing leucoencephalitis. Lancet, *1*:980-981, 1967.

35. Freeman, J. M., Magoffin, R. L., Lennette, E. H., Herndon, R. M.: Additional evidence of the relation between subacute inclusion body encephalitis and measles virus. Lancet, *2*:129-131, 1967.

36. Legg, N. J.: Virus antibodies in subacute sclerosing panencephalitis. Brit. Med. J., *3*:350-352, 1967.

37. Périer, O., Thiry, L., Vanderhaeghen, J. J., and Pelc, S.: Attempts at experimental transmission and electron microscopic observations in subacute sclerosing panencephalitis. Neurology, *18*:138-143, 1968.

PART II

Viral Infections in Which Muscular Manifestations Predominate

physiognomy, has perfectly clear-cut characteristics. Most of the facts observed in the course of other viral infections, so varied and so complex, contrast with this relatively simple schematic evolution. An infection such as mumps has multiple clinical aspects ranging from pluriglandular involvement and neurological localizations to inapparent forms.

With poliomyelitis, which, as is well known, can also assume many forms, from fatal to inapparent, a new fact appears: the possibility of reinfections by a virus of the same type, despite the existence of an immunity that is sufficient to protect against central nervous system involvement. These reinfections are manifested simply by a brief elimination of virus, a rise in the level of the specific neutralizing antibodies (immune response of secondary type), and a reappearance of complement-fixing antibodies. These possibilities are, moreover, taken advantage of in successive revaccinations, for example with live attenuated antipoliomyelitis vaccine.

Finally, certain respiratory infections, especially the common cold, recur indefinitely and often several times a year in the same subject. One reason for this is that colds are produced by a very large number of viruses with different antigenic characteristics, each creating its own type-specific immunity; but other factors doubtless intervene, such as insufficient protective action of the general defense mechanisms against this infection, the evolution of which remains local. This could be the case in the recurrent infections due to *Myxovirus parainfluenzae* viruses or to respiratory syncytial viruses of the same serotype.

Other infections raise an entirely different problem. It is known that the first herpes infection regularly induces production of neutralizing antibodies, the level of which is reinforced by clinical or subclinical infections that recur from infancy. However, the adult, despite an apparently stable level of antibodies, sometimes presents recurrent, more or less frequent lesions of labial herpes. The mechanism of this latent infection with repeated acute manifestations still remains poorly explained. Certain factors that can cause recurrences are known: menstruation, fatigue, and certain bacterial infections such as pneumonia or meningococcosis. It is supposed that the weakness of action of the neutralizing antibodies is due to the manner of propagation peculiar to this virus or else to the absence of immunoglobulins with local action (IgA).

The relationships that man thus establishes with the herpes virus recall in certain ways those that can sometimes be revealed in infections by the cytomegalovirus. It is known, in fact, that besides the perinatal disease, almost always fatal, there exist minor or inapparent forms in the older child and in the adult. In these cases, the presence of the virus in the saliva and, above all, in the urine has been demonstrated for 18 to 32 months, while the presence of complement-fixing antibodies indicates the existence of serological reactions. Genuine chronic infections are involved that are capable, on occurrence of an immunological deficit (massive therapeutic irradiation for organ grafts, marasmus in malignant infections), of yielding massive invasion of the organism by the virus.

Even more insidious are certain latent infections manifesting themselves neither by acute incidents nor by virus elimination in the excreta. Thus, when fragments of adenoidal tissue are placed in tissue culture, in nearly 90 per cent of cases one finds adenovirus producing no detectable clinical manifestation whatever. These latent viruses generally give rise to the appearance of specific antibodies. However, as we shall see in Chapter 44, this is not always the case.

These different aspects of viral infection reveal the extent to which the presence of virus or the presence of neutralizing antibodies can, according to the infection in question and according to the dates and the conditions of sampling, present different meanings. The existence of immunological reactions can indicate an acute infection, a long-since-cured infection, a chronic infection, or even a latent infection. The elimination of a virus in the secretions or the excretions can occur in a patient, in a subject in the incubation phase of the disease, in a convalescent patient (and from the example of poliomyelitis it is known that the virus carrier state can extend over several weeks), in a chronically infected individual (e.g., a subject with infection by the cytomegalic inclusion virus), or, lastly, in a healthy individual who has had a subclinical or asymptomatic infection (such as the enteroviruses, mumps virus, or rubella virus can produce). Thus, all the types of carriers are found: those who are in the incubation period of the disease, those who are convalescent, and, lastly, the chronic carriers. The "healthy carrier"—that is to say, a person harboring a virus without presenting pathological manifestations—can be a convalescent or a chronically infected subject; he may or may not eliminate viruses, he may or may not act as a contaminator, and he may or may not have responded to the infection by a defense reaction, in particular by antibody production; lastly, he can, under certain circumstances, pass from the stage of healthy carrier to that of ill person.

To the study of these phenomena must be added that required when superinfection by a different virus occurs in the course of a first infection by a given virus, or when a bacterial superinfection occurs.

If the term interference is generally applied to a phenomenon inhibiting viral multiplication, this is because, in fact, the implantation of a first virus in the human organism most often creates, by various mechanisms, of which interferon production is the most important, a resistance against all new viral invasion. Nonetheless, in certain rare cases the first virus can permit and even favor the implantation of a second virus by a phenomenon that could be called "stimulating interference." It was in regard to the relationships between poliomyelitis viruses and Coxsackie A that these facts were revealed by Dalldorf in the mouse. It has not been proved that they also exist in man. Nevertheless, descriptions have been made of mixed infections by enteroviruses (poliovirus and ECHO virus or poliovirus and Coxsackie virus) or by respiratory viruses (adenovirus and *Myxovirus parainfluenzae* or *influenzae*) in the course of which it can be extremely difficult to determine the part attributable to each in the lesions observed. Thus there can arise—though relatively rarely—etiological problems that are very difficult to solve.

Bacterial superinfections in the course of cutaneous or respiratory viral diseases are, on the other hand, frequent, well known, and feared by practicing physicians, who generally attribute to them the high mortality of certain epidemics, particularly of measles and influenza. The destruction of cutaneous or mucosal coverings by different viruses explains the rapidly extensive implantation of infections by streptococci in smallpox, by *Haemophilus influenzae,* staphylococci, or pneumococci in influenza, and by streptococci or pneumococci in measles. The edema,

hyperemia, and vascular disorders further favor their spread. The exact role of bacterial superinfection in the serious or fatal course of these viral diseases is, however, poorly specified and doubtless less important than has been believed. The widespread use of antibiotics and of systematic bacteriological controls has made it possible to verify the existence of deadly influenza epidemics in the absence of any bacterial superinfection. The same is true for measles, and these notions should be kept in mind in order to moderate preventive antibiotic therapy in such cases.

SIGNS, SYMPTOMS, AND METHODS OF DIAGNOSIS

The general considerations discussed in preceding sections inspire the spirit and the structure of this book, which comprises the study of viral infections classified by organ system, as in all treatises of pathology. Since the clinical picture usually involves varied localizations, the predominant manifestation will determine the place attributed in our classification of the diseases. In each case the clinical study will be completed by a description of the laboratory methods of diagnosis, then by the epidemiology, and, lastly, by the problems of prophylaxis and treatment.

CLINICAL DESCRIPTION

The clinical description of the signs and symptoms observed and the study of the elements of clinical diagnosis should be considered from the outset.

Certain clinical pictures are perfectly clear-cut and known to every physician, as for example those of the eruptive fevers or of mumps or of poliomyelitis. Along with a simple summary of their characteristics, it will be important to add to the traditional concepts the contributions of recent work.

In other cases, the clinical picture of the viral disease is either less clear-cut or less well known: exanthema subitum or epidemic megalerythema, for example; in such cases a complete clinical study is required, including all the elements of a clinical differential diagnosis.

In still other numerous cases, the clinical picture appears identical for several viral infections that are extremely different from one another: certain encephalitides or myelitides, certain cutaneous eruptions, certain inflammations of the respiratory or the digestive tract, and the meningitides with clear fluid are striking examples. In these cases, our task will be a closer study of the patient and a more thorough analysis of the clinical signs and symptoms in order to help the physician make or propose an etiological diagnosis and to orient the virologist toward the search for a particular virus or group of viruses. In the diagnosis, for example, between a pharyngitis of viral origin and a streptococcal infection, it is to be remembered that hoarseness is a valid sign; the ancients said that scarlet fever does not like the larynx, and Rammelkamp, studying streptococcal infections, declared he had never observed a case of hoarseness in streptococcic pharyngitis. Another example: among the myelitides, poliomyelitis can be distinguished by a symptomatology that indicates the elective involvement of the cells of the striomotor column of the anterior horn of the spinal cord and of the brain stem. Yet another example: the highly individual lesions that certain Coxsackie viruses provoke on the pharyngeal mucosa permit the identification of herpangina.

Thus refinement of the clinical examination can in many cases be fruitful even though, in the very cases we have cited, the concordance between a given virus and a given disease is not always perfect. Thus certain diseases due to Coxsackie virus are very much like poliomyelitis. In other cases, it is only the virologist who can define the disease by establishing its etiology. An important factor must be recalled here: the physician who suspects a viral disease that is directly transmissible from man to man must concern himself with the persons around the patient — those in the family, school, military unit, village or town, region, or even larger units. The investigations must be pursued far enough to detect the disease in all its forms, not only evident but also inapparent or atypical; some well-known examples are "aseptic" meningitis or slight digestive disturbances among the neighbors of the poliomyelitis patient, and encephalitis in the course of a mumps epidemic. They demonstrate both the essential role of the clinician and the method of work of the practitioner. Need it be repeated that the fundamental task of the family doctor is not only to examine his patient but also to be concerned with the state of health of all those around him?

Under these circumstances, the virologist's help will be as useful for recognition of the virus in the patients presenting various clinical manifestations as for detection of inapparent spread by healthy carriers. This necessity is all the greater because certain epidemics are linked to the spread and the simultaneous pathogenic action of several viruses. Epidemics of poliomyelitis accompanied by meningitides and even paralysis due to other viruses (Coxsackie among others) are a typical example of this phenomenon.

It is hence through a combination of clinical, epidemiological, and virological work that a correct diagnosis becomes possible. From this fact arises the necessity of describing in the first part of each chapter of this book the characteristics of the epidemic as the clinician observes it. If the virologist is to be really helpful he should be given samples not only from the patient or patients but from the persons around the patient — family, schoolmates, military population, and so forth. This association of familial and social medicine with individual medicine is imperative today, necessitating close contact between family doctors and public health physicians and (let us insist on the point) teamwork guided by the practitioner.

SAMPLES

The second part of each chapter contains precise directions concerning the samples that are most useful in each case (spinal fluid, nasal or pharyngeal mucus, urine, fecal matter, skin crust, or fluid from cutaneous blisters), and the biopsies recommended in each circumstance. The best times for blood sampling in view of the different serodiagnoses should be thoroughly known. The directions for sampling, storage, and transportation to the laboratory should be followed with care. If a single element of this program is poorly understood or poorly executed, the laboratory may be subjected to useless and exhausting research — for example, serial passages to detect a virus that was destroyed by an improper temperature or pH, isolations of viruses without significance from samples taken too late, titrations of noninterpretable antibodies. Under these circumstances, the diagnosis remains uncertain and the epidemiological investigation fails.

As concerns the laboratory work (culture, inoculation, search for and titration of antibodies, and so forth), we shall provide in this book only the summary indications that the practitioner must know. We shall give references for more complete information on these subjects to treatises on virology. On the other hand, the interpretation of laboratory results will be discussed in some detail. Indeed, at this point great difficulties can arise. Many pathogenic viruses are widespread in human groups, and occult immunization is frequent in healthy carriers, so that the discovery of a virus in an individual does not mean that the disease he manifests is due to the action of this virus. Moreover, the fact that the subject possesses antibodies (neutralizing, hemagglutinating, and so forth) to a virus does not prove, either, its pathogenic role in particular circumstances. A rapid rise in the antibody level must be demonstrated by successive tests before it can be concluded that a given virus has just infected the subject whose blood is being examined. Occasionally, it is possible to use the techniques of fluorescent microscopy, which in certain cases reveal viruses in the very tissue they have infected — e.g., in the nasal mucus. Or a search will be made for the characteristic cellular inclusions, as, for example, cytoplasmic inclusions in the altered ciliated cells collected by nasal swabbing or, more frequently, in the urinary sediment. These are merely examples to show the multiplicity of methods of virological exploration. One must interpret all results with great caution, for a single positive test result rarely suffices to establish a diagnosis.

The possible causes of error that can invalidate the results reported should never be neglected. Is it certain that the isolated virus originated from the patient and not from the living tissue on which it has been cultivated or from the animal into which it has been inoculated? Inversely, what value is to be attributed to a negative result of a search for a virus? Are the conditions of sampling and the techniques utilized those most favorable for its isolation? It must be remembered that the phenomenon of hemagglutination inhibition can be provoked by nonspecific factors or, to give still another example, that a rise in antibodies can be due to an anamnestic reaction when the patient has already undergone infections by viruses closely related to the virus in question. It would be possible to give many more examples of the need for a severely critical spirit in the interpretation of results. The clinician and the virologist should discuss such questions together so as to conclude only in function of study of the patient, of the epidemic, of the virus concerned, and of the reactions of the patient and his human environment.

BIOLOGICAL DIAGNOSIS

These indications show the importance of the biological diagnosis to which the third part of each chapter is devoted and which comprises (1) identification of the virus isolated and (2) the serodiagnostic methods.

We shall consider in this work only the techniques most generally employed. Many others that are utilized in research work have not yet found a practical application in biological diagnosis. It must be thoroughly understood that this biological diagnosis is founded on delicate techniques requiring excellent standardization of all the reagents; each reagent can, if it is not of good quality and perfectly titrated, be a cause of error that only well-equipped laboratories and highly experienced specialists will know how to avoid.

Presence and Identification of the Virus. The product to be studied, after proper sampling, conservation, and preparation according to the type of virus to be sought and the material available, is inoculated either into an animal (newborn mouse, adult mouse, guinea pig, rabbit) or into cells or tissues in culture.

Numerous systems of cell culture are utilized in virology; they can be of human or animal origin, established from adult or amniotic or embryonic cells. The cell cultures can originate directly from the tissue sampled. They are then *primary cultures: explant* cultures that utilize the entire tissue fragment, from which the cells migrate in the liquid culture medium and multiply there, or cultures *in monocellular layers* that, after dislocation of the tissues by appropriate means, employ suspensions of selected cells. They can result in *cell lines* such as those already long maintained in the laboratory and which furnish cells of unstable heteroploid* karyotype. The evolution of such lines is theoretically infinite; to this category belong HeLa, KB and Hep 2 cells, which originated in different human cancers and now have continued to reproduce in laboratories for more than ten years. Lastly, they can be established from human diploid strains. In contrast to the cell lines, which can be considered "immortal,"

---

*Diploid: involving 2N chromosomes; heteroploid: involving a number of chromosomes different from 2N.

these strains have an evolution that is limited in time. Their origin is embryonic and they furnish cells of stable diploid character, that is to say, equipped with a fixed number of chromosomes characteristic of their human origin.* Each laboratory has at its disposal a variety of animals to inoculate and cellular systems and can, with this material, isolate with varying chances of success a greater or lesser variety of viruses. For each type of virus there is one preferable system of several. No system is genuinely specific for a given virus, and under certain circumstances less efficacious systems can be substituted. Therefore the clinician, in his interpretation of results, should take into account the materials at the disposal of the laboratory and should appraise, with the virologist's help, the value of each result, be it negative or positive.

In a certain number of instances, the presence of virus manifests itself by the appearance of pathological phenomena: disease in the animal, histological lesions in one or another organ, appearance of characteristic lesions on the chorioallantoic membrane of the hen's egg, appearance of lesions (commonly called cytopathogenic effect) in cell culture. These phenomena are generally not pathognomonic, but they orient the virologist toward a particular family of viruses for which he will seek other elements of differentiation. Staining, either in sections obtained from infected animals or in slides of inoculated tissue culture, can demonstrate cellular modifications: giant cells, plasmoids, inclusions, that is to say, structured elements of the nucleus or the cytoplasm, sometimes of viral nature, sometimes sequelae or manifestations of toxicity more or less specific in regard to the metabolic disturbances induced by the virus in the cell that it infects.

It is the *serological methods,* however, specific and quantitative, which usually permit the identification of the viruses isolated. These are primarily techniques of neutraliza-tion, hemagglutination, and hemadsorption. The principles of these methods will be discussed in the section on serological diagnosis; the complement-fixation technique is used less often.

In the last few years a new method, as remarkable for its specificity as for the rapidity with which results are obtained, has been applied to the early diagnosis of viral infections: this is the immunofluorescence method described by Coons in 1950. It is based on marking specific antibodies by fluorescent compounds. Thus marked, the antibodies fix themselves, within the very cell infected, either on the viral antigen itself or on certain of its constituent elements. It is thus possible, under ultraviolet light, to reveal the presence of a specific viral material within the infected cells. The practical application of this method is at present limited to a small number of human virus diseases; among them are the respiratory tract diseases, in which direct search is made for the virus, or for germs similar to viruses, in the nasopharyngeal secretions or the sputum (influenza, ornithosis-psittacosis, Eaton's "atypical pneumonia," respiratory syncytial virus infection). The viral diseases with cutaneous localizations also furnish a material easy to use, e.g., slides from blisters of herpes, smallpox, and vaccinia. For the diseases demanding urgent diagnosis, it is possible to track down the virus with fluorescent antibodies in organs of inoculated laboratory animals, e.g., the mouse brain for rabies, or in tissue cultures, e.g., those infected with poliomyelitis. This remarkable method at present can be used only by specially equipped laboratories; its application will doubtless expand greatly, in particular for revealing viruses that cannot be detected directly by the lesions they provoke.

Furthermore, viruses exist that, in the course of the first inoculation into the animal or in tissue cultures, yield no detectable effect. Systematic *blind passages* permitting either adaptation or multiplication of the virus are then necessary. These techniques of serial passage should be submitted to rigorous criticism before the lesions observed are interpreted. Thus numerous primary cultures (in particular those established from monkey kidney cells) are frequently contaminated by latent viruses peculiar to the animal of their origin. Cell lines often harbor mycoplasma. Adult animals and even embryos can also be carriers of different more or less latent viruses.

---

*During a meeting held at WHO Headquarters July 24, 1962, the following terminology was adopted: a "cell line" is a population of cells that develops in vitro by reseeding for an indefinite time but without conserving the number of chromosomes characteristic of the tissue from which it derives; a "cell strain" is a population of cells that develops in vitro by repeated reseedings but that possesses a limited life span and that conserves the chromosomal karyotype characteristic of the tissue from which it derives.

Lastly, contamination may occur from the laboratory personnel, who may be eliminating virus (herpes, respiratory viruses, enteroviruses, and so forth).

Finally, viruses exist that, whatever the number of passages, multiply without provoking any detectable effect, particularly in cell cultures. Such is the case, for example, for the rubella virus, which can be detected in tissue culture only by the interference phenomenon. In this case the cells are seeded first with the product studied, viral multiplication provokes interferon formation, and the cell culture becomes insensitive to the inoculation of a virus cytopathogenic for the cellular system.

Techniques of such complexity can hardly be used unless the virologist and the clinician agree in the first place on the clinical interpretation and on the necessity for and the orientation of the biological investigations. The isolation and identification of viruses require a perfect collaboration — this cannot be repeated too often — between the physician and the biologist, for the virologist must have at his disposal both correctly handled samples and the information necessary to orient his research. The situation is such today that systematic biological study in a great number of directions is impossible.

In addition, although certain identifications can be made rapidly, for example that of poliovirus, which for a well-run laboratory requires three to four days, others take longer, for example those of nonpoliomyelitic enteroviruses revealed in tissue culture, for which the numerous neutralizing sera specific for each type must be tested successively.

Thus in each case it will be necessary to judge the interest of the research, the extent of the effort required for a precise virological diagnosis, and whether the results will still be of any value when they are finally obtained.

The significance of a virus isolation depends on the clinical circumstances, on the ubiquity of the virus identified, and on the nature of the sample from which it is isolated.

The presence of a virus in a tissue fragment, in the cerebrospinal fluid, or in a liquid discharge generally affirms not only an actual infection but also the direct participation of the virus in the lesions in which it is found. On the other hand, the presence of a virus in the blood or urine, the nasopharyngeal secretions, the stools, or the respiratory or digestive mucosa, though it signifies an infection, does not affirm the etiological role of the virus.

As a matter of fact, the demonstration of viremia, which is very exceptional and very difficult, would at the most prove that the infection is in full evolution. Any connection between the clinical manifestations and the virological results must thus be confirmed either by indisputable clinical signs (poliomyelitic paralysis, for example) or by precise epidemiological demonstrations, such as the coincidence in several subjects of the same pathological signs and the same virological results, or by the elimination, by means of the appropriate serological tests, of all other concomitant infections that might cause the same symptoms.

When the patient's serum shows a positive serological reaction to the virus identified, the diagnosis is confirmed and, if the samples have been taken at the proper times, the date of infection is fixed. Serological tests are thus necessary elements in the biological diagnosis; under certain conditions that we shall specify and if the type of virus is indicated by the clinical or epidemiological data, the diagnosis can be made by results of serological tests alone.

Serological Diagnosis. Infection by viruses causes the formation and the presence in the blood of antibodies comparable to those found in bacterial diseases: (1) neutralizing antibodies, (2) complement-fixing antibodies, and (3) agglutinating antibodies.

Often these reactions take on their interest from their conjoint results and the comparative study of the evolution of each of the antibodies.

The principles of the reactions most commonly employed for the diagnosis of viral diseases will be discussed here briefly.

COMPLEMENT-FIXATION REACTION. This reaction is more useful for the viral diseases than for the acute diseases due to bacteria. It is easy to perform. Its positivity and its level are of great importance. To utilize it correctly, several samples must be obtained over a period of weeks. If the curve rises and then falls, the infection is both undeniable and recent. Indeed, the antibodies that fix complement present a transitory character which makes them evidence of the infection itself, in contrast to neutralizing and hemagglutinating antibodies, which are more durable and evolve in parallel with immunity. The complement-fixing antibodies usually appear early — even during the first days of the infection — and disappear in a variable, but generally limited time; they have in particular this precise character in the course of influenza, since they disappear in three months in almost all subjects. In particularly favorable conditions, this reaction thus permits the diagnosis of a viral infection even when virus isolation is difficult or problematical.

It should be remembered that this reaction must be applied under very rigorous conditions if it is to have real value. Antigens must be sufficiently powerful and devoid of anticomplementary power; tests must always be made in the presence of a valid reference serum permitting the comparison of results.

At the minimum, two or three serum samples are required. The first, the *early serum,* is taken immediately after onset of the disease; then a second is taken from the tenth to the twentieth day after the onset of the disease, and finally a third toward the thirtieth day; these are the *late sera.* These figures are not applicable in all circumstances, as we shall see.

When the antibody titer increases at least fourfold between the early serum and a late serum, this increase is a strong element in support of the diagnosis. In certain viral diseases, as will be seen further on, contrary to the rule, the complement-fixing antibodies appear late and their level rises late. When antibodies appear initially in the first late serum, a third sample (thirtieth to sixtieth day, for example) is indicated to see if there is a significant rise in the antibody level. In other circumstances, successive samplings will demonstrate during convalescence a lowering of the level of these antibodies after a transitory rise, and this curve will be significant. If only a single sample can be taken, its value in each case should be estimated in terms of the clinical and epidemiological picture.

It should be recalled that the time required for disappearance of complement-fixing antibodies differs notably according to both the virus and the subject. In adenovirus infections, for example, high titers can persist a year, and in poliomyelitis it has been possible to detect them for two years. Lastly, in measles they seem to persist as long as the neutralizing antibodies. Complement-fixing antibodies hence do not have absolutely the same significance for each type of viral infection.

Furthermore, in some cases these antibodies are not specific for a virus type but only for the group to which the virus belongs. This is the case for the adenoviruses. Hence the clinician must judge whether the diagnosis of adenovirosis suffices or whether it is necessary, particularly in an epidemiological investigation, to ascertain the virus type involved.

The values of the levels also vary with the diseases in question, as will be indicated in connection with each possibility. Then again, subjects vaccinated with live virus vaccines can, for a certain time, elaborate complement-fixing antibodies for the germ that was inoculated.

It is clear that the clinician should constantly seek the virologist's advice, as much in order to decide on the samples and their timing as to appraise the significance of the results obtained. He will recognize the usual value of the complement-fixation test for demonstration of a recent infection while considering this reaction as only one of the elements in the diagnosis.

REACTION OF VIRUS NEUTRALIZATION. Serum containing neutralizing antibodies, if mixed with the corresponding virus, hinders, under defined conditions, the formation in the sensitive animal of lesions produced by the virus. This is the case for the nerve lesions in poliomyelitis of the monkey, for the muscle lesions in Coxsackie virus infections of the suckling mouse, for the alterations produced in embryonated hen's egg by the poxviruses or myxoviruses, or, finally, for the cytopathogenic effect on tissue culture.

Unlike the complement-fixing antibodies, neutralizing antibodies persist well beyond the disease and are evidence of acquired immunity. Thus their mere presence cannot permit a diagnosis of recent viral infection. On the other hand, if their first appearance is noted or a fourfold or greater rise over the initial titer is detected in a few days, a recent infection can be seriously considered.

These antibodies are specific for virus type and do not generally produce cross-reactions, i.e., responses to different types of viruses. Nonetheless, an already immunized subject can, on infection by a serologically related virus, show an anamnestic reaction so that the rise in titer of the previously acquired antibodies is even greater than that of the antibodies linked to the present infection. Hence, here as well the practitioner must consult the virologist to interpret results. Often a complement-fixation test or a virus search must be added to the neutralization test to confirm the diagnosis.

Carrying out a neutralization reaction requires the preparation of a stable virus suspension, the titration of this suspension and the preparation of the sera to be studied. As is always the case in serological diagnosis, tests are run on the sera under consideration, a reference serum, and a normal serum or negative control serum.

Among the variants of neutralization tests, the most commonly used in virology involves mixing constant quantities of virus with decreasing quantities of diluted serum in equal volumes. More rarely, the dilutions are effected on the virus or on both the virus and the serum.

These techniques permit titration of neutralizing antibodies. This titration is more or less precise according to the dilutions utilized; titers are comparable from one laboratory to another only to the extent that the reference sera are identical.

In certain cases, a single dilution of serum is placed in the presence of a fixed quantity of virus, a procedure which indicates only the presence or absence of antibodies at the serum dilution considered. Such a simplified method is often utilized to study the distribution of persons with antibodies in a given population or to search for subjects lacking antibodies for some virus.

Titrations are, on the other hand, indispensable for tracing a curve of antibodies and for diagnosis of recent infection. They are also indispensable in the appraisal of the value of a vaccination. Indeed, it is important to determine not only the conversion rate, i.e., the percentage of subjects who have acquired antibodies, but also the titers of antibodies obtained, the curve of their evolution, and, most important, their persistence. Such longitudinal studies can be effected only if the possibility of inapparent infections is taken into account. That is to say, often two series of tests must be associated; for example, the complement-fixation test, which specifies the presence or absence of intercurrent infections, and the neutralization, which gives evidence of the degree of immunization. Such an association was utilized, for example, when we studied the effects of inactivated-virus vaccine against poliomyelitis in collectivities of children in the Paris region.[27] It was also utilized by Voroshilova et al.[33] to appraise both the persistence of immunity and the possibility of reinfection by the attenuated-virus vaccine against poliomyelitis in Moscow.

HEMAGGLUTINATION AND HEMADSORPTION — HEMAGGLUTINATION INHIBITION.

The hemagglutination tests are based on the fact that certain viruses possess the capacity to agglutinate red cells and that the specific antibodies inhibit this hemagglutination.* Most of these viruses can also confer on the tissues they infect the property of adsorbing certain red cells.† These two reactions, hemagglutination and hemadsorption, are utilized for the identification of viruses, but only the hemagglutination-inhibition reaction is at present employed for clinical serological diagnosis. The ability of the patient's serum to prevent the reaction is determined, the final titer obtained being the greatest serum dilution still sufficient to prevent the hemagglutination by a suspension of virus so calculated as to contain, according to cases, 4 or 8 hemagglutinating units.

Like the neutralization reaction, the hemagglutination-inhibition reactions remain positive longer than the complement-fixation reaction. The mere presence of antibodies inhibiting hemagglutination hence does not constitute proof of a recent infection; but the appearance of these antibodies or a significant increase in their titer suggests a recent infection. The tests can be considered clearly positive only when they reveal an appearance of antibodies at a sufficient titer — 16 at the least — or an increase such that the titer of the late serum is eight times that of the early serum.

The reading of hemagglutination-inhibition reactions is not always easy. The virologist must eliminate the causes of error; he must standardize his reagents, particularly the antigen, which has to be of very good quality; and he must introduce into the test a reference serum. Under good conditions, however, this test is very useful, especially because, like the complement-fixation test, it is rapidly executed.

In systematic serological investigations, all the tests mentioned are useful, as they reveal the existence of a previous infection. Likewise, for the study of certain vaccinations, such as vaccination against measles, the choice of subjects not having had previous infection, the establishment of the conversion rate, and the surveillance of the immunity acquired are accomplished by tests of hemagglutination inhibition.

---

*This phenomenon was revealed by Hirst[29] for the influenza virus.

†Described by Vogel and Shelokov[32] in 1957.

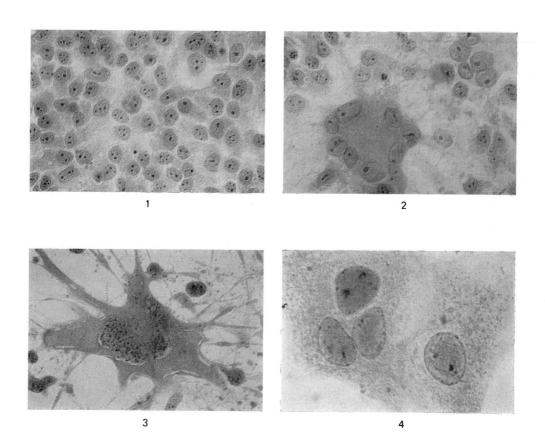

1

2

3

4

See Introduction, page 14.

1. Normal HeLa cells. (Courtesy of the Merieux Institute.)

2. Cytopathogenic effect of measles virus on HeLa cells. A multinucleated giant cell and intranuclear inclusion bodies. (Courtesy of the Merieux Institute.)

3. Cytopathogenic effect of a hyperattenuated measles virus on chick fibroblasts. Giant multinucleated spindle cell with a large inclusion almost filling the entire cytoplasm. (Courtesy of the Merieux Institute.)

4. Cytopathogenic effect of a human herpes virus on monkey kidney cells: an intranuclear inclusion. (Courtesy of the Merieux Institute.)

EPIDEMIOLOGY

The clinical domain is not separable from epidemiology, particularly in the field of virology; in this field its importance is such that it is necessary to recall certain definitions and certain principles. Epidemiology goes far beyond the framework of the more or less extensive investigation conducted around one or several cases. It includes the study of the world distribution of a disease over the years, of the distribution of cases according to given geographical, chronological, and occupational sectors. It requires a patient search for its conditions of appearance, for its areas of predilection and their characteristics (regions or countries, latitude, longitude, population, fauna, flora, geology), for the dates (year, month, periods, and evolution through the centuries), for the characteristics of the human beings that it involves (race, sex, age, residence, socioeconomic status, profession, education, marital status, composition of the family, and so on). Lastly, it requires the establishment of numerical data that will permit prospective or retrospective investigations that can verify the correlations under consideration.

It must be recalled that the term epidemiology, created for infectious diseases that sweep down suddenly "upon the people" ($\delta\eta\mu\text{os}$), was later extended to all the diseases in which the study of distribution contributes new and useful concepts.

Whether or not they do actually have any infectious agent at their origin, numerous diseases present general problems in common such as the identification of cases and the revelation of the circumstances that account for the development or the disappearance of morbidity. The case distribution, if it differs significantly from what would be expected by chance, suggests the role of systematic factors the etiological importance of which can be measured. This comparison, which brings to bear the methods of statistics, has progressively made of epidemiology a rigorous discipline. It has shown itself to be fruitful in establishing risk factors in cancerology, cardiology, and so forth. It has renovated the epidemiology of infectious diseases by making it possible to specify the role of those elements that constitute the "terrain" and that render one subject more or less sensitive than another to the same aggression of a live pathogenic agent.

Epidemiology hence never limits itself to study of the evolving outbreaks usually designated as epidemics. It embraces all cases of a disease, whether they develop in epidemic, endemic, or sporadic form. It embraces the study not only of evident forms but also of unusual and even of inapparent forms of the disease, here again, seeking, by the study of their distribution, the factors that cause the appearance or aggravation of the disease or its various manifestations.

As concerns viral infections, when the essential etiological agent, if not perfectly known, is at least well identified, then epidemiology takes in, along with the study of the patients and of the more or less apparently infected subjects, that of the virus itself, its mode of life, the environments in which it reproduces and develops, and the conditions of its spread in man and outside the body of man. The immunological investigations, the systematic searches for virus in populations in good health and the detection of healthy carriers and reservoirs of virus, permit the resolution of certain epidemiological problems. It must be added that the term epidemiology is sometimes, by extension of its meaning, applied to the animal and even to the vegetable worlds. Indeed, for certain viral infections common to man and animals, rabies for example, epidemiology in its broadest sense permits an over-all view of the distribution of the disease.

All these elements being taken into account, epidemiology, using the numerical data provided by the clinician and the virologist and the research subjects that they propose, approaches its third field of activity: the experimental investigation of various prophylactic and therapeutic methods. That is to say, epidemiology aids the clinician not only in making his diagnosis but also in appraising suggested measures against viral diseases.

DESCRIPTIVE EPIDEMIOLOGY

To study the distribution of cases, it is necessary to appraise their frequency. Frequency can be defined in different ways, particularly, as *incidence* and *prevalence*.

The *incidence* is the number of new cases during the period studied. This number is given in terms of total population at risk. This ratio can be multiplied by 100, 1000, or 10,000, according to the population unit that is most interesting to consider; thus comparisons can be made between populations of differing sizes, and the evolution of a given disease can be followed over the years. Most epidemiological studies of both viral and nonviral diseases are based on the incidence.

The *prevalence* is of much less interest in the diseases of brief duration. It includes both the new and the old cases. The instantaneous prevalence indicates the number of cases existing at a given moment (point prevalence rate), while the total prevalence indicates the total number of cases existing during a given period (period prevalence rate). This approach is particularly adapted to the study of illnesses that occur in outbreaks over successive years.

The interest and value of these data depend on the manner in which they are established. For the infectious diseases, the sources are usually the registration of diseases with obligatory declaration, hospital registration, and inquiries among either physicians or families. The regular notification of diseases with obligatory declaration ought to be considered one of the most important roles of the medical practitioner. This role is not always appraised at its proper value. In France, cases of smallpox are well reported. The same has been true within the last few years for poliomyelitis. This was not always true, and the development of morbidity curves for poliomyelitis is difficult to estimate: in particular, the increase in the number of cases of poliomyelitis during the last ten years before vaccination is not clearly demonstrated.

Other diseases remain neglected: for example, in Australia the number of births of mongoloid infants was compared during a given period with the incidence of epidemic hepatitis nine months before, but few countries are at present capable of comparing their results with these data. Likewise, England is, to our knowledge, the only country that furnishes valid statistics on measles morbidity.

The notification of illnesses of viral origin should, in a certain number of cases, be backed up by virological investigations. For poliomyelitis, especially the nonparalytic forms, laboratory confirmation is of great interest; it at least permits specification of the virus type involved. For a great many other illnesses, particularly influenza, these systematic investigations are indispensable.

The absence, insufficiency, or poor quality of these notifications render useless all

associated research. Thus, to establish the number of fatal cases of a disease (case fatality) or the frequency of complications or of certain clinical aspects, one must first know the total number of cases. It is also necessary to be certain that the clinical aspect or the complication stated has been correctly identified. The common recourse to hospital statistics in the hope, sometimes fallacious, that the diagnosis will be more precise does not resolve the problem, since the hospital sample is not representative of any particular fraction of the population.

Inquiries directed to physicians require a particular sanitary organization. The English system of public health service, by permitting precise definition of the clientele of each physician, is well adapted to this type of research. Lastly, inquiries in families are difficult except in the very limited number of illnesses marked, as in the case of measles, by easily distinguished features.

Despite all these difficulties and reservations, a certain number of interesting data have already been established. They will, with the more precise study of epidemics, make it possible someday to trace the general aspects of viral diseases in man.

EPIDEMICS OF VIRAL DISEASES

Any significant increase in the number of cases of a given disease can be called an epidemic; nevertheless, one must specify what is to be considered a significant increase and how the illness in question is characterized.

In viral infection, the etiological factor is the virus responsible, and all the cases enumerated, whatever the clinical aspect, should be attached to the same virus type.

It is obvious that laboratory studies are not obligatory in all cases; they are not indispensable for the diagnosis of measles or varicella. Nevertheless, the unusual forms, as well as the illnesses that lack a pathognomonic character, require virological diagnosis.

On the other hand, the carriers of virus detected during an epidemic cannot be added in the count of the epidemic itself unless they present the clinical and serological signs compatible with the diagnosis in question.

We shall hence reserve the term *epidemic* for viral spread involving the appearance of a number, variable but grouped, of major or minor illnesses. The term *viral spread* corresponds to a purely virological concept based on laboratory results that specify, in a given population, the percentage of healthy carriers of germs and the length and the extent of this carrier state.

Thus the distinctive characteristics of each of the cases constituting an epidemic can theoretically be defined in a general way. This is not the case when it comes to specifying the minimum number of cases that would be considered to constitute a genuine epidemic.

Usually, the current incidence of the illness is compared with the incidence in the same population during the same period of the year over several recent "nonepidemic" years. In fact, it is occasionally difficult to establish what is accepted as a "nonepidemic situation."

For smallpox, the nonepidemic situation in our countries is the absence of any case. The appearance of a single case is considered a veritable epidemic menace, implying all the imperative preventive measures. Two or three cases constitute a genuine epidemic. This example is all the more valid because a single case of smallpox in a more or less receptive population indeed represents, potentially, the source of a dramatic dissemination of this deadly infection.

An identical situation is going to arise for all the diseases which will be eradicated in the years to come. Thus, as a result of the remarkable decrease in poliomyelitis in many countries, the occurrence of three or four cases together, which five years earlier would have been considered a low number, is now looked on as an epidemic. Thus the definition of an epidemic should depend not only on the number of cases that occurred in recent years but also on the prophylactic or therapeutic progress and the results legitimately to be expected of it, to establish the limit number of cases beyond which the word epidemic should be applied.

SOURCES OF VIRUSES; CONTAMINATION; OUTBREAK AND DIFFUSION OF EPIDEMICS

All modes of contamination can be found in viral infections: direct inoculation, alimentary infection, and respiratory contamination. Contamination by inoculation can occur during transfusions (serum hepatitis), injections (poliomyelitis due to insufficiently inactivated vaccines or "syringe diseases"),

trauma (wrestler's herpes), bites or scratches by animals (rabies), or insect bites (arbovirus infections). Alimentary infections can be due to water, to eating fresh vegetables raw, or to eating shellfish contaminated by the virus or viruses of epidemic hepatitis; these impurities may be introduced by waste water, by manipulations by contaminated subjects, or by vectors, such as flies. Respiratory contamination can come directly from the patient by means of Flügge's droplets (influenza, measles) or from the bedding or the clothing of a patient (smallpox).

The mode of contamination depends on the characteristics of the virus itself, on its conditions of survival and reproduction, as well as on the reservoirs of virus.

Man is known to be only an occasional and aberrant host for the rabies virus, the survival and the propagation of which depends on different animals, especially the dog and the wolf. Certain arboviruses are accidentally transmitted to man from reservoirs constituted by wild animals (birds, rodents, monkeys) through a whole series of relay hosts (migratory birds) and vectors (wild, then domestic arthropods).

In the Occidental world the viruses most often encountered are in general transmitted from man to man; even the fly seems to play only a minimal role. Contamination of the air, the water, the soil, and foods is important here. Thus the distinction is established between the hand-borne and the air-borne infections (to use the expressions of Marcel Lelong). While it is generally agreed that influenza, the rhinopharyngo-tracheo-bronchitis diseases, and the viral pneumonopathies are air-borne and linked to the inhalation of viral particles exhaled by infected persons, the route of contamination in other viral diseases such as poliomyelitis remains the object of controversy. The abundant elimination of the virus by the intestine and the contamination by ingested virus vaccines are not proofs sufficient to exclude the possibility of air-borne infection, which for epidemiological reasons appears to us more likely in most cases. The recently demonstrated elimination of measles virus in the urine does not modify the traditional notion of air-borne contamination in measles.

The possibilities of interhuman contamination thus depend on the modalities of viral elimination: the routes adopted, the quantities of virus eliminated by each route, and the characteristics of transmissibility and of virulence kept or lost by viruses. They determine, in turn, the extent of viral spread, the outbreak, the development, and the arrest of epidemics.

Epidemics hence depend both on ability of the virus to spread and on its pathogenicity, factors whose influence depends on the environment.

If we take as an example a virus with constant characteristics, such as measles, the outbreak and the epidemic spread depend almost exclusively on the proportion of receptive subjects. Thus in England and Wales, where the annual number of cases is regularly registered, the outbreaks are regular, every two years, the interval between them being long enough to bring forward a sufficient contingent of subjects without acquired protection.

Other viruses such as the poliomyelitis viruses, however, are not of equal pathogenicity. In the countries where poliomyelitis is endemic, many subjects are immunized by inapparent infections, and the newborn can thus acquire an active immunity occasionally even under the cover of maternal antibodies. However, epidemic outbreaks can be observed under two very different circumstances: either as the result of the massive introduction of unprotected individuals, which was the case for the American troops stationed in Southeast Asia or the Eastern Mediterranean during World War II, or as the result of an increase in the pathogenic power of the viruses, which seems clearly to have been the case for certain epidemics observed recently in Africa and less recently in Europe.

It is difficult to ascertain whether the variations in pathogenicity and in ability to spread are always strictly linked. In the worst epidemics, it seems highly probable that these two factors increase together. Inversely, most of the live attenuated viruses utilized for vaccination (poliomyelitis, measles, rubella), if they implant themselves well in the vaccinated subject, generally spread rather poorly or not at all in the human surroundings, a fact which tends to prove that the ability to spread has been attenuated at the same time as the pathogenicity. This is, however, perhaps not always the case, and other factors doubtless modify the ability to spread without reducing the pathogenicity. Thus the lesser spread of measles attenuated

by seroprophylaxis might be linked simply to the reduced degree of the catarrh.

Rarer but more brutal in their effects are the antigenic variations of viruses. Such variations are well known among the influenza viruses and have been responsible for the severe pandemics against which the previously acquired immunities do not protect. Thus in the winter of 1957-1958 the influenza originating in Asia invaded America and Europe, not encountering along its passage enough individuals protected against the A_2 virus. The numerous episodes of influenza in the preceding years had conferred only immunities specific for viruses antigenically different from the Asian virus.

Theoretically, epidemics cease when the spread of the virus runs into a barrier of immunized subjects. Although this phenomenon has been verified as general, it is also true that during full viral spread, even when the population concerned still comprises a certain number of subjects without detectable specific protection, the diffusion process halts spontaneously. In the course of the Asian influenza epidemic, there were several successive outbreaks in the same human group. Likewise, in studying the spread of poliomyelitis viruses in collectivities of children, we were able to verify that approximately 2 per cent of subjects lacking detectable homotypical neutralizing antibodies were not contaminated and did not present virus in their stools any more than antibodies in their blood.[28]

Finally, it is well known that despite massive ingestion of attenuated viruses, the oral poliomyelitis vaccine does not implant itself in all cases, refusing to infect and hence to immunize an appreciable, although usually very minimal, percentage of subjects. This resistance to spontaneous or voluntary infection is usually explained by the phenomena of interference. In fact, it has been possible to demonstrate, during studies of attenuated antipoliomyelitis vaccine, that certain enteroviruses or adenoviruses present in the organism at the moment of vaccination are capable of preventing to some extent the implantation of this concurrent virus. It is possible that, likewise, certain epidemics wane because of the chance spread of another virus with either apparent or totally inapparent clinical manifestations.

These interference phenomena doubtless do not explain all failures of viral implantation or spread. Nonspecific resistance factors, for the most part temporary, have been suggested, but these phenomena have not so far been well analyzed. In another connection, if viruses can increase in their pathogenicity spontaneously, it is possible that the reverse process can also occur spontaneously, though proof of such a possibility has not yet been furnished.

ANALYTICAL AND
EXPERIMENTAL EPIDEMIOLOGY

The investigations based on precise data try to determine the factors provoking, propagating, and finally limiting or arresting epidemics. These data are of very diverse origin. The investigations naturally take into account the facts observed by the clinicians and epidemiologists, such as the role of age at first vaccination against smallpox in the appearance of encephalitic complications, or the influence of trauma or of muscular fatigue on the localizations of paralysis in acute anterior poliomyelitis. They also utilize facts established by research in fundamental virology, the influence of temperature or pH on the intracellular multiplication of viruses or the conditions of appearance of defense mechanisms, specific or not.

Such investigations can be directed toward revealing an etiological factor. Thus certain research on the role of viral factors in disturbances of embryonic development is based on prospective studies which permit the establishment of correlations between the acquisition of some type of specific immunity by the pregnant woman and the existence of pathological manifestations in the newborn.

Only by such investigations can a therapeutic or prophylactic effect be revealed, analyzed, and measured. The reader will remember, for example, that the first trials of poliomyelitis vaccination were made with double-blind investigations in which neither the subject participating in the investigation nor the observer knew whether the product injected was the vaccine itself or a placebo.

In all cases, the correct procedure should be established after careful study of the objectives, account being taken of both medical ethics and the material working conditions. There should always be a control group chosen by lot from the subjects previously chosen to participate, and the two groups should be comparable as regards not only the conditions under which they are subjected to the risk under study but also the conditions under which the observations are made. In the case of viral diseases, laboratory tests can give objective evidence of infection and its date of appearance. They are utilized, for example, to demonstrate, during a prophylactic trial aiming to reduce the clinical manifestations of some viral disease, that the two groups—controls and treated subjects—have in fact undergone the same infection, as evidenced by the appearance of specific antibodies. In other cases, they will be utilized to demonstrate that the appearance of particular clinical manifestation coincides with greater or lesser frequency with a particular infection. The quality of the criteria, the conditions, and the objectives will determine the number of subjects required and the choice of mathematical tests that will indicate whether the differences between the two groups are significant.

In summary, such investigations require the participation of virologists to specify the conditions of sample taking and to furnish laboratory tests that can be interpreted clearly, of clinicians who are painstaking in their objective analysis of signs and symptoms, and finally of statisticians, who, with the help of the others, can plan the investigation properly and interpret its results.

On the basis of these general concepts, the practitioner will be able to organize the investigations that will permit him to add to the clinical observations the elements of epidemiology that can help to orient the virological research. These general concepts will also enable him to understand the preventive action that he will need to accomplish in collaboration with the health authorities.

PROBLEMS OF PROPHYLAXIS
AND THERAPY

The struggle against viral infections is dominated by our knowledge but also by our ignorance concerning the life of the virus, its modes of transmission, and the reactions of those it infects. It is agreed that the virus cannot multiply outside the living cell it penetrates, but little is known concerning the behavior of the viral particle outside the body—in the air, on the ground, in the water, or in the body of insect vectors such as the fly. The possibility of its persistence is known, and there are a few data on the chemical or physical factors (heat, cold, light, dryness) that, in nature and not in the laboratory, can shorten or favor this persistence. There is some slight knowledge of modes of contagion (air, insects, hands, contaminated foods, and so forth). Finally, certain aspects of human reactions according to the virus, its pathway of introduction, and so forth, are known.

Certain conclusions can be drawn concerning (1) public and particularly environmental hygiene, (2) personal hygiene, (3) collective public health measures, (4) methods of passive and active immunization, and (5) specific therapy.

PUBLIC HYGIENE

In the past, sanitary measures concerning the environment—the disinfection of premises, furnishings, clothing, bedding, and dishes—played an important role during epidemics or in the prevention of familial infections. The interest accorded at present to these measures has not diminished. However, at least in the countries where the living standard is high, the general cleanliness is such that it is not necessary to insist on these measures. Besides, we believe less, in certain cases, in indirect contagion by objects and premises than in a more direct interhuman contagion.

It is only for certain viral infections that these measures remain of major importance. Thus the clothing and the bedding of subjects with smallpox contain large quantities of virus that is secreted from the mouth and the respiratory tract during the initial stage of

the disease[38] and from the cutaneous lesions themselves during later stages. Likewise, the role of insects in the transmission of arbovirus infections is so well known that we need only mention it, especially as this will be discussed further on.

Usually we are concerned more with possible viral contamination of foods, drinking water, and milk. Thus the survival of poliomyelitis virus in waste water gives rise to the suspicion that, as with the typhoid fevers, drinking water or river water may become contaminated. However, poliomyelitis epidemics due to contaminated foods have never been confirmed in the laboratory, and indirect contamination plays only a slight role in the spread of this essentially interhuman disease.

Numerous epidemiological facts indicate that epidemic hepatitis is transmitted by shellfish or by raw green vegetables. Here again, however, although virological arguments are lacking for want of appropriate techniques, healthy carriers (the frequency of such carriers is still unknown) doubtless play an important if not dominant role (cf. Chapter 24).

As for flies, which are so frequently mentioned as vectors of virus, in all cases in which it has been possible to pinpoint their role, particularly for the enteroviruses or trachoma, they have appeared to be more witnesses of than participants in viral spread.

Whatever the case may be, and even if these factors do not play a decisive role in public health, it is important to rid waste water and other wastes of the pathogenic viruses they may contain. The addition of chlorine or ozone to water already purified by physical-chemical means effectively elimi-

Table 4. *Effectiveness of Various Antiseptics Against Viruses*

	QUATERNARY AMMONIUM	HYPOCHLORITE (200 PPM)	ETHYL ALCOHOL (70%)	PHENOL (5%)	IODINE
Viruses with envelopes					
Poxviruses, herpes viruses, myxoviruses	+	+	+	+	+
Viruses without envelopes					
Adenoviruses, reoviruses	+	+	+	+	+
Picornaviruses	−	+	+	+	+

nates not only bacteria but also viruses. With the doses commonly used, it is exceptional to isolate viruses from drinking water.

Table 4 shows the action of a few antiseptics. One remark, however, is called for: when the virus is intracellular or in the presence of a high proportion of organic matter, as is the case in the laboratory for the destruction of culture media, the efficacy of most of the antiseptics is greatly diminished. For each product to be disinfected there is thus a particular problem as regards the choice, the concentration, and the time of action of the antiseptic.

INDIVIDUAL AND FAMILIAL HYGIENE

Even more than measures of public hygiene, measures of individual hygiene demand a precise knowledge of viral physiology. Even though they have a limited scope, they can be of major importance. What are some of the factors that can favor the infection or its pathological evolution—factors for which some action is possible for each individual?

The dramatic character that measles occasionally takes on in patients with leukemia is known. Everything possible should be done to prevent measles in such patients or to attenuate the infection with immunoglobulins. It is also known that either the introduction of corticosteroid treatment or its abrupt arrest can turn varicella, which is usually so benign, into a grave disease. This problem is discussed at length in Chapter 30. Experiments have shown that corticosteroids have an aggravating effect in animals infected with various viruses; this is why all vaccinations with live viruses are contraindicated in subjects undergoing such treatment.

Finally, trauma and muscular fatigue are known to play a role in the neurological localizations of poliomyelitis. That is why during epidemics certain surgical operations, such as tonsillectomy, and certain vaccinations, such as that with adsorbed vaccine against whooping cough, are put off, and violent physical effort, particularly in sports, is discouraged.

Other infections are so dangerous at particular times and under defined conditions that they should be the object of exceptionally rigorous preventive measures. This is the case for herpes in the newborn, who should at birth be removed from all risk of contamination by other persons, especially his mother, although he may have been contaminated during delivery. Similarly, because rubella is so dangerous to the human embryo and fetus, the physician would be justified in prescribing contraceptives in case of danger of an epidemic, not to mention the more specific preventive measures that will be discussed in the appropriate chapter.

Many other factors play a role in viral diseases, but they are difficult to analyze and uncertain in their consequences. Thus extensive research on the seasonal incidence of poliomyelitis did not lead to any prophylactic method. The brilliant results of vaccination have perhaps stopped this line of research, but a vaster domain remains, that of the respiratory viral diseases, many of which undergo an autumn-winter recrudescence. Is the ancient fear of exposure to cold and fog justified? Certain epidemiological investigations[45] seem to have confirmed the role of atmospheric conditions in coryza and the usefulness of individual precautions. The low temperatures act not only in terms of their absolute value but also in terms of the temperatures normal for the season. Their most decisive moment of action is two to four days before the appearance of the first signs.[45] Although such demonstrations may renew our interest in protection against cold, particularly for fragile or predisposed subjects, they provide at the most only an accessory means of prevention, of limited range and of questionable value (cf. Chapter 40).

The essential task, in the absence of methods of immunization or effective chemoprophylaxis, is to reduce the risks of contamination: disinfection of hands, of linen, of toilet objects, and of waste material for the infections with possible digestive transmission such as epidemic hepatitis; and the use of face masks, frequently changed, for the highly epidemic viral diseases with aerial transmission such as influenza, the mask being used not only to prevent the dissemination of infectious particles by patients but also as a barrier behind which new subjects can protect their respiratory tracts.

PUBLIC HEALTH MEASURES

The first point, and the major one, is regular notification of cases. Although we have already stressed the importance of this measure, it is fitting to come back to it. Indeed, aside from the general epidemiological indications they provide, notifications, if they are precise, rapid, well grouped, and well studied, permit the application of public health measures at the opportune time.

The most effective of such measures (when they exist) are unquestionably those involving specific prophylaxis. We will discuss them in greater detail in the section on individual protection, but the institution of such measures belongs rightly to the medical authorities charged with protecting the community when it is menaced by an epidemic.

Associated with specific prophylaxis in a limited number of cases are measures of quarantine. Two of the six human diseases governed in this matter by international legislation are linked to a viral agent; they are yellow fever and smallpox.

On the other hand, for most of the common diseases of children, isolation measures are passing into disuse or are relaxed because of their lack of efficacy. Thus most authors agree that it is pointless to close the schools. As a matter of fact, when the schools are closed, the pupils continue to circulate and, left more or less on their own, risk spreading the disease in environments other than the school, particularly to very young children, who are at times more fragile than the school children. In addition, in certain cases healthy carriers or ill subjects have already spread the virus widely by the time closing of the schools is proposed.

Comparable problems are posed by outbreaks of viral diseases in nursery schools, where most closures during epidemic periods would be for financial or psychological reasons.

Measures involving suspension from school have recently been relaxed and correspond generally to the period of real evolution of the disease. The suspension of subjects in contact with the patient is still too rigidly practiced in some places; the distinction is sometimes made between immune and receptive subjects. Thus brothers or sisters of children with poliomyelitis have been inconsiderately made to remain at home, where they multiply the family's difficulties, even though the poliomyelitis viruses are already widespread in the establishment from which they are excluded.

It might be more rational in certain cases temporarily to forbid gatherings that assemble populations of different origins, or to change their site. It would not be logical to establish, in an area where there is a poliomyelitis epidemic, a summer camp in which the children and personnel are not all correctly vaccinated. It would be equally illogical to permit all the youngsters of a city to encounter, in the only urban swimming pool, the inhabitants of a neighborhood in which there is an outbreak of epidemic hepatitis, poliomyelitis, or conjunctivitis.

Finally, the problem of transfusion hepatitis is known, as are the difficulties that it creates in blood banks and in regard to the effective sterilization of injection apparatus.

INDIVIDUAL PROPHYLAXIS

These are the prophylactic measures conferring on individuals an effective immunity, be it passive (immunoglobulins) or active (vaccination); this is, in fact, the most effective protection.

Two types of viral infections must be distinguished here. There are those such as smallpox, measles, poliomyelitis, yellow fever, equine encephalitis, and epidemic hepatitis which confer durable and solid immunity; in consequence, they may respond well to measures of individual prophylaxis. Others, in particular the respiratory viral diseases, confer a less valid immunity, and the complexity of the antigens involved and their variability, in influenza for example, make the results of vaccinations more problematical.

The Immunoglobulins. It is in the prophylaxis of measles that the gamma globulins have most clearly and most effectively demonstrated their possibilities. They have thus replaced convalescent serum. The two modes of action, seroprevention and seroattenuation, have been perfectly analyzed.[37] In 1950, it was by systematic utilization of gamma globulins that Straus[49] was able to arrest deadly epidemics of measles among displaced persons. In the nurseries of the Paris region in 1963, the level of protection conferred by gamma globulins on 2044 children in contact with measles was estimated at 96 per cent.[36] It is nevertheless likely that vaccination against measles, because of its superior duration of action and lesser cost, will replace methods of passive immunization.

On the other hand, for hepatitis (both epidemic and transfusion-transmitted) the gamma globulins remain valuable. The length of their action is fairly remarkable, since in the course of hepatitis epidemics a dose of

0.12 ml. per kilogram of body weight has assured protection for at least four months. Above all, attenuation is involved: systematic hepatic tests revealed that the number of anicteric forms was not modified[41, 46] and hence the spread of the disease remains identical.

The same is true for mumps, since, in the course of a systematic blind study, Baron et al.[35] noted a reduction in both number and gravity of cases, while the percentage of seroconversions was identical in the subjects having received gamma globulins and in the controls.

Even in those infections in which gamma globulins can act, their effectiveness is determined by their specificity, their dosage, and the time of their injection in relation to the moment of contamination. When the time of contact can be ascertained, for example when the subject has been exposed to a typical case of measles, the chronology is easy to establish and the results are clear. But when the disease can be spread by healthy carriers and when the stage of the infection and its spontaneous evolution are unknown, the results with gamma globulins are problematical and disappointing. This has been observed countless times in attempts at passive immunization during epidemics of poliomyelitis or even of rubella.

The Vaccines. The advantage of the vaccines is that they protect the individual for a long time. Their disadvantage is that there is a certain lapse of time, varying between several days and several weeks, before a solid immunity is established; however, this period is always shorter on revaccination.

There exist, essentially, two types of vaccines: live vaccines and inactivated vaccines.

The *live vaccines* contain either a virus homologous to that to be combated after artificial attenuation in the laboratory (oral poliomyelitis vaccine, live measles vaccine, yellow fever vaccine) or a closely related virus (smallpox vaccine).

The *inactivated vaccines* do not contain living infectious particles (injectable poliomyelitis vaccine, for example).

An intermediate type is represented by the present vaccine against rabies, in which only the greatest part of the infectious particles is inactivated by phenol.

Vaccination with live virus theoretically offers four possibilities of accidents: (1) A serious disease may appear unexpectedly in place of the benign disease normally caused by the vaccination, (vaccinial encephalitis after smallpox vaccination). (2) Because of individual sensitivity or lowered resistance (leukemia, agammaglobulinemia) a normally attenuated virus may cause serious disturbances. (3) With the vaccinated subjects acting as centers of viral dissemination, the virus might undergo serial passages that would cause it to regain its virulence. (4) The vaccine might contain foreign agents possibly pathogenic for man.

To know whether these dangers are real, it is essential to calculate the frequency of the incidents and to appraise their variations. Thus it is necessary to follow vaccinated subjects carefully, to report cases to the health authorities, and to undertake immunological or virological research.

This work has been accomplished in the United States since 1961 for oral poliomyelitis vaccine. It should also be done for all the countries that utilize this type of vaccine and for all the live virus vaccines, including the smallpox vaccine.

The risk of pathogenic agents in the vaccine, exemplified by the demonstration of the SV 40 virus in poliomyelitis vaccine or of viruses of avian leukoses in the yellow fever or smallpox vaccines prepared in the embryonated egg, is theoretically eliminated (for the known viruses) by the strict standards of manufacture and control imposed by the national or international authorities.

There remain the unknown viruses that are not revealed by present techniques: here the risks can only be hypothetical. It is because of this fourth uncontrollable risk that certain physicians prefer, when they have the choice, an inactivated vaccine to a live vaccine. It is owing to the first three risks that physicians generally hesitate to give two different live vaccines at one time. In order to decrease accidents of vaccination it has been proposed that in certain cases attenuated virus be given with gamma globulins or inactivated vaccine be given before attenuated vaccine.

With the inactivated virus vaccines the risks are mainly of allergic type, the greater antigenic load necessary for immunization being taken into account. The risks are, however, lesser, in as much as it is possible to purify this inert material further. This almost total innocuousness makes it possible to give several vaccines at once, such as poliomyelitis vaccine, tetanus and diphtheria toxoids, and whooping cough vaccine.

Since the purpose of vaccination is effective and lasting protection, however, the choice between attenuated and inactivated vaccines must be based on a comparison of the risks incurred and the effectiveness of each type of vaccine. The decision whether vaccination should be undertaken on an individual or community scale should also be based on such considerations.

The effectiveness of a vaccination can be appraised serologically and epidemiologically. Serologically, one determines the conversion rate or, more explicitly, the percentage of subjects acquiring specific immunity, the titer of antibodies obtained, and the persistence of these antibodies. Epidemiologically, one can calculate the protection level conferred by the vaccination during an epidemic period, and, in a more general manner, one can follow the evolution of morbidity curves and of spontaneous viral spread.

It is generally accepted that proper vaccination should give a conversion rate of at least 90 per cent. The titer of antibodies obtained depends on the viral infection combated, the vaccine chosen, the type of antibodies sought, and the techniques utilized to titrate them. Thus, after poliomyelitis vaccination, neutralizing antibodies at the level of 1/16 are considered mediocre, while levels above 1/256 are excellent; in contrast, after a single injection of live measles vaccine, the appearance of antibodies inhibiting hemagglutination at a level above 1/20 is the sign of a sufficient immunity.

To judge both the serological conversion and the duration of immunity after vaccination, it is necessary to eliminate intercurrent inapparent infections. This is sometimes difficult, as for example in appraising the efficacy of vaccination against poliomyelitis in a highly endemic zone.

Whatever may be their antigenic value, viral vaccinations should generally be repeated: the total vaccination program actually consists of an initial vaccination that creates immunity or the beginning of immunity, and booster vaccinations that reinforce and prolong it. The number and the timing of these boosters depend on the quality of the vaccines utilized (see Chapter 4).

The primary vaccination with inactivated vaccine requires two or three injections that complete each other and permit the establishment of a sufficient initial immunity. The first vaccination with a live attenuated virus theoretically requires only one scarification (smallpox), injection (measles), or oral intake (poliomyelitis). With oral intake, however, there is the chance that the virus administered may not implant itself, particularly in the presence of rival viruses (enteroviruses or adenoviruses), which may cause an interference phenomenon. This is why many authors prefer to give the primary dose of attenuated poliomyelitis vaccine several times, to be sure it "takes."

Aside from the interference phenomenon, the other reasons for failures of vaccinations of all types remain unknown. It is hard to understand why the same product injected in the same manner causes the appearance of antibodies in the majority of cases but does not cause any apparent immune response in 5 or 10 per cent of cases. Sometimes it is merely that the response is too weak to be detected, in which case it will be reinforced and hence made detectable by the booster dose, but in other cases the absence of immune response is absolute and resists repeated boosters. It is then said that the vaccine has insufficient antigenic power, but the phenomena covered by this phrase are hardly specified and the problem remains open.

Calculation of the protection rate during an epidemic period is an excellent means of verifying the efficacy of a vaccine: it is usually about 90 per cent. The ideal vaccination, however, also reduces the risk of epidemics, a result indicated not only by a reduction in the general morbidity but also by a decrease in or even the disappearance of spontaneous viral spread, the outcome of the process being, ideally, the eradication of the disease. This goal requires a vaccine of excellent quality that protects not only against the disease but also against inapparent infections when they exist. It also requires that a certain percentage of the population be vaccinated. This percentage would vary according to the epidemiology of the natural strains but would have to be high enough so that, when wild strains of viruses are introduced into the community, they cannot find receptive subjects to transmit them: thus those who have been vaccinated protect those who have not.

Vaccination is a civic duty that, depending on the population, will be voluntarily accepted or legally imposed. Only those vaccinations that protect against a dread disease at the price of an insignificant risk can be made obligatory.

In other cases, the viral disease is dangerous only for certain well-defined segments of the population: rubella for pregnant women, mumps for men after puberty, measles for young children in closed communities and in developing countries, influenza in subjects with respiratory insufficiency. An effective vaccination is unquestionably indicated in all these cases.

Likewise, it may be useful to protect civilians and military personnel against illnesses that do not cause a serious disease but that do cause a more or less prolonged immobilization or loss of time from work. Obviously, however, the vaccine must be totally innocuous, and careful epidemiological and immunological studies should be available that guarantee that the benign illness averted at one period in life will not represent a danger later on, at a time when it might be infinitely more dangerous.

SPECIFIC THERAPY

Therapy specific for viral diseases is still in its beginnings, and usually the only treatment available is symptomatic: treatment of pain, of motor disturbances, and of fever. The prophylaxis of bacterial super-infections is also necessary, although, as indicated elsewhere in this book, use of antibiotics with this intention has led to pointless and even dangerous use of these invaluable therapeutic agents.

It seemed to us interesting to show, in the pages to follow, the directions of current research and the first results of experimental trials. The interest of the ideas that have inspired these works, and the hopes elicited by the studies in vitro, in the animal, or even in man, justify, it seems to us, this brief account.

The research on specific therapy takes two directions: amplification of the organism's natural means of defense, and chemotherapy.

Interferon. Just as specific gamma globulins can, if given early enough, hinder diffusion of the virus by the blood route, so interferon can prevent development of the virus within the cells. Gamma globulins fail in the majority of therapeutic trials during viral illnesses: their time of action is too short, limited to the extracellular stage, an early and generally brief stage of the viral infection. Interferon shows greater promise. It is not specific for a given virus; with a few isolated exceptions it acts on almost all viruses. Nevertheless, to be effective it should

be given in sufficient quantity to the cells that will be affected before they are invaded by the pathogenic agent. In addition, a relative cellular specificity requires, in man, the use of interferon of human or, at the very least, simian origin.

The intradermal injection of rabbit interferon hinders the development of vaccinial lesions in this animal; similarly, the ocular instillation of interferon arrests vaccinial lesions on the cornea. The administration of interferon in the form of aerosols to mice reduces mortality significantly when these animals are subsequently infected by the influenza virus. The endogenous interferon that is induced by inoculating mice intravenously with the Newcastle disease virus protects these animals against the subsequent intracerebral inoculation of an arbovirus.

The problem thus is to provide, at the proper time and site for each type of viral infection, a sufficient quantity of an effective interferon of exogenous or even of endogenous origin. The results obtained to the present writing are far from satisfactory: while a marked reduction of the cutaneous lesion of primary smallpox vaccination has been obtained in man by use of interferon from the monkey, the protective action in regard to vaccinial lesions of the cornea is more limited, and the preventive action in regard to the common cold is nil. Despite the great hopes for interferon and the work that it has given rise to, the details of its fabrication in sufficient quantities and of its application still remain to be worked out.

Antiviral Chemotherapy. The research work in antiviral chemotherapy encounters great difficulties because of the close links uniting viruses with human cells. As we have seen earlier, the virus utilizes the molecular precursors, the enzymes, the energy of the cell. It is hence very difficult to act on one without interfering with the other. It is, however, likely that antiviral agents that do not disturb cellular life will be found.

During recent years a great number of substances have been put to trial, mostly in cell cultures, a few in animals, and fewer still in man. Theoretically, these specific inhibitors act during any one of the extracellular and intracellular periods of the viral infection: before fixation on the cellular membrane, at the moment of penetration into the cell, on denudation of the nucleic acid, during each of the stages of the transmission of the genetic code and of the synthesis of the new viral constituents. In fact, as we have seen, the exact mechanism of this long series of phenomena is still not clearly known for each type of virus, and the choice of the products to be tested must be based on fragmentary data. This also means that the mode of action of these various inhibitors is not always clear.

THE ANTIMETABOLITES. The idea is to furnish the cell with amino acids, glucides, purine or pyrimidine bases, and nucleosides analogous to those necessary to the life of the virus in the hope that, once disturbed in its structure, the virus will no longer be able to survive or to multiply.

Amino Acids. Parafluorophenylalanine, β-phenylserine, and L-*canavanine* have an antiviral action limited to infected cell cultures. The abundance of phenylalanine, tyrosine, or arginine in animal tissues prevents these antimetabolites from acting in vivo.

Purine, Pyrimidine, and Nucleoside. As these bases exist in the normal cell, the analogs should interfere with the viruses at different doses or should selectively inhibit enzymatic reactions indispensable to formation of the viruses.

Diazouracil prevents poliomyelitis in the mouse but not in the monkey.

In the *synthetic nucleosides* the methyl radical ($-CH_3$) of thymidine is replaced by a halogen as shown in the formula below.

Since these are thymidine analogs destined to form fraudulent desoxyribonucleic acids, they act only on the DNA viruses. The Rous sarcoma virus, which is an RNA virus, is an exception (Force and Stewart, 1964).

FUDR (5-fluoro-2'-deoxyuridine) inhibits the synthesis of the enzymes DNA polymerase, thymidine kinase, and thymidilate kinase; the vaccinia virus does not reproduce in its presence, but the NP and LS antigens appear notwithstanding. The cytopathogenic power of the herpes and varicella viruses is not hindered, unlike that of the adenoviruses. A related compound, 5-trifluoromethyl-2'-deoxyuridine, may act on the herpetic keratitis of the rabbit provoked by strains resistant to IUDR.

BUDR (5-bromo-2'-deoxyuridine) is incorporated into the viral DNA in place of thymidine but does not hinder appearance of cytopathogenicity. A large number of non-infectious or ill-formed particles appear under its influence. Herpetic or vaccinial viruses resistant to BUDR are easily observed.

IUDR (5-iodo-2'-deoxyuridine) was first tried in the animal and in man as an antineoplastic agent. The risk of a teratogenic effect caused its systemic use to be reserved for very serious diseases. It has been used for the local treatment of herpetic or vaccinial keratitis thanks to the work of Kaufman. Its action is the more clear-cut the more often the applications are repeated. In the rabbit, intrarachidian injection of IUDR did not prevent development of herpes encephalitis. On the other hand, in a human case of laboratory-proved herpes encephalitis, Evans et al. claim to have obtained an improvement in 36 hours followed by cure with sequelae by administering 1.50 gm. of IUDR in saline-dextrose solution and repeating this treatment two days later.

The fraudulent DNA is manufactured at the same time as the protein, but it hinders the assemblage, and under the electron microscope a great number of particles are seen that lack an envelope.

1-β D-*Arabinofuranosylcytosine* acts on the DNA viruses (pox, herpes) but not on adenoviruses by inhibiting in the cells undergoing active multiplication the synthesis of deoxycytidylic acid and perhaps of phos-

R= CH₃ = Thymidine
F = FUD
I = IUD
Br = BUD

phokinase. Mutants resistant to cytosine arabinoside are not observed. Despite the toxicity of the product, even administered locally, experimental herpetic keratitis of the rabbit could be cured or greatly retarded.

THE DERIVATIVES OF BENZIMIDAZOLE, GUANIDINE, AND BIGUANIDE. Research was undertaken on different compounds derived from benzimidazole owing to their structural similarity to the purines. Thompson, and Tamm and co-workers at Rockefeller Institute have studied, among others, the (α-hydroxybenzyl)-benzionidazole.

HBB 2 (α-hydroxybenzyl)-benzimidazole does not inactivate poliomyelitis virus in vitro but has a hightly selective action on the ECHO and Coxsackie B viruses.

HBB

It acts during the eclipse phase of the virus and, as in antibacterial chemotherapy, during the longest part of the exponential multiplication of the virus. The frequent appearance of resistant mutants explains its lack of effectiveness in the animal.

Guanidine, $\begin{matrix} NH_2 \\ \diagdown \\ C \mathrel{=\!=\!=} NHCl, \text{ in con-} \\ \diagup \\ NH_2 \end{matrix}$

trast to HBB, has a more marked selective action on the multiplication of poliomyelitis virus than on that of ECHO and Coxsackie B viruses. Both HBB and guanidine have made it possible to establish subgroups within the vast group of enteroviruses (see Chapter 3 for more details). The poxviruses, the myxoviruses, and the arboviruses are not sensitive to it. The mechanism of action is similar to that of HBB; guanidine impedes the adsorption not of the virus but of the RNA-polymerase that is necessary to its synthesis. Trials in the monkey at subtoxic dosage had seemed promising in diminishing poliomyelitis lesions, but the appearance of resistant mutants makes its clinical use in man unlikely. HBB and guanidine administered together have a synergistic effect owing to the lesser number of resistant mutants.

The biguanide ABOB has been widely used for influenza, herpes zoster, and varicella. Such use has been possible only because of its slight toxicity. This toxicity is nonetheless disproportionate, with the uncertain results of animal or human experimentation.

ABOB

THIOSEMICARBAZONE. The action of the thiosemicarbazones on the tuberculosis bacillus, known since 1950, led Thompson et al. to search for a possible antiviral activity. Among the derivatives, isatin β seems particularly interesting for the vaccinia or smallpox viruses, whereas it is inactive on the enteroviruses, the myxoviruses, the arboviruses, the herpes virus, and the rabies virus. In the mouse treated preventively or even in the three days following intracerebral inoculation of vaccinia virus, the infectious titer is reduced by 10 to 100 times and a good number of animals are protected against certain death.

N-Methylisatin-β-thiosemicarbazone

In the rabbit, the product has little action on the dermal vaccinia infection.

Various applications have been made in man to prevent the appearance of smallpox in contacts or to cure children with vaccinial complications (progressive vaccinia). Other derivatives must be found, however, for nauseous disturbances, occasionally very severe, hinder regular absorption of the product by the patients.

ANTIBIOTICS AND POLYSACCHARIDES. *Statolon (M 1758)* is a polyanionic polysaccharide containing glucose, galactose, arabinose, xylose, rhamnose, galactosamine, and glycuronic acid. It is extracted from cultures of *Penicillium stoloniferum.*

It is not toxic in cell culture or in the animal and exerts its action on various arboviruses, poliomyelitis viruses types I to III, the rhinoviruses, Coxsackie A 21 virus, and Rous chicken sarcoma virus. This product is not virucidal, and its effect on viruses is thought to be caused by the fact that it makes the cells secrete interferon; it is not, however, understood why it does not act on the DNA viruses under these conditions.

Helenine is a ribonucleoprotein that contains the fundamental bases (guanine, cytosine, adenine, uracil) and is extracted from *Penicillium funiculosum*. It inhibits poliovirus II and ECHO virus 9 in cell culture. Its slight toxicity has permitted its preventive use in infection of the mouse by the Columbia SK encephalomyelitis virus and in that of the monkey by the poliomyelitis virus.

Cyclopin, derived from *Penicillium cyclopum*, inhibits various arboviruses of groups A and B, but has not acted on five enteroviruses, the herpes virus, and the adenoviruses.

Distamycin, synthesized by *Streptomyces distallicus,* is not virucidal and does not impede, either, the adsorption of virus to the surface of cells. Administered one day after the cutaneous or corneal inoculation of vaccinia virus to the rabbit, it can lead to recovery by reducing the number of infectious particles and the cytopathogenicity. A beneficial effect has also been shown on herpetic keratitis, the gravity of which was lessened.

Actinomycin D is an antibiotic extracted from *Streptomyces antibioticus*. It has antibacterial, antiviral, and antitumoral activity. The mechanism of action of this product has been particularly well studied. It is thought to act by blocking the synthesis of the RNA manufactured under control of the cellular DNA. The most sensitive viruses are those whose development requires the synthesis of messenger RNA: the poxviruses, the reoviruses, and also the influenza virus. The viruses that can themselves serve as messenger, having only a single strand of ribonucleic acid, are not affected (poliovirus, arbovirus, parainfluenzae). The action of actinomycin D on the poxviruses in ovo has not been confirmed in vivo (it is much too toxic in the animal).

Mitomycin C also has an antitumoral action by blocking the synthesis of cellular DNA and that of poxvirus (vaccinia). This antibiotic is thought to act by soldering the two strands of the cellular DNA.

Gliotoxin is an antibiotic produced by different molds. It has an inhibitory effect in vitro against various RNA viruses. This product has been reported to exert a marked antiviral effect in monkeys infected with poliomyelitis by the intramuscular route and in mice and puppies with influenza.

Ketoaldehyde

OTHER PRODUCTS. *Ketoaldehyde (xenalamine)* was administered by Magrassi within 24 hours of inoculation by the nasal route into the mouse of a very weak dose of influenza virus. This product was reported not only to increase survival but also to reduce the viral infectious titer at the lung level. This product, which is active in cell culture, has also been reported to have a certain local effect on herpetic keratitis of the rabbit, but it does not act by the systemic route on herpetic encephalitis. Thus far the clinical results have not confirmed the initial hopes.

1-Adamantanamine is a symmetrical amine that is thought to slow down the adsorption and the penetration of different strains of influenza A virus and of the rubella virus; on the other hand, the influenza B, parainfluenzae 2 and 3, and mumps viruses are not sensitive to it. Mice inoculated with influenza A virus by the peritoneal route and treated shortly before or shortly afterwards with this product present infections less severe than the controls. With 200 mg. per day over ten to 13 days, Wendel reduced the rate of influenza infections from 77 to 31 per cent in 794 prisoners. Appleyard obtained a similar reduction in volunteers inoculated by the nasal route with the influenza A_2 virus by administering a dose of 300 mg. per os 20 hours beforehand followed by 200 mg. per day (in two fractions) for five days.

Sulfoniazide (isonicotinyl hydrazonotoluene-*m*-sulfonic acid) has been utilized with success in the treatment of tuberculosis. It can, in heavy dosage in the rabbit, prevent the lesions of vaccinia if it is administered one day before the inoculation.

Most of this account reports very recent work or techniques; it is hence possible that certain facts or hypotheses may be contradicted in the years to come. Nonetheless, these important chemical research works do not have a merely speculative aspect: all the problems of cancer and of viral chemotherapy loom in the background. The results are still modest indeed, but they have, notwithstanding, the most enthralling interest. The abundance of publications shows clearly the importance attributed to the problems raised. In a brief general review, it has been impossible for us to cite all the works and all the authors.

REFERENCES

VIRUSES: DESCRIPTION

1. Caspar, D. L. D.: Design principles in virus particle construction. In: Horsfall, F. L., and Tamm, I. (eds.): Viral and Rickettsial Infections of Man. Ed. 4. Philadelphia, Lippincott, 1965, pp. 51-93.
2. Dales, S.: Penetration of animal viruses into cells. Progr. Med. Virol., 7:1-43, 1965.
3. Franklin, R. M.: Significance of lipids in animal viruses. Progr. Med. Virol., 4:1-53, 1962.
4. Green, M.: Chemistry and structure of animal virus particles. Amer. J. Med., 38:651-668, 1965.
5. Jacob, F., and Monod, J.: Genetic regulatory mechanism in the synthesis of proteins. J. Molec. Biol., 3:318, 1961.
6. Joklik, W. K.: The molecular basis of the viral eclipse phase. Progr. Med. Virol, 7:44-96, 1965.
7. Joklik, W. K.: The poxviruses. Bact. Rev., 30:33-66, 1966.
8. Lwoff, A., Horne, R., and Tournier, P.: A system of viruses. Cold Spring Harbor Symp. Quant. Biol., 27:51-55, 1962; C.R. Acad Sci. 254:4225, 1962.
9. Mayor, H. D., and Jamison, R. M.: Morphology of small particles and subviral components. Progr. Med. Virol., 8:183-213, 1965.
10. Melnick, J. L., and McCombs, R. M.: Classification and nomenclature of animal viruses, 1966. Progr. Med. Virol., 8:400-409, 1966.
11. Wagner, R. R.: Interferon. Amer. J. Med., 38: 726-737, 1965.
12. Walker, D. L.: Viral carrier state in animal cell culture. Progr. Med. Virol., 6:111-148, 1964.
13. Waterson, A. P.: The significance of viral structure. Arch. Ges. Virusforsch., 15:275-300, 1965.

GENERAL PHENOMENA OF RESISTANCE TO VIRAL INFECTION

14. Bellanti, J. A., and Artenstein, M. S.: Mechanisms of immunity and resistance to virus infections. Pediat. Clin. N. Amer., 11:549-561, 1964.
15. Bellanti, J. A., Artenstein, M. S., and Buescher, E. L.: Characterization of virus neutralizing antibodies in human serum and nasal secretions. J. Immun., 94:344-351, 1965.
16. Buffe, D., and Burtin, P.: Localisation des chaînes légères des immunoglobulines humaines dans les cellules lymphoïdes. Ann. Inst. Pasteur, 110: (Suppl. 3) 49-52, 1966.
17. Cohen, S.: Antibodies—structure and biological function. Proc. Roy. Soc. Med., 60:589-591, 1967.
18. Downie, A. W.: Pathways of virus infection. In: Smith, W. (ed.): Mechanisms of Virus Infection. New York, Academic Press, 1963, pp. 101-152.

19. Enders, J. F.: A consideration of the mechanisms of resistance to viral infection based on recent studies of the agents of measles and poliomyelitis. Trans. Coll. Physicians Phila., 28:68-79, 1960.
20. Fahey, J. L.: Antibodies and immunoglobulins. I. Structure and function. J.A.M.A., 194:71-73, 1965.
21. Fahey, J. L.: Antibodies and immunoglobulins. II. Normal development and changes in disease. J.A.M.A., 194:255-258, 1965.
22. Janeway, C. A.: The immunological system of the child. I. Development of immunity in the child. II. Immunological deficiency states. Arch. Dis. Child., 41:358-365, 366-374, 1966.
23. Kaplan, K. C., Catsoulis, E. A., and Franklin, E. C.: Maternal-foetal transfer of human immune globulins and fragments in rabbits. Immunology, 8:354-359, 1965.
24. Paupe, J., and Meyer, M.: Les moyens de défense du nouveau-né contre l'infection. XXIème Congrès de l' Association des Pédiatres de Langue Française. Expansion Scientifique Française, Paris, 1967, Vol. 3, pp. 141-276.
25. Suter, E., and Ramseier, K.: Cellular reactions in infection. Advances Immun., 4:117-173, 1964.
26. West, C. D., Hong, R., and Holland, N. H.: Immunoglobulin levels from the newborn period to adulthood and in immunoglobulin deficiency states. J. Clin. Invest., 41:2054-2064, 1962.

CLINICAL DESCRIPTIONS AND METHODS OF DIAGNOSIS. EPIDEMIOLOGY

27. Celers, J., Lazar, P., Drouhet, V., Boue, A., Zourbas, J., Said, G., and Drai, M.: Remarques sur les méthodes utilisées pour le contrôle du pouvoir antigénique de lots de vaccin antipoliomyélitique inactive. Rev. Franç. Etud. Clin. Biol., 3:260-270, 1963.
28. Debré, R.: Transmission de la poliomyélite. In: Journées Pédiatriques. Paris, E. Lanord, 1960. pp. 185-196.
29. Hirst, G. K.: The agglutination of red cells by allantoic fluid of chick embryos infected with influenza virus. Science, 94:22-23, 1941.
30. Schwartz, D.: Les méthodes de recherche en épidémiologie. Bull. Inst. Nat. Santé, 21:25-32, 1966.
31. Sohier, R.: La réaction de fixation du complément en virologie. Sa valeur et ses limites pour le diagnostic et pour les enquêtes épidémiologiques. Bull. Soc. Med. Hop. Paris, 115:1273-1280, 1964.
32. Vogel, J., and Shelokov, A.: Adsorption-hemagglutination test for influenza virus in monkey kidney tissue culture. Science, 126:358-359, 1957.
33. Voroshilova, M. K., et al.: Serological survey of children in Moscow for antibody to polioviruses, 1961 and 1962. Bull. WHO, 32:317-329, 1965.

PROBLEMS OF PROPHYLAXIS AND THERAPY

34. Appleyard, G.: Chemotherapy of viral infections. Brit. Med. Bull., 23:114, 1967.
35. Baron, S., Barnet, E. V., Goldsmith, R. S., Silbergeld, S., Ehrmantraut, W. R., Boyland, J. E., and Burch, B. L.: Prophylaxis of infections by gamma globulin. Amer. J. Hyg., 79:186-195, 1964.

36. Celers, J.: Problèmes de santé publique posés par la rougeole dans les pays favorisés. Séminaire du Centre International de l' Enfance. Juin. 1964. Arch. Ges. Virusforsch., *16*:1-5, 5-18, 1965.

37. Debré, R., and Joannon, P.: La rougeole. Epidémiologie, Immunologie, Prophylaxie. Paris, Masson et Cie, 1926.

38. Downie, A. W., Meiklejohn, M., Vincent, L. S., Rao, A. R., Sundara Babu, B. U., and Kempe, C. H.: The recovery of smallpox virus from patients and their environment in a smallpox hospital. Bull. WHO, *33*:615-622, 1965.

39. Evans, A. D., Gray, O. P., Miller, M. H., Verrier, E. R., Weeks, R. D., and Wells, C. E. C.: Herpes simplex encephalitis treated with intravenous idoxuridine. Brit. Med. J., *1*:407-410, 1967.

40. Falcoff, E., Falcoff, R., Fournier, F., and Chany, C.: Production en masse, purification partielle et caracterisation d'un interferon destiné à des essais thérapeutiques humains. Ann. Inst. Pasteur, *111*:562-584, 1966.

41. Gamma-globulin prophylaxis of hepatitis. Lancet, *2*:674, 1965.

42. Finter, N. B.: Interferons. In: Neuberger and Tatum (eds.): Frontiers of Biology. Vol. 2. Amsterdam, North-Holland Publishing Co., 1966.

43. Kaufman, H. E.: Problems in virus chemotherapy. Prog. Med. Virol., *7*:116-159, 1965.

44. Larin, N. M., Copping, M. P., and Herbst Laier, R. H.: Antiviral activity of gliotoxin. Chemotherapia, *10*:12-23, 1965.

45. Lidwell, O. M.: The epidemiology of the common cold. IV. The effect of weather. J. Hyg., *63*:427-439, 1965.

46. Mirick, G. S., Ward, R., and McCollum, R. W.: Modification of post-transfusion hepatitis by gamma-globulin. New Eng. J. Med., *273*:59-65, 1965.

47. Recueil International de législation sanitaire. *10*:196-258, 1959.

48. Shope, R. E.: An antiviral substance from Penicillium funiculosum. J. Exp. Med. *123*:213-227, 1966.

49. Straus, P.: Les gamma-globulines et la médecine des enfants. Seminaire sur les Gammaglobulines et la Medine des Enfants. Centre International de l' Enfance. Paris, Masson et Cie, 1955, pp. 241-248.

50. Tamm, I., and Eggers, H. J.: Biochemistry of virus reproduction. Amer. J. Med., *38*:678-698, 1965.

51. Werner, G. H., and Maral, R.: Problèmes actuels de la chimiothérapie antivirale. Actualités Pharm., *21*:133-173, 1963.

PART I

Viral Infections in Which Neurological Manifestations Predominate

DISEASES OF THE PERIPHERAL MOTOR NEURONS

1

Acute Anterior Poliomyelitis (Infantile Paralysis)

By S. THIEFFRY and E. FARKAS

INTRODUCTION

Poliomyelitis occupies a unique place among viral diseases. It is the only one to be so well known in all its clinical aspects. The names of Heine (1840) and Medin (1887) are rightly linked with its clinical description. Its anatomopathology has been thoroughly described since its predilection for the anterior gray columns of the spinal cord was stressed by Vulpian. It was the first infectious disease of the central nervous system to be transmitted experimentally to the monkey. Finally, it is with polioviruses that J. F. Enders and his co-workers, T. H. Weller and F. C. Robbins, made the discovery which opened the way to modern virological research and the effective vaccines not only against poliomyelitis but also against other viral diseases.

Poliomyelitis presents a wide spectrum of clinical disorder. Clinicians have long suspected that this disease did not invariably result in paralysis and that it was able to appear as a generalized illness without any involvement of the nervous system that could be discerned by the examining physician. This suspicion has been transformed into certainty by the virological investigations which have been carried out in nonparalytic forms of the disease.

The neurological catastrophes produced by polioviruses demonstrate their selective attack on the peripheral motor neurons by the damage to and preferential destruction of the ganglion cells of the anterior horns of the spinal cord. In a more general way the track left by the passage of poliovirus in the central nervous system is the destruction of the cells of the descending striomotor column of the anterior horn of the spinal cord and of its homolog in the bulbopontopeduncular region which constitutes the sites of origin of the motor cranial nerves. For the clinician, this results in a nicely defined symptomatology, characterized by lower motor neuron paralyses as opposed to those of upper motor neuron origin. The very name of acute anterior poliomyelitis encompasses perfectly the primary and essential lesion of the illness.

But for a long time, even before the infectious nature and viral cause of infantile paralysis had been observed, even before complete anatomical and experimental studies had been undertaken, it had become clear that this lesion could not explain every feature of the disease. "Typical" infantile paralysis includes, at least from the time of onset, a series of signs and symptoms which may be explained only by a more diffuse neuronal lesion, spreading widely above and around the anterior horn of the spinal cord, and by a constant meningeal reaction. "Typical" infantile paralysis regularly includes, in varying degrees of severity, an associated meningitis and certain features of "polio-encephalitis."

A general clinical picture stems from this which evolves in a characteristic enough way for an alert physician to make the correct diagnosis without the aid of the virologist. It is this clinical picture which will be described here.

CLINICAL PICTURE OF POLIOMYELITIS

We will discuss later, in appropriate sections, those less well recognized forms of poliomyelitis which have been included in the clinical picture only following virological, immunological, and epidemiological studies. These are the pure meningeal and the encephalitic varieties.

The paralytic forms will be described under their main headings, taking into account those localizations which may endanger the patient's life.

TYPICAL SPINAL FORM

Three phases may be distinguished in the evolution of infantile paralysis: (1) the phase of incubation, occurring between the moment of infection (nearly always unknown) and the frank onset of illness; (2) the invasive, or preparalytic phase, occurring from the first signs of illness until the appearance of paralysis; and (3) the paralytic phase.

The Phase of Incubation. The average duration of incubation is not known. We suspect that a period of ten days is common, although the possibility of longer incubation periods (35 to 40 days) must be borne in mind.* The period during which the patient incubates the virus is usually asymptomatic. Nevertheless, careful analysis of clinical findings shows that it is not unusual to find minor manifestations—the minor illness described by Paul and Russell—doubtless due to virus already present in the body, which form the first phase of the illness. These manifestations consist of fever, sore throat, pharyngitis, nausea, vomiting, abdominal pain,

diarrhea, rarely aching pains, or simply abnormal sensations of fatigue or a change of character.

Indeed, the picture is not very characteristic and, even at the height of an epidemic, the correct diagnosis becomes the less easy when there are no clinical or biological signs of damage to the nervous system.

This minor illness occurs 15 to 20 days before the clinical onset of poliomyelitis. Occasionally, it precedes it by only a few days. To recapitulate the progress of the disease, we see, in turn, first a febrile attack, corresponding to the "minor illness," then a period which is free from fever, then a second febrile episode which coincides with the clearest manifestation of the "major illness." For this mode of onset is reserved the title of "diphasic."

Invasive or Preparalytic Phase. Whether it has been preceded a few weeks earlier by an episode of illness, whether it assumes a classically diphasic mode of onset, or whether the disease arises *de novo,* a time comes when clinical poliomyelitis shows its face with the unmistakable features of a disease of the nervous system.

The onset is abrupt, almost to the minute, generally at the end of the day. From the first hours of the illness, the patient complains of headache and almost always he vomits. From this time on, for several days, events progress in a sufficiently characteristic way to direct the diagnosis, when one is aware of the symptomatology of this period or alerted during the presence of an epidemic. Fever is constant and is rarely very elevated. It persists throughout the invasive phase and even beyond. The facies is drawn, often with rapid alterations in color. Very frequently, fluctuations in consciousness are observed in the patient. These take the form of an onset of semicoma or of sleepiness, from which the child may be easily distracted by simple stimuli, rapidly regaining all his lucidity to reply with precision to questions. Convulsions are exceptional.

The patient is anxious and complains of headache, pain in his neck (which is sometimes held in the attitude of torticollis), and also pains in all his limbs, especially his back. This low back ache may be of all degrees of severity, from a mild discomfort to an agonizing pain which immobilizes the patient. This pain is exaggerated by changes of position. It may radiate to the thighs in a symmetrical fashion. Sometimes these pains are localized

---

*The question of episodes of paralytic poliomyelitis which have been induced by intercurrent causes (trauma, muscular exertion, encephalography) is relevant here. It is possible that an illness which was evolving subclinically is thus made manifest in a paralytic form (i.e., "exteriorized").

to one limb or to the neighborhood of the joints, with a resulting false impression of rheumatism or even of osteomyelitis. These spontaneous pains sometimes result in a rigid posture which may simulate paralysis.

If these spontaneous pains are only mild, on examination the physician may accentuate them or make them appear by attempts to move the limbs. In doing this, the physician may be able to reassure himself that there is no paralysis but, in fact, a limitation of movement caused by reaction to pain as soon as muscle groups or individual muscles are stretched. The phenomenon of painful muscular tension may be demonstrated by straightening the angle of the foot to the leg, by separating the thighs, and by raising the arm into the horizontal position.

When we try to make the patient sit up, holding him by his shoulders, we observe that he lets his head fall back and places his arms behind to hold himself upright (the tripod sign). At length, he is unable to hold his trunk vertically, owing to violent pain with spasm of the paravertebral muscles.

Of all the clinical procedures which may be used to show pain upon muscular stretching, the most sensitive and the earliest to become positive is the maneuver of Lasègue*; in this, passive elevation of the leg above the level of the bed produces, almost immediately, a fixed spasm on extending the muscles of this thigh, together with intolerable pain which prevents any elevation above a very limited angle. We should mention that, initially, the painful responses to the passive stretching of muscle groups are remarkably symmetrical and bear no relation to the paralyses which eventually appear.

This painful syndrome, clear to the observer, is without doubt most important during this period of the illness. For the clinician, it may mask or complicate the assessment of the meningeal syndrome, with which confusion is often made. However, neck stiffness and Kernig's sign are found in half of the cases seen. Kernig's sign may be difficult to distinguish from that of Lasègue. In Kernig's sign, passive elevation of the leg above the plane of the bed provokes, beyond a certain angle, marked flexion of the knee, with spasm of the posterior thigh muscles. Pain appears at the same time as the spasm or perhaps afterwards, whereas in Lasègue's sign intolerable pain precedes and accompanies spasm during extension. The tendon reflexes are, at this time, rarely altered and, on the contrary, are often brisk.

Abdominal crises are frequent (such pain may suggest appendicitis). Constipation is usually seen, together with meteorism and, occasionally, visible peristalsis in the epigastric area.

The physician must be aware of the frequency of bladder dysfunction, unrelated to disturbances in consciousness. This may result in retention of urine, necessitating catheterization. These problems are transitory and are no longer met with after about ten days.

To the common signs which have just been detailed and described because of their value in diagnosis and which bear witness to a very diffuse attack on the nervous system, one must add others of secondary diagnostic interest, which apparently vary in differing epidemics. These are: profuse vomiting, diarrhea, pharyngitis, sore throat, coryza, and signs of upper respiratory tract infection.

The phase of preparalytic invasion is of variable duration. Usually of three or four days, it may be shorter and last no more than 36 or 48 hours. Very rarely it may be absent. In exceptional cases, it may be prolonged for eight or even 14 days.

In infantile paralysis, there does not seem to be any correlation between the severity of the initial symptoms and the gravity of the ensuing paralysis. Even more, if the diagnosis of this disease has been suspected during this period, it is not possible to assert that paralysis will eventually result and that this case of poliomyelitis will not be abortive.

The Phase of Acute Paralysis. With the appearance of paralyses begins a new stage in the disease, which now is unmistakably a disease of the nervous system. Stripping off the overlying symptomatology, the motor paralysis makes it clear that the clinical picture represents primarily a disease of the motor neurons of the anterior horn.

The onset of paralysis is abrupt, and the physician observes it after several days of illness. There is some doubt about the reality of "morning paralysis" (whose description has been attributed to West). More typically, it is at the height of a febrile and painful period that the patient notices the paralyses or when one observes their onset and their extension. Contrary to widespread opinion,

---

*Charles Lasègue (1816-1883) has had his name attached to "Lasègue's sign," characteristic of sciatica, a disorder concerning which he wrote nothing.

ascending paralysis (Landry) is the exception and, indeed, the paralyses do not follow each other in any systematic order. In about three days, all the muscles that are destined to become paralyzed have, in fact, become so: a fresh site of paralysis is rarely seen at one week after the onset.

The onset of paralysis does not necessarily coincide with the disappearance of the infectious phase of illness nor with that of the painful syndrome, which may persist for a number of weeks. In contrast to this persistence, the clinical picture of meningism disappears quite rapidly.

In the usual form of infantile paralysis, the distribution of the paralyses is very variable, as capricious as the spread of the virus throughout the area served by the striomotor gray matter. Nevertheless, a preference may be seen for muscles receiving their innervation from the cervical and lumbar enlargements.

There is no muscle which has not been attacked, and the disease has been observed in every site. All combinations of paralysis may be seen: quadriplegia, paraplegia, diplegia, monoplegia, a solitary muscular group, several muscles, one muscle, or one muscular fasciculus. We may only draw attention to the facts that the lower limbs are more frequently affected, that the tibialis anterior and the deltoid muscles are most frequently attacked, that the paralyses of poliomyelitis are usually asymmetrical when two limbs are affected, and that they may vary greatly in degree from one muscle to another in the same limb.

In examining and assessing a case of poliomyelitis, it is thus essential to evaluate deficiencies in muscular power and not those in the corresponding nerve or spinal root.

The paralyses of poliomyelitis bear the hallmark of an attack on the anterior horn cells and on the lower motor neuron.

1. The tendon reflexes are abolished in the paralyzed regions and sometimes in those areas which have, apparently, been spared.

2. Changes in muscular tone are found — hypotonia — although this characteristic may be masked for some time by the persistence of pain.

3. Vasomotor disturbances are encountered almost uniformly and very soon after the onset.

4. Muscular atrophy is an early and important phenomenon.

5. Electrical reactions (reaction on stimulation, detection of action potentials, speed of conduction) show results compatible with the presence of denervation.

To these positive, constant, and harmonious signs must be added negative signs which are as important, viz., the absence of pyramidal signs (except in some very unusual reported cases) and the absence of objective evidence of impaired sensation.

The tendency toward recovery of poliomyelitic paralysis is well recognized. It is unusual for a certain amount of recovery not to occur, even in the most severe forms of the disease. This recovery shows itself early and persists for some years following the acute phase of the disease. One of the important objectives in the treatment of the illness is to be fully prepared to exploit and encourage this spontaneous improvement.

The sequelae in an attack of poliomyelitis vary greatly from one patient to another.

In practice, it is not until the end of the first month that one may have even an approximate idea of the prognosis and be in a position to discuss a program of re-education. Details of a program are determined by a very detailed schedule of the evolution of muscular weaknesses, their distribution, the areas affected, and the severity. Certain sites of paralyses, notably those which endanger the stability of the vertebral column, are especially important. The greatest problems are found in poliomyelitis in young children (scoliosis, contractures, disturbances of growth, muscular atrophy).

In a consideration of the typical form of spinal infantile paralysis, which has just been under discussion, we must include among the sequelae a varying degree of disability whose repercussions on the life and occupation of the individual can never be forgotten. Without taking into account the problems of social and educational readjustment of the child, and considering only the indisputable infirmity which stems from the disease, we may guess that 7 per cent of patients will never be able to earn their living and that 75 per cent will have reduced capacity for work.

SPINAL FORM WITH PARALYSIS OF THE RESPIRATORY MUSCLES

Among the various types of poliomyelitis, we must give a special place to those accompanied by paralysis of the respiratory muscles. These follow an attack of the virus on the nuclei, situated in the cervical and dorsal spinal column (From C-3 to D-12), which supply the principal and accessory respiratory muscles. This grave event generally accompanies severe poliomyelitis affecting the four limbs and trunk and, in particular, the abdominal muscles. But this is not invariably the case, so much so that it is essential to examine systematically the integrity of the respiratory musculature and its function in all cases of poliomyelitis. This should be done on three muscular levels: intercostal, diaphragmatic, and abdominal. This investigation is the more important as those physiological signs which betray respiratory insufficiency do not always occur immediately. These signs are excessively rapid respiration, loss of the power to cough, use of the accessory muscles of respiration, and cyanosis.

Any paralysis, even if localized, of the respiratory muscles, endangers the life of the patient to a greater or lesser degree, especially if the diaphragm is concerned. Left to itself, such a situation is likely to deteriorate gradually or more abruptly into asphyxia, pulmonary embarrassment, and collapse.

The subsequent progress of each patient depends upon the speedy help which one may bring by artificial respiration and also on the quality of care which may be available in a specialized center. The great technical advances during the past 15 years have considerably reduced the mortality (previously very high) of these respiratory forms of the disease. This has been achieved by protecting the patient from the threat of infectious and mechanical accidents regularly associated with this type of pulmonary hypoventilation.

The great progress in reëducative physiotherapy of the respiratory musculature has also reduced the frequency and severity of the sequelae of respiratory paralysis, but without removing completely the bedrock of respiratory disability. These patients are handicapped at the same time by their paralyses and by their respiratory disability, which obliges them to have permanent or intermittent assistance with their ventilation.

BRAIN-STEM POLIOMYELITIS

We describe under this heading cases of poliomyelitis which are remarkable for the predominance of viral lesions in the supramedullary gray matter of the brain stem and in the striomotor formations of medulla, pons,

and cerebral peduncles. At this level, as at the level of the spinal cord, the lesions of poliomyelitis are found primarily in the nuclei of the motor cranial nerves (III, V, VI, VII, IX, X, XI, XII). However, the initial inflammation around the areas of neuronal destruction spreads readily into other neuronal elements of the cerebral axis and also into the regions immediately above the subthalamic area, in particular the parasympathetic nuclei close to the cranial nerves and those of the reticular substance. In extreme cases, this results in a fairly typical picture which is associated with paralyses of some of the cranial nerves together with sympathetic and parasympathetic disturbances, and with deep disturbances in the state of awareness and even in consciousness.

The frequency of such forms of poliomyelitis is perhaps greater in some epidemics than in others. It does not seem to be related to age, and it is not clearly related to a particular type of virus. The phase of invasion of this type of poliomyelitis often shows nothing unusual beyond pharyngeal phenomena and a frequency of sore throat or more exactly of a reddening with edema of the pharynx and of the uvula.

In 90 per cent of cases, the brain-stem localization coincides with spinal paralysis, perhaps widespread, perhaps predominantly localized to the muscles of the shoulders, of the upper limbs, or of the diaphragm.

Nevertheless, some forms are remarkably localized. The clearest example is given by the isolated facial paralysis which is apparently frequent in some epidemics of poliomyelitis. Pharyngeal palsy may also be isolated, but usually it accompanies individual paralyses of the roots of the upper limbs. It is these brain-stem forms in which we occasionally observe, in all their clarity, certain autonomic disturbances, which are otherwise often only outlined in the spinal forms of the disease.

The most remarkable are disturbances in the respiratory rhythm; irregularities, pauses, sighs, arrhythmia, asynchrony of the muscles of respiration, use of the alae-nasae muscles, and, in extreme cases, the patient's complete inability to control his respiratory rhythm and amplitude.

Circulatory disturbances are more difficult to observe and are only of clear value in the absence of respiratory insufficiency: tachycardia, arrhythmia, variations in blood pressure, collapse. Vasomotor and secretory disturbances are common: alternations of flushing and pallor of the skin, especially in the face, attacks of sweating often provoked by examination, increased lachrymal and salivary secretion.

Disturbances of consciousness may proceed to the stage of coma. Increasing sleepiness often marks the onset of the illness. One must be aware of the possibility of hallucinations *("hallucinose pedonculaire")*.

When this collection of autonomic symptoms is not combined with a hyperthermia which strikes down the patient with catastrophic suddenness by acute pulmonary edema, collapse, or hemorrhage, or other brutal accident, it is remarkable to see symptoms become less distinct and disappear in about ten days.

All the motor cranial nerves may be involved, but the gravity and frequency of involvement vary. Trigeminal paralyses are unusual.

Paralyses of the eye muscles (VI and III) are not common. Against this, there is an array of abnormal eye movements, nystagmus, dissociation of eye movements, spasmodic tremors, and even paralysis of lateral gaze. Unilateral or bilateral facial palsies do not possess any particular characteristics. Their long-term prognosis is uncertain. Lesions of the XIIth cranial nerves are not exceptional.

Of all the paralyses of the cranial nerves, by far the most frequent and the most severe are those which alter the mechanism of swallowing through damage to the nucleus ambiguus. These usually consist of a paralysis of the pharyngeal constrictors and the soft palate, which local examination allows one to diagnose accurately. But, in fact, there are functional signs which disclose this important lesion. The first in onset are choking, fits of coughing after drinking, and, frequently, the return of fluid through the nose.

With surprising rapidity, attacks of asphyxia and pulmonary embarrassment due to pharyngeal stasis and obstruction occur, together with flooding and descending infection of the bronchial alveolar tree. Even alone, paralysis of swallowing may lead to death or at the very least to severe respiratory complications.

On the other hand, of all the paralyses produced by poliomyelitis, that of swallowing has the most pronounced tendency to complete cure. Its treatment is relatively easy: postural drainage, systematic pharyngeal aspirations, and, above all, the cessation of oral feeding, the necessary nutrition being provided by the parenteral route. When this battery of measures is prolonged as long as necessary, until the careful resumption of feeding through a gastric tube after some weeks or months, recovery normally follows.

Laryngeal paralysis may be met in poliomyelitis. We may suspect this when sudden attacks of suffocation occur, starting in the initial period of the illness. Later on, their symptomatology becomes lost in the general picture of respiratory distress, and their treatment is difficult.

Taken together, the brain-stem forms of poliomyelitis have lost the character of desperate severity with which they were generally associated until very recently. The true measure of their seriousness is in the immediate threat which they hold over the control of the autonomic functions. Against this, there is no longer any doubt that, if the patient is able to pass through the initial critical phase, we may hope for recovery, sometimes complete. At present, granted that all the methods of respiratory and circulatory resuscitation are available and are under adequate biochemical and clinical control, it is not an exaggeration to say that one may be able to save the life of almost all of these patients.

DISCUSSION: CLINICAL ASPECTS OF DIAGNOSIS

The diagnosis of the paralytic forms of poliomyelitis is not always obvious, but it is usually possible by clinical means alone, especially when one has reason to suppose that there is an epidemic in the neighborhood.

Poliomyelitis, in spite of its variety and the varieties of localization, possesses fundamental signs of the attack on the peripheral neurons, and an infective phase which is very characteristic.

One must also add that the examination of the cerebrospinal fluid is of particular interest in showing, constantly, that there is an associated meningitis. This concept is of such importance that we must doubt the diagnosis if it is lacking. This constant meningeal reaction is of variable intensity; independent of the gravity of the disease, it is found in all forms, even those in which there is very little paralysis, or in those which abort without any paralysis being detectable. Meningeal reaction, therefore, constitutes a confirmatory sign of the disease and is ultimately one of the best means of checking the clinical diagnosis. Simultaneous changes in the cytology and biochemistry of the cerebrospinal fluid enable one to give a schematic description. A notable increase in the total cell count is found from the first hours of the illness; it is at a maximum during the first two days but rarely exceeds 400 cells per cubic millimeter. It begins to fall from the beginning of the third day but remains at a lower level until the second week of the disease, on an average about 15 cells per cubic millimeter, at about the tenth day.

The cellular contents of the cerebrospinal fluid change. A pure polymorphonuclear leukocytosis may be found during the first two or three days (even mimicking a puriform aseptic meningitis), and then lymphocytes appear to replace the polymorphonuclear leukocytes. Histiocytes are present in the cerebrospinal fluid during the first two weeks of the disease.

The change in the level of albumen in the cerebrospinal fluid is characteristic. Elevated during the first week parallel with the cell count (50 to 70 mg. per 100 ml.), the level falls toward the tenth day to become secondarily raised toward the third week, sometimes attaining a high level, 100 to 400 mg. per 100 ml. Thus an albuminocytological dissociation is found during this phase of the disease which is very constant and slow to disappear, sometimes lasting several months. Methodical analysis of the clinical signs and examination of the cerebrospinal fluid, taken together, usually allow one to affirm with a great degree of certainty the diagnosis of paralysis due to poliovirus.

We must also remember possible confusion in the initial period, above all with disease of the joints in an infant or of the bones and joints in the baby. There may be confusion with tuberculous meningitis or even with cerebrospinal meningitis. As against this, one must clearly distinguish poliomyelitis from other diseases of the nervous system. The other acute myelitides whose initial picture may be comparable distinguish themselves by the existence of pyramidal signs, disturbances of sensation, and lasting disturbances of the sphincters. Some of the myelitides are only one element in neurological complications of some of the

exanthemata. A most frequent error, but nevertheless avoidable, concerns the radiculoneuritides (described in Chapter 5). There is no evidence that the virus of poliomyelitis may cause these.

In practice it is only the polioviruses which create the picture of infantile paralysis which has been described. Virological investigation, which in clinical practice is no longer indispensable, has demonstrated this general rule superabundantly. The role of the other enteroviruses is very small. It deserves to be discussed with care and to be made the object of special attention in a separate critical discussion where virological arguments carry more weight than clinical observations.

PATHOLOGICAL ANATOMY

Acute paralytic anterior poliomyelitis is a meningoencephalomyelitis in which lesions are found mainly in the neuroganglion cells of the anterior horn of the spinal cord. On macroscopic examination, the gray matter of the cord appears congested and hemorrhagic.

The histological picture, perfectly described by Bodian, varies according to the time relationship between the death of the patient and the beginning of his illness.

In the early stages, *inflammatory phenomena* dominate the scene. These are characterized by an infiltration of polymorphonuclear leukocytes, lymphocytes, and histiocytes, which is both perivascular and diffuse. A congestion of all the small vessels, acellular exudates, and petechial hemorrhages accompany this cellular infiltration. Although always present from the beginning of the illness, parenchymous alterations may be masked at this stage by the intensity of the inflammatory reaction. These consist of a more or less intense chromatolysis of the neurons which may reach the stage of complete necrosis of the nervous cells with formation of neuronophagic nodules. The parenchymatous lesions concern essentially the peripheral motor neurons situated in the anterior horns of the spinal cord.

After some days have passed, the infiltrate now includes lymphocytes, plasmocytes, and microglia. The polymorphonuclear leukocytes have disappeared. The perivascular inflammation is more noticeable and the interstitial infiltrate more nodular, as prolific elements accumulate and take the place of degenerate neurons. Neurons may show signs of damage without being completely destroyed, and around these satellitosis will be the most frequently found lesion. These pathological processes are reversible and recovery is likely. In experimental poliomyelitis in animals, acidophilic intranuclear inclusions of Cowdry's type II (not occupying all the nucleus and not crowding out the nucleolus) have been observed, but they are practically never found in human poliomyelitis.

In cases lasting for two or three weeks or more, the motor neurons are rarefied or may have even completely disappeared, while those in which the lesions are completely reversible have practically recovered their normal appearance. Inflammatory phenomena have diminished, but perivascular inflammation may be found even after a number of weeks of illness. In the areas where the inflammatory and parenchymatous lesions have resulted in massive tissue destruction there are found actual cavities with accumulations of compound granular phagocytic corpuscles, cavities which are followed by gliofibrillary organization.

Wallerian degeneration is found along those nerve fibers whose central neuron has been destroyed. Atrophy now appears in all the muscle fibers belonging to the motor units which have lost their nerve cells. This is an atrophy which produces the classical appearance of neurogenic atrophy in islets, in which groups of fibers of normal size are found side by side with groups of fibers which have completely atrophied.

Localization of lesions along the course of the nervous system is characteristic. Lesions predominate in the gray substance of the cord and are maximal in the cervical and lumbar enlargements, while the sacral spinal cord is, in general, spared.

But often inflammatory and parenchymatous lesions are unrelated. Thus neuronal destruction predominates in the anterior horn cells and may also be observed in the nuclei of Clarke's column, while the neurons of the posterior horns and lateral horn cells are constantly spared in spite of the frequent existence of significant inflammatory infiltrations. Those lesions found above the level of the spinal cord are mainly in the reticular substance, with their maximal distribution in the pontomedullary region, seat of the respiratory centers, in the nuclei of the motor and sensory cranial nerves, as well as in the roof nuclei of the fourth ventricle, the *substantia nigra,* the *locus caeruleus,* the hypo-

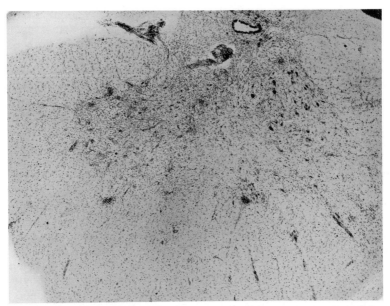

Figure 1-1.   Poliomyelitis. Photomicrograph of hemisection of dorsal spinal cord, showing disappearance of neurons in the anterior horn—although the cells in Clarke's column are spared—inflammatory changes, glial proliferation, and neuronophagic nodules. Nissl's stain.

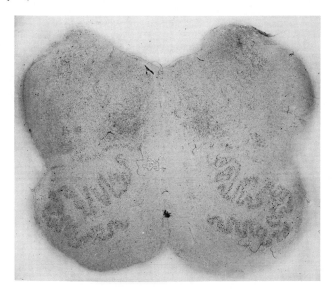

Figure 1-2. Poliomyelitis. Photomicrograph of medulla oblongata, showing two symmetrical areas of inflammation in the reticular substance. Nissl's stain.

thalamus, the thalamus, and the ascending frontal gyrus. The dentate nucleus of the cerebellum, the cortex of the vermis, the red nucleus, and the globus pallidum are less frequently affected. In general, lesions above the cord level are mainly of an inflammatory nature, but neuronal destruction can be observed in the brain stem forms attacking the motor nuclei of the cranial nerves, the reticular substance, and to a lesser degree the nuclei of the eighth nerve. But parenchymatous damage is only exceptionally found in these nuclei, at any rate to the massive degree so frequently found in the anterior horn cells.

The lesions of acute anterior paralytic poliomyelitis are virtually always localized to the gray substance, the white substance itself being spared, whereas in cases of acute myelitis the lesions, either of perivenous type (when they occur in the course of an eruptive fever) or of inflammatory or necrotic type (as in herpes zoster), occur in both the white and the gray substances.

Involvement of the meninges by inflammatory phenomena is constant in poliomyelitis; the spinal ganglia and those of the cranial nerves, in particular the Gasserian ganglion, may be infiltrated.

Apart from the nervous system, inflammatory changes have been observed in the myocardium in 14 per cent of observations in fatal cases (Ludden and Edwards).

Anatomical data give account of the symptomatology and clinical evolution of poliomyelitis. Paralyses of the peripheral type indeed result from the selective destruction of peripheral motor neurons. The partial or complete regression of the symptomatology which is observed in the acute phase of the illness may be explained by the functional repair of neurons which have not suffered irreversible lesions, or possibly by the regression of inflammatory phenomena which were responsible for a transient hindrance only to cellular function.

Thus the essentially reversible character of the central respiratory lesions, of the vasomotor lesions, and of the diverse encephalitic and meningeal manifestations may be explained as resulting from the nature of lesions above cord level which are almost always purely inflammatory.

Finally, late recovery may be attributed to the reinnervation of those muscular fibers which have lost their neuronal innervation by intact nerve fibers originating from preserved neurons.

BIBLIOGRAPHY

1. Bodian, D.: Virus and host factors determining the nature and severity of lesions and of clinical manifestations. In: 2nd International Poliomyelitis Conference. Philadelphia, J. B. Lippincott Company, 1952, pp. 61-87.
2. Bowden, R. E. M.: Some recent studies of skeletal muscle in anterior poliomyelitis and other neuromuscular disorders in man and the experimental animal. In: 2nd International Poliomyelitis Con-

ference. Philadelphia, J. B. Lippincott Company, 1952, pp. 95-99.

3. Cowdry, E. V.: Problem of intranuclear inclusions in virus diseases. Arch. Path., *18*:527-542, 1934.

4. Debré, R., et al.: Poliomyelitis. Geneva, World Health Organization, 1955.

5. Debré, R., and Thieffry, S.: Poliomyélite antérieure aiguë – Traitement. In: E. M. C. Mal. Inf., Paris, 1964.

6. Ludden, T. E., and Edwards, J. E.: Carditis in poliomyelitis; anatomic study of thirty-five cases and review of literature. Amer. J. Path. 25:357-373, 1949.

7. Thieffry, S., and Arthuis, M.: Poliomyélite antérieure aiguë (maladie de Heine-Médin). Symptomes et diagnostic. In: E. M. C. Mal. Inf., Paris, 1964.

8. Van Bogaert, L.: Poliomyélite antérieure aiguë. Handbuch der Speziellen Pathologischen Anatomie und Histologie. Berlin, Springer-Verlag, 1956, Vol. 13, part 2, pp. 243-297.

9. Wohlfart, S., and Wohlfart, G.: Mikroskopische Untersuchungen und progressiven Muskelatrophien unter besonderer Rusksichtnahme auf Ruckenmark muskelbefunde. Acta Med. Scand., Suppl. 63, pp. 1-137, 1937.

10. Wohlfart, G.: Regenerative phenomena of muscular innervation in poliomyelitis and amyotrophic lateral sclerosis. Nord. Med., *54*:1075-1078, 1955.

2

Paralysis Due to Enteroviruses Other Than Polioviruses

By S. THIEFFRY

Insofar as it is easy to describe unequivocally the varying clinical appearances and the diverse neurological manifestations which we may attribute with complete confidence to poliovirus infection, to the same extent we find difficulty in identifying, defining, and outlining the parts played by other enteroviruses in the pathology of neurological disease.

Against the thousands of cases of paralysis caused without any doubt by poliomyelitis, we may place a few handfuls of neurological illnesses which sufficiently resemble poliomyelitis for the clinicians to confuse them with this disease and from which enteroviruses are, or may be, recovered which are not polioviruses (i.e., Coxsackie and ECHO viruses). The true prevalence of these poliomyelitis-like illnesses is, in fact, impossible to determine from the results of systematic virological studies or from a thorough search of reported observations. The planned enquiries which allow the necessary synthesis of clinical and virological information are very rare.

Having expressed these general reservations, we may say that virological studies have yielded the conclusion that, in the course of epidemics, a certain number of cases of paralysis may be attributable not to poliovirus, but to other enteroviruses. When investigators have searched for an association between Coxsackie virus infection and paralysis, they have found a very variable frequency, from 0.5 per cent to 19 per cent, but these figures indicate only a statistical coincidence between the clinical manifestation and the presence of virus.

The prevalence of cases of "poliomyelitis" attributable to viruses other than poliovirus is indeed very low when one accepts this diagnosis only in the presence of certain conditions. These are: clinical manifestations of the type habitually found in infantile paralysis, proof of the presence of a virus in the body with corresponding serological reactions, and the absence of an accompanying genuine poliovirus infection. When systematic enquiry is made in the light of these criteria, a noticeable reduction appears in the number of authentic neurological illnesses which are indeed produced exclusively by enteroviruses other than poliovirus. We may cite two examples: Grist, in a virological study of individuals with "poliomyelitic" paralyses seen in Scotland over a period of seven years, recovered 315 enteroviruses. Among these, polioviruses were found on 289 occasions and an enterovirus other than poliovirus on 26 occasions (including two incidents in which the infection was mixed). Among the 24 cases which were attributed at first to infection with an enterovirus other than poliovirus, critical analysis left only four cases where the intervention of poliovirus was excluded and where the illness could be attributed to infection by Coxsackie A7 virus.

Thieffry and his colleagues examined 473 cases of acute nervous system infection by enteroviruses and found on 12 occasions evidence of a Coxsackie or ECHO virus. In seven cases alone was it certain that these viruses had been responsible for the neurological illness. These included acute ataxia, encephalitis, meningitis, and discrete paralyses; the viruses responsible were ECHO 6, Coxsackie B5, and Coxsackie B6 viruses.

It is with these considerations in mind that we indicate in the following list the types of different enteroviruses incriminated in pseudopoliomyelitis. Among them, Coxsackie A7 virus may be accorded a ranking position.

    ECHO viruses: types 1, 2, 4, 6, 9, 11, 12, 13, 14, 16, 30

    Coxsackie A virus: types 2, 4, 7, 9, 23

    Coxsackie B virus: types 2, 3, 4, 5, 6

Having read the relevant literature, we are convinced that, even for experienced clinicians, the differential diagnosis is very difficult (if not impossible) if we take account of the intrinsic nature of the paralysis alone. A few peculiarities in the anatomical distribution or in the clinical course of the disease have been described, but these are subject to dispute. It is doubtful whether facial paralysis is more frequent than in poliomyelitis, when one is aware of the prevalence of this feature during certain epidemics. Indeed, there are reports of considerable variations in the sites of paralysis: one or more limbs, abdominal muscles, eyes, tongue, pharynx — that is to say, the same dispersion and variety as seen in typical poliomyelitis.

Writers have stressed the lack of initial severity, the habitual light touch of these infections, and their tendency to complete cure without sequelae. But they also find definite sequelae with atrophy, quite certainly comparable to typical poliomyelitis. Furthermore, this benign reputation appears quite a relative one, for fatalities have followed infection with Coxsackie viruses B2, B7, and A7 and with ECHO 2 virus.

The clinical progress of these fatal cases is exactly the same as in those of brain-stem poliomyelitis or of poliomyelitis with respiratory paralysis and gives rise to the same therapeutic difficulties.

It is necessary to warn the clinician against the temptation to assign too much importance to a solitary result of virological examination, and it is vital to recall the rarity of "poliomyelitis" caused by enteroviruses other than poliovirus. In practice, it is wise, in the face of such a discovery, to examine the possible significance of the findings (coincidence or, above all, coexistence with poliovirus). For the clinician, one must contrast the constant affinity of poliovirus for the nervous system with the inconstant and occasional or weak affinity of other enteroviruses for the same tissues of the body.

Such thoughts do not go as far as to exclude absolutely the mediation of other enteroviruses in the pathology of the nervous system, but merely to limit the frequency of such events. From our point of view, we feel that there is value in the study, during an epidemic period, of cases of transient weakness or paralysis occurring in some individuals out of a population which has been massively infected by an enterovirus, provided that such a clinical study is backed up by a parallel serological investigation. Such was the case during the epidemics of meningitis due to ECHO 6 virus and again in the disease caused by ECHO 9 virus. We must still remember that Sabin found only five mild cases of the type which we have been considering among thousands of sick persons in the Milwaukee epidemic. In the case of epidemics due to ECHO 4 virus, the proportion was even smaller. Nevertheless, the agreement between epidemiological and virological studies leaves no doubt as to the reality of "poliomyelitis" due to ECHO virus.

We may remark that, up to the present date, no one has observed epidemics of paralytic disease due to Coxsackie viruses and all the cases seen have been sporadic. Among the agents responsible for paralytic disease, a particular place must without doubt be reserved for Coxsackie A7 virus for clinical, anatomopathological, and experimental reasons.

To end this chapter, which has been devoted to lower motor neuron paralyses, we must record that the part played by enteroviruses other than poliovirus, if it is not negligible, is certainly very limited and out of all comparison with the virus responsible for the disease of Heine and Medin. In other chapters will be found details of epidemiology and other clinical manifestations of these enteroviruses other than poliovirus.

3

Enteroviruses

THE ENTEROVIRUSES: DEFINITION AND PROPERTIES

by V. Drouhet

Because they have many characteristics in common, polioviruses, Coxsackie viruses, and ECHO viruses are considered to belong to the same group, named enteroviruses by a committee created by the National Foundation for Infantile Paralysis (1957).[6] The enteroviruses are associated with a wide range of clinical syndromes (see p. 80).

The enteroviruses belong to a larger group which, under the name picornaviruses (1963),[41] includes the rhinoviruses and enteroviruses. These small viruses (Andrews' naniviruses) have ribonucleic acid as their infectious nucleic acid (see p. 11). At present the enteroviruses have 62 antigenically distinct prototypes: 3 types of poliovirus, 30 types of ECHO virus, 23 types of Coxsackie A, and 6 types of Coxsackie B.

Certain antigenic types are no longer considered to be ECHO viruses. Thus, ECHO virus 10 is a member of the more recently constituted reovirus group, and ECHO 28 has been reclassified in the rhinovirus group. Nonetheless, the number of enteroviruses is ever increasing. A special commission is in charge of their antigenic study and of classifying new prototypes. All ECHO viruses have the capacity to multiply in the human alimentary tract with or without signs or symptoms. They have similar epidemiologic characteristics and the same seasonal occurrence. The biochemical and biophysical data obtained have enabled biologists to determine the physical and chemical properties common to enteroviruses.

PHYSICAL AND CHEMICAL PROPERTIES OF ENTEROVIRUSES

The dimensions of enteroviruses have been studied by various methods: filtration through gradocol membranes of known porosity,[3] sedimentation in the ultracentrifuge, and direct electron microscopic examination of purified preparations and determination of the rate of inactivation by ionizing radiation.[2] By correlating the information gained by these methods and by chemical analysis it is possible to obtain a precise idea of the structure of enteroviruses.

The use of tissue cultures has made it possible to obtain larger amounts of viruses. Using this source and filtration through a gradocol membrane of known porosity, Sabin et al. (1954)[47] and Schwerdt and Schaffer (1955)[49] determined polioviruses to be about 25 mμ in diameter.

Coxsackie and ECHO viruses have also been studied in the same way, and their diameters also range between 25 and 29 mμ.[39] Direct electron microscopic examination of purified preparations has confirmed the preceding data;[37, 50, 53] Mattern and du Buy in 1956[37] and Schwerdt in 1957[50] obtained crystallized polioviruses and Coxsackie viruses which, under the electron microscope, appear as spherical particles 28 mμ in diameter.

The purified viruses are constituted of nucleoproteins characterized by absorption in the ultraviolet spectrum. It has since been determined that the infectious unit of polioviruses consists of 20 to 25 per cent RNA; the rest is a protein.[48] Colter et al. (1957)[5] and Alexander et al. (1958)[1] separated the RNA from the protein and succeeded in infecting cell cultures with the RNA alone. Rouhanded[46] obtained RNA from ECHO viruses types 1, 5, 7, 8, 11, 12, 19, 25, and 26.

Finch and Klug,[13] examining polioviruses, found that the protein has an icosahedral symmetry.

The virion, or viral particle, of enteroviruses contains a single type of nucleic acid, ribonucleic acid, which forms its genetic material. The capsid consists of a symmetrical arrangement of protein constituents, grouped in capsomeres, arranged on the surface of an icosahedral-type geometric figure (cubic symmetry). In 1962, Lwoff et al.[32] took the molecular characteristic of the infectious particle as the basis for classification. Each variety of virus is defined by the total number and structure of capsomeres located on its surface (p. 11). Unlike other viruses, whose envelopes contain lipids, the capsid of the enteroviruses is bare.

Whereas RNA is the infectious particle of the virus, the external protein plays several roles: it protects against the action of tissue nucleases (ribonuclease), it facilitates penetration into the cell, and above all it is responsible for the antigenic properties of the virus, provoking the formation of the serum and tissue antibodies which induce immunity in the infected organism. The amino acid composition of this protein is known.[30]

The viral particle has no lipid envelope and is not susceptible to treatment with ether, alcohol, or phenol, but it is sensitive to oxidizing agents such as iodine, chlorine, and formol. This observation was applied in the preparation of formol-inactivated antipoliomyelitis vaccine.

It is worth mentioning that Gevaudan and Charrel[16] and Kelly and Sanderson[23] found that total inactivation of enteroviruses is not realized under the usual conditions of disinfection of urban water supplies (concentration of residual chlorine 0.2 ppm for a 10-minute contact at pH 7.0). Accordingly, longer contacts and higher concentrations of residual chlorine would be required.

The infecting power slowly decreases at +4° C., but when the viruses are stored in a 50 per cent buffered glycerin solution they keep for months or even years. The viral titer of stools can be maintained unchanged for eight years or more at −70° C.

The bivalent metallic ions Ca^{++} and Mg^{++} stabilize enteroviruses for one to three hours at 50° C. This property has found a practical application in the preparation of live vaccine on cultures of monkey kidney cells which often contain a high concentration of vacuoling virus. The vacuoling virus SV 40 is easily inactivated by means of MgCl$_2$, to which the polioviruses are not sensitive. Moreover, MgCl$_2$ permits preservation of the poliomyelitis vaccine for six months to one year at +4° C.

Another remarkable property of enteroviruses in their stability at pH 3.0.[31, 44] This property distinguishes between the enteroviruses and the rhinoviruses, which do not possess this stability in acid media.[24]

The enteroviruses are inactivated by ultraviolet rays and by bombardment with high energy electrons.

INHIBITION BY CHEMICAL MEANS

Many antiviral substances have been used on polioviruses in vivo and in vitro. 5-Fluorouracil, which is an antimetabolite, is included in poliovirus RNA in the form of 5-fluorouridylic acid, but this abnormal RNA does not differ from the natural virus in any biological property.

Halogenous compounds of benzimidazole and α-hydroxybenzyl-2-benzimidazole (HBB) exhibit inhibitory activity with regard to polioviruses.[11] The influence of HBB is exerted in RNA biosynthesis. At noncytotoxic concentrations HBB inhibits in varying degrees the multiplication of poliovirus types I, II, and III and of ECHO types 1 through 29, with the exception of types 22, 23, and 28. HBB also fails to inhibit Coxsackie viruses types A7, A11, A13, A16, and A18.

The observations made by A. and M. Lwoff in 1961 and 1962[33, 34] concerning the influence of urea on multiplication of polioviruses in KB cells are of great interest. The higher the maintenance temperature of the cultures, the more marked is this inhibitory effect. Guanidine also has an inhibitory influence, and in many respects its activity can be compared with that of HBB.

N'N'-anhydrobis-(β-hydroxyethyl)biguanide hydrochloride (ABOB) is a generally well-tolerated product which was used in many clinical trials against viral infections but which proved without effect.

To return to the general subject of the physicochemical properties of the enteroviruses, the search for such properties is imperative when a new virus is introduced into the group, but they are of little help in diagnosis, which is based essentially upon pathogenicity, cultural characteristics, and antigenicity.

BIOLOGICAL PROPERTIES

PATHOGENICITY

The three types of poliovirus are characterized by their pathogenicity for the central nervous system of primates, while pathogenicity for suckling mice is characteristic of Coxsackie viruses. ECHO viruses are cytopathogenic for monkey kidney cells and are not virulent for the animal. However, classification criteria are not absolute, since some strains have mixed characteristics. In the present classification, for instance, certain strains of ECHO virus type 9, isolated in 1956 in Europe, prove virulent for newborn mice and thus behave like Coxsackie viruses. Dalldorf designated them Coxsackie A23. They were subsequently re-placed in the ECHO group, owing to the fact that the prototype strain and other strains are not immediately pathogenic for newborn mice.

Coxsackie virus A7, besides having the characteristic properties of its group, is also neuropathogenic for monkeys. Therefore, it was regarded by Russian authors as a fourth type of poliovirus until American research workers identified it as Coxsackie A7.[18]

CULTURAL CHARACTERISTICS

The in vitro multiplication of enteroviruses in cell cultures produces a cellular degeneration called the *cytopathogenic effect*. Since 1949, when Enders made that important demonstration for the polioviruses, cell cultures have become to virologists what "inanimate" culture media are to bacteriologists.

The cytopathogenic effect, first described by Enders for poliovirus, seems characteristic of all the other enteroviruses. It is easily observed under the microscope without preparation and is characterized by degeneration of the cells, which become round and birefringent and separate from one another. Impaired cells become detached from the cell layer in the culture medium, and finally only a few cell fragments remain on the tube wall. Special techniques of fixation and staining on glass slides permit further observations concerning certain peculiarities. The infected cells are round; in the cytoplasm an acidophilic mass is noted which is due to virus multiplication in the cytoplasm. The nucleus, displaced to the cell periphery, shows early eosinophilic inclusions; then it becomes more and more pyknotic and eccentric. However, it seems that ECHO viruses types 22 and 23 do not produce this sequence of events.[51, 57]

Because of their wide sensitivity spectrum, primary cultures of monkey kidney cells are usually used for the isolation of polioviruses and viruses of the ECHO group and Coxsackie B and A9. The species of monkey used for these cultures is important. *Macacus rhesus* and *Macacus cynomolgus* monkeys are most often used, but the African monkeys such as *Cercopithecus aethiops sabaeus*[10] or *tantalus*, *Cercopithecus pygerythrus*, and the "papio" baboon can also be utilized; on the other hand, use of the African monkey *Erythrocebus patas* is of little help in revealing ECHO viruses and Coxsackie virus A9.[19] Many human cell cultures are also successfully utilized for polioviruses. ECHO type 21 is isolated more easily on amniotic

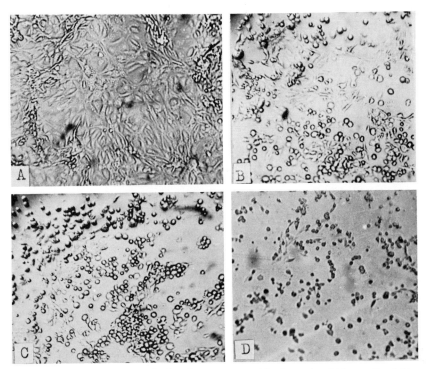

Figure 3-1. Cytopathogenic effect of poliovirus I on unprepared fresh monkey kidney cells. *A*, Normal cell culture; *B*, appearance of birefringent round cells; *C*, 48 hours after inoculation, the impaired cells separate from the cell layer; *D*, 75 per cent of the cell layer is destroyed.

cells. Coxsackie viruses A9, 11, 13, 15, 18, and 21 have a cytopathogenic effect in human amniotic cells.[27, 28, 56] After several passages all types have been adapted to amniotic cells except types 1, 4, 5, 6, 19, and 22. The stable human cell lines, such as HeLa, Hep2, and KB, which are sensitive to the multiplication of polioviruses and Coxsackie B and A4, 11, 13, 15, 18, and 21,[52] are not suitable for the isolation of ECHO viruses.

Coxsackie virus A7 was successfully adapted to monkey kidney cell cultures by Habel and Loomis.[18] For the isolation of viruses from pathological products it is necessary to use the most sensitive cells; however, the adaptation of strains to another cellular system is, from the practical point of view, of great advantage for it permits serological tests on the more usual types of cell cultures.

Some enteroviruses produce plaques of dead cells when they are in contact with a layer of cells cultivated in a Petri dish and covered with agar. The presence of these plaques is revealed by their failure to take up vital stains which color the living cells. Study of the shape, size, and outline of the plaques

gives information which is useful in distinguishing between polioviruses, Coxsackie viruses, and ECHO viruses.[19] The plaques induced by Coxsackie viruses on monkey kidney cells are large and round, similar to those produced by polioviruses but less transparent.

ECHO viruses produce two types of plaques on kidney cells of Patas monkeys. Types 22, 23, 24, and 25 produce small and irregular plaques, whereas types 7, 12, and 19 produce larger, round, irregular plaques. All ECHO viruses except type 21 induce plaques on kidney cells of Rhesus monkeys.

This plaque method is also used to separate two different viruses from one another, to purify strains after the virus has been titrated, and in the biological diagnosis of some types of ECHO virus infections.

The search for and the identification of an enterovirus require many techniques which have been considerably perfected and simplified during past years. The possibility of cultivating viruses in vitro and the facility of obtaining cell cultures and pathological samples free from microbial con-

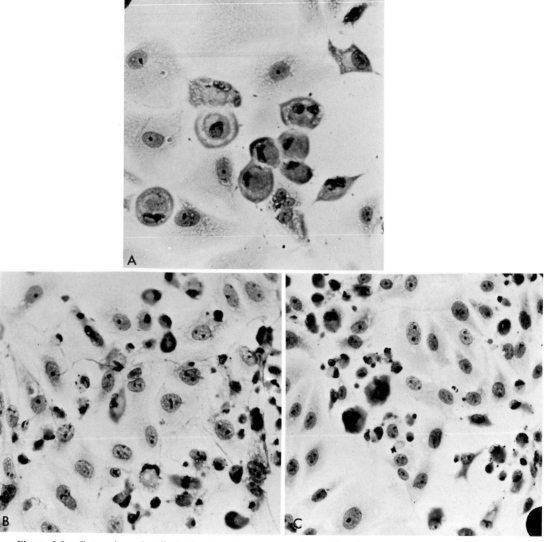

Figure 3-2. Cytopathogenic effect of enteroviruses on monkey cell cultures (May-Grünwald-Giemsa stain on glass slide). *A*, Poliomyelitis virus: round cells, excentric pyknotic nucleus, and paranuclear acidophil mass. *B*, ECHO 7 virus: similar cytopathogenic appearance, with various stages of cellular degeneration. *C*, Coxsackie B1 virus: appearance similar to that of the preceding viruses.

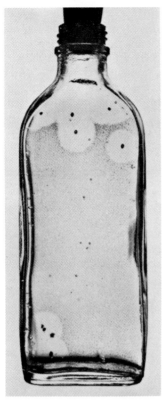

Figure 3-3. Clear, round, regular-outlined plaques, made by poliovirus I 4 days after inoculation (rhesus monkey kidney cells in monocellular layer under gelose).

tamination through the use of antibiotics account for the great progress made in that field.

ANTIGENICITY

Because of their protein structure, enteroviruses possess antigenic properties. Antigens are determined by their capacity to induce the formation of antibodies, and antibodies by their property of specifically reacting with the antigen which induced them. The chemical nature of antigens conditions this specificity.

The poliovirus antigens have been studied by means of centrifugation and sedimentation analysis (Mayer et al.[38]), by diffusion and precipitation in agar (Le Bouvier[26]), and by complement fixation (Hummeler and associates[20, 21]). At present, it is known that polioviruses have at least two type-specific and distinct antigens: antigen C, which reacts with the sera of persons in the acute phase of the disease, and antigen D, detectable only in sera obtained during con-

valescence. Antigen D is heavier than C and has infectious activity. Antigen D is found in larger amounts; it is type specific and seems to be linked to the complete viral agent. It is the antigen which reacts in the neutralization reaction and on which immunologic classification depends, while antigen C has no infectious properties. Antigen D, when heated or exposed to ultraviolet light, is transformed into antigen C. The proportion of the two antigens determines the antibody response. Their presence is revealed by the complement-fixation reaction, but pure sera prepared from fraction C do not contain any virus-neutralizing antibodies.

With antipoliomyelitis sera, the antigens form two distinct lines of precipitation in agar.

Basis of Serological Methods of Diagnosis. It occurs in serological practice that the same antibody is involved in several reactions.

NEUTRALIZING ANTIBODIES. Seroneutralization is based upon the capacity of antibodies to inactivate the infectivity of the virus. The neutralizing antibodies block a phase of the infectious cycle without inactivating the virus irreversibly. The neutralization reaction permits identification of the virus if the immune serum is known, or it permits discovery of small amounts of neutralizing antibodies in human serum, with a diagnostic or epidemiological purpose, if the virus is known.

Reference antisera have confirmed the serological homogeneity of the virus prototypes and have also revealed the existence of antigenic relations among the various serotypes. With polioviruses, a weak antigenic cross reaction can be observed between type I and type II and sometimes even with type III. Infection with type I causes the formation at very low titer of type II antibodies. The studies concerning Coxsackie viruses show a relation between types A15 and A18, as well as between B1 and B5. The antigenic cross reaction between ECHO viruses types 1 and 8 makes their serological identification so difficult that they are at present considered identical. The ECHO type 12 antiserum neutralizes ECHO I weakly. The same difficulty arises for types 23 and 22, between which antigenic cross reaction may be rather strong. A weaker reciprocal neutralization is obtained between ECHO types 11 and 19. Prototypes of ECHO 4 induce only a weak antibody response and the antisera neutralize the prototype strain only slightly or not at all in the generally used tests.

But Melnick, utilizing plaques reduction, obtained more significant neutralization results. Not all strains of the same type have the same antigenic activity; in particular, some ECHO virus strains such as type 6 are only partly neutralized by the prototype serum. This partial neutralization permits determination of strains of intermediate type to which is allotted a number with a prime superscript. The revelation of intratypic antigens by Wenner et al.,[55] MacBride,[35] Gard,[14] and Wecker[54] has proved to be extremely useful in epidemiology. The sera neutralize the homologous virus more rapidly and in larger amount than the homotypic strain. Techniques utilizing these intratypic antigens are used to distinguish between virulent strains and attenuated strains of the same type of poliovirus.

COMPLEMENT-FIXING ANTIBODIES. The enteroviruses have no *group antigen* permitting rapid identification. However, the complement-fixing reaction reveals heterologous antibodies more readily than the neutralization test and suggests the possibility of common complement-fixing antigens among various types of viruses of the same group (poliomyelitis, ECHO, or Coxsackie) and even antigenic crossings between the various types of the three groups of enteroviruses.[12, 29, 36, 42, 43]

Neva and Malone[40] have observed antibodies to ECHO 16 antigen following human infections with ECHO types 6, 9, and 20 and with Coxsackie B3.

Antibodies to poliovirus type I have been detected after an infection with ECHO virus 6 or 9 or Coxsackie viruses.

Heterologous antibodies are more frequently produced when the viral antigen used to immunize the animal has been inactivated by heat, formalin, or ultraviolet light than when live virus is used. If the serum to be tested contains antibodies, they form, with the viral antigen, an antigen-antibody complex which fixes complement, thus preventing hemolysis of red blood cells, added thereafter, by the hemolytic serum (indicator system).

IMMUNOFLUORESCENCE. The technique of immunofluorescence is based on the observation by Coons and Kaplan[7] in 1950 that it is possible to make an antigen-antibody complex visible under ultraviolet light if the antibody has been labeled previously with a fluorescent dye. As a matter of fact,

the antibody globulins can be chemically conjugated with fluorescent compounds without losing their immunologic properties; they then selectively fix themselves on their specific antigen, which is the virus itself or its constituent protein elements. In the case of the enteroviruses the antigen-antibody complex is within the cytoplasm of infected cells.

Immunofluorescence is applicable to identification of antigens by means of a known serum. It was proposed as a method for rapid diagnosis of enteroviruses from fecal samples and from inoculated monkey kidney cells; the polioviruses are revealed by immunofluorescence at an early stage, prior to the appearance of cytopathogenic effect.[4] Brown[4] also succeeded in demonstrating ECHO and Coxsackie viruses in autopsy specimens. Kisuma, using the indirect immunofluorescence technique with an anticomplement serum, has shown viral antigen in desquamated cells in the sediment of centrifuged urine of patients with aseptic meningitis caused by Coxsackie virus B5.

The immunofluorescence inhibition technique, which has very limited applications in serology, consists of a possible blocking of the antigen by means of a serum used in a first

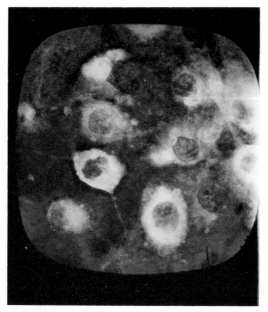

Figure 3-4. Monkey kidney cells in poliovirus I-infected culture, 16 hours after inoculation. Granular fluorescence in the cytoplasm. (Indirect fluorescent antibody technique.)

stage and supposed to contain antibodies. The fluorescent specific antibody, which is added later on, is incapable of fixing the antigen if it is blocked and, consequently, is incapable of revealing it.

HEMAGGLUTINATION INHIBITION. The hemagglutinins of human group O cells were first shown with ECHO viruses in 1957 by Goldfield et al.[17] Since then, much work has been directed to this study.[8, 9, 25]

About one-third of ECHO viruses possess hemagglutinating properties: types 3, 6, 7, 11, 12, 13, 18, 19, 20, 21, 22, and 29. The hemagglutinins of some strains are very labile, which accounts for the inconstant character observed with strains of the same ECHO virus type: 6, 13, 18, 20, 21, 22, and 29. Gaudin et al.[15] indicated the agglutinating capacity of types 1 and 20 for trypsin-treated human red blood cells, and of types 4, 7, and 12 for some monkey red blood cells.

It is supposed that the ECHO virus hemagglutinin is linked to the viral particle. Its behavior with respect to the mucoprotein receptors is not determined, but it is known that this receptor is not abolished.

The hemagglutinating properties of some ECHO virus strains permit distinction between the various types of ECHO viruses and, as a consequence, help to identify them by the usual methods of neutralization of the cytopathogenic effect.

Such an agglutination is not due to any immunologic phenomena, but it can be used to detect the presence of a virus in a suspension with the corresponding antibody and also in serum to detect the presence of antibodies corresponding to the agglutinating virus. If the virus combines with its antibody, the agglutination of human group O cells subsequently introduced into the mixture is inhibited. The inhibition is immunologically specific; the reaction of hemagglutination inhibition represents a particular category of neutralization.

Among the works bearing on Coxsackie viruses, those of Goldfield[17] reported in 1957 should be mentioned. He was the first to reveal the hemagglutinating properties of Coxsackie B3.

The Coxsackie viruses possessing hemagglutinins are types A20, 21, and 24.[22, 45]

Human cord blood is recommended to reveal the hemagglutinin of some types B, which does not appear with adult human red blood cells.

BIBLIOGRAPHY

1. Alexander, H. E., Koch, G., Mountain, M., Sprunt, K., and Van Damme, O.: Infectivity of ribonucleic acid of poliovirus on HeLa cell monolayers. Virology, 5:172, 1958.
2. Benyesh, M., Pollard, E. C., Opton, E. M., Black, F. L., Bellamy, W. D., and Melnick, J. L.: Size and structure of ECHO, poliomyelitis and measles virus determined by ionizing radiation and ultrafiltration. Virology, 5:266-274, 1968.
3. Breese, S. S., Jr., and Briefs, A.: Certain physical properties of a herpangina strain and a pleurodynia strain of Coxsackie virus. Proc. Soc. Exp. Biol. Med., 83:119-122, 1953.
4. Brown, G. C.: Fluorescent antibody techniques for the diagnosis of enteric infections. Arch. Ges. Virusforsch., 13:30, 1963.
5. Colter, J. S., Bird, H. H., Moyer, A. W., and Brown, R. A.: Infectivity of ribonucleic acid isolated from virus-infected tissues. Virology, 4:522, 1957.
6. Committee on the Enteroviruses, National Foundation for Infantile Paralysis, N.Y.: The enteroviruses. Amer. J. Public Health, 47:1556, 1957.
7. Coons, A. H., and Kaplan, M. H.: Localization of antigen in tissue cells. II. Improvements in a method for the detection of antigen by means of fluorescent antibody. J. Exp. Med., 91:1-14, 1950.
8. Dardanoni, L., and Zaffiro, P.: Sul potere emoagglutinante di virus appartenenti al gruppo. ECHO. Boll. Ist. Sieroter. Milan., 37:346, 1958.
9. Dardanoni, L., and Zaffiro, P.: Identificazione di virus ECHO a mezzo della reazione de emoagglutino inibizione. Boll. Ist. Sieroter. Milan., 38:11, 1959.
10. Drouhet, V.: Etude comparative de la sensibilité des cultures de tissu rénal de *Cercopithecus aethiops sabaeus* et de *Macacus philippinensis* aux virus polio et aux autres virus entériques humains. Ann. Inst. Past., 89:666-671, 1955.
11. Eggers, H., and Tamm, I.: Spectrum and characteristics of the virus inhibitory action of 2 (α hydroxybenzyl) benzimidazol. J. Exp. Med., 113:657, 1961.
12. Federici, E. E., Lerner, A. M., and Abelman, W. H.: Observation on the course of Coxsackie A9 myocarditis in C 3 H mice (28 136). Proc. Soc. Exp. Biol. Med., 112:672, 1963.
13. Finch, J. T., and Klug, A.: Structure of poliomyelitis virus. Nature, 183:1709, 1959.
14. Gard, S.: Immunological strain specificity within type I poliovirus. Bull. WHO, 22:235, 1960.
15. Gaudin, O. G., Barral, A. M., and Sohier, R.: Hémagglutination par certains types de virus ECHO. I. Etude de quelques caractères des hémagglutinines. Ann. Inst. Past., 104:313, 1963.
16. Gevaudan, P., and Charrel, J.: Survie du virus Coxsackie dans différentes eaux. Rev. Path. Gen., 747:391-399, 1963.
17. Goldfield, M., Srihonse, S., and Fox, J. P.: Hemagglutinins associated with certain human enteric viruses. Proc. Soc. Exp. Biol. Med., 96:788, 1957.
18. Habel, K., and Loomis, L. N.: Coxsackie A7 virus and the Russian "polio virus type 4." Proc. Soc. Exp. Biol. Med., 95:597, 1957.
19. Hsiung, G. D., and Melnick, J. L.: Comparative susceptibility of kidney cells from different mon-

key species to enteric viruses (polio, Coxsackie and ECHO groups). J. Immunol., *78*:137-146, 1957.

20. Hummeler, K., and Hamparian, V. V.: Studies on the complement fixing antigens of poliomyelitis. I. Demonstration of type and group specific antigens in native and heated viral preparations. J. Immunol., *81*:499, 1958.

21. Hummeler, K., and Tumilowicz, J. J.: Studies on the complement fixing antigens of poliomyelitis. II. Preparation of type specific anti N and anti H indicator sera. J. Immunol., *84*:630, 1960.

22. Johnson, K. M., Bloom, H. H., Rosen, L., Mufson, M. A., and Chanock, R. M.: Hemagglutination by Coe virus. Virology, *13*:373, 1961.

23. Kelly, S., and Sanderson, N.: The effect of chlorine in water on enteric viruses. Amer. J. Public Health, *48*:1323-1334, 1958.

24. Ketler, A., Hamparian, V. V., and Hilleman, M. R.: Characterization and classification of ECHO 28. Rhino-virus coryzavirus agents (27 662). Proc. Soc. Exp. Biol. Med., *110*:821, 1962.

25. Lahelle, O.: Capacity of certain ECHO virus 6 strains to cause hemagglutination. Virology, *5*: 110, 1958.

26. Le Bouvier, G. L.: Poliovirus D and C antigens: their differentiation and measurement by precipitation in agar. Brit. J. Exper. Path., *40*:453, 1959.

27. Lehman-Grube, F., and Syverton, J. T.: Pathogenicity for suckling mice of Coxsackie viruses adapted to human amnion cells. J. Exp. Med., *113*:811, 1961.

28. Lenahan, M., and Wenner, H. A.: Propagation of group A Coxsackie virus in primary human amnion cells. I. Cytopathogenic changes produced by 5 more serotypes. Proc. Soc. Exp. Biol. Med., *107*: 544, 1961.

29. Lennette, E. H., Schmidt, N. J., and Magoffin, R. L.: Observations on the complement fixing antibody response to poliovirus in patients with certain Coxsackie and ECHO virus infections. J. Immunol., *86*:552, 1961.

30. Levintow, L., and Darnell, J. E.: A simplified procedure for purification of large amounts of poliovirus: characterization and amino-acid analysis of type 1 poliovirus. J. Biol. Chem., *235*:70, 1960.

31. Loring, H. S., and Schwerdt, C. E.: Studies of purification of poliomyelitis virus at pH stability range of MVA strain. Proc. Soc. Exp. Biol. Med., *57*: 173, 1944.

32. Lwoff, A., Horne, R. W., and Tournier, P.: Un système des virus. C. R. Acad. Sci., *254*:4225-4227, 1962.

33. Lwoff, A., and Lwoff, M.: Les évènements cycliques du cycle viral. I. Effets de la température. II. Les effets de l'eau lourde. III. Discussion. Ann. Inst. Past., *101*:469; 478; 490; 1961.

34. Lwoff, A., and Lwoff, M.: Inhibition de la multiplication du poliovirus par l'urée considérée comme substance thermomimétique. C. R. Acad. Sci., *254*:771, 1962.

35. MacBride, W. D.: Antigenic analysis of poliovirus by kinetic studies of serum neutralization. Virology, *7*:45, 1959.

36. MacIntosh, E. G. S., and Sommerville, R. G.: An analysis of 24 strains of ECHO virus type 7. Arch. Ges. Virusforsch., *9*:261, 1959.

37. Mattern, C. F. T., and duBuy, H.: Purification and crystallization of Coxsackie virus. Science, *123*: 1037-1038, 1956.

38. Mayer, M. M., Rapp, H. J., Roizman, B., Klein, S. W., Cowan, K. M., Lukens, D., Schwerdt, C. E., Schaffer, F. L., and Charney, J.: The purification of poliomyelitis virus as studied by complement fixation. J. Immunol., *78*:435, 1957.

39. Melnick, J. L., Rhian, M., Warren, J., and Breese, S. S., Jr.: The size of Coxsackie viruses and Lansing poliomyelitis virus determined by sedimentation and ultrafiltration. J. Immunol., *67*:151-162, 1951.

40. Neva, F. A., and Malone, M. F.: Specific and cross reactions by complement fixation with Boston exanthem disease virus (ECHO 16). J. Immunol., *83*:645, 1959.

41. Panel for Picornaviruses: Picornaviruses: Classification of nine new types. Science, *141*:153, 1963.

42. Philipson, L., and Chopin, P. W.: On the role of virus sulfhydryl groups in the attachment of enteroviruses to erythrocytes. J. Exp. Med., *112*:455, 1960.

43. Riggs, J. L., and Brown, G. C.: Differentiation of active and passive poliomyelitis antibodies in human sera by indirect immunofluorescence. J. Immunol., *89*:868, 1962.

44. Robinson, L. K.: Effect of heat and of pH on strains of Coxsackie virus. Proc. Soc. Exp. Biol. Med., *75*:580, 1950.

45. Rosen, J., and Kern, J.: Hemagglutination and hemagglutination-inhibition with Coxsackie B viruses. Proc. Soc. Exp. Biol. Med., *107*:626-628, 1961.

46. Rouhandeh, H.: Facilitation of infection of monkey kidney cells with certain Picornavirus ribonucleic acids. Ann. N.Y. Acad. Sci., *101*:398, 1962.

47. Sabin, A. B., Hennessen, W. A., and Warren, J.: Ultrafiltration and electron microscopy of three types of poliomyelitis virus propagated in tissue-culture. Proc. Soc. Exp. Biol. Med., *85*:359, 1954.

48. Schaffer, F. L., and Schwerdt, C. E.: Purification and properties of polioviruses. Advances in Virus Res., *6*:159, 1959.

49. Schwerdt, C. E., and Schaffer, F. L.: Some physical and chemical properties of purified poliomyelitis virus preparations: biology of poliomyelitis. Ann. N.Y. Acad. Sci., *61*:740, 1955.

50. Schwerdt, C. E.: Physical and chemical characteristics of purified poliomyelitis virus. Special publications of N.Y. Acad. Sci., *5*:157-166, 1957.

51. Shaver, D. N., Barron, A. L., and Karzon, D. T.: Distinctive cytopathology of ECHO viruses type 22 and 23. Proc. Soc. Exp. Biol. Med., *106*:648, 1961.

52. Sickles, G. M., Mutterer, M., Feorine, P., and Plager, H.: Recently classified types of Coxsackie virus, group A. Behaviour in tissue culture. Proc. Soc. Exp. Biol. Med., *90*:529-531, 1955.

53. Taylor, A. R., and MacCormick, M. J.: Electron microscopy of poliomyelitis virus. Yale J. Biol. Med., *28*:589-597, 1956.

54. Wecker, E.: A simple test for serodifferentiation of poliovirus strains within the same type. Virology, *10*:376, 1960.

55. Wenner, H. A., Kamitsuka, P., and Lenahan, M.: A comparative study of type 2 poliomyelitis viruses. II. Antigenic differences relating to 18 type 2 strains. J. Immunol., *77*:220, 1956.

56. Wenner, H. A., and Lenahan, M. F.: Propagation of group A Coxsackie viruses in tissue cultures. II. Some interactions between virus and mammalian cells. Yale J. Biol. Med., *34*:421, 1961-62.
57. Wigand, R., and Sabin, A. B.: Properties of ECHO types 22, 23 and 24 viruses. Arch. Ges. Virusforsch., *11*:224, 1961.

LABORATORY DIAGNOSIS OF ENTEROVIRUS INFECTIONS

by V. Drouhet

The pathogenic role of polioviruses has been known for a long time, while that of ECHO and Coxsackie viruses has been confirmed only recently by virological, immunological, epidemiological, and even experimental evidence.

It has been possible to correlate the clinical manifestations due to infection with certain enteroviruses during epidemics with a single prevailing type of virus.

The presence of the virus during the acute period of the disease and a significant increase in antibodies against the virus during the progression of the disease are laboratory criteria indispensable for diagnosis.

The presence of the virus in the cerebrospinal fluid in cases of lymphocytic meningitis is evidence of its etiological role.

It is also necessary to establish that well-known viruses that are capable of causing the same clinical syndromes are not involved.

In order to demonstrate the etiological association, it is sometimes necessary to show that the same virus is present in subjects in contact with the patient, especially young subjects, or to search for epidemics in the patient's environment.

The laboratory methods and techniques utilized in the diagnosis of enterovirus infections are based on (1) virological methods: the isolation and the identification of the single virus; and (2) serological methods: the search for neutralizing antibodies, complement-fixing antibodies, and antibodies inhibiting hemagglutination.

It is imperative to take samples carefully and to provide information which will permit choice of the most appropriate diagnostic techniques.

VIROLOGIC DIAGNOSIS

COLLECTION OF SAMPLES

Materials employed to isolate the virus are: stools, rectal and pharyngeal samples, blood, cerebrospinal fluid, urine, tissue biopsies, and necropsy samples.

Stools. Stools are one of the most important sources of enteroviruses because of the abundant and prolonged fecal elimination of the virus. As a rule, the virus is present in the feces up to the tenth day of the disease. Later, the amount of virus decreases and its elimination is intermittent, with some variation from one patient to another. In exceptional cases, the virus has been isolated from stools six to seven weeks after the onset of the disease. However, the isolation of enterovirus, poliovirus, or other viruses from stools taken immediately after the patient's admission is much more valid and rules out a possible hospital infection.

A single stool sample taken at the onset of the disease is usually sufficient to isolate the virus, but the success is increased by taking several successive stool samples. A small amount of feces suffices for these investigations.

Fecal samples are also obtained from persons in contact with the patient and from apparently healthy persons when an epidemiologic investigation is aimed at revealing a viral etiology.

Rectal Swabs. A sterile swab, moistened with buffered Hank's solution (buffered physiological solution, with mineral salts, glucose, and pH color indicator), is introduced deeply into the rectum in order to take a little feces. It is then placed in a tube containing 2 ml. of Hank's solution with antibiotics (500 units penicillin, 2.5 mg. streptomycin, and 50 units nystatin per milliliter). This easy process can replace use of stool samples in some cases. We occasionally use it in epidemiological investigations.

Pharyngeal Swabs. A sterile swab, previously moistened with Hank's solution, must be placed in contact with the tonsils and the posterior wall of the pharynx in order to bring back not only mucus but also cell fragments. It is then treated like the rectal swabs.

It is advisable to restrict use of pharyngeal swabs to the first five to seven days of the disease or for special epidemiological investigations. The amount of virus in the pharynx is small, and it is always desirable to search for the virus in the stools as well.

Poliovirus has been isolated from the throat only for a few days[8] after the onset of the disease; ECHO virus 11 has been found in the throat from the third to the ninth day[21] after experimental inoculation when clinical signs had appeared between the second and the fourth days.

In epidemiological investigations, to estimate the viral distribution and its duration, several series of pharyngeal and fecal samples are taken from the same subjects at regular intervals (five to 10 days).

Blood.   The blood is obtained by venipuncture with sterilized instruments. The sterile blood is quickly sent to the laboratory, where it is allowed to clot at room temperature for 24 hours and is then sent to the specialized laboratory where the serum is aseptically removed. If unclotted blood is desired, heparin solution (200 I.U. per milliliter) is placed in the syringe and the sample is sent immediately to the specialized laboratory.

According to Bodian, in poliomyelitis viremia occurs from the second to the fifth day before paralysis appears. This is rarely seen with other enteroviruses. However, during an epidemic due to ECHO virus 9, Wigand and Sabin[30] isolated the virus from the blood of a contact subject 36 hours before the onset of the disease, in only one out of six cases in which isolation from blood was attempted 24 hours after the onset of the disease, and in none of 22 cases in which samples were taken two to six days after the onset of the disease.

Neva and Zuffante[19] isolated ECHO virus 16 from a blood sample obtained two days after the onset of the disease. ECHO virus 6 was isolated from blood by Francis and Ceballos[5]; Medearis and Kramer[15] proved the existence of ECHO virus 18 viremia in the case of febrile exanthema; and Munk and Nasemann[17] demonstrated ECHO virus 4 viremia and Klein et al.[12] ECHO virus 11 viremia in cases of gastroenteritis.

Coxsackie A3, A6, and B2 were revealed in blood samples taken from Egyptian children during the febrile period of the disease.[27]

Coxsackie B2 was isolated from a patient's blood three days after the onset of the disease and five days before the meningeal signs appeared.[7] Later, Utz and Shelokov[28]

revealed the presence of Coxsackie virus in the blood.

Cerebrospinal Fluid.   The cerebrospinal fluid is aseptically collected in a tube and must be sent to the specialized laboratory as soon as possible. Isolations are obtained very early in the course of meningitis, with a higher frequency during the febrile period of the disease, before neutralizing antibodies can be detected in the blood.

The isolation of the virus from the cerebrospinal fluid is seldom mentioned in the case of poliomyelitis. Bodian isolated it in a paralytic case of poliomyelitis a few hours before death. However, in infections with ECHO types 2, 4, 5, 6, 9, 11, 14, 15, 16, 18, and 19 and with Coxsackie B and A9,[28] the virus is found in the cerebrospinal fluid.

During epidemics, the virus has occasionally been isolated from cerebrospinal fluid of patients with meningeal signs even when there was no leukocytosis of the cerebrospinal fluid.

Urine.   Urine samples aseptically taken are immediately inoculated into culture tubes or stored at $-20°$ C. Only Coxsackie B viruses have been found in urine.[28]

Tissue Biopsies.   Polioviruses were first isolated by Jungeblut[9] from muscle samples. Lepine, in the course of an epidemic myalgia, isolated Coxsackie viruses in biopsy samples from paralyzed muscles.

The biopsy samples may also be used for histological examination. Coxsackie viruses cause a fairly characteristic myositis.

Necropsy Samples.   It is easier to take samples for virological investigations at the same time as those intended for pathological tests. It is known that histopathological tests can confirm the presence of characteristic lesions or of cytoplasmic or intranuclear inclusions—a finding which, although it does not have absolute value for diagnosis, is nevertheless of great help in interpreting the results.

The samples for virus isolation must be obtained three to seven hours after death. Sterile instruments must be employed for each organ, and the tissue fragments from each organ must be kept separately in sterile Petri dishes. The origin of the sample must be noted on each dish.

When autopsy is not possible, organ paracentesis should be made by use of trocars passing through the occipital orifice or a small trepanning orifice so as to obtain fragments of neuraxis, or by use of viscerotomes to remove fragments of liver or lung. The organ samples must be brought to the virology laboratory as soon as possible. If they must be mailed it is advisable to place the fragments in sterilized flasks containing a few milliliters of glycerin buffered at pH 7.1.

If death has occurred within seven to 10 days after onset of the disease, the following samples should be taken: small (2-cc.) fragments from the cerebral trunk, the optic layers, and the spinal cord (cervical and lumbar); one fragment of skeletal muscle and of cardiac muscle; some pericardial fluid; the mesenteric ganglia and the tonsils; the content of an intestinal loop, especially if a search for virus in the stools was not made while the patient was living.

Virological confirmation in the fatal cases of poliomyelitis is a well-established procedure. Isolation of virus is attempted from either the central nervous system or the cerebrospinal fluid, as well as from the cardiac muscle and the mesenteric ganglia.

Fatalities caused by Coxsackie or ECHO virus infections are less frequently reported.

Virological studies have been done in some cases. According to Steigman and co-workers,[25, 26] ECHO viruses 2 and 11 are responsible for fatal cases following generalized paralysis. Chumakov et al.[3] reported a fatal case which occurred after paralysis due to a Coxsackie A7 infection.

Kalter et al.,[10] in a comprehensive virological study of cases of paralysis, isolated Coxsackie B3 from the cerebrospinal fluid in a fatal case.

Coxsackie B3 is believed to be responsible for the fatal cases of meningoencephalitis in newborn children,[11] and, more recently, Coxsackie viruses B have been isolated in several cases from the cardiac muscle in cases of fibroelastosis in newborn children.

Let us recall here that Coxsackie viruses A4 and A8 are associated with sudden death in children and that Coxsackie A9 was isolated by Lerner and associates[13, 14] during an epidemic from the lung of a patient who died of pneumonia, clinically diagnosed and confirmed by pathological examination.

ECHO virus 9 was isolated by Verlinde and Wilterdink[29] from the spinal cord of a boy who died of encephalitis. In the same sample, Pette et al.[20] showed the presence of a poliovirus. However, in spite of this association, the high titer of ECHO virus 9 seems to make its pathogenic role unquestionable with respect to the central nervous system.

HANDLING OF SAMPLES

Storage. The samples for virus isolations must not be subjected to any great change in temperature. Fortunately, the

Table 3-1. *Samples for the Isolation of Enteroviruses**

Virus	SECRETIONS, EXCRETIONS				VESICLES, MUCOUS LESIONS	ORGANIC FLUIDS		BIOPSY		NECROPSY SPECIMENS		
	Nose	*Throat*	*Stools*	*Urine*		*Blood*	*C.S.F.*	*Muscle*	*C.N.S.*	*Ganglia, Tonsils*	*Cardiac Muscle*	*Lung*
Polio I II III	++	+	+			+	++	++	+	+	++	
Coxsackie A	21	21			2, 3, 4, 5, 8, 9, 10, 16	3, 6	9	2	2, 7, 9			9
B		+	+	+	2, 3, 5	2	1, 2, 3, 4, 5, 6	1 to 5	3	+	4	
Echo	4, 11, 28	+	+			9	4, 6 9, 11 16, 18	2, 4, 5, 6, 9, 11, 14, 15, 16, 18, 19		9		

*The figures represent the types of virus most currently isolated up to now.
+Isolated in exceptional instances.

enteroviruses are hardy and can be carried and preserved without difficulty.

In the case of enteroviruses present in the stools, viruses can survive a long time — several days at 4° C. — but with samples from the throat and cerebrospinal fluid, in which the amount of virus is smaller, the virus is more likely to survive at low temperature — anywhere from the −7° C. available with a freezer to the −60° to −70° C. obtainable with frozen carbon dioxide (dry ice). Suitable apparatus must be available for dry ice. However, it is easy to obtain dry ice in large towns, although it is not always delivered daily.

It is often preferable to have the samples placed in a thermos flask containing some ice and carried to the virology laboratory. If this is not possible, the sample can be mailed at room temperature provided it has not been previously frozen.

Sending to Laboratory. CHOICE OF VESSELS. The vessels must be solid, preferably transparent, and perfectly closed. Perfect sealing protects from possible deterioration by CO_2 when dry ice is used or from contamination by water when ice is used.

As a rule, a rubber-stoppered penicillin flask is used, with the stopper carefully wrapped twice with adhesive tape, or a flask with an ordinary stopper fixed by adhesive tape. The vessel should be made of glass, for plastic is difficult to sterilize and does not withstand freezing well.

MARKING OF VESSELS. The best process consists in using a band of adhesive tape and writing on it with pencil or with a ballpoint pen; in this way, the inscription will not be damaged by water or other fluids and the label will not fall off. An ordinary label, filled out in pencil and covered with transparent adhesive tape, can also be used. It is advisable to place the vessel in a small plastic bag, tied with a rubber band or a string.

The following information should be written on the label: the name of the patient, the date when the sample was taken, and the origin of the sample. The name of the hospital, the clinic and the department, and the name and address of the physician sending the samples should also be given.

All the samples must be accompanied by a slip giving further information regarding the clinical examination, other tests made, and the suspected organism. It is important that the date on which the disease appeared, the patient's temperature, and whether an epidemic may have existed in the environment be given. This information is very important for a valid interpretation of the results. As a rule, such slips are provided by the laboratory.

PACKING CONDITIONS. It is advisable to send the samples by messenger, since they reach the laboratory sooner and can be maintained at low temperature in a thermos flask, with ice or with dry ice. When sent by mail, samples should be placed in a wood or a metal box, hermetically closed. Wood shavings or paper should be placed between the glass vessel and the wood or metal box to prevent breakage and to avoid infection of postal employees.

In warm weather, refrigeration is necessary. In this case, the wood or metal box is lined with cork or glass fiber and encloses another box made of cork or of plastic. Ice cream packing cases can be purchased for this purpose. In the plastic box, dry ice must be added. Two kilograms of dry ice last for 24 hours. It is sometimes preferable to put the tube with the sample in dry ice and then in a plastic bag, which is then put in the plastic box. The latter is itself placed in the large insulating case with an opening to allow the carbon dioxide gas to escape.

One can also use wide-necked thermos flasks in which pieces of dry ice are placed around the sample tubes. A small opening must be made in the cork to allow the carbon dioxide to escape. In both cases, the parcel must be protected against shock (crumpled paper is adequate). It is advisable to label the parcel "fragile," "keep cool," and "urgent."

INTERPRETATION OF VIROLOGICAL STUDY RESULTS

At present, most virology laboratories utilize cell cultures to isolate enteroviruses. This method is good for isolation of polioviruses, Coxsackie B and A9, and ECHO viruses, but it is not reliable to isolate most Coxsackie A viruses, for which inoculation of newborn mice is the method of choice (see chapter on Coxsackie A).

Sometimes, the clinical information and the cytopathogenic effect obtained help to identify the virus. Seroneutralization of the cytopathogenic effect on various cell systems or seroneutralization by inoculation into newborn mice are the methods most frequently used. While isolation and identification of polioviruses are currently done, this is not always so for other enteroviruses because identification is often expensive owing to the large number of reference sera required. The slip accompanying the results should mention the cell cultures utilized for isolation. This information is especially useful in the negative cases and may account for some failures of isolation; thus the comparatively limited value of a negative result, which may be due to the fact that the cells used do not allow the virus in question to multiply (for instance, HeLa cells with respect to ECHO viruses).

A poliovirus type may be identified within two to four days by the isolation-identification technique. This is not the case with other enteroviruses which most laboratories identify in stages. The first stage is the isolation of a virus, which must then be identified. A second sample of blood is required for this purpose, and the clinician is advised that it may take from one to three weeks to identify an enterovirus other than poliovirus.

In general, when an enterovirus has been isolated and identified from a patient with typical symptoms, isolation of the virus may be sufficient. However, recourse to the laboratory is most frequent when the disease has not presented a typical form and the etiology is variable. In this case the isolation of the virus does not necessarily mean that the causative agent has been found. Enterovirus infections are very common, especially in children, and elimination of the virus in the stools lasts for some months after the initial infection. It is therefore very difficult to establish a cause-and-effect relationship between the virus isolated and the syndrome observed in the patient.

Sometimes a double infection is revealed, but in most cases only the virus that multiplies more rapidly is found.

SEROLOGICAL DIAGNOSIS

Search for specific antibodies in the patient's blood is among the most important tests used to incriminate the virus isolated as the etiological agent. The appearance of specific antibodies or an increase in their titer must be detected with great care, it being taken into consideration that enteroviruses may be widespread in the surrounding population.

Whatever the technique used, samplings, storage, and delivery of serum to the laboratory are subject to the same requirements.

COLLECTION OF SAMPLES

From 3 to 5 ml. of blood is usually obtained by venipuncture. Blood can also be obtained by puncturing the finger tip, but under such conditions bacterial contamination often interferes with the serological reactions.

All kinds of processes have been suggested for drawing blood: use of a vacuum tube with a needle, use of a test tube with a cork and a needle through it provided with a glass tube temporarily stoppered up with cotton, which permits air to enter. Most often blood is drawn best by means of a sterile syringe provided with a short-beveled needle of wide diameter.

The blood is then transferred into a sterile test tube. If delivery to the virology laboratory occurs within 36 hours, the blood is likely to be in a satisfactory state when it gets there. It is advisable to leave the blood at room temperature; it should not be placed in the refrigerator, to avoid hemolysis. The serum is collected as soon as possible after coagulation and retraction of the clot. The amount of blood to be taken depends, first, upon the number of reactions and on the number of antigens to be used. As a rule, the quantity of blood should not be less than 5 ml. When the various serological reactions cannot be carried out at the same laboratory, a larger amount of blood should be provided, and distributed in several sterile tubes. In some cases it is possible to distribute the serum in several tubes, which is undoubtedly less expensive.

It should be kept in mind that sera stored for several days at room temperature very quickly become anticomplementary, which is a major drawback for the complement-fixation reaction.

Repeated serum samples are required in order to obtain interpretable results. The first sample must be obtained as soon as possible after the onset of the disease, if possible before the second day and not later than the fifth day.

The second sample must be obtained between seven and 15 days after the first. Sometimes a third sample is required if the first two were taken too close together. The aim is to show either the appearance of antibodies or a significant increase in antibody titer in the second sample. If the first blood sample has been taken too late, the second must be taken at least 10 days after the first, since, if the appearance of antibodies cannot be observed, it is necessary to observe at least a fourfold increase over the initial titer to establish that the infection was recent. If the titers are similar in the two samples one must look for a decrease in antibody titer in a third sample taken much later.

Often, only one blood sample can be taken. If it is an early one, it probably will not provide valid information, but if it is a later sample, a high titer of antibodies may signify a recent infection. Lastly, if a late sample shows no antibody, the hypothesis of infection by the virus searched for can be eliminated.

HANDLING OF SAMPLES

The best storage method is to freeze the sera immediately and to send them to the specialized laboratory. When freezing cannot be done, the serum is sent to the laboratory as rapidly as possible.

When whole blood is sent it is preferable to replace the cotton stopper with a rubber stopper. The same precaution should be taken with frozen serum. If the serum is frozen, dry ice in a thermos flask must be provided. One should not forget the adhesive tape label, directly placed on the tube and giving the patient's name and the date the sample was drawn. A slip bearing the necessary clinical data (date the disease appeared, whether sample is a first or a second bleeding) and all information useful to the investigation to be undertaken, should be included.

LABORATORY PROCEDURES

At present, various seriological techniques are available to the clinician. Those most commonly used involve the search for neutralizing antibodies and for complement-fixing antibodies, as well as joint virological and serological tests. Other techniques, such as those involving flocculation and precipitation, hemagglutination inhibition, and immunofluorescence, are, however, used in some laboratories to reveal antibodies.

Search for Neutralizing Antibodies. To reveal antibodies, the patient's serum is used to neutralize either a reference virus maintained in the laboratory or the virus isolated from the patient. The latter technique is most often used in sporadic infections, especially since sera are likely to exhibit higher antibody titers when tested against the homologous virus than when tested against a prototype strain. Nevertheless, in epidemiological investigations use of a reference virus is preferable.

The protective activity of a serum sample is determined by inoculating the serum-virus mixture either into an animal (inhibition of pathogenicity) or into cell cultures (inhibition of cytopathogenicity). The neutralizing action of the serum is expressed as the highest dilution which inhibits the infectious power of a known viral suspension (constant dose of virus) or by the lowering of a virus titer (variable quantity) by an undiluted serum. In order to interpret the results, it is desirable to know whether this search was carried out on both sera in the same test series.

Three tests can be applied to the technique of neutralization on cell cultures: the neutralization of the cytopathogenic effect (described in the preceding paragraph); the color test; or the plaque reduction technique.

In the color test, viral activity is indicated by pH variations, which reveal the metabolic changes in the cell cultures. The pH of the culture medium is indicated by phenol red; an acid pH means that the cells are alive and have metabolized the glucose present in the culture medium. This is due to the inactivation of the virus by the neutralizing antibodies. An alkaline pH reveals that the cells are disrupted by the viral infection, which could not be inhibited by the serum because it lacks antibodies. The color test is widely used for epidemiologic investigations, since it reveals small amounts of antibodies. A further advantage is its rapidity. However, it is difficult to apply to slow-growing viruses, such as ECHO 14, 16, 22, 23, and 24.

The assay of plaque reduction by antibodies has its origin in the ability of some viruses to form plaques in cell media. This test, which can indicate small amounts of antibodies, is very expensive. However, it is the only technique which demonstrates the neutralizing antibodies to ECHO 4, a virus with low antigenic power. The method using disks impregnated with serum is a modification of the latter test. It was successfully applied to epidemiological studies on polioviruses. It is a useful method because the whole blood is taken from the finger tip, which, in mass studies, saves much time.

INTERPRETATION OF RESULTS OF TESTS FOR NEUTRALIZING ANTIBODIES. *Neutralizing Antibodies in Poliomyelitis.* With very rare exceptions, homotypic and heterotypic antibodies are present in the first blood sample from patients with poliomyelitis induced by a virus of a known type. The heterotypic neutralizing antibodies should be regarded as secondary and due to antigenic crossing. Their titer is low, they are labile, and in most cases they disappear very rapidly (Table 3-2).

Most normal subjects above a certain age have at least one type of neutralizing antibody, despite lack of history of clinical manifestations of poliomyelitis. This fact has been proved by numerous systematic studies in a wide variety of geographic areas (see Chapter 4). Consequently, the early presence of neutralizing antibodies in the patient's blood is in itself of no diagnostic value. A negative result after several days' paralysis is of primary importance and under these precise conditions may permit differential diagnosis. When the presence of neutralizing antibodies is not informative, the comparative titration of neutralizing antibodies in two sera makes it possible to observe a significant increase in titer. The appearance of neutralizing antibodies in the course of a poliomyelitis infection is very rapid and the maximal titer is quickly reached.

Although the presence of neutralizing antibodies in the patient's blood, even at a low titer, seems to affect the multiplication of the virus in the rhinopharynx, it does not stop elimination of virus in the stools. Neutralizing antibodies at a moderate titer do not prevent infection of the digestive tract, but they shorten the infection and the elimination of the virus in the stools does not last as long.

Neutralizing Antibodies in Infections Caused by Enteroviruses Other than Poliovirus. Contrary to what occurs in poliomyelitis infections, in other enterovirus infections the neutralizing antibodies appear later and the increase in the antibody titer is evident in the second or third blood sample. The titer of antibodies rapidly decreases three weeks after natural infection with ECHO 11 in children and after approximately seven weeks in experimental infection in adults.[21]

The titer of neutralizing antibodies for ECHO 16 is from two to four times lower one year after infection, but after that period the antibody titer remains constant, in any event for six years.[18]

The appearance and the persistence of neutralizing, complement-fixing, and hemagglutination-inhibiting antibodies were studied in 24 cases of ECHO 6 lymphocytic meningitis.[2] The neutralizing antibodies were significantly increased in 96 per cent of the cases, while the complement-fixing and hemagglutination-inhibiting antibodies increased in only 67 per cent of the cases. The three types of antibodies reached maximal titer toward the second week of the disease. The neutralizing antibodies persisted for about three years. The hemagglutination-inhibiting antibodies rapidly decreased, but they persisted at a low titer for three years. The complement-fixing antibodies disappeared after the third week. The neutralizing antibodies were specific, whereas the complement-fixing ones indicated heterotypic relations among ECHO viruses 6, 4, and 9.

Clarke et al.,[4] studying antibodies neutralizing the homologous virus in cases of aseptic meningitis occurring in Toronto in 1957 proved that in most cases the titer of

Table 3-2. *Poliovirus-Neutralizing Antibodies Found in Serum in Two Examples of Type I Poliomyelitis*

VIRUS ISOLATED FROM STOOLS	DAY OF DISEASE	TITER OF ANTIBODIES TO POLIOVIRUS TYPE		
		I	II	III
Type I	8	1/1024	1/2	0
	22	1/512	0	0
Type I	2	1/4	0	0
	16	1/512	1/2	0
	21	1/512	0	0

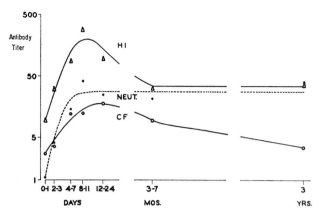

Figure 3-5. Neutralizing, complement-fixing and hemagglutination-inhibiting antibodies consecutive to an ECHO 6 infection in man. (From Russel, R. M., et al.: J. Immunol., *88*:47, 1962.)

neutralizing antibodies increases to at least four times the initial value (Table 3-3).

The search for neutralizing antibodies by the usual techniques of neutralization of cytopathogenic effect has been made easier by the adaptation of some Coxsackie A viruses to cell cultures. In particular, the adaptation by Habel and Loomis[6] of Coxsackie A7 to monkey kidney cells has been of great use, in view of the pathogenicity of this virus type for man.

Search for Complement-Fixing Antibodies. The search for complement-fixing antibodies, which is less helpful for diagnosis because of heterotypic responses and of the absence of definite identification of the virus type, may be really useful in some cases, since it is inexpensive and easy to carry out.

Complement-Fixing Antibodies in Poliomyelitis. In poliomyelitis, two antigens are used: living antigens and heated antigens. In most cases, use of the living antigens makes it possible to note the appearance of and to estimate a significant increase in antibodies; moreover, heterotypic responses are less frequent.

The results are more easily interpreted if the virus is isolated, because fairly often the titer of heterotypic antibodies in patients is higher than the homotypic titer; it is possible to observe the appearance of heterotypic antibodies while homotypic antibodies are still absent. This is particularly true in infections due to poliovirus of type I; on the other hand, infections caused by type III more rarely induce the appearance of type I antibodies. Heterotypic type II antibodies are observed in most infections with types I and III.

Infections caused by enteroviruses other than poliovirus also induce the appearance of antibodies reacting with poliovirus antigens in the complement-fixation test (see earlier in this chapter). In a single blood sample, a titer equal to or higher than 1/64 reveals a recent infection in most cases.

In absence of virus isolation, the complement-fixation reaction reveals the appearance and the significant increase of antibodies whereas the neutralization test seldom reveals the appearance of antibodies (most often, they are unchanged in the second sam-

Table 3-3. *Titers of Antibodies Neutralizing the Homologous Virus Isolated from Stools in Some Examples of Enterovirus Infection**

Virus Isolated	Day of Disease[†]		Acute Period	Recovery Period
ECHO 6	2	29	1/8	1/128
	3	17	1/2	1/128
ECHO 9	4	23	1/2	1/32
	3	27	1/4	1/128
Coxsackie A9	2	24	1/2	1/32
Coxsackie B3	5	20	1/2	1/16
	4	58	1/4	1/128

*Data from Clarke et al.[4]
†Early and late sample.

Table 3-4. *Comparison of Neutralizing and Complement-Fixing Antibodies in Three Examples During Various Stages of Poliomyelitis Infection*

Virus Isolated	Day of Disease	Neutralizing Antibodies			Complement-Fixing Antibodies		
		I	II	III	I	II	III
Type I	2	1/4	0	0	0	0	0
	16	1/512	1/2	0	1/16	1/2	0
	21	1/512	0	0	1/16	1/2	0
Type II	6	1/2	1/2	0	0	1/2	1/8
	20	1/2	1/128	1/8	0	1/16	1/4
Type III	8	0	0	1/512	0	1/8	1/64
	26	0	0	1/512	0	1/4	1/128

ple). On the other hand, heterologous reactions are much less frequent with the neutralization reaction while they are present in the first serum sample at very low titer (Table 3-4).

The complement-fixing antibodies appear from the third to the fourth day of the disease. Their titer increases until the 30th day or even the 45th and then decreases during the following six to ten months and persists for one year and occasionally one and one-half years.

In epidemiologic investigations the complement-fixation test permits study of the frequency of recent inapparent infections. It is less often positive than the neutralization reaction.

One should bear in mind that in vaccinated children with a recent infection the complement-fixing antibodies appear extremely fast and the heterotypic responses are very intense. Vaccination with living vaccine induces the formation of neutralizing antibodies as well as complement-fixing antibodies.

Complement-Fixing Antibodies in Infections Caused by Enteroviruses Other Than Polioviruses. A major drawback in searching for complement-fixing antibodies in infections due to ECHO and Coxsackie viruses is the increase in heterologous antibodies in the course of spontaneous infections (see the first section of this chapter).

Associated Virological and Serological Tests: Their Diagnostic Values. From the virological-serological point of view, there is no way to differentiate a major poliomyelitis infection from a minor infection or even from an inapparent infection (Fig. 3-6). Since polioviruses are widely distributed, it is possible to observe by chance serological results positive for polioviruses in diseases not due to this virus. The chance of finding the virus in the stools prior to the tenth day of the disease are about 90 to 100 per cent. Neutralizing antibodies are present from the first signs of the disease, and their presence in a patient's serum suggests but does not confirm a case of poliomyelitis. The observation of both virus in the stools and neutralizing antibodies in the serum is of great value in diagnosing a recent infection, but actually tells us only that an infection has occurred recently. A negative virological result is a strong argument against a diagnosis of poliomyelitis, and the absence of neutralizing antibodies in a late serum sample is sufficient to rule out such a diagnosis.

The isolation of virus in the cerebrospinal fluid is of great importance for the diagnosis of ECHO and Coxsackie virus infections. One can say that a neurological condition is due to ECHO or Coxsackie enteroviruses when the virus is recovered from the stools and the corresponding antibodies are present in the blood, and when virological and serological tests do not reveal recent infection by poliovirus.

Other Serological Methods. Several serological methods are less commonly used.

THE FLOCCULATION REACTION. The flocculation reaction has been experimentally applied to enteroviruses. It is a difficult test which requires purified and concentrated antigens. It is a microflocculation test which can be observed either in fluid medium or in gel. The percentage of heterologous reactions is low, but the early presence of flocculating antibodies does not permit a rise in antibody titer to be shown. These antibodies disappear rapidly. Schmidt and Lennette[24] recom-

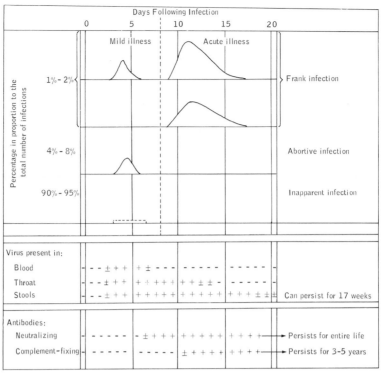

Figure 3-6. Diagram of clinical and subclinical forms of poliomyelitis illustrating the presence of the virus and antibodies in relation to the evolution of the illness. The shaded parts indicate the period of fever.

mended that flocculation and complement-fixation reactions be carried out jointly. This association would reportedly establish a serologic diagnosis in 83 per cent of the cases of poliovirus infections as compared to 75 per cent when both complement-fixation and neutralization reactions are carried out.

THE HEMAGGLUTINATION-INHIBITION REACTION. The value of the hemagglutination-inhibition reaction cannot be asserted because, at present, there is no valid technique for a suitable treatment of the sera. Moreover, only some ECHO and Coxsackie viruses possess hemagglutinating capacity.

THE IMMUNOFLUORESCENCE TECHNIQUE. Many authors have confirmed the possibility of applying the indirect immunofluorescence technique to enteroviruses. Riggs and Brown[22] and Brown[1] used it to search for the three types of poliovirus-specific antibodies and found it to be type-specific. The frequency of antibodies in convalescent patients or in vaccinated children is higher than that indicated by the neutralization technique. Muller and Klein[16] successfully utilized immunofluorescence by means of anticomplement sera in a case of Echo 9 meningitis.

BIBLIOGRAPHY

1. Brown, G. C.: Fluorescent antibody techniques for the diagnosis of enteric infections. Arch. Ges. Virusforsch., *13*:30, 1963.
2. Bussel, R. M., Karzon, P. T., Barron, A. L., and Hall, F. T.: Hemagglutination-inhibiting, complement-fixing and neutralizing antibody responses in ECHO 6 infection, including studies on heterotypic responses. J. Immunol., *88*:47, 1962.
3. Chumakov, M. M., Voroshilova, M. K., Zhevandrova, V. I., Mironova, L. L., Itzelis, F. I., and Robinson, I. A.: Vydelenie i izuchenie IV immunologicheskogo tipa virus poliomielita. (Isolation and investigation of the IV immunological type of poliomyelitis virus). Probl. Virol., *1*:16-19, 1956.
4. Clarke, M., Hunter, M., McNaughton, G. A., Von Seydlitz, D., and Rhodes, A. J.: Seasonal aseptic meningitis caused by Coxsackie and ECHO viruses, Toronto, 1957. Canadian Med. Assn. J., *81*:5, 1959.
5. Francis, R. D., and Ceballos, R.: Viremia in ECHO 6 type virus infection. Proc. Soc. Exp. Biol. Med., *101*:479, 1959.
6. Habel, K., and Loomis, L. N.: Coxsackie A7 virus and the Russian "poliovirus type 4." Proc. Soc. Exp. Biol. Med., *95*:597, 1957.
7. Habel, K., Silverberg, R. J., and Shelokov, A.: Isolation of enteric viruses from cases of aseptic meningitis. Ann. N.Y. Acad. Sci., 67:223-229, 1957.
8. Howe, H. A., and Wilson, J. L.: In: Viral and Rickettsial Infections of Man. (T. M. Rivers and F. I.

Horsfall, eds.) Lippincott, Philadelphia, 1958, p. 432.

9. Jungeblut, C. W.: Newer knowledge on the pathogenesis of poliomyelitis. J. Pediat., *37*:109-128, 1950.

10. Kalter, S., Page, M., and Suggs, M.: Study of specimens submitted for poliomyelitis diagnosis January 1956–June 1957. Read before American Association of Immunologists, Philadephia, April 15, 1958; Summary in C.D.C. Poliomyelitis-Surveillance Report. No. 138, April 1958)

11. Kibrick, S., and Benirschke, K.: Acute aseptic myocarditis and meningo-encaphalitis in the newborn child infected with Coxsackie virus group B, type 3. New Eng. J. Med., *255*:883-889, 1956.

12. Klein, J. O., Lerner, A. M., and Finland, M.: Acute gastroenteritis associated with ECHO virus type 11. Amer. J. Med. Sci., *240*:749, 1960.

13. Lerner, A. M., Klein, J. O., Levin, S. H., and Finland, M.: Infections due to Coxsackie virus group A type 9 in Boston 1959 with special reference to exanthema and pneumonia. New Eng. J. Med., *263*:1265, 1960.

14. Lerner, A. M., Klein, J. O., and Finland, M.: A laboratory outbreak of infections with Coxsackie virus group A, type 9. New Eng. J. Med., *263*: 1302-1304, 1960.

15. Medearis, D. N., Jr., and Kramer, R. A.: Exanthem associated with ECHO virus type 18 viremia. J. Pediat., *55*:367, 1959.

16. Muller, F. von, and Klein, P.: Fluoreszenz serologische Darstellung der Komplementbindung auf Virus-Anti-Körper-Komplexe in der Gewebckultur. Deutsche Med. Wschr., *84*:2195, 1959.

17. Munk, K. K., and Nasemann, T.: Untersuchungen über die Ätiologie der in Süddeutschland beobachteten Fälle des variablen infektiösen Exanthems: Isolierung eines ECHO-Virus. Klin. Wschr. *37*:371, 1959.

18. Neva, F. A., and Malone, M. F.: Persistence of antibodies to ECHO 16 viruses following Boston exanthem disease. Proc. Soc. Exp. Biol. Med., *102*: 233-235, 1959.

19. Neva, F. A., and Zuffante, S. M.: Agents isolated from Boston exanthem disease during 1954 in Pittsburgh. J. Lab. Clin. Med., *50*:712, 1957.

20. Pette, H., Maass, G., Valenciano, L., and Mannweiler, K.: Zur Frage der Neuropathogenität von enteroviren experimentelle untersuchungen zur Neuropathogenität verschiedener Stämme von ECHO 9 virus. Arch. Ges. Virusforsch., *10*:408, 1960.

21. Philipson, L.: Experiments in human adults with a recently isolated virus associated with respiratory disease. Arch. Ges. Virusforsch., *77*:318-331, 1958b.

22. Riggs, J. L., and Brown, G. C.: Differentiation of active and passive poliomyelitis antibodies in human sera by indirect immunofluorescence. J. Immunol., *89*:868, 1962.

23. Sabin, A. B., Krumbiegel, E. R., and Wigand, R.: ECHO type 9 virus disease. Virologically controlled clinical and epidemiologic observations during 1957 epidemic in Milwaukee. A.M.A.J. Dis. Child., *96*:197, 1958.

24. Schmidt, N. J., and Lennette, E. M.: A microflocculation test for poliomyelitis. Amer. J. Hyg., *70*:51, 1959.

25. Steigman, A. J., Kokko, V. P., and Silverberg, R. J.: Unusual properties of a virus isolated from the spinal cord of a child with fatal poliomyelitis. A.M.A.J. Dis. Child., *86*:509, 1953.

26. Steigman, A. J., and Lipton, M. M.: Fatal bulbospinal paralytic poliomyelitis due to ECHO 11 virus. J.A.M.A., *174*:178, 1960.

27. Taylor, R. M.: A report on the isolation of unidentified viruses from human blood and mosquitoes. Atti VI Congr. Intern. Microbiol. II, *108*:236-240, 1953.

28. Utz, J. P., and Shelokov, A. J.: Coxsackie virus infection. Presence of virus in blood, urine and cerebrospinal fluid. J.A.M.A., *168*:264, 1958.

29. Verlinde, J. D., and Wilterdink, J. B.: Neuropathogenicity of non polio enteroviruses with special reference to ECHO 9 virus. Folia Psychiat. (Neerl.), *61*:670, 1958.

30. Wigand, R., and Sabin, A. B.: Properties of epidemic strains of ECHO type 9 virus and observations on the nature of human infection. Arch. Ges. Virusforsch., *11*:683-707, 1962.

CLINICAL SYNDROMES ASSOCIATED WITH ENTEROVIRUSES

by V. Drouhet

Clinical Syndrome	Enterovirus Types	Isolations from Parenteral Sources	Outbreaks
Paralytic diseases	Polio I, II, III Cox. A2, 4, 7, 9, 23 Cox. B2, 3, 4, 5 ECHO 1, 2, 4, 6, 7, 9, 11, 14, 16, 18, 30 (12, 13)	7 (CNS) 5 (CSF) 2, 3 (CSF) 2 (CNS) 6 (blood)	I, II, III A7

Encephalitis and meningo-encephalitis	Polio I, II, III
	Cox. A2, 5, 6, 7, 9
	Cox. B2, 3, 5
	
	ECHO 1, 2, 6, 9, 11, 19
		A7
		B5 ⎫ electro-
		   ⎬ encephalo-
		   ⎪ graphic
		ECHO 1, 6, 9, 11 ⎭ changes
		ECHO 2, 9 (fatal cases)	

Cerebellar ataxias	Polio I, II, III ECHO 1, 9		
Aseptic meningitis	Polio I, II, III Cox. A1, 2, 3, 4, 5, 6, 7, 9, 10, 14, 16, 22, 23, 24 Cox. B1, 2, 3, 4, 5 (6?) ECHO 1, 2, 3, 4, 5, 6, 7, 9, 11, 12, 13, 14, 15, 16, 17, 18, 19, 20, 21, 22, 24, 25, 30, 31, 32	I, II, III 1, 2, 4, 5, 6, 7, 9, 10, 14, 16, 22, 24 (CSF) 1, 2, 3, 4, 5 (CSF) 2, 4, 5, 6, 7, 9, 11, 14, 15, 16, 17, 18, 19, 20, 23, 30, 31 (CSF)	I, II, III A7, 9 B1, 2, 3, 4, 5 4, 6, 9, 11, 16, 30
Meningoeruptive syndromes	Cox. A9, 23 ECHO 4, 9, 6, 14, 16, 18		4, 6, 9, 16
Epidemic myalgia	Cox. B1, 2, 3, 4, 5		B1, 2, 3, 4, 5
Conjunctivitis	Cox. A9, 10, 16 Cox. B5 ECHO 1, 4, 6, 9, 16, 20, 28		
Respiratory syndromes Upper respiratory illnesses	Cox. A9, 10, 21, 24 Cox. B2, 3, 5 ECHO 1, 2, 3, 6, 7, 19, 20, 4, 11, 25, 28		
Croup	Cox. A9 Cox. B5 ECHO 11		
Lower respiratory illnesses (pneumopathies)	Cox. A9, 16 Cox. B4, 5 ECHO 9, 19, 20	A9 (lungs)	
Respiratory and gastro-enteric syndromes	ECHO 8 (= type 1) 11, 19, 20		
Gastrointestinal syndromes Enanthem	ECHO 9		
Vesicular Enanthem	Cox. A9 Cox. B2, 3, 5 ECHO 6, 9, 16		
Lymphonodular pharyngitis	Cox. A10		
Vesicular stomatitis	Cox. A16		
Herpangina	Cox. A1, 2, 3, 4, 5, 6, 8, 10, 22		
Parotitis	ECHO 9	ECHO 9 (saliva)	
Hepatitis	Cox. A4, 9 Cox. B3, 4, 5 ECHO 4, 9	A4 (blood), 9 (liver) B5 (liver)	

CLINICAL SYNDROME	ENTEROVIRUS TYPES	ISOLATIONS FROM PARENTERAL SOURCES	OUTBREAKS
Enteritis (diarrhea)	Cox. A9 ECHO 2, 6, 7, 8 (= 1), 9, 11, 12, 13, 14, 18, 19, 22, 23, 24		ECHO 2, 11, 14, 18
Cardiovascular syndromes Myocarditis	Cox. B1, 2, 3, 4, 5		
Pericarditis	Cox. A1 (?) Cox. B1, 2, 3, 4, 5 ECHO (8, 9, 19) ?	B2, 3, 4 (pericardial fluid)	
Lymphadenopathy	Cox. A5, 6, 9, 16 Cox. B5 ECHO 2, 4, 9, 16, 20		
Splenomegaly	Cox. B5 ECHO 9		
Vulvitis	Cox. A10		
Orchitis	Cox. B5 ECHO 9	B5 (testis biopsy)	

Cutaneous Syndromes
  Rashes
  (maculopapular exan-
  them various erythema)
	Polio I, III
	Cox. A2, 4, 5, 9, 16
	Cox. B1, 3, 4, 5
	ECHO 16, 9, 6, 4
	      1, 2, 3, 5, 7, 11, 12, 14, 18,
	      19
		4, 6, 9, 16 (blood)
		18 (blood)
			A4, 9, 16
			B5
			2, 4, 9, 11, 16

Vesicular dermatitis	Cox. A5, 9, 16 Cox. B3, 5 ECHO 4, 5, 9, 11, 12	16 5 4, 11	
Petechiae	Cox. A9 Cox. B3 ECHO 4, 9		
Neonatal infection: encephalomyocarditis	Cox. A16 Cox. B3, 4	blood and heart muscle blood and heart muscle	

4

Poliomyelitis

POLIOMYELITIS: PHYSIOPATHOLOGY

by R. DEBRÉ

In spite of numerous and extensive investigations, we are familiar only with the appearance of poliovirus in the rhinopharynx and oropharynx at the onset of infection, its constant and prompt appearance in the intestine, evidence of its presence in blood, lymph nodes, and nervous system, and the serological reactions which it may induce and whose appearance bears witness to a solid and lasting immunity. That is to say, we know where it multiplies and which cells it destroys, but the precise spot where the virus gains entry, the pathways by which it chooses to spread throughout the body, even the reasons for its disappearance from the nervous system, remain subject to discussion, and the schemata which are most often adopted still contain a portion of hypothesis and interpretation.

ROUTE OF ENTRY

We now know that the virus, or rather the viruses, of poliomyelitis, are able to disperse through human communities abruptly and without warning for reasons of which we are completely ignorant. In Denmark, for example, there were 381 cases of poliomyelitis in 1951, and 5667 cases in 1952. These epidemics with their sudden onset are widely disseminated, and a proportion of the population consequently harbors the virus, with subclinical infection and antibody production.

In the same way, in sporadic cases, the family and contacts of the patients are, to a considerable degree, infected and this infection is detectable at the very moment when the first case of illness appears. Spread among human communities, with large geographic, social, and seasonal variations, is thus both intense and rapid, notably in children and particularly in the youngest. A great proportion of these become infected simultaneously and spread the virus widely among their contacts.

How does this dissemination take place? How does it check itself? How does virus penetrate the body of an individual exposed to infection? At present, we can give no definite answers to these questions.

Our own figures, confirming known facts, indicate that examination of 300 stool specimens from poliomyelitic patients showed detectable virus in 95 to 100 per cent of cases. This gives an undeniable diagnostic value to such examinations, although its interest may be, in most cases, retrospective (owing to the time necessary for laboratory studies).

In these patients, as in the numerous individuals suffering from occult infections, fecal excretion persists for many weeks (average, two months.) The amount of virus particles excreted is also remarkable, for this may reach 10^4 to 10^5 infectious particles per gram of feces.

Such fecal excretion explains readily the fact that virus has been found on the hands of carriers of these organisms and, above all, the presence, confirmed in all places with a remarkable frequency and abundance, of virus in sewage water or, in a more general way, in waste water. If we add to these facts the remarkable survival of virus in this environment, in spite of cleansing operations, its eventual presence in drinking water, and its transport by insects and birds, we can understand that the general idea of spread by the oral route could be accepted, whether this is carried out via food, water, milk, or contaminated hands.

Nevertheless, epidemiological studies suggest further hypotheses. No convincing proof of an epidemic mediated by tap or river water, milk, or food has ever been given, in spite of attempts to demonstrate this. The way that viruses spread in communities, in the population of a town, in infants, in a residential nursery, in school children, in hospital patients, or in members of a family, suggests airborne spread more than contamination of fecal origin, as is well recognized in typhoid fever or cholera. The spread of poliomyelitis resembles much more that of measles or influenza. In the latter, spread is airborne by droplets (Flügge) and entry is essentially through the nasal passages during respiration, the virus then crossing the junction of pulmonary and gastrointestinal tracts.

May not the viruses of poliomyelitis normally follow the same routes as those of influenza or measles, even if the cells in which they finally come to rest are different?

In poliomyelitis, at the onset of paralysis, investigation of specimens taken from the oropharyngeal mucous membrane surfaces shows that virus was identified in 50 to 60 per cent of cases. We have been able to confirm these figures in 25 children observed during the first ten days of the disease.

In another series of investigations, in 16 children affected by poliomyelitis, we attempted to demonstrate virus in specimens taken with great care from nasal cavities and conjunctival mucosa. Swabs and aspirations were taken at the same time as those throat swabs which later proved to be positive, that is to say between the third and eighteenth days after the onset of paralysis. We were unable to recover virus either from the nasal or ocular mucosae or from the nasal and lacrimal sections that we examined. These findings agree with those of other workers, notably Sabin. Negative as they are, and without denying their relative value, they do not definitely exclude the possibility of entry via these routes. Indeed, these specimens were taken after the onset of clinical signs and so are clearly situated, in time, after the moment of viral penetration.

Conversely, we know from experience with attenuated virus vaccine that oral entry is feasible in man. But is this artificial infection comparable to the natural one?

Furthermore, a rather unusual site of entry has impressed us as worthy of study, following the work of our colleague Karola Papp,[12] who has investigated the entry of measles virus via the conjunctiva and seems to have confirmed this possibility (demonstrating in particular that, in an environment contaminated with measles virus, the wearing of spectacles may protect the infant against infection). We proceeded to inoculate poliovirus into the conjunctival sac of cynomolgus monkeys, thus producing infection following a procedure which, to our knowledge, has not previously been used. Our experiment demonstrated that we could use the ocular route to infect cynomolgus monkeys with poliovirus. Under experimental conditions, using a very virulent strain, we were able to observe paralytic infections and inapparent infections (nevertheless resulting in immunity) following inoculation. Virus was not detectable at the site of inoculation, was found rarely in the nasal fossae, and, having once entered the body, became implanted in the intestinal mucosae, allowing prolonged fecal excretion.

In the case of the eye, at any rate, the entry of virus may, therefore, not be revealed by growth at the site of entry. Doubtless, the conditions of this experiment are such that we may not extrapolate the results and apply them to natural infection in man. Nevertheless, we must distinguish the site of entry from the site of implantation.

We know that the nasal route was recognized very early as a possible route of infection in man. The first writers considered that poliovirus was able to attack only the nervous system thanks to direct propagation in nervous tissues (neuroprobasia). Early experiments, using the nasal route, confirmed

this hypothesis (paralysis of monkeys, recovery of virus from the olfactory bulb (Landsteiner and Levaditi,[11] Flexner and Lewis,[9] Flexner and Clark[8]). Later, Sabin[13] discovered in the same way characteristic histological lesions in the olfactory bulb of the monkey on the fourth day following infection. The possibility of infecting the monkey through differing pathways has since been shown, by use of oral, subcutaneous, intraperitoneal, intracerebral, and intraspinal routes; in these differing cases, virus is constantly found in the feces.

Today, general opinion is in favor of entry by the oral route; the absence of results when one looks for virus in the nasal mucosa, the frequent presence from the onset in the oropharynx, the example of vaccination via the oral route, appear to be arguments in favor of this route of entry. Bodian and Horstmann[2] write that it is generally believed that the entry of the virus is via the upper alimentary passages and its exit is by the same route and through the lower gastrointestinal tract, entry via the nasal route being an explanation now abandoned. Sabin agrees with these conclusions.

It appears justifiable for us to accept this opinion but with some reservations, for it confuses penetration of the virus with implantation. All that appears proved to us is the initial implantation in the lymphoid tissue of the digestive mucosa (tonsils, oropharynx, Peyer's patches in the intestine), but such implantation does not demonstrate that nasal penetration (the more likely in view of epidemiological data) must be excluded. In summary, the propagation of infection by fecal, alimentary, or handborne origin has not been demonstrated, any more than airborne infection by the respiratory route has been excluded.

SPREAD OF THE ORGANISM

Having entered the body and then penetrated the intestinal tract and in particular the intestinal lymphoid tissue, which routes does the virus take to invade the nervous system?

Bodian in demonstrating the existence of a viremic phase, introduced a concept, new at that time, concerning the dissemination of the virus. The idea thus put forward was of a viremic phase with secondary localization in the nervous system. According to

Bodian's schema, the virus enters via the mouth and replicates initially in the pharynx, in the tonsils, and in the Peyer's patches of the intestine. From the lymphoid tissue, it spreads on the surface of the mucosa, where it multiplies extensively and is excreted in the stools. In addition, it enters the blood. This hematogenous infection is responsible for infection of different organs, of which the nervous system is particularly sensitive to its action.

Sabin adopted a slightly different explanation. He considers that the virus replicates in the superficial epithelial cells of the oropharyngeal mucosa and in the cells of the intestine. By and large, all the intestinal mucosa becomes infected and the virus is then absorbed by the lymphatic system, which then decants it into the blood. From the latter source comes the final penetration into sensory and sympathetic ganglia, from which the virus is able to invade the corresponding territories of the central nervous system. Observing virus distribution and titer in the previremic period, Wenner[15] found it to be present initially in the oropharyngeal and ileal tissues, but he found it difficult to specify whether the initial multiplication of virus took place in the epithelial or in the mesenchymal cells of these tissues.

The pathogenesis of poliomyelitis was explained in still a different way by Faber. The regional nerve ganglia absorb virus through their terminations in the bucopharyngeal and intestinal mucosa. Virus multiplies in these regional nerve ganglia, then invades the throat and the intestine by centrifugal spread, and, by centripetal flow, the central nervous system. Viremia, according to Faber, may also directly infect the spinal cord. Nevertheless, he considers that in certain conditions, direct contamination through the peripheral nervous pathways is possible.

Indeed, the replication of virus in the intestinal tract and its early passage into the blood during the preparalytic phase of the disease (presymptomatic viremia) is a concept which is well founded and verified in man. Infection of the nervous system via the blood seems likely. Is it the only route of entry to the central nervous system, or does transmission along nerve fibers play a part? We do not know enough at the present to answer this question definitively. Nevertheless, the behavior of man following immunization, when virus may be implanted in the intestine but does not spread, allows us to presume that humoral antibodies have the prevention of viremia as an essential role, thus avoiding invasion of the central nervous system. If the presence of humoral antibodies before infection, even in relatively small quantity, may thus protect the central nervous system and allow serious illness to be avoided, the most common natural fact yet remains obscure, namely, the frequency with which virus multiplies in the intestines and the rarity of clinically evident poliomyelitis. Does a limited infection in most subjects induce the immediate production of antibodies adequate to prevent viremia (and thus, ultimately, the infection of ganglia and subsequent dissemination along the nervous pathways), while a more massive natural infection overcomes this natural defense? Here individual characteristics come into play, the "predisposing factors" of age in particular. And here, secondary causes come into the field, such as trauma, muscular and neurological fatigue, and the role of subcutaneous or intramuscular injections. We will refer to these later on.

In every case, we must add to these variable host factors those factors pertaining to the virus itself. It is well known that polioviruses differ, not only in their antigenic constituents but also in so far as these characteristics relate to immunity, that is to say, their capacity for implantation and invasion (virulence). Should we not also add the possible function of the viral flora in the infected person, the role of interference which may inhibit or, alternatively, may be favorable? The study of the viral interreactions which we suspect in mixed epidemics (poliovirus and Coxsackie virus) is far from complete.

INVASION OF THE NERVOUS SYSTEM

The distribution of lesions in the nervous system is remarkably constant both in man and in monkey (cf. pathological anatomy, in Chapter 1). They are of two types: destruction of motor neurons and inflammatory reactions, which both unite in the production of the clinical picture (cf. Chapter 1).

The relationships between the two types of lesion and the mechanism of the inflammatory reactions are poorly understood. According to Bodian, the primary lesions are neuronal; they are certainly able to appear in the absence of inflammatory changes.

Moreover, they are associated (in the experimental animal) with high virus titers, thus appearing to connote virus replication in the affected cell. Inflammatory reaction follows, secondary to the neuronal lesion. Nevertheless, severe inflammatory reactions of poliomyelitis are not always associated with massive nerve cell destruction. Some writers have considered the possibility of virus multiplication outside the neurons, in particular in the neuroglia. Others envisage a toxic effect of poliovirus.

We must stress that anatomical lesions may be found in subclinical forms of the disease, in particular in the monkey, in which careful and systematic examination of the nervous system has shown neuronal and inflammatory lesions in the cord and in the brain stem, although the animals had not shown the slightest corresponding clinical signs. In the same way, subclinical neurological lesions are found in man.

Such data show that the intensity of anatomical lesions must reach a certain critical point before they can manifest themselves. They also show that the boundary between apparent and inapparent forms of disease is not always easy to define. Finally, they show that the presence of detectable antibodies in the blood is not the only factor which intervenes to stop the pathological process. Other factors exist in the nervous system itself. In the animal which has been inoculated intracerebrally, no appreciable neutralizing antibody response can be detected, yet, nevertheless, the decrease in virus concentration occurs in the same way as in the course of natural infection or in experimental infection via the oral route. It seems likely, therefore, that inhibiting factors here play a part, whether they be nonspecific or local tissue antibodies such as IgA (whose role, it is true, has not yet been demonstrated).

Whatever the obscurities of the physiopathological problems, some discussion should be devoted to the predisposing causes.

PREDISPOSITIONS TO ILLNESS

The best known predisposition is age. If it is needless to stress infancy, as the very name infantile paralysis implies its importance, we must still stress two features: the frequency, too long ignored, of poliomyelitis in infants of less than two years of age, and the increasing proportion of adolescents and young men compared with children during the past few years; thus, in Copenhagen, patients of 15 years of age and above composed 20 per cent of the total in 1934, 27 per cent in 1937, 44 per cent in 1942, and 53 per cent in 1944. These data, in the countries where such surveys were made, are unrelated to the age distribution of the population. Furthermore, poliomyelitis is more often severe in the adult or the adolescent than in the child. Involvement of the upper part of the central nervous system and death are relatively more frequent in adults.

The sex-linked predisposition is very curious (Weinstein); in children there is an excess of males, and in adults a slight excess of females, among whom, in addition, the disease appears to be milder than in men. Severe forms are most frequently found in the fourth decade. These considerations must not be overlooked when one is introducing the practice of vaccination into a country.

Familial susceptibility, impressive in a few exceptional cases, does not appear to play a part of great importance.

Pregnancy appears to play a predisposing and aggravating role. Abortion may be induced when poliomyelitis occurs at an early stage in pregnancy. According to their extent or distribution, lesions in the mother give rise to obstetric difficulties or to anoxemia in the infant at birth. Poliomyelitic involvement of the infant is relatively rare, although transplacental spread of poliovirus has been demonstrated at varying stages of pregnancy. In general, the children are normal at birth, without signs of paralysis and without any abnormalities attributable to poliomyelitis. It even seems that a certain number of them may be capable of producing an inapparent form of poliomyelitis with an active immune response. Nevertheless, cases of paralytic neonatal poliomyelitis occur, possibly acquired at the very moment of birth, possibly at a time so near to this that they can be due only to intrauterine infection (see Chapter 61).

Various traumatic factors (shocks, operations, fatigue, muscular exercise, prolonged bathing, excessive sunbathing) have been studied as predisposing causes. The role of some peripheral traumas is, furthermore, so clear that they appear, in some instances, to have favored not only the diffusion of virus but also the localization of its action in the nervous system to the region corresponding to the damaged areas. Tonsillectomy is particularly notorious in this respect and appears, when it has been performed recently, to give cause for fear of brain stem distribution of poliomyelitis. Does tonsillectomy carry the same risk when it has been performed long before the risk of infection? Some figures lead us to think so.

The problem of injections, especially of vaccines—particularly pertussis—considered as predisposing and localizing factors, remains a subject for dispute. The role of muscular fatigue, sports, and sea and river bathing and swimming has not been clearly explained. The possibility of the predisposing role of these factors should lead us to give suitable advice during epidemics and to add bed rest to this when, in the course of an epidemic, we suspect (by the presence of fatigue, fever, sore throat, or gastrointestinal disorders) the preparalytic phase of the disease.

BIBLIOGRAPHY

1. Bodian, D.: Virus and host factors determining the nature and severity of lesions and of clinical manifestations. *In*: Papers and discussions presented at the Second International Poliomyelitis Conference. Philadelphia, Lippincott, 1952, pp. 61-87.
2. Bodian, D., and Horstmann, D. M.: Poliovirus. *In:* Horsfall, F. L., and Tamm, I. (eds.): Viral and Rickettsial Infections of Man. 4th ed. Philadelphia, Lippincott, 1965, pp. 438-442.
3. Craig, D. E., and Brown, G. C.: The relationship between poliomyelitis antibody and virus excretion from the pharynx and anus of orally infected monkeys. Amer. J. Hyg., 69:1, 1959.
4. Debré, R., Boué, A., Drouhet, V., and Bargeton, E.: Etudes expérimentales chez le singe Cynomolgus de la pénétration dans l'organisme du virus poliomyélitique pulvérisé par voie nasale. C.R. Acad. Sci. Paris, 257:330-333, 1963.
5. Debré, R., Drouhet, V., Boué, A., and Bargeton, E.: Etude de l'infection poliomyélitique expérimentale chez les singes porteurs d'anticorps neutralisants. C. R. Acad. Sci. Paris, 257:571-576, 1963.
6. Debré, R., Bargeton, E., Drouhet, V., and Boué, A.: Etudes expérimentales chez le singe Cynomolgus de la pénétration dans l'organisme du virus poliomyélitique inoculé dans le cul-de-sac conjonctival. C.R. Acad. Sci. Paris, 257:814-817, 1963.
7. Faber, H. K.: The evolution of poliomyelitic infection. Pediatrics, 17:278, 1956.
8. Flexner, S., and Clark, P. F.: A note on the mode of infection in epidemic poliomyelitis. Proc. Soc. Exp. Biol., 10:1, 1912.
9. Flexner, S., and Lewis, P. A.: Epidemic poliomyelitis in monkeys. A mode of spontaneous infection. J.A.M.A., 54:1140, 1910.
10. Kelly, S. M., and Sanderson, W. W.: The effect of chlorine in water on enteric viruses. II. The effect of combined chlorine on poliomyelitis and Coxsackie viruses. Amer. J. Public Health, 50:14, 1960.
11. Landsteiner, K., and Levaditi, C.: La transmission de la paralysie infantile aux singes. C.R. Soc. Biol., 67:592, 1909.
12. Papp, K.: The eye as the portal of entry of infections. Bull. Hyg., 34:969, 1959.
13. Sabin, A.: The olfactory bulb in human poliomyelitis. Amer. J. Dis. Child., 60:1313, 1940.
14. Sabin, A.: Pathogenesis of poliomyelitis. Reappraisal in the light of new data. Science, 123:1151, 1956.
15. Wehrle, P. F., Reichert, R., Carbonaro, O., and Portnoy, B.: Influence of prior active immunization on the presence of poliomyelitis virus in pharynx and stools of family contacts of patients with paralytic poliomyelitis. Pediatrics, 21:353 1958.
16. Wenner, H. A.: The pathogenesis of poliomyelitis; sites of multiplication of poliovirus in cynomolgus monkeys after alimentary infection. Arch. Virusforsch. 9:537, 1959.
17. Weinstein, L.: Influence of age and sex on susceptibility and clinical manifestations in poliomyelitis. New Eng. J. Med., 257:47-52, 1957.

POLIOMYELITIS: EPIDEMIOLOGY

by J. Celers

The history of poliomyelitis has been marked by three phases: the first, purely clinical, began in 1789[32] with the description of the disease in the child; the second, or virological phase, began with reproduction of the disease in monkeys, the identification of three different types of poliomyelitis virus, and, above all, the numerous laboratory studies made possible by Enders' discovery (see Introduction); finally the third, or prophylactic phase, has developed since the general application of antipoliomyelitis vaccination. In the light of these three successive phases "infantile medullary paralysis," a morbid entity that had been described by Heine, gradually was superseded by poliomyelitis infection, at first clinically evident with its meningeal manifestations, or simply pyretic, then totally inapparent, and subsequently voluntary as a result of vaccination.

This paper is an attempt to describe the main epidemiological features before the vaccination era, with regard to both the clinical and the virological aspects.

POLIOMYELITIS THROUGHOUT THE WORLD BEFORE VACCINATION

The History of Age in Poliomyelitis

The history of poliomyelitis began with its description as a children's or infant's disease. In 1836, when Bell reported a case of poliomyelitis in the daughter of an English clergyman of St. Helena, he noted that an epidemic fever had simultaneously affected all the children of the island between three and five years of age, with after-effects of "disorders of growth" in the body and limbs.[32]

In 1911, in Cincinnati, 83 per cent of the paralyses due to poliomyelitis occurred in children below five years of age; in 1916, in New York, 79 per cent belonged to this same age group. From 1911 to 1913, in the Swedish towns of Stockholm, Göteborg, and Malmö, 63 per cent of the cases were to be found in children below five years of age.[39,40]

An explanation of this fact is provided by serological studies which show the extreme susceptibility of the child to poliomyelitis viruses. Indeed, the infant can be infected by poliomyelitis virus within the first few days of its life; this infection is reflected in some of the curves of the development of neutralizing antibodies according to age; it can be seen that a high percentage of children possess antibodies at an age when the passive antibodies of maternal origin should normally have completely disappeared. In France, in 1955, 25 per cent of the children between nine and 12 months of age already possessed type I antibodies, and, if one arbitrarily prolongs the second, ascending,

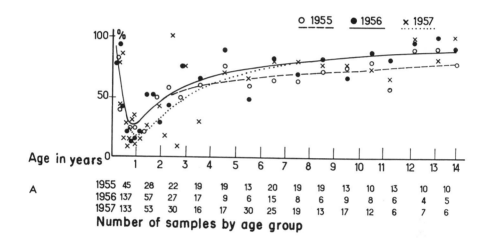

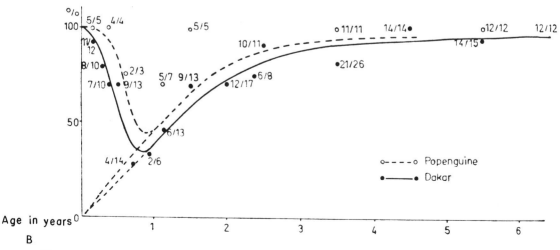

Figure 4-1. Age distribution in the acquisition of type I neutralizing antibodies; *A*, in France, *B*, in Africa. (From Said, G., et al.: Sem. Hop. Paris *35*:1362, 1959.)

portion of the curve of acquisition of type I neutralizing antibodies toward its origin, it will be seen that they begin to appear at birth.[8] Even more conclusive observations can be drawn from the curves established for the children of the region of Dakar, Africa (Fig. 4-1).[43]

Similarly, the systematic search for poliovirus in the stools of healthy infants reveals their relative frequency in very young infants. In Great Britain, 28,797 samples of stools were examined from the spring of 1957 to the autumn of 1959; these samples were from children five years of age and under presenting no pathological symptoms. During the first year of the survey, which was a year of high morbidity from poliomyelitis, the incidence of positive specimens was 15 in 1000 for all the children examined and 11.25 in 1000 for those less than one year of age.[46]

The human body seems to be susceptible from the first few days of life, but the chances of the poliomyelitis virus to meet possible hosts vary greatly. The reasons for these variations generally are not known, and, although a seasonal factor was very soon recognized, and more recently a factor related to "living conditions," in actual fact most epidemics occur and then disappear without any apparent explanation.

SEASONAL NATURE OF POLIOMYELITIS IN TEMPERATE CLIMATES

In France, since 1943, the morbidity rate per 100,000 inhabitants has been maximal from July to September and minimal from January to March.[22] Similar phenomena are to be found in all the nontropical countries of the Northern hemisphere, e.g., Greece, Italy, Japan, the United States, Denmark,[26] Holland,[49] and Switzerland.[37]

On the other hand, in the Southern hemisphere, Argentine, Brazil, Chili, South Africa, and Australia show an increase in the number of cases of poliomyelitis from December on, the highest rates occurring between January and May. Between these two extremes, the tropical regions show a regular distribution in the number of cases declared throughout the year.[26]

The seasonal variations in the morbidity rates in temperate countries reflect the seasonal variations in the spread of the polio-

myelitis virus. The most important investigations concerning this subject are those already mentioned of the laboratories of the National Health Service in Great Britain.[46] In 1957, a year of high morbidity, the highest number of cases of poliomyelitis were reported in the 30th to 37th weeks of the year. This period is also that when the highest incidence of poliomyelitis virus was demonstrated among healthy children: 24 to 32 positive results in 1000 as against 3.97 between the 14th and 17th weeks of the same year.

In an attempt to explain the influence of season or climate the following factors have been studied individually or simultaneously: temperature, relative indoor and outdoor degrees of humidity, rainfall, vapor pressure, and light. It is, however, difficult to compare the epidemiological and meteorological data, which often give contradictory results.[45,47,25] Certainly, not all the meteorological factors vary simultaneously in the same way; some factors occurring at the same time may have different or even opposite effects. Furthermore, other seasonal factors more or less related to climate, such as bathing or the concentration of the population on the beaches or at holiday resorts, may intervene to the same extent as the meteorological factors themselves. Nevertheless, certain meteorological phenomena play an essential part in the survival and spread of poliomyelitis viruses. Hemmes et al.[19] have shown, for example, that a relatively high degree of humidity inside a house favors the survival of the poliomyelitis virus atomized in the air, whereas it impedes that of influenza. This relative intramural humidity reaches its peak during the warm season, the period of the epidemic outbreaks of poliomyelitis, as opposed to the lowest incidence in winter, the season of influenza, when the air of houses is dry. In addition to these notions concerning the relative humidity, Harper suggests other variables such as temperature and the chemical composition of the medium.[17]

Hence meteorological factors appear to play a certain part in the seasonal spread of the poliomyelitis virus. It should also be emphasized that they probably play a major part in the almost permanent spread of the poliomyelitis virus in tropical or subtropical climates. They have recently been somewhat masked by the increasing number of observations that demonstrate the evolution of poliomyelitis according to living conditions. Their importance should, however, be taken into consideration, but no doubt it varies relatively from one epidemic to another.

LIVING CONDITIONS AND POLIOMYELITIS

The most remarkable epidemiological phenomenon during the ten years prior to the widespread use of vaccination was the evolution observed in the distribution of poliomyelitis disease according to age.

In 1913, Frost observed that, although the number of cases recorded among children below three years of age formed 60 to 70 per cent of the total number of cases reported in American cities, these comprised only 42 per cent of the cases in Massachusetts and 24 to 27 per cent in Minnesota and Iowa.

During the First International Conference on Poliomyelitis, Sabin[39] submitted a detailed study of this problem. In an attempt to eliminate the causes of error related to possible variations in the age of the populations (a more or less high percentage of young subjects depending on the period and country) and those due to the virologically unconfirmed outbursts of mild forms of poliomyelitis, he mentioned, as far as possible, only the paralytic forms and gave age-specific rates. By comparing the three major epidemics of New York in 1916, 1931, and 1944, he was able to demonstrate a progressive change in the distribution of the cases according to age. In 1916 the highest number of cases per 100,000 inhabitants occurred in the age group birth to four years. Between five and nine years of age this figure did not attain even a quarter of the previous one; it then decreased rapidly. In 1931, the figures observed for 100,000 inhabitants in the age groups birth to four years and five to nine years were almost comparable. In 1944, however, the highest number of cases per 100,000 inhabitants occurred in the age group five to six years; it was then twice that observed in the age group birth to four years. Thus in New York in 1944, the most affected portion of the population was again composed of children, but of an older age group than in 1916: essentially those five to nine years of age.

In Sweden, however, the evolution has been even more rapid. Whereas from 1905 to 1950 epidemics recurred fairly regularly,

the deviation toward higher age groups was even more marked. Indeed, as demonstrated by Olin,[33] if one compares the number of cases of paralytic poliomyelitis per 100,000 subjects of the same age during two periods remotely separated from each other, but which have comparable morbidity rates — 1905 on the one hand, and 1935-1945 on the other — then there exists a reduction by about one-third in the number of cases for the age group birth to three years; an increase to twice the number of cases for the age group fifteen to 25 years; and an increase to three times the number of cases for persons over 25 years of age. This evolution is continuous and proceeds regularly during the two intermediary periods.

Elsewhere, however, the highest rates are still observed among young children. For example, in England and Wales from 1950 to 1957[28] the incidence rates of paralytic poliomyelitis per 100,000 inhabitants below five years of age consistently remained above that observed for the five-to-ten-year age group, and represents more than two times those reported after ten years of age. Similarly in France in 1957, the year of the highest morbidity from poliomyelitis, for 4109 cases reported the morbidity rates per 100,000 inhabitants were 25.2 for subjects under one year old; 48.8 for those one to four years; 26.2 for those five to nine years; 12.5 for those 10 to 14 years; and 10.4 for those 15 to 19 years old. In still other places infants provide the majority of cases of poliomyelitic paralysis. In Italy from 1905 to 1953[37] the rates reported per 100,000 inhabitants were ten times higher for children below five years of age than for children five to ten years of age. In Ceylon up until 1950, and in Japan in 1947, 70 to 75 per cent of the cases affected children less than three years of age. In Panama, in 1951, the first extensive epidemic caused 56 per cent of the cases among children less than two years of age and 81 per cent among children less than five years of age.[16]

Corresponding to the evolution of morbidity there is an evolution of immunity, not so much with time, since it is impossible to establish percentages of acquired antibodies according to age for the beginning of the 19th century, but an evolution in space, progressing from those countries where poliomyelitis is still an infant's disease to those where it has become an adults' disease.

In France, which is a country that has an intermediate position, we established the antibody curves in 1955-1956-1957 in children hospitalized in Tours, Nantes, Rouen, and Le Havre.[8] From the 1500 sera examined it appears that, at two years of age, 50 per cent of the children possess at least one type of antibody, and at seven years of age this same percentage is reached for the three different types of antibodies. Between 14 and 15 years of age over 90 per cent of the children possess at least one type of antibody and 70 per cent possess the three different types. That is to say that the curve of acquisition is steep, reducing the risk of infection from paralytic poliomyelitis by half after seven years of age.

This risk decreases even more rapidly in countries of Asia, Africa, or America where poliomyelitis remains an infection of the younger child. For example, in Dakar[43] 50 per cent of the infants possess at least one type of antibody as early as at one year of age, and the three types at three years of age. On the other hand, in Sweden, where poliomyelitis has become a disease of the older child and adult, this risk remains the same at a much older age since it is only between 10 and 15 years that 50 per cent of the children begin to acquire a natural protection as reflected by the appearance of a neutralizing type of antibody.[34]

To this delayed acquisition of immunity and this wider range of susceptible subjects corresponds an increase in the incidence of poliomyelitis, these three phenomena being interdependent and closely related to different living conditions most obviously reflected by the infant mortality rate—defined as the number of deaths during the first year of life per 1000 live births.

Payne et al.[38] demonstrated that a low infant mortality rate corresponds to a higher incidence of poliomyelitis and vice versa. The figures reported show, in countries where the mortality rate is over 100, an average incidence of poliomyelitis of less than 1 in 100,000; in countries where the mortality rate is between 50 and 100, an average incidence of poliomyelitis of 2 to 6; and in countries where the mortality rate is less than 50, an incidence of over 10.

These three groups of countries correspond to the three different age groups of poliomyelitis. In the first, where the infant mortality is high, poliomyelitis is almost exclusively a disease of the very young child.

In the second group, where the infant mortality rate is less dramatic, it is a disease of the older child. Finally, in the third group, where the infant mortality rate is low, it is mainly a disease of the older child or adult. It is conceivable that in the places where health measures protect the infant against all forms of aggression, even viral, the chances of acquiring antipoliomyelitis immunity in the first months of life may be lacking, hence a more or less important prolongation of the risk of poliomyelitis infection over the following years.

On the other hand, it is less evident that with this shift of poliomyelitis toward older ages there is a corresponding increase in the absolute number of cases. As Paul himself noted,[36] the relationship between the morbidity rate of poliomyelitis and health conditions may give rise to a number of possibilities. For instance, the simple fact that in certain areas where poliomyelitis appears to be a minor problem and where the conditions of sanitation are primitive the means of detecting and reporting the cases of poliomyelitis are limited, so that the figures given are far below the true values. Similarly, in other countries where poliomyelitis has been duly recognized, the necessity for strict notification of cases became apparent to the medical practitioner only when an efficient means of protection, i.e., vaccination, was introduced. Finally, considerable variations are provided by the sometimes numerous and unverified reports of nonparalytic forms of unconfirmed etiology.

It is therefore advisable to be cautious about the morbidity rates from poliomyelitis reported in countries having insufficient health services and in those where the medical personnel have not long been interested in problems of public health. In fact, if one considers two well-organized countries such as Sweden and the United States, the increase in the number of cases of poliomyelitis is not apparent during the past few decades in spite of the well-defined shift of the age of patients.[33, 39]

INCREASES IN THE INCIDENCE RATE OF POLIOMYELITIS CAUSED BY FACTORS OTHER THAN SEASONAL AND SOCIOECONOMIC

The annual morbidity rates declared before the introduction of vaccination, both in the United States and in different Euro-

Table 4-1. *Paralytic Poliomyelitis: Annual Number of Notified Cases**

Year	Denmark	France	Italy	England and Wales	Sweden	United States
1950	308	1979	2034	**5565**	–	33,300
1951	20	1493	2867	1529	551	28,386
1952	**2450**	1665	2708	2747	492	**57,879**
1953	695	1834	**5010**	2976	**5090**	35,592
1954	72	1534	3404	1319	1009	38,476
1955	25	1834	2685	**3712**	486	28,985
1956	34	1150	3485	1717	551	15,140
1957	26	**4109**	4452	**3177**	250	5485
1958	94	1647	**8377**	1419	192	5787
1959	27	2566	4241	739	25	8425
1960	22	1664	3555	257	9	3190

*Figures in boldface represent epidemic years.

pean countries, reveal their sudden multiplication by 2, 4, or even 10 in certain years. These outbreaks occur sometimes fairly regularly, sometimes in an isolated manner, and always without any obvious relationship from one country to the other (Table 4-1).

Outbreaks of this type have occurred for example in 1950, in 1955, and in 1957 in England and Wales; in 1952 in Denmark and the United States; in 1953 and 1958 in Italy; in 1953 in Sweden; in 1957 in France.

These sudden epidemic variations are still more apparent within the country when local morbidity rates are given per province, per district, or per department. Such examples are found in France,[4] Germany, Sweden, Yugoslavia, Austria, and England.

These epidemic outbreaks are usually linked with the degree of herd immunity existing in the studied population. Each important viral spread, during apparent infections, but particularly during multiple accompanying inapparent infections, results in a high percentage of immune subjects; these latter not only are protected but may also protect their contacts, since they do not spread the new homotypic epidemic strains well. For a certain number of years after an epidemic it is likely that few subjects will become immunized; thus the number of susceptible individuals will gradually increase with the new births. Only when the susceptible individuals attain a sufficient percentage can a new epidemic outbreak occur. These hypotheses are supported by the periodicity of recurrent epidemics sometimes observed: a periodicity of about five years in Czechoslovakia[44] and five to eight years in Sweden.[33]

However, such precise periodicity is not observed on all morbidity curves. Furthermore, systematic serological studies carried out in some countries demonstrated the almost permanent spread of viruses. In France[8] we were able to observe, in the years 1955-1956-1957, among children examined in the same towns, belonging to the same social milieu, and subdivided into similar age groups, an almost perfect superimposition of the curves of antibodies I and III during three successive years. The only well-defined variation was in the case of Type II which, during the year 1955, seemed to have disappeared almost totally, and reappeared the following year; this happened without any modification in the poliomyelitis morbidity rate. Similarly, in Dakar and the Senegal, a serological survey performed in 1957, a year when there was no epidemic and three years after the last epidemic, showed the persistence and intensity of viral spread.[43]

Thus the absence of viral spread and the resulting absence of immunization for the major part of the population do not suffice to explain sudden epidemic outbreaks. Another factor also intervenes which is likely to act even within a population exhibiting a high percentage of spontaneous immunization. This factor, which may or may not add to the absence of natural protection so that it periodically raises the poliomyelitis morbidity rate in countries such as Sweden, is the only factor that may cause serious epidemics in highly endemic regions: namely, an increase in pathogenicity.

Indeed, within any given type, wild strains occur spontaneously with considerable variations of their pathogenicity, thus causing, when the pathogenicity increases, a sudden increase not of the number of poliomyelitis infections but of their pathological manifestations, whether paralytic or meningeal. Variations of this type in the virulence of strains isolated either from patients or from healthy subjects without any known contact with infected patients have been demonstrated in monkeys by Sabin on several occasions.[40, 42] They have also been reproduced experimentally in an attempt to obtain the nonpathogenic strains having a strong immunizing effect which form the basis for the production of live vaccine.

Thus numerous factors intervene in the spontaneous development of poliomyelitis: the viruses themselves, their characteristics, their variations, as well as the host, i.e., man, his susceptibility and his means of protection, whether natural or artificial.

TRANSMISSION OF POLIOMYELITIS

Sources of the Virus

"When one realizes that every individual, not only infected with poliomyelitis but even simply a carrier of the germ, is capable of eliminating such a quantity of the virus for several weeks in the stools that it may exceed 10,000 to 100,000 units per gram of stools, it is not very surprising that this germ is easily found in the sewage and drinking water."[9] In 1957, in 308 samples of sewage water, Kelly found the poliomyelitis virus alone in 21 per cent of the samples and associated with the Coxsackie virus in 13 per cent of the samples.[24]

It is not surprising either that the germ is taken up and transported by flies, or picked up by certain birds such as sea gulls, or may even be found in oysters, since it survives in sea water.[18] But it is not clear whether this wide spread of the poliomyelitis virus in nature plays a part with regard to human infection, of which the spreading seems to be a consequence rather than a cause. Indeed, the studies performed on waste waters and flies are usually contemporary with or following epidemics, and the number and duration of the positive results essentially reflect the intensity of the viral elimination by man.[13, 30] Campaigns for the destruction of insects in order to reduce the number of flies or even eliminate them do not seem to have reduced the incidence of poliomyelitis. The epidemics reported to have arisen from bad food, particularly milk or cream, have not been confirmed virologically[15] and may well be explained by interhuman contaminations from inapparent infections.

However, one cannot definitely exclude the part played by these different vectors in the occurrence of sporadic cases, as the starting point of epidemics, or as a complementary and minor factor in their development.

Man does not require an intermediary host in order to transmit poliomyelitis; he is himself both contaminator and reservoir of the virus.

Interhuman Transmission

The importance of interhuman transmission is clearly observed during studies of viral spread among communities of young children. Numerous surveys have shown that when a child is infected with poliomyelitis nearly all his age-mates are contaminated too.[1, 27, 30, 48] This contamination is not immediately massive; it occurs from one child to another, day after day, rapidly affecting all the children in the same room, week after week or even month after month when there are several rooms in the institution or when the occupants change during the epidemic. Between April and June, 1957, we were thus able to observe the spread of the poliomyelitis virus to the three floors of a pavilion for children below three years of age.[7] Another example occurred in a resident-nursery in Basel,[1] where the epidemic was prolonged for five months.

Susceptibility

All the studies which have shown massive contamination of 80 to 90 per cent of the population were made among young children. In fact, when the population in contact with patients consists of individuals of various ages, the results are far less regular. Intrafamily surveys demonstrate the more or less high incidence of positive results according to age; e.g., in 31 families comprising 38 patients and 148 contacts, the results were positive in 97 per cent of the subjects under four years of age, 67 per cent of the subjects five to nine years of age, 43 per cent of those 10 to

19 years of age, and 20 per cent of those over 20 years of age.[2] Hence the role of age with regard to the possibility of infection by the poliomyelitis virus is obvious.

Other factors have been studied, such as interference phenomena and individual factors,[19] but previously acquired immunity plays the major role: it explains to a certain extent the difference observed in terms of age. Thus in a remarkable study carried out on over 100 families submitted to repeated systematic sampling it was shown that among 277 immune subjects in contact with poliomyelitis virus carriers, infection was absent in 216 subjects having a mean titer of homotypic neutralizing antibodies of 1/160. Infection, with a significant increase in the titer of the homotypic neutralizing antibodies, was noted in 61 subjects who had a mean titer of 1/40 prior to exposure to the virus.[14]

Even more accurate results confirming these data were obtained by means of experimental contaminations obtained with live attenuated vaccine. We shall have occasion to mention these in the section concerning this type of vaccination.

MODES OF INFECTION

This subject is treated under the heading Physiopathology, earlier in this chapter.

BIBLIOGRAPHY

1. Bamatter, F., et al.: Epidémie de poliomyélite dans une pouponnière. Etude clinique et virologique. Schweiz. Med. Wschr., *91*:1604-1612, 1961.
2. Bhatt, P., et al.: Extent of infection with poliomyelitis virus in household associates of clinical cases as determined serologically and by virus isolation using tissue culture methods. Amer. J. Hyg., *1*:287-301, 1955.
3. Bodian, D.: Poliovirus in chimpanzee tissues after virus feeding. Amer. J. Hyg., *64*:181-197, 1956.
4. Celers, J.: La poliomyélite en Europe: épidémiologie et immunité naturelle. Ann. Soc. Belg. Med. Trop., *28*:817-840, 1958.
5. Celers, J., et al.: Etudes immunologiques sur la poliomyélite. 3. Recherche de facteurs liés à l'acquisition des anticorps antipoliomyélitiques. Rev. Immun. (Paris), *22*:530-545, 1958.
6. Celers, J., et al.: Etudes immunologiques sur la poliomyélite. IV. Dépistage des anticorps neutralisant les trois virus poliomyélitiques chez quelques étudiants parisiens. Confrontation des résultats sérologiques et de certains éléments du mode de vie. Rev. Immun. (Paris), *23*:299-311, 1959.
7. Celers, J., et al.: Etude de la diffusion de virus polio-

myélitiques parmi des enfants en milieu hospitalier. Bull. Inst. Nat. Hyg., *14*:505-521, 1959.
8. Debré, R., et al.: Résultats de trois années d' études sérologiques comparatives sur la poliomyélite dans quatre villes de France. Bull. Inst. Nat. Hyg., *14*:493-503, 1959.
9. Debré, R.: Transmission de la poliomyélite. Journées Pediat., Paris, E. Lanord, 1960, pp. 185-196.
10. Debré, R., et al.: Pénétration du virus de la poliomyélite et cheminement dans le corps de l'animal infecté. Essais expérimentaux sur le singe Cynomolgus. Rev. Fran. Etud. Clin. Biol., *9*:27-37, 1964.
11. Debré, R., et al.: Implantation et diffusion du vaccin vivant poliomyélitique administré par voie nasale et par voie orale. Bull. Acad. Nat. Med. (Paris), *150*:412-418, 1966.
12. Dick, G. W. A.: Poliomyelitis. Lect. Scient. Basis Med., *7*:426-450, 1957.
13. Downey, T. W.: Polioviruses and flies: studies on epidemiology of enteroviruses in an urban area. Yale J. Biol. Med., *4*:341-352, 1963.
14. Fox, J. P.: Studies on the development of natural immunity to poliomyelitis in Louisiana. 1. Overall plan, methods and observations as to patterns of seroimmunity in the study group. Amer. J. Hyg., *65*:344-363, 1957.
15. Gear, J. H. S.: The extrahuman sources of poliomyelitis. 2nd International Poliomyelitis Conference. Philadelphia, J. B. Lippincott Company, 1952, pp. 343-354.
16. Gear, J. H. S.: La poliomyélite dans les régions insuffisamment développées. In Debré, R., et al.: Poliomyélitis. Geneva, World Health Organization, 1955, pp. 31-59.
17. Harper, G. J.: The influence of environment on the survival of airborne virus particles in the laboratory. Séminaire sur l'epidémiologie et la prévention de certaines maladies à virus entériques et respiratoires. Centre International de l'Enfance. Arch. Ges. Virusforsch., *13*:64-71, 1965.
18. Hedström, C. E., et al.: An experimental study on oysters as virus carriers. Amer. J. Hyg., *79*:134-142, 1964.
19. Hemmes, J. H., et al.: Virus survival as a seasonal factor in influenza and poliomyelitis. Nature, *188*:430-431, 1960.
20. Horstmann, D.: The clinical epidemiology of poliomyelitis. Ann. Int. Med., *43*:526-533, 1955.
21. Institut National d'Hygiène: Incidence du sexe et de l'âge sur la morbidité et la mortalité par maladies infectieuses en 1957. Bull. Inst. Nat. Hyg., *13*:1061-1080, 1958.
22. Institut National de la Santé et de la Recherche Médicale: Evolution générale de la morbidité. Bull. Inst. Nat. Sante, *20*:223-242, 1965.
23. Isacson, P., et al.: Environmental studies of endemic enteric virus infections. 2. Poliovirus infections in household units. Amer. J. Hyg., *65*:29-42, 1957.
24. Kelly, S., et al.: Poliomyelitis and other enteric viruses in sewage. Amer. J. Public Health, *47*:72-77, 1957.
25. Lawrence, E. N.: Importance of meteorological factors to the incidence of poliomyelitis. Brit. J. Prev. Soc. Med., *16*:46-48, 1962.
26. Van Loghem, J. J.: Poliomyelitis and photoperiodicity. Lancet, *7204*:706-708, 1961.
27. Maass, G., et al.: Virologische Umgebungsuntersuchungen während einer Poliomyelitis-Epidemie

in einem Kinderheim. Die Ergebnisse im Verlauf der Epidemie und ihre Bedeutung für seuchen-hygienische Maasnahmen. Deutsch. Med. Wschr., *84*:2026-2030, 1959.

28. Martin, W. J.: Statistical aspects of poliomyelitis in England and Wales in recent years. Bull. Minist. Health, *18*:54-64, 1959.

29. Meenan, P. N., et al.: Polioviruses in the upper respiratory tract of household contacts. Lancet, *7314*:907-908, 1963.

30. Melnick, J. L.: Isolation of poliomyelitis virus from single species of flies collected during an urban epidemic. Amer. J. Hyg., *49*:8-16, 1949.

31. Murphy, A. M., et al.: Poliovirus in an infant's home. Med. J. Aust., *2*:46-48, 1963.

32. The National Foundation for Infantile Paralysis: A Bibliography of Infantile Paralysis: 1789-1949. 2nd edition, Philadelphia, J. B. Lippincott Company, 1951.

33. Olin, G.: The epidemiologic pattern of poliomyelitis in Sweden from 1905 to 1950. In: 2nd International Poliomyelitis Conference. Philadelphia, J. B. Lippincott Company, 1952, pp. 367-375.

34. Organisation Mondiale de la Santé (World Health Organization): Série de Rapports Techniques — Comité d'Experts de la Poliomyélite. Deuxième Rapport. Geneva, 1958.

35. Paul, J. R.: Epidémiologie de la poliomyélite. In Debré, R., et al.: Poliomyelitis. Geneva, World Health Organization, 1955, pp. 9-30.

36. Paul, J. R.: Endemic and epidemic trends of polio-myelitis in Central and South America. Bull. WHO, *19*:747-758, 1958.

37. Payne, A. M. M.: Poliomyelitis as a world problem. In: 3rd International Poliomyelitis Conference. Philadelphia, J. B. Lippincott Company, 1955, pp. 393-400.

38. Payne, A. M. M., et al.: Poliomyelitis in 1954. Contribution to the series of similar statistical studies which have appeared since 1935 in the epidemiological publications of W.H.O. Bull. WHO, *15*: 43-121, 1956.

39. Sabin, A. B.: Epidemiologic patterns of poliomyelitis in different parts of the world. In 1st International Poliomyelitis Conference. Philadelphia, J. B. Lippincott Company, 1949, pp. 3-33.

40. Sabin, A. B.: Poliomyelitis virus of low virulence in patients with epidemic of "summer grippe or sore throat." Amer. J. Hyg., *49*:176-193, 1949.

41. Sabin, A. B.: Transmission of poliomyelitis virus: analysis of differing interpretations and concepts, practical implications. Chicago Med. Soc. Bull., *54*:163-171, 1951.

42. Sabin, A. B.: Properties and behavior of orally administered attenuated poliovirus vaccine. In 4th International Poliomyelitis Conference. Phila-delphia, J. B. Lippincott Company, 1958, pp. 124-135.

43. Said, G., et al.: Etude des anticorps neutralisant les virus de la poliomyélite chez trois groupes d'en-fants africains de la région de Dakar. Paris, *35*: 1362, 1959.

44. Skovranek, V.: Vaccination avec vaccins inactivé et vivant antipoliomyélitiques en Tchécoslovaquie. Courrier, *10*:229-235, 1960.

45. Spicer, C. C.: Influence of some meterorological factors in the incidence of poliomyelitis. Brit. J. Prev. Soc. Med., *13*:139-144, 1959.

46. Spicer, C. C.: The incidence of poliomyelitis virus in normal children aged 0-5 years. A report on a study by the Public Health Laboratory Service and local health authorities. J. Hyg., *59*:143-159, 1961.

47. Spicer, C. C.: Comments on Mr. E. N. Lawrence's paper on poliomyelitis and meteorological factors. Brit. J. Prev. Soc. Med., *16*:49-50, 1962.

48. Svedmyr, A., et al.: Infections with poliovirus types 2 and 3 in day nurseries and an orphanage. Acta Paediat. (Stockholm), *47*:46-55, 1958.

49. Verlinde, J. D.: Epidemiology of enteroviral infections. T. Soc. Geneesko., *37*:255-263, 1959.

50. Wenner, H. A., et al.: Primary sites of virus multi-plications following intramuscular inoculation of poliomyelitis virus in Cynomolgus monkeys. Virology, *3*:429-443, 1957.

POLIOMYELITIS: PROPHYLAXIS

by J. CELERS

At present there is no specific therapy for poliomyelitis. Hence we can deal only with the problems of prophylaxis. Until 1954 the only procedure used was the injection of gamma globulins; since then a new era of vaccination has presented new possibilities.

THE GAMMA GLOBULINS

The literature contains many reports on the protective power of passive antibodies with regard to experimental poliomyelitis. These investigations specify the various factors likely to influence this protective effect, e.g., strain of virus, infecting dose, mode of inoculation, time at which the antibodies are administered. In particular they show that the gamma globulins, when injected immediately before the oral intake of polio-myelitis virus, protect the chimpanzee against the appearance of lesions of the spinal cord — without, however, impeding either the immune reactions of the animal, especially the formation of antibodies, or the elimination of the poliomyelitis virus in the feces.[3,4,5]

An extensive study was carried out by Hammon in approximately 55,000 human subjects in three epidemic foci in which approximately 50 per cent received gamma globulins and 50 per cent a placebo; during the week following the injection risk of paralysis for the subjects who had received passive antibodies significantly diminished.[18]

A method of this type is difficult to apply on a large scale in view of the difficulty of delimiting the number of subjects who are both susceptible and in danger of infection, the relatively short period of effectiveness of passive antibodies, and the uncertainty of the exact time of exposure.

Although greatly outdistanced by the possibilities offered by systematic vaccination, the gamma globulins nevertheless retain one indication: the immediate protection of subjects in danger of poliomyelitis infection and for whom there exists a contraindication for vaccination with the live vaccine. This could be the case during an intrahospital epidemic for subjects suffering from acute diseases or who are on corticosteroid therapy. The doses advised are of the order of 3 to 5 ml. per 10 kg. body weight of standard gamma globulins.

INACTIVATED
VIRUS VACCINE

Inactivated poliovirus vaccine consists of an aqueous suspension of human poliovirus types I, II, and III, grown in monkey-kidney tissue cultures and inactivated by a suitable method.

The usual inactivating agent used is formaldehyde, but, depending on the country and the producers, numerous variations have been reported, the main differences being in the strain of virus, in the methods of inactivation and filtration, in the agents used for preservation, and in the adjuvants used.

These variations result from the dismay following the first incidents in 1955 after vaccination with an inactivated vaccine; from the difficulties of obtaining a perfectly regular production that corresponds to the normal standards of safety and efficaciousness; and finally from a legitimate need for improvement. They explain the fact that the World Health Organization has been obliged to establish a standard international reference preparation, samples of which have been deposited at the Statens Seruminstitut at Copenhagen and may be sent to the National Control Laboratories, which are enabled to effectuate thus in parallel the tests of efficacy chosen (a wide range of tests exists on the monkey, guinea pig, chick, or other) with the vaccine to be tested and the reference vaccine.[34]

MODE OF ACTION

Inactivated virus vaccine constitutes an antigenic mass to which the organism responds by producing neutralizing antibodies the titer and duration of which will depend on several factors: the antigenic power of the vaccine, i.e., its quality and the amount administered, the number of injections, and the spacing between them. Salk,[47] who was the first to perfect inactivated virus vaccine against poliomyelitis, clearly demonstrated that (1) three small repeated doses are clearly more effective than a single dose, even if the single dose is larger than the sum of the three doses, this observation being, moreover, in agreement with that of Ramon concerning the anatoxins; and (2) the response in antibodies is far better when the three injections are spaced out over a period of seven months instead of being performed every four weeks. Consequently, in order to obtain protection with a single dose it is necessary to use larger quantities of a particularly effective vaccine; that for vaccinations employing three doses injected at only four-week intervals, as for example in the case of triple or quadruple associated vaccinations (diphtheria-tetanus-poliomyelitis or diphtheria-tetanus-pertussis-poliomyelitis), a vaccine of excellent quality would need to be available.

It should be added that the booster effect of later injections depends, above all, on the primary response to immunization; hence the quality of this primary vaccination affects the patient's whole future.

SAFETY

In the spring of 1955, in the two months following the injection of the vaccine prepared by Cutter Laboratories, 94 cases of poliomyelitis were ascertained among vaccinated subjects and 166 among contacts. These were attributed to the insufficient inactivation of a particularly virulent strain of the type I virus.[31] Since then the standardized methods of production and control imposed ensure complete safety from accidents of this type.

The more recent discovery of an agent not inactivated by formalin that is oncogenous for certain newborn laboratory animals again gave rise to some concern. However it does not seem that since 1955 in the United States the frequency of malignant diseases has been any higher in the subjects who received injections of vaccine containing this virus (SV 40).[14] It is no doubt still too early to estimate this effect, but the concern was such that at present every precaution is taken to avert such risks.

Hence the only incidents that can be apprehended are those of the allergic type: medicamentous, to antibiotics such as penicillin* or streptomycin; or more complex allergies due to the protein material itself. With regard to the latter, various types have been described: cutaneous reactions, attacks of asthma, and, very exceptionally, pronounced hyperthermic reactions at times accompanied by neurological manifestations, e.g., encephalopathies and polyarticuloneuritis of uncertain mechanism and debatable etiology.

EFFECTIVENESS

The efficacy of inactivated vaccine may be estimated by three different methods: the serological response, the level of protection during an epidemic, and the effect on the epidemiology.

According to Salk,[47] the inactivated vaccine should be of such a capacity that following the administration of two doses only, one month apart, the appearance of neutralizing antibodies should be observed in at least 75 per cent of children with no previous or concomitant spontaneous poliomyelitis infection. The vaccine produced in Sweden,[15] even after two doses, yields a conversion rate of 92 per cent for type I and 100 per cent for types II and III, and after three doses, a 100 per cent conversion rate for all three types. The inquiry carried out by the Medical Research Council in 1957 in Great Britain under the same conditions produced the same excellent results,[28, 29] with a geometric mean for the titers of neutralizing antibodies of 72 for type I, 282 for type II, and 101 for type III.

Unfortunately these results are far from being achieved and are certainly not achieved regularly by most of the producers. Gard tested two batches of vaccine imported to Sweden and was able to observe the appearance of neutralizing antibodies after two injections in 20 and 35 per cent of the subjects respectively.[15]

---

*Kanamycin is now substituted for penicillin in some vaccines.

In 1960 in Cincinnati, Sabin et al.[44] observed, depending on the age group and socioeconomic background, in children of less than six years of age who had received three doses of Salk vaccine, percentages of neutralizing antibodies varying from 57 to 88 per cent for type I, from 70 to 98 per cent for type II, and from 70 to 87 per cent for type III. Results as mediocre were also reported by Ashkenazi and Melnick in Houston in 1961-1962.[2] Hence it is not very surprising that the levels of protection during a period of epidemic are extremely variable.

For the United States, in 1959, the level of protection during an epidemic was estimated by Langmuir to be between 82 and 93 per cent for subjects who had received three injections of inactivated vaccine, and between 86 and 96 per cent for subjects who had received four injections. However, in this same year, 1959, during the epidemic in Massachussetts, among the 49 cases recorded in patients between five and fourteen years of age, 77.5 per cent had had three vaccine injections.[25] Although it is possible to blame the mediocrity of the batches of vaccine used in this state, and legitimate to count on the nonrepetition of such accidents, nevertheless, in 1963, 20 per cent of the cases of poliomyelitis in the United States and 18 per cent of those in Canada occurred in subjects who had received at least three doses of inactivated vaccine.[8]

Furthermore, the inactivated vaccine does not generally afford protection against digestive infection by the poliomyelitis virus and hence does not modify the extraordinary interhuman spreading of this pathogenic agent among individuals or groups of individuals who are insufficiently or badly vaccinated. This explanation accounts for epidemics in the United States in 1958,[51] in Israel[52] and in Sweden[1] in 1961, and in France in 1963.[10]

Despite these few setbacks the inactivated virus vaccine has made it possible to obtain remarkable results in the fight against poliomyelitis. In the United States, the mortality rate, which from 1950 to 1954 varied between 18.5 and 37.2 per 100,000, progressively decreased to 9.1 in 1956, 3.3 in 1958, and 1.8 in 1960. In the United Kingdom it varied from 4 to 18 before 1955, but during the three years 1959, 1960, and 1961 it was between 0.6 and 1.7. Finally, in Sweden, where the average morbidity index was 16 before adoption of vaccination, figures of less than 1 were reported as early as 1959, and since 1963 poliomyelitis has almost completely disappeared, results which incontestably, because of their permanent nature, may be attributed to inactivated vaccine alone.

LIVE ATTENUATED VIRUS VACCINE

The live attentuated virus vaccine or, more simply, the oral vaccine, is a preparation of live attenuated poliovirus containing any one type or any combination of the three types.

On February 27, 1950, poliomyelitis vaccine composed of attenuated live germs was for the first time administered orally to a human being, a 6-year-old boy. This type II vaccine had been prepared by Koprowski and was obtained by successive passages in the cotton rat; the oral administration to the child produced no ill effects, and the presence of neutralizing antibodies for type II was later demonstrated.

Numerous tests for attenuation have been attempted by carrying out successive passages with various types of poliomyelitis not only in the cotton rat but also in the hamster and chick embryo. The discovery of Enders et al. which made it possible to culture and select the different strains of poliomyelitis virus in tissue culture helped to intensify and accelerate these research investigations. Several strains of poliovirus, attenuated by tissue culture, have been devised and used since 1957 in different countries, particularly those prepared by Koprowski, Lederle, and Sabin.

At present it is the Sabin strains that are the most currently used. Only these strains will be dealt with here. Monkeys of well-defined species, carefully selected and supervised, provide the renal tissue for the production of the vaccine. The present conditions of production and control have been established according to extremely strict requirements.

MODE OF ACTION

The purpose of the ingestion of attenuated strains is to reproduce the natural process of poliomyelitis infection in man, a process that consists of the implantation and multiplication of the vaccinal viruses in the digestive tract and the production of neutralizing antibodies and of complement-fixing antibodies. This viral multiplication takes place in the nasopharyngeal region and in the alimentary tract; this is reflected by excretion of virus in the nasopharyngeal secretions and stools.

The fecal elimination is by far the most abundant and lasting; on an average it spreads over four to six weeks, but may be prolonged for three months. The maximum excretion occurs between the seventh and twentieth days after vaccination, at which time the concentration per gram of feces may attain 10^4 to 10^6 $TCID_{50}$ of virus. The intensity and duration of this excretion depends on the conditions of implantation, doses, strains, and type of virus.

The nasopharyngeal excretion is of shorter duration and more variable. Nevertheless, type I virus has been found following the oral intake of a monovalent homotype vaccine until the twenty-second day in pharyngeal swabs and the eighteenth day in nasal swabs.[11] Moreover, these are not limiting figures, the sampling having been arbitrarily stopped at this date. As in the case of fecal excretion, the nasopharyngeal elimination depends on the conditions of implantation, doses, strains, and type of virus.[20]

Viral multiplication may be demonstrated less than 24 hours after the oral intake of the vaccine. It is indispensable for the appearance of complement-fixing antibodies, which reflect infection, and of neutralizing antibodies, which reflect immunity. The latter may be ascertained between the seventh and tenth days,[42] sometimes later. The levels obtained progressively increase to reach a maximum between the twentieth and sixtieth day. They show a moderate but significant decrease one year after the vaccinal intake. If the vaccinal immunity is identical with natural immunity it should persist for a long period. But it is extremely difficult to foresee the behavior of these antibodies, either because the majority of authors prefer giving systematic booster doses, or because reported results do not consider possible inapparent infections. It should be mentioned, however, that the persistence of antibodies for over four years after vaccination has been verified in a limited number of cases.[39] Furthermore, between the first and the second years following vaccination with two doses of trivalent vaccine the fall in the titer of the postvaccinal antibodies is very slight and the children may even retain, unmodified, titers that are relatively low.[7]

Sabin is of the opinion that, besides this process of general immunization there is a local resistance of the alimentary tract. In fact he has been able to demonstrate that subjects previously infected with poliomyelitis virus do not accept the implantation of a vaccinal virus of the same type either as frequently or as lastingly as nonimmunized subjects.[41] This relative resistance to reinfection is identical whether the initial infection is natural or simply related to the intake of an attenuated virus. Inversely, subjects vaccinated by the injection of inactivated vaccine behave under these circumstances in the same way as nonimmunized subjects.

The mechanism of this phenomenon is not perfectly clear. It was thought that it was simply consequential to general immunization: the neutralizing serum antibodies transude through the digestive mucosa in sufficient quantity to inhibit viral multiplication. In fact, during natural infection Howe[21] was able to demonstrate, in patients and contacts, that there was an inverse relationship between the quantity of neutralizing antibodies in the blood and the titer of poliomyelitis virus in the tonsils, the anterior buccal cavity, and the feces. The titers of inhibiting antibodies are relatively high, since levels higher than or equal to 1/625 have been found, and it is conceivable that the inactivated vaccine, which rarely produces titers as high as these, and especially high titers that are prolonged over a certain period of time, would generally not be able to prevent infection of the organism by poliovirus.

Sabin disagrees entirely with regard to the above concept. He has in fact revaccinated at the age of six months children who at birth showed abundant viral elimination following vaccination by type I vaccine, without, however, producing neutralizing antibodies in sufficient levels to be detectable at three months of age. In these subjects, and in contrast to the situation in children who have not been previously vaccinated, the second oral intake of vaccine is followed only by a transitory multiplication or none at all. Hence he concludes that there is a

local resistance, independent of the phenomena of general immunity.[46]

The substratum of this local resistance is not known. The coproantibodies inconstantly discovered in the stools[23, 24, 26, 27] seem to play an occasional role. But, above all, this local resistance is inconstant and irregular. As already mentioned, multiplication of the vaccinal virus, just as in the case of natural infection, causes the appearance of transitory complement-fixing antibodies. After revaccination with live vaccine (i.e., after the successive intake of three monovalent vaccines, followed by one trivalent vaccine, then revaccination by a bivalent vaccine, and lastly by a trivalent vaccine) Voroshilova et al.[50] found in 106 children complement-fixing antibodies with antigen I, II and III for 42, 43, and 44 per cent of them, respectively. These observations suggest that, in spite of repeated doses, reinfection is possible and hence the local resistance created by the previous vaccinations is far from absolute.

SAFETY

The live attenuated virus vaccine, like all vaccines that contain a live germ, presents three problems: the risk of insufficient attenuation of the vaccinal strain itself, of the recurrence of pathogenicity following a series of passages between the vaccinated subjects and contacts, and of the presence of other pathogenic agents besides the vaccinal strain which are less sensitive to the processes of attenuation used.

Risk of Insufficient Attenuation. The answer to the first of these questions is provided by the surveys organized since 1961 in the United States by the Special Advisory Committee on Oral Poliovirus Vaccine. All the incidents observed among vaccinated subjects are recorded and submitted to a double clinical and virological test. For an incident to be attributable to a live vaccine, the following criteria should be fulfilled: (a) an onset of illness between four and 30 days following feeding of the specific vaccine, with an onset of paralysis not sooner than six days after the feeding; (b) significant residual lower motor neuron paralysis; (c) laboratory data not inconsistent with respect to multiplication of the vaccine virus fed; (d) no evidence of upper motor neuron disease, definite sensory loss, or progression or recurrence of paralytic illness one month or more after onset.

It should be emphasized that these criteria do not enable one to confirm the vaccinal etiology of the incidents observed but simply allow one not to eliminate it. Indeed it is impossible, in vivo, to provide proof that a neurological accident is related to the presence of a vaccinal virus. It would be necessary to demonstrate the presence of the virus in the lesion or at least in the cerebrospinal fluid, whereas the only place where it can easily be searched for and found, i.e., the stools, is just the place where it should be found in any case after an efficient vaccination: its presence therefore is only a criterion of vaccination. On the other hand, the demonstration of another virus that is pathogenic to the nervous system, and particularly a natural poliomyelitis virus, enables one to eliminate a vaccinal etiology.

On the basis of the criteria defined above, the Special Advisory Committee on Oral Poliovaccine in 1962 calculated the risks to be 1 per 4.4 million subjects vaccinated with type I and 1 per 1.4 million subjects vaccinated with type III.

For 1963, after intensification of the vaccination campaigns and distribution of more than 100 million doses of live vaccine, the risks appeared to be even less: 1 per 6 million subjects vaccinated with type I, 1 per 2.5 million subjects vaccinated with type III, and 1 per 50 million subjects vaccinated with type II.

In England and Wales, where similar criteria have been applied, the survey for the years 1962 to 1964, during which 18 million doses of trivalent vaccine were distributed, established the frequency of accidental poliomyelitis-like paralysis as 1 per 4.5 million doses.[30] Here again, no proof was provided of the vaccinal etiology of the accidents, and only the chronological sequence of the facts substantiated these.

Such are the possible risks related to the oral intake of a live attenuated vaccine against poliomyelitis; they have been established from the facts observed under present epidemiological conditions. There is nothing that confirms that they are real, nor that they are nonexistent. But it should be emphasized that these risks are extremely small in comparison with the considerable benefit of a vaccination which promises the complete disappearance of poliomyelitis.

Risk of Recovery of Neurovirulence. The risk of recovery of neurovirulence during successive passages in man at present appears to be still lower. Indeed, contrary to general opinion, the vaccinal virus, whether its diffusion is looked for or feared, does not spread very easily among contacts of vaccinated subjects. Gelfand and co-workers have presented two series of research studies,[16,17] one with the three different types of monovalent vaccine in 56 family units, the other with the monovalent type III vaccine in two urban groups in southern Louisiana. In both groups the conclusions were identical: only approximately 50 per cent of the homotypic negative subjects in contact with live virus-vaccinated subjects were found to be infected by the vaccinal strain. Most of these infections were short-lived, causing a viral excretion that was so slight and transitory that it could not serve as a subsequent source of contamination. The infections were even insufficient to provoke the production of antibodies in the affected subjects. Similar results were found with the live type I vaccine in day-nurseries in the Paris region.[11] Hence, not only does the live vaccine spread so slightly that it can hardly be responsible for passages in series, but it is even generally incapable of conferring simply an efficient protection to the subjects living in contact with the vaccinated persons.

Hence no studies have been made of the strains eliminated after several successive spontaneous contaminations. On the other hand, Smorodintsev et al.[48] succeeded in artificially inducing a series of passages in volunteer children from extracts of stools redistributed to them. Tests of neurovirulence in the monkey were performed from the stools eliminated during eight successive passages, and the results showed that there were variations in this neurovirulence but these were very slight and there was never a continuous progression.

The Special Advisory Committee on Oral Poliovirus Vaccine, from 1961 to 1963 inclusive, was never able to demonstrate the possibility of poliomyelitis contagion by transmission of the virus through vaccinated subjects. The observations made in England and Wales from 1962 to 1964 confirm these results. However, during the first 29 weeks of 1967, in the United States, although no cases of poliomyelitis were reported in recipients of oral polio vaccine, two cases occurred in adults whose children had received oral polio vaccine 28 and 35 days, respectively, before the onset of illness. These two cases were both attributable to type II poliovirus and a "vaccine-like" type was isolated from a stool specimen of one patient.

Risk of Contamination with Other Viruses. The possibility of contamination of the live attenuated vaccine by viral agents that have been unknown up to now and that may be pathogenic to man was suddenly revealed with the isolation in 1960[49] of the simian virus no. 40 (SV 40) from certain monkey-kidney tissue cultures of batches of live vaccine and even from batches of vaccine inactivated by formalin and heat.

It is known that this virus SV 40 is capable of causing the appearance of tumors in the newborn hamster. Its pathogenicity in man has not been demonstrated until now, neither following injections performed four years earlier with inactivated virus vaccine, nor following the oral intake of the vaccine. All the batches of vaccine placed at the public's disposal are tested for the absence of this virus as well as for all other known agents.

There remains the hypothetical risk of the presence of an unknown virus, undetectable by present techniques. It has yet to be proved that this risk is higher in the case of the live vaccine than it is for the injection of an inactivated vaccine.

EFFECTIVENESS

The problem of effectiveness of the live vaccine is essentially governed by its possibilities of implantation and multiplication. Apart from certain special cases which we shall deal with later on, the acquisition of immunity is directly related to the development of an infection due to the vaccinal virus in the tonsils and the digestive tract. Now, in some cases the vaccinal virus is purely and simply eliminated. The great majority of these failures of vaccination can be explained by a phenomenon of interference, i.e., competition between viruses.

Interference of Vaccinal Viruses with One Another. First of all the vaccinal viruses compete among themselves: when the three types of vaccine are given simultaneously and in equal amounts, it is the type II virus that dominates. Generally it is the only one to multiply and cause production of antibodies. After type II, type III virus is the one that multiplies the best; type I has the most

chance of being eliminated by the others. But it is infinitely more practical and advantageous to have a trivalent vaccine at one's disposal. Hence it is necessary to solve this problem. Two solutions have been devised for this purpose: the repetition of doses, and an adjustment of the respective amounts of each type.

For the usual vaccination, i.e., when there is enough time, the ideal is to give three doses six or, better, nine weeks apart. The vaccinal viruses which multiply during the first intake thus have time to be eliminated and to leave room for the strains which have not been able to establish themselves. If one shortens the time between the two intakes, e.g., to four weeks, then these chances are decreased slightly. If they are more spaced out, this prolongation favors the vaccinal process, but vaccination takes longer and the time when complete immunity becomes certain is delayed.

It also seems very important to adjust the respective proportions of each of the different types of virus present in the vaccine. The French vaccine in use at present consists of approximately 1 million TCD_{50} of type I, 300,000 TCD_{50} of type III, and only 10,000 TCD_{50} of type II. Under these conditions the conversion rates obtained for each one of the three types are distinctly higher than 90 per cent.

Interference by Natural Strains of Poliomyelitis Virus. Interference by natural strains of poliomyelitis virus is always to be feared in regions where the spontaneous spread of this virus is endemic. This presents a particularly severe but interesting problem during a period of epidemic. In fact, if vaccination takes place sufficiently early it can forestall infection by the epidemic strain and provoke the establishment of a vaccinal strain that is able to compete effectively with the pathogenic viruses. When the vaccinal virus multiplies abundantly in the tonsils and alimentary tract it prevents infection by the wild strain, thus protecting not only the vaccinated subject but also his contacts, since it sets up a barrier to the spread of the epidemic.

If, on the other hand, vaccination with the live vaccine is performed too late in a subject already infected by an epidemic strain, it is generally unable to dislodge its opponent. The substitution of the vaccinal strain for the epidemic strain can be ascertained only rarely. This occurred in children who, although carriers of a wild strain, had not yet acquired homotypic neutralizing antibodies.[10] Very often the attempt at vaccination fails, and in subjects who are in the incubation period of poliomyelitis this failure is marked by the evolution of poliomyelitis. These cases of poliomyelitis, when paralysis occurs before the sixth day, may be attributed without hesitation to a natural infection. After this date the laboratory may sometimes be able to distinguish the epidemic strain from a vaccinal strain of the same type by means of appropriate techniques (e.g., intratypic serodifferentiation test: identification of the strains by genetic markers involving conditions of culture such as temperature or pH). In this way, during the epidemic at Saint-Brieuc (France), we identified the epidemic strain SB 27 in five subjects vaccinated from three to nine days prior to the first symptoms.[10]

Hence the possibility of poliomyelitis occurring in vaccinated subjects during a period of epidemic should clearly be considered, and, apart from malicious or simply erroneous interpretations, there is a risk that the vaccine could be incriminated in some cases. But this possibility would be all the more reduced when the vaccination is performed under the best conditions, which are the most favorable to the vaccinal virus in combating the spread of the epidemic. It is necessary to act quickly, i.e., to vaccinate before the epidemic has had time to manifest itself, and, if necessary, to confirm *a posteriori* the reality of the viral spread by examining the stools, sampled before vaccination, of children who have been in contact with the first clinical cases. It is necessary to distribute the first dose within two or three days, at a maximum, no matter what the size of the population requiring vaccination. It is necessary to repeat the vaccinal intake within a short period of time (eight to ten days), a second dose being certainly indispensable and a third dose useful so as to palliate any failures of vaccination not related to the presence of the epidemic strain. Vaccination should be as widespread as possible in view of the rapidity of spread of the epidemic strain, and any dangerous possible sources of infection should be given priority, such as children, especially young children.

Under these circumstances it is certain, although sometimes difficult to prove, that vaccination with a live vaccine is able to stem an epidemic.

Interference by Nonpoliomyelitic Viruses. It is highly probable that the application of strict vaccination will gradually eliminate the problem of competition between the natural and vaccinal poliomyelitis viruses. But there are other viruses which are also capable of preventing the establishment of vaccinal strains.

Ramos-Alvarez et al. were the first to relate the failures of vaccination observed in Mexico[40] to interference phenomena by nonpoliomyelitic enteroviruses. The exact list of viruses other than the poliomyelitis viruses liable to interfere with the live vaccine has not been established. Under certain precise circumstances it has been possible to incriminate the following: Coxsackie B4,[13] Coxsackie B5,[16] Coxsackie A7,[32] ECHO 15,[12] ECHO 12,[35] and others; ECHO 14[22] was not found to be responsible. In fact the problem is extremely complex, as the factors which enable a virus to interfere with a vaccinal strain are linked not only to its individual characteristics, i.e., its type, but also to the stage and standing of the infection, to the number of viral units present, and to the specific reactions of the infected organism. Thus a given virus, if in a phase of intense multiplication, offers resistance to the establishment of the vaccinal strain, whereas it would allow the vaccinal strain to develop normally if it happened to be in its terminal phase of infection. Hence it is extremely difficult to foresee for each individual the chances of establishment of the vaccinal strains, even on the supposition that the distribution of the enteroviruses would be known at the time of the oral intake of the vaccine. Furthermore, not only the enteroviruses but also the adenoviruses are capable of interfering with the vaccinal strain, a fact which eliminates the possibility of choosing the best period for distributing the live vaccine, the spread of the adenoviruses and enteroviruses occurring throughout the year.

In point of fact the practical solution to this extremely complex problem was found to be relatively simple; it suffices, as proved by Sabin in Toluca, to repeat the oral intake of live vaccine at intervals of six to nine weeks.[43] Indeed, between the intakes the nasopharyngeal and intestinal flora have time to become transformed, thus enabling the implantation of the vaccinal strains to take place at the second or third attempt. Thus the general rules for an effective vaccination remain unchanged, and here again we encounter the same principles mentioned at the beginning of this chapter.

Other Causes of Failure. Besides the essential failures due to the phenomena of interference, two other particular facts should be mentioned: the possibility of un-explained failures despite very precise viro-logical investigations and the possibility of immunological unresponsiveness of the new-born infant.

The unexplained failures are reported in studies including systematic examina-tion of the viral flora in nasopharyngeal samples and in stools prior to vaccination and in the days following it. Excretion of the vac-cinal virus is almost nil or very transitory despite the absence of viruses other than the poliomyelitis viruses detectable in tissue culture and by inoculation to newborn mice.[12, 20] These failures are known to occur not only following the intake of live vaccine but also during the spread of natural strains of poliomyelitis. They appear to be temporary, and the subsequent oral intake of live vaccine generally has the desired effect.

The problem with regard to newborn infants is a particular one, since the establish-ment of the vaccinal strain, though it takes place without difficulty in infants who lack a high titer of passive antibodies of maternal origin (≤ 128), nevertheless provokes the ap-pearance of active antibodies in only 40 per cent of the cases. This dissociation between visual multiplication and the immune response may perhaps be explained by a delay in ma-turity; this latter, however, is not constant. It is not due to a phenomenon of immune tolerance, since subsequent attempts at vac-cination with the same techniques succeed; it even probably facilitates immunization by secondary vaccination.[46] As will be seen further on, in the second to third month the infant responds to vaccination with atten-uated vaccine just as well as the older child.

Live attenuated virus vaccines are widely used: since 1959 in the U.S.S.R., Poland, and Hungary; since 1960 in East Germany and Czechoslovakia, Yugoslavia, Albania, and Bulgaria; since 1961 in Rumania, Austria, Switzerland, the United States, and Japan; since 1962 in West Germany and the United Kingdom; since 1963 in Belgium, Italy, and Denmark; and since 1964 in Spain. The morbidity rate for poliomyelitis per 100,000 inhabitants has been less than 0.10

since 1961 in Czechoslovakia, East Germany, and Hungary; since 1962 in Finland; and since 1963 in Poland. But it is particularly interesting to trace the development of this morbidity rate in countries such as the United States, where the inactivated vaccine was first used before the attenuated vaccine was adopted. This morbidity rate, which was over 20 from 1950 to 1954, was seen to decrease gradually to below 2 in 1960; there were 3190 cases in that year. The campaign for vaccination with live vaccine began in 1961, and the morbidity rate then dropped to less than 1; it has remained below 0.10 since 1964, with 121 cases for 1964 and 59 cases for 1965.

THE PLACE OF ANTIPOLIOMYELITIS VACCINATION IN THE VACCINATION CALENDAR

The place of the antipoliomyelitis vac-cination in the vaccination calendar depends on the age at which there is a risk of paralysis by poliomyelitis and also on the possibilities of immunization with the type of vaccine employed.

The risk of paralysis by poliomyelitis may be estimated by studying the data on immunity and the morbidity curves. It is well known that, at birth, a child inherits passive neutralizing antibodies at a titer that is approx-imately the same as that of the mother. The titer of these transmitted antibodies subse-quently decreases, and it is estimated that their half-life is 30 to 45 days, i.e., every 30 to 45 days the titer decreases by half. Hence the duration of protection of the newborn infant depends on the titer of the maternal anti-bodies, which in turn depends on the spon-taneous infections and reinfections which the mother has experienced as well as the vac-cinations received. From a survey performed in the Paris region in 1960-1961, it appeared that, among 75 nonvaccinated pregnant women, the titer of neutralizing antibodies was less than or equal to $1/64$ in 43 subjects with regard to type I, in 32 for type II, and in 50 for type III. It can be deduced that 50 to 60 per cent of their children would no longer be protected against type I or type III from age three months on. We verified this in 25 of these subjects.

In France, in 1957, the year of the highest morbidity from poliomyelitis, there was a total of 4109 cases, 198 of which occurred in children less than one year of age. They were distributed as follows: 5 per cent of the patients were less than three months old, 22 per cent were three to six months, 37 per cent were six to nine months, and 36 per cent were nine to 12 months. Hence already at the age of three months, it is certain, under the epidemiological conditions established in France from 1957 to 1961, that the infant deprived of maternal antibodies begins to run the risk of paralysis, and it is at this age that vaccination should be undertaken. Whether variations of a few weeks may be made in this date depends on whether maternal immunity has been reinforced by antipoliomyelitis vaccination and on the conditions of spread of the natural strains of poliomyelitis. But it appears to be indispensable to protect the child in an active manner as early as possible after birth.

Attempts at vaccination with inactivated vaccine during the first few months of life are countered by the presence of maternal antibodies. In a group of 24 children from five to 48 weeks of age, Hillary observed that in all the children who possessed maternal antibodies to type I at a titer equal to, or higher than, 1/16 vaccination was unsuccessful with regard to this type.[19] However, a booster injection six months later is sufficient in itself to complete vaccination. Perkins[36] obtained identical results, but it should be noted that during the six months following the initial vaccination or preceding the booster injection the children remain poorly protected, and most authors prefer to wait six months and begin poliomyelitis vaccination with an inactivated vaccine that is effective immediately. As far as the attenuated poliomyelitis vaccine is concerned, the presence of maternal antibodies creates a weaker obstacle. It is only when the titer is over 1/128 that this presence becomes an obstacle to acquisition of immunity.[46] Thus this vaccination can be performed as early as the capacity for response of the newborn infant to immunization will allow, i.e., from the second or third month.[9]

Poliomyelitis vaccination should be included in the vaccination calendar of the child without modifying the compulsory protection against other diseases, in particular diphtheria, tetanus, and whooping cough. The triple diphtheria, tetanus, and poliomyelitis vaccine presents no practical problem; each of its constitutents retains the same antigenic capacity as when each is administered separately.

On the other hand, a tetravalent diphtheria, tetanus, poliomyelitis, and whooping cough vaccination presents more difficulties because of the unstable nature of the whooping cough component. The reduction in vaccinating property of the whooping cough component has been calculated by Pittman to be approximately 6 per cent per month.[37] This reduction is far more rapid when the samples are kept in the usual conditions of variable temperature. On the other hand, mixing at the time of injection produces no modification in the quality of the antigens; that is why certain manufacturers have made available materials that, without manipulations, can be mixed in the syringe. The only problem that remains is that of the intrinsic value of the poliomyelitis and whooping cough components.

The attenuated poliomyelitis vaccine can be given at the same time as the mixed diphtheria and tetanus vaccines or the triple diphtheria, tetanus, whooping cough vaccine, by oral administration on the same day as the injection.

BIBLIOGRAPHY

1. Anden, T., and Lycke, E.: An outbreak of poliomyelitis in a partially vaccinated population. The epidemic in Gothenburg in 1961. Acta Path. Microbiol. Scand., *57*:75-80, 1963.
2. Ashkenazi, A. E., and Melnick, J. L.: Poliomyelitis antibody levels of young children in Houston, 1961-1962. Existence of susceptible pockets in an area using Salk vaccine of high effectiveness. Texas Rep. Biol. Med., *20*:550-554, 1962.
3. Bodian, D.: Experimental studies on passive immunization against poliomyelitis. I. Protection with human gamma globulin against intramuscular inoculation and combined passive and active immunization. Amer. J. Hyg., *54*:132-143, 1951.
4. Bodian, D.: Experimental studies on passive immunization against poliomyelitis. II. The prophylactic effect of human gamma globulin on paralytic poliomyelitis in Cynomolgus monkeys after virus feeding. Amer. J. Hyg., *56*:78-89, 1952.
5. Bodian, D.: Experimental studies on passive immunization against poliomyelitis. III. Passive-active immunization and pathogenesis after virus feeding in chimpanzees. Amer. J. Hyg., *58*:81-100, 1953.
6. Brown, G. C.: Immunologic response of infants to combined inactivated measles-poliomyelitis vaccine. Séminaire sur l' Epidémiologie de la rougeole et de la rubéole. Arch. Ges. Virusforsch., *16*: 353-357, 1965.
7. Cabasso, V. J., Nozell, H., Ruegsegger, J. M., and Cox, H. R.: Poliovirus antibody two years after oral trivalent vaccine (Sabin strains). J.A.M.A., *190*:248-250, 1964.
8. Communicable Disease Center: Poliomyelitis Sur-

veillance. United States Public Health Service, 1964.

9. Debré, R., Celers, J., and Drouhet, V.: Vaccination antipoliomyélitique par voie orale avec le vaccine à virus atténués (souches Sabin) à partir de l'âge de 3 mois. C. R. Acad. Sci., *254*:195-199, 1962.

10. Debré, R., et al.: Essai d'interpretation de quelques observations et recherches au cours d'une épidémie de poliomyélite de type I ayant donné lieu à une campagne de vaccination par vaccin vivant homotypique. Bull. WHO, *33*:593-606, 1965.

11. Debré, R., et al.: Implantation et diffusion du vaccin poliomyélitique administré par voie nasale et par voie orale. Bull. Acad. Nat. Med. (Paris), *150*:412-418, 1966.

12. Drouhet, V., et al.: Multiplication dans le tractus digestif des trois souches poliomyélitiques atténuées (type Sabin) aprés vaccination orale. Sa relation avec l'état immunitaire préexistant et la réponse sérologique. Rev. Franc. Etud. Clin. Biol., *10*:381-393, 1965.

13. Feldman, R. A., Holguin, A. H., and Gelfand, H. M.: Oral poliovirus vaccination in children: A study suggesting enterovirus interference. Pediatrics, *33*:526-533, 1964.

14. Fraumenei, J. F., Ederer, F., and Miller, R. W.: An evaluation of the carcinogenicity of SV 40 in man. J.A.M.A., *185*:713-718, 1963.

15. Gard, S.: Vaccination against poliomyelitis in Sweden. Association Européenne de la Poliomyélite et das Maladies Associées. 7th Symposium. Paris, Masson et Cie, 1962, pp. 59-64.

16. Gelfand, H. M., et al.: Intrafamilial and interfamilial spread of living vaccine strains of polioviruses. J.A.M.A., *170*:2039-2048, 1959.

17. Gelfand, H. M., et al.: The spread of living attenuated strains of polioviruses in two communities in Southern Louisiana. Amer. J. Public Health, *50*:767-778, 1960.

18. Hammon, W. M., et al.: Evaluation of Red Cross gamma globulin as a prophylactic agent for poliomyelitis. 4. Final report of results based on clinical diagnosis. J.A.M.A., *151*:1272-1285, 1953.

19. Hillary, I. B.: Antibody response in infants to the poliomyelitis component of a quadruple vaccine. Brit. Med. J., *1*:1098-1102, 1962.

20. Horstmann, D. M., et al.: Viremia in infants vaccinated with oral poliovirus vaccine (Sabin). Amer. J. Hyg., *79*:47-63, 1964.

21. Howe, H. A.: The quantitation of poliomyelitis virus in the human alimentary tract with reference to coexisting levels of homologous serum neutralizing antibody. Amer. J. Hyg. *75*:1-17, 1962.

22. Ingram, V. G.: Behavior of Sabin type 1 attenuated poliovirus in an infant population infected with ECHO 14 virus. Pediatrics, *29*:174-180, 1962.

23. Kawakami, K., Tatsumi, H., Tatsumi, M., and Kono, R.: Studies on poliovirus coproantibody. I. Neutralizing antibodies in feces of children following Sabin oral poliovirus vaccination. Amer. J. Epidemiol., *83*:1-13, 1966.

24. Kono, R., Ikawa, S., Yaoi, H., Hamada, C., Ashirara, Y., and Kawakami, K.: Studies on poliovirus coproantibody. II. Characterization of neutralizing substance in fecal extracts. Amer. J. Epidemiol., *83*:14-23, 1966.

25. Langmuir, A. D.: Inactivated virus vaccines: protective efficacy. In: 5th International Poliomyelitis Conference. Philadelphia, J. B. Lippincott Company, 1961, pp. 105-113.

26. Lipton, M. M., and Steigman, A. J.: Human coproantibody against poliovirus. J. Infect. Dis., *112*: 51-66, 1963.

27. Masson, A. M., Rogala, E., and Rolland, D.: Neutralizing antibodies in faecal extracts during poliomyelitis live vaccine immunization. Canad. J. Public Health, *56*:276-280, 1965.

28. Medical Research Council: Antigenic activity of British poliomyelitis vaccine. Brit. Med. J., *1*: 366-368, 1957.

29. Medical Research Council: Serological response of children to a third dose of poliomyelitis vaccine. Brit. Med. J., *2*:1207-1209, 1957.

30. Miller, D. L., and Galbraith, N. S.: Surveillance of the safety of oral poliomyelitis vaccine in England and Wales, 1962-4. Brit. Med. J., *2*:504-509, 1965.

31. Nathanson, N., and Langmuir, A. D.: The Cutter incident: poliomyelitis following formaldehyde-inactivated poliovirus vaccinations in the United States during the spring of 1955. 1. Background. 2. Relationship of poliomyelitis to Cutter vaccine. 3. Comparison of the clinical character of vaccinated and contact cases occurring after use of high rate lots of Cutter vaccine. Amer. J. Hyg., *78*:16-81, 1963.

32. Netter, R., Drouhet, V., Grist, N. R., and Delpy, J.: Epidémie de poliomyélite de type I en France et emploi du vaccin homotypique (Sabin L Sc 2 ab). III. Etude des virus entériques non poliomyélitiques isolés avant et aprés vaccination. Prédominance du virus Coxsackie A 7. Arch. Ges. Virusforsch., *18*:72-79, 1966.

33. Organisation mondiale de la Santé (World Health Organization): Série de Rapports Techniques Comité d'Experts de la Poliomyélite. Troisième Rapport. Geneva, 1960.

34. Organisation Mondiale de la Santé (World Health Organization): Série de rapports techniques. Normes pour les Substances Biologiques. Rapport d'un Groupe d'Études. Geneva, 1966.

35. Paul, J. R., et al. An oral poliovirus vaccine trial in Costa Rica. Bull. WHO, *26*:311-329, 1962.

36. Perkins, F. T., Yetts, R., and Gaisford, W.: Polio myelitis immunization in infants in the presence of maternally transmitted antibody. Brit. Med. J., *1*:404-406, 1961.

37. Pittman, M.: Instability of pertussis-vaccine component in quadruple antigen vaccine. Diphtheria and tetanus toxoids and pertussis and poliomyelitis vaccines. J.A.M.A., *181*:25-30, 1962.

38. Plotkin, S. A., et al. Persistence of antibodies after vaccination with living attenuated poliovirus. J.A.M.A., *170*:8-12, 1959.

39. Przesmycki, F., and Dobrowolska, H.: A virological and serological poliomyelitis survey in Poland 1963. Association Européenne de la Poliomyélite et des Maladies Associées. 10th Symposium. Paris, Masson et Cie, 1965, pp. 150-153.

40. Ramos-Alvarez, M., Gomez-Santos, F., Rangel, R. L., and Mayes, O.: Viral and serological studies in children immunized with live poliovirus vaccine. Preliminary report of a large trial conducted in Mexico. In: 1st International Conference on Live Poliovirus vaccines. Washington, Pan American Sanitary Bureau, 1959, pp. 483-496.

41. Sabin, A. B.: Behaviour of chimpanzee-avirulent

poliomyelitis viruses in experimentally infected human volunteers. Brit. Med. J., *2*:160-162, 1955.

42. Sabin, A. B.: Properties and behavior of orally attenuated poliovirus vaccine. J.A.M.A., *164*:1216-1223, 1957.
43. Sabin, A. B., et al.: Live, orally given poliovirus vaccine. Effects of rapid mass immunization on population under conditions of massive enteric infection with other viruses. J.A.M.A., *173*:1521-1526, 1960.
44. Sabin, A. B., et al.: Community-wide use of oral poliovirus vaccine. Effectiveness of the Cincinnati program. Amer. J. Dis. Child., *101*:546-567, 1961.
45. Sabin, A. B.: Oral poliovirus vaccine. Recent results and recommendations for optimum use. Roy. Soc. Health J., *82*:51-59, 1962.
46. Sabin, A. B., et al.: Effect of oral poliovirus vaccine in newborn children. I. Excretion of virus after ingestion of large doses of type I or of mixture of all 3 types, in relation to level of placentally transmitted antibody. II. Intestinal resistance and antibody response at 6 months in children fed type I vaccine at birth. Pediatrics, *31*:623-640, 641-650, 1963.
47. Salk, J. E.: Poliomyelitis: Control. In: Rivers, T. M., and Horsfall, F. M. (eds.): Viral and Rickettsial Infections of Man. 3rd ed. Philadelphia, J. B. Lippincott Company, 1959, pp. 499-518.
48. Smorodintsev, A. A., et al.: Results of a study of the reactogenic and immunogenic properties of live antipoliomyelitis vaccine. Bull. WHO, *20*:1053-1074, 1959.
49. Sweet, B. H., and Hilleman, M. R.: Vacuolating Virus SV 40. Proc. Soc. Exp. Biol. Med., *105*:420-427, 1960.
50. Voroshilova, M. K., et al.: Serological survey of children in Moscow for antibody to polioviruses, 1961 and 1962. Bull. WHO, *32*:317-329, 1965.
51. Wehrle, P. F.: Recent developments in the epidemiology of poliomyelitis. Chicago Med. Soc. Bull., *61*:60-66, 1958.
52. Yofe, J., et al.: An outbreak of poliomyelitis in Israël in 1961 and the use of attenuated type 1 vaccine in its control. Amer. J. Hyg., *76*:225-238, 1962.

DISEASES OF THE PERIPHERAL NERVOUS SYSTEM

5

Diseases of the
Peripheral Nervous System

By   S. THIEFFRY

Viruses play but a very small part in the pathology of the peripheral nervous system, and the frequency of primary or secondary viral infections of the central nervous system makes an obvious contrast with the rarity with which similar pathological processes are found in the peripheral nervous system.

The description of the peripheral neuropathy most frequently encountered — radiculoneuritis — will be kept brief, therefore, in order to contrast it with poliomyelitis.

In the great majority of these cases, we find a well-defined illness, characterized by clinical and biological features and by the course it takes. This is the polyradiculoneuritis with clinical recovery, in which the albuminocytological dissociation of Guillain and Barré (1916) is found.

It normally begins without prodromal symptoms, often without fever, and is characterized by paralyses which progress in their extent by fresh attacks on new areas (often ascending extensions of the same lesion). These paralyses are not always complete and are, on the other hand, diffuse and symmetrical and eventually involve the cranial nerves. The tendon reflexes are absent. Disturbances of deep or superficial sensation are often found. From the beginning of the illness, the cerebrospinal fluid is abnormal. A constant observation is the striking increase in albumin without any corresponding

cellular reaction. These cases of radiculoneuritis may threaten life when certain anatomical areas (diaphragm, intercostal muscles, muscles of deglutition) are affected and respiratory function is impaired. Prompt measures of resuscitation have an effect which is disproportionately increased by the fact that the disease has a spontaneous tendency to remit and to resolve without sequel. Thus, the radiculoneuritides of the Guillain-Barré type may be contrasted from every point of view with poliomyelitis, an illness with which they are often confused.

Radiculoneuritis of this type presents, in most cases, as a primary illness without obvious or detectable etiology, in spite of all the research which has been undertaken. In particular, no evidence of a viral etiology has, so far, been given, although it has often been suggested.

However, there exist some cases of viral primary radiculoneuritis different from Guillain-Barré's syndrome in that no albuminocytologic dissociation is encountered. As a matter of fact, there is, in these forms, constant hypercytosis of the cerebrospinal fluid. Some of these forms may be seasonal and epidemic. They have been particularly well studied by Schaltenbrand and Bammer in the Würzburg area. Virological diagnosis was established by the existence of a tick bite at the onset of the disease and of neutralizing antibodies against the virus of Central European spring-summer encephalitis. Lastly, a virus related to but different from this encephalitis virus was isolated in one case from a patient's cerebrospinal fluid and from ticks of that region.

Cases of polyradiculoneuritis have also been reported after monkey bites. They are due to herpes virus simiae (B virus), which was isolated from patients.

Besides these cases of radiculoneuritis in which the peripheral involvement is primary, there exist some uncommon forms occurring in the course of viral diseases such as measles, rubella, chickenpox, vaccinia, herpes zoster, mumps, and infectious hepatitis. Again we must remark, in order to stress even more strongly the rarity of such conditions, that these are more often instances of meningomyeloradiculitis or of encephaloradiculitis than of strictly peripheral involvement.

BIBLIOGRAPHY

1. Guillain, G., Barré, J. A., and Strohl, A.: Sur un syndrome de radiculonévrite avec hyperalbuminose du liquide céphalo-rachidien sans réaction cellulaire. Bull. Soc. Med. Hôp. Paris, *40*:1462-1470, 1916.
2. Schaltenbrand, G., and Bammer, H.: La clinique et le traitement des polynévrites inflammatoires ou séreuses aigues. Rev. Neurol., *115*:753-810, 1966.

ENCEPHALITIDES, ENCEPHALOPATHIES, AND MENINGOENCEPHALITIDES

6

Encephalitides and Encephalopathies Arising in the Course of Virus Infections: General Anatomical Considerations

By E. FARKAS

Anatomical study of the nervous system in patients who had shown signs of encephalitis during the course of virus infections rarely permits an anatomical diagnosis of encephalitis. Usually the lesions discovered on examination of the nervous system are not specific. They consist of acute encephalopathic reactions such as may be observed in the course of infectious diseases with commonplace organisms or during the course of a number of metabolic disorders; there are no traces of inflammatory change.

The presence of inflammatory changes is, however, a prerequisite for the anatomical confirmation of a diagnosis of encephalitis. Furthermore, the present definition of encephalitis is purely anatomical and demands the presence of inflammatory changes in the cerebrospinal axis. On the other hand, inflammatory phenomena may always be found during the course of degenerative or toxic conditions as well as in the center of tumors and in areas of softening of vascular origin.

It is therefore essential to take these inflammatory changes into account with other tissue reactions before deciding whether the inflammation is secondary to some other condition, whether it is symptomatic (Spatz), or whether it is indeed an autonomous inflammatory disease. It is only when a certain amount of independence may be attributed to the inflammatory phenomena that a label of encephalitis is justified. *The viral encephalitides* are, in conformity with the morphological criteria adopted above, inflammatory diseases of the cerebrospinal axis produced by direct action of a virus on neurological tissues. These inflammatory phenomena may spread in the meningeal spaces, resulting in the histological picture of a meningoencephalitis, and in the cord, in which case there is a meningomyeloencephalitis. The neuropathological appearance of these encephalomyelitides varies according to the nature of the pathogenic virus responsible.

Encephalitides agreeing with the current

anatomical definitions (given above) do not necessarily pertain directly to a viral etiology. Thus, *the postinfectious encephalitides of perivenous type* which arise during the course of the exanthemata, influenza, and so forth are apparently related not to the direct action of a virus on the brain but to mechanisms as yet unknown, for which the hypothesis of allergic reaction has been invoked. Moreover, the lesions are invariably identical in these encephalitides, whichever virus may have been the cause of the illness during which they arose.

THE VIRUS ENCEPHALOMYELITIDES SENSU STRICTO

These are characterized by (1) the presence of inflammatory phenomena, (2) the parenchymatous changes resulting from the cytopathogenic effect of the virus, and, finally, (3) the distribution of lesions, which varies in the case of each type of encephalitis.

INFLAMMATORY PHENOMENA

Inflammation of the type described in general anatomopathological terms, adapted to neuropathology by Nissl, Spielmeyer, Spatz, Pette, and Lhermitte, may be considered a process of vascular reaction, more or less localized, with an accompanying glial proliferation.

The vascular reaction process is marked predominantly by an infiltration of the perivascular spaces by elements of mesodermal origin, which sometimes invade the cerebral parenchyma. These cellular perivascular infiltrations are known as "perivascularities." The infiltrating cells are of a number of types: polymorphonuclear leukocytes, lymphocytes, plasmocytes, and histiocytes. Some derive from the circulating blood, having crossed the vascular barrier by diapedesis, and some are formed by proliferation from the vascular adventitia. With this cellular infiltration are often found hyperemia, exudates of plasma or sera, and even gross hemorrhages.

The glial proliferation involves primarily the microglia, cells of reticuloendothelial origin, which adopt characteristic rod cell forms in the proliferating elements. These altered microglia may be looked upon as general reactions of the cerebral mesenchyma. A proliferation of the astrocytes—cells of ectodermal origin—often accompanies that of the microglia. The oligodendroglia play only a small part in these inflammatory phenomena. This glial proliferation may be distributed diffusely in the inflammatory foci or may be localized, in which case it takes on the typical appearance of glial nodules.

LESIONS IN THE PARENCHYMA

Although these alterations may be considered secondary to the inflammatory phenomena in encephalitides of bacterial etiology, they are also seen in viral encephalomyelitis, in which they are a primary feature which may precede the inflammatory changes. These diseases are therefore to be considered not only as protective gliomesodermal processes of a purely inflammatory nature, but also as an expression of a series of direct interactions between the virus and the cerebral parenchyma.

Parenchymal damage is demonstrated, in the main, by neuronal alterations induced by the cytopathic effect of the virus on the nerve cells. These changes may be reversible, such as chromatolysis, or may result in the death of the neuron, which is then engulfed by glial cells whose proliferation around the altered cells produces the typical appearance of a neuronophagic nodule.

In some viral encephalitides, virus proliferation in the nerve cells or in glial cells results in the formation of *intranuclear or intracytoplasmic inclusion bodies*. The acidophilic intranuclear inclusion bodies have been classified by Cowdry into two groups, A and B.

Inclusions of type A, the commonest, are seen in herpes simplex, herpes zoster, cytomegalic inclusion disease, some of the exanthemata, and panencephalitis (the viral origin of which is as yet uncertain). They occupy part or all of the nucleus, crowding out the nucleolus and the chromatin against the nuclear membrane; they are often surrounded by a clear halo. Their structure seen under the light microscope is sometimes homogeneous, sometimes granular. Morgan and his colleagues, using the electron microscope, have studied such inclusions appearing in the course of infections with herpes virus and have shown that the homogeneous forms are packed with virus particles, while these are not present in the granular forms. Brihaye, working with histochemical methods, considers that only the young homogeneous inclusion bodies are rich in

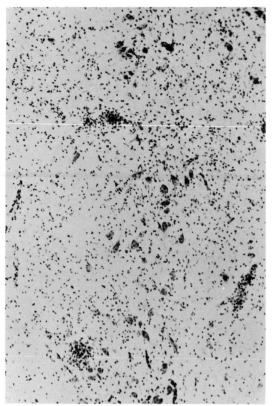

Figure 6-1. Encephalomyelitis (probably of Central European type). Photomicrograph of locus niger showing neuronophagic nodules, diffuse glial proliferation, and "perivascularites." Nissl's stain.

Figure 6-2. Encephalomyelitis (probably of Central European type). Photomicrograph of occipital cortex, showing glial proliferation in the deep layers of the cortex. Nissl's stain × 55.

nucleic acid. We may therefore conclude that these inclusions do not indicate strongly the presence of living virus particles in the cell and that they can represent only one type of cellular reaction—a degenerative cellular reaction following virus attack.

Type B inclusion bodies are sometimes multiple. They are homogeneous in appearance, spherical, and on account of their small size do not push back the nucleolus. Their presence has been observed in poliomyelitis in monkeys and, above all, in experimental equine encephalomyelitis. The viral nature of these latter inclusions is debated.

Finally, there are specific acidophilic intracytoplasmic inclusions—the Negri bodies described in rabies. Sourander could not demonstrate the presence of nucleic acids in these bodies by histochemical methods, and this author concluded that these represent, quite simply, a cytoplasmic reaction to virus infection.

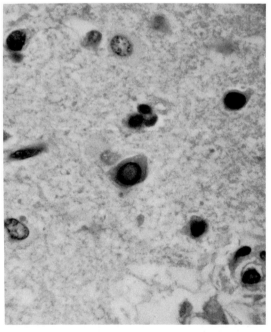

Figure 6-3. Subacute sclerosing leukoencephalitis. Photomicrograph of cortex showing an intranuclear inclusion body of Cowdry's type A in the nucleus of an affected neuron, with the chromatin pushed out to the periphery of the nucleus. Hematoxylin and eosin × 1600.

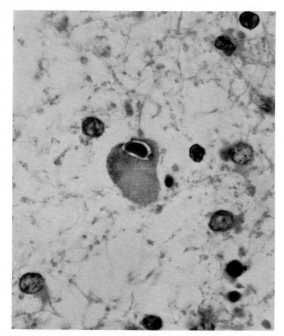

Figure 6-4. Cytomegalic inclusion disease. Photomicrograph of amygdaloid nucleus, showing an intranuclear inclusion body, surrounded by a clear halo and small intracytoplasmic inclusion bodies, in a hypertrophied neuron. Hematoxylin and eosin × 1600.

DISTRIBUTION OF LESIONS

The great affinity of viruses for neurons explains why the lesions in most of the virus encephalomyelitides known at present are localized essentially at the level of the gray matter—the center of the neurons—and are therefore *polioencephalitides.*

Poliomyelitis, other enterovirus diseases of the nervous system, rabies, herpes B encephalitis, or arthropod-borne encephalitides, such as St. Louis encephalitis, Japanese B encephalitis, louping ill, Murray Valley encephalitis, Central European encephalitis, Russian spring-summer encephalitis, Far-East encephalitis, and to a lesser degree the equine encephalitides, are, in fact, polioencephalitides.

But these viruses do not possess identical affinities for all the neurons of the nervous system. Thus, lesions are not found everywhere throughout the gray matter, and in each one of the polioencephalitides an individual pattern of lesions occurs which is more or less characteristic.

An anatomical survey of the lesions often enables us to attach a diagnostic label

to the encephalitis under observation. Thus, for example, in poliomyelitis the anterior horn cells are preferentially attacked, while those of the cortex and central gray nuclei are typically affected in Japanese encephalitis, and those of the locus Niger in von Economo's encephalitis (for which a virus has not yet been identified).

This localization of pathological changes to a particular area, differing for each virus under study, probably depends upon the metabolic structure of the nervous tissues (Seitelberger). Biochemical, histochemical, and cytochemical research in recent years has shown that in fact there exists a complex biochemical structure in the nervous system, varying from one formation to another, which is modified during the course of maturation and corresponds, on the whole, to the anatomical and functional structures which have been delineated by classical histological and neurophysiological studies.

Parenchymatous lesions may sometimes preferentially affect the white substance and lead to demyelinization, a condition which is then known as *leukoencephalitis,* or the lesions may affect the gray and white matter simultaneously, in which case the condition is known as *panencephalitis.*

The only panencephalitides in which a viral etiology is now recognized without doubt are herpes encephalitis, in which the lesions are found in the temporobasal cortex and in the underlying white matter, and, to a lesser degree, Western equine encephalitis, in which the lesions can be found also in the white matter (on the whole, however, areas of necrosis secondary to patches of arteritis are more constantly observed in the course of this disease, rather than parenchymatous changes directly resulting from the original viral infection).

There remains a group of panencephalitides such as acute necrotizing encephalitis and the subacute sclerosing leukoencephalitis of Van Bogaert, nowadays identified with the inclusion encephalitis described by Dawson—the viral origin of which, although likely, has not yet been definitely established. These diseases are described in another chapter.

One must always remember that the parenchymatous damage suffered during viral encephalitis, whether in neurons or in myelin sheaths, is not always due to the cytopathogenic effect of the virus. The damage may be mediated just as effectively by disturbances in vascular permeability and by the hemodynamic alterations inherent in inflammatory processes. In this case, there are inflammatory necroses of a secondary type, such as are observed in bacteriological encephalitis. These secondary parenchymatous necroses may interfere with the specific distribution of the lesions of the virus encephalitis and may often obscure the picture.

DIFFUSE MENINGOENCEPHALITIDES

These meningoencephalitides are purely inflammatory diseases of the central nervous system in which, by contrast with encephalomyelitis, as defined, lesions in the parenchyma are totally lacking. Inflammatory phenomena are here found only in the cerebral mesenchyma (that is to say, the meninges and blood vessels), which is infiltrated by lymphocytes and also by plasmocytes. Glial proliferation is absent or is, in general, moderate. The attack on the meninges, in these conditions, is probably a primary phenomenon, and invasion of the nervous tissues is secondary to spread along the vascular arborizations.

These lymphocytic meningoencephalitides were described long ago by von Economo, then by Jellinger and Seitelberger, and by Macchi and his colleagues in the course of epidemics of influenza, of infectious mononucleosis, and also of certain enterovirus infections. Similarly, they were able to demonstrate the neuropathological picture of rubella encephalitis and of measles encephalitis (Adams and colleagues). The onset of these meningoencephalitides has been discussed; sometimes they appear as primary virus illnesses (Jacob) and sometimes as secondary manifestations of a recognized infection.

It seems, therefore, that the purely inflammatory nature of encephalitis, in the absence of any parenchymatous lesion, does not exclude the possibility of a direct viral etiology. Much work suggests that inflammatory phenomena and parenchymatous lesions, although both determined by the presence of virus in nervous tissue, do not result from identical physiopathological mechanisms.

Thus, the work of Sabin (using immunofluorescent techniques) demonstrated con-

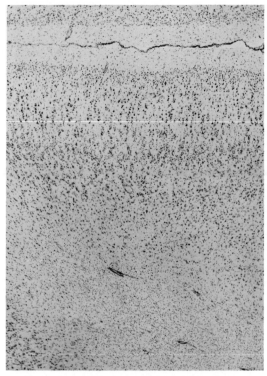

Figure 6-5. Infectious mononucleosis. Photomicrograph of cortex, showing widespread lymphocytic meningoencephalitis, with inflammatory infiltration of the meninges and in the perivascular spaces. Nissl's stain × 80.

vincingly that herpes virus was able to multiply in neurons which showed no cellular abnormality and that the distribution of inflammatory and necrotic lesions bore no relation to that of the virus. This spatial dissociation between parenchymatous lesions and inflammatory phenomena is also found in numerous encephalomyelitides, in poliomyelitis for example (see Chapter 1A). The study of multifocal leukoencephalopathy described by Aström et al. yields, in this respect, valuable data. This demyelinating disease—in which there is no evidence of an inflammatory process—occurs in patients suffering from Hodgkin's disease, lymphosarcoma, lymphoid or myeloid leukemia, or carcinomatosis, or in very aged patients. The viral origin of this disease has been demonstrated by Zu Rhein and Chou, who produced electron microscopic evidence for the presence of a virus of the papova group in the intraglial inclusion bodies commonly encountered in this disease. It seems, therefore, that in these patients the absence of inflammation indicates an immunological incompetence, or even an abatement of allergic reactions, a weakness which allows viruses which are normally nonpathogenic for the human nervous system to reach the brain and produce a cytopathic effect, visible at the level of the glial cells.

In the light of these observations, inflammatory changes appear therefore as immunologic phenomena, determined by the presence of virus but different in their mechanism from the viral cytopathic effects.

POSTINFECTIOUS ENCEPHALITIS OF THE PERIVENOUS TYPE

This disease, which carries the name of perivenous leukoencephalopathy, follows Jennerian vaccination, exanthematous diseases in childhood, influenza, infectious mononucleosis, and also vaccination against rabies. The perivenous encephalitides occupy an anatomical level which is always the same, whatever has been the cause of the infection during which they appeared. Microglial proliferation, perivenous demyelinization, and a preferential localization of the lesions in the white substance of the brain characterize this condition (see Chapter 9, under the heading General Anatomical Observations).

These encephalitides have been considered to have a neuroallergic etiology, not merely for clinical and virological reasons (see Chapter 9) but also on grounds of similarity between the anatomical picture in the postinfectious encephalitides and that of the accidents occurring during vaccination against rabies. Remlinger, as far back as 1929, suspected that the source of these accidents lay in the injected material which forms the substrate of the rabies virus, that is to say, nervous tissue, since the lesions observed were not those of rabies virus infection.

The experiences of Rivers and Schwentker, Ferraro and Jervis, Kabat et al., and Halpern et al. have confirmed this point of view, as these authors have been able to reproduce in the animal the exact lesions of perivenous encephalitis by repeated injections of brain substance with Freund's adjuvant.

It is but a small step to the conclusion that postinfectious encephalitis denotes an allergic type of reaction of the nervous tissues to viral allergens. As the lesions of experimental allergic encephalomyelitis vary according to the type of experimental animal, the applications of experimental observations to human pathology remain rather tentative. Study of the early lesions of experimental allergic encephalitis (Waksman and Adams) shows that a perivenous infiltration of mononuclear cells forms the first stage of the illness

(Text continued on Page 120)

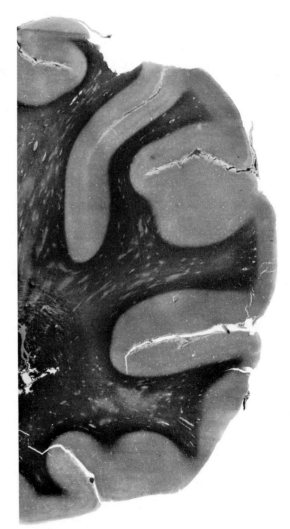

Figure 6-6. Perivenous encephalitis. Close-up photograph of cerebral hemisphere, showing an area of perivascular demyelination. Loyez' stain.

Table 6-1. *Diseases or Infections Common to all Countries in Which the Etiological Agent is Known.*

Associated Disease or Infection		Virus Recovered from the Central Nervous system or Cerebrospinal Fluid*	Anatomical Features		
Clinical Diagnosis	*Responsible Virus*		*Type*	*Distribution*	*Inclusion Bodies in the Central Nervous System*
Poliomyelitis	Poliovirus types I, II, III	+	(1) Meningomyeloencephalitis	(1) Gray matter (anterior horn cells of spinal cord and dorsal part of the brain stem)	No
	ECHO viruses types 2, 9, 11	+	(1) Meningomyeloencephalitis (2) Meningomyeloencephalitis		No
	Coxsackie A viruses types 2, 7, 9	+			No
	Coxsackie B viruses types 1, 5	+	(2) Meningomyeloencephalitis	(2) Widespread in the gray matter	No
Herpes	Herpes virus hominis	+	Necrotizing encephalitis	Widespread, mainly in the temporal lobes	Intranuclear
Cytomegalic inclusion disease	Cytomegalovirus	+	Encephalitis	Mainly observed around the ventricles	Intranuclear and intracytoplasmic
Mumps	Mumps virus	+	3 possible aspects but very few anatomical descriptions: (1) Postinfectious leukoencephalitis of perivenous type (2) Lymphocytic meningoencephalitis (3) Acute encephalopathy		No
Influenza	Influenza virus	+ (Type A)		(1) White matter (perivenous distribution) (2) Widespread	No
Measles	Measles virus	−	3 possible aspects in order of frequency:		No

Disease	Virus	Virus isolation	Anatomical forms	Distribution of lesions	Inclusion bodies
Chickenpox (Varicella)	Zoster-varicella virus	—	(1) Postinfectious leukoencephalitis of perivenous type; (2) Acute encephalopathy (especially during the first two years of life); (3) Meningoencephalitis	(1) Mainly in the white matter; perivenous and subcortical distribution; cerebellar predominance in chickenpox, spinal cord predominance in measles and vaccinia. (3) Widespread	(N.B. Inclusion bodies have been described, but without any virological confirmation.) No (N.B. Inclusion bodies have been observed in posterior root ganglia.)
Smallpox (Variola)	Smallpox (variola) virus				No
Vaccinia	Vaccinia virus	(Recoveries of virus during vaccinial septicemia)			No
Rubella	Rubella virus	Recoveries of virus in cases of congenital rubella	3 possible presentations, but very few anatomical descriptions: (1) Meningoencephalitis (2) Postinfectious leukoencephalitis of perivenous type (3) Acute encephalopathy	(1) Widespread (2) White matter (perivenous distribution)	No
Adenovirus infection	Adenovirus	(Type 7a)	2 possible aspects but very few anatomical descriptions: (1) Acute encephalopathy (2) Meningoencephalitis	(2) Widespread	No

*Viruses not yet isolated in situ or not related to the central nervous system lesions.

Table 6-2. *Diseases or Infections Occurring in Particular Climatic Zones, Regions, or Living Conditions and in Which the Etiological Agent is Known*

ASSOCIATED DISEASE OR INFECTION		VIRUS RECOVERED FROM CENTRAL NERVOUS SYSTEM TISSUE OR FROM CEREBROSPINAL FLUID*	ANATOMICAL FEATURES		
Clinical Diagnosis	*Responsible Virus*		*Type*	*Distribution*	*Inclusion Bodies in the Central Nervous System*
Rabies	Rabies virus	+	Encephalomyelitis	Gray matter (Ammon's horn)	Intracytoplasmic (Negri bodies)
Vaccination against rabies	??	−	Postinfectious leukoencephalitis of perivenous type	White matter (perivenous distribution)	No
Epidemic equine encephalitides	Arbovirus group A				
Venezuelan	Vee virus	−	Encephalomyelitis	Gray matter, but with some lesions in the white matter in the case of Vee	No

Disease	Virus				
Western	WEE virus	+			No
Eastern	EEE virus	+			No
Other epidemic encephalitides	Arbovirus group B				
St. Louis encephalitis	SLE virus	+	See following table	See following table	No
Japanese B encephalitis	JE virus	+			No
Murray Valley	MVE virus	+		Gray matter (mainly in the cortex and the basal ganglia in the case of JE, and in the anterior horn cells of the spinal cord and in the brain stem in the case of central European encephalitis).	No
West Nile	WN virus	−	Encephalomyelitis		No
Tick-borne (or central European spring-summer)	TBE virus	+			No
Louping Ill	Louping Ill virus	+			No
Herpes B encephalitis	Herpes virus B (or simian herpes virus)	+	Encephalomyelitis	Widespread	Intranuclear
Lymphocytic choriomeningitis	LCM virus	+	Lymphocytic meningo-encephalitis	Widespread	No

*Virus not yet isolated in situ or not related to the central nervous system lesions.

Table 6-3. *Diseases in Which the Etiological Agent, Presumed To Be Viral, Has Not Yet Been Identified*

Associated Disease or Infection	Morphological or Virological Features Suggesting a Viral Lesion of the Central Nervous System	Anatomical Features		
Clinical Diagnosis	*Responsible Virus*	*Type*	*Distribution*	*Inclusion Bodies in the Central Nervous System*
Exanthem subitum	?	2 possible types:		No
		(1) Postinfectious leuko-encephalopathy of perivenous type	White matter (perivenous distribution)	
		(2) Acute encephalopathy		
Infectious mononucleosis	?	Meningoencephalitis	Widespread	No
Cat-scratch disease	?	Encephalopathy (very few anatomical descriptions)		No

Encephalitis lethargica	?	0 (Herpes virus recovered ?)	Encephalomyelitis	Gray matter, predominantly in the mesencephalon, especially in the locus niger	No
Van Bogaert's subacute sclerosing encephalitis	?	Virus-like particles seen on electron microscopy	Encephalitis	Widespread, mainly in the white matter	Intranuclear (inconstant)
Acute necrotizing encephalitis	?	Isolation of herpes simplex virus in 1/3 of cases	Meningo-encephalitis	Widespread, mainly in the gray matter	Intranuclear (inconstant)
In the course of chronic infections in patients with immunological deficiency syndromes.	?	Particles resembling papovaviruses in glial cells visible on electron microscopy	Multifocal Leukoencephalopathy	White matter	Intranuclear inclusions in glial cells
Kuru	?	Disease passed to chimpanzees by inoculation of human brain		Distribution similar to the group of diseases typified by hereditary cerebellar ataxia	No

and that demyelinization is confined strictly to those parenchymal zones which have been infiltrated by these cellular elements. It is interesting to observe that the lesions of Hurst's hemorrhagic leukoencephalitis, generally considered to be a subacute variety of postinfectious encephalitis, are identical with the early lesions of experimental allergic encephalitis. Some recent findings throw new light on the relationships existing between viral infection, inflammation, and allergic reactions.

Hotchin has observed that the intracerebral injection of lymphocytic-choriomeningitis virus produces no histological changes in newborn mice or in adult mice who were thymectomized at birth. In these mice, histological lesions of an inflammatory type appear when lymphocytes from normal adult mice are injected. It seems, therefore, that lymphocytic choriomeningitis may be considered an allergic disease, in spite of the presence of virus in the brain, and that the inflammatory changes demonstrate this allergic reaction. The pathological changes observed in the encephalitides, whether primary or secondary to a recognized infection, are always considered, therefore, to be controlled by, although in variable propor-

tions, the direct effect of the virus on the one hand and host reactions on the other.

ACUTE ENCEPHALOPATHIES OCCURRING IN THE COURSE OF VIRUS INFECTIONS

The acute encephalopathies are essentially functional cerebral syndromes in which no inflammatory changes can be seen. Those anatomical changes which can be observed in these syndromes are devoid of any specificity and are most frequently determined by cerebral edema. This shows itself by an increase in the weight of the brain, flattening of the convolutions, temporal and tonsillar hernia with collapse of the ventricles, and, on histological examination, spongiosis of the white matter and engorgement of the meninges and perivascular spaces by acellular exudates. Less frequently, congestion of the blood vessels and hemorrhages dominate the neuropathological picture—changes which were formerly known under the title of hemorrhagic encephalitis. Nonspecific degenerative changes of the neurons may be seen; these sometimes have an anoxic type of distribu-

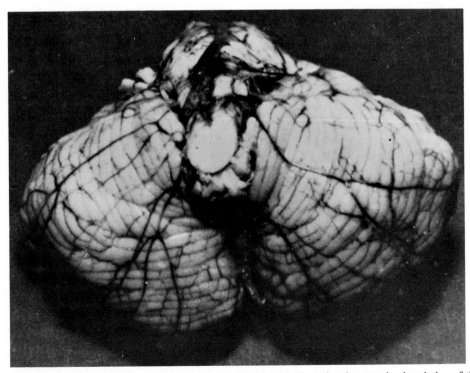

Figure 6-7.   Acute encephalopathy. Close-up photograph of cerebellum showing massive herniation of the amygdaloid bodies.

Figure 6-8. Acute encephalopathy. Photomicrograph of corpus callosium, showing edema and spongiosis in the white matter. Hematoxylin and eosin × 75.

tion. The glial reaction is generally moderate. The changes observed demonstrate a pathological process which affects both permeability and tone of the cerebral vessels.

Sometimes, in spite of a dramatic clinical picture, no anatomical changes may be noticed.

The encephalopathic reaction is found very frequently in small infants. Indeed, it is the only postinfectious cerebral manifestation which is seen at that age after Jennerian vaccination and the exanthemata. It may, in the same way, come on in the course of other virus infections, such as mumps, influenza, and adenovirus infections, and, by the same token, in infectious diseases caused by bacteria (scarlet fever, whooping cough).

The etiology of these complications of virus infections which have an encephalopathic nature is unknown. The possibility has been put forward that microbial toxins cause these disturbances in the course of other infectious diseases; as a result several writers, such as Lyon et al., have used the term "acute toxic encephalopathy" to describe these conditions.

BIBLIOGRAPHY

1. Aström, K. E., Mancall, E. L., and Richardson, E. P., Jr.: Progressive multifocal leuko-encephalopathy; a hitherto unrecognized complication of chronic lymphatic leukaemia and Hodgkin's disease. Brain, *81*:93-111, 1958.
2. Brihaye, J.: Etude des encéphalites herpétiques et des encéphalites nécrosantes aiguës. Acta Neur. Psychiat. Belg., *59*:1-114, 1959.
3. Cowdry, E. V.: Problem of intranuclear inclusions in virus diseases. Arch. Path., *18*:527-542, 1934.
4. Dawson, J. R., Jr.: Cellular inclusions in cerebral lesions of lethargic encephalitis. Amer. J. Path., *9*:7-16, 1933.
5. Ferraro, A., and Jervis, G. A.: Experimental disseminated encephalopathy in monkey. Arch. Neur. Psychiat., *43*:195, 1940.
6. Halpern, B. N., Bertrand, I., and Lhermitte, F.: L'encéphalomyélite allergique expérimentale. Presse Med., *58*:684-687, 1950.
7. Jacob, H.: Neuropathology of virus diseases of the central nervous system. Deutsch. Z. Nervenheilk., *182*:472-491, 1961.
8. Kabat, E. A., Wolf, A., and Bezer, A. E.: Rapid production of acute disseminated encephalomyelitis in rhesus monkeys by injection of brain tissue with adjuvants. Science, *104*:362-363, 1946.
9. Lhermitte, F.: Les leucoencéphalites. Paris, Editions Medicales Flammarion, 1950.
10. Lyon, G., Dodge, P. R., and Adams, R. D.: The acute encephalopathies of obscure origin in infants and children. Brain, *84*:680-708, 1961.
11. Macchi, G., et al.: *In* Symposium Anvers, 1959.
12. Morgan, C., Ellison, S. A., Rose, H. M., and Moore, D. H.: Electron microscopic examination of inclusion bodies of herpes simplex virus. Proc. Soc. Exp. Biol. Med., *82*:454-457, 1953.
13. Nissl, F.: *In:* Histol. Histopath. Arb. Jana, 1904.
14. Pette, H., and Kalm, H.: *In:* Hdb. d. Inneren Med. Berlin, Springer-Verlag, 1953.
15. Remlinger, P.: C.R. Soc. Biol., pp. 82-1098, 1919.
16. Rivers, T. M., and Schwentker, F. F.: Encephalomyelitis accompanied by myelin destruction experimentally produced in monkeys. J. Exp. Med., *61*:689-702, 1935.
17. Sabin, A. B.: Fatal B virus encephalomyelitis in a physician working with monkeys. J. Clin. Invest., *28*:808, 1949 (abstract).
18. Spatz, H.: *In:* Hdb. d. Geisteskr. Berlin, Springer-Verlag, 1930.
19. Spielmeyer, W.: *In:* Histop. des Nervensystems. Berlin, Springer-Verlag, 1922.
20. Van Bogaert, L.: Une leucoencéphalite sclérosante subaiguë. J. Neurol. Neurosurg. Psychiat., *8*: 101-120, 1945.
21. Waksman, B. H., and Adams, R. D.: A histologic study of the early lesion in experimental allergic encephalomyelitis in the guinea pig and rabbit. Amer. J. Path., *41*:135-162, 1962.
22. Zu Rhein, G. M., and Chou, S. M.: Assoc. Res. Nerv. Ment. Dis., 1968, in press.

7

The Clinical Diagnosis of the Encephalitides and Acute Encephalopathies Occurring in the Course of the Common Virus Infections of Childhood

By S. THIEFFRY

Study of the central nervous system accidents that may occur in the course of virus infections is not easy. Before describing them in detail, let us outline their exact limits, their nature, and their general clinical manifestations.

These disorders are generally described together under the name of encephalitides, meningoencephalitides, or, if one has reason to believe that the spinal cord is also involved, encephalomyelitides.

These accidents are particularly likely to occur in children. This obvious preference is easily explained. First, the common viral infections, in particular the exanthemata, are contracted predominantly in childhood. Second, the child's brain, because of its immaturity, is vulnerable to damage from extrinsic or intrinsic insults that would be inconsequential at another age.

The pediatrician thus frequently finds himself confronted with acute cerebral accidents of sudden onset occurring in a child who has normally been in good health and free from chronic infection of the nervous system; these events may or may not follow a definite infectious disease.

These dramatic acute cerebral accidents include varying proportions of disturbances of consciousness, convulsions, signs of a diffuse or localized attack on the nervous system (upper or lower motor neuron lesions, extrapyramidal syndrome, cerebellar signs), and possibly psychic disturbances. In this general picture of acute or subacute cerebral injury, disturbances of consciousness and convulsions usually dominate the scene.

Faced with an acute cerebral syndrome which compromises communicative function in such an abrupt fashion and often alters vegetative function irremediably, when the etiological circumstances render an infectious etiology likely, the physician often thinks of the term encephalitis and, for want of a better diagnosis, the diagnosis of encephalitis is made.

This approach is not correct. However little one studies these situations, it is easy to demonstrate that, in fact, not every acute cerebral syndrome is encephalitis. On the contrary — and we must insist on this — such a picture has little chance of reflecting an authentic encephalitis. Encephalitis is a very rare disease, in spite of an erroneous opinion which is too widely spread among medical men. Clinical-anatomical study shows that most of these acute cerebral syndromes are provoked by completely different factors from encephalitis: diffuse circulatory disturbances, vascular alterations, and status epilepticus. It is better to apply the term acute encephalopathy to this clinical picture if one does not wish to empty the term encephalitis of its precise meaning.

In the strict sense of the word, encephalitis, whatever its etiology, is produced by inflammatory lesions of the cerebral parenchyma. Their aspect is described in Chapter 4. The lesions of encephalitis always include two essential elements: an inflammatory perivascular exudate, and a microglial proliferation which may be diffuse or localized. Thus encephalitis possesses an anatomical mark of differentiation. It is one of the modes of reaction of the brain to external insult, usually infectious.

With this process we must contrast others which compromise the blood supply of the brain, the intracranial circulation, and which reflect a general or local humoral disequilibrium, giving rise to functional difficulties or to lesions which do not possess any inflammatory element. They may be described separately under the term "encephalopathy."

This distinction is of prime importance. To confuse all the febrile encephalopathies under the term of "encephalitis" not only constitutes a nosological error but also may lead to prognostic and therapeutic errors which might have serious consequences.

To approach the problem of the acute encephalitides of childhood (as we have just defined them), we must remember, first that they are illnesses which are, at present, rare or very rare in Western Europe and that they correspond to a precise anatomical phenomenon, inflammation of the cerebral parenchyma. What complicates the diagnosis of encephalitis for the clinician is the absence of specificity in the clinical picture throughout or at least at the beginning of the evolution. This makes them difficult to distinguish from the functional encephalopathies, which are frequent in the course of infectious diseases of childhood and may, moreover, be associated with true encephalitides.

Diagnosis is particularly difficult and is very often gainsaid by the anatomical findings when an acute cerebral syndrome appears *de novo* without any clear hint as to its etiology.

In the absence of circumstantial evidence or of indisputable virological evidence, the clinical diagnosis of encephalitis at present remains only a probability, from which arises the major interest of undertaking clinical, epidemiological, and virological research in this domain.

The problem is, in principle, easier to resolve when the cerebral accident occurs during and as a complication of an infectious disease, often an exanthem. Encephalitis is then a well-recognized possibility. Nevertheless, even in circumstances favorable to the clinician, caution must prevail, for not all the "parainfectious" cerebral accidents are attributable to specific perivenous encephalitis.

Even though encephalitis has long been acknowledged and justly held to be the main cause of these acute cerebral accidents, today we know that a noninflammatory encephalopathic process shares with this true encephalitis the responsibility.

The outline and warning given in the preceding paragraphs bring out the complexity of the problem. The necessity to reserve for the term encephalitis a precise clinical and anatomical significance might almost forbid the clinician from diagnosing this disease during the lifetime of the patient. This is of course absurd. Fortunately the diagnosis may be made more or less confidently according to circumstances. We will see, for example, that the clinical picture of certain encephalitides secondary to an infectious state is sometimes characteristic enough.

In contrast, this is not so when the acute cerebral syndrome appears clinically as the primitive disease. The physician is then confronted with an isolated cerebral syndrome of brutal onset which may correspond to diverse pathogenic processes. The illness evolves for a number of days, during which it may be possible to carry out objective neurological examinations, to obtain biological reports, and to analyze electroencephalographic tracings. Facets in the clinical picture become clearer in the course of the disease, and certain symptomatological groupings appear. Opinion on the precise nature of a cerebral accident may then crystallize, little by little, after some days spent in collecting pieces of information, in treating symptoms, and in methodically correcting all the metabolic abnormalities which may be met.

It is from this pragmatic viewpoint that we must begin the study of acute cerebral syndromes, if we wish not to remain content with an impression alone but to make sure of the necessary factual knowledge. We must remember that, during the initial period, the clinical picture is more or less the same, whether the disease is encephalopathy or encephalitis. Also to be kept in mind is the fact that an encephalopathy is much more likely than an authentic primary encephalitis. A last point not to be lost from sight is that often enough the diagnosis of encephalitis will be made or confirmed only retrospectively by elimination after all possible hypotheses have been examined critically. It is always from this practical viewpoint of the clinician that we outline the general character of the *encephalopathies* in contrast with those of the *encephalitides*.

The encephalopathies are provoked by a great variety of processes: toxic states, general metabolic disorders (in particular, hypo- or hyperosmolarity of the plasma), infectious vasculitis (arteritis or cerebral phlebitis). But above all, they may express an explosive vasomotor reaction to a variety of pathogenic agents or factors involving the whole cerebral circulatory system and giving a true diffuse circulatory encephalosis. This last type is the only one which deserves to be studied and described in this chapter dedicated to the cerebral manifestations of virus diseases.

Circulatory encephalosis and encephalitis are the two principal aspects of the cerebral accidents which occur with human virus infections. Particularly good examples of this double response are observed in measles and vaccinia.

If genuine encephalitis is due in the first place to a viral disease—which is, in fact, the sole known cause—circulatory encephalosis is in itself only a mode of reaction proper to the nervous system of the child and without etiological specificity. It is an anatomico-clinical syndrome produced by a reaction to very diverse insults, among which may be found virus infections.

DEFINITIONS

CIRCULATORY ENCEPHALOPATHY

The syndrome of circulatory encephalopathy occurs predominantly during the first years of life and is by far the most frequent cause of the acute cerebral syndromes. It has been described under the names of "acute encephalopathy of indeterminate origin," "acute toxic encephalopathy," "primary acute circulatory encephalopathy," or "acute hemodynamic brain," or under the unfortunate title of "congestive hemorrhagic

encephalitis in the course of the infections of infancy." In fact, it manifests clinically as a process of dilatation of the entire cerebrovascular tree (circulatory encephalopathy) and gross edema of the whole brain, which is often herniated through the foramen magnum and the temporal cleft (the weight of the brain increases by 15 to 25 per cent). Histologically, spongiosis of the white matter and perivascular exudates devoid of cells are found, together with anoxic changes of the nerve cells. But we do not find any inflammatory element which permits us to speak of encephalitis.

The onset is extremely sudden, whether it occurs in a completely healthy patient or during or after a transient insignificant infection. From the onset, fever, coma, severe and subintrant convulsions, or status epilepticus are associated with this condition.

Neurological signs are inconstant or diminished, never localized. The spinal fluid shows only minor abnormalities. The optic fundus is sometimes abnormal.

In the electroencephalogram, the normal rhythm is replaced by diffuse slow waves of large amplitude without signs of particular localization, and the tracing flattens very rapidly until all electrical activity disappears. Death occurs within a few days by collapse, without any remission.

Patients with this syndrome may possibly survive, but with very severe neuropsychiatric sequelae.

The cause for this illness is not usually found. Without doubt, this syndrome has been shown to be linked to a viral cause in some cases (measles, vaccinia, adenovirus infection) and systemic virological research would be desirable. Its characteristic and always unique appearance and its relentless progress, scarcely modified by any treatment, enable one to contrast it fairly clearly with encephalitis, either immediately after the onset of illness or, at most, after a few days.

ACUTE ENCEPHALITIS

The acute encephalitides normally commence with convulsions, abnormalities of consciousness, or psychiatric disturbances of rapid onset. Headache and meningism are frequent. Fever is usual and may precede neurological signs by several days. Not uncommonly, convulsions and neurological signs are localized (e.g., hemiplegia).

After a few days, the picture becomes clearer and changes: abnormalities of consciousness, obnubilation, coma, extension of neurological signs, appearance of fresh motor signs (pyramidal, extrapyramidal, cerebellar) or psychological signs (delirium, confusion, excitement). All this symptomatology is curiously variable and so confirms the impression of an evolving diffuse cerebral disease.

Usually, or at least in the early stages, infectious signs are present. The spinal fluid is rarely normal, and a moderate lymphocytosis and elevation of the protein level in the cerebrospinal fluid are usual. The level of sugar remains normal.

The electroencephalogram gives information which is not specific but is useful in the differential diagnosis. Taken as a whole, the tracings are always bilaterally abnormal and diffuse during the first days, overcharged with spikes of high voltage. These tend to become more regular, at least for short periods, and sometimes even suggest focal discharges. But the tracing varies from one case to another and also from one day to another in the course of the same illness. This is a very important sign in the diagnosis of encephalitis, as it differs from the constant and inexorable deterioration found in circulatory encephalopathy.

We must add that in other encephalopathies (of metabolic origin, for example) the tracing quickly returns to its normal character once the cerebral functions have been reestablished. In encephalitis, on the other hand, the tracing, weeks and months later, still shows abnormalities or demonstrates epileptic foci.

The course of encephalitis is very variable and defies prognosis. The period of severe illness is usually about ten days, after which it is not uncommon to see the illness terminate or improve. This period also marks the point after which it is uncommon to observe fresh neurological manifestations.

On the other hand, however, the course of the disease is often fatal after a few days or months, and the designation of "acute" is applicable more to the mode of onset than to the duration of the illness, which is often prolonged, thanks to present-day methods of resuscitation. The use of these methods is warranted because spectacular transformation of the situation can occur after all hope of recovery has been abandoned; recovery may eventually occur in favorable cases, however severe the initial illness appeared.

Motor or mental sequelae or convulsions may occur; they may be very selective, as, for example, disturbances of memory.

The general picture of acute encephalitis which we have shown indicates that diagnosis may be made on a number of points. Its features have been contrasted with those of circulatory encephalopathy in so far as these concern the mode of onset, the major signs, the course, and the results of clinicobiological examinations (cerebrospinal fluid, electroencephalogram).

These two types of illness may be encountered in the pathology of virus diseases of the brain, either disclosing a viral infection, which will be then particularly difficult to identify without the help of specialized investigations, or presenting as catastrophes occurring in the course of a viral illness. It is necessary to distinguish the one from the other.

The excessive stress laid on encephalitis by the majority of clinicians, and the confusion still prevalent between encephalopathy and encephalitis, not only are regrettable on scientific grounds, but have considerable importance in subsequent prognosis. Circulatory encephalopathy still retains, despite all therapeutic efforts, a grave prognosis. Acute encephalitis often offers hopes of survival and recovery.

In either case, and in view of the real difficulties in differentiating them, we are obliged to put into operation without delay all means of resuscitation which may enable the patient to overcome the critical initial phase of the illness.

Medical treatment, *sensu stricto,* is summarized in the use of anticonvulsive drugs, cardiovascular stimulants (should they be necessary), and antibiotics (should they appear to be useful).

It is impossible at present to venture an opinion on the indications or efficacy of corticosteroid drugs.

8

Encephalitides Caused by Enteroviruses

By S. THIEFFRY

The clinician who has had occasion to examine, from the onset of their illnesses, a large number of persons stricken with infantile paralysis becomes familiar with a rich symptomatology due to involvement of areas of the nervous system other than that of the anterior horn alone to which poliomyelitis owes its name.

Pathologists have for a long time drawn attention to the extreme diffusion of inflammatory and even neuronal lesions spreading beyond the territories of predilection. Thus, many cases of poliomyelitis that are otherwise quite usual appear to the clinician to have a transient encephalitic aspect. For the pathologist, the concept of poliomyelitic encephalitis is an accepted fact.

These remarks, interesting though they may be, have only a limited application in practice, for they are but vague hints which should not distract our attention from the fundamental paralytic symptomatology of Heine-Medin disease.

For many years, the attention of clinicians was held by certain acute diseases of the nervous system which bore a cerebral symptomatology justifying the diagnosis of encephalitis; these diseases were very different from the usual type of poliomyelitis but nevertheless had to be attached to poliomyelitis. The incorporation in poliomyelitis of forms so atypical has been proposed on the basis of epidemiological arguments (cases seen in context of an epidemic, instances of familial cases), clinical grounds (association

with typical paralysis), or suggestive course of the illness (disappearance of encephalitic signs and persistence of typical paralyses). This accumulation of evidence adds up to a conviction but not an absolute certainty. However, the existence of encephalitic forms of poliomyelitis has now been demonstrated indisputably. Some of these forms, such as acute ataxia, bear such an individual character that their diagnosis is immediately evident. In other cases, the precise diagnosis does not come to mind as the picture is so unusual— and is the more so owing to the unobtrusiveness or masked quality of the paralytic lesions.

THE ATAXIC FORM OF POLIOMYELITIS

This was described perfectly by Medin in 1898.[5] About 50 descriptions of such cases have been made, from which emerges a picture which is almost unique.

The onset is often abrupt, marked by an infectious illness which does not differ in any way from that of typical poliomyelitis. Neurological signs always appear abruptly and reach their height at the onset or perhaps after two or three days. Tremor is the most important sign. It involves the whole body, and by its intensity makes walking or sitting impossible without support. It becomes more marked on examination, on emotion, and in the course of movement. This is only one of the signs, but the most obvious one, of a cerebellar syndrome, at the same time static and dynamic, from which one may discern more or less easily other elements, such as hypermetria and passivity. Speech is often affected.

Other motor signs are noticed. These include abnormal movements of the limbs, particularly massive motor discharges. One of the most striking manifestations, opsoclonia, affects eye movements, often to an extreme degree; this consists of a slow rhythmical ocular tremor with similar excursions in all directions; the slow rhythm shows its greatest amplitude on midline fixation.

The usual paralyses of poliomyelitis are absent or are unobtrusive or regressive (limb-root or facial paralysis).

This complex neurological syndrome is associated with a moderate infectious syndrome and the usual painful and meningitic symptoms of poliomyelitis. The same abnormalities are found in the cerebrospinal fluid as in usual poliomyelitis.

The prognosis of these forms is excellent, as Médin indicated long ago. All patients recover without any sequelae within one month. Occasionally the ataxia is transitory. In that case it marks the onset of the illness and frank paralyses follow, but even in these cases it is curious to observe that they are commonly benign forms in which the paralyses are of limited extent and tend to improve.

There is no anatomical documentation for these ataxic forms, but we may remark that on anatomical examinations in fatal cases of poliomyelitis, lesions in the cerebellum are observed in 77 per cent of the cases, with preferential localization in the dentate nucleus, the roof nucleus, and the vermiform cortex. There are inflammatory lesions and also neuronal alterations. The observer may well be surprised at the relative rarity of clinical manifestations corresponding to these pathological lesions.

OTHER ENCEPHALITIC FORMS OF POLIOMYELITIS

Other encephalitic forms, although undisputable, are even rarer than the ataxias of Medin, and their study rests on but a few observations. Their symptomatology is so unusual that the clinician is not able to give appropriate weight to signs which are much more commonly found in the usual course of poliomyelitis: somnolence, torpor, peripheral paralyses, the infection syndrome, and clinical and biological meningism.

We may enumerate four clinical types of which the characteristic elements are the following:

1. A generalized extreme hypotonia, but with reflexes preserved. Development of this hypotonia and its coexistence with an akinetic mutism enable one to interpret this syndrome as a global akinetic syndrome. The only clinical observation indicating poliomyelitis is a bilateral facial paralysis which tends to disappear.

2. Attacks of tonic contractions, interspersed with tremor, which involve in particular the musculature of the mouth and pharynx and which are partially influenced by voluntary movements.

3. Intermittent spasm of the facial muscles and limbs, with or without coma, lasting for five days to three weeks.

4. Complete parkinsonian syndrome: plastic hypertonia, exaggeration of postural reflexes, cogwheel rigidity, preservation of attitudes, immobile facies, monotonous and jerky voice, excessive salivation, and disturbances of emotional expression.

We have therefore shown that the symptomatology of poliomyelitis may at times be dominated in the initial period of illness by extrapyramidal manifestations. These manifestations are superimposed on the usual picture of the disease and do not necessarily imply a particularly severe type of illness. The fate of the patient is decided by the extent and by the distribution of these paralyses and not by encephalitic accidents. On the contrary, these latter disappear in a few days or weeks without leaving any sequel peculiar to them.

To what appears to be a general rule, we must at present contrast an exception, since one case reported supports the concept of sequelae of parkinsonian type.

ROLE OF OTHER ENTEROVIRUSES

Complete laboratory investigations have not shown any relation of the prevalence of these encephalitic forms to epidemics of any particular type of virus. It is thus in order to include a chapter on the encephalitic forms of Heine-Medin disease, brief though it may be. We may also indicate that poliomyelitis viruses are not the only enteroviruses which may provoke these unusual clinical events. Even less commonly, similar manifestations have been observed in infections with Coxsackie and ECHO viruses.

In the course of the epidemic of ECHO 9 virus in Milwaukee, besides several paralytic cases, other rare and transitory neurological manifestations were observed: choreiform movements and coma, instability on walking, vertigo, or nystagmus.

Sporadic manifestations have been reported; a picture of encephalitis with choreoathetosis, extrapyramidal syndromes with hallucinations, and acute ataxia which is transitory and improves spontaneously (Coxsackie A7, ECHO 1).

Isolated as they are, and not often confirmed by every possible immunological proof, these scattered observations nevertheless deserve to attract attention and justify new systematic research.

BIBLIOGRAPHY

1. Alajouanine, T., Mignot, H., and Mozziconacci, P.: Un syndrome parkinsonien peut-il reconnaître la maladie de Heine-Medin comme étiologie? Rev. Neurol., *72*:66-69, 1939.
2. Drouhet, V.: Sur le diagnostic virologique et sérologique des infections á entérovirus. Path. Biol., *8*:17-28, 1960.
3. Grist, N. R.: An outbreak of "paralytic poliomyelitis" due to Coxsackie A7 virus. Association Européenne de la Poliomyelite et des Maladies Associées. 7th Symposium. Paris, Masson et Cie, 1962, pp. 211-215.
4. Marinesco, G., Draganesco, S., and Grigoresco, D.: Sur un cas de parkinsonisme post-encéphalitique survenu chez un ancien poliomyélitique. Rev. Neurol., *2*:102-104, 1929.
5. Medin, O.: L'état aigu de la paralysie infantile. Arch. Med. Enf., *1*:257-279; 321-343, 1898.
6. Sabin, A. B., Krumbiegel, E. R., and Wigand, R.: ECHO type 9 virus disease. Virologically controlled clinical and epidemiologic observations during 1957 epidemic in Milwaukee with notes on concurrent similar diseases associated with Coxsackie and other ECHO viruses. A.M.A. J. Dis. Child. *96*:197-219, 1958.
7. Thieffry, S.: Entérovirus (poliomyélite, Coxsackie, E.C.H.O.) et maladies du système nerveux. Révision critique et expérience personnelle. Rev. Neurol., *108*:753-776, 1963.

9

Encephalitis in the Common Exanthemata of Childhood

By S. THIEFFRY AND E. FARKAS

The notion that cerebral mishaps occur during the common infantile exanthemata has been well recognized for a long while.

The concept of encephalitis arose during their study, was accepted by clinicians, and led to the description of an unusual inflammation of the brain, eventually described under the title of diffuse perivenous leukoencephalitis. That name recalls the predilection of the lesions for scattered areas in the circumference of the veins of the white matter. The end-product of these inflammatory lesions is a perivascular parenchymatous infiltration with patchy demyelinization in areas which tend to become confluent.

Pari passu with the development of these lesions, a clinical illness develops whose general appearance, without being specific, is sufficiently definite to enable one to accept such a diagnosis readily.

We may discern a common clinical picture in all the leukoencephalitides, although some particular characteristics are associated with particular causative diseases.

But, as has already been suggested, it is of great importance to distinguish the perivascular leukoencephalitides from other cerebral accidents which may occur during an episode of an exanthematous disease.

Leukoencephalitis, in contrast to other brain-damaging processes, is exclusively encountered in the group of viral diseases of which the exanthemata are most typical, but other types may also be met with (in influenza, mumps, and infectious mononucleosis, for example).

A prime characteristic deserves attention: this is the identical physiopathological process, whatever the causative virus.

A second point in the history deserves attention: the encephalitides present to the clinician as accidents in the evolution of exanthemata. They do not begin simultaneously with the rash or the first signs of illness but appear some days later, the period being more or less fixed for each disease. This concept, extremely valuable for diagnostic purposes, must nevertheless be modified somewhat by the fact that such encephalitis may be of precocious onset and may even occur before the rash; there exist some observations of such cases. Even more, the systematic use of the electroencephalograph in the course of diseases such as measles has revealed the truly remarkable frequency of latent changes in uncomplicated cases of measles. It is therefore possible that encephalitic attacks may be much more frequent than is apparent and that we only observe clinical effects later and in cases where the anatomical process has been sufficiently powerful to produce them.

However this may be, the resemblance of the histopathological reactions, the time relationships of the accidents, and the general appearance of the clinical manifestations, independent of the identity of the causative virus, have raised the problem of the mechanism of the leukoencephalitides.

It is difficult to believe that they are the consequence of a direct attack of the virus on the brain. The virus is not isolated from the brain or the cerebrospinal fluid. And one would expect in accord with this hypothesis, to observe groups of cases of encephalitis in the course of an epidemic or, for example, after sessions of collective jennerian vaccination. Finally, one would imagine that episodes of encephalitis would then be more frequent at the stage of initial viremia.

The hypothesis of an individual reaction of an allergic type has been put forward, to deal with these objections and to take into account the very low frequency of encephalitides when compared with the extremely widespread distribution of the responsible viruses. This postulated allergic reaction consists of a local cellular reaction resulting from a conflict between the antigen and the antibodies already developed by the initial illness. This tentative immunological explanation is supported by the analogies between human leukoencephalitis and so-called experimental allergic encephalomyelitis, produced by injection, generally of white matter with adjuvants favoring antibody formation. This pathological problem will doubtless be resolved by investigations concerning the detection of virus *in situ* and histological study of cellular structures and constituent parts and their distribution.

GENERAL ANATOMICAL OBSERVATIONS

There is a multiple anatomical basis for the cerebral manifestations of the common exanthematous illnesses of childhood. Indeed, Jacob distinguishes anatomical variations of four different types in these illnesses: perivenous encephalitis, diffuse lymphoplasmocytic encephalitis, serous exudative encephalitis, and congestive and hemorrhagic encephalitis. With the definitions adopted and described earlier, the two latter categories—serous exudative encephalitis and congestive and hemorrhagic encephalitis—do not include gliomesodermal proliferative phenomena but only hemodynamic changes and lesions in the vascular permeabilities and will be considered together as encephalopathic reactions.

We will therefore consider only three types of anatomical lesions encountered in the course of exanthemata.

PERIVENOUS ENCEPHALITIS

This was described in 1926 by Turnbull and McIntosh in infants who had been vaccinated against smallpox. Numerous similar cases occurring in other vaccinated children were studied subsequently in Holland by Bouman and Bok, by Boowdisk-Bastiansee, and recently by de Vries.

An identical anatomical picture to that of perivenous encephalitis following Jennerian vaccination has been observed subsequently in the course of cerebral complications following chickenpox, measles, smallpox, and rubella. Lesions of this type have similarly been described, apart from the exanthemata, in the case of influenzal encephalitis, mumps, and infectious mononucleosis, and in the cerebral complications following antirabies vaccination.

Macroscopic Changes. The macroscopic changes of these cases of encephalitis are discrete and consist of a congestive and hemorrhagic appearance of the white matter with a constant presence in this area of small grayish areas with a perivascular distribution.

Histological Changes. Inflammatory infiltration at the level of the meninges and in the depth of the nervous tissue is not found, and the proliferative phenomena of the vascular mesenchymal tissues are relatively limited, with only a discrete lymphoplasmocyte infiltration in the perivascular spaces. As against this, the *microglial proliferation* reveals here a primordial character, and its perivascular distribution is pathognomonic. The mesodermal reaction being minimal or absent, the cellular infiltration, owing to its glial nature, is localized, not in the level of the Virchow-Robin spaces, but in the depth of the perivascular nervous tissue. This microglial proliferation, which often assumes

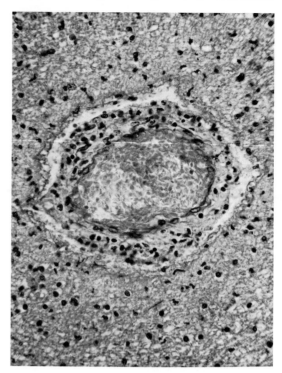

Figure 9-2. Perivenous encephalitis. Microphotograph showing moderate inflammatory infiltration in the adventitia, and glial proliferation within nervous tissue and around the blood vessels, with numerous rod-shaped microglial elements. Hematoxylin and eosin stain.

a syncytial appearance, attains its maximum intensity around the venous walls and diminishes in proportion as one gets farther away from these.

Parenchymatous Changes. These involve, in the first instance, the myelin and the cylindrical axons surrounding the veins. In fact, zones of perivenous demyelination are observed in all cases in which the disease process has been under way for 48 hours or more. Inside these zones of demyelination, the axon cylinders are damaged and phagocytes of microglial or adventitial origin, full of debris and products of myelin degeneration, may be seen. As against this, neuronal changes, *sensu stricto,* are muted and always remain in the background of the anatomical picture.

Distribution of Lesions. Lesions clearly predominate in the white matter, but their distribution depends more upon the cerebral venous circulation than on the anatomy of the neuronal tissues (Finley; Lhermitte). The lesions seem to group themselves around veins of medium and large caliber and so

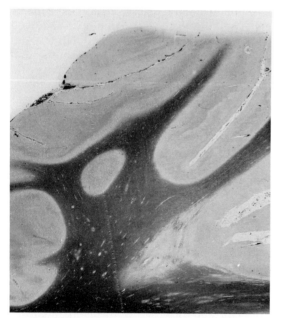

Figure 9-1. Perivenous encephalitis, showing an area of subcortical perivascular demyelination. Cerebral hemisphere, close-up view. Loyez' stain.

appear surrounding the veins of the deep layers of the cortex and those of the white matter and, very frequently, around the large veins situated in the neighborhood of the lateral ventricles. They are absent from the superficial cortical layers whose blood is drained toward the meninges by very small venules. In the same way, at the level of the cerebral peduncles, the cerebellum, and the medulla, microglial infiltration and demyelination are respectively paramedian, situated in the central convolutions of the cerebellum, and have, at the level of the medulla, a radial distribution, mainly under the pia, in accordance with the regional venous topography.

Development of Lesions. In rapidly developing types of illness, by the second or third day, a transitory mesodermal reaction was observed by Walthard and Adams et al.[1] in postmeasles encephalitis. In subacute forms with only a few days' history (Wohlwill, Greenfield), perivenous demyelination is obvious and proliferative phenomena are purely glial, with numerous phagocytic granular bodies already present in the demyelinated areas. Finally, at the stage of organization (Walthard, Malamud) the microglial proliferation is moderate or absent and there exist diffuse demyelinated areas formed by the confluence of small perivenous lesions.

Allergic Nature. The allergic nature of these perivenous microglial encephalitides, whose anatomical substrata are identical whatever the nature of the causal affection, has already been described. This pathogenic interpretation has value only as a hypothesis, for the lesions observed in experimental allergic encephalomyelitis in animals are never exactly of the same type as those seen in the perivenous encephalitis in man.

DIFFUSE PLASMOCYTIC ENCEPHALITIS OF EXANTHEMATA

An infiltration with lymphoplasmocytes may be observed during the onset of genuine perivenous encephalitis, as shown by the observation of Walthard of lymphoplasmocytic perivascular infiltrates and glial perivenous proliferation coexisting in an infant that died from measles encephalitis developing over 24 hours.

There also exist lymphoplasmocytic encephalitides with isolated proliferation of the meningeal and vascular mesenchyma, and no microglial reaction, or perivenous demyelination, in spite of an illness which lasts some days. Jacob reports some isolated lymphoplasmocytic forms after jennerian vaccination and, in the same way, Pfeiffer, Wiegand, and Davison and Friedfeld described analogous anatomical forms in cases of postrubella encephalitis. Pfeiffer considered the possibility of a viral etiology in those cases of lymphoplasmocytic meningoencephalitis which occur in the course of exanthematic disease. Some arguments in favor of a viral etiology occurring in certain instances of postmeasles encephalitis have been put forward by Adams et al. These authors found intranuclear and intracytoplasmic inclusion bodies in the central nervous system of patients dying from postmeasles encephalitis and also giant cells identical to those described by Hecht and Ciaccio in measles pneumonia and by Enders and Peebles in tissue cultures inoculated with measles virus. Furthermore, the presence of inclusion bodies in postmeasles encephalitis had already been described by Wohlwill in 1928.

We may remark here that, in the series of cases reported by Adams et al., inclusion bodies were also found on four occasions in children who presented the neuropathological picture of perivenous encephalitis, but without any infiltration with leukocytes or plasmocytes. Must we invoke, to explain these facts, a double origin for the changes which we observe? Does the presence of virus in the nervous system produce inclusion bodies, with a later "allergic" process leading to a perivenous encephalitis, or must we resurrect the hypothesis of direct viral origin in certain instances of postmeasles perivenous encephalitis?

THE ENCEPHALOPATHIC REACTION DURING THE COURSE OF EXANTHEMATA

In many observations, the neuropathological examination of patients who have presented with cerebral complications in the course of different exanthemata fails to reveal the presence of any gliomesenchymal inflammatory phenomenon. The lesions we observe are purely encephalopathic, comprising vascular congestion with stasis, with or without an erythrocytic diapedesis and an acellular extravasation of serum or plasma. We are in this case describing lesions which at one and the same time involve the tone and the permeability of the cerebral vessels, being able to create, through the ischemia and the edema which they produce, degenerative parenchymatous changes.

The usual macroscopic appearance of these acute encephalopathies is a cerebral edema with areas of more or less significant involvement. These acute encephalopathic reactions, still called hemodynamic by van Bogaert, are nonspecific functional vascular syndromes which, according to the definitions which we have adopted, are certainly not of an encephalitic nature, since they do not result in inflammatory changes.

Encephalopathic reactions were described by van Bogaert in 1932 in subacute forms of postmeasles encephalitis. This author considered that these were the initial stage of a true perivenous encephalitis, with death occurring during the first 24 hours in these cases.

However, many subsequent findings confirm the work of Jacob, of de Vries, and also of Dolgopol and van Bogaert that the acute encephalopathic reactions are not representative of the initial stage of perivenous encephalitis, since they have been observed after illnesses whose course varied from a few days to more than one month.

This viewpoint is confirmed by the report by de Vries on three patients with post-vaccinal encephalitis who died 24 to 48 hours after the onset of neurological signs and whose postmortem examinations showed, even at this early stage, the characteristic changes of glioperivenous encephalitis.

The encephalopathic reaction must therefore be considered as a type of reaction that is autonomous and never as the initial stage of a microglial encephalitis.

De Vries, in Holland, in a systematic study of 62 fatalities following neurological complications of smallpox vaccination, remarked that, in infants under two years of age, the anatomical picture of perivenous encephalitis was always absent; modifications of an encephalopathic type were constantly observed in his patients. The absence of lesions of the type of glioperivenous encephalitis in young infants has also been confirmed in the course of the cerebral manifestations of measles (Dagnelie et al., Musser and Hauser) as well as in those of chickenpox (Zimmermann and Yannet). Changes of an encephalopathic type are therefore the usual anatomical substrate of the cerebral complications of exanthemata in the young infant. Exceptionally, we may find in these patients, associated with hemodynamic illness, the presence of sudanophilic perivascular lipids. In the absence of any disintegration of the myelin, we may consider that these lipids have crossed the vascular walls following the peripheral disturbance of the blood-brain barrier, which we know to be vulnerable in the young infant.

At present, we do not propose any valid explanation to account for the particular vulnerability of the nervous tissues in immature subjects subjected to attack by the viruses of the exanthemata. The inability of the infantile brain to develop allergic manifestations has been discussed in this connection.

In any case, the record of neuropathological changes differing from perivenous encephalitis, such as the lymphoplasmocytic forms and the encephalopathic reactions, so frequent in the young infant, indicate that, beyond the ultimate allergic mechanisms, other factors must be considered in the etiology of the cerebral lesions arising during the exanthemata.

GENERAL CLINICAL OBSERVATIONS

A discussion of the clinical aspects of the leukoencephalitides follows. We will not describe at wearisome length all the signs which may occur, but will attempt to indicate which diagnostic elements deserve to be considered and finally accepted. The elements of positive diagnosis must follow from the remarks concerning differential diagnosis.

Acute leukoencephalitis occurs during an eruptive disease that was of no particular gravity, occasionally already in the convalescent phase and following a normal course.

The illness has an abrupt onset and appears grave from the beginning. The temperature rises to 40° C. or higher. Convulsions occur which are localized or generalized, single or repeated, occasionally frequent but generally short in duration and not leaving the patient in the complete coma between convulsions that arouses the fear of status epilepticus. Disturbances of consciousness may range between obnubilation and light or even deep coma.

The first hours or days are dominated by signs of a global and widespread involvement of the nervous system, without very precise localizing signs, but sometimes with tonic contractions of the muscles of the body displaying decerebrate or decorticate attitudes. Autonomic disturbances are severe and variable (fever, cardiac irregularities, vasomotor disturbances, respiratory irregularities). Variations in consciousness are usual but in different degrees; agitated coma is frequent, and mental confusion and hallucinatory episodes are not unusual. On the other hand, deep coma is unusual. Convulsions may be repeated, of varying types and frequencies, rarely localized to the same areas.

After a few days, more precise and localized neurological signs may be demonstrable upon systematic examination. These develop fairly rapidly and are not necessarily accompanied by deep diminution of consciousness or vigilance. These neurological signs are extremely diverse: they include deficiency syndromes with unilateral or bilateral lesions of the pyramidal tract, abolition or exaggeration of reflexes, Babinski's reflex, hypertonia of trunk or limbs, choreic or dystonic movements, cranial nerve palsies, disturbances of ocular movements, trismus, disturbances of micturition, cortical blindness, akinetic mutism, and so forth.

On the other hand, it is exceptional for encephalitis to produce a frank meningeal symptomatology, although a detectable biological meningeal reaction in fact always occurs, so that the presence of a normal cerebrospinal fluid must arouse doubt as to the diagnosis of leukoencephalitis. Usually, there are from one dozen to several dozens of lymphocytic cells and an excess of protein of 0.40 to 1 gm. per 100 ml. without any changes in chlorides or sugar. We must remember that, in exceptional cases, a puriform meningeal reaction with unaltered polymorphonuclear leukocytes may mark the onset of certain types of encephalitis and may mistakenly be taken for suppurative meningitis.

We therefore soon find ourselves faced with a complex clinical situation that suggests a widespread lesion involving cerebral function. But, significantly, the signs vary from one examination to another, from one day to another. This fluctuation in symptomatology, combined with variations in the state of consciousness and temperature, is doubtless one of the strongest arguments for a diagnosis of leukoencephalitis. This characteristic period lasts, on an average, about ten days, during which the situation seems to deteriorate, with a frequent regularity, but the temptation to accept a definite prognosis must be resisted. After about ten days there are generally no fresh symptoms, and once this point has been passed, favorable outcome is almost certain.

When death occurs it is usually during the first days as the result of progressive and rapid changes in the autonomic system: disturbances in swallowing, changes in the respiratory rhythm, pulmonary embarrassment, hyperthermia, circulatory collapse, and deepening coma.

When the illness progresses favorably, a gradual improvement is seen. The convulsions become less frequent and disappear. Neurological signs, apparently firmly installed, disappear, although some persist. Consciousness returns. Here again, one must refrain from giving a firm prognosis too hastily, for surprising recoveries may be seen weeks and even months after the onset of the illness. The most tenacious symptoms are those concerned with intellectual functions, particularly memory.

All in all, we must look at acute leukoencephalitis with relatively qualified optimism (especially in contrast with vascular encephalopathy) while recalling that, although cases that appeared hopeless may be cured completely without a trace. Nevertheless the possibility of sequelae must not be forgotten. Neurological disturbances persist fairly frequently: abnormal movements, ocular paralyses, and, above all, convulsive episodes. In the psychological and intellectual spheres, the patient may retain disturbances of character and behavior and intellectual disturbances hindering or impeding educational or social adaptation.

SOME CLINICAL FEATURES

The exanthematic leukoencephalitides present suddenly and severely, with many varied symptoms and fluctuating neurological manifestations, the total picture showing clearly the degree and distribution of the inflammatory process. But we must recall some variations or attenuations of this general picture. They concern either the intensity of the cerebral reaction or the topographical predominance of the inflammatory lesions of the neuraxis.

The general picture may be *attenuated* and reduced to a slight diminution in the state of consciousness, to discrete convulsive episodes, or to isolated and transitory changes in reflexes and muscular tone. Study of the cerebrospinal fluid and electroencephalographic tracings are then of great value in diagnosis.

Two particular distributions may give the illness a particular appearance; cerebellar lesions and lesions in the spinal cord. In fact, it is preferable to speak of symptomatic dominances.

Cerebellar involvement provides a picture of the acute ataxic syndrome of which encephalitis is one possible etiology. It manifests, to a variable degree, but often very violently, the disturbances in balance and especially in motor function resulting from cerebellar incoördination (rombergism, drunken gait, tremors, hypermetria, incoördination). These incidents, particularly when due to chickenpox, normally regress and disappear in a few days or weeks.

Acute myelitis begins abruptly or after some prodromal symptoms which make confusion with poliomyelitis possible up to the moment when doubt is resolved by the observation of sensory changes, pyramidal signs, and sphincteric disturbances. These symptoms often produce the picture of acute transverse myelitis. The prognosis is variable and very difficult to make. All eventualities may be encountered, from complete recovery to a persisting flaccid paralysis with atrophy (indicating necrosis of a segment underlying the main lesion). The diagnosis of myelitis is an urgent indication for those measures of nursing and treatment (physiotherapy, careful attention to the bladder) which have transformed and improved the progression of the condition and its unfavorable prognosis.

The diagnosis of the acute encephalitides, in spite of the particular circumstances of their onset, is neither simple nor easy, notwithstanding the too-widespread notions to the contrary.

They must be carefully differentiated from the other cerebral manifestations which may complicate the exanthemata, directly or indirectly. The difficulties, first in the diagnosis and later in the prognosis, must not be underestimated.

In formulating the diagnosis and the immediate and later prognosis, *electroencephalographic investigation* plays a very important role. The tracings display, when taken together, the degree of spread, the dissemination and the variation, and the longitudinal evolution of encephalitis. At the time of onset, they are generally composed of large, irregular, high-voltage waves in the delta band, irregular waves already modified

for short periods to rhythmic delta waves or to lower-voltage theta waves. This tracing is not usually influenced by stimulation. Against this background of general dysrhythmia, more or less numerous acute episodes sometimes occur. Finally, when the progress of the disease is favorable, improvement is demonstrated by the appearance of changes on stimulation. Slow dysrhythmia reappears only intermittently, with alternating rhythmical theta waves or complete flattening. The alpha rhythms reappear little by little, but spikes of theta waves may exist for a long time with unilateral predominance, especially in the posterior areas.

Indeed, we must usually wait weeks and sometimes months before a return to normal rhythm or normal reactivity to stimulation occurs. Even in the most favorable clinical circumstances it is wise not to relax this electroencephalographic surveillance, as epileptic foci may appear, above all in the temporal lobes, even after the tracing has been unchanged for a long period.

DIFFERENTIAL DIAGNOSIS

In taking care to make the diagnosis of encephalitis only in the light of clear knowledge, it is prudent to accept this diagnosis only after systematic examination and for weighty reasons even if circumstantial evidence seems to demand such a diagnosis.

1. In fact, exanthemata often occur in young children at the age of predilection for febrile convulsions. The distinction between such a simple and banal incident and a grave and rare encephalitis is, in fact, initially very difficult and even impossible, for, at the onset of the cases, paralytic phenomena are frequent and the electroencephalograms themselves do not differ. Only the ultimate progress, the results of lumbar puncture and the later electroencephalogram allow one to decide.

2. On the other hand, the exanthemata, by themselves or frequently through *superinfection* with pyogenic bacteria, may introduce cerebral accidents distinct from leukoencephalitis, such as meningitides or cerebrovascular accidents, among which intracranial phlebitis has long been recognized.

Certain inflammatory lesions of the cerebral veins which are complicated by considerable edema produce a picture very close to that of the encephalitides in which the localizing signs so important for diagnosis run the risk of being misinterpreted.

3. Finally, we have stressed in the preceding chapter the frequency and importance of the syndrome of *circulatory encephalopathy,* which must be excluded from the classification of encephalitis. It is probable, furthermore, that a certain number of extremely grave episodes described as acute encephalitis, especially those that follow vaccination against smallpox, are indeed encephalopathies of this type. The clinical distinction is not easy. Nevertheless, we must retain, as favoring a diagnosis of circulatory encephalopathy, the sudden onset with repeated convulsions *ab initio,* subintrant and without even a partial return of consciousness, relentless onset of profound progressive coma, the absence of localizing neurological signs, and the normal character of the cerebrospinal fluid. The initial electroencephalogram shows a slow dysrhythmia, very rapidly replaced by a level tracing or one devoid of any activity at all. The prognosis of these encephalopathies is grave in the extreme, and, if the sick person does not die in a few days, a marasmic state with very severe neurological and, above all, psychological sequelae commences without any real ultimate improvement. Thus if encephalitis and encephalopathy resemble each other in their early stages, in general evolution they are sufficiently distinct and even divergent to permit their differentiation by the clinician. These general remarks are applicable to the majority of cerebral accidents which may appear during the exanthemata.

ETIOLOGICAL PATTERNS

POSTVACCINIAL ENCEPHALITIS

This is the most important of the complications of vaccination against smallpox. It is even more so as it is scarcely foreseeable and as we have only the most sketchy of ideas concerning its prevention and its conditions of appearance and other determining factors. Even group studies possessing a statistical value reveal differences which are scarcely explainable.

It is probable that these anomalies stem in part from the fact that diagnostic criteria concerning true encephalitis are fairly imprecise and embrace all the accidents attributed to smallpox vaccination (which

themselves are often independent of or not directly dependent on such vaccination).

There is general agreement that encephalitis complicates, in the main, primary vaccination. In those cases following revaccination, it usually occurs in patients with a strong local reaction at the site of vaccination, leading one to consider an immunological deficiency.

The predisposing role of a preëxisting cerebral lesion is probable: thus it is very wise not to vaccinate individuals with brain injury and children who have previously had convulsions. It is likely that the risk lies more in a febrile convulsive reaction than in the induction of an authentic encephalitis.

The basic factor is the age of the vaccinated subject. All statistics have shown that the frequency of encephalitis following vaccination clearly is much greater (from 1.5 to 12 times) after the age of four years. After the age of four years, it is very difficult to state that this risk regularly occurs or is attenuated above a certain age. For ages below four years, comparison of different statistics reveals discrepancies. Thus, for example, some indicate equality or a frequency increasing from year to year, whereas others, like those of Griffith, suggest for Great Britain, a frequency of encephalitis which is greater following vaccination before the age of 1 year (0.154 per 10,000) than between one and four years (0.019). This paradoxical idea probably can be explained by the fact that those vaccination accidents in the first year which are often diagnosed as acute encephalitis are, in fact, diffuse reactive circulatory encephalopathies. It has been pointed out earlier that the immature brain has a general nonspecific reaction, consisting of convulsions, to all forms of insult, whatever the etiology, and particularly to fever.

These general remarks concerning the age of primary vaccination and the sensitivity of certain subjects lead us to suggest some precautions or actions which may avoid neurological complications. It is difficult to affirm the innocuousness of attenuated vaccines, and equally difficult to appreciate the value of preventive injections of gamma globulin. Nevertheless, the work of Nanning concerning its use in young recruits in the Dutch Army suggests that a very significant reduction in nervous complications can be produced (1 in 17,500 against 1 in 4000).

On the whole, and for the clinician, it is certain that one may contrast two types of cerebral accident and two principal features which superimpose themselves fairly strictly on the general remarks which have been made concerning the baby and the toddler. This distinction, which clearly must include exceptions and emendations, is in conformity with postmortem anatomical studies.

In the older infant, a genuine encephalitis or an encephalomyelitis is the most frequently observed accident. The date of onset is near the seventh or fourteenth day following inoculation. Extreme limits may be taken as between four and 18 days. The illness unfolds itself in the acute fashion described earlier, with the usual symptomatic fluctuations found in leukoencephalitis, the same grave picture, and the usual uncertainties of immediate prognosis and of secondary and late sequelae.

In the infant, postvaccinial cerebral accidents usually have different characteristics. They occur toward the ninth day, at a time when one often finds a febrile reaction following vaccination. The onset is extremely abrupt, and the child immediately slips into a deep coma with superimposed convulsions and in most cases never recovers from this state. One finds only unlocalized global neurological signs and especially respiratory and circulatory disturbances. Death within a few days is the usual end. The anatomical lesions are not those of encephalitis but those of "hemodynamic brain." When survival occurs, this diffuse circulatory encephalopathy leaves neuropsychiatric sequelae of extreme gravity.

Even by analyzing the statistics concerning vaccinial encephalitis, it is very difficult to differentiate between the two types of accident, of which one—genuine encephalitis—stems directly from vaccination and the other follows a vaccinial reaction. Taken together, mortality is as high as 20 to 50 per cent and very grave sequelae are usually observed. However, complete recovery occurs in a quarter of cases.

Detailed statistical studies, in which one may analyze cases occurring in infancy, show the particularly serious prognosis of such cases (50 per cent mortality before one year of age), confirming the exceptional seriousness of circulatory encephalopathy, which allows little chance of survival or improvement, when compared with the encephalitides, which carry a less grave immediate prognosis and considerable possibilities of improvement or even of complete recovery.

MEASLES ENCEPHALITIS

Measles is complicated with encephalitis in about one in 1000 cases, which is not negligible. This figure concerns only the unmistakable forms which are clinically evident. We must recall that systematic studies have revealed the relative frequency of abnormalities in electroencephalographic tracing in normal measles, as well as in subclinical meningeal reactions. It is possible that this common illness is responsible for late neurological sequelae (convulsions) following subclinical encephalitis. There do not appear to be any definite predisposing factors: general seriousness of the illness, intensity of the rash, age, type of epidemic, individual predisposition—none of these seems to have much importance. Of greater importance is the date of onset, which is toward the fourth or fifth day following the onset of the rash. It rarely occurs earlier or later. Nevertheless there exist exceptional cases, with onset during the period of invasion.

Encephalitis makes its appearance known by a return of or increase in fever, and the illness unfolds with the general symptomatology which has been described earlier. It is one of the encephalitides which present the most varying and changing symptoms (pyramidal signs, cerebellar signs, abnormal movements, lesions of the cranial nerves). Medullary lesions are rather frequent. Disturbances of consciousness are often marked, and coma with sympathetic disturbances is an index of immediate gravity. In about 10 per cent of cases, death occurs in a few days, but normally after about a week of critical illness an improvement is seen and from then the general evolution is as has been described. Of all the encephalitides, this is, perhaps, the one which, in spite of apparent extreme gravity, is likely to improve after some weeks or months, although the neurological lesions may have appeared to be severe and irrecoverable.

On the whole, the prognosis of measles encephalitis (taking into account its relatively common frequency, itself related to the wide spread of measles) appears to be relatively unfavorable, 20 to 40 per cent of patients having neurological or psychological sequelae.

Special attention must be paid to late convulsive sequelae which apparently bear no relation to the illness. The electroencephalographic anomalies indeed take some while to disappear, from whence follows the routine of periodic follow-up examinations during the two years following suspected neurological manifestations and the systematic treatment of the ill child with anticonvulsive therapy until the tracing has regained normality.

CHICKENPOX ENCEPHALITIS

Perhaps of all the encephalitides which follow the exanthemata, chickenpox encephalitis alone possesses the clinical peculiarity of a cerebellar symptomatology. It is also distinguished, in this type of cerebellar ataxia, by a habitual lack of severity. These peculiarities make one suspect that it should not be included in the general classification of the leukoencephalitides. Nevertheless, the frequent conjunction of other minor neurological signs which are extracerebellar, and on occasion the appearance of the typical picture of a diffuse encephalitis, makes one think, in spite of the absence of anatomical observations, that cerebellar encephalitis does not differ fundamentally from the other exanthematous leukoencephalitides.

This complication appears on the second to ninth day following the eruption of the rash. This delay is only approximate, and we have seen cases of encephalitis occur a few days before the onset of the rash. There is no clear relationship between the intensity of the rash or its character and nervous complications. It is particularly difficult to state whether a genuine encephalitis plays a large part in the unfavorable evolution of cases of chickenpox which occur while the patient is under treatment with corticosteroids.

The most frequently seen picture is an acute ataxia of sudden onset with or without a recrudescence of pyrexia. The cerebellar symptomatology is quite pronounced (hypermetria, tremor, astasia, and incoördination). The cerebrospinal fluid and the electroencephalogram are slightly abnormal.

Recovery usually occurs within a few weeks without any sequelae.

RUBELLA ENCEPHALITIS

Cerebral manifestations undoubtedly occur during the course of rubella. Nevertheless, they are very rare, although it is possible that some cases are not correctly diagnosed on account of the frequent atypical picture presented by rubella, an illness which often is difficult for the clinician to recognize or to identify.

The onset occurs after the usual period which typifies the appearance of the postexanthematous encephalitides (two to five days after the rash). The general symptomatology is not very different from that of the other encephalitides occurring in the exanthemata, including a meningeal reaction and, in those cases where such observations have been feasible, compatible changes in the electroencephalogram. Because so few cases have been studied, it is difficult to attribute with confidence any particular weight to these findings.

It is possible, moreover, on the basis of anatomical studies, that certain fatal cerebral manifestations in the course of rubella are compatible more with anoxic encephalopathy than with a genuine leukoencephalitis.

CEREBRAL MANIFESTATIONS OF EXANTHEM SUBITUM

These accidents are observed with relative frequency in this illness and particularly during epidemics.

Indeed, they have not the stereotyped character which one meets in the illnesses previously described, and they are differentiated from these by their time of onset during the initial febrile phase and before the onset of the rash.

A number of types of manifestation have been described: a discrete meningeal syndrome confirmed by a cellular reaction and a moderate increase of protein in the cerebrospinal fluid, or a convulsive episode coinciding with a brief spell of hyperthermia and without clinical or electroencephalographic sequelae, or a much graver picture of coma and convulsions with prostration, progressing to hemiplegia and definitive sequelae. The abrupt onset, the severity, and the clinical and electroencephalographic symptomatology mark this as a circulatory encephalopathy or a vascular accident rather than a leukoencephalitis with disseminated lesions. The onset in the preëruptive phase strengthens this hypothesis.

BIBLIOGRAPHY

1. Adams, J. M., Baird, E., and Filloy, L. D.: Inclusion bodies in measles encephalitis. J.A.M.A., *195*: 290, 1966.
2. Bouman, L., and Bok, S. K.: Die Histopathologie der Encephalitis post vaccinationen. Z. Ges. Neurol. Psych., *3*:495, 1927.
3. Davison, C., and Friedfeld, L.: Acute encepha-

lomyelitis following German measles. Amer. J. Dis. Child., *55*:496, 1938.

4. Dagnelie, J., Dubois, R., Fonteyne, P., Ley, R. A., Meunier, M., and van Bogaert, L.: Les encéphalites nonsuppurées de l'enfance, rapport anatomopathologique. J. Belge Neurol. Psychiat, *32*:547-674, 1932.

5. De Vries, E.: Post Vaccinial Perivenous Encephalitis. New York, American Elsevier Publishing Co., 1959.

6. Enders, F., and Peebles, T. C.: Propagation in tissue cultures of cytopathogenic agents. Proc. Soc. Exp. Biol. Med., *86*:277, 1954.

7. Finley, K. H.: Central nervous system involvement by viruses. Int. J. Neurol., *1*:256, 1960.

8. Greenfield, J. G.: Pathology of measles encephalomyelitis. Brain, *52*:171, 1929.

9. Griffith, W.: Symposium on immunization in childhood. Brit. Med. J., *2*:1342-1346, 1959.

10. Hecht, V.: Die riesenzellenpneumonie im Kindesalter. Beitr. Path. Anat., *48*:263, 1910.

11. Holliday, P. B.: Preeruptive neurologic complications of the common contagious diseases: Rubella, rubeola, roseola and varicella. J. Pediat., *36*:185-198, 1950.

12. Jacob, H.: On the different course of postinfectious encephalitis and encephalopathy. Proceedings of the 2nd Congress of Neuropathology. London, 1955, p. 197.

13. Jacob, H.: Zur klinisch-neuropathologischen Differentialdiagnose zwischen parainfektiösen (und postvaccinalen) Encephalitiden und akuten sporadischen, panleukoencephalitiden. Arch. Psychiat., *197*:507, 1958.

14. Joseph, R., Ribierre, M., Job, J. C., and Gabilan, J.: Les complications nerveuses de l'exanthème subit. Sem. hôp. Paris, *34*:546, 1958.

15. Keyzer, J. L.: Encéphalite vaccinale. *In:* Vaccinations contre les maladies contagieuses de l'enfance. Paris, Centre International de l'Enfance, 1952, pp. 131-137.

16. Lhermitte, F.: Les leucoencéphalites. Paris, Flammarion, 1950.

17. Malamud, N.: Sequelae of postmeasles encephalomyelitis. Arch. Neurol. Psychiat., *41*:943, 1939.

18. Margairaz, A., Barois, A., and Christophe, P.: Les complications neurologiques de la rougeole (à propos de 53 observations dont 49 méningoencéphalitis). Rev. Neuropsychiat. Infant., *10*:601-611, 1962.

19. Musser, J. H., and Hauser, G. H.: Encephalitis as a complication of measles. J.A.M.A., *90*:1267, 1928.

20. Nanning, W.: Prophylactic effect of antivaccinia gamma-globulin against post-vaccinal encephalitis. Bull. W.H.O., *27*:317-324, 1962.

21. Pfeiffer, J.: Über eine in der grauen Substanz sich ausbreitenden Encephalitis nach Rubeolen. Arch. Psychiat. Neurol., *93*:337, 1955.

22. Radl, H.: Encephalitis und Myelitis bei Rubeolen. Kinderaerztl. Prax., *28*:151-154, 1960.

23. Riley, H. D.: Encephalitis complicating attenuated rubeola. A.M.A. J. Dis. Child., *95*:270-275, 1958.

24. Turnbull, H. M., and Mc Intosh, J.: Encephalomyelitis following vaccination. Brit. J. Exp. Path., *7*:181, 1926.

25. van Bogaert, L.: Essai d'interprétation des manifestations nerveuses observées au cours de la maladie sérique et des maladies éruptives. Rev. Neurol., *1*:26, 1932.

26. van Bogaert, L.: Über funktionelle Kreislaufstörungen des Zentralnervensystems und das Problem der postvaccinalen Encephalitis. Arch. Psychiat., *185*:482, 1950.

27. Walthard, B.: Encephalitis nach Masern. Z. Ges. Neurol. Psychiat., *157*:100, 1937.

28. Walthard, K. M.: Spätstadium einer Encephalitis nack Massern. Z. Neurol., *124*:176, 1930.

29. Wiegand, H.: Tödliche Encephalomyelitis nach Röteln. Z. Neurol., *173*:448, 1941.

30. Wohlwill, F.: Über Encephalomyelitis bei Masern. Z. Ges. Neurol. Psychiat., *112*:20, 1928.

31. Zimmerman, H., and Yannet, C.: Nonsuppurative encephalomyelitis accompanying chickenpox. Arch. Neurol., *26*:322, 1931.

10

Rabies

By M. BALTAZARD

THE DISEASE

HUMAN RABIES

The prodromal signs of rabies are most often discrete, when they are not completely lacking. Fever, cephalalgia, exaggerated emotional responses, despondence, insomnia, and the sensation of deep malaise are not necessarily characteristic. Two signs alone are pathognomic. The earliest and the surest of these, but also the most inconsistent, is a tingling and lancing sensation at the scarred-over bite, with or without true pain, a paresthesia which tends to spread, particularly in the case of a bite on one of the limbs; it is accompanied in some instances by reddening, and even slight swelling. The most consistent but a later-appearing sign is a state of anxiety that gives the rabid patient a characteristic facial expression. The profound anxiety is very different from that seen in highly nervous people, the "false rabid" person presenting the "nervous hydrophobia" syndrome (see the section on diagnosis). The anxiety of the rabid patient does not respond to reasoning or stop with tranquilizers; it is not a psychological phenomenon but one of the signs of encephalitic involvement.

The prodromal signs can last for several days, but usually after a few hours the first symptoms appear that no longer leave room for doubt. Cephalalgia intensifies, nausea begins, and repeated dizzy spells occur, while the anxiety increases to the point of becoming intolerable. Spasmodic excitation and extreme hypersensitivity develop very quickly: spasms of the respiratory tract, reflecting bulbar involvement, muscular spasms, and fibrillation of the face are soon followed by the classic laryngopharyngeal spasms which unerringly identify the disease. Hydrophobia appears, being due to laryngopharyngeal spasms but even more to extreme erethism. Noise and light become unbearable for the patient, and a hallucinatory state of excitation is followed by signs of acute excitement or by convulsions. The physician must avoid the appearance of these latter signs by having the patient transferred to a specialized center, if this has not been done already. At first these signs appear intermittently, with periods when the patient becomes quiet and often remains voluntarily immobile, fearing a new crisis. However, even if one takes advantage of these calm intervals, transfer of the patient is very difficult, for the least excitement brings on a new crisis.

This series of signs marking the onset of disease is rarely incomplete. In about one quarter of the cases paralysis occurs as well: Landry-type syndrome or paralysis limited to a group of muscles or the bitten limb. In rare cases this paralysis is the first sign of disease.

It does not seem necessary to review the later evolution of the disease or the agony of the rabid patient, which has been well known since Trousseau and which is only an aggravation of the presenting signs. Today's arsenal of hypnotics, analgesics, sedatives, neuroleptics, and curarizing agents should permit us to avert the most horrible aspects of the progression of this disease. In survival centers, generalized convulsive crises, fits of madness, barking, biting, terror, and asphyxia, and, even more, the awful lucidity of this long agony, should give way to a peaceful coma.

ANIMAL RABIES

In the absence of a veterinarian, the doctor will often have to diagnose the disease in the animal, a diagnosis which governs his actions with respect to the bitten person (see the section on prophylaxis and treatment).

Rabies in the dog appears after a 20- to 50-day incubation period (25 days on the average). Only rarely is this period longer (up to a year) or shorter (a week in very young dogs). The warning signs are the same as in man: fever, unrest, despondency, prostration in some, extreme nervousness and aggressiveness in others, anxiety in all. The expression of the eyes is, here again, characteristic. Paresthesia around the bite can occur, as in man. It is not rare to see a dog bite, even to the bone, the wounded foot or thigh. After two or three days, the first symptoms appear. As in man, the earliest is a laryngopharyngeal spasm which is evidenced by a hoarseness and a particular rhythm of the barks, and by extreme difficulty and then true inhibition of swallowing. A state of excitation quickly develops which is reflected by fits of madness and convulsive spasms separated, as in man, by phases of depression.

Again, as in man, in about one-quarter of the cases a paralysis appears early that changes this clinical picture to such an extent that for a long time a distinction was made between this paralytic rabies, so-called "mute rabies," and "raving madness," because the dog does not bark and the paralysis calms him. However, the paralyzed dog can at any moment enter into a phase of excitation and bite. He is thus particularly dangerous to his owner and, especially to children, who, out of pity, care for him and caress him, often putting their hands in his mouth to try to remove from his throat the bone which they suppose is responsible for his spasms.

Both forms evolve rapidly (two to five days). If he has not been put in a cage, the rabid dog always escapes and runs through the streets or countryside biting everything that comes in reach of his teeth. He no longer eats but continues to drink (hydrophobia does not exist in animals) and becomes considerably thinner; his eyes are wild; he howls and is shaken by spasms which become more and more frequent. Finally he lies down to die, biting for the last time whoever comes to help him. In the paralyzed dog, death comes more quickly, most often being due to asphyxia. The continuous, particularly intense flow of saliva makes this terminal phase very dangerous if diagnosis has not yet, as is frequent, been made.

Unlike man, the dog does not necessarily die from rabies. Cases of healing (Levaditi's autosterilizing neuroinfection) are, however, extremely rare, and this possibility is not taken into account in the regulations for the observation of animals (see the section on prophylaxis and treatment).

Rabies in the cat follows about the same course. The cat, however, does not bite spontaneously, and in the agitated form does not tend to bouts of biting as does the dog. In herbivorous animals the signs of rabies are often discrete, and the disease is not usually recognized except when the diseased animal bites. The physician practically never sees rabies in wild animals: these animals are almost always killed and, if they are captured, cannot easily be kept under observation.

THE RABIES VIRUS

CLASSIFICATION

The rabies virus is difficult to classify. The current tendency on the part of most authors is to relate it to myxoviruses, with which it has several characteristics in common: morphology, sensitivity to ether and acids, the ribonucleic nature of its nucleoprotein component, and extracellular migration of the virus particles. However, it differs in other characteristics, including the appearance and location of virions in the cell, the absence of hemagglutinating and hemadsorption properties, and so forth.

MORPHOLOGY

The dimensions of the virus particles were ascertained in 1936 by ultrafiltration on graduated Elford membranes; this information has now been confirmed by electron microscopic study of animal brains and, in recent years, even more clearly in tissue

cultures. The virions have roughly the shape of a bullet (at least the short forms) and have a rounded or ogival form at one extremity, being flattened at the other. The diameter is more or less constant (60 to 80 mμ), but its length varies (115 to more than 300 mμ). In tissue culture, the shorter forms seem to be related to the "fixed" viruses, while only the "street" strains of virus are thought to give longer forms. If confirmed, these morphological differences, noted earlier by ultrafiltration data, should be interesting in that they would prove that "fixed" viruses are true mutants of "street" viruses.

"STREET" AND "FIXED" VIRUSES

The term "street virus" applies to all viruses isolated in nature. This term, which dates from the time when the dog was considered to be the reservoir of infection, now covers all viruses isolated from domestic as well as from wild animals. In fact, after much controversy as to the differences which could exist on the one hand between the rabies viruses in different parts of the world and, on the other hand, between the viruses of domestic animals and those of wild animals (in particular the viruses of wolves), often qualified as "reinforced" viruses, it seems that currently one can affirm that all rabies viruses in nature are the same.

The "fixed" viruses are creations of the laboratory, and it was Pasteur himself who chose the word to designate the virus which he was first to obtain by repeatedly passing the street virus from one rabbit brain to another. It was the "fixed" virus that he used for the prevention of the disease in man and which, at this writing (early 1967) after 2065 passages in the rabbit at the Pasteur Institute, remains the most widely used in the world in the preparation of antirabies vaccines.

The fixed viruses are distinguished from the street viruses precisely by the fixedness of their pathogenic character. The length of the incubation period in the rabbit inoculated intracerebrally is considerably shortened, being four to ten days (six days for the Pasteur Institute virus) instead of the 15 to 30 days for the street viruses. Becoming fixed after a certain number of passages, it remains perfectly constant under identical conditions of climate, technique, and breed of rabbit used. Similarly, the duration and symptomatology of the disease in the rabbit become immutable. Paralysis is a regular occurrence; its form and time of appearance are fixed. Under similar experimental conditions the pathogenicity remains unchanged during the passages. The average infective dose (LD50) after intracerebral inoculation remains the same. When it is subcutaneously incubated, the pathogenicity of the fixed virus is practically nil. This property doubtless came into play in Pasteur's preventive treatment of man and continues to play an important role which, in our opinion, has not been sufficiently pointed out. Finally, the fixed viruses do not produce the Negri bodies characteristic of the street viruses, but only peculiar acidophilic nuclear lesions (see the section on pathological anatomy).

Of course, this model suffers exceptions which the artifacts of experimentation have created. However, it is of consistent practical value in identifying the rabies virus in question in case of a failure in the treatment of man (see the section on laboratory diagnosis).

PROPERTIES

The properties of the rabies virus which are of interest to the practitioner are those which concern its fragility in the extracellular environment and the practical consequences of that fragility. The virus in its free, extracellular state—as it very likely occurs in the virulent saliva—has a very poor resistance compared to the intracellular virus, especially that in the neural cells. This fragility of the free virus, its sensitivity to air, to light, and to nearly all antiseptics makes obligatory the thorough cleansing of wounds, now recognized as an urgent step in preventive treatment, and absolutely forbids suturing except after careful cleansing. Suturing is too often a veritable reflex on the part of many practitioners, particularly in the case of mutilating face wounds, but in rabies it is the most dangerous possible treatment (see the section on preventive treatment).

On the other hand, the resistance of the virus in nerve cells is such that the virus can still be isolated from buried corpses after several weeks and from cerebral material liquefied by putrefaction. Simple refrigeration and transportation in ice suffice for sending to specialized laboratories the samples necessary for identification of the virus and even for its inoculation into animals (see the next section).

LABORATORY DIAGNOSIS

SPECIMENS

Practically speaking, the diagnosis of rabies can be made only *post mortem* in the laboratory, and solely in a specialized laboratory.

In Man. Laboratory confirmation is solely of retrospective interest and is only rarely necessary to confirm the clinical diagnosis in atypical cases or in those cases in which the question of identification of the virus arises following antirabies treatment.

In theory, the laboratory should receive the whole brain with the cerebellum and the medulla oblongata, and, if possible, the superior portion of the spinal cord, a dissection which requires the trepanning of the whole calvarium and which is both destructive to the cadaver and dangerous to the operator. If the family refuses the autopsy or if the practitioner is not equipped for it without running risks, there remains the possibiliy of puncture biopsy, a procedure which we have used successfully and which is acceptable to the family and without danger to the operator. The scalp is incised with a bistoury in the center of the occiput. A hole is made with a trepan or a simple carpenter's wimble of a caliber sufficient to allow the introduction of the biggest trocar at the operator's disposal. This trocar is gently pushed along the long axis of the head. After the dura mater has been crossed, which is easily perceived by the hand holding the trocar, the mandrel is withdrawn and the cannula alone is pushed obliquely in the horizontal plane to the right or to the left in the direction of the frontal angle in such a way that it has the greatest chance of crossing the area of Ammon's horn, which is the richest in virus. When it strikes the frontal wall, the cannula is withdrawn in one motion. It then contains a cylinder of cerebral material taken from different parts of the encephalon. The instrument is most easily sent directly to the laboratory in a thermos with ice, without any attempt to take the material out of the cannula. The transethmoidal puncture described by Beytout et al., which is done with the same type of trocar, is even less damaging, since it is done via the nostril without leaving a trace, but it does not allow sampling of all parts of the brain.

In Animals. On the other hand, laboratory diagnosis in a dead or dying animal is a current practice and an urgent one, since it dictates the preventive treatment of wounds and the veterinarian's prophylactic measures (see the section on prophylaxis and treatment). In the absence of a veterinarian, and because of the urgency, the doctor himself will often have to do the necessary biopsies to be sent immediately to the laboratory.

The technique is simple and requires a minimum of precaution: a pair of thick gloves and a knife with which to cut the neck at the thorax, the knife being strong enough to separate the cervical vertebrae. No contamination is to be feared for the operator, even by spattered blood. However, it is preferable to wear glasses. The head thus taken is to be sent to the laboratory in an ice-filled container as quickly as possible. If the operator does not have any ice on hand, or if long delays in delivery are foreseen, the head should be submerged in a container filled with glycerin, which retards putrefaction without harm to the rabies virus.

TECHNIQUES

Indeed, while putrefaction is of little hindrance to the laboratory in the isolation of the virus, whose resistance has previously been discussed (see the preceding section on the rabies virus), it may falsify results of the two techniques which are currently used in rapid diagnosis of rabies: the search for Negri bodies (see the section on pathological anatomy) by direct staining, and the detection of virulent elements by use of immunofluorescent techniques.

The first technique, applied to smears of brain matter in order to gain time (confirmation later being given by histological sections), preferably uses the Sellers stain, a combination, mixed just before use, of alcoholic solutions of methylene blue and basic fuchsin which brings out Negri bodies as bright red against a purplish-pink background. The second technique, similarly applied to smears or impression preparations of brain or salivary glands, is based on the "attraction" of antibodies by antigens: the globulins from hyperimmune serum, conjugated with (or marked by) fluorescein isothiocyanate, fasten to the virulent elements, particularly the Negri bodies. Examination with a special microscope reveals the latter as brilliant spots on a greenish-black background, while the non-infected smears appear uniformly fluorescent. When these methods give negative results, diagnosis should be made on histo-logical sections of various samples of the same specimen. Inoculation of susceptible animals (intracerebrally in the mouse or rabbit) is also indicated in order to eliminate, in the case of a man recently treated or of a dog recently vaccinated with living fixed virus, the possibility of an infection by this virus, a possibility which is sometimes raised by authorities.

The details of these techniques, as well as all other laboratory techniques relevant to rabies, can be found in the recent treatises of Lépine or of Netter and in the manual of the World Health Organization on laboratory techniques in rabies.

INTERPRETATION

The doctor does not have to wait for laboratory results, even though they may be quickly available (less than 24 hours), to decide upon his course of action concerning the patient (see the section on prophylaxis and treatment). In the absence of a veterinarian, positive results from the laboratory require the physician to notify the authorities so that they can take the necessary prophylactic measures. Negative laboratory results allow him to delay this action while waiting for confirmation by histological studies and inoculation of laboratory animals.

EPIDEMIOLOGY

DEFINITION

We use the word "epidemiology" here in its English sense, that is to say, covering all that concerns the life of the virus in nature. As concerns rabies, the term ought to be epizootology or, better, enzootology. In fact, while we hardly like the word "zoonosis," which has been badly abused, it must be recognized that rabies is a zoonosis-type infection, proper to animals, which only accidentally affects man, who plays no role in its natural cycle.

GEOGRAPHIC DISTRIBUTION

The infection can practically be considered world-wide. Presently, except for a few countries such as England, Ireland, Australia, and New Zealand, which are protected by their insular position against any invasion of wild rabies and by harsh quarantine laws on the importation of animals as possible carriers of infection, the list of "countries free of rabies" in the last WHO report is extremely short. Moreover, most of these have been "freed" relatively recently and probably only temporarily.

In fact, in recent years, a recrudescence and an important spread of rabies have occurred the world over.* A better knowledge of the infection of wild animals and systematic search for this infection in a number of countries have permitted an estimate of its gravity.

WILD RABIES

Vast campaigns have been organized against rabies among wild animals. Besides the direct danger that they represent to man, rabid wild animals are the real mode by which the infection is spread and, without any doubt, are the only permanent reservoir from which epizootics among domestic animals arise or are reborn.

Wolves, coyotes, foxes, civets, badgers, mongooses, polecats, weasels, raccoons, skunks, civet cats, martens, and, in general, all wild carnivores can be found to be infected in the wild. The latest information published shows the size of this wild reservoir in countries where rabies is established. West Germany, for example, considered by the countries of Europe which are free of rabies as the most dangerous current source, certainly seems to have been invaded by the infection only during the last war as a result of the prevailing disorder, the confiscation of arms, and the evacuation of populations. The first statistics (1950) reported 1170 confirmed cases of rabies in animals, the number of cases being higher in foxes (690) and badgers (105) than among domestic animals (112 dogs). Recent statistics showed 2660 cases among wild animals (2071 of them in foxes) as opposed to 726 among domestic animals (dogs, cats, sheep, cows, horses, and pigs). Systematic research undertaken in the wild certainly influences this numerical increase: recently West Germany reported true epizootics among herds of forest deer, victims of the enzootic among wild carnivores.

In Czechoslovakia's western provinces

of Bohemia-Moravia, a study made in the first six months of 1964 indicated that 42 foxes out of 91 examined, two badgers out of six, and a lone captured marten were all infected with rabies. These figures illustrate well the density of infection in the wild and the seriousness of the problem which it poses. Of 22 deer captured in these enzootic regions, three were found to be infected, as was one of two stags examined. Of 16 muskrats (or Canadian beavers, transplanted by man to Europe and numerous others in the wild state in these same regions), two were positive. At the same time, for domestic animals in these provinces that were suspect because they were biters, the figures are completely different: only five dogs of 110 examined, five cats of 51, and one sheep were positive for rabies. These figures illustrate the primacy of the wild reservoir.

In the United States, where the problem of rabies remains very serious, the importance of the wild reservoir becomes more evident each year. The latest statistics published for all of the states show that the number of cases detected among wild animals, in a systematic investigation, has increased over the number of cases found among domestic animals, which are subject to extensive preventive vaccination campaigns. Among these infected wild animals, the fox heads the list, with about 50 per cent of the cases, but skunks represent almost 30 per cent. A recent study, limited to skunks in the state of Ohio during an epizootic period, showed that 62 per cent of 502 animals examined were infected.

Thus it seems certain that wild animals, in the countries where the infection is inveterate, constitute the natural reservoir for virus and that rabies is connected with the carnivores alone. While cases have been seen in other, noncarnivorous wild animals (e.g., cervidae, rodents, sciuridae), their rarity shows fairly well that these animals are only occasional victims of rabid carnivores and do not play any role in the cycle of rabies.*

---

*Wild rabies has recently crossed the Rhine: infected foxes have been found in Belgium and Luxembourg. It has now penetrated France, where the first infected fox was detected in March, 1968.

---

*A surprising work, the results of which, however, seem unassailable, was done in 1966 in Thailand (P. C. Smith et al., Nature, *217*:954, 1968). A systematic investigation by inoculation of ground-up brain into newborn mice revealed the infection in five species of rats and two species of bandicoots at a level sometimes as high as 7.9 per cent of rodents captured in nature. This work raises anew the question of the reservoir of wild rodents, a capital question since wild rodents are the principal prey of carnivores.

Indeed, one must class apart the case, limited to Central and South America alone, of the large blood-sucking bats, the vampires. Can these vampires, which bite cattle and Equidae in order to gorge themselves with blood, thereby transmitting rabies, be the reservoir of virus in these regions? The relation of these flying animals with infected wild carnivores is practically nil. On the other hand, the virus does not circulate in the blood of rabid horses and cattle. Can the vampires maintain the virus themselves, among themselves? It was in these bats that, for the first time among wild mammals, silent prolonged forms of the infection were discovered, seemingly healthy vampires being capable of excreting virus in their saliva for several months.

Other non-blood-sucking bats in Brazil (frugivores or insectivores) had been found to be similarly infected, but always when there was contact with vampires. One can indeed understand the extraordinary interest awakened by the identification in 1953 of the virus in insectivorous bats in Florida, United States, where vampire bats do not exist. Later, the virus was found in several species (some of which were living in huge colonies in caves) in several southern and western states as far north as Canada. Five cases of human rabies contracted from bats have been reported in the United States. As with the vampires of Central and South America, asymptomatic forms have been observed. The virus was isolated from interscapular brown fat of bats of which neither the salivary glands nor the brain were infected. The possibility that these animals serve as virus reservoirs was immediately considered, but extensive studies undertaken in the areas of Europe, Asia, and Africa in which rabies is enzootic have, until now, given positive results only in Turkey, Yugoslavia, and Thailand, and these results still require confirmation.* On the other hand, in the laboratory it is practically impossible to obtain transmission by biting from infected bats to healthy bats or laboratory animals. However, extensive epizootics have been shown to exist in the caves of the southern United States. Following the appearance of two cases of rabies in man contracted in these caves without bites from the bats, an experiment performed with such rigor that it seems unassailable showed that in such highly infected caves virus transmission can occur through the air, thanks to the humidity, which favors the formation of a true aerosol.

The greatest interest of these studies on bats has been to draw attention to the "latent" forms of infection. The bats which can have such forms do not, it seems, come in contact with carnivores, although in the United States some statistical analyses do tend to show a relationship between the incidence of rabies among foxes and among bats. On the other hand, if wild rodents, being the basic food of carnivores and living in close contact with them, were to have such latent forms of rabies, they could give a permanence to the disease which, until now, could not be accounted for in terms of transmission of the infection by biting between carnivores, whose sensitivity to the disease (moreover in general poorly known) would be assumed to condemn them to a rapid death. However, none of the studies done so far on the wild rodent populations of several countries where the disease is enzootic among carnivores has shown the presence of infection, latent or not, in these rodents. Similarly, research on the possible persistence of virus in acarians, insects, coleopters, and necrophagous insects in the burrows of these animals have been negative.

As we have mentioned, the role of reservoir of the wild rabies virus should without a doubt be attributed to carnivores alone.* In spite of the difficulty of capturing and observing these animals, and, even more, of experimenting on them, it is among them that one must systematically look for the species, undoubtedly different according to the region, whose natural resistance to the infection is sufficient to permit them to harbor it in a latent form long enough to insure its perennial nature.† Current research in the United States seems to show that in this country skunks and opossums could present this type of infection.

RABIES AMONG DOMESTIC ANIMALS

While knowledge of rabies among wild animals is more interesting in terms of introduction and durability of infection, it is

---

*This confirmation has been given for Thailand (P. C. Smith et al. Nature, *216*:384, 1967) where the very important question arises concerning rodents as a virus reservoir (see note on p. 143).

---

*See footnote, left column.

†P. C. Smith et al. seem to have revealed the existence of this form in the rodent *Bandicota indica*, with presence of the virus in the salivary glands.

rabies in domestic animals with which the physician has to deal most often. In fact, in those countries where wild rabies is most prevalent, even in those where the way of life puts man and wild animals most in contact, the danger a man runs of being attacked by these carnivores remains very limited. None of these countries has, to our knowledge, reported a percentage of bites by wild animals higher than 20 per cent of the total incidence of biting, even during the most active years. An attack on man by a timid and mistrustful animal such as the fox, even a rabid fox, is exceptional. Attack by the fearful and fleeing jackal is rare, even in the countries where jackals abound. The wolf, powerful and afraid of nothing, represents a danger to man which, in Iran for example, we have been able to observe but which remains very limited.

It is therefore domestic animals, forming a link between wild animals and man, that play the primary role. Indeed, these have more contact with wild animals than is apparent: Dogs, above all, in their wanderings during hunts and, in many countries, the great mass of stray dogs, especially in suburban areas; cats in their nocturnal vagabonding; even herbivorous animals (cattle, cows and particularly calves, buffalo, sheep, goats, horses, camels, donkeys, and mules), especially in countries where herds move to and fro in the fields, wandering or spending the night in the pasture—all of these animals have many contacts with wild animals.

In practically all countries, the fox is primarily responsible for the passage of infection to domestic animals. This is because it is the most numerous of the wild carnivores and because the fox's way of life brings him in contact with the human habitat and domestic animals, particularly with cats at night; this explains the frequency of feline rabies in countries where infection is frequent among foxes (e.g., West Germany). A rabid fox is also likely to bite domestic herbivores at night in the pasture.

However, rabies in herbivorous animals, despite its frequency in certain countries such as the United States, where it is considered a real economic pest, is not dangerous to man. Herbivorous animals (except the camel) have no natural tendency to bite, and the figures show that the number of people treated for bites of such animals in all countries remains extremely low. The same is true for rabies in the cat, whose sharp teeth can inoculate the virus in the most dangerous manner, but who bites only occasionally, even when made aggressive by rabies.

Thus to the dog falls the primary role in the transmission of rabies to man, first because of his close contact, second because he bites by nature and because he is most often stricken with furious rabies, during which he will attack even his owner, and last because, before dying or being killed, he will almost always have bitten numerous domestic animals around him, especially other dogs.

In all countries, male dogs are most often stricken because of their fighting instincts. The young are the most susceptible to infection. In a dense population of dogs, epizootics can last for a long time by transmission from dog to dog. The incubation of the disease is variable and can be long. In dogs bitten by the same rabid animal, this period has varied between 15 days and three months. In addition, it is not impossible that the dog could present "defective" forms of rabies with healing, or "chronic" or "recurrent" rabies, or even "inapparent" rabies. True canine enzootics sometimes seem to exist, and, in Morocco for example, the very numerous stray dogs have been accused of playing the role of virus reservoir. However, no parallel study to support this contention has been done among wild carnivores, particularly the jackals, which are as numerous in Morocco as in other countries where their role as a reservoir has been duly demonstrated, and which live in close contact with stray dogs.

In fact, it seems that rabies cannot be maintained for a long time in a canine population and that the seeding of infection in countries free of the disease cannot be the result of the importation of an infected dog, but only of the penetration and spreading of rabies from one wild carnivorous animal to the next.

HUMAN RABIES

The usual means of infection of man is a bite by a rabid animal. But the virulent saliva can penetrate in other ways: scratches from a cat, which constantly licks its paws and which has a greater tendency to scratch than to bite. Such scratches are classically considered dangerous. Licking of skin abrasions or of the mucosa is similarly dangerous. The conjunctiva is the elective pathway, and sprays of saliva in the eyes and even on undamaged mucosa represent a source of contamination not to be neglected. The blood and urine of infected animals, and even the milk, can occasionally be virulent and penetrate via the conjunctiva or mucosa. It is possible that certain human cases (like those from the bats in caves in the United States) are due to such means of contamination.

These pathways and means of virus inoculation should not be ignored, for the physician will often have to deal with patients who, wishing to help a sick animal, have put their hands in its mouth during laryngopharyngeal spasms to remove from its throat the bone which they believe responsible for these spasms. Others will have been licked by a paralyzed dog, whose mildness and quiet agony left them unaware of the nature of the disease. Finally, others will have been brutally scratched when trying to take in their arms their cat which has hidden for hours under the furniture.

However, it is for bites that the immense majority of patients come to consult a physician. In areas where rabies is enzootic, all biting animals should be suspect, even the sick squirrel found by a child, tamed mongooses, mice, even birds, and especially bats.

The probability that a man will become infected by the bite of a rabid animal is not, however, absolute. In Iran, we were able to observe large groups of peasants attacked at the same time by the same rabid wolf (one wolf bit 32 people), presenting serious wounds, who remained untreated or arrived too late to benefit from treatment. Only 60 per cent of those bitten on the head and 30 per cent, at most, of those bitten on the trunk or on the limbs contracted rabies.

Among those bitten by dogs (although observation of a group as large as the aforementioned has never been made) and among those bitten by cats, the percentages are even lower yet, the wounds being less serious and less deep.

DIAGNOSIS

HUMAN RABIES

Early diagnosis of the disease, which is important in other infections because it permits a prognosis and decisions as to treatment, is unfortunately not of as much interest in rabies, since this disease is inevitably fatal and since there is no treatment which can arrest its evolution.

However, early diagnosis is necessary since, as we have seen (under the heading The Disease), the patient cannot be kept at home and must be hospitalized immediately, if possible in an artificial survival center, where at least the horrible symptomatology of the disease can be suppressed, a symptomatology which the patient's lucidity makes even more horrible (see the section on treatment).

In virtually all cases, diagnosis is ascertained at once by the patient himself by exact recall of the contaminating incident; moreover, bites, even scarred-over, are easily identifiable. Many patients have also received preventive antirabies treatment. Only exceptionally will the idea of rabies infection fail to arise: in very young children, for example, in primitive people, or in the very rare cases of contamination by unusual means from an apparently healthy animal (licking, via the mucosa or conjunctiva).

Finally, in the case of a very long incubation period, it could happen that the patient would totally forget the contaminating incident. These cases are, however, exceptional. Early statistics show that incubation periods longer than three months represent not more than 15 per cent of the cases, and cases of very long incubation (a year or more), during which time the accident could have been forgotten, are extremely rare (1.2 per cent according to the most recent statistics). The average length of incubation for rabies is in fact from 15 to 55 days, cases of very short incubation (less than 15 days) also being rare.

In fact, early diagnosis, which is necessary, is most often obtained through the patient himself, who consults a physician as soon as the first signs appear, subtle as these may be. Few people, even the most courageous, even the most primitive, following contamination, have not studied their case in some layman's medical handbook or have not heard some terrifying story, usually legendary, about the tragic fate which awaits them. This is one of the factors which contributes to rabies' frightening reputation. During this incubation period, whose length has been exaggerated because of the rare cases of particularly long incubation, the patient, although his wounds have long since scarred over and despite any confidence he may have in the preventive treatment he is following, never stops watching for the slightest symptom, which he has learned to recognize often better even than the doctor he consults. All those who have headed an antirabies treatment center are familiar with this psychological factor and the nervous state into which it can put certain patients, a state which, it seems, has a bad influence on the effects of preventive treatment. However, this "nervous hydrophobia" subsides with administration of neuroleptics.

In other respects, early diagnosis is based solely on subjective symptoms: premonitory fever at first and, when present, peculiar sensations around the wound, excitability, despondence, insomnia, and then the almost pathognomonic anxiety. Later diagnosis is based on characteristic objective signs, essentially laryngopharyngeal spasms and hyperesthesia, and then convulsions and paralysis when they occur (see the section on The Disease). Usually, there is no room for doubt in making the diagnosis. Only the paralytic form, which may have no accompanying signs, might present an unresolvable diagnostic problem if the patient is incapable of answering questions.

The need for differential diagnosis practically never arises. The only possibility would be tetanus "from the bite," but its incubation period is much shorter than that of rabies. Certain poisons and some forms of encephalitis or acute myelitis might be thought to bring on the Landry syndrome, and even poliomyelitis might be confused with the pure paralytic forms of rabies, but these are exceptional. The furious or convulsive form, seen in the terminal stages, will sometimes lead to the erroneous referral of a patient to a psychiatric service. "Nervous hydrophobia" cannot lead the physician astray for long.

Finally, in the fortunately rare complications in patients bitten and subjected to antirabies treatment, differential diagnosis may be necessary between rabies and the paralytic complications of the vaccination (see the section on Prophylaxis and Treatment), the symptomatology of which is almost always limited to an often painful paraplegia which should regress rapidly. In exceptional cases in which the paralysis persists or spreads, resulting in death, without other clinical signs of rabies (complications attributable to the living fixed virus in the vaccine), diagnosis should be made by the laboratory by histological examination of brain samples and inoculation of susceptible animals.

ANIMAL RABIES

The sooner the diagnosis is made the greater will be the chances of preventing the animal from biting and, particularly for the dog, from launching himself on a disastrous final wandering which increases the chances of spreading the infection (see the sections on The Disease and Epidemiology). Such early diagnosis is based on the unrest, despondence, and prostration of an ordinarily very energetic animal or on the aggressiveness and extreme nervousness of an ordinarily very calm animal. In an area where rabies is enzootic, the knowledge of these signs is indispensable not only to the doctor but to all animal owners. All animals whose behavior becomes even unusual should immediately be put under observation in a very strong cage which, when the objective signs appear, permits diagnosis without danger, after which one can safely wait for death, which is necessary for the quality of the specimens (see the next section).

PATHOGENESIS; PATHOLOGICAL ANATOMY; PHYSIOPATHOLOGY

INTRODUCTION OF THE VIRUS

Usually, the rabies virus multiplies only in nerve cells. Although current tissue culture techniques have made possible proliferation on a number of cell types (e.g., fibroblasts), it seems that in vivo the inoculated virus can develop only in the neural filaments, the nerves, or the neural trunks. When these have been injured by a bite, viral multiplication is particularly rapid, a fact which governs the urgency of the treatment of wounds (see the section on Prophylaxis and Treatment).

MIGRATION AND MULTIPLICATION

The virus propagates solely by way of the nerves in a centripetal direction (Levaditi's neuroprobasia). At present no other pathway (the blood particularly) seems to be incriminated. The virus, once it gets to the nerve centers, multiplies there, creating lesions which will result in rabies encephalitis. The combined times of these processes, migration and multiplication, represent the length of the incubation period. Migration can be very rapid: virus inoculated into the masseter muscle or by nasal instillation can be recovered in the brain as early as four days later. The rapidity of this invasion does not seem to be related to the distance covered by the virus from the bite to the brain, but rather to the amount of innervation of the region, that is to say, to the possibility of immediate "fixation" and multiplication of the virus, and to the size of the pathways available. If it is true that face wounds have the shortest incubation periods, it is because they most often involve nerves or neural trunks of a large caliber, while scalp wounds, for example, could have a longer incubation period than a leg wound touching on the popliteal nerve. Rabies develops more often and more quickly from penetrating finger wounds than from wounds affecting muscles of the buttocks or trunk, which are less richly innervated.

This also explains the fact that a virus of slight aggressiveness, like the fixed viruses, when introduced subcutaneously into very poorly innervated tissue, never causes rabies (an undoubtedly valuable property, as we have mentioned, in the use of living vaccines injected under the skin or into the abdominal panniculus adiposus), whereas the same virus, in infinitely weaker doses, causes rabies when inoculated into richly innervated derma.

Like migration, multiplication of virus in the brain can be very rapid. It is accompanied by a diffusion, this time centrifugal, and a generalization to the whole nervous system: axons, neural trunks, and peripheral nerves (Nicolau's septineuritis). This generalization, prior to the spreading of encephalitic lesions, explains the fact that the virus can appear in the saliva several days before the first symptoms become manifest, an important notion which makes it necessary to put apparently healthy but biting animals under observation (see the section on Prophylaxis and Treatment). Viral multiplication in the brain can be slow, with a true latent period. It seems that the exceptionally long incubation periods are due to such a phenomenon and not to a slow or retarded migration of the virus from the point of inoculation.

LESIONS

No specific macroscopic lesions of the neural centers and organs are observed. However, considerable lesions are detected under the microscope, namely, (1) nonspecific lesions existing in all cases of encephalitis, such as perivascular inflammatory lesions, nodules of microglial proliferation, neuronic changes, and degeneration of the axons; and (2) specific pathological manifestations (Negri bodies and oxyphilic nuclear lesions).

Nonspecific lesions are localized, in the common forms, to the ganglia of the cranial nerves, the spinal ganglia, the medulla oblongata, the hypothalamus, the cerebral and cerebellar cortex, the spinal cord, and the peripheral nerves in decreasing intensity; they prevail, in the paralytic forms, in the latter two areas.

Specific changes, Negri bodies in particular, are observed mainly in the areas where inflammatory manifestations are mild: in the pyramidal cells of Ammon's horn, the neurons of the neighboring temporal cortex, and, lastly, in Purkinje's cells of the cerebellum.

Negri Bodies. Negri bodies are, as we have said (see the section on Laboratory Diagnosis), characteristic of the street virus. They occur only rarely and in small numbers in fixed virus infections, and their absence, in cases of clinically confirmed rabies, requires the inoculation of laboratory animals in order to identify the virus in question (see Laboratory Diagnosis). Negri bodies are oval or rounded elements in the cytoplasm of nerve cells. Their size, which seems to vary with the age of the elements, can reach 20 and even 30 μ. Their number, which can be very great, since all neurons can contain one or more, similarly varies with the age of the infection; this necessitates putting any suspect animal under observation until death. Indeed, in animals killed early, e.g., those having forms of the disease with a short incubation period and rapid evolution, Negri bodies can be overlooked or very difficult to find because of their small number and size. Specifically stained by special methods, these bodies have a corpuscular "internal structure" in which, however, even with the electron microscope, complete virus particles cannot be found. The nature of these bodies, long debated since they could be confounded with protozoa, is now recognized as being specific. Identification of the proteins, of the RNA, and particularly of rabies antigen in the Negri bodies seems to indicate that they are due to an abortive viral duplication or to specific defense mechanisms of the cell.

Nuclear Lesions. These lesions exist in street virus infections as well as in fixed virus infections, but in the latter case, because of their abundance and the absence of Negri bodies, they represent the specific element of microscopic diagnosis. Lépine, who discovered them with Sautter, describes them as "oxyphilic lesions in profoundly modified, pyknotic neural cells; in an acidophilic mass which represents vestiges of the nucleus, heaps of oval or rounded corpuscles are seen, irregular in size, hyperchromatic, mostly basophilic, and some of which are highly acidophilic."

PHYSIOPATHOLOGY

The pathological processes and death, the inevitable end of this disease, certainly seem to be due to the marked impairment of neural cells and particularly of neurons of the encephalon and medulla oblongata. However, in man and even more often in animals, these lesions are apparently not a sufficient explanation for death. The recent discovery, using complement fixation, of a complex soluble antigen in virus-free material obtained by high-speed centrifugation, may add something to our knowledge of the physiopathology of this infection.

IMMUNOLOGICAL RESPONSES

Immunological study of rabies in man is based solely on the discovery of neutralizing antibodies in the blood. This technique is used largely to evaluate horse sera prepared for the prevention of human disease, sera in which one tries to have the highest possible titer of neutralizing antibodies whose antiviral action is certain. Experience has shown, however, that the level of neutralizing antibodies does not faithfully indicate the state of immunity. Numerous horses, after immunization, are perfectly able to resist inoculations of massive doses of living virus without producing a usable serum. In laboratory animals, in which the most severe tests can be done intracerebrally, the resistance of vaccinated animals can be as great in those having no evident antibodies in the blood as in those who have a high titer of them.

Studies done by a group of laboratories on numerous sera sampled at the Pasteur Institute of Iran from a group of people bitten by a rabid wolf have shown that some survivors had only a very low titer of antibodies, while one of the patients who died from rabies had a very high level.

This method of titrating neutralizing antibodies, the only one applicable in studying human responses to immunization with antirabies vaccine, allows only an approximation; in animals, however, immunization can be studied with precision by intracerebrally testing with the same batch of virus and using series of mice vaccinated with different doses or, more exactly, with various dilutions of a vaccine to be titrated. This "Habel test," interpretable statistically, is perfectly reliable.

PROPHYLAXIS AND TREATMENT

PROPHYLAXIS

Long-term prophylaxis is the veterinarian's domain: it includes fighting against the wild reservoirs in enzootic areas, quarantine, campaigns warning animal owners, and systematic and repeated preventive vaccination of dogs and cats.

In man, preventive vaccination should be applied only to persons constantly in danger of infection in enzootic regions: veterinarians, animal pound employees, forest rangers, and so forth. The vaccines used for this immunization are the same as those for preventive treatment. The last WHO Expert Committee on Rabies recommended the following posology for this vaccination: "Such immunization may consist of a short course of 2 to 3 injections of a potent anti-rabies vaccine, preferably of a non-nervous-tissue type, at one month intervals, followed by a booster injection of vaccine six months later.... Further booster injections should be administered at intervals of one to three years as long as the exposed person remains at risk..."

The immediate prophylaxis in the absence of or before the arrival of a veterinarian will often be the responsibility of the physician. Concomitant to putting the biting animal under observation in a solid cage, he should require the authorities to tie up or cage all animals (even those vaccinated) that have been bitten or that are suspected of having been bitten or, better yet, all animals within the widest radius possible that show any wounds, however recent. Observations of the biting animal should last at least ten days.

If signs of rabies appear, the period of observation should be extended, if circumstances allow, until the death of the animal, thus giving the laboratory maximum chances for making a diagnosis (see the sections on Laboratory Diagnosis and Pathological Anatomy).

In the event of a positive diagnosis for the biting animal, the physician should advise slaughtering all unvaccinated animals that have been bitten or that have been wounded. This is the surest measure, but it cannot be made obligatory. In case of a refusal on the part of owners, vaccination of these animals should be required, as well as continued observation of the caged or chained animals for a minimum of two months. Previously vaccinated animals do not have to be sacrificed. They should be revaccinated and kept under observation for a month.

PREVENTIVE TREATMENT

The WHO Expert Committee on Rabies, at each of its meetings, regularly revises its table of indications for and means of this treatment. Table 10-1 reproduces the revision of June, 1965.

For the practitioners' use, this table can be commented upon as follows:

Treatment of Wounds. The first and most urgent measure is cleansing of the wounds, sores, and scratches. This is so efficacious that a person with scratches and abrasions contaminated by the saliva of a definitely rabid animal need not be subjected to antirabies treatment if the damaged skin has been carefully washed with soap and abundantly rinsed immediately after contamination. In the enzootic areas, this notion should be widely publicized among animal owners by the authorities, since the sooner washing is done the more effective it is; it should always be done immediately, on the spot, by the victim or someone with him. If, however, the patient comes to the doctor with uncleansed wounds, the doctor, before doing anything else, ought to cleanse the wounds all the more carefully considering the delay in arrival of his patient. One of the best techniques, particularly for deep and anfractuous wounds, is to clean them with jets from a large glass syringe or a ball syringe. Under no circumstances should the wounds be sutured unless they have been thoroughly cleansed first (see the section on the Rabies Virus).

Seroprevention. The second most urgent action on the part of the physician is to use antirabies serum. The Expert Committee limits this to certain cases for fear of complications of serum therapy. However, in countries where serotherapy complications are rare and where very few people receive preventive serum inoculations for other infections, there is an advantage in extending the benefit of seroprevention to all those bitten for whom vaccine treatment cannot be started immediately either because the animal is under observation or because the victim has to be taken to a far-off treatment center. With the protection of antirabies serum, the wounded can wait without danger.*

Local application (see Table 10-1, A1b (iii) and A2a) is not easy if the serum is in liquid form, and powdered sera or globulins are not yet currently used. Infiltration (A2b) around anfractuous or bruised bites is very painful, and prior injection of an anesthesic is, in itself, painful. Finally, the action of the serum *in loco* is not better than that of serum injected by the usual intramuscular pathway, which is, therefore, the preferred route. With current sera, however, this injection requires a large volume (40 to 60 ml.) and, when the practitioner is fearful of complications or does not have enough serum on hand (for example, in case of many bitten patients), he must resort to local infiltration.

Besides its immediate action on the virus, the antirabies serum has the advantage of convenience. In its lyophilized form it can be kept for years in a simple household refrigerator and for months at ordinary temperatures. All doctors and all health centers can, therefore, be provided with it.

Antirabies Vaccination. Last comes the question of preventive treatment with the antirabies vaccine. In many countries, this treatment fortunately has not yet been decentralized, and the practitioner's only role is to send the victim, under the protection of antirabies serum, as has just been described, to a specialized center. This must be done

---

*The "interference effect" mentioned by the Expert Committee (note 1 of Table 10-1B) has been confirmed: the antirabies serum "blocks" the active immune response to the vaccine. The general tendency is hence to retard vaccine treatment for at least 24 hours: the first dose of vaccine is not injected "at the same time" as the serum, as was recommended by the Expert Committee (note 2 of Table 10-1B) but 24 hours later.

immediately if the rabid animal has escaped, has been killed, or is an unknown animal which has disappeared, or as soon as signs of rabies appear in a biting animal that has been taken under observation. In this last case, in practice, the patient can remain at home, thanks to the protection given by serum, until the death of the animal, the head of which will be sent to the specialized center.

On the other hand, other countries, particularly those where antirabies vaccine has been made available commercially, have left the responsibility of treatment to the practitioner. In our opinion, this is regrettable, since it poses difficult problems for the doctor. The first is the choice of vaccine, a choice not so much between similar brands as between preparations based on totally different, even opposed principles: so-called living vaccines or so-called inactivated vaccines, according to the terminology used by the Expert Committee itself. It must be said that this terminology is unfortunate, for, while among the so-called living vaccines there are some which are really alive (Flury vaccine, LEP and HEP; Kelev K vaccine, which is not recommended for preventive treatment in man; and rabies viruses modified by passages in chicken embryos, lyophilized, and not treated with an "inactivating" agent), the other "living" vaccines (Fermi-type vaccine), prepared with classic strains of fixed virus treated with phenol, contain living virus only in so far as they have been transported and preserved in the cold (or immediately lyophilized) to prevent the continued action of the phenol.

Among the so-called inactivated vaccines, those of the Semple type, which are the most commonly used, differ according to the manufacturer and, even more important, according to the mode of preservation. Some, even though prepared according to the Semple technique, still contain living virus if they have been lyophilized or transported and preserved in the cold, but no longer contain living virus if, as is most frequently the case, the vaccines have been transported and kept in a liquid state with no special precautions. Other Semple-type vaccines are prepared in such a way that they no longer contain living virus (by prolongation of heating at 37° C., for example). Finally, vaccine prepared on duck embryos and "inactivated" by β-propiolactone does not contain living virus either.

In fact, owing to voluntarily imprecise terminology such as "inactivated," the old argument about living and killed vaccines arises and the Pasteur technique is again questioned. Certainly nobody doubts the principle. "Inactivated" vaccines are used only to avert complications during treatment, which are most often attributed to the presence of living virus. Nevertheless, the use of these "inactivated" vaccines has not eliminated these complications. Vaccines prepared on duck embryos, which should eliminate "paralyzing factor" since they contain neither living virus nor cerebral material, do not avert them.*

If the specialists of antirabies institutes themselves still hesitate about choosing a vaccine, choice must be all the more difficult for the practitioner, especially if there is a complication or failure of treatment, because it is to him that complaints are made and not to the manufacturer.

The indications for treatment are also difficult. To renounce treatment when it is useless is a heavy responsibility which requires much practical experience and knowledge. Furthermore, "decentralization" of treatment always leads to a considerable increase in the number of people treated, and since treatment, as we have seen, is not without risk, this is profitable only for the vaccine manufacturers.

The decision concerning the duration of treatment is also delicate. Pushed to complaisance by psychological factors difficult to escape, the physician will tend to shorten treatment. Even in antirabies institutes, where defense against such factors is easier, treatment of only five or seven days is too frequently practiced. Paradoxically, the greatest number of complications seem to arise from these foreshortened treatments.

Finally, antirabies treatment must indisputably be accompanied by physical and mental rest as complete as possible, this being very difficult to obtain when a patient remains at home.

To summarize, since seroprevention now allows the patient to be sent, in all

---

*Vaccines prepared from tissue culture preparations, concerning which it is hoped that they will eliminate nervous system accidents, are not yet perfected sufficiently to be available. On the other hand, the new vaccines with a basis of cerebral matter of newborn mice or rats, besides the exceptional antigenic potency they show, seem to be devoid of "paralytic factor."

Table 10-1.   *Indications for and Means of Preventive Treatment of Rabies, as Recommended by the WHO Expert Committee on Rabies, June, 1965.*

A. Local Treatment of Wounds Involving Possible Exposure to Rabies

(1) Recommended in all exposures

(a) First-aid treatment

Immediate washing and flushing with soap and water, detergent or water alone (recommended procedure in all bite wounds including those unrelated to possible exposure to rabies).

(b) Treatment by or under direction of a physician

(i) Adequate cleansing of the wound.
(ii) Thorough treatment with 20% soap solution and/or the application of a quaternary ammonium compound or other substance of proven lethal effect on the rabies virus.[1]
(iii) Topical application of antirabies serum or its liquid or powdered globulin preparation (optional).
(iv) Administration, where indicated, of antitetanus procedures and of antibiotics and drugs to control infections other than rabies.
(v) Suturing of wound not advised.

(2) Additional local treatment for severe exposure only

(a) Topical application of antirabies serum or its liquid or powdered globulin preparation.
(b) Infiltration of antirabies serum around the wound.

---

[1]Where soap has been used to clean wounds, all traces of it should be removed before the application of quaternary ammonium compounds because soap neutralizes the activity of such compounds.

Benzalkonium chloride in a 1% concentration, has been demonstrated to be effective in the local treatment of wounds in guinea pigs infected with rabies virus. It should be noted that at this concentration quaternary ammonium compounds may exert a deleterious effect on tissues.

Compounds that have been demonstrated to have a specific lethal effect on rabies virus *in vitro* (different assay systems in mice) include the following:

Quaternary ammonium compounds

0.1% (1 : 1000) benzalkonium chloride = mixture of alkylbenzyldimethylammonium chlorides
0.1% (1 : 1000) cetrimonium bromide = hexadecyltrimethylammonium bromide
1.0% (1 : 100) Hyamine 2389 = mixture containing 40% of methyldodecylbenzyltrimethylammonium chloride and 10% of methyl-dodecylxylylene bis(trimethylammonium chloride)
1.0% (1 : 100) methyl benzethonium chloride = benzyldimethyl {2-{2-[p-(1,1,3,3-tetramethylbutyl)tolyloxy]ethoxy}ethyl}ammonium chloride
1.0% (1 : 100) benzethonium chloride = benzyldimethyl{2-[2-(p-1,1,3,3,-tetramethylbutylphenoxy)ethoxy]ethyl}ammonium chloride
1.0% (1 : 100) SKF 11831 = p-phenylphenacylhexamethylenetetrammonium bromide.

Other substances

43-70% ethanol; tincture of thiomersal; tincture of iodine and up to 0.01% (1 : 10,000) aqueous solutions of iodine; 1% to 2% soap solutions.

B. Specific Systemic Treatment

NATURE OF EXPOSURE	STATUS OF BITING ANIMAL (IRRESPECTIVE OF WHETHER VACCINATED OR NOT)		RECOMMENDED TREATMENT
	AT TIME OF EXPOSURE	DURING OBSERVATION PERIOD OF TEN DAYS	
I. No lesions ; indirect contact	Rabid	—	None
II. Licks:			
(1) unabraded skin	Rabid	—	None
(2) abraded skin, scratches and unabraded or abraded mucosa	*(a)* healthy	Clinical signs of rabies or proven rabid (laboratory)	Start vaccine[1] at first signs of rabies in the biting animal
	(b) signs suggestive of rabies	Healthy	Start vaccine[1] immediately ; stop treatment if animal is normal on fifth day after exposure
	(c) rabid, escaped, killed or unknown	—	Start vaccine[1] immediately

B. **Specific Systemic Treatment** *(Continued)*

| NATURE OF EXPOSURE | STATUS OF BITING ANIMAL (IRRESPECTIVE OF WHETHER VACCINATED OR NOT) | | RECOMMENDED TREATMENT |
	AT TIME OF EXPOSURE	DURING OBSERVATION PERIOD OF TEN DAYS	
III. Bites:			
(1) mild exposure	(a) healthy	Clinical signs of rabies or proven rabid (laboratory)	Start vaccine[1,2] at first signs of rabies in the biting animal
	(b) signs suggestive of rabies	Healthy	Start vaccine[1] immediately; stop treatment if animal is normal on fifth day after exposure
	(c) rabid, escaped, killed or unknown	–	Start vaccine[1,2] immediately
	(d) wild (wolf, jackal, fox, bat, etc.)	–	Serum[2] immediately, followed by a course of vaccine[1]
(2) severe exposure (multiple, or face, head, finger or neck bites)	(a) healthy	Clinical signs of rabies or proven rabid (laboratory)	Serum- immediately; start vaccine[1] at first sign of rabies in the biting animal
	(b) signs suggestive of rabies	Healthy	Serum[2] immediately, followed by vaccine ; vaccine may be stopped if animal is normal on fifth day after exposure
	(c) rabid, escaped, killed or unknown		
	(d) wild (wolf, jackal, pariah dog, fox, bat, etc.)	–	Serum[2] immediately, followed by vaccine[1]

[1]Practice varies concerning the volume of vaccine per dose and the number of doses recommended in a given situation. In general, the equivalent of at least 2 ml of a 5% tissue emulsion should be given subcutaneously daily for 14 consecutive days. Many laboratories use 20 to 30 doses in severe exposures. To ensure the production and maintenance of high levels of serum-neutralizing antibodies, booster doses should be given at 10 days and at 20 or more days following the last daily dose of vaccine in *all* cases. This is especially important if antirabies serum has been used, in order to overcome the interference effect.

[2]In all severe exposures and in all cases of unprovoked wild animal bites, antirabies serum or its globulin fractions together with vaccine should be employed. This is considered by the Committee as the *best* specific treatment available for the post-exposure prophylaxis of rabies in man. Although experience indicates that vaccine alone is sufficient for mild exposures, there is no doubt that here also the combined serum-vaccine treatment will give the best protection. However, both the serum and the vaccine can cause deleterious reactions. Moreover, the combined therapy is more expensive; its use in mild exposures is therefore considered optional. As with vaccine alone, it is important to start combined serum and vaccine treatment as early as possible after exposure, but serum should still be used no matter what the time interval. Serum should be given in a single dose (40 IU per kg of body weight) and the first dose of vaccine inoculated at the same time. Sensitivity to the serum must be determined before its administration.

safety and without hurry, to a specialized center, it certainly seems that the practitioner does best to free himself in this way of all responsibility for the treatment. He will thus undertake only the responsibility of giving the necessary boosters upon the patient's return to his home, a necessity insisted upon by the Expert Committee (see Table 10-1).†

Complications of Preventive Treatment. Complications of seroprevention are "seral

†Recently, new failures of antirabies treatment with protracted incubation in patients duly treated by serum and vaccine have confirmed the absolute necessity of booster injections in *all* cases, as directed by the WHO Expert Committee. The current general trend sets the time of these booster injections 20 to 60 days after the end of treatment; a third booster after four months should be given in all cases possible.

reactions" on the part of persons sensitive to heterologous sera. These reactions can be avoided by questioning the patient and performing intradermal or ophthalmic sensitivity tests. If the test result is positive, a strong dose of an antihistamine should be administered before injection of the serum and several times during the following days. Certain countries where seral reactions are frequent (up to 20 per cent of those treated), including serious anaphylactic shock, have undertaken the production of "antirabies immune human gamma globulin."

Much more serious, but fortunately very rare, are the other complications of vaccine treatment. Occurring usually during the second week of treatment, these accidents cause a neuritic syndrome (radial, cubital, sciatic, and so forth) or, more often, myelitis with paresis of the lower limbs and sphincteric disturbances, of which the most serious type ends in complete paraplegia with sphincteric retention. Most often, these complications have a favorable evolution. The paresis or paralysis regresses in a few weeks, and there are no after-effects. True paraplegia can, however, be definitive, or, worse still (fortunately in exceptional cases) it can develop into the Landry syndrome, spreading toward the upper spinal cord, reaching the medulla oblongata, and causing death.

The cause of these reactions during anti-rabies vaccination is unknown. They may be due to phenomena of an allergic nature which "falsify" the organism's reaction with respect to the rabies virus introduced. However, as seen, the so-called inactivated vaccines, i.e., those not containing living virus, can also cause paralysis.

Statistically speaking, these reactions are, as we have said, very rare. At the time when world statistics on rabies were compiled, their frequency was evaluated as one per 5000 to 6000 persons treated. In fact, this frequency varies considerably from country to country. Practically nonexistent among people in primitive living conditions, these complications of vaccination seem to be more numerous the better the standard of living. The last WHO Expert Committee on Rabies recognized "that it is impossible at present to determine the basis of these apparent differences, but any consideration must take into account such host factors as the population involved, physiological state of the individual, species of animals used in vaccine production, method of virus inactivation and posology. The incidence of these complications is sufficiently high in certain areas of the world to justify further efforts to eliminate the factors responsible." These efforts are principally made on the use of vaccine prepared from the brains of suckling animals which are, as the last WHO Expert Committee wrote, "apparently free from the paralytic factor." The multiplication of the fixed rabies virus in tissue culture gives hope, moreover, that vaccines from cultures could be used.

Finally, it seems that recent attempts to treat these paralytic complications with corticosteroids and ACTH have been very successful, especially against the appearance of Landry syndromes, thus eliminating fatal complications.

CURATIVE TREATMENT

As yet, there is no specific treatment for rabies once it has declared itself. Presently, the only hope, based on the fact that, experimentally, the infection can be "auto-sterilizing," is to keep the patient alive artificially. The attempts of Thiodet's clinical research group in Algeria on man maintained in "artificial survival" using a method perfected by Thiéry on animals (electroshock and massive serotherapy) merit close attention.

The treatment of symptoms is, as we have seen, best accomplished at a specialized center. Barbiturates should be administered by the physician as soon as the first symptoms appear in order to facilitate immediate transfer of the patient to one of these centers.

BIBLIOGRAPHY

1. Beytout, D., et al.: Une technique de viscérotomie pour l'étude post mortem des encéphalites: la ponction viscérotomie transnasale. Bull. Soc. Path. Exot., *57*:52, 1964.
2. Janssens, P. G., and Mortelmans, J.: La rage. Ann. Soc. Belg. Med. Trop., *43*:893, 1963.
3. Lépine, P.: Techniques de laboratoire en virologie humaine (la rage). Paris, Masson et Cie, 1964.
4. Netter, R.: La rage. *In*: Sohier, R.: Diagnostic des maladies à virus. Paris, Flammarion et Cie, 1964.
5. Organisation Mondiale de la Santé (World Health Organization): Série de Rapports Techniques. Comité d' Experts de la Rage. Cinquième Rapport. Geneva, 1966.
6. Organisation Mondiale de la Santé (World Health Organization): La Rage Techniques de Laboratoire. 2nd edition. Geneva, in press.
7. Thiéry, G.: [Theoretical and practical considerations on a curative treatment of known rabies.] C.R. Acad. Sci., *252*:4219, 1961.
8. Thiodet, J., et al.: [Therapeutic trials in diagnosed rabies in man, using the combined methods of respiratory resuscitation, electroshock and intensive serotherapy.] Presse Med., *71*:172, 1963.

11
Encephalitides Due To Arboviruses

INTRODUCTION

by C. HANNOUN

A certain number of encephalitides are due to viruses of the arbovirus family. This family, which comprises more than 250 different viruses of which 63 have been isolated from man, present no clinical unity, since the manifestations provoked by these agents may be acute febrile syndromes (cf. Chapter 58), hemorrhagic fevers (cf. Chapter 47), or involvement of the central nervous system, not to mention the always possible inapparent infections. Among the most important arbovirus infections are the meningoencephalitides, encephalitides, and encephalomyelitides provoked by viruses belonging to different groups of the same family. The principal members are, in Group A: equine encephalitides (Eastern, Western and Venezuelan); in Group B: tick-borne encephalitis, Japanese encephalitis, Murrary Valley encephalitis, and St. Louis encephalitis; in the California group: California encephalitis.

Moreover, owing to the potential neurotropism of arboviruses, easily demonstrated by experimental inoculation into the young mouse, which always leads to a fatal encephalitis, in many illnesses belonging to the two other clinical types (febrile and hemorrhagic), signs of central nervous system involvement may appear. But these manifestations are inconstant and, although their agents are occasionally responsible for genuine epidemic episodes (due to West Nile virus, for example) they will be treated in another chapter of this book.

JAPANESE ENCEPHALITIS

by HIROTSUGU SHIRAKI

In Japan, encephalitis japonica prevails in midsummer from July to October and is particularly prevalent in August and September. It still represents one of the severest diseases caused by the arboviruses. The mortality rate is exceedingly high, ranging from 24 to 92 per cent in the period 1924-1960,[14] and a majority of survivors, especially children, develop severe neuropsychic sequelae, although a slight recovery can be expected during the protracted clinical course.[6-11] The details of the past and present status of the clinical, pathological, and epidemiological features of the disease—which will be described here only briefly—have already been published by us.[30, 33] More detailed information about the prognosis of survivors during the past 15 years,[10,11] and about the essential pathomorphological features, from autopsy of chronic cases,[12, 13, 31, 37] has since been accumulated, and it thus becomes possible to propose a relationship between the clinical and pathological features of the disease. Furthermore, the recent advances in the fluorescent antibody technique for both clinical diagnosis[20, 21] and experimentation[18, 19, 34] permit more reliable early diagnosis and give a clue for understanding the etiology and pathogenesis of the disease.

EPIDEMIOLOGY OF JAPANESE ENCEPHALITIS IN HUMANS AND ANIMALS

Since 1873, both endemic and epidemic outbreaks of the disease have occurred in Japan every year. The severest epidemics occurred in 1924, 1935, and 1948, the interval between epidemics ranging from 11 to 13 years.[14] Many feared that Japan might have a fourth great epidemic following the same periodicity. However, in the past, outbreaks of the disease actually differed from area to area and from year to year. For example, as indicated in Figure 11-1, in the southwestern districts the disease was endemic each year, and occasionally epidemics developed. The outbreak in 1961, on the other hand, was conspicuous in the northeastern districts, where there had been only one outstanding outbreak in the past, in 1948 (Figure 11-1*B*).[14] In Hokkaido, the northernmost island, a few suspicious cases had been reported sporadically before World War II. During the severest epidemic, which attacked the whole

territory of Japan in 1948, three years after the war, the greatest epizootic occurred in Hokkaido as well. Five humans and 789 horses developed the disease, which was, however, exclusively confined to the southwestern district of the island.[22, 23] However, a gradual shifting of the disease process, i.e., development of neutralizing antibody among both horses and humans, outbreak of an epizootic, and development of protective immunity of aged horses, took place thereafter, and apparent infection is now widespread over the whole island.[17,22,23] Thus there exists no virgin area for viral invasion in all Japan.

Among humans, the morbidity rate of the disease for each age group has been changing year by year. Before 1935, the oldest group was most susceptible, whereas after 1935 the infection rate among children, particularly preschoolers, gradually increased, the 31 to 40-year age group showed the lowest rate, and among persons over 50 years of age the rate again increased.[16] During the past 10 years or so, vaccination has been adminis-

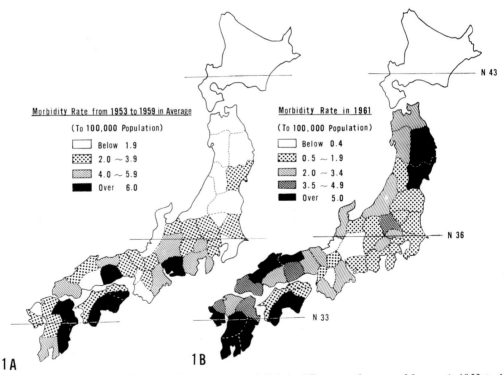

Figure 11-1. Human morbidity rate of Japanese encephalitis in different prefectures of Japan. *A*, 1953 to 1959 (average). In southwestern districts, constant endemics each year and occasional epidemics. No outstanding outbreak in Hokkaido, northernmost island (see Fig. 11-2), although small-scale definite outbreaks had been occurring since 1939. *B*, Disease outbreak in 1961, predominant in northeastern districts, where no outstanding outbreaks had been observed since 1948. (Modified from Hirayama.[14])

tered energetically, particularly to children, among whom the disease incidence tends to decrease year by year. The question has been raised whether both adults and aged people should be vaccinated, since the present vaccines still contain a minimal amount of nervous tissue of animals and, thus, a complication of vaccination of an "allergic" encephalomyelitic type might occur.

The infectious pathways of the disease during both epidemic and nonepidemic seasons are summarized in Figure 11-2. The vector of the disease has now definitely been concluded to be mosquitoes, particularly *Culex tritaeniorhynchus*,[3, 24, 25, 26] while the amplifiers and reservoirs are pig, night heron, and others.[4, 5, 24] How the virus survives the winter is still unknown.

CLINICAL FEATURES OF JAPANESE ENCEPHALITIS IN HUMANS

ACUTE STAGE

Typical Type (Fig. 11-3).[15, 33] The onset of the disease is rather abrupt, initiated by fever and headache, followed by nausea and vomiting. Abdominal pain and diarrhea are frequent in infants. On the second day of the illness the temperature reaches 39° C. and patients develop slight meningitic signs; cerebral complications are exceptional. On the third day the temperature reaches 40° C., consciousness becomes disturbed, and such signs as psychomotor excitement, lack of facial expression, muscular rigidity, involuntary movements, pathological reflexes, and motor palsy occasionally occur. On the fourth to fifth day impaired consciousness accompanied by neuropsychic abnormalities becomes more pronounced. Oculomotor or facial palsy is fairly common. In mild to moderate cases the fever tends to subside from the sixth day, and the aforementioned disturbances tend to improve and disappear, as a rule, after ten to 14 days. In severe cases death occurs with a high temperature of 42° C. on the fourth to the seventh day, or, if death does not occur, cerebral complications continue during the subsequent stage, and cardiac weakness due to pneumonia develops during the afebrile stage. Consequently, severe sequelae remain, particularly in infants and patients with a temperature of over 41.5° C. The prognosis for each disturbance varies from case to case, psychic disturb-

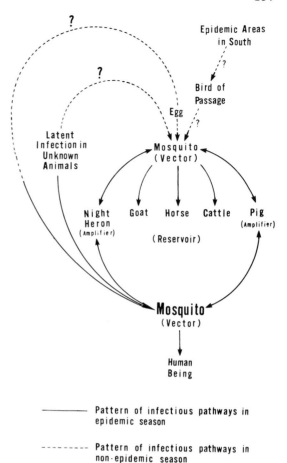

Figure 11-2. Schematic pattern of presumed infectious pathways of Japanese encephalitis during both epidemic and nonepidemic seasons. See text for explanation. (Modified from Ôya.[24])

ance prevailing in some instances and neurological signs and symptoms in others. The occurrence of each disturbance varies day by day and frequently fluctuates.

Meningitic Type (Figure 11-3).[15, 33] Vomiting and neck stiffness develop, and there is pleocytosis of over 500 per milliliter of cerebrospinal fluid. Cerebral focal or psychic disturbances, as a rule, do not occur, except for an occasional slight degree of impaired consciousness. No sequelae remain.

Abortive Type (Fig. 11-3).[15, 33] This type is milder than the meningitic type. No clear-cut or even minimal meningitic signs are encountered, and fever, headache, and occasional vomiting subside rapidly. The disease is often misdiagnosed as a common cold, and definite diagnosis is made only by serological examinations or lumbar puncture.

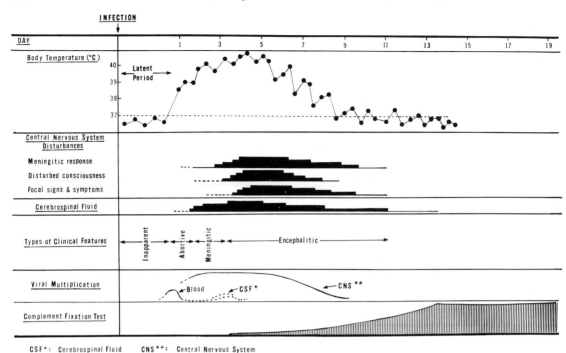

CSF*: Cerebrospinal Fluid   CNS**: Central Nervous System

Figure 11-3. Schematic pattern of various forms of the disease and their relationship to virus isolation and immunological response. See text for explanation. (Modified from Ishii.[15])

Inapparent Infection (Fig. 11-3).[33] Inapparent infection which can be detected only by serological examination is important, and develops both spontaneously and experimentally in rabbits, guinea pigs, and pigs, in which apparent infection never occurs.[16] Although the exact incidence is difficult to determine, about 10 per cent of Japanese children become infected annually, and 500 to 1000 inapparent infections occur for each apparent infection; comparison can be made with the depth of an iceberg beneath the sea.[2, 35] This infection has now become widespread not only among humans but also among other mammals and birds.

Atypical types.[15, 33] A majority of patients with the *bulboparetic type of infection* develop cerebral complications of the brain stem type from the initial stage. In a ten-year-old boy whose disease was of four days' duration, the encephalitic processes were mainly confined to the pontine region and virus was isolated. *Spinal cord involvement* occurred at the onset of the disease in a 23-year-old female and certain pyramidal signs remained one month later. Moderate pleocytosis in the cerebrospinal fluid developed, and the titer of complement-fixing antibody to Japanese

encephalitis virus ranged from $1/4$ to $1/64$. *Severe trauma,* such as a car accident, was identified in 17 patients among a total of 200. In 1948, in seven patients (0.8 per cent) the disease developed within one day of severe trauma, which may possibly indicate a provoking factor in the disease onset.

Diagnosis.[1, 15, 33] Isolation of the virus from cerebrospinal fluid and blood is extremely difficult even during the initial stage. Virus can be isolated from brain tissue of adult mice on the fourth through the seventh days of illness (Fig. 11-3 and Table 11-1). A titer higher than $1/4$ of complement-fixing antibodies during the recovery stage is considered a positive result, and a titer higher than $1/16$ alone may be diagnostic for the disease. However, positive conversion of the serological finding takes a long time and is not suitable for early diagnosis.

Kusano et al.[20, 21] recently applied the fluorescent antibody technique to autopsy specimens of human brains (Fig. 11-11). They compared the results with those of virus isolation and routine neuropathological examinations and found that the fluorescent antibody technique is much more reliable than the virus isolation test. Besides, this method

Table 11-1. *Isolation of Virus of Japanese Encephalitis from Brain and Fluids of Human Patients Inoculated to Adult Mice Brain at Different Days of Illness**

DAY	BRAIN	CEREBRO-SPINAL FLUID	BLOOD
2	–	1/19	1/10
3	0/1	1/50	1/22
4	5/8	2/40	2/27
5	12/19	0/13	1/18
6	9/17	0/4	0/7
7	10/19	0/2	0/2
8	3/12	–	–
9	1/8	–	–
10	1/5	–	–
11-14	0/6	–	–
15-20	1/4	–	–

*Modified from Ishii.[15] The denominator indicates the total number of animals examined; the numerator indicates the number positive. A dash means no information.

is simple and fast and thus has an advantage over routine histopathological examination.

Clinical-epidemiological diagnosis, however, still has significance, particularly during the acute stage, for delineating the following points: characteristics of the disease outbreak during each year and in each district, its preferential occurrence in different age groups in each district and year, its seasonal occurrence, and cerebrospinal fluid findings. Among the latter, pleocytosis, consisting mainly of polymorphonuclear leukocytes during the initial stage and of mononuclear cells during the fifth to the seventh days, is encountered in a great majority of cases. Ishi[15] pointed out that there were only three patients with a cell count below 15 per milliliter, and the virus was isolated from two, and that slight pleocytosis is accompanied, as a rule, by severe clinical manifestations.

PROTRACTED COURSE (SUBACUTE TO SUBCHRONIC)

The 117 patients with neuropsychiatric disturbances among the 628 patients admitted during the great epidemic in Tokyo, in 1948, were followed up for one to four months by Goto et al.[33] and Tatetsu,[36] who divided them into nine main groups. The largest and most important group, those with psychomotor abnormality, can be further divided into six subgroups.

Psychomotor Abnormality.[33, 36] On the basis of various primary disturbances, six subgroups have been determined, comprising both obligatory and facultative disturbances:

1. Hyperkinetic group: tremor, chorea, wriggling and tossing, and agitated motions of the limbs make up the obligatory syndrome, combined with almost all other primary disturbances as facultative symptoms.

2. Akinetic-hypokinetic group: obligatory syndrome consists of akinesia-hypokinesia; identity disturbance, forced laughing, and talkativeness do not develop.

3. Mixed hyperkinetic and akinetic-hypokinetic groups: almost all other primary disturbances occur as facultative symptoms.

4. Parkinsonian group: impulsive wandering, lack of inhibition, hypokinesia, and abulia make up the obligatory syndrome, combined with infantile behavior, identity disturbance, delusion, paroxysmal neuropsychic symptoms, and neurological deficits such as are seen in parkinsonism.

5. Mixed hyperkinetic and parkinsonian groups.

6. Catatonic group: both hyperkinetic and parkinsonian symptoms develop alternately, combined with negativism, catalepsia, echolalia, stereotypy, and mannered behavior as facultative symptoms.

The psychomotor abnormality is further combined with somatic and neurological deficits: vegetative dysfunctions, such as hypersalivation, hyperhidrosis, polydipsia, polyuria, hypertrichosis, fever, somnolence, sleeplessness, sleep perversion, motor paralysis, hyperreflexia, pathological reflexes, convergent ocular paresis, and meningitic responses.

Miscellaneous Abnormalities.[33, 36] (1) Some degree of *disturbance of intellectual functions* is found in almost all patients with psychomotor abnormality. (2) An *apathetic-hypobulic-abulic disturbance* occurs, including as well hypokinesia, slow movement and speech, and lack of facial expression, always combined with impaired memory or amnesia; this disturbance persists for 20 to 40 days. (3) *Amnesia or Korsakov's syndrome* persists for 43 to 312 days (average, 127 days). (4) *Delirium-clouded consciousness* persists for 38 to 311 days or more. (5) *Delusion* can be either secondary to experiences in the delirious state or primary, with or without amnesia. In one case motor and sensory aphasia, alexia, agraphia, and perseveration prevail, while in another, amnesic aphasia and paraphasia. Four patients complained of fatigability, amnesia, headache, malaise, and sleeplessness.

TRANSITIONAL STAGE FROM PROTRACTED TO CHRONIC COURSE

The aforementioned 117 patients and others have been further followed by Goto,[6, 33] who lays emphasis particularly on two obligatory syndromes, *hyperkinesia and hypokinesia*. Both are among the subgroups of psychomotor abnormality mentioned before, and the type determines the prognosis for survivors. The prognosis for hyperkinesia, which subsides an average of 30 days after the onset of the illness, is in general benign, while that of hypokinesia, which persists for 16 to 525 days (average, 60 days) is as a rule malignant, and severe sequelae remain occasionally. A gradual shifting of neurological disturbances to manifestations of psychic abnormalities occurs at this stage. For example, in the hyperkinetic group neurological disorders at the acute stage, such as involuntary movements, wriggling, tossing, and agitation, subside, and subsequently psychic impairments, such as restlessness, lack of inhibition, and intellectual disturbance, become more and more pronounced. In the hypokinetic group, on the other hand, akinesia or hypokinesia subside and there is a gradual shift to hypobulia or abulia.

NEUROPSYCHIATRIC SEQUELAE DURING THE CHRONIC STAGE

The aforementioned patients and others have been followed for three to 15 years by Goto.[7-11, 33] The colorful neuropsychic abnormalities at the earlier stages tend to improve slowly and to be almost fixed after three years.

One hundred forty-three unselected patients and 40 patients selected because they showed severe disturbances at the acute stage were followed for five years;[6, 7, 33] 55 with neuropsychic sequelae at the fifth year were followed for the subsequent five years;[8, 9, 33] and 43 of these 55 were followed for the subsequent five years.[10, 11]

As indicated in Tables 11-2 and 11-3, among 40 patients who had severe disturbances in the acute stage, and survived it, death occurred in four and sequelae were observed in 35 during the next five years; thus,

only one survivor developed no sequelae. Even among 143 unselected patients only 21.6 per cent developed no sequelae. During the subsequent five years a certain improvement of sequelae could be observed, but the mortality rate of children became important. No further deaths or improvement of sequelae occurred during the next five years, and thus, the data at the fifteenth year were exactly the same as those at the tenth year.

Classification.[6-11, 33] Elementary neuropsychic sequelae of various degrees were observed in nearly 100 per cent of the survivors in the selected group after five years and in a great majority of the patients in the unselected group.

Neurological sequelae were observed in a majority of survivors and were particularly severe in those below ten years of age. The sequelae, in decreasing order of incidence, were as follows: muscle hypertonia, motor paresis, lack of facial expression, abnormal tendon reflexes, primitive reflexes, ocular paresis, pathological reflex responses, contracture, tremor, involuntary movements, and convulsion. Each sequela persisted at the tenth-year observation, although minimal improvement did occur, and remained essentially unchanged at the fifteenth year. Among them lack of facial expression or mask-like facies was characteristic.

A parkinsonian syndrome developed even during the protracted stage in 17 per cent of the severe cases, 11.6 per cent at the fifth year, 13.5 per cent at the tenth year, and 12 per cent at the fifteenth year. This, however, can be differentiated from that of von Economo's encephalitis by the following points: it is mild in its expression, there is a low incidence of ocular and vegetative disturbances and tremor, disease onset is earlier, and the clinical course is stationary, with occasional improvement. Such paroxysmal symptoms as convulsions, episodic disturbances of consciousness, fugues, and psychoses were observed in a minority of the survivors at the fifth year, but were more or less increased at the tenth and fifteenth years. Children under ten years of age occasionally died in status epilepticus.

Abnormalities of motility, impulse, and will essentially originated from the psychomotor abnormality at the protracted stage. These were divided into two main groups, hyperkinesia and hypokinesia. In hyperkinesia, a gradual shifting of motor abnormalities to psychic ones; i.e., involuntary movements,

Table 11-2. *Outcome of Japanese Encephalitis in Survivors Five, Ten, and Fifteen Years After Acute Illness**

	5 YEARS AFTER ACUTE ILLNESS		10 YEARS AFTER ACUTE ILLNESS	15 YEARS AFTER ACUTE ILLNESS
	SELECTED GROUP:	UNSELECTED GROUP:	SELECTED GROUP:	SELECTED GROUP:
	40 CASES WITH SEVERE DISTURB-ANCES AT ACUTE STAGE	143 CASES	55 SURVIVORS WITH SEQUELAE AT 5TH YEAR OBSERVATION	43 SURVIVORS WITH SEQUELAE AT 10TH YEAR OBSERVATION
OUTCOME	NUMBER (%)	NUMBER (%)	NUMBER (%)	NUMBER (%)
Death	4 (10.0)	4 (2.7)	4 (7.2)	0 (0)
Sequelae	35 (87.5)	108 (75.5)	44 (80.0)	36 (83.7)
No sequelae	1 (2.5)	31 (21.6)	7 (12.7)	7 (16.3)

*Modified from Goto[7, 8, 11]

wriggling, and tossing shifted to impulsive wandering and restlessness, while in hypokinesia the akinesia or hypokinesia shifted to hypobulia and abulia. These disturbances progressed until the end of the third year and subsequently tended to become fixed gradually. A minimal improvement of restlessness and abulia was observed at the tenth- and fifteenth-year observations, while the catatonic syndrome disappeared. Among *abnormalities of emotion,* easy weeping and laughing, which tended to improve until the end of the fifth year, did not show any further improvement at the tenth year. All survivors at the fifth year showed some degree of *impairment of intellectual function,* which remained unchanged or minimally improved at the tenth and fifteenth years; this impairment was particularly severe in children. *Personality changes* were observed in all survivors. Infantile behavior, such as impulsive wandering, restlessness, talkativeness, vio-

lence, impudence, egocentricity, overfamiliarity, carefreeness, and lability, prevailed in the selected group and in infants, and had its origin in hyperkinesia. Rigid behavioral disorders, on the other hand, were more pronounced in adults. These personality changes improved slightly over 15 years.

Several combinations of the aforementioned primary sequelae could be differentiated: neurological and intellectual disturbances, personality changes intermediate between these personality changes characteristic of the parkinsonism following von Economo's encephalitis, and psychotic disturbances.

Among the psychotic disturbances, a few exceptional cases are worth mentioning. In a few survivors with certain neuropsychiatric sequelae exacerbations occasionally occurred in which both identity disturbance and delusion developed. For example, 12 years after the acute illness one patient de-

Table 11-3. *Calculated Prognosis of Japanese Encephalitis for Survivors at Fifth, Tenth, and Fifteenth Year Observations**

OUTCOME	5 YEARS AFTER ACUTE ILLNESS (%)	10 YEARS AFTER ACUTE ILLNESS (%)	15 YEARS AFTER ACUTE ILLNESS (%)
Death	2.7	8.1	8.1
Sequelae	75.5	60.4	60.4
No sequelae	21.6	31.1	31.1

*From Goto.[10]

veloped an exacerbation of wandering, excitement, and anxiety. Identity disturbance and delusion occurred simultaneously, lasted for two years, and disappeared. The incubation period of psychiatric disturbances with or without impaired consciousness varied from cases to case, ranging from six to 16 years, while the duration ranged from six months to two years. A majority of the disturbances closely resemble schizophrenia, but the patients' contact with reality is, as a rule, comparatively well preserved.

Social Prognosis[8-11, 33]   The social prognosis for survivors is, as a rule, poor. Children in particular showed severe disturbances in school. Adults were more or less disturbed in their family and social lives, but less so than children. At the tenth-year observation, only eight among 46 survivors showed a slight improvement; three were hospitalized with impulsive excitement. At the fifteenth-year observation, two showed antisocial behavior.

NEUROPATHOLOGY OF JAPANESE ENCEPHALITIS IN HUMANS

ACUTE STAGE (25 CASES OF THREE TO NINE DAYS' DURATION)[30-33]

Perivascular cell cuffs, cellular nodules (neuronophages), and *rarefied necrotic foci* are among the main characteristics. *Cell cuffs,* consisting of lymphocytes, polymorphonuclear leukocytes, and mononuclear cells, develop in dilated perivenous spaces and migrate slightly into periadventitial parenchyma (Fig. 11-4C and E). Leukocytes prevail at the earliest stage and subside rapidly thereafter. A less pronounced focal meningitic response occurs (Fig. 11-4A and D). In horses killed even earlier—after one to two days—leukocytic migration in both meninges and cerebral parenchyma far exceeds that noted in humans (Fig. 11-5A and B). *Cellular nodules,* both compact and loose, consisting mainly of activated rod cells and to a lesser extent polymorphonuclear leukocytes, generally develop around capillary walls (Fig. 11-4A-E). Neuronophages of ischemia-shrunken nerve cells are independent of cellular nodules; subsequently, however, they tend to coalesce and become difficult to differentiate from the nodules. The lesions mentioned occur concurrently in all

cases. They are predominant in different cortical layers and subcortical gray matter, far less pronounced in pericornual white matter, widespread from cerebrum to spinal cord, and generally speaking most pronounced in Ammon's horn, the thalamic nuclei, and the substantia nigra.

Round or oval, *rarefied necrotic foci* are multiple, of different sizes, sharply demarcated, and restricted to gray matter. They tend to coalesce and occur, as a rule, in close relationship to arteriolar or precapillary walls (Fig. 11-6A and B). Foci are characterized by spongy tissue disruption, nerve cell disintegration, and ischemia-degenerated remainders. Some leukocytes and cellular debris are visible centrally, but inflammatory cells never infiltrate central vessel walls. They are predominant in deeper cortical layers, but they never or rarely occur in the molecular layer, except in the cerebellum. These foci are in general severe in Ammon's horn, followed by temporal, frontal, and parietal cortices; they are slight to moderate in insular, occipital, and cerebellar areas. The severest foci are found in the thalamic nuclei, of which the lateral, intralaminar, dorsomedial, and pulvinar are most susceptible. The substantia nigra is also severely involved, and the striatum and pallidum are damaged as well. No lesions occur in the brain stem and spinal cord, except for the red nucleus and pontine basis, as far as our materials are concerned. The necrotic foci are differentiated from the cellular nodules and perivascular cell cuffs in both their nature and their distribution, and they are absent in a few instances.

Tissue damage due to circulatory disturbances, such as diapedesis hemorrhage, plasma or fibrin transudation, and pseudolamellar cortical deterioration, are occasionally combined and found in the thalamic nuclei, the cerebral cortices and meninges, or rarely the white matter.

SUBACUTE STAGE (FIVE CASES OF 11 TO 18 DAYS' DURATION)[30-33]

Cellular elements consisting of activated rod and phagocytic cells laden with byproducts of myelin breakdown and tiny pseudocalcareous particles are mobilized in necrotic foci and diffused in the parenchyma, while perivascular cell cuffs and cellular nodules become less conspicuous. Plasma cells intermingled with lymphocytes accumulate around the veins, and migrate

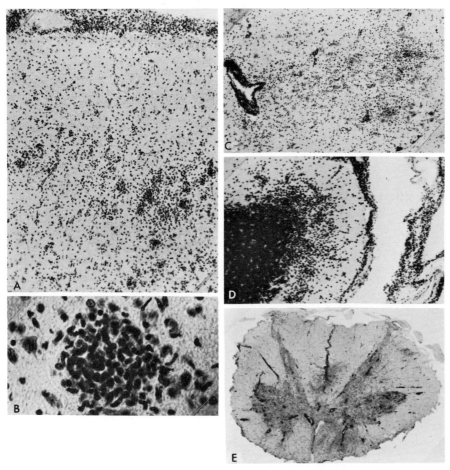

Figure 11-4. Acute stage. *A* (7-year-old male, 6 days' duration). Hippocampal cortex. Slight meningitic response, multiple coalescent cellular nodules of a compact nature, and diffuse cellular increase in the parenchyma. ×86. *B* (73-year-old female, 7 days' duration). Frontal cortex. Compact cellular nodule consisting mainly of activated rod cells. ×460. *C* (16-year-old male, 4 days' duration). Compact zone of substantia nigra. Pronounced perivenous cell cuffs, loose coalescent cellular nodules, diffuse cell proliferation in the parenchyma, and well-preserved pigmented cells. ×55. *D* (10-year-old female, 4 days' duration). Cerebellar cortex. Slight meningitic response, coalescent cellular nodules in the molecular layer, neuronophagia to Purkinje cells, and well-preserved granule cells. ×80. *E* (7-year-old female, 5 days' duration). Cervical cord. Perivascular cell cuffs, coalescent cellular nodules, and diffuse cell proliferation in the entire gray matter, predominant in the anterolateral horns, less in the white matter. ×9.0. (*A-E*, thionine.)

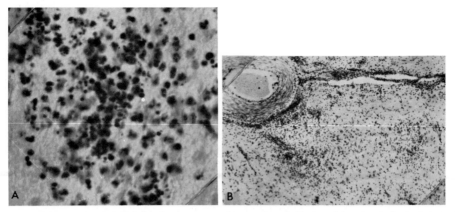

Figure 11-5. Japanese encephalitis in the horse; earliest stage. *A* (1-year-old male, 1 day's duration). Frontal cortex. Meningitic response, cellular nodules both compact and loose, and shadow-like shrunken nerve cells. ×40. *B.* Higher magnification of the cellular nodule in *A*. A great majority of infiltrated cells consisting of polymorphonuclear leukocytes. ×480. (*A* and *B*, thionine.)

around the adventitia to a slight degree. Widespread cortical deterioration resulting from circulatory disturbance is manifested particularly from the wall of the gyrus to the depth of the sulci, while necrotic foci with increased cellularity are concurrently visible within the former lesion (Fig. 11-7*D*).

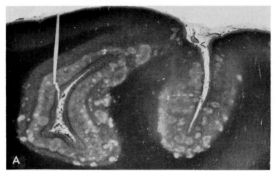

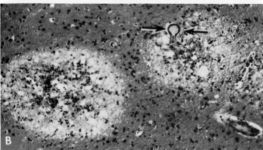

Figure 11-6. Acute stage. *A* (15-year-old male, 4 days' duration). Different-sized multiple coalesced rarefied necrotic foci predominant at the interwall and valley of sulci, and restricted to the frontal cortices. ×5.0. *B* (17-year-old female, 7 days' duration). Two adjacent necrotic foci with central cell mobilization. One of them is close to the vessel wall (arrows). (*A* and *B*, hematoxylin and eosin.)

SUBCHRONIC STAGE (NINE CASES OF 30 TO 138 DAYS' DURATION)

A tendency of the necrotic foci to coalesce becomes more and more pronounced, and a softening, spongy, or cystic character prevails (Fig. 11-7*A*). Foci contain a large number of fat-laden cells and a variable number of multinuclear giant cells of Langhans type, which prevail in thalamic nuclei and occasionally in deteriorated cortices (Fig. 11-7*B*). Gliomesenchymal proliferation is pronounced in advanced foci. Pigmented cells of substantia nigra are severely disintegrated, a large number of phagocytic cells laden with melanin pigments are mobilized, and the former finally disappear to some degree (Fig. 11-7*C*). So far, rarefied necrotic foci are irreversible and can play an important role in the development of severe neuropsychiatric sequelae in survivors. A majority of both perivascular cell cuffs and cellular nodules, on the other hand, is essentially reversible and can subside at this stage. For example, activated rod cells and minimal perivascular cell cuffs are diffusely or focally encountered, while nerve cells are well preserved in cerebral cortices, the inferior olivary nucleus, and the anterior horn of the spinal cord, all of which are preferential sites of both foci during the acute stage.

Further accentuation of sequelae of the illness can be attributed to circulatory disturbances, and particularly to impairment of the blood-brain barrier, which, as mentioned, develops during the acute to subacute stages and continues in the subchronic stage. For

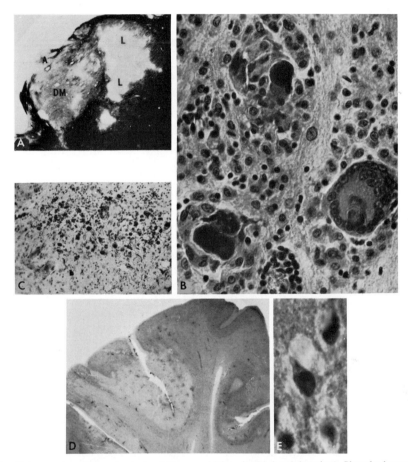

Figure 11-7.   Subacute to subchronic stage. *A* (3-year-old female, 33 days' duration). Sharply demarcated, confluent large softening lesion in the lateral thalamus (L) and smaller ones in the dorsomedial (DM) and anterior (A) nuclei. ×2.1. *B* (15-year-old female, 37 days' duration). Deteriorated lateral thalamic nucleus. Pseudocalcareous concretions of a concentric nature phagocytosed by multinuclear giant cells of Langhans type. ×460. *C* (45-year-old male, 30 days' duration). Compact zone of substantia nigra. A large number of phagocytic cells laden with melanin pigments derived from damaged pigmented cells. Both activated rod and astrocytic nuclei in the parenchyma. ×80. *D* (8-year-old male, 11 days' duration). Frontal gyri. Widespread confluent cortical deterioration containing multiple necrotic foci with increased cellularity predominant from the interwall to the valley of sulci. ×2.2. *E* (8-year-old male, 31 days' duration). Remaining nerve cells in the cortical deterioration similar to that in *D* are shrunken by ischemia. ×1100. (*A*, Sugamo myelin; *B* and *E*, hematoxylin and eosin; *C* and *D*, thionine.)

example, widespread cortical deterioration with ischemia-shrunken nerve cells is shown in Figure 11-7*D* and *E*, and fresh hemorrhages or plasma transudation of recent origin are seen not only in cortices but also in white matter. These foci were most impressive in the patient with disease of 138 days' duration, in whom exceedingly widespread demyelination and gliosis were pronounced in the cerebral white matter bilaterally (Fig. 11-8*A*) and cortical deterioration with cavity formation was widespread as well. An intimal proliferation, particularly of meningeal arteries, was observed diffusely, falling into an abnormal range considering the age of the patient (nine years) and was closely related to recent pseudolamellar cortical deterioration (Fig. 11-8*B*). A smaller number of fresh ring hemorrhages were still visible in the white matter of both cerebrum and brain stem (Fig. 11-8*C*). In addition, diffuse or patchy foci in both striatum and globus pallidus may to a greater or lesser degree be correlated with the process of cardiopulmonary arrest due to the severe pneumonia signs observed from the beginning of the illness.

So far, two main processes, i.e., the primary disease and circulatory disturbances of various origins, can concurrently or co-operatively play important roles in the development of widespread lesions in both gray and white matter from the acute to the subchronic stage.

CHRONIC STAGE (SIX CASES OF EIGHT TO 40 YEARS' DURATION)[12, 13, 31, 37]

In four cases (cases 1 to 4 in Table 11-4) Japanese encephalitis was definitely proved clinically and serologically during the acute stage, while in two instances (cases 5 and 6 in Table 11-4), it was proved post mortem. The essential pathomorphological characteristics at this stage can be divided into the following three groups:

1. Residue of Lesions from the Acute Through the Subchronic Stage. Severely scarred foci with gliomesenchymal proliferation, focal cavity formation, calcified remainders of nerve cells, and deposition of pseudocalcareous concretions in varying numbers were found in the thalamic nuclei in all cases examined. These lesions were bilateral except for case 1, in which the right side was severely involved and the left side only minimally involved (Figs. 11-9*A* and 11-10*A* and *B*). Among the thalamic nuclei,

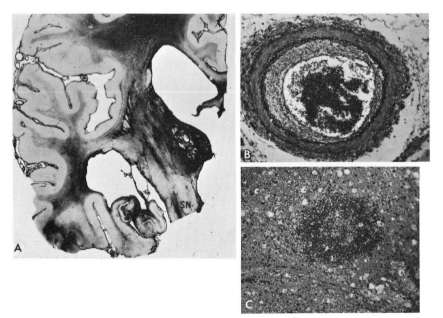

Figure 11-8.   Subchronic stage. *A* (9-year-old female, 138 days' duration). Widespread diffuse gliosis, slight to severe, in almost the entire white matter, and intense in the basal ganglia, substantia nigra (SN), and entire thalamic nuclei, with focal cavity formation. ×1.2. *B,* Moderate intimal proliferation of the meningeal artery. ×83. *C,* Fresh ring hemorrhage in the pyramidal tract of pontine basis. ×110. (*A,* Holzer; *B* and *C,* hematoxylin and eosin.)

Previous History of Japanese Encephalitis*

Case Number, Age at Autopsy (Yr.), Sex	Acute Stage Date (Age, Yr.)	Period of Hospitalization	Serological Data	Sequelae at Discharge	Subsequent Main Clinical Features	Cause of Death	Complications	Total Duration of Illness (Yr.)	Main Neuropathological Features
Definite Group									
1 17, M	August 1950 (4)	20 days	CF 1/16	Infantile speech, left hemiparesis, mental retardation, petit mal	Left spastic paresis, right rigidity 1+, slurred speech, muscular atrophy and ankylosis of left foot joint, hyperreflexes (1 ≧ r), convulsions 2+, severe imbecility, slow, hypokinesia, violent behavior	Fever, emaciation	–	12	Right hemisphere atrophy, particularly fronto-temporal, residue of necrotic foci of right substantia nigra, scar formation of right intralaminar thalamic nucleus and right superior frontal gyrus
2 22, M	August 1950 (7)	30 days	Identified	0	No neurological sequelae, convulsions 3+, occasional epileptic status, debility, trickiness, quarrelsomeness, occasional episodes of restlessness, wandering, violent and cruel behavior	Pneumonia after epileptic status	Pneumonia	15	Diffusely distributed deteriorated foci with two-nucleus nerve cells and 1+ perivascular cell cuffs in bilateral thalamic nuclei, deteriorated substantia nigra 1+, left ulegyric parieto-occipital gyri
3 18, M	August 1955 (10)	50 days	HI 1/640 (1/4)	Amnesia, knee jerk ↑	Right hemiparesis 1+, right Jacksonian convulsion 1+ since 17 yr.-old, debility, lack of spontaneity, mutistic, slow	Brain tumor	Left parietal meningioma	8	Scar formation and 3+ calcareous deposition of bilateral thalamic nuclei, deteriorated substantia nigra 1-2+, perivascular cell cuffs and intimal proliferation around tumor mass 3+
4 36, M	August 1941 (12)	15 days	Identified	0	In July, 1957 (28 yr.-old), disease returned. In October, fever (40° C.), incomplete paraplegia, slurred speech, difficulty of excretion, slowly progressed and admitted in October, 1960; in July, 1961, auditory hallucination, delusion, suicide attempt, rigidity ↑, pathological reflexes, dysarthria, forced laughing and crying, involuntary movements	General weakness	–	11	Old foci of bilateral thalamic nuclei and substantia nigra, cellular nodules of recent origin predominant in brain stem and cerebellum, perivascular cell cuffs 1-2+, two-nucleus nerve cells of Purkinje cell layer and hypoglossal nucleus, diffuse rod activation in cerebral cortices
Indefinite Group									
5 19, M	Summer 1935 (3)	–	–	–	Right hemiparesis 1+, slurred speech, convulsion 3+, idiocy, epileptoid character, negativism, autistic, progressed to fetus-like posture	General weakness	–	16	Diffusely distributed deteriorated foci with gliosis, calcareous deposition, and two-nucleus nerve cells in bilateral thalamic nuclei, gliosis and cellular nodules of substantia nigra, cystic formation of frontal cortices
6 42, F	August 1922 (2)	–	–	Mental retardation	Convulsion 3+, disturbed gait since 23 yr. old, complete paraplegia, hypokinesia, slow, rigidity ↑, dysarthria, pathological reflexes, imbecility, violent behavior, negativism, fetus-like posture	General weakness	Lung tuberculosis, cerebral arteriosclerosis	40	Left ulegyric parietal gyri, scar formation, calcareous deposition and two-nucleus nerve cells of bilateral thalami (1 > r), disintegration of substantia nigra 1+, disintegration of Ammon's horn, cerebellar cortex and inferior olivary nucleus 3+

* Reported by Shiraki,[31] Hamada,[12, 13] and Totsuka.[37]
0 = negative, 1+ = slight, 2+ = moderate, 3+ = high, – = no information, ↑ = increased, CF = complement-fixation test, HI = hemagglutination-inhibition test.

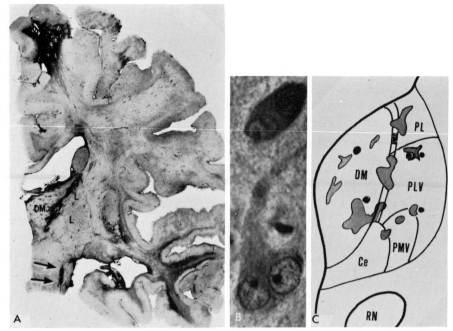

Figure 11-9.   Chronic stage. *A* (case 1 in Table 11-4). Right hemisphere. Intense gliosis in the intralaminar, dorsal portion of the lateral (L) and dorsomedial (DM) thalamic nuclei, Ammon's horn, substantia nigra (arrows), and both cortices and white matter of the superior frontal gyri. *B* (case 2 in Table 11-4). Dorsal portion of lateral thalamic nucleus. Closely adjacent two nerve cells apparently with two nuclei. ×1000. *C* (case 5 in Table 11-4). Schematic distribution pattern of two-nucleus nerve cells (black dot) to incomplete necrotic foci (dark gray areas) in thalamic nuclei. See text for explanation. Thalamic nuclei: DM—dorsomedial, PL—posterior part of dorsolateral, PLV—posterolateral part of ventral, PMV—posteromedial part of ventral, Med—intralaminar, Ce—centromedianus. RN, red nucleus. (*A*, Holzer; *B*, thionine.)

the intralaminar and medial part of the pulvinar are the most severely and consistently affected, followed by the dorsomedial and dorsolateral.[12] The substantia nigra, cerebral cortices, white matter, and other areas are naturally involved as well, but less severely and consistently, and sometimes the lesions are unilateral (Figs. 11-9*A*). During the chronic stage the thalamic nuclei are the most important site of involvements which can be attributed to both rarefied necrotic foci and circulatory disturbances occurring during the acute through the subchronic stages. The distribution pattern of the foci at this stage generally corresponds with that at the previous stage.

2. Active Tissue Responses Presumably Related to the Disease Process.   A fair number of nerve cells with two nuclei were found in three cases and exclusively confined to the areas adjacent to the severely scarred thalamic lesions (Fig. 11-9*B*). The distribution pattern and actual number of these unusual nerve cells are schematically illustrated in Figure 11-9*C*.[12] Minimal to slight perivascu-

lar cell cuffs of lymphocytic nature and a very few clear cut cellular nodules were found in the thalamic nuclei, substantia nigra (Fig. 11-10*E* and *F*), and elsewhere in all cases. In case 4,[37] on the other hand, a fairly large number of perivascular cell cuffs and cellular nodules of recent origin were widespread in the diencephalon, brain stem, and cerebellar cortex (Fig. 11-10*C*), while activated rod cells were diffusely distributed in the cerebral cortices. Nerve cells with two nuclei were again visible in the Purkinje cell layer (Fig. 11-10*C* and *D*) and hypoglossal nucleus. The significance of these findings will be discussed in the next section.

3. Tissue Damage due to "Krampfschädigung."   In all cases except case 4, convulsive seizures developed at the chronic stage. Thus, the development of so-called "Krampfschädigung"—i.e., pseudolamellar cerebral cortical deterioration of a comparatively recent origin, circumscribed cerebellar sclerosis, deterioration and sclerosis of the olivary nucleus, and so forth—can be expected and actually observed in some instances. The

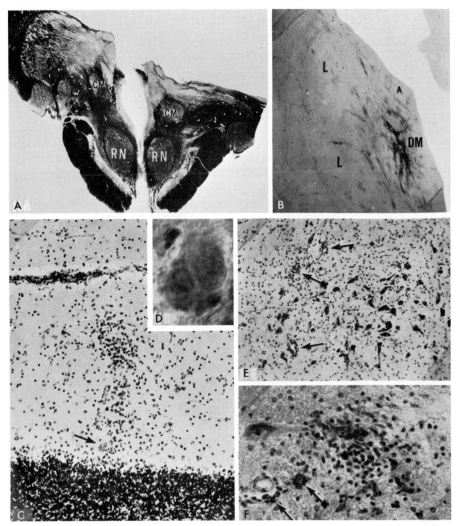

Figure 11-10. Chronic stage. *A* (case 3 in Table 11-4). Caudal part of thalamic nuclei and midbrain. Severely atrophic demyelinated lesions bilaterally in the dorsomedial part of thalamic nuclei, predominant on right. CM: centrum medianum; RN: red nucleus. ×1.5. *B* (same case as in *A*). Marble-like intense gliosis predominant in the dorsomedial (DM) and less pronounced in the lateral (L) and anterior (A) thalamic nuclei. ×2.7. *C* (case 4 in Table 11-4). Cerebellar cortex. Cellular nodule of a comparatively compact nature in the molecular layer and minimal lymphocytic infiltration in the meninges. ×130. *D*, Higher magnification of the Purkinje cell apparently with two nuclei indicated by arrow in *C*. ×900. *E* (case 5 in Table 11-4). Cranial portion of compact zone of substantia nigra. Slight perivascular cell cuffs (arrows), tiny cellular nodule (arrow with cross), diffuse proliferation of glial nuclei, and well-preserved pigmented cells. ×80. *F*, Higher magnification of *E*. Slight perivascular cell cuffs (arrow), calcified pigmented cell (arrow with cross), and cellular nodule of a comparatively compact nature. ×306. (*A*, Woelcke myelin; *B*, Holzer; *C* and *D*, hematoxylin and eosin; *E* and *F*, thionine.)

developmental mechanism of diffuse or patchy ulegyric foci in both cerebral cortices and white matter (Fig. 11-9*A*) is sometimes difficult to interpret. These lesions can result from "Krampfschädigung" alone, but, as illustrated in Figure 11-8*A*, foci in the white matter can also be caused by the process of Japanese encephalitis at the subchronic stage; in the case illustrated (138 days' duration) convulsive seizures never occurred.

RELATIONSHIP BETWEEN CLINICAL AND PATHOLOGICAL FINDINGS IN JAPANESE ENCEPHALITIS IN HUMANS

When there are clinical manifestations of meningitic involvement, some degree of histopathological meningitis occurs as well. The histopathological response, however, is generally milder than the clinical manifestations and indicates that meningitic involvement can subside comparatively rapidly even at the acute stage. Actually, in horses killed after one or two days of illness, a large number of polymorphonuclear leukocytes are found to have infiltrated into the meninges; this finding corresponds well with a conspicuous pleocytosis during the earliest stage of the disease. Parkinsonian features can possibly be attributed to severe damage of the substantia nigra and partial damage of the basal ganglia. Involuntary movements are closely related to severe damage of the striatum, pallidum, or certain thalamic nuclei. When hyperkinesia occurs with certain involuntary motions, such as wriggling, tossing, or agitated movement, an irritative process from cortical lesions together with involvement of the basal ganglia may be responsible. Brain stem lesions can result in dysarthria, dysphasia, dysphonia, ocular paresis, pupil stiffness, and so forth.

Many or most of the perivascular cell cuffs and cellular nodules are reversible, their reversal corresponding to a gradual improvement of the clinical manifestations during the protracted stage. Rarefied necrotic foci, on the other hand, are irreversible and can have great significance in the occurrence of severe neuropsychiatric sequelae in survivors. As mentioned before, in regard to the mechanism whereby additional sequelae develop, another possibility, i.e., circulatory disturbances of both cerebral and general origin, should be considered: impairment of the blood-brain barrier, due to such factors as hemorrhage, fibrin or plasma transudation, or serophagic process, can persist continuously from the acute to the subchronic stage, widespread not only in gray matter but also in white matter, particularly during the protracted stage, and can cause severe tissue necrosis. Actually, the rarefied necrotic foci may also result from a circulatory disturbance: severe cardiopulmonary arrest mainly due to a severe pneumonia process, most frequently encountered at the protracted stage, can impair cerebral circulation and leave behind certain lesions of basal ganglia, cerebral cortices, and other areas.

There is no doubt that the severe lesions of the subchronic to chronic periods correspond well with the drastic sequelae observed in long-term survivors. Thalamic lesions were the most common and severe finding; moreover, they were bilateral except

in one case. They may play an important role in an interpretation of the behavioral disorders of long-term survivors, particularly the emotional disturbances, since the thalamic foci are predominant in dorsomedial, dorsolateral, and occasionally anterior nuclei, which may represent a more recent origin, both ontogenetically and phylogenetically, and are correlated with psychic functions. However, since ulegyric lesions of various degrees are visible concurrently in both cerebral cortices and white matter, a final conclusion cannot be drawn at present.

With regard to a further increase of sequelae, a serious question arises whether chronic infection, exacerbation, or reinfection can occur during the chronic stage. As mentioned before, in three chronic cases nerve cells with two nuclei were found in the thalamic nuclei but not in other regions. Considering the high incidence of this finding, together with minimal to slight perivascular cell cuffs and a few but clear-cut cellular nodules in the thalamus, substantia nigra, and elsewhere in all chronic cases, the presence of nerve cells with two nuclei is not coincidental, nor does it represent a congenital malformation process, but it may develop during the long-term clinical course. Of interest in this connection are the findings in case 4 (Table 11-4). The patient had the disease as a 12-year-old but without sequelae. Sixteen years later he developed high fever, and three months later, paraplegia. Brain stem involvement and a schizophrenic syndrome followed, and he died four years and three months later. Histopathologically, the old foci were predominant in both thalamus and substantia nigra, while a fairly large number of cellular nodules and perivascular cell cuffs of recent origin were widespread in the brain stem, cerebellar molecular layer, and basal ganglia and less pronounced in the cerebral cortices, with a diffuse rod cell activation. The distribution pattern and nature of these foci corresponds more or less with those of Japanese encephalitis at the acute stage. In addition, nerve cells with two nuclei were again visible.

As mentioned in the section on clinical features of the disease, severe trauma can trigger the disease, while in a few survivors a certain progression or occasionally an exacerbation simulating schizophrenia can occur during the long-term clinical course.

In view of these clinical experiences, as well as the pathomorphological characteristics of case 4 and of others at the chronic stage, several questions arise: Is this a true exacerbation or reinfection with the virus of Japanese encephalitis or other viruses, or is it only a symptomatic inflammation with slow degradation of nervous tissue? If the former is true, how long can the virus survive in the central nervous system or viscera of survivors? Can attenuated Japanese encephalitis virus in the form of latent or chronic infection survive for a long period, and how can such a virus be isolated or identified? What is the mechanism of exacerbation or reinfection? A careful systematic survey of survivors from different aspects, e.g., clinical, epidemiological, morphological, immunological, and virological, can answer these questions eventually.

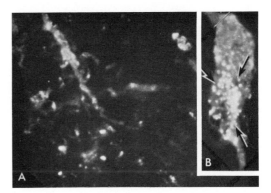

Figure 11-11. Thalamic nucleus of human patient treated with fluorescent antibody technique. (reported by Kusano et al.[20, 21]). *A,* Greenish-blue virus antigens abundant in both the cytoplasm and dendritic processes of nerve cells. *B,* Higher magnification of one nerve cell. Similar to *A;* yellowish granules are of lipid nature and represent an autofluorescence (arrows).

EXPERIMENTAL JAPANESE ENCEPHALITIS IN ANIMALS

Kusano[18, 19] recently applied the fluorescent antibody technique to 100 litters of newborn mice and almost the same number of adult mice inoculated intraperitoneally or intracerebrally with 10^3 to 10^5 baby mouse lethal units of Japanese encephalitis virus, and Shiraki et al.[34] compared the data with data obtained in experimental induction of herpes simplex and rabies virus infections. The following findings were obtained with the suckling mice: the Japanese encephalitis virus replicates almost exclusively in both cytoplasm and processes of nerve cells, though less prominently than in humans (Fig. 11-11*A* and *B*) and monkeys (Fig. 11-12*F*), in which nearly half the brain develops an intense fluorescence (Fig. 11-12*D*). In suckling mice virus antigens, appearing as tiny aggregated particles, first show up in the cerebral cortex, hippocampus, and cerebellum two or three days after inoculation; they appear in the brain stem after a delay and in the spinal cord only weakly and after a long delay. In visceral organs the virus antigens are strictly confined to Auerbach's or Meissner's plexus (Fig. 11-12*A*) and a few spindle-shaped cells of subcutaneous tissue and periosteum (Fig. 11-12*B* and *C*), becoming apparent within 24 hours after inoculation. In adult mice, on the other hand, fluorescence does not appear in visceral organs. There is

a widespread infection of the central nervous system, where virus antigens appear six or seven days after inoculation; antigens are never visible in the ependyma, choroid plexus, meninges, blood vessels, and perivascular cell cuffs (Fig. 11-12*E*). So far, it appears that the Japanese encephalitis virus is largely neurotropic, as compared with herpes simplex and rabies viruses, and it is highly probable that the infection is blood borne, since early involvement of the brain is prominent even after infection has been induced at a peripheral site and despite the paucity of infection outside the nervous system.

This neurotropism of the Japanese encephalitis virus, particularly to nerve cells, was again noted with the electron microscope by Oyanagi,[27–29] who inoculated intracerebrally a 1/10 dilution of infected mouse brain containing LD_{10} of Japanese encephalitis virus into adult mice. Data on both treated and control animals were carefully processed. At 72 and 92 hours after inoculation, spherical dense particles, 38 to 45 mμ in diameter, consisting of a thin marginal limiting membrane, a narrow outer zone with low electron density, and a central core with high electron density, 25 mμ to 30 mμ in diameter, were visible in varying numbers in the Golgi vesicles and vacuoles as well as in the rough and smooth endoplasmic reticulum of cytoplasm of nerve cells. Oyanagi concluded that these could be Japanese encephalitis virus particles. They were never encountered in glial cells and capillary walls (Fig. 11-13*A* and *B*).

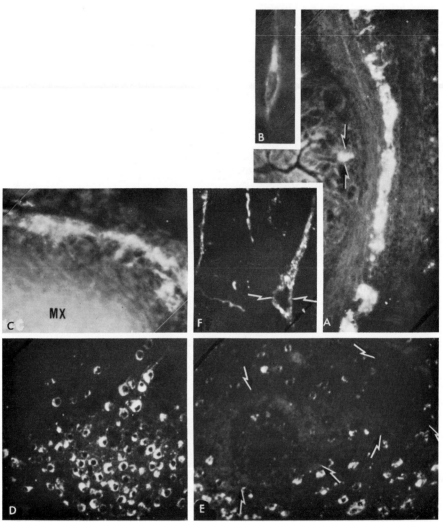

Figure 11-12. Experimental Japanese encephalitis treated with fluorescent antibody technique (reported by Kusano, Shiraki, et al.[18, 19, 34]) *A* (2-day-old mouse, intraperitoneal inoculation, 2 days' duration). Small intestine. Virus antigens confined to both Auerbach's and Meissner's plexi (arrows). ×150. *B* (2-day-old mouse, intraperitoneal inoculation, 1 day's duration). Spindle-shaped cell in the subcutaneous tissue containing cytoplasmic virus antigens. ×600. *C* (2-day-old mouse, intraperitoneal inoculation, 2 days' duration). Virus antigens in the spindle-shaped cells of periosteum of the maxilla (MX). Blue autofluorescence of the bone. ×300. *D* (3-day-old mouse, intraperitoneal inoculation, 2 days' duration). Cerebral cortex. Focal fluorescence of both the cytoplasm and processes of nerve cells. ×150. *E* (4-week-old mouse, intracerebral inoculation, 3 days' duration). Cerebral cortex. A fair number of nerve cells containing virus antigens and their lack in two perivascular cell cuffs (arrows). ×150. *F* (monkey, intracerebral inoculation, 10 days' duration). Anterior horn of lumbar cord. Virus antigens predominant in both the cytoplasm and processes of pyramidal cells and lacking in the nucleus (arrows). ×250.

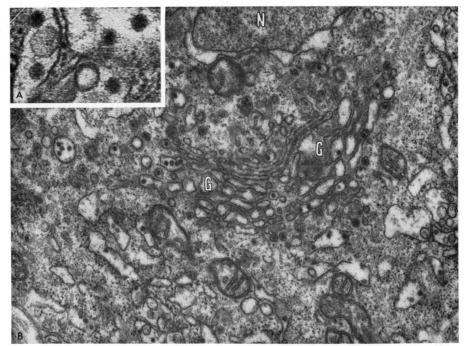

Figure 11-13. Experimental Japanese encephalitis in mouse; electron microscopic observation (reported by Oyanagi[27–29]). *A*, Golgi apparatus (G) of cortical nerve cell 72 hours after inoculation of virus particles. The latter are visible mainly in endoplasmic reticulum. N, nucleus. ×50,000. *B*, Higher magnification of *A*. Diameter of virus particles is, as a rule, 40 mμ; the particles consist of central nucleoid 25 mμ in diameter, marginal narrow viroplasm with low electron density, and outermost limiting membrane. ×100,000.

CONTROL AND TREATMENT OF JAPANESE ENCEPHALITIS IN HUMANS

Control of the disease is difficult, since it is now widespread not only in humans but also in mammals and birds, and the details of reservoirs or vectors of virus in winter are still unknown. Vaccination against the disease is therefore necessary. Many Japanese scientists agree that purified inactivated mouse brain type vaccines are effective, definitely in horses and less so in humans. The vaccines, however, still contain a small amount of mouse brain tissue, and there is thus the possibility of an "allergic" encephalomyelitis. A commission for a large-scale systematic survey of vaccination against Japanese encephalitis was organized in 1964, and thorough investigations were carried out in different ways. For example, 50,000 individuals of different ages and in different districts inoculated with both old and recent vaccines of mouse brain type were carefully followed up by neurologists in 1965, but no complica-

tion of an "allergic" nature developed. There were a very few suspicious cases, particularly in infants, two of whom came to autopsy, and neuropathological findings indicating acute circulatory disturbances of an ischemic nature but not of an "allergic" one have been reported to date. The possibilities of a tissue culture vaccine, as well as the optimal dosage, time, site, and number of inoculations are now under systemic investigation.

No definitely effective treatment for patients during the acute stage has been reported to date. Active treatment for both general and cerebral circulatory disturbances during the acute through the protracted stages could to some extent prevent the development of severe neuropsychic sequelae, since, as mentioned, the histopathological damage develops in the acute and subsequent stages. The details of the effectiveness of thalamotomy in Parkinsonism as well as of amygdalatomy in behavioral disorders of the survivors have been mentioned in our previous publication.[33]

BIBLIOGRAPHY

1. Abe, M., and Ishii, K.: Clinical features and diagnosis of encephalitis japonica with especial reference to complement fixation test. Nihon Iji Shinpo, *1477*, 3-11, 1952 (Japanese edition).
2. Bawell, M. B., Duel, R. E. J., Matsumoto, M., and Sabin, A. B.: Status and significance of inapparent infection with virus of Japanese B encephalitis in Japan in 1946. Amer. J. Hyg., *51*:1-12, 1950.
3. Buescher, E. L.: Arthropod-borne encephalitis in Japan and Southeast Asia. Amer. J. Public Health, *46*:597-600, 1956.
4. Buescher, E. L., Scherer, W. F., Rosenberg, M. Z., Gresser, I., Hardy, J. L., and Bullock, H. R.: Ecologic studies of Japanese encephalitis virus in Japan. II. Mosquito infection. Amer. J. Trop. Med. *8*:651-664, 1959.
5. Buescher, E. L., and Scherer, W. F.: Ecologic studies of Japanese encephalitis virus in Japan. IX. Epidemiologic correlations and conclusions. Amer. J. Trop. Med. *8*:719-722, 1959.
6. Goto, A.: Prognosis of Japanese encephalitis. Follow-up study of the patients in 1948 and 1949. Psychiat. Neurol. Jap., *54*:722-735, 1953 (Japanese edition).
7. Goto, A.: Follow-up study of long duration on Japanese encephalitis. Psychiat. Neurol. Jap., *59*:147-182, 1957 (Japanese edition).
8. Goto, A.: A long duration follow-up study of Japanese encephalitis. Psychiat. Neurol. Jap., *64*:236-266, 1962 (Japanese edition).
9. Goto, A.: Sequelae of encephalitis japonica. Saishin Igaku, *17*:1321-1325, 1962 (Japanese edition).
10. Goto, A.: A long term follow-up study of encephalitis japonica: Prognostic observation of 43 personal cases fifteen years after the onset. Psychiat. Neurol. Jap., *68*:44-59, 1966 (Japanese edition).
11. Goto, A.: Clinic of encephalitis japonica with especial reference to neuropsychic sequelae and prognosis. Symposium on viral encephalitides in the Japanese, Tokyo, April 7, 1966. Psychiat. Neurol. Jap., *68*:130-131, 1966 (Japanese edition).
12. Hamada, S.: Pathology of encephalitis japonica at chronic stage. Symposium on viral encephalitides in the Japanese, Tokyo, April 7, 1966. Psychiat. Neurol. Jap., *68*:131-132, 1966 (Japanese edition).
13. Hamada, S., and Ishii, T.: A histopathological study of the residual disturbances after Japanese B encephalitis. Psychiat. Neurol. Jap., *68*:60-78, 1966 (Japanese edition).
14. Hirayama, T.: Epidemiology of encephalitis japonica. Saishin Igaku, *17*:1272-1280, 1962 (Japanese edition).
15. Ishii, K.: Encephalitis japonica from clinical viewpoint. Saishin Igaku, *17*:1312-1320, 1962 (Japanese edition).
16. Kawakita, Y.: Encephalitis japonica. Medical Microbiology, Virology. Tokyo, Igaku Shoin, 1961, pp. 482-519 (Japanese edition).
17. Kitaoka, M., and Arbor Virus Study Group: Seroepidemiology of Japanese B encephalitis in Hokkaido. Seminar on Japanese B encephalitis and other arthropod-borne virus infections. World Health Organization, Tokyo, 1962.
18. Kusano, N.: Studies on the pathogenesis of Japanese encephalitis. Acta pathol. Jap., *14*:207-209, 1964 (Japanese edition).
19. Kusano, N.: Morphopathogenesis of encephalitis japonica. Symposium on fluorescent antibody technique and viral encephalomyelitides. Adv. Neurol. Sci., *9*:3-4, 1965 (Japanese edition).
20. Kusano, N.: Fluorescent antibody technique and Japanese encephalitis. Symposium on viral encephalitides in the Japanese, Tokyo, April 7, 1966. Psychiat. Neurol. Jap., *68*:300, 1966 (Japanese edition).
21. Kusano, N., Aoyama, Y., and Kawamura, A.: The diagnosis of Japanese encephalitis by means of fluorescent antibody technique in autopsy cases. Second Colloquium on Actual Encephalitides. Warsaw, September 15, 1965. To be published by Polish Academy of Science.
22. Miura, T.: Age distribution of neutralizing antibodies against Japanese B encephalitis and poliomyelitis (Lansing) viruses among the peoples in northern part of Japan. Jap. J. Bact., *5*:313-317, 1950 (Japanese edition).
23. Miura, T., and Kitaoka, M.: Immunological epidemiology of Japanese encephalitis in Hokkaido. Virus, *5*:62-73, 1955 (Japanese edition).
24. Ôya, A.: Epidemiology of encephalitis japonica with especial reference to mosquitoes. Saishin Igaku, *17*:1281-1284, 1962 (Japanese edition).
25. Ôya, A.: Mosquitoes and virus of encephalitis japonica. Science, *32*:28-33, 1962 (Japanese edition).
26. Ôya, A., and Kitaoka, M.: Epidemiology of arbor animal virus infections in Japan. Recent Review Med. Biol., *1*:483-495, 1960 (Japanese edition).
27. Oyanagi, S.: An electron microscope study on the fine structure of cerebral cortex in the mouse infected with Japanese encephalitis virus. Niigata Igakukkai Zasshi, *79*:461-468, 1965 (Japanese edition).
28. Oyanagi, S.: An electron microscopic study on the fine structure of cerebral cortex in the mouse infected with Japanese encephalitis virus. Second Colloquium on Actual Encephalitides. Warsaw, September 15, 1965. To be published by Polish Academy of Science.
29. Oyanagi, S.: Electron microscopic observation of central nervous system of mouse infected experimentally with Japanese encephalitis virus. Symposium on viral encephalitides in the Japanese. Tokyo, April 7, 1966. Psychiat. Neurol. Jap., *68*:132-133, 1966 (Japanese edition).
30. Shiraki, H.: Neuropathology of encephalitis japonica with especial reference to the material at the great epidemic in 1948, Tokyo. Saishin Igaku, *17*: 1285-1311, 1962 (Japanese edition).
31. Shiraki, H.: The neuropathology of encephalitis japonica in humans especially from subchronic to chronic stage. Second Colloquium on Actual Encephalitides. Warsaw, September 15, 1965. To be published by Polish Academy of Science.
32. Shiraki, H.: Pathology of encephalitis japonica from acute to subchronic stage. Symposium on viral encephalitides in the Japanese, Tokyo, April 7, 1966. Psychiat. Neurol. Jap., *68*:130-131, 1966 (Japanese edition).
33. Shiraki, H., Goto, A., and Narabayashi, H.: État passé et présent de l'encéphalite japonaise au Japon. Rev. Neurol., *108*:633-696, 1963.
34. Shiraki, H., Yamamoto, T., Otani, S., Kusano, N., and Aoyama, Y.: Comparative study of experi-

mental herpes simplex, rabies and Japanese encephalitis demonstrated by fluorescent antibody method. Second Colloquium on Actual Encephalitides. Warsaw, September 15, 1965. To be published by Polish Academy of Science.

35. Southham, C. M.: Serologic studies of encephalitis in Japan. II. Inapparent infections by Japanese B encephalitis virus. J. Infect. Dis., *99*:163-169, 1956.
36. Tatetsu, S.: Mental and neurological symptoms after the acute stage of Japanese B encephalitis. Psychiat. Neurol. Jap., *52*:183-199, 1951 (Japanese edition).
37. Totsuka, S.: Neuropathology of one autopsy case of Japanese encephalitis at chronic stage. Discussion at Symposium on viral encephalitides in the Japanese, Tokyo, April 7, 1966.

AMERICAN ENCEPHALITIDES

by C. Hannoun

Severe encephalitides occur on the American continent and particularly in the United States, some especially among children and others especially in old people. They are caused by a variety of different viruses among which are the three equine encephalitis viruses (Western, WEE; Eastern, EEE; and Venezuelan, VEE), that of St. Louis encephalitis (SLE) and that of California encephalitis. Though the incidence of these infections varies considerably from year to year and from one region to another, they present an important public health problem, as the number of notified cases each year is often high (Table 11-5). Recent years have seen a recrudescence of activity of some of these viruses, while improved methods for their specific diagnosis have brought about a better understanding of the virus etiology of infections of the central nervous system. It is difficult, for lack of precise data, to evaluate in what percentage of cases the correct diagnosis has been made, but it is certain that when antigens of the above-named arboviruses have been included among the specific reagents used in serological examinations the corresponding viruses have been found to play an important role in human disease. For example, of 1014 cases of human encephalitis notified in eight states in 1956, 87 were caused by arboviruses; and, in the whole of the United States, of 2410 notified cases in 1962, 270 were due to arboviruses (Table 11-6). It should be noted that during this period California encephalitis was not systematically looked for and is not included in these figures, and it is possible that other arboviruses, not yet identified, were responsible for a further number of undiagnosed cases. Besides these, imported cases of encephalitis have occurred when the patient was infected with a virus prevalent in another part of the world, as happened in 1956 when a man en route from Okinawa manifested, the day after his arrival in San Francisco, typical Japanese encephalitis. The importance of such observations lies in the fact that some regions of the United States are potentially receptive to the circulation of this virus because of their climate and their mosquito population.

EQUINE ENCEPHALITIDES

Equine encephalitides or encephalomyelitides are typical anthropozoonoses which affect man, the horse (from which the virus was first isolated, hence the name), and some species of birds such as pheasants. The causative viruses also cause inapparent infections in a variety of other bird species and these form the reservoirs and disseminators of the virus in nature.

Western Equine Encephalitis (WEE)

Of the three equine encephalitis viruses, that of Western equine encephalitis is the most widespread in the United States. It was first isolated in California (Meyer et al., 1930) and though for many years it was identified only in the western and north central states ("west of the Mississippi"), it is now known to occur throughout the country, particularly on the East Coast from Massachusetts to Florida, as well as in Canada and in Central and South America. However, the human disease has been found only in North America and in Brazil. It is interesting that, although in the United States the virus is found in nearly all the states, the disease in man is rare on the East Coast, and, for this reason, it was discovered only much later.

The Disease in Man. Most people infected by WEE virus show no clinical illness or at least no symptoms of involvement of the central nervous system. The proportion with serological evidence of the infection may be high in a region where the disease is rare or

Table 11-5. *Human Cases of Arbovirus Encephalitis Notified in the United States, 1955 to 1962*

	WEE	EEE	SLE	TOTAL
1955	37	15	107	159
1956	47	15	563	625
1957	35	5	147	187
1958	141	2	94	237
1959	14	36	118	168
1960	21	3	21	45
1961	27	1	42	70
1962	17	0	253	270

even unknown, a finding not uncommon with arboviruses. But WEE is also capable of producing severe illness, especially in the young child.

The disease presents with high fever and somnolence. The other manifestations differ in the adult and the child. Adults show lethargy, stiffness of the neck and back, and often mental confusion, even temporary coma; however, recovery is usually rapid and complete. In children, on the other hand, the severity is inversely proportional to age; the disease provokes convulsions, vomiting, and signs of excitation. Mortality is high in certain epidemics; children who recover are usually left with serious physical and mental handicaps.

Epidemiology. The first vector incriminated was *Culex tarsalis* from which the virus

Table 11-6. *Etiology of Infectious Encephalitis in the United States in 1956*

	1956 (8 STATES)		1962
Arbovirus		87	270
Postinfection following		523	1008
Mumps	332	358	
Measles	91	337	
Chickenpox	20	76	
Influenza	0	40	
Other viruses		7	7
Etiology unknown	397		1125
Total	1014		2410

was isolated for the first time in 1941 and re- peatedly since then, especially in California where the group under the direction of Reeves has pursued thorough studies on the ecological cycle of the WEE virus in this mosquito. This vector bites chiefly domestic and wild birds but also attacks rodents, horses, and man. It is thus a good agent for disseminating the virus both in the reservoir and in the susceptible species. However, east of the Mississippi, this mosquito is not found, a fact probably ex- plaining why the incidence of the disease is very different there. In the East the virus has been isolated chiefly from *Culiseta melanura* and in several less abundant species of *Culex* (among which *pipiens*), *Aedes,* and even *Anopheles.*

The virus has also been isolated fre- quently from the blood of various wild birds, first in California and then in other zones of activity of the virus. These birds are often sedentary, like the common sparrow, and belong to many different species, a fact suggesting that there is no species specificity. Antibodies against the virus can be found in a high percentage of these birds. The role of birds was suspected from the beginning, since from the onset of the mosquito season the virus was detected close by or at a great dis- tance. The experimental inoculation of virus into various species of birds demonstrated that birds in general, but especially young birds, were affected but that infection took place with a period of viremia lasting several days, with virus titers clearly high enough to infect *Culex tarsalis*. Domestic birds, chickens in particular, have commonly been found to have antibodies against WEE, and the virus has often been isolated from them in epizootic zones. One reason may be the intimate gre- gariousness in which they are raised; in a chicken house infection becomes universal shortly after introduction of the virus. Poultry have consequently been used by epidemi- ologists to study the activity of the virus by the "sentinel animal" or "indicator animal" method which consists in placing, or selecting in a chosen area, a few groups of ten or 20 chickens on farms where they would be ex- posed to normal environmental conditions and particularly to mosquitoes. Antibody de- terminations are made at the beginning of the season to ensure that all the birds lack anti- bodies, and subsequently blood is taken at regular intervals, monthly for example, for further antibody titrations. Thus at a certain

period in the year serological conversions are detected which indicate that infection by the virus has occurred. Virus isolation can then be attempted from the same poultry run or from mosquitoes, and the chronology of the stages of virus circulation is established by following the increase in the number of posi- tive results. The introduction of virus among poultry is usually noted at the middle or end of spring. Human cases begin to occur later in the summer.

Considerable research has been done on the question of the survival of virus during winter, a question which applies to the major- ity of arboviruses and one which has been studied particularly, although not completely answered, in the case of WEE. A possible explanation for the survival of the virus is that *C. tarsalis* can hibernate, and mosquitoes infected in autumn are able to overwinter, sheltered in holes in rocks, and survive to start the cycle again in the spring. Several workers have isolated virus from mosquitoes caught in the open in winter. However, whether this event is exceptional or plays a real part in the conservation of the virus is not easy to discern. Another hypothesis is based on ob- servations by Reeves, who showed that ex- perimentally infected birds could harbor the virus for periods up to ten months. Physio- logical factors, hormonal for example, could allow the reappearance of virus lying latent in certain organs. Another possibility is that some cold-blooded animal species such as snakes, or species which hibernate, such as some rodents, may harbor the virus in low titers throughout the winter, but with the re- turn of warm weather present a viremia. In support of this last hypothesis may be the recovery of virus from snakes experimentally infected and kept under natural temperature conditions and the isolation of virus from rodents in winter.

EASTERN EQUINE ENCEPHALITIS (EEE)

This virus was first isolated from the brain of a horse which died from encephalitis (Ten Broek and Merrill, 1933). It was soon found to be responsible for disease in horses throughout the eastern and southeastern states and all along the Atlantic Coast from Massa- chusetts to Florida and the Gulf of Mexico to Texas. The virus has also been isolated in Argentina, Central America, and the West

Indies. In the horse, the disease is always severe and may be fulminating, usually causing death in 24 to 48 hours.

The Disease in Man. The disease in man is often serious, particularly in children. The clinical picture is similar to that of the encephalitis caused by other arboviruses but tends to run a more acute course with more severe symptoms. Death often occurs before the fifth day, and the children that survive are left with serious physical and mental sequelae. In the adult the disease is less severe and recovery occurs without sequelae. Inapparent infections are common.

The virus is transmitted by certain common species of mosquitoes, most frequently belonging to the genera *Culex* and *Aedes*. The main hosts are wild birds, even small birds like starlings and sparrows, and domestic birds. Pheasants in particular are highly susceptible and present severe clinical illness: epizootics occur on pheasant breeding farms every year; the vector in this case is *Culiseta melanura*. This mosquito rarely bites mammals and is probably not responsible for the transmission of the virus to either man or horses. There may be methods of spread other than those usual with arboviruses: it is very likely that the virus spreads directly from pheasant to pheasant without the aid of mosquitoes. Another possibility is that of mechanical transmission by other parasites such as acarians; mechanical transmission has been demonstrated. It appears that the primary source of virus in a pheasant colony is exterior (wild birds), with mosquito transmission; but thereafter ensues a secondary cycle within the group, the topographical and chronological characteristics of which indicate the possibility of transmission by direct contact.

The hypothesis of an annual introduction of virus by birds returning from migration has been studied, and certain facts raise doubt as to its likelihood. In particular, it has been shown in Louisiana that virus is present in wild birds two months before the arrival of flocks of birds from the south. It is thus more likely that the virus persists through the winter as has been shown by the isolation of virus from rodents which could thus form the winter reservoir of the virus.

VENEZUELAN EQUINE ENCEPHALITIS (VEE)

The third variety of equine encephalitis was discovered in 1938. The virus was iso-lated from horses dying of a fulminating encephalitis and was soon found to be different from the other two viruses although classified as a member of the same serological group.

In man the disease found in Venezuela, Colombia, and Panama appears in two forms. One is a fairly mild generalized illness, rarely fatal, and the other presents as a severe encephalitis with a 10 per cent case fatality rate. VEE virus is dangerous to handle, and many laboratory infections have occurred in different countries. For this reason several laboratories prepare for their staff a vaccine which is neither completely effective nor sufficiently innocuous.

The virus has been isolated from several species of mosquitoes, among which are *Aedes serratus* and *Psorophora ferox*. Birds seem to be the usual reservoir; the infection is inapparent but accompanied by a high titered viremia lasting some time. However, it is particularly important to note that this virus may also be transmitted by other means. Contamination by direct contact between horses has been demonstrated, and laboratory infections have probably been due to aerosols of virulent suspensions.

ST. LOUIS ENCEPHALITIS (SLE)

St. Louis encephalitis was recognized as a disease entity during an epidemic in St. Louis, Missouri, in 1933, when the virus was isolated for the first time. It has subsequently been found frequently in the United States either in widespread epidemics or as sporadic cases in states where the virus was known to exist. It is a disease that holds an important place in the pathology specific to the United States and represents a significant proportion of the notified cases of encephalitis.

The geographical distribution of SLE covers most of the southern states in the United States: Arizona (1952), California (1945-1950), Florida (1952), Kentucky (1955), Texas (1957), and Colorado (1959). In Florida, one of the most affected states, SLE was first identified in Miami in 1952; in 1957 one case was notified and a cluster of cases in 1958; epidemics appeared in 1959 and 1961 and were followed in 1962 by an epidemic with 250 notified cases and at least 42 deaths. Between 1955 and 1962 the number of confirmed cases notified in man attained 1345. Since 1962 new and widespread epidemics have occurred, including a particularly severe one in Houston, Texas, in 1964, which involved more than 700 people with at least 32 deaths. The same year epidemics were notified in the states of Tennessee, Kentucky, Illinois, Ohio, Pennsylvania, and New Jersey. In 1966 the worst epidemics were again in Texas, in Dallas and Corpus Christi. It is difficult to know whether the disease existed before 1933 since its clinical aspects do not suffice to provide a specific diagnosis and laboratory tests have entered current practice in only fairly recent years. It is likely that many cases of encephalitis due to the SLE virus were not identified and that numerous cases still escape notification. SLE virus has also been isolated from mosquitoes and wild birds in Trinidad and in Jamaica, where it has caused cases of encephalitis in man, and from mosquitoes in Panama. Serological studies in Mexico, Colombia, Brazil, and Argentina suggest the possibility of its extension farther to the south of the American continent.

CLINICAL ASPECTS

As with most arbovirus infections, the number of inapparent cases greatly outnumbers the clinical ones. During large epidemics studied with care the estimated proportion of the total population involved could attain 60 or 70 per cent while the number of notified cases remained limited. Other estimates have suggested a ratio of subclinical to clinical cases of about 64 to 1. A second degree of gravity is represented by the so-called "benign" form of the disease, not often diagnosed, which may attract attention during an epidemic owing either to surveillance measures or to the anxiety of the exposed population. These forms are limited to a short febrile, influenza-like illness with headache and aching stiffness. Recovery is complete within a few days.

However, in some patients infection with SLE virus produces a more serious picture. The clinical picture is that of encephalitis, meningoencephalitis, or viral encephalomyelitis. The clinical condition was described at the time of original recognition of the disease and more recently by a group of clinicians and virologists in Houston during the 1964 epidemic (Melnick et al., 1965).

The clinical form most typical of SLE is abrupt onset with headache, fever, and vomiting, followed rapidly by evidence of involvement of the central nervous system. In the adult the disease provokes disturbance of cerebral functions, lethargy in particular, stiffness at the nape of the neck, and a mononuclear reaction in the cerebrospinal fluid (50 to 100 cells per cubic millimeter, with lymphocytes predominating). Fever lasts for four to eight days, reaching temperatures of 39 to 41° C. (102.2 to 105.8° F.). Neurological symptoms are usually more marked in aged patients who occasionally present particularly serious forms with coma or hyperexcitability. In certain cases the tendon reflexes are altered, and often pareses or even flaccid paralyses and tremors of the limbs and the lips occur. The protein content of the cerebrospinal fluid varies between 25 and 500 mg. per ml., usually being from 50 to 100 mg. per ml. during the first week of illness and sometimes a little higher in the second week.

In most cases the electroencephalogram shows a moderate or severe diffuse encephalopathy, sometimes associated with focal lesions. There is no evident correlation between the extent of the electroencephalographic changes and the clinical severity of the illness.

There are often signs of involvement of other organs indicating a probable generalization of the infection to almost the entire organism, with a polymorphonuclear leukocytosis, high transaminase levels, radiological anomalies suggesting acute pneumonia, and alterations in the electrocardiogram. These manifestations may be due to a reactivation of a previously compensated pathological condition.

Case fatality rates vary considerably from epidemic to epidemic and also depend on the way in which clinical cases are diagnosed. The meticulous investigation of mild cases not requiring hospitalization and those found only by serological examination increases the morbidity rate and lowers correspondingly the case fatality rate. However, as a rule, this rate lies between 10 and 25 per cent. The fatal cases are chiefly in patients aged over 50, and in those with coma from the onset (the prognosis in this second case is very poor, with only about 50 per cent of survivals). A marked cellular response in the cerebrospinal fluid with a count of 100 cells or more indicates a better prognosis than when the count is low. The cause of death is usually the encephalitis itself, but death is sometimes due to bacterial complications, to pulmonary embolisms, or to hemorrhages in various sites.

Although the disease is serious principally in aged adults, it also involves children. In over one half of cases in children, the disease is very mild. As in the adult, the onset is abrupt; the fever appears at the same time as headache, nausea, and a moderate to profound lethargy. The illness lasts an average of seven days with other possible symptoms such as stiffness of the nape of the neck, anorexia, ataxia, vertigo, and irritability. There are physical signs of meningeal irritation, exaggerated tendon reflexes, and altered sensory perception. Recovery is rapid in mild cases, but in others the neurological disturbances may last for over six weeks.

In children, the differential diagnosis from other virus encephalopathies can be difficult, especially from those due to enteroviruses, or adenoviruses, or even mumps virus. The clinical picture is not distinct enough to allow an etiological diagnosis, which must depend on the results of specific laboratory investigations.

PATHOLOGY

The main pathological changes seen in the nervous system in fatal cases of SLE are (Suzuki and Phillips, 1966): degeneration of the neurons, perineural or perivascular proliferation of the microglia, and perivascular mononuclear infiltration.

The lesions in nerve cells vary from chromatolysis of the swollen nuclei and the phagocytosis of neurons to the complete destruction and the disappearance of the cells. The most severe lesions are found in the substantia nigra, with loss of pigment and phagocytosis by the microglia. The degeneration of neurons or the proliferation of microglia is found in the anterior horn cells as well. Similar lesions are found in the thalamus, cerebellum, cerebral cortex, and corpus striatum. Inflammatory perivascular infiltration is seen throughout the brain substance and the subarachnoid space. A few perivascular hemorrhages and petechiae are occasionally found in the anterior horn cells as terminal signs.

SEQUELAE

Recovery from the immediate consequences of the disease may, however, be followed later by neurological and psychological changes. In a retrospective study of the sequelae in 96 patients two to five years after SLE, Azar and Lawton found that these survivors of this disease had had an abnormally high accident rate (falls, motor accidents, and so on) during the immediate convalescent period and in the months following. These accidents were attributed to defects in sensory perception or to disturbances of equilibrium. Long-term effects were most often psychological, for example, irritability and instability.

DIAGNOSIS

As for the other arboviruses, the etiological diagnosis is made from the results of two types of examination: attempts at virus isolation and the interpretation of the results of three serological tests: hemagglutination inhibition (HI), complement fixation (CF), and serum neutralization (SN).

Virus isolation is not of much practical use in diagnosis of a single case, since it is difficult and time-consuming, as it usually is in virus diseases. By contrast, the HI and CF tests are currently used, and criteria for the interpretation of results have been established by the Communicable Diseases Center of the United States Public Health Service.

Confirmed cases are those that show a fourfold or greater increase or decrease in titer between two successive serum samples from the patient by either HI or CF; or which have a titer of 1:320 or more by HI or 1:16 or more by CF in any single sample of serum.

Presumed cases are those in which the increase or decrease in titer is only twofold or in which the titers in a single serum sample are only 1:20 to 1:160 by HI or 1:8 by CF.

Doubtful cases are those in which antibody titers are less than 1:20 by HI or 1:8 by CF during the first 21 days of illness.

In regions where the virus of SLE is prevalent, these tests should be systematically practiced at the same time as those for the other viruses in laboratory investigation of every case of encephalitis of supposed viral origin. In this way, besides the frank epidemics, a small number of sporadic cases can be detected every summer.

EPIDEMIOLOGY

As with other arboviruses, SLE virus has a natural cycle involving vertebrates, in this case birds, and arthropod vectors, here mosquitoes, most commonly of the genus *Culex.* But the precise mechanisms vary widely from one region to another.

In California the cycle is essentially rural, and human cases are usually sporadic without any sizable epidemic waves. The main vector is *C. tarsalis* which also transmits WEE virus and which particularly attacks birds. This mosquito propagates the virus in flocks of wild and domestic birds among which the spread is so extensive that at the end of the season the majority have acquired antibody. It is equally able to bite man and in this way transmit the disease. This cycle is favored in California by the abundance of birds and by the profusion of mosquitoes breeding especially in reservoirs and irrigation canals.

In contrast, in eastern states (Florida) and those of the Midwest the virus causes localized outbreaks of considerable magnitude, most often in towns. The mosquito vectors are *C. pipiens* and *C. quinquefasciatus,* and the vertebrate species implicated are domestic and urban birds which permit a sufficiently ample source of virus. The main natural reservoirs are not precisely known; they may be these same domestic or urban birds, but also wild birds which could accidentally introduce the virus into towns where swarms of mosquitoes can breed in drains, in waste water, or in pools of stagnant rain water. In recent years the vector in several epidemics in Florida has been found to be *C. nigripalpus,* a species of mosquito which is both anthropophilic and ornithophilic.

Outside the United States, the virus has been found in the West Indies and in some countries of South America where, however, it does not cause epidemics and where the situation is of an endemoenzootic type. It is possible that the virus is introduced once or annually by the many species of migratory birds which arrive in the south of the United States in spring on their way from the tropics.

The only way to tackle the problem of control is by attempt to eliminate the mosquito vectors. Measures have been successfully applied in California where there is strict inspection of all irrigation installations and specific treatment is applied as soon as larvae appear. In towns the fight against *C. pipiens* can be a means to prevent or stop epidemics of encephalitis. No satisfactory vaccine has been developed against the virus. Yellow fever vaccine is not effective even though the virus belongs to the same serological group.

CALIFORNIA ENCEPHALITIS

The history of research on the virus of California encephalitis is a typical example of the slow progress of knowledge concerning viruses "in search of a disease" which have kept laboratory workers busy for the last 20 years. In 1943 and 1944 a new virus was isolated in California by Hammon, Reeves, and Sather from homogenates of pools of mosquitoes of the species *Culex tarsalis* and *Aedes melanimon.* The same research workers demonstrated the experimental transmission of virus from one animal to another by *A. melanimon.* Antibodies were found in a number of animal species such as the rabbit and various small rodents, but not in birds. Then in 1945 a significant antibody response against the California virus was detected in three human cases of encephalitis which occurred in the region where the mosquitoes had been captured. During the same period a study of 188 patients convalescing from various neurological illnesses hospitalized in this region revealed 11 per cent with neutralizing antibodies for the virus. In another similar investigation by the Public Health Laboratory of the State of California, of 292 patients 8 per cent showed positive reactions. The term "virus of California encephalitis" began to be used by some authors though others, still unconvinced, more cautiously called it the "California virus." During the following years new isolations of the virus were made, notably in Texas in 1958 from *Anopheles pseudopunctipennis,* and in Montana in 1959 from ticks (*Haemaphysalis leporispalustris* and *Dermacentor andersoni),* and from a snowshoe hare. Serological surveys revealed antibody to the virus in the human population of several states.

Since 1943 similar but not identical viruses have been isolated from both mosquitoes and man in other parts of the world: Trivittatus (United States), Guaroa (Colombia), Tahyna (Czechoslovakia), Melao (Trinidad), and Lumbo (Africa). The significance of California virus and of these others of the same family remained in suspense for some 20 years since proof of their pathogenicity for man had not been conclusively demonstrated.

Interest in the problem was revived in 1963 in the course of a systematic study by a group of workers in the state of Wisconsin of arbovirus encephalitis in that state. They found neutralizing antibody to this virus in sera of 51 of 144 men employed in parks and forest reservations. Although these men gave no history of any recent clinical illness, these results indicated that there must be a rural focus of activity of the California virus in the area (Thompson and Evans, 1965). Subsequent studies of groups of persons similarly employed gave positive results in from 10 to 34 per cent; of the deer examined in the same forests, 50 per cent had antibodies for the virus. Research in the same state was then extended to an investigation of clinical cases of encephalitis; significant increases in antibody levels were found in several cases among children.

Finally the same team of workers, encouraged by these results, attempted virus isolation from various matter sampled in earlier cases and stored under refrigeration "on the off chance" that they might be of use. Thus in 1964 these investigators succeeded in isolating a strain of virus from the brain of a 4 year old child who had died of encephalitis in September, 1960. This virus was identified as a strain of the California virus. It had taken 20 years to establish the name "California encephalitis virus."

Since then, more sustained attention has been paid to the etiological diagnosis in epidemics of encephalitis, and, in the United States, laboratory tests now include, besides the classical laboratory tests for WEE, EEE, and SLE viruses, those utilizing the antigens of California encephalitis virus. In the autumn of 1964, ten cases at least were diagnosed in Indiana in children aged between four and 16 years (nine boys and one girl). Since then, the known geographical distribution of California encephalitis has increased year by year. The disease is specially severe in children but the number of subclinical cases is always relatively high in comparison with clinical cases. The regions where the virus is endemic are the forests of the central states in the United States and Canada. The persons most exposed to the risk are those living in close proximity to the forest, since the mosquitoes have a somewhat short range.

This virus has an interest greater than simply that of providing an etiological diagnosis in a small proportion of cases of encephalitis in North America. A number of other viruses serologically related to it have been found elsewhere, notably Tahyna virus which has been particularly studied in Czechoslovakia, France, Italy, and other European countries. As with the virus of California

encephalitis before 1964, the role of Tahyna virus in human and animal disease, although suspected, is still uncertain. Positive serological responses have been found in many different sorts of illness, in infections of the respiratory tract, neurological syndromes, involvement of the lymphatic glands, joints, and circulatory and cardiac systems. It is possible that all these data, surveillance in endemic areas, and the detailed study of suspected cases by virological and immunological methods will one day clarify the role of Tahyna virus.

BIBLIOGRAPHY

1. Azar, G. J., and Lawton, A. H.: Saint Louis encephalitis sequelae and accidents. Public Health Rep., *81*:133-137, 1966.
2. Hammon, W. M., and Reeves, W. C.: California encephalitis virus. 1. Evidence of natural infection in man and other animals. Calif. Med., 77:303-309, 1952.
3. Hammon, W. M., Reeves, W. C., and Sather, G.: California encephalitis virus. 2. Isolations and attempts to identify and characterize the agent. J. Immun., 69:493-510, 1952.
4. Melnick, J. L.: Epidemic Saint Louis encephalitis (SLE) in Houston, 1964. J.A.M.A., *193*:139-146, 1965.
5. Meyer, K. F., Haring, C. M., and Howitt, B.: The etiology of epizootic encephalomyelitis in horses in the San Joaquin Valley. Science, 74:227-228, 1930.
6. Reeves, W. C., and Hammon, W. M.: The changing picture of encephalitis in the Yakima Valley. J. Infect. Dis., *90*:291-301, 1952.
7. Suzuki, M., and Phillips, C. A.: Saint Louis Encephalitis. Arch. Path., *81*:47-54, 1966.
8. Ten Broeck, C., and Merrill, M. H.: A serological difference between eastern and western equine encephalomyelitis virus. Proc. Soc. Exp. Biol. Med., *31*:217-220, 1933.
9. Thompson, W. H., and Evans, A. S.: California encephalitis virus studies in Wisconsin. Amer. J. Epidem., *81*:230-244, 1965.

TICK-BORNE ENCEPHALITIDES

by E. OSETOWSKA

HISTORICAL NOTE

The last epidemic waves of von Economo encephalitis and the first cases of tick-borne encephalitis must have coincided in time. Thus von Economo's disease invaded Europe between 1917 and 1926,[6, 49] whereas cases of tick-borne encephalitis are thought to have been observed in Austria[51] in 1927 and around

1930-1934 in Russia.[23] On the other hand, sheep encephalitis or "louping ill," known for over 150 years in Scotland,[65] did not attract attention either before or after as a disease transmissible to man. The isolation and identification of the viruses responsible were made much later and, according to Clarke[12] in the following order:

1931 — Scotland — "louping ill"
1937 — U.S.S.R. — verno-estival encephalitis or Far Eastern encephalitis
1940 — U.S.S.R. — "Bialorus" strain
1947 — U.S.S.R. — Kubin strain
1948 — Czechoslovakia
1953 — U.S.S.R. — biphasic fever
1954 — Poland — two different but apparently related strains[59]
1953 — Austria
1958 — Sweden
1959 — Finland
1953 — Yugoslavia
1955-1959 — Germany
1956 — Rumania[16]
1952 — Hungary[50]

To our knowledge, this encephalitis remains unknown in certain countries of Western Europe; we know of no reports from France, Spain, Portugal, or Italy. In England, the only cases known represent isolated forms arising in relation to contact with sheep. The Belgian cases collected as suspect by Ludo van Bogaert[7] were not confirmed by anatomical verification.

The research concerning, and the classification of, the tick-borne encephalitis viruses isolated rapidly made it obvious that in the territories of Central Europe, Western Russia, and Far Eastern Russia there exist several strains of virus, related by their serological properties, a fact enabling Casals[9, 10] to assemble them into classes or serological groups.

According to the data of the Prague Symposium (1962), there occur in these areas the Central European encephalitis (CEE) virus, including the virus of biphasic meningo-encephalitis and that of the encephalitis contracted from drinking raw milk; and the "louping ill" virus known in Great Britain and the virus of spring-summer encephalitis also widespread in Central Europe as well as the U.S.S.R.; all belong to Casals' group B.[10]

A commentary must be made on the terminology of the Russian encephalitides since, at a certain period, it was believed that there were several of them. Chumakov[11] and his followers maintained the existence of a single encephalitis due to one and the same virus involving both Western and Far Eastern Russia.

Chumakov's opinion was accepted by Fourth Session of the Academy of Medical Sciences of the U.S.S.R.[29] Zilber[76, 77] defended a different opinion and expressed it again in 1962. According to his view, the virus of Far Eastern encephalitis differs from that of CEE. Particularly, in Far Eastern encephalitis epidemics, case fatality rate is 30 per cent, whereas it is from 5 to 15 per cent in the European epidemics. The paralyses due to the Far Eastern virus are irreversible for the most part; the vector of the virus is different: in the Far East, *Ixodes persulcatus,* in Europe, *Ixodes ricinus.* Nonetheless Chumakov's opinion has been generally accepted and, for example, Polish textbooks of clinical neurology in their 1961 edition[27, 28] refer to a single tick-borne or spring-summer encephalitis "still called by Occidental authors Far Eastern encephalitis."[28]

Thorough studies have demonstrated the identity of the 11 strains of CEE virus in epidemics in Eastern Europe. At the same time, without Casals' classification being entirely discarded, antigenic differences have been shown between the viruses of the tick-borne encephalitis complex.

These differences distinguish, for example:

1. the "louping ill" virus, with its distribution in Great Britain;
2. the CEE virus, represented geographically in Central Europe and Occidental U.S.S.R.;
3. the virus of Omsk (U.S.S.R.) hemorrhagic fever, which has no nervous system repercussions;
4. the virus of Russian Far Eastern spring-summer encephalitis, particularly linked to the Eastern region of Russia.[12, 76]

This observation has closed the discussion concerning the existence of two viruses in Russia. The similar characteristics within the entire group enable tick-borne encephalitis to be considered as a single anatomicoclinical entity without the subtle differences between its causal agents being lost from sight.

EPIDEMIOLOGY

The arbor-viruses, now denominated arboviruses, owe their name to their vectors: arthropods. The nature of these vectors and that of the animal reservoir of the virus are responsible for the fact that the infection is grouped in foci. These foci are located in the forest regions in which the ticks and the animal reservoirs of virus find shelter. The host or reservoir of virus is usually comprised of rodents such as hares, mice, wild rats, and so forth.[37] The virus circulates within the focus between the reservoir animal, tick vector, and infected animal.[75] The animal parasite, the tick, being a vector common to the animal and to man, can contribute permanently to the acquisition of new hosts.[59, 75] The virus absorbed by the tick with the animal's blood multiplies and is diffused within the tick, reaching its salivary glands and ovaries. The female transmits the virus to its progeny by the transovarian route.[26, 75] The migration of the tick-bearing animals can result in the propagation of the virosis; this propagation can moreover be increased by the passage of epidemics across neighboring frontiers because of natural conditions, as is the case for the frontiers between Russia, Poland, Czechoslovakia, and so forth. Once a biological equilibrium between the virus and the immunological state of the population has been reached, the epidemic dies away and the disease thereafter appears only in the form of isolated cases, but always linked to the focus, which is then called endemic.[17]

The spring and summer occurrence of the disease is also in accordance with the biology of the tick. The outbreak of cases between the months of May and September, with a peak in June, coincides with the period of greatest vitality of the adult forms of ticks.[59, 75]

The relative geographical stability of the disease seems strange if it is compared with the serological grouping (group B of Casals) established between viruses originating in regions widely distant from each other. This group includes Kyasanur Forest disease in India, the Omsk virus, "louping ill" virus, and so on. The serological relationships between these viruses seem all the more bizarre for the fact that, among the viruses mentioned, only the CEE virus, that of spring-summer encephalitis, and that of "louping ill" are responsible for a disease of the nervous system in the strict sense. The Omsk virus and the Kyasanur virus provoke, under natural conditions, fevers with hemorrhagic eruptions. Nonetheless, these last two viruses, under experimental conditions, are capable of producing in the laboratory mouse an enceph-

alitis with characteristics similar to those due to the virus of the encephalitis complex.[57]

PATHOGENESIS

There are two ways in which man can be infected by tick-borne encephalitis: the blood and the alimentary routes. The first is involved after tick bite; the second is the result of absorbing raw milk of cows or goats that are reservoirs of virus.[4, 17, 26, 76] During 48 hours, under experimental conditions, after the bite of the tick, the virus multiplies to the point of producing a diffuse viremia. The penetration of the central nervous system by the virus can occur by the blood,[1] by the lymphatic route,[43] and by the peripheral nerves.

Kornyey[38] underlined heavily this last-mentioned possibility. Albrecht[1] in investigations based on the immunofluorescence method, revealed the presence of the virus in the sympathetic and parasympathetic ganglia, at the same time as in the blood vessels, after subcutaneous inoculation. To be noted in particular is that virus was absent from the vascular endothelia. By what pathway the virus penetrates the vascular bed and reaches the nerve cells has not been elucidated. According to Malkova,[43] the lymphatic route prevails over that of the blood. It seems that when the infection is alimentary the virus passes through the intestinal walls and first reaches the lymph nodes. Then it passes into the blood, and the infection of the central nervous system occurs in the same way as after tick bite.[52] Albrecht[1] emphasizes the fact that the presence of virus in the lymph nodes is never accompanied by its presence at the level of the spleen. Pogodina[58] affirmed the presence of the virus in the feces, but this result was not confirmed by the Austrian investigators.[52] In conclusion, it seems that the hematogenous pathway may well be the most common route to cerebral infection, the lymphatic routes and those of the peripheral nerves appearing to be supplementary or perhaps pathways of junction.

Our own research[57] confirmed the fact observed by Albrecht[1] as concerns the absence of virus in the endothelia and the other layers of the blood vessel walls. After pentration of the brain, the virus is found immediately in the neurons. However, later inflammatory infiltration is found at the blood vessel level; the hypothesis of Jacob[32] that the virus, in transversing the hematoencephalitic barrier, disturbs its equilibrium irreversibly should be considered.

NEUROPATHOLOGY

According to the data of the Russian investigators,[11, 30, 31, 45, 70, 71] the differences in the anatomical aspect between the spring-summer encephalitides and the tick-borne encephalitides of Central Europe are slight. The topography of the lesions is characterized by the "spotty accumulation" ("fleckförmige Kontinuierlische Polioencephalitis") either at the level of the cortex and the nuclei of the diencephalon, or at the level of the brain stem nuclei and of the medulla oblongata, and spinal cord.[67]

In the cerebral cortex a certain predilection may be noted for the frontal-central circumvolutions, with a decrease in involvement toward the parieto-occipital region. The temporal circumvolutions and the region of the hippocampus with Ammon's horn are almost invariably involved. The underlying white matter is almost entirely spared, the lesions attaining their extinction point at the junction of the white and the gray matter.

In basal nuclei the lesions are concentrated preferentially at the level of the lentiform nucleus, putamen, and globus pallidus, without any distinct preference for one or the other.[62] The thalamus is the site of an inflammatory process more often in its laterocentral areas, although in certain cases a predilection of the lesions for the median nuclei has been noted.[55, 62] The subthalamic region, the mesencephalon at the level of the locus niger, the pons, the medulla oblongata, and the cerebellum are obligatorily involved.

At the medullary level, the lesions of the gray matter are comparable to those in poliomyelitis with the difference that their extent is greater toward the posterior horns and that they also constitute infiltrations of the white matter. As a rule, the cervical medullary level is the only one involved, but the lesions occasionally also involve the lumbar level or even the spinal cord in its entire length. The intravertebral ganglia often present inflammatory lesions. The meninges are exempt from characteristic lesions; edema and lymphocytic (rarely lymphoplasmocytic) infiltrations are seen, in some cases perivascular and in others disseminated.[14, 15, 78]

In the spring-summer forms, the especially prominent involvement of the spinal cord is typical, but it is also seen in some cases of tick-borne CEE virosis. The cerebral topography of tick-borne encephalitis is summarized in Figure 11-14, which is adapted from Haymaker.[25] The clinical variations result from a difference in intensity of the lesions at the different levels under consideration.

The pathological process is similar in all cases; it differs quantitatively according to the period of the disease. In the early phase, known almost exclusively through experimental data,[1, 5, 19, 32, 44, 62, 64] the predominant element is the neuronal involvement related to parasitism by the virus in the nerve cell. This necrobiotic phase culminates in the destruction of several neurons, at which point the inflammatory phase commences.

The inflammation is characterized by the presence of gliomesenchymal nodules around the dead neurons, of diffuse glial plaques, and of perivascular infiltrations. The perivascular infiltrations are discrete, most often of lymphocytic composition (Fig. 11-15), exceptionally with polymorphonuclear leukocytes, and, from time to time, participation of plasmo-

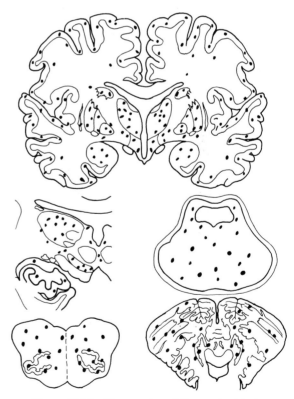

Figure 11-14. Topography of the cerebral lesions of tick-borne encephalitis.(Adapted from Haymaker, W.: Mosquito-borne encephalitides. In: Encephalitides. Bogaert, L. van, et al. (eds.). New York, American Elsevier, 1961, pp. 38-56.)

Fig. 11-15   Fig. 11-16

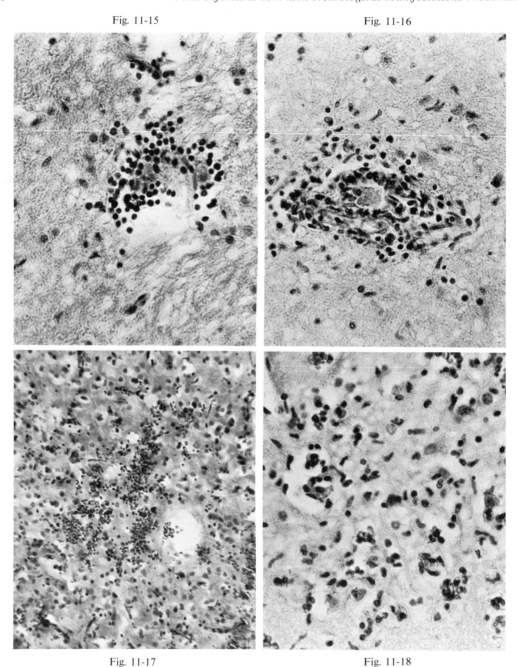

Fig. 11-17   Fig. 11-18

Figure 11-15. Lymphocytic perivascular infiltration. Paraffin section; hematoxylin-eosin stain; × 300. (From Osetowska, E.: Diagnostic neuropathologique d'encéphalite à tiques en Pologne. Neuropat. Pol., *4*:401-410, 1966.)

Figure 11-16. The afflux of microglia in short-rod shaped form. Paraffin section; hematoxylin-eosin stain; × 300. (From Osetowska, E.: Diagnostic neuropathologique d'encéphalite à tiques en Pologne. Neuropat. Pol., *4*:401-410, 1966.)

Figure 11-17. Small intracortical perivascular hemorrhages, frozen section; hematoxylin-eosin stain; × 300. (From Osetowska, E.: Diagnostic neuropathologique d'encéphalite à tiques en Pologne. Neuropat. Pol., *4*:401-410, 1966.)

Figure 11-18. Spongiosis of the cortex partially covered over by the microglia. Transition image with rarefaction necrosis. Paraffin section; hematoxylin-eosin stain; × 300. (From Osetowska, E.: Diagnostic neuropathologique d'encéphalite à tiques en Pologne. Neuropat. Pol., *4*:401-410, 1966.)

cytes. The afflux of rod-shaped microglial cells in the neighborhood of the vessels is characteristic (Fig. 11-16). Extravasations of blood are rare but occur particularly in the brain cortex (Fig. 11-17). Also among the neurons of the cortex, accumulation of microglia on a rarified background (Fig. 11-18) may appear, as the transition image between the necrosis of rarefaction and the diffuse microglial plaque. These diffuse plaques resemble microglial nodules of unusually large size; they are most often seen among the neurons of the pons, the circumvolutions of the inferior olivary nucleus, and the nerve cells of the dentate nucleus (Figs. 11-19, 11-20, and 11-21).

The necroses of rarefaction, lacking all cellular elements, are less often seen in tick-borne and verno-estival encephalitis (Fig. 11-22). They are highly characteristic of Japanese B encephalitis and of all the best-known encephalitides due to viruses of Casals' group A.[10, 49]

The presence of eosinophilic intranuclear inclusions has been strongly emphasized by the Russian authors.[70, 71] A critical review of the problem was first contributed by Bethlem,[3] and then by all the literature concerning inclusions in the different forms of present-day encephalitides.

The neuropathological differential diagnosis is all the more important because it often remains the only precise element of the diagnosis.[47] Theoretically the differential diagnosis includes von Economo's encephalitis lethargica; in practice it involves especially poliomyelitis, rabies, and the encephalitides due to other arboviruses and to enteroviruses other than poliovirus.

In typical von Economo encephalitis the cerebral picture differs in the extent of the lesions at the various cerebral levels and in the involvement of the cerebellar cortex, but this difference is by no means certain, particularly as regards involvement of the cerebellar cortex. To our knowledge,[49, 56] von Economo encephalitis is no longer encountered in the Western hemisphere.

The most difficult problem is the differentiation from poliomyelitis. The cortical involvement, the prevalence of olivary lesions, and the extensiveness of the process in the cerebellar cortex yield the most characteristic indications. Nonetheless, in certain cases, this differential diagnosis can be made only by highly specialized research workers[31, 33, 62] and, in other cases, it may even be impossible.[24, 39]

The encephalitides provoked by certain strains of Coxsackie or ECHO viruses are rarely fatal. Their pathologic anatomy is practically unknown; the few autopsies made have failed to reveal typical characteristics.

Rabies can usually be distinguished owing to a typical anamnesis. The finding of Negri inclusion bodies, which are absent in only 5 per cent of cases, facilitates the diagnosis. Moreover tick-borne encephalitis in its low form, poliomyelitis, and rabies belong to the same group of polioencephalitides characterized by Spatz spots[67] which we mentioned earlier.

The differentiation from the other arbovirus encephalitides is possible;[56] moreover, the risk of error is further reduced in proportion to the geographic autonomy, to the fidelity to a particular geographic distribution, of these different forms of encephalitis.

CLINICAL STUDIES

The literature dealing with the clinical aspects of tick-borne encephalitis may be divided into two periods: that of the severe epidemics recurring up to 1953-1954 and that of sporadic cases arising in endemic foci. In Poland clinical case reports were made by Falkiewicz,[18] Goralski,[20-22] Szajna,[69] and Kamieniecka et al.[34] Thereafter there appear only more or less isolated reports.[8, 46] We shall not recapitulate the literature of Central Europe, which the reader can find remarkably well assembled and compared in the work of Seitelberger and Jellinger.[62] It is nonetheless important to mention that tick-borne encephalitis appears relatively often in Western Germany.[53, 54] The first German case reports of tick-borne encephalitis authenticated by neuropathological investigation go back to approximately 1940.[47] We shall not go into detail, either, in regard to the Czechoslovakian literature concerning which a rich bibliographical source is available in the work of Henner and Hazal.[26] The Russian works also had their classical period with the discoveries of the viruses by Chumakov[11] and Zilber.[77] The usual clinical picture is summarized by Sepp et al.[63] But since these first works, tick-borne encephalitis reappears regularly in the Russian medical journals with new particular characteristics described in connection with more or less sporadic cases.[2, 35, 42, 48, 60, 73, 74]

If the patient does not arrive at the hospital already in a state of obnubilation, the clinical diagnosis begins with a *study of his*

Fig. 11-19   Fig. 11-20

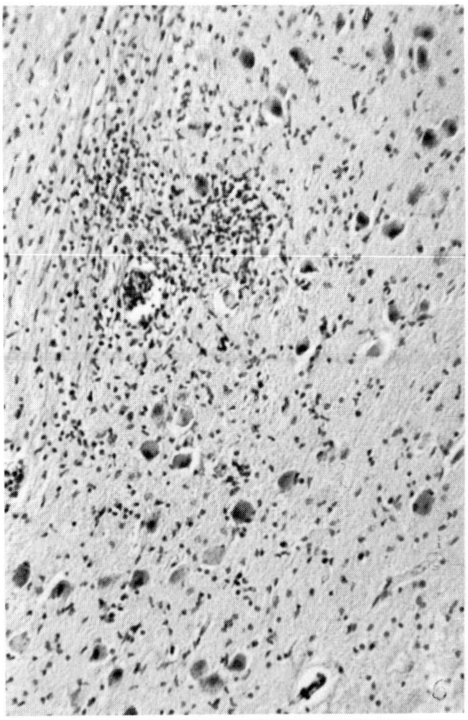

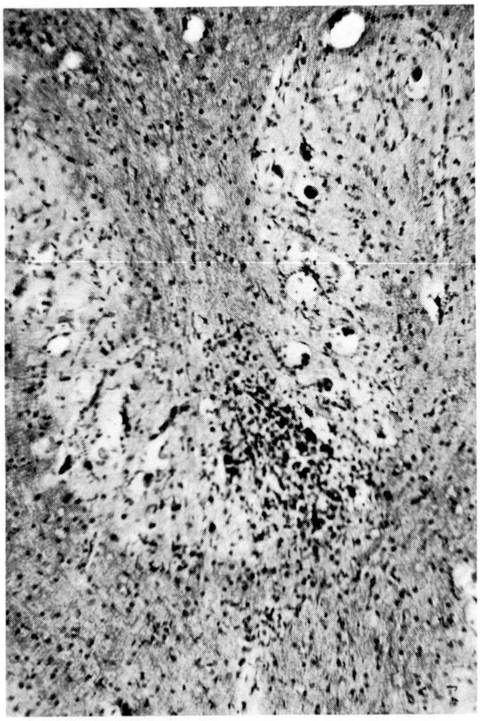

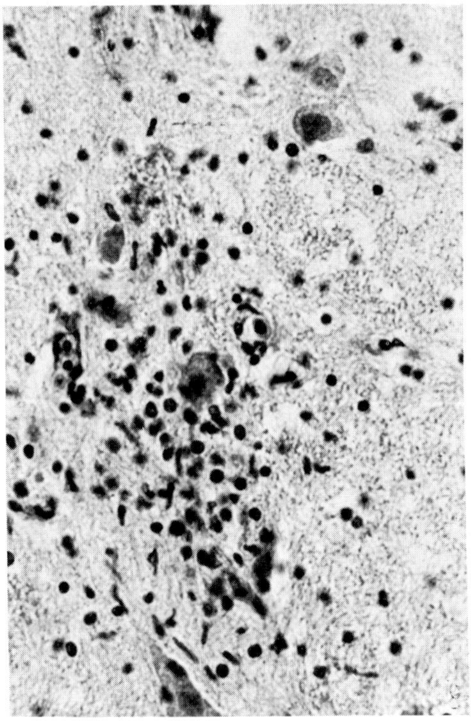

Fig. 11-21 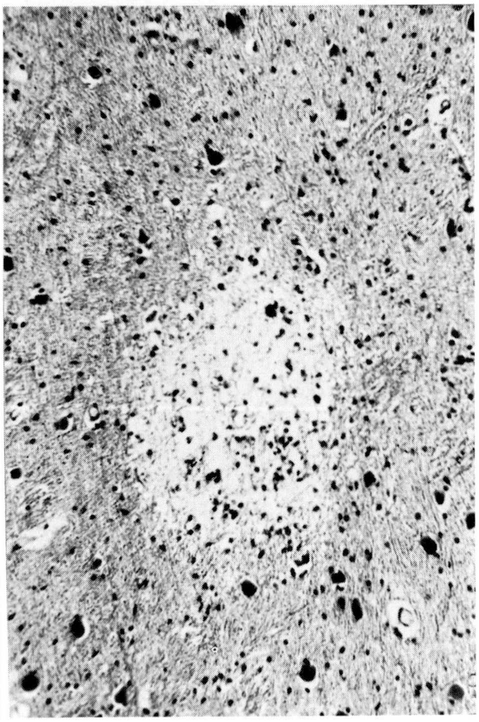   Fig. 11-22

Figure 11-19. Microglial plaque at the level of the pons. Paraffin section; × 300.

Figure 11-20. Microglial plaque among the cells of the inferior olive. Frozen section; hematoxylin-eosin stain; × 100.

Figure 11-21. Formation of a gliomesenchymal neuronophagic nodule at the level of the dentate nucleus. Paraffin section; hematoxylin-eosin stain; × 400. (From Osetowska, E.: Diagnostic neuropathologique d'encéphalite à tiques en Pologne. Neuropat. Pol., *4*:401-410, 1966.)

Figure 11-22. "Empty"-type necrosis typical of the mesencephalic level. Paraffin section; hematoxylin-eosin stain; × 150.

history, in which the three following points are of decisive importance: the season, the geographical location, and the bite by tick or the presence of a tick on the skin or in the clothing. In accord with the biological data on the tick, the encephalitis may be contracted in spring, summer or early autumn (not later, in general, than September). The geographical location of the inoculation usually corresponds to work premises: in forests or in the fields of forest regions; the isolated cases are found as a rule among participants of weekend outings in forests in which tick-borne encephalitis is epidemic. In Poland, for example, the Mazury lake region is among those that attract visitors by their picturesqueness.[22]

The bite or the presence of the tick may be evident and immediately discovered. However, often no traces are found. The bite of the tick responsible for Central European encephalitis, *Ixodes ricinus,* does not generally provoke any great dermatological reaction, in contrast to that observed with other ticks that provoke considerable erythema.[61] The only exception is the skin inflammation after bite by *Ixodes ricinus* described by Goralski.[21] The transmission of the CEE virus by other arthropods (mosquitoes, fleas) is discussed but highly dubious.[72]

Most often, the disease evolves in two phases. *The first phase* corresponds to that of generalized viremia. It can pass unnoticed or be very discrete, especially in the rural population, robust and inattentive to general malaise. The clinical manifestations of this first period are ill characterized by an influenzal state or a simple chill. The fever oscillates between 38 and 39° C. (100.4 and 102.2° F.); it is accompanied by a few articular or muscular pains. In certain cases, however, as early as this phase, some meningeal signs or obnubilation appears, immediately drawing attention to the central nervous system.

Almost always there are also vegetative disturbances such as hypertension and tachycardia, usually unsuspected by the patient.[68] These disturbances can evolve independently from the other clinical signs and occur even if this first period takes an inconspicuous form.

The initial phase lasts approximately a week. The apparently free interval between this beginning and the encephalitic phase *sensu stricto* also lasts almost a week. This second period does not correspond to a complete remission. The most sensitive patients feel weakened with more or less defined malaise.

Sometimes, especially during epidemics, the initial phase alone appears to constitute the entire disease. Only the blood antibody titer will permit later diagnosis in these cases.

The clinical aspects of the *encephalitic* or *nervous* phase may be classified according to the following syndromes: cerebromeningeal, brain stem, ascending spinal (Landry-type paralysis), and spinoperipheral. Between these syndromes, there exist transitional forms.

The encephalitic phase is expressed by recurrent fever, a state of obnubilation, and disseminated or focal signs.

The *cerebromeningeal* and *brain stem* forms are the most redoubtable. The disturbances of consciousness, isolated paralyses or hemiplegias, crises of epilepsy, hyperkinesia, and the Kozewnikow[40] type of partial continuous epilepsy constitute the essential elements. The patient slips gradually into coma.

In the brain stem form there predominate signs of involvement of the cranial nerves and the vegetative centers: disturbances of respiration, of cardiac rhythm, and of deglutition, and spinal paralyses, affecting particularly the shoulder muscles and the upper limbs.

It seems that these forms are considered characteristic of Far Eastern encephalitis. Both of them, nonetheless, are encountered in epidemics in Western Russia and Central Europe. Magazanik[42] in the Ural epidemic or epidemic of the frontier between European and Asiatic Russia, observed 101 patients of whom 22 per cent presented a pseudopoliomyelitic form with Kozewnikow epilepsy, 17 per cent with hemiplegias of the central type, and in 13 patients, from the onset, an evolution toward chronicity, with symptoms suggestive of amyotrophic lateral sclerosis. Renne[60] and Kantor[35] have emphasized the existence of multiple hyperkinesias. Similar aspects have also been observed in Poland and in Czechoslovakia.[18, 21, 26, 36, 69]

The *Landry ascendent* form is well known for the rapidity of its clinical evolution and its unfavorable prognosis.

The *spinoperipheral syndromes* with minimal cerebral involvement generally yield transitory sequelae.

Mitrochina[48] observed 71 children in whom the cerebromeningeal forms with biphasic fever predominated. It should be emphasized that this type of manifestation is exceptional, tick-borne encephalitis being theoretically a disease of adults with an average age of 38 years.[51]

The tick-borne disease contracted by the alimentary route is usually benign, with a biphasic evolution in almost all cases.[58] The nervous phase, observed with remarkable thoroughness by Henner and Hanzal[26] during an epidemic in Rozniava, resembles to the point of creating a possibility of diagnostic error von Economo's encephalitis lethargica, with exaggerated somnolence, disturbances of the intra-orbital muscles, "oily" face, and so forth. This epidemic affected 200 persons, in all with a favorable outcome.

SEQUELAE

It is difficult for us to make a statement concerning the prognosis in the forms evolving from their onset toward chronicity. We know them primarily through reading the Russian literature, in which the texts are not explicit about the length of time of observation.

The evolution of the Polish cases has never been very long. According to the American investigation,[66] most of the symptoms disappear in a few months to two or three years in the case of both arbovirus A encephalitides and those of Central Europe and the Far East.

Goralski's personal case report[22] is especially interesting because the patient and the physician were one and the same. The encephalitis was contracted during an excursion on one of the Mazury lakes. Goralski mentions a certain state of fatigue close to depression and trembling of the hands. These symptoms diminished gradually and disappeared in a few months.

The peripheral paralyses in the forms due to CEE virus all tend to disappearance. The parkinsonian syndrome, relatively infrequent, regresses after several months with recovery *ad integrum.*[56]

Zilber[76] affirmed without exception that the paralyses observed in the patients of the Far East leave severe sequelae comparable to those of poliomyelitis.

DIAGNOSIS

Serological tests have considerable value for the diagnosis. According to Libikova[41] and Moritsch[51] the methods of complement fixation and of agglutination inhibition can be considered absolutely trustworthy. The first

blood specimen should be taken during the viremia phase, the second from seven to 23 days later. The antibody titers increase during this period by as much as four times. In certain positive cases the titers reach the figures of 1:64 to 1:2048.[41]

Isolation of the virus from the patient's blood is possible in the viremic phase.

In the cases of alimentary origin isolation of the virus is in fact impossible and the antibody level rises but slowly.

The other laboratory data are of no diagnostic value. However, the investigator may find an increase in blood sugar level and, in the urine, traces or levels slightly more elevated of albumin and of urobilinogen.

The blood leukocyte level is fairly often above normal; the cerebrospinal fluid shows a pleocytosis with a number of cellular elements ranging from a few to several hundreds. These elements may be constituted at the onset of polymorphonuclear cells, but, with the evolution of the encephalitis, the lymphocytes become much more numerous than the polymorphonuclear cells, which later on disappear.

DIFFERENTIAL DIAGNOSIS

Theoretically, the differential diagnosis arises in the same conditions as on neuropathological examination. In fact, if the results of the serological tests are available, no difficulty exists.

In the countries in which the existence of arbovirus encephalitis is established, the patient's history and the clinical picture contribute arguments essential to the diagnosis.

If the patient with encephalitis represents the first case to be reported in the region or if he has contracted the disease in another region, the differentiation from poliomyelitis becomes really difficult. The usual differences between the age groups struck by one or the other of the two diseases is enlightening in an epidemic situation, although this element is of less diagnostic utility in isolated cases. The polyradiculomyelitides and polyradiculitides of unknown origin differ more or less by the whole clinical picture and its context.

TREATMENT

No specific treatment is available. At present the physician disposes of only palli-

ative treatment used to lessen the consequences of the symptoms. The Russian physicians propose an antiencephalic serum. In
high-risk cases, such as in a laboratory infection,[74] this therapeutic attempt failed, as did
other attempts.

Vaccination against tick-borne encephalitis has been begun experimentally in Prague.[13]

BIBLIOGRAPHY

1. Albrecht, P.: Pathogenesis of experimental infection with tick-borne encephalitis virus. Introductory lecture. In: Symposia ČSAU. Biology of viruses of the tick-borne encephalitis complex. Praha, Czechoslovak Academy of Sciences, 1962, pp. 247-257.
2. Belman, Ch. L.: Woprosy lokalizacij w klinike kleszczowego encefalita. Ž. Nieuropat. Psich., 63:1670-1672, 1963.
3. Bethlem, J.: The significance of inclusion bodies in virus meningo-encephalitis. In: Virus Meningo-Encephalitis. Ciba Foundation Study Group No. 7. London, J. & A. Churchill, 1961, pp. 84-86.
4. Blaskovic, D.: Some aspects of the epidemiology and prevention of tick-borne encephalitis. In: Symposia ČSAU. Biology of viruses of the tick-borne encephalitis complex. Praha, Czechoslovak Academy of Sciences, 1962, pp. 25-31.
5. Bodian, D.: The virus, the nerve cell and paralysis. A study of experimental poliomyelitis in the spinal cord. Bull. Johns Hopkins Hosp., 83:1-107, 1948.
6. Bogaert, L. van: Encéphalite léthargique type A (maladie d'Economo). Handb. spez. path. Anat. Histol. Henke-Lubarsch-Scholz. Berlin, Springer, 1958, 13, IIA, pp. 313-361.
7. Bogaert, L. van: Aspects cliniques des méningo-encéphalites actuelles d'origine inconnue mais dites virales en Europe Occidentale. Encéphale, 5:1267-1293, 1956.
8. Borzuchowska, A., and Jezyna, Cz.: Przypadek kleszczowego zapalenia mozgu. Przegl. Lek., 19:195-197, 1963.
9. Casals, J.: In: Viral Encephalitis. Fields, W. S., and Blattner, R. J. (eds.). Springfield, Ill., Charles C Thomas, 1958, pp. 5-22.
10. Casals, J.: Antigenic relationships among arthropod-borne viruses, effect on diagnosis and cross immunity. Introductory lecture. In: Symposia ČSAU. Biology of viruses of the tick-borne encephalitis complex. Praha, Czechoslovak Academy of Sciences, 1962, 53-66.
11. Chumakov, M. P.: Wirusnyje Nieuroinfekcyj. Klin. Mied., 27:3-10, 1949.
12. Clarke, D. H.: Antigenic relationships among viruses of the tick-borne encephalitis complex as studied by antibody absorption and agar gel precipitin techniques. In: Symposia ČSAU. Biology of viruses of the tick-borne encephalitis complex. Praha, Czechoslovak Academy of Sciences, 1962, pp. 67-75.
13. Daneš, L., and Benda, R.: Evaluation of the immunogenic efficiency of a tick-borne encephalitis virus vaccine. In: Symposia ČSAU. Biology of viruses of the tick-borne encephalitis complex. Praha, Czechoslovak Academy of Sciences, 1962, pp. 354-357.
14. Denk, H., and Kovac, W.: Zur Entwicklung des morphologischen Bildes der experimentellen FSEM (Frühsommer-Encephalomyelitis) der weissen Maus. Acta Neuropath., 7:1, 62-69, 1966.
15. Denk, H., and Kovac, W.: Die experimentelle Frühsommer-Encephalomyelitis (FSEM) der weissen Maus. Acta Neuropath. 7:162-174, 1966.
16. Draganescu, S., and Draganescu, N.: Sur la nature et l'aspect clinico-morphologique des encéphalites virotiques primitives actuellement observées dans la république populaire roumaine. Encéphalite Actuelles. Sofia, L'Académie Bulgare des Sciences, 1964.
17. Draganescu, N., and Popescu, G.: Recherches clinico-épidemiologiques et sérologiques dans certains foyers d'encéphalite par le virus à tiques de la République socialiste de Roumanie. Neuropat. Pol., 4:333-344, 1966.
18. Falkiewicz, S.: Klinika kleszczowego zapalenia mózgu. Postepy Hig. Med. Dośw., 8:47-54, 1954.
19. Fischer, J., and Bardoš, V.: The influence of the concentration of the virus of Czechoslovak tick-borne encephalitis on the dynamics of the histopathological inflammatory changes in the central nervous system in mice. Acta Univ. Carol. Med., 7:461-468, 1959.
20. Goralski, H.: Epidemia wirusowego zakażenia układu nerwowego w województwie olsztyńskim. Pol. Tyg. Lek., 10:3-12, 1955.
21. Goralski, H.: Epidemia kleszczowego zapalenia mózgu (encephalitis ixodica) w województwie olsztynskim. Neurol. Neurochir. Psychiat. Pol., 6:429-440, 1956.
22. Goralski, H.: Une epidémie d'encéphalite à tiques en Pologne. World Neurol., 2:336-342, 1961.
23. Graschenenkow, N. I.: Tick-borne encephalitis in the USSR. Bull. WHO, 30:187-196, 1964.
24. Grinschgl, G.: Grenzen der Klinischen Differential-diagnostik neurotroper Viruserkrankungen. Wien. Z. Nervenheilk., 12:434-451, 1956.
25. Haymaker, W.: Mosquito-borne encephalitides. In: Encephalitides. Bogaert, L. van et al. (eds.). New York, American Elsevier, 1961, pp. 38-56.
26. Henner, K., and Hanzal, F.: Encéphalite tchécoslovaque à tiques tableau clinique, diagnostic et traitement. Rev. Neurol., 96:384-408, 1957.
27. Herman, E.: Choroby zapalne mózgu. In: Choroby układu nerwowego pod red. W. Jakimowicza (ed.). Warszawa, PZWL, Vol. II, p. 5, 1952.
28. Herman, E.: Kleszczowe zapalenie mózgu. In: Neurologia Kliniczna. W. Jakimowicza (ed.). Warszawa, PZWL, 1961, pp. 159-161.
29. Herman, E., and Przesmycki, F.: Choroby wirusowe układu nerwowego. Warszawa, PZWL, 1954.
30. Ivanowa, L. M.: Aperçu épidémiologique bref de l'encéphalite à tiques et sa prophylaxie en République socialiste soviétique russe. Encéphalites Actuelles. Sofia, L'Académie Bulgare des Sciences, 1964.
31. Jabotynski, J. M.: Distinctions morphologiques entre les infections neurovirales à caractère antigenique proche ou identique. Neuropat. Pol., 4:359-366, 1966.
32. Jacob, H.: Neuropathologie der Viruserkrankungen des Zentralnervensystems. Deutsch. Z. Nervenheilk., 182:472-431, 1961.
33. Jellinger, K., and Kovac, W.: Beitrag zur Neuropathologie der Frühsommer-Meningoencephalomyelitis. Path. Microbiol., 23:375-391, 1960.

34. Kamieniecka, Z., Kirkowska, I., and Szajna, M.: Badania nad zapaleniem mózgu kleszczowym. IV. Ocena stanu zdrowia ozdrowiencow po zapaleniu mózgu kleszczowym. Przegl, Epidem., *8*:226-228, 1954.

35. Kantor, W. M.: O niektórych giperkineticzeskich sindramach pri kleszczowom encefalitic. Ż. Niewropat. Psichiat., *61*:48-51, 1961.

36. Kirkowska, I., Kamieniecka, Z., and Szajna, W.: Kleszczowe zapalenie mózgu. Neurol. Neurochir. Psychiat. Pol., *4*:281-292, 1954.

37. Kolman, J. M., and Havlik, O.: Vy'zkum přènásěcu a reservoárii prirodnim ohnisku nákaz. Česk. hyg. epidem. mikrobiol. imun., *3*:74-78, 1954.

38. Környey, S.: Zur vergleichenden Pathologie der Zeckenencephalitis. Verh. Deutsch. Ges. Inn. Med., *61*:231-235, 1955.

39. Kornyey S.: Zur histologischem Differentialdiagnose von Encephalomyelitiden (über die Bedeutung der Knötchenbildung in den unteren Oliven). Stud. Cercet. Neurol. (Extras), *9*:505-511, 1964.

40. Kożewnikow, A. J.: Osowyj wid kortikalnoj epilepsi. Gosudarstwiemoje izdatielstwo Medicinskoj literatury, 1952.

41. Libiková, H., Kroö, A., and Tesřová, J.: Immunogenesis of tick-borne encephalitis correlated to the development of clinical of the infection. Neuropat. Pol., *4*:321-328, 1966

42. Magazanik, S. S.: Klinika i leczenie progredientnych form kleszczewego encefalita na Urale. Ż. Niewropat. Psichiat., *62*:277-281, 1962.

43. Málková, D.: Role of the lymphatic and blood circulation in the distribution of tick-borne encephalitis virus in the organism of susceptible and non-susceptible animal. In: symposia ČSAU. Biology of viruses of the tick-borne encephalitis complex. Praha, Czechoslovak Academy of Sciences, 1962, pp. 271-274.

44. Manuelides, E. E.: General histopathological aspects of some experimental viral encephalitides. Handb. spez. path. Anat. Histol. Henke-Lubarsch-Scholz. Berlin, Springer, 1958, 13, IIA, pp. 209-243.

45. Mielnikow, C., and Makonkova, A. G.: Patomorphologie de la variation occidentele de l'encéphalite à tiques. Ż. Niewropat. Psichiat., *58*:1349-1353, 1958.

46. Migdalska-Kassurowa, B.: Kleszczowe zapalenie mózgu z omówieniem 16-stu własnych przypadków. Przegl. Epidem., *17*:277-286, 1963.

47. Minauf, M., and Tateishi, J.: Über einen Fall Frühjahr-Sommer-Encephalomyelitis. Acta Neuropath., *7*:349-356, 1967.

48. Mitrochina, P. A.: Osobiennosti kliniki kleszczewogo encefalita diestkowo worzrasta. Ż. Niewropat. Psichiat., *62*:978-980, 1962.

49. Mollaret, J., and Schneider, J.: Classification épidémiologique et virologique des encéphalites humaines. Les encéphalites á virus. Paris, Masson et Cie, 1963.

50. Mólnar, E.: Vorkommen von neutralisierenden Antikörpern gegen Zechen encephalitis bei asetischen Meningitiden in Ungarn. Encéphalites Actuelles. Sofia, L'Academie Bulgare des Sciences, 1964.

51. Moritsch, H.: Diagnostic procedures in human cases of TBE. Neuropat. Pol., *4*:313-318, 1966.

52. Moritsch, H., and Kovac, W.: Investigation on pathogenesis of alimentary infection with tick-borne encephalitis virus in mice. In: Symposia ČSAU.

Biology viruses of the tick-borne encephalitis complex. Praha, Czechoslovak Academy of Sciences, 1962, pp. 283, 285.

53. Müller, W.: Orientierende Untersuchung über die Zeckenaktivität in der Umgebung von Würzburg während der Vegetationsperiode des Jahres 1965. Deutsch. Z. Nervenheilk., *189*:259-270, 1966.

54. Müller, W., and Türk, B.: Geographische und jahreszeitliche Verteilung von Krankheitsbildern mit möglicher Arthropodenätiologie. Deutsch. Z. Nervenheilk., *189*:240-258, 1966.

55. Osetowska, E.: Diagnostic neuropathologique d'encéphalite à tiques en Pologne. Neuropat. Pol., *4*:401-410, 1966.

56. Osetowska, E.: L'encéphalite d'Economo et les encéphalites Arbor. Acta Neurol. Belg., *67*:172-197, 1967.

57. Osetowska, E., and Wróblewska-Mularczyk, Z.: Neuropatologia doswiad-czalnego zapalenia kleszczowego mózgu. Neuropat. Pol., *2*:231-244, *4*:63-82, 1966.

58. Pogodina, V. V.: The course of alimentary infection and development of immunity in tick-borne encephalitis. In: Symposia ČSAU. Biology of viruses of the tick-borne encephalitis complex. Praha, Czechoslovak Academy of Sciences, pp. 275-281, 1962.

59. Przesmycki, E., Taytsch, Z., Semkow, R., and Walentynowicz-Stańczyk, R.: Badania nad zapaleniem mózgu kleszczowym. Przegl. Epidem., *8*:203-214, 1954.

60. Renne, T. F.: O niekotorych giperkineticzeskich formach wiesen-neletniego encefalitis. Ż. Niewropat. Psichiat., *61*:52-55, 1961.

61. Schaltenbrand, G.: Durch Arthropoden übertragene Infektionen der Haut und des Nervensystems. München Med. Wschr., *32*:1557-1562, 1966.

62. Seitelberger, F., and Jellinger, K.: Neuropathologie der Zeckenencephalitis. Neuropat. Pol., *4*:367-400, 1966.

63. Sepp, E. K., Cuker, M. B., and Szmidt, E. W.: Newrńyje bolezni kleszczowoj encefalit (wiesnnyjeletnyj). Medgiz. Moskwa, pp. 392-397, 1950.

64. Simon, J., Slonim, D., and Zavadova, H.: Experimentelle Untersuchungen von klinischen und subklinischen Formen der Zeckenencephalitis an unterschiedlich empfänglich Wirten. Acta Neuropath., *7*:70-78, 1966; 89-100, 1966; *8*:24-34, 35-46, 1967.

65. Slonim, D.: The tick-borne encephalitis complex. In: Virus Meningo-Encephalitis. Ciba Foundation Study Group No. 7. London, J. & A. Churchill, 1961, pp. 59-67.

66. Smadel, J. E., Bailey, P., and Baker, A. B.: Sequelae of the arthropod-borne encephalitides. Neurology, *8*:873-895, 1958.

67. Spatz, H.: Encephalitis. In: Handb. d. Geisteskrankheiten (Bumke). Bd. 11, Spez. Teil VII, S. 157, Berlin, Springer, 1930.

68. Stille, W., and Banke, J.: Zechenencephalitis in Westdeutschland. München Med. Wschr., *107*:370-374, 1965.

69. Szajna, M.: Badania nad zapaleniem mózgu kleszczowym. III. Obraz kliniczny kleszczowego zapalenia mózgu w N. Przegl. Epidem., *8*:219-224, 1954.

70. Szeni, R. M., and Drobyszewskaja, A. J.: Morfologija dalniewostocznogo kleszczewogo encefalita. Vop. Med. Virus., *1*:302-316, 1948.

71. Szubladze, A. K., Margulis, M. S., and Galiainowicz, C. J.: Eksperymentalnyj ostryj rassiejannyj encefalomielit u obiezian, wyzwanyj wirusom piernicznowo ostrowo encefalomielita człó-wieka. Vop. Med. Virus., *1*:284-301, 1948.

72. Taytsch, Z. F., and Wróblewska, Z.: Badanie naturalnego ogniska zapalenia mózgu w puszczy Bielowieskiej. Przegl. Epidem., *12*:339-353, 1958.

73. Vizen, E. M.: Ob atipicznych formach kleszczewogo encefalita. Z. Niewropat. Psichiat., *63*L1462-1467, 1963.

74. Vizen, E. M., and Knieziew, A. N.: Sluczaj laboratornogo zarazenija czolowieka wirusom kleszczewogo encefalita. Z. Niewropat. Psichiat., *62*:333-338, 1962.

75. Wróblewska-Mularczykowa, Z.: Arbor-Wirusy (wirusy zapalenia mózgu i inne przenoszone przez stawonogi). Zarys wirusologii praktycznej. Warszawa, PZWL, 1963, pp. 234-264.

76. Zilber, L. A.: Pathogenicity of Far East and Western (Eüropean) tick-borne encephalitis viruses in sheep and monkeys. In: Symposia CSAU. Biology of viruses of the tick-borne encephalitis complex. Praha, Czechoslovak Academy of Sciences, 1962, pp. 260-264.

77. Zilber, L. A.: Predwatitelnyje itogi iznaczenija encefalita w Bielorussii. Vop. Med. Virus., *1*:275-283, 1948.

12

Lethargic Encephalitis or von Economo's Disease

By R. DEBRÉ

INTRODUCTION AND HISTORY

The history of von Economo's disease, also called lethargic encephalitis or A encephalitis, is extremely peculiar. The physicians who observed epidemics of this illness from 1915 to 1926 did not doubt its specific nature. The epidemic which at that time spread over the whole world affected a great number of subjects. The disease presented a characteristic clinical picture, and different types of cases were concurrently observed in hospitals. As von Economo pointed out, every practitioner in most European and American countries and in Australia observed several patients and identified the disease with certainty. This is significant for both the wide spread of the disease and its peculiar characteristics. A certain degree of epidemic coincidence and resemblance to the typical form made it possible to attribute to the same pathogenic agent very specific morbid symptoms, among them epidemic hiccup.

The disease was striking not only in its clinical picture in the acute phase but also in the severity of its motor and mental sequelae. One of the most important after-effects was the Parkinson syndrome. It was thought at that time that the saliva of these patients with postencephalitic parkinsonism might be capable of causing infection. Such a concept foreshadowed today's thinking on the prolonged action of viruses fixed in the nervous system and capable of determining new progressive disturbances long after the acute invasion period; it also foreshadowed present thinking on the possibility of virus elimination through the secretions of affected subjects, who act as a true reservoir of germs (cf. Chapter 19).

It was impossible at the time to carry out a conclusive etiological study, and more recent, far-reaching virological studies carried out at the time of other epidemics of encephalitis could not shed any light on von Economo's encephalitis. The fact remains, however, that a very big world-wide epidemic of an autonomous encephalitis developed for nearly 10 years and then disappeared almost completely. For the last 40 years, conclusive observations have been published only for individual cases.

Everything leads to the conclusion that this disease is autonomous: its specific picture and its striking spread in both hemispheres. Its comprehensive clinical characteristics, both anatomopathological and epidemiological, point very strongly to a virus disease in spite of the complete absence of laboratory evidence.

Because it is useful to know about this historical event, which was very suggestive as to the general pathological effects of viruses, because sporadic cases must still be identified today—however, exceptional they may be—and, finally, because the possibility of an epidemic flareup is not excluded, we shall sum up in this paper the essential notions on lethargic encephalitis or von Economo's disease. This is all the more important, because its description has been excluded—mistakenly, we believe—from modern virological treatises.

Cruchet, Moutier, and Calmettes (from Bordeaux) published in 1917 a paper on 40 cases of subacute encephalomyelitis that had been observed since the end of 1915. The disease was characterized by weariness, headaches, dullness of facial expression, torpor, loss of weight, sometimes fever, and a number of nervous disorders, particularly mental disorders, choreal movements, ptosis, cerebellar signs, and, primarily, ocular signs. A few days after the communication by these authors, von Economo described in Vienna, upon observation of 11 cases seen during the last months of 1916, six of which were fatal, a disease characterized mainly by lethargy, paralyses of cranial nerves and primarily ocular nerves, and fever. A little later, Netter noted the appearance of this disease in Paris and recalled the striking and picturesque description (Albrecht in 1706) of earlier epidemics of the same morbid type. He also gave an excellent preview of the numerous clinical forms which were little by little to be identified in France. Abundant world-wide literature was to round out later the clinical and anatomical description of the disease.

Thus, encountered in southwest France from 1915 to 1917, then in Austria during the winter of 1916-1917, the disease appeared in Paris in winter, 1917-1918, in England in spring, 1918, and in Italy. In Portugal, the disease appeared in February, 1919, and it appeared the same year in Finland, Norway, Denmark, Belgium, Holland, and Switzerland. In 1920, it was noted in Poland, Spain, and Rumania. India was affected in the winter of 1919 and North Africa in the same year. It would seem that the disease appeared in Australia as early as 1917. It was first noted on the east coast of the United States in 1918, and it reached the west coast in October, 1919. The disease invaded Uruguay and Peru the same year. It appeared in Brazil in 1920. During the winter of 1919-1920, the description of many cases was published in Belgium, Algeria, Greece, Italy, Latin America, and the United States. The disease was now world-wide.

In each country, the disease took its course in fairly spaced outbreaks of long duration and wide spread; between these outbreaks, it was kept alive by sporadic cases. Epidemics showed a clear seasonal trend (spring and primarily winter). Beginning with 1926, the pandemic stopped and sporadic cases became infrequent. It has practically never been encountered since 1930. Some authors think that the disease disappeared completely. A few cases, however, are still reported in various countries (United Kingdom, U.S.S.R., Germany). In view of the fact that there exists no specific test and that no identifiable virus has been detected, diagnosis today, as 50 years ago, rests on clinical characteristics and, possibly, anatomopathological features.

EPIDEMIOLOGY

The disease developed during the world pandemic in the form of isolated cases more or less densely distributed in each community. Family cases were infrequent. The centers of infection became active in winter or in spring; they became quiescent in summer and quite often became active again the next winter. Other centers of infection were found in other communities. The number of people affected was quite considerable, and many mild and atypical forms of the disease were difficult to identify. The general aspect and the epidemic distribution were reminiscent of poliomyelitis. Such modes of transmission as arthropods, various insects, food, and water were eliminated one by one. The idea of interhuman transmission, more likely airborne (Flügge droplets) than handborne (fecal origin), gained considerable credence. It was thought that healthy germ carriers or latently infected subjects served as an intermediary link between the centers of viral outbreaks and reservoirs of virus during quiescent periods. It was also thought that in certain areas – of which there were many – most persons were infected by the supposed virus.

The disease affected mainly persons between 30 and 50 years of age, but many children and adolescents were also involved. The proportion of patients from ten to 20 years of age was estimated at approximately 25 per cent. It seemed that males were affected in a greater proportion than females.

VIRUS

Levaditi and Harvier thought in 1920 that they had isolated a virus that was transmissible in series. This virus was soon identified with that of herpes. In some ten other cases of lethargic encephalitis the same herpes virus was isolated by other authors. Various hypotheses were then envisaged: the disease was provoked by a specifically active herpes virus; it was a superinfection by the herpes virus; or a laboratory error was involved. No conclusion was arrived at at the time, and it is still a complete mystery today – all the more so because, as in the course of recent cases which appear to be clinically authentic, no virus was detected and no serological reaction obtained. Thus, although the virus origin of von Economo's disease remains highly probable and the nature of the virus must be specific, nothing further is known today about the etiology.

CLINICAL DESCRIPTION

Lethargic encephalitis is characterized by a threefold set of symptoms: somnolence or lethargy; paralysis or paresis of mesocephalic nerves and, primarily, of the motor oculi; and an infectious febrile condition.

The incubation period is ill defined, and a duration of ten days was fixed without proof. The start of the disease is sometimes progressive: psychic and physical asthenia, intense headaches, and fever. Alternatively, the onset may be violent, with headaches, vomiting, a clearly infectious syndrome, and a remarkable state of somnolence from the very beginning. Finally, and more infrequently, the disease takes an apoplectic form at the start, with coma and convulsive crises.

The acute period of illness is dominated by sleep. Von Economo wrote, "It is a kind of sleeping sickness which may range from mere drowsiness to deepest coma." Generally speaking, the sleeping subject wakes up when disturbed, gives the right answers to questions directed to him, obeys orders, gets up, eats unaided, and sometimes falls asleep in the middle of his meal. Certain patients may continue to discharge their duties with varying degrees of efficiency, but they fall asleep at the first opportunity (ambulatory forms described by Sicard). Another feature of encephalitic sleep is that it is not continuous. Quite often, it takes the form of several short naps during the day. The patients get up several times a day, carry out some routine activity, are overcome by sleep, and return to bed. To daylight drowsiness is added either normal night sleep or nocturnal insomnia (inversion of the nyctohemeral cycle). Sleep sometimes comes suddenly and invincibly, interrupting the course of some activity, to the point that an object held by the patient may escape his hands. More rarely, sleep becomes a true state of lethargy. Patients remain absolutely immobile with closed eyes and relaxed features. When called, they reply by fluttering their eyelids or by soundlessly moving their lips. Quite incapable of eating by themselves, they must be tube-fed. Some patients keep their eyes wide open, in a state of lucid catatonic stupor. Some of these patients are capable of keeping up indefinitely uncomfortable postures imposed on them by the observer. There is a common element to all forms of this lethargic condition: slowness of ideation and lack of movement flexibility.

OCULAR DISORDERS

Ocular disorders are the most frequent of the many nervous symptoms accompanying sleep disturbances. These disorders have a considerable polymorphic range; their nature is variable and evolves rapidly in the same patient. Paralyses of the third pair of cranial nerves occur most frequently. Ptosis is an essential feature caused by the impairment of the eyelid retractor muscle. This is usually one of the first signs, which may remain unheeded because of drowsiness. Indeed, it is perfectly possible to speak in connection with lethargic encephalitis of paralytic ptosis affecting simultaneously both eyes, which may remain the sole ocular symptom or be accompanied by a paralysis of the oculomotor muscles.

The affection of the motor muscles of the eyeball is shown by more or less pronounced functional and physical symptoms according to the degree of paralysis. There are patients who consult a physician merely because of double vision. Those are attenuated forms. More usually, both eyes show, to different degrees, concurrent parallel disturbances of their external muscles. Disorders of internal muscles are less marked; however, accommodation paresis is more frequent. It is bilateral and it starts early and suddenly. It may continue for months. The impairment of parallel movements concerns vertical movements of raising and lowering, or horizontal or lateral movements. Most often, a limitation of movements in a determined zone is involved rather than complete paralysis. Nystagmic movements may appear in certain positions of the eyeball. *Oculogyric attacks* are very characteristic. During the attack, the eyeballs assume an abnormal position which is almost always one of forced elevation (syndrome of eyes raised to the ceiling); this phase may or may not be preceded by a phase of lowering the eyeballs. Other phenomena, such as retraction of the upper eyelids and holding the head in hyperextension, may accompany an oculogyric attack. Fixity of look with a straight forward immobilization of the eyeballs has been noted more rarely. These symptoms evolve fitfully, starting suddenly and stopping abruptly within a few minutes to several hours. The attacks occur at variable periods of the evolution of the disease. They may continue for years. They are of great importance, because they seem to be characteristic for this type of encephalitis. They have not been described in the many subsequent epidemics of greatly varied types of encephalitis and should be considered pathognomonic.

Ocular disturbances, whatever the degree of their intensity, are nearly constant. They are encountered in all simple or ambulatory forms of the disease; they are its essential or at least most striking symptom, which is sometimes merely limited to a convergence or accommodation paralysis.

In general, ocular muscle disturbances improve progressively. They actually disappear completely in cases in which encephalitis does not evolve toward Parkinson's disease. When this evolution does take place, they may continue in a more or less limited or attenuated manner; among them oculogyric crises and discrete convergence paralysis are the most frequent.

IMPAIRMENT OF THE DIFFERENT ZONES CONTROLLED BY CRANIAL NERVES

The symptoms of these impairments are unilateral or bilateral facial paralysis of the peripheral type, and involvement of the trigeminal nerve, either sensory (facial neuralgia) or motor, accompanied by impairment of tongue and lip movements and of mastication, by vestibular disturbances, or by, less frequently, tongue atrophy and impairment of mixed nerves or bulbar centers; these forms may be compared to bulbar forms of the disease, accompanied by swallowing and respiratory disturbances and attacks of tachypnea.

DISTURBANCES OF THE PERIPHERAL MOTOR SYSTEM

Algomyoclonia. The algomyoclonic syndrome (Sicard) encountered during the French epidemic in 1920 was observed in a number of countries in subsequent years; later, it became infrequent. At the outset there are intense, throbbing, lightning pains, not unlike tabes or thalamic pains. These pains first affect the neck and the nape of the neck and then extend to the arms before spreading to the whole body. Five to seven days later myoclonus begins — sudden, brief, and explosive muscular contractions. Sometimes the contractions are rhythmically synchronized in the different muscles affected and sometimes they are arrythmical; sometimes they are divided and localized and sometimes massive and global. Myoclonus may occur at almost any site but the preferential localizations are face, neck, shoulders, abdomen, and diaphragm; most often it is accompanied by hiccup.

Myoclonus generally abates, and then disappears approximately a month later.

Psychic disturbances may then appear; they evolve toward mental confusion or a dreamlike state which develops into coma, with vegetative disturbances that are occasionally severe.

Choreal Syndrome. After an acute and very rapid start a state of grand chorea sets in with involuntary, disorderly, and arrhythmical gesticulations involving mainly neck and head, rotating, balancing, and bowing movements affecting to a lesser degree the limbs, the trunk, and the abdomen and presenting a picture of particularly intense chorea. After a prolonged convalescence cure is possible.

Slower movements, resembling athetosis, may be observed, as well as curious cases of bradykinesia—slow rhythmic movements, very wide, with big oscillations, repeated every two or every four seconds.

Disturbances of Muscular Tonus (Hypertonic Syndromes). Tonus disorders in encephalitic patients are either of the hypotonic type (von Economo) or, more usually, of the extrapyramidal hypertonic type. This hypertonicity, together with the hypersomnia, imparts to patients an atonic facial expression which looks like a set rigid mask, a ramrod bearing, and a slow stiff gait.

These tonus disturbances may be expressed by torticollis, scolioses, and torsion spasms. Although acute parkinsonian forms have been observed when the clinical picture was dominated by an early Parkinson's syndrome, they were less frequent than retarded parkinsonian symptoms.

Mental Syndromes. Disorders of vigil function seem to provide the common substrate for a large number of mental disturbances, such as confused dreamy states and delirious outbreaks. Mental disorders generally appear rather suddenly in young subjects, amidst the course of infectious symptoms, but primarily in the middle of a more or less pronounced state of somnolence. There is disorientation as to time and space, indifferent dumbness, dazed vacancy occasionally interrupted by agitation, and expression of delirious ideas on some visual and terrifying subject such as zoopsia with occupation-derived hallucinations, and even fugues.

ELEMENTS COMMON TO DIFFERENT SYNDROMES

Fever has been observed in all these cases. Occasionally it is rather high, but in general the temperature fluctuates around 38° C. and its degree is not connected with the severity of the disease. Fever is usually transient, lasting from one week to one month. Digestive disorders include nausea, vomiting, and constipation. Rapid denutrition has sometimes been noted, accompanied by a more or less high level of azotemia. Sympathetic disorders are both frequent and intense: violent blushing at the slightest emotion, sweating, sialorrhea.

CEREBROSPINAL FLUID

Lumbar puncture yields a clear fluid which usually shows a slight excess of proteins. The cerebrospinal fluid pressure is sometimes elevated. Hyperglycorrhachia, which is considered an important symptom by certain authors, is unusual. Xanthochromia, the presence of which leads to diagnostic errors (meningeal hemorrhages due to a variety of causes), has also been mentioned.

At the outset of the encephalitis the number of cells (predominantly mononuclear) in the cerebrospinal fluid may be a little high; it may continue increasing during the first days. In half the cases the cell count fluctuates around 10 per milliliter; it may sometimes rise to more than 100 and may reach 300. Subsequently, this figure decreases and more or less rapidly attains a normal level. This decrease is not final, and new outbreaks of pleocytosis may occur.

EVOLUTION

The evolution of the disease is extremely variable. Sometimes, after a few days of fever, drowsiness, and motor disturbances, the patient succumbs to the depth of the coma. Alternatively, the evolution may drag out for several weeks, then, little by little, symptoms are attenuated and fade away; again, it may last several months, with the subject passing progressively from the period of illness to the phase of after-effects. Frequently it is possible to distinguish clearly between an initial phase, a period of typical illness, a more or less protracted phase of remission, sometimes very protracted indeed, and then the appearance of after-effects.

AFTER-EFFECTS

The study of the after-effects of lethargic encephalitis poses a fundamental theoretical problem. Are they, according to the definition of this term, a consequence of lesions that occurred during the initial phase and left a durable or definitive trace, or are they a tardy evolutionary process connected with the persistence of the virus in the organism? This problem will be considered later.

It should be noted immediately that in the years following upon the epidemics of 1917 to 1926, Netter called attention to the possibility that the disease might be transmitted through the infected saliva of patients with parkinsonism who had been ill with lethargic encephalitis a few years before.

Be that as it may, the same stress should be put on the number, the variety, and the diverse associations of after-effects as on the varied clinical forms during the acute period of illness.

The after-effects consist of attacks of headache, various sleep disturbances, and continuation or appearance of oculomotor disorders, either permanent or paroxysmal. Mental disorders, either intellectual or psychic, may appear within several months or several years following the illness. The most important and characteristic element of the 1917-1926 epidemic was the establishment of a more or less complete parkinsonian syndrome of varying severity, evolving by a succession of outbreaks and very comparable to idiopathic Parkinson's disease.

Postencephalitic Parkinson Syndrome. The postencephalitic Parkinson syndrome is very frequent. It appears mainly after the oculolethargic forms of the disease. It is very difficult to establish an accurate ratio of this after-effect, because mild parkinsonian symptomatology may elude the observer or because it is associated with more obvious aftereffects which have caused it to be missed. Some contend that this syndrome appears in half of the cases, others that its rate attains 80 per cent. There is also an opinion that parkinsonism is a constant phenomenon, at least in its outline form, after von Economo's encephalitis.

Most often, there is a certain interval between the acute period and the beginning of Parkinson's syndrome, which may last from several months to five years. In rare cases latency may exceed 15 or even 20 years, although in these cases the slow and progressive nature of the syndrome makes the date of onset extremely debatable. This syndrome may reproduce the essential clinical picture of idiopathic Parkinson's disease: hypertonicity, akinesia, stiffness of aspect (dystonia of posture), sialorrhea and watering eyes, various vegetative disturbances, as well as more or less severe changes in the mental condition (bradyphrenia, melancholia, and so forth).

As a rule, the evolution of the postencephalitic Parkinson's syndrome is progressive and very slow, leading only after a long time to confinement to bed. Some of these patients have fixed or barely evolving forms of the disease. There have even been descriptions of regressive and curable postencephalitic forms of Parkinson's disease.

In their valuable survey, Duvoisin and Yahr mentioned in 1965 that 49 patients with Parkinson's disease which could be reasonably connected with von Economo's encephalitis were observed from January, 1962, to July, 1964, at the specialized clinic of Columbia-Presbyterian Medical Center. Only seven of these 49 cases seemed dubious to the authors. Almost all had been affected before 1940, a few of them between 1940 and 1950, and perhaps two after 1950. This group doubtless represents survivors of the 1920-1926 epidemic.

For most neurologists, postencephalitic parkinsonism should be distinguished from idiopathic Parkinson's disease. The latter, the etiology of which remains a mystery (except for certain cases which seem to be connected with cerebral arteriosclerosis, although coincidence or association remain possible in such cases), affects elderly subjects, whereas postencephalitic parkinsonism attacks young people. This phenomenon appeared striking to the clinicians of 50 years ago. Moreover, postencephalitic parkinsonism evolves even more slowly (protracted forms) and has a symptomatology less distinct (discrete forms) or less complete than idiopathic Parkinson's disease. It is often asymmetric and is frequently accompanied by peculiar nervous disorders which are characteristic for this type of encephalitis: dystonia, torsion spasms, and, more particularly, oculogyric fits. Some authors even believe this association of oculogyric fits with the Parkinson's syndrome to be characteristic of von Economo's encephalitis.* Indeed, the numerous sporadic or epidemic cases of encephalitis described in recent years all over the world occasionally show a parkinsonian syndrome among their after-effects, but this is very infrequent, as demonstrated recently by Duvoisin and Yahr: Japanese or

---

*As mentioned by Duvoisin and Yahr, only intoxication by phenothiazine may lead to such oculogyric fits.

B encephalitis, St. Louis encephalitis, Eastern and Western equine encephalitis, and the tick-borne encephalitis of Central Europe are rare if not nonexistent causes of true parkinsonian syndrome. If the description of some of them, as well as that of very exceptional cases of encephalitis induced by poliomyelitis and measles or chickenpox, contains syndromes of stiffness and trembling, these are early, little-developed, barely outlined symptoms which are most often transient and do not show themselves as true parkinsonian syndromes, such as only von Economo's encephalitis seems capable of producing.

The question was raised about a possible link between epidemic influenza and Parkinson's disease; however, the coincidence of influenza epidemics with the picture of von Economo's disease, the lighter forms of which are occasionally labeled as "flu," prevents any valid conclusion or leads rather to the speculation that Parkinson's disease was the consequence of von Economo's encephalitis which had not been diagnosed at the acute stage. Furthermore, the possibility of very simple, very brief, and almost latent cases of von Economo's disease may suggest that certain cases of Parkinson's disease have been caused by this type of encephalitis, although this is impossible to prove.

At any rate, toward the end of the big epidemic, the majority of cases of Parkinson's syndrome were certainly the consequence of von Economo's disease. Little by little, this percentage decreased. Dimsdale indicated that in various London neurological clinics postencephalitic Parkinson's syndrome represented two-thirds of all cases of parkinsonism observed from 1920 to 1930; only half of the cases observed from 1931 to 1942 were of that origin. The author thought that this was the case partly because of the decline of lethargic encephalitis after 1926 and its almost total disappearance later than 1940, and partly because toward the end of this pandemic parkinsonian aftereffects had become less frequent in subjects affected by von Economo's encephalitis. Today, a few subjects may still survive who were affected after the 1917-1926 pandemic, but they will soon have disappeared.

FORMS ENCOUNTERED IN CHILDREN AND ADOLESCENTS

Lethargic encephalitis causes after-effects in children and adolescents that have strongly impressed observers. These after-effects include not merely a rigidity syndrome with a whole train of the disorders observed in Parkinson's disease (juvenile postencephalitic Parkinson's disease), often accompanied by muscle tone disorders (torticollis), abnormal movements (tics, and so forth), and oculogyric fits (ocular paralyses), but in addition, disturbances of sleep, character, and behavior and pyschological disturbances which have been abundantly commented upon. Thus, certain children put to bed at their habitual evening hour do not fall asleep. They display an unusual agitation, turn about in bed, throw the pillow and the blankets aside, sit up, and lie down again. Quite often, they cannot control their saliva and soil all objects around them. They make faces and jump out of bed. Others carry out activities that they were incapable of performing during the day, because of muscular rigidity. This phase of agitation continues for hours on end, and it is only in the middle of the night that the child finally settles down and falls asleep.

Other children and adolescents constantly sleep in the daytime and are ceaselessly agitated at night. Moreover, mutations are possible between the two conditions. None of this variety of disorders is continual. At certain periods and for several months they are intense; then they disappear, only to reappear after some time.

Certain subjects show signs of psychomotor agitation such as garrulousness, logorrhea, and even coprolalia. They display at the same time a lack of psychic stability and tendencies to repeated fugues and to kleptomania.

This curious mixture of motor and neurovegetative disturbances and psychic disorders may either coincide with or appear at different phases of the postencephalitic period. The evolution is variable. Complete cure without after-effects is possible. The continuation of psychic and behavior disorders is equally possible and may be followed by a tendency to delinquency: kleptomania, violence, and even criminal assault devoid of all logical motivation.

During the 1917-1926 epidemic, the most varied clinical forms of the disease were observed concurrently, as well as the different types of impairments in different age groups. This clinical polymorphism was not the least peculiar feature of this pandemic.

HICCUP

Another remarkable fact: observers had noted hiccup in the same areas, and were obviously led to connect it with the myoclonic forms of encephalitis. Patients who first had a localized, light rhinopharyngeal infection had, after 24 to 48 hours, uncontrollable and incessant bouts of hiccup which never stopped in their waking state and hindered their falling asleep. Hiccup ceased completely during sleep, and started again with awakening. There was no other significant symptom except a little fever and weariness and also a saburral condition of the digestive tract, nervous irritation, and anxiety. Hiccup definitively disappeared after two or three days, most often after a phase of sleep. Epidemic hiccup was almost always perfectly harmless, but a few cases were complicated by lethargic encephalitis but never, it seems, by parkinsonism.

The etiological identity between epidemic encephalitis and epidemic hiccup rests on the epidemic coincidence and the symptomatological association (hiccup in lethargic encephalitis and, inversely, disturbances reminiscent of lethargic encephalitis in certain cases of epidemic hiccup). From the history of medicine we learn that epidemics of hiccup were observed in the past and taken for hysterical manifestations. The nature of epidemic hiccup is hence not completely elucidated.

PROGNOSIS

The prognosis of lethargic encephalitis, seen in the absolute, is rather severe. The general mortality due to this disease has been assessed at anywhere from 30 to 60 per cent. It is likely, however, that these figures are exaggerated because many mild cases and ambulatory forms were not recognized. It is difficult to assess the frequency of serious after-effects. This has been held to be 50 to 80 per cent. These figures are undoubtedly too high, again because of the frequency of mild forms during an epidemic when many cases were not identified.

It should be noted that in spite of an abundant symptomatology, alarming nervous disturbances, and a gravely impaired general condition, cure is possible—all prognoses notwithstanding—perhaps even complete and definitive cure.

DIAGNOSIS

Even in periods of epidemic the diagnosis of von Economo's encephalitis met with serious difficulties: tuberculous meningitis, which was frequent at the time of the epidemic, cerebral tumors, cerebral circulatory disturbances, typhoid fever, somnolent forms of poliomyelitis, various symptoms of neurosis and psychosis, different choreas and, displays of pithiatism are often quite difficult to distinguish from von Economo's encephalitis. Mild forms were all the more easily mistaken for "flu" because an influenza epidemic coincided with that of lethargic encephalitis. Today, it is differential diagnosis between different forms of virus encephalitis that raises serious problems. Attention should be called to the possibility of sporadic cases or small groups of cases, and all epidemiological notions and all knowledge of clinical differences will have to be brought to bear to direct the diagnosis. Laboratory tests—all negative so far—will help to make it accurate.

TREATMENT

Use of serum of persons convalescing from encephalitis was recommended during the acute stage of the disease, as were therapeutic shocks and fixation abscesses. All these methods are useless. Only sedatives when needed and nutritional support are necessary. Maintenance of a sound condition of the skin and the mucous membranes and of hydration is also important. Physiotherapy and psychotherapy may be necessary to alleviate the different motor and psychic after-effects. The administration of drugs useful against parkinsonism, such as atropine, Artane (trihexyphenidyl), and Isomadrin (1 - phenyl - 1 - cyclohexyl - 3 - pyrrolidino - 1-propanol chlorhydrate), may also be indicated.

PATHOLOGICAL ANATOMY
(by E. FARKAS)

All lesions inflicted by lethargic encephalitis as described by von Economo (1929) and by Marie and Tretiakoff have the anatomical characteristics of virus encephalitides (cf. Chapter 6: General Anatomical Considerations). Indeed, neuropathological examination reveals (1) the presence of inflammatory mesodermic infiltrates which are at once perivascular and diffuse, accompanied by an often nodular glial proliferation; (2) primary parenchymatous changes, often without relation to the localization of inflammatory phenomena; these changes consist of neuronic degeneration of variable severity, which may go as far as the death of the neuron and the formation of neuronophagic nodules; and (3) a specific topography of lesions within the cerebrospinal axis.

The distribution of lesions caused by von Economo's encephalitis is indeed pathognomonic; it involves almost exclusively the gray matter. Its intensity is at its maximum at the dorsal part of the mesencephalon and predominates at the level of substantia nigra (Tretiakoff), in the periaqueductal region, and the nuclei of the third pair of cranial nerves. From the mesencephalic region the lesions spread upward with diminishing intensity toward the hypothalamus, the walls of the third ventricle, the median nuclei of the thalamus and the pulvinar, the massa intermedia, and the lower parts of the globus pallidus.

They also extend below the mesencephalic region and involve the dorsal part of the brain stem, the floor of the fourth ventricle, the locus ceruleus, and certain nuclei of the cranial pairs in this region, especially those of the eighth and tenth pairs. The dentate and the fastigial nuclei of the cerebellum may also be affected, as well as the anterior horn of the spinal cord.

The inflammatory meningeal lesions are in general very discrete and the intensity of parenchymatous changes leads only quite exceptionally to complete necrotic lesions with a massive formation of granular bodies. Certain typical cases acquire a pronounced hemorrhagic form.

In verified cases of postencephalitic Parkinson's disease, the lesions observed represent the after-effects of changes during the acute phase. They are characterized by neuronic rarefaction which is especially noticeable in the substantia nigra and to a lesser extent in the hypothalamic region, in the pallidum, and exceptionally, at the level of the anterior horn of the spinal cord. This neuronic rarefaction is accompanied by astrocytic gliosis and fibrillary degeneration of certain neurons, not unlike that observed in Alzheimer's disease.

CONCLUSION

Von Economo's lethargic encephalitis or A encephalitis is a morbid entity with characteristic symptomatology and pathological anatomy. It spread as a pandemic for less than ten years and then disappeared almost completely. Certain isolated cases or small groups of cases—up to 60 or 70—are still described now and then, particularly in the United Kingdom (Leigh in 1946, Bickerstaff and Cloake in 1951, Barret, Gardner, and McFarlan in 1952, Brewis and Neubauer in 1948 and 1954; cited by Espir[4]). Espir and Spalding[4] described three cases among British soldiers stationed in West Germany, where no other cases seem to have occurred. Rudaja observed 43 patients at the Medical Institute of Vinitsa whom he believed to have been affected by this disease. There is therefore every reason to keep this disease in mind even today and to be able to diagnose it on the basis of its characteristic symptomatology.

The history of this curious disease would be incomplete if we did not recall that it has played a role—often a revolutionary one—in medical thinking. For the first time, except for rabies, the medical world observed the occurrence, most probably under the influence of a virus, of motor, intellectual, and psychic disturbances corresponding to well-defined lesions of the cerebral nervous system. The peculiar nature and the variability of symptoms were remarkable, extending from lethargy to hiccup, from manic outbreaks to Parkinson's syndrome, from oculogyric fits to juvenile delinquency. It is undoubtedly the behavior disturbances which struck physicians most, when they observed fugues, illegal acts, and psychic changes of neurotic, psychotic, and hysterical types as a sequel of an encephalitis epidemic. Postencephalitic parkinsonism, which is so remarkable in relatively young subjects, posed the possibility of the viral origin of all Parkinsonian syndromes, including the so-called idiopathic Parkinson's disease. The assertion that contamination occurred through the saliva of parkinsonian patients raised the problem of the prolonged persistence of the infecting virus and its role during the evolution of the alleged after-effects, which rather implies a chronic viral infection of the brain, remaining latent for a lengthy period.

It is not unlikely that all these sometimes forgotten lessons will be remembered one day.

BIBLIOGRAPHY

1. Blattner, R. J.: Encephalitis lethargica, type A encephalitis, Von Economo's disease (comments on current literature). J. Pediat., *49*:370-372, 1956.
2. Duvoisin, R. C., and Yahr, M. D.: Encephalitis and parkinsonism. Arch. Neurol., *12*:239, 1965.
3. Eadie, M. J., Sutherland, J. M., and Doherty, R. L.: Encephalitis in etiology of parkinsonism in Australia. Arch. Neurol., *12*:240-245, 1965.
4. Espir, M. L. E., and Spalding, J. M. K.: Three recent cases of encephalitis lethargica. Brit. Med. J., *1*: 1142-1144, 1956.
5. Marie, P., and Tretiakoff, C.: Anatomie pathologique de l'encéphalite léthargique. Ann. Med., *7*:1, 1920.
6. Rudaja, B. I.: Le tableau clinique de la forme léthargique de l'encéphalite épidémique actuelle. 2nd Nevropat. Psikhiat. Korsakov, *64*:334-339, 1964.
7. Thieffry, S.: Les manifestations extrapyramidales de la maladie de Heine-Medin. Journees. Pédiat., pp. 115-124, 1961.
8. Trétiakoff, C.: Contribution à l'étude de l'anatomie pathologique du locus niger avec quelques déductions relatives à pathogénie des troubles du tonus musculaire et de la maladie de Parkinson. Thèse de Paris, 1919.
9. Warembourg, H.: Syndrôme parkinsonien. Séquelle d'une poliomyélite aiguë à forme d'encéphalite léthargique chez un enfant de 20 mois. Sem. Hop., *38*:2299-2307, 1962.

13

Encephalitides and Encephalopathies of Probable Viral Origin

By E. FARKAS AND S. THIEFFRY

The viral etiology of a number of disorders of the central nervous system, although suspected, has not yet been demonstrated convincingly.

There are, in fact, many arguments in favor of a viral origin in subacute sclerosing leukoencephalitis (also known as subacute inclusion body encephalitis), in temporobasal necrotizing encephalitis, and in multifocal leukoencephalopathy.

These arguments are: (1) the frequent presence, in these cases, of intranuclear inclusion bodies in the nervous system; (2) the discovery, through the electron microscope, of structures reminiscent of viral particles in glial cells; and, finally, (3) the recovery, albeit inconstantly, of viruses from the brains of patients suffering from acute temporobasal necrotizing encephalitis.

The force of these arguments made it seem useful to us to mention these conditions briefly in the chapter devoted to viruses in which neurological manifestations predominate.

SUBACUTE INCLUSION BODY ENCEPHALITIS OF DAWSON[3, 4] OR SUBACUTE SCLEROSING LEUKOENCEPHALOPATHY OF VAN BOGAERT[8] (See also Chapter 19)

Clinical Picture

The clinical characteristics and the course of the disease in subacute sclerosing leukoencephalopathy are often sufficiently clear for a diagnosis to be made during the lifetime of the patient.

The onset is sometimes acute but more often subacute. The first manifestations, related to deficiencies in perception as yet barely obvious, are psychological in nature and suggest pyschiatric disturbances (unexplained deterioration in work and in scholastic achievement, disturbances in conduct and behavior).

Differing and variable signs in the pyramidal and extrapyramidal tracts may be discovered on clinical examination, but the sign that is most typical of the disease consists of rhythmic involuntary movements of spontaneous onset, limited in each patient to certain parts of the body (limbs, eyes, trunk) and sometimes following each other in stereotyped waves with a fairly constant rhythm. The moment in the course of the disease when they appear varies greatly, but that case in which they never appear is exceptional. If they occur very early in the disease, they may immediately lead to diagnosis.

The electroencephalogram may indicate, besides nonspecific changes, an item of great value in reaching a diagnosis: the appearance of periodic complexes consisting of slow waves of large amplitude which occur in groups and recur with a constant form. These complexes sometimes synchronize perfectly with the involuntary movements observed clinically.

The changes in the cerebrospinal fluid are typical of the disease: an initial increase in cells and a lasting increase in albumin.

The irrevocable course of the disease, which remains uninfluenced by any treatment at present in use, is toward progressive psychological and motor deterioration and unconsciousness in a complex neurological picture finally ending in cachexia. The disease lasts, on an average, from six to 18 months; some forms, apparently arrested, may last for some years, with the patient in a marasmic state.

PATHOLOGICAL ANATOMY

From the histological point of view, the lesions are those of a subacute encephalitis with perivascular lymphoplasmocytic infiltration and with microglial and macroglial proliferation involving both the white and the gray substance. The parenchymatous lesions have a similar panencephalic distribution.

At the Level of the White Matter. At this level, the lesions consist of a demyelination of the usual type of varying degree, with sudanophilic products of breakdown. Fibrillary gliosis is often out of proportion to the severity of the demyelination. The demyelinating process involves almost exclusively the white matter in the cerebral and cerebellar hemispheres.

At the Level of the Gray Matter. At the level of the gray matter there is neuronal degeneration with occasional diffuse necrotic areas. The severity of degeneration varies with the individual case and, in general, is related to the degree of inflammatory infiltration. Neuronal lesions may dominate the neuropathological picture, lesions in the white matter then appearing minor, as in the cases described by Dawson,[3, 4] Brain,[2] Greenfield and Russell, and others. Conversely, neuronal lesions may be very patchy in the cortex, their presence being demonstrated by a few neuronophagic nodules; the lesions in the white matter then predominate. These cases then appear as genuine leukoencephalitides, which explains the terminology used by van Bogaert (1945).[8] Proliferation of microglia in short rods is almost always observed in the cortex, even in the absence of any neuronal change.

Lesions in the gray matter are mainly found in the cortex of the cerebral hemisphere,

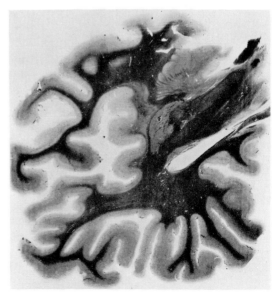

Figure 13-1. Subacute inclusion body encephalitis, Close-up view of cerebral hemisphere, showing widespread disappearance of myelin. Loyez' stain × 1.6.

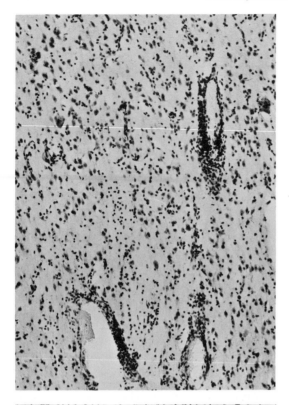

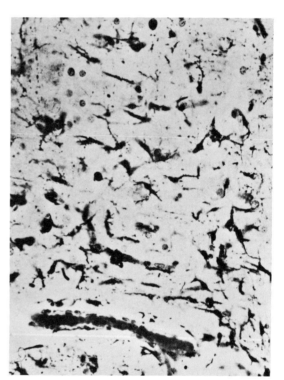

Figure 13-2. Subacute inclusion body encephalitis. Photomicrograph of thalamus, showing perivascular inflammatory changes. Nissl's stain × 140.

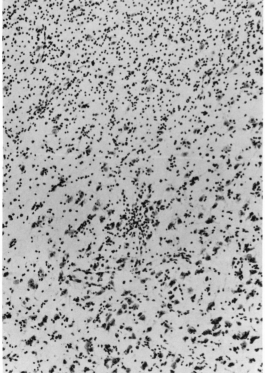

Figure 13-3. Subacute inclusion body encephalitis. Silver impregnation for microglia. Photomicrograph of cortex showing diffuse microglial proliferation.

Figure 13-4. Subacute inclusion body encephalitis. Photomicrograph of cortex and underlying white matter, showing nodular glial proliferation in the cortex with widespread glial proliferation in the underlying white matter. Nissl's stain × 140.

the thalamus, and the base of the ventral part of the brain stem, showing there a predilection for the nuclei of the pons. Conversely, the dorsal part of the brain stem, the cerebellar cortex, the hypothalamus, the subthalamic area, and the lenticular formations are most frequently spared.

Inclusion Bodies. In a great number of cases in which the course of the disease has not been too long, acidophilic inclusion bodies of type A have been observed. The short-lived appearance of these inclusion bodies was established by the observations of Bouteille et al.,[1] who saw these cellular formations disappear over a period of a month and a half, during the course of repeated cerebral biopsies; this was confirmed by the complete absence of inclusion bodies at postmortem examination. These inclusions take up part or the whole of the nucleus and may be homogeneous or granular. They are often surrounded by a clear halo and by a corona of chromatin which has been pushed out, with the nucleolus, to the periphery of the nucleus. They are found either in the nuclei of more or less damaged neurons in the gray

matter, or in the nuclei of the oligoglial cells in the white matter.

Observations made by electron microscopy have shown structures which look like the particles seen in tissue cultures infected with measles virus or in the course of development of polyoma virus[1] or else particles of 500 to 800 Å in diameter in astrocytes or in neurons which stain with osmium tetroxide and which appear to be genuine virus particles.[5, 6, 7]

Still more recently, it has been shown that the particles thus revealed could be colored by antimeasles antibodies marked with fluorescein. Hence it would seem most likely that a myxovirus immunologically related to measles virus is involved (see Chapter 19 and Measles: Virological Study and Prophylaxis in Chapter 27).

ACUTE NECROTIZING ENCEPHALITIS

This condition was defined by van Bogaert et al. in 1955.[14]

CLINICAL PICTURE

Although clinical observations of acute necrotizing encephalitis suggest a common etiology, it is not sufficiently characteristic for the disease to be identified. The speed of development (death in one or two weeks) scarcely allows one to undertake specific investigations to eliminate more common diseases (abscess, tumors, vascular accidents) with closely similar symptoms and signs. In all cases, after an initial febrile episode, often called "influenza," the following picture appears: severe disturbances in consciousness, psychiatric upsets, neurological signs of localization to one hemisphere (hemiplegia, aphasia), abnormal movements, and temporal epilepsy; meningism is frequent, and a meningeal reaction in the cerebrospinal fluid (cells and protein) is a constant.

The electroencephalogram is almost invariably altered, but in a nonspecific fashion.

PATHOLOGICAL ANATOMY

The anatomical diagnosis can be made by a gross examination of the brain, as the cortex has a softened consistency which may be moved over the deeper formations, which

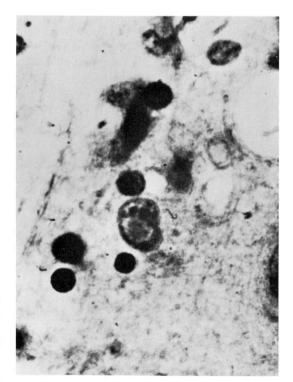

Figure 13-5. Subacute inclusion body encephalitis. Photomicrograph of pontine nucleus, showing intranuclear inclusion body of Cowdry's type A in a neuron. Hematoxylin and eosin.

have a firmer consistency. In most cases, this softening is found mainly in the temporobasal areas.

From a histological point of view, we find a meningoencephalitis characterized by intense inflammatory changes, perivascular as well as diffuse, associated with glial proliferation and massive necrosis of the cortical parenchyma; this necrosis can lead to true cavitation. These lesions are found mainly in the cortex of the hemispheres and are most marked in the temporal, orbital, insular, and rhinencephalic structures. These inflammatory phenomena also involve the white matter, especially in the areas underlying cortical lesions. Massive edema and hemorrhages frequently accompany the inflammatory and necrotic changes. They may spread into the white substance, producing spongiosis and considerable demyelinization.

These lesions are often asymmetrical, sometimes exclusively unilateral, with displacement of the median line and temporal herniation on the side of the lesions.

The resemblance of these histopathological findings and their distribution to those observed in herpes simplex encephalitis is reinforced by the presence of type A inclusions in 46 out of 59 cases of acute necrotizing encephalitis described by Bennett and his colleagues.[9]

In these 59 characteristic cases, herpes virus was looked for on 20 occasions and was demonstrated in the central nervous system in 13. It is therefore certain that at least some of the acute necrotizing encephalitides are due to herpes virus. Furthermore, Périer and Vanderhaeghen[12] have shown, under the electron microscope, structures in the intranuclear inclusions which resemble those observed by Morgan et al.[11] in cell culture infections with herpes virus.

However, encephalitides of this type have been described in which, in spite of a careful examination, herpes virus was not demonstrable in the nervous tissues. Furthermore, authentic cases of acute necrotizing encephalitis may be associated with the syndrome of Harada (Pingault[13]), with cases of hepatitis which were certainly not herpetic in origin (unpublished observations), and with lymphocytic choriomeningitis.

We may therefore support the viewpoint of van Bogaert,[14] according to whom the anatomical lesions of acute necrotizing encephalitis are not invariably associated with herpes virus infection. These encephalitides correspond to an anatomical type which is very characteristic, but probably not arising from a single etiology.

MULTIFOCAL PROGRESSIVE LEUKOENCEPHALOPATHY

This disease was first described by Aström et al. in 1958.[15] It is found in patients suffering from carcinomatosis, lymphosarcoma, generalized reticuloses, or lymphatic or myeloid leukemias, or in patients whose general state of health is very poor. Sometimes the neurological symptoms precede any other pathological changes.

CLINICAL PICTURE

The diagnosis of this disease may be considered when a picture of encephalopathy with a subacute course develops rapidly in a patient suffering from one of the neoplastic diseases mentioned above.

This encephalopathy includes disturbances of alertness and of consciousness,

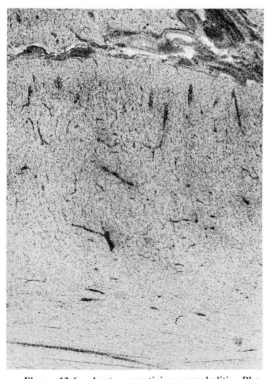

Figure 13-6. Acute necrotizing encephalitis. Photomicrograph of cerebral cortex, showing neuronal rarefaction, massive inflammatory changes, perivascular and diffuse, mainly in the cortex, and "perivascularites," more discrete in the deep white matter. There are inflammatory infiltrates in the arachnoid and pia mater. Nissl's stain × 32.

intellectual deterioration, paralysis, and bilateral abnormal movements, variable and asymmetrical. Signs which bring to mind a peripheral paralysis are encountered. Generally this picture steadily deteriorates until death occurs on an average, six months after the first clinical signs.

One observation (Tessa Heldley-White and colleagues) describes remission and even regressions in the course of the disease in one patient who survived for five years.

PATHOLOGICAL ANATOMY

Anatomical examination shows areas of demyelination in the white matter of the cerebral hemispheres and, rarely, in that of the brain stem and the cerebellum. These areas are of variable size, sometimes confluent, and at different stages of disintegration.

Demyelination is of a sudanophilic type, and numerous granular bodies packed with lipids (Scharlack positive) are scattered throughout the areas where the myelin sheaths have disappeared. The axons are relatively spared, inflammatory phenomena being practically always absent. In the demyelinated areas there are hypertrophic nuclei, very basophilic, which seem to belong to oligodendroglia. In these areas, the astrocytes are similarly hypertrophied, with multiple and misshapen nuclei. These abnormal glial cells contain acidophilic or amphophilic intranuclear inclusions of type A. Zu Rhein and Chou[17] and Silverman and Rubenstein[16], who studied these inclusions under the electron microscope, showed virus particles similar in morphology to the viruses of the papova group.

If the hypothesis of the viral origin of this disease were confirmed, it would be established that, on the one hand, viruses which are usually nonpathogenic for nervous tissues may become so in patients who have lost their immunological capacity and, on the other, that infectious diseases due to the effect of a virus on the brain do not necessarily include the presence of inflammatory phenomena.

BIBLIOGRAPHY

SUBACUTE INCLUSION BODY ENCEPHALITIS OF DAWSON

1. Bouteille, M., Fontaine, C., Vedrenne, C., and Delarue, J.: Sur un cas d'encéphalite subaigue à inclusions. Etude anatomique et ultrastructurale. Rev. Neurol., *4*:454, 1965.
2. Brain, R. W., Greenfield, J. G., and Russel, D.: Subacute inclusion encephalitis. Brain, *71*:365, 1948.
3. Dawson, J. R.: Cellular inclusions in cerebral lesions of lethargic encephalitis. Amer. J. Path., *9*: 7, 1933.
4. Dawson, J. R.: Cellular inclusions in cerebral lesions of epidemic encephalitis. Arch. Neurol. Psychiat., *31*:685, 1934.
5. Gonatas, N. K.: Subacute sclerosing leucoencephalitis: Electron microscopic and cytochemical observations in a cerebral biopsy. J. Neuropath. Exp. Neurol., *25*:177, 1966.
6. Périer, O., and Vanderhaeghen, J. J.: Indications étiologiques apportées par la microscopie électronique dans certaines encéphalites humaines. Rev. Neurol., *115*:250, 1966.
7. Tellez-Nagel, I., and Harter, D. H.: Subacute sclerosing of leucoencephalitis. J. Neuropath. Exp. Neurol., *25*:560, 1966.
8. van Bogaert, L.: Une leucoencéphalite sclérosante subaiguë. J. Neurol. Neurosurg. Psychiat., *8*: 101, 1945.

ACUTE NECROTIZING ENCEPHALITIS

9. Bennett, D. R., Zu Rhein, G. M., and Roberts, T. S.: Acute necrotizing encephalitis. Arch. Neurol. *6*:26, 1962.
10. Flament-Durand, J., Capon, A., and Coërs, C.: Etude anatomoclinique de 5 cas d'encéphalite nécrosante aiguë. Rev. Neurol., *113*:503, 1965.
11. Morgan, C., Rose, H. M., Holden, M., and Jones, E. P.: Electron microscopic observations on the development of herpes simplex virus. J. Exp. Med., *110*:643, 1959.
12. Périer, O., and Vanderhaeghen, J. J.: Leucoencéphalite sclérosante subaiguë à inclusions. Rev. Neurol., *115*:252, 1966.
13. Pingault, C.: Contribution à l'étude de la maladie de Harada. Thèse de Lyon, 1963.
14. van Bogaert, L., Radermecker, J., and Devos, J.: Sur une observation mortelle d'encéphalite aiguë nécrosante. Rev. Neurol., *92*:329, 1955.

MULTIFOCAL PROGRESSIVE LEUKOENCEPHALOPATHY

15. Aström, K. E., Mancall, E. L., and Richardson, E. P.: Progressive multifocal leukoencephalopathy. Brain, *81*:93, 1958.
16. Silverman, L., and Rubinstein, L. J.: Electron microscopic observations on a case of progressive multifocal leukoencephalopathy. Acta Neuropath., *5*:215, 1965.
17. Zu Rhein, G. M., and Chou, S. M.: Particles resembling papova viruses in human cerebral demyelinating disease. Science, *148*:1477, 1965.

14

The Common Viral, So-Called Aseptic Meningitides

By S. THIEFFRY

From long association, clinicians have become familiar with an acute infectious syndrome encountered predominantly in infants and which includes fever, headache, clinical signs of meningitis (especially neck stiffness), and an increased number of cells, mainly lymphocytes, in the cerebrospinal fluid; this syndrome tends to regress spontaneously and result in a complete cure.

A variety of labels, each of which emphasizes one or another of these characteristics, has been proposed for this disease: serous meningitis, acute aseptic meningitis, abacterial meningitis, benign lymphocytic meningitis, and idiopathic meningitis with a clear cerebrospinal fluid.

Much, if not all, of the history and study of these meningitides has been written in the margin of that of tuberculous meningitis, from which the differential diagnosis is of great importance.

The revolution brought by chemotherapy and antibiotics to tuberculosis has drastically altered the attitude of the physician confronted by a case of meningitis with a clear cerebrospinal fluid. Formerly, the most frequent etiology was tubercular, and other, nontuberculous, diagnoses were the exception. Today the disappearance, for all practical purposes, of tuberculous meningitis brings the abacterial meningitides into the first rank of importance—at the risk, we must stress, of forgetting a possible tuberculous etiology.

The fact must be recalled clearly that all meningitides with clear cerebrospinal fluids must, in every circumstance, be studied by all possible methods, with all the resources of clinician and laboratory, in order to exclude tuberculosis. We must also recall the number of occasions when Koch's bacillus and a virus occur together in the same patient.

In any case, this group of meningitides with a clear cerebrospinal fluid, which clinically present a well-defined individuality, very rapidly show that they have a diverse etiology. A list of the responsible pathogenic agents tends to become extremely lengthy. In particular cases, a definite etiology may be suspected or confirmed at the bedside. More frequently, the etiology may be found only by examination in a specialized laboratory. Even in these conditions, extensive hospital statistics derived from accurate sources show that, up to recent years, half of these meningitides remained undiagnosed.

But without any doubt, in the course of the past 20 years, with the arrival and practice of clinical virology, the notion of a viral origin of the acute "cryptogenic" aseptic meningitides with clear cerebrospinal fluids has been increasingly investigated and increasingly often confirmed. This rule is verified little by little as new procedures of culture or identification have become available to the clinician, and it is probable that, with further progress, the proportion of undiagnosed cases will steadily diminish.

In spite of some variations or anomalies, clinical observations are very uniform and agree without ambiguity in describing the usual picture of viral meningitis. Whether it is epidemic or sporadic, the disease begins either abruptly with headache, fever, vomiting, and signs of meningitis, or more gradually with only general symptoms in the early stages (slight fever, anorexia, malaise, sore throat) and, after a more or less complete remission for a few days, clear meningeal symptoms with a frank rise in temperature, which may often reach 102 to 105° F. Meningeal signs are more or less intense and include headache, changes in consciousness and in state of awareness, and sometimes spontaneous stiffness of the neck and the trunk. Signs of meningism may be observed with more or less ease or clarity (Kernig's sign, Brudzinski's sign, and especially neck stiffness). Convulsions are exceptional, and significant or long-lasting signs of nervous system lesions are not found. In this context, it should be borne in mind that the often applied designation of meningoencephalitis is not exact for nothing in the course of the illness, nor any anatomical argument confirms the hypothesis of damage to the cerebral parenchyma. Any electroencephalographic changes which may be demonstrable are associated with meningitis and disappear upon recovery. Throughout the acute phase, the fever may assume a diphasic or triphasic curve.

This general picture may vary in its intensity and its duration, as is verifiable during epidemics. Thus, in the Iowa epidemic, during which 329 cases were notified, the illness lasted from three days to three weeks, and temperatures varied from 97.9° F. to 104.3° F. It is during the course of the period of definite meningitis that we have the best chance of making those observations eminently valuable for the clinical diagnosis: e.g., exanthem or enanthem and muscular pains.

In spite of the apparent gravity in some cases, in which disturbances of consciousness deepen as far as coma, the course of the disease is favorable. The syndrome dissociates and disappears in a few days or sometimes a few weeks. In some cases slight headache, irritability, and asthenia may persist but finally go away. A relapse is possible but, in the end, recovery takes place without any sequelae.

Changes in the cerebrospinal fluid occur immediately and at the same time as the onset of the clinical syndrome of meningitis. The usual pattern is a lymphocytic pleocytosis, with cell counts ranging from a few cells to 500 to 1000 cells per cubic millimeter or more; on the other hand, the level of albumin is moderately increased (0.30 to 0.60) and that of sugar normal or slightly subnormal.

These biochemical characteristics are valuable in the differential diagnosis from tuberculous meningitis, in which, in particular, the level of sugar falls quickly. We may note also that, in benign lymphocytic meningitis, the cellular reaction reaches its height immediately and thereafter tends to decrease in a regular fashion, while more frequently the lymphocytosis in tuberculous meningitis is variable and may increase. Another peculiarity must be mentioned, which may prove a source of error with microbial meningitides. Fairly frequently, if the lumbar puncture has been performed in the first hours of illness, the increase in cell count is found to be exclusively in the polymorphonuclear leukocyte element and the abundance of cells gives a cloudy appearance to the cerebrospinal fluid. An aspectic, purulent-looking meningitis with unaltered polymorphonuclears is observed. This pattern rapidly disappears, but up to the fifth day remains mixed; lymphocytes quickly replace the polymorphonuclear cells. In this context, we must recall the problem of the "decapitated" pyogenic meningitides already treated with antibiotics before the first lumbar puncture. In fact, differentiation in these cases is made easier by the observation that the polymorphonuclear leukocytes which one sees are modified, unlike those found in aseptic meningitis, and that there is generally a significant increase in the albumin content of the cerebrospinal fluid.

The general picture of the acute abacterial meningitides with clear cerebrospinal fluid shows little characteristic change and does not indicate, per se, any precise etiological designation. When one meets a sporadic case, without any other hint as to diagnosis, its precise etiology will be determined only through laboratory work. As against this, in the context of a large epidemic or even of one of average size or small scale, the discovery, perhaps in contacts, perhaps in the patient himself, of other symptoms may assume from the onset a considerable value in leading to the diagnosis. As often happens in epidemiology, the collection of a group of symptoms or signs in different patients from the same community takes on a quite definite value. It is with this in mind that we will review some of the surrounding circumstances where a precise etiology may be suggested, accepted, or confirmed in accord with the clinical facts alone.

MUMPS

As we know, clinically latent meningeal reaction in this disease is almost constant.

Frank meningitis may appear before, during or after the parotitis and may also form the only apparent clinical manifestation of the disease. It is often found in a familial environment or in schools or in the armed forces. Some peculiarities should be remembered: the intensity of headache and vomiting, the bradycardia, the very considerable increase in cerebrospinal fluid pressure, and, above all, the significant pleocytosis, with several hundreds (even thousands) of lymphocytic cells. These cells disappear very slowly, and a complete return to normal often takes six weeks; occasionally symptoms recur during this period. Mumps meningitis is one of the longest in duration, is often the most violent, and is one of the rare diseases which, even in its uncomplicated form, may bring in its wake a grave, early, and irrevocable complication: deafness (see Chapter 57).

We must remember that a well-defined picture of encephalitis in the course of mumps has been described on very rare occasions. These crises seem to be related either to a perivenous leukoencephalitis or sometimes to a meningoencephalitis. It seems likely that many of the cases reported under these designations ought, in fact, to be reallocated among the encephalopathies (see Chapters 6 and 7).

POLIOMYELITIS

This is one of the well-known causes of benign meningitis. All recent statistics indicate that the frequency varies according to the epidemic, the season, and the orientation and degree of specialization of the laboratory pursuing the virological investigation. Indeed, we may pose the question of the actual frequency of pure poliomyelitic meningitis and ask whether it is not being overestimated. By careful clinical analysis, we may persuade ourselves that, very often, the symptomatology of these cases includes other features indicating damage to the nervous system itself (for example, very slight diminution in muscle strength, abolition or diminution of a reflex, retention of urine) and which may lead us to assign them rather to the class of nonparalytic or abortive poliomyelitis. This is only a nosological quibble which stresses the uniformity of the meningeal reaction in Heine-Medin's disease. Epidemiological ideas play a very important role in the etiological diagnosis, the cases of meningitis generally appearing at the same time and in the same population as the cases of confirmed paralysis.

OTHER ENTEROVIRUSES

Other enteroviruses may also be responsible for acute benign aseptic meningitis. In some clinical circumstances, the diagnosis may be put forward but cannot be confirmed until virological tests have been made. These are indispensable in sporadic cases.

THE ECHO VIRUSES

The ECHO viruses certainly form the most important group and the best defined (by a meningeal syndrome accompanied by a rash).

Many so-called summer epidemics of illnesses associating a rash with meningeal symptom have been reported. At least five types of virus have been held responsible (ECHO 9, 4, 16, 18, 2).

ECHO 9. ECHO 9 virus disease is, from this point of view, the most manifest. Its spread and extension are astonishing. The disease is benign. After an incubation period of three to five days, the onset is rapid or insidious with headache, vomiting, sore throat, muscle pains, and fever. This first "minor" phase may comprise the complete illness, but in 36 to 60 per cent of cases, after a period of apparent calm, a second phase arrives, uniformly febrile, in which meningeal signs and, frequently, abdominal pains are found. This period lasts for five to ten days. A rash breaks out at the onset or only during the second phase. The rash is seen more frequently when the subject is very young and may persist (an important observation) throughout the whole febrile period.

This rash is maculopapular and is composed of small lesions from 2 to 4 mm. in diameter, which are pale red, then a darker shade of red. It is found on the face, neck, thorax, trunk, and extremities. It does not result in desquamation and does not itch. Rarely, it is petechial and may then suggest meningococcemia. An enanthem, taking the form of very discrete lesions, from 1 to 2 mm. in diameter, grayish white in color, has been observed on the pillars of the tonsils and the buccal mucosa and sometimes on the tongue.

Even in cases in which clinical signs are

minimal, it is usual to find significant changes in the cerebrospinal fluid for eight to 12 days after the onset of the illness. The number of white cells varies from a minimum of 20 or 150 to 1500 and even 3000; in cases of high counts confusion may occur with purulent meningitis.

ECHO 4. Epidemics of ECHO 4 virus are much less frequent. Epidemics of meningitis have been described in the United States, South Africa, Australia, Sweden, and Switzerland. One of their particular features is the frequency of relapse at intervals of five to ten days. Most frequently, the signs are not sufficiently characteristic (e.g., cervical adenopathy, photophobia) to lead one to consider a specific viral disease. In the Australian epidemic, a fleeting rash was mentioned in only two cases out of 263. By contrast, in the Swedish epidemics, a rubella-like exanthem accompanied the meningitis in most cases.

Other ECHO Viruses. It goes without saying that, by themselves, the rashes which have been observed do not have sufficiently specific characteristics to be of any value in diagnosis, save in certain epidemiological situations. In sporadic cases, they may only urge one to seek a viral etiology, especially in the ECHO group. Thus we know of several cases of meningitis due to ECHO 2, 9, 14, and 18 which were accompanied by a rash. Conversely, ECHO 6 and ECHO 11, which have been responsible for major epidemics of lymphocytic meningitis in numerous parts of the world, have not up to now produced a rash. Likewise, in the sporadic cases attributed to ECHO 2, 3, 5, 7, 8, 12, 13, 14, 16, 18, 19, 21, 22, and 23, the disease consisted solely of an amicrobial acute meningitis, without any other element which could be used for diagnosis. Furthermore, in an important epidemic of so-called Boston exanthem due to ECHO 16 virus and marked by unusually coherent symptomatology there was no mention of meningitis. In contrast, this ECHO 16 has been isolated from patients with meningitis (wrongly diagnosed as nonparalytic poliomyelitis) but during this little epidemic no rash was observed.

From this very simplified outline, it is possible to extract one concept: a number of ECHO viruses present a significantly clear meningotropism.

THE COXSACKIE VIRUSES

Coxsackie B Viruses. In this group, from the point of view of the nonmicrobial acute meningitides caused by viruses, the most striking, originally, was Bornholm disease, still known as epidemic myalgia, "bamble disease," devil's grip, acute epidemic muscular rheumatism, intermittent diaphragmatic spasm, and pleurodynia; all these are names which highlight its major symptom. This disease occurs in large epidemics in which Coxsackie B1, 2, 3, 4, and 5 viruses are recognized as responsible. These epidemics occur in August or September, attacking individuals of every age, including young infants. One must, in view of the predominant sign — muscular pain — recall the suddenness of the onset and the habitual benign character of the disease, but one must also bear in mind the possibility of early or late relapse. To this very unusual picture is added a frank or subclinical early or late meningitis (five to nine days after the clinical onset). This disease is mentioned here because at times, particularly in infants, the meningitis is clinically isolated and may arise and evolve without pleurodynia, and may then form the whole illness. Thus, in the course of an epidemic in the United States, myalgia occurred in only 40 per cent of patients with meningitis.

Coxsackie A Viruses. The viruses of the Coxsackie A group may produce the same clinical picture. Types A7 and A9 are most frequently responsible for lymphocytic meningitis; more rarely mentioned are types A2, 3, 4, 5, 6, and 23.

OTHER VIRUSES

The role of other viruses in the etiology of isolated, benign, clinically primitive meningitis is inconspicuous. When they produce neurological accidents, these viruses seem to be responsible for meningoencephalitis or meningoradiculitis rather than a simple meningitis (herpes, respiratory viruses, hepatitis). Among hematological disorders, acute epidemic lymphocytosis (the disease described by Carl Smith) presents the possibility of meningeal forms.

15

Epidemiology of the ECHO Viruses

By V. DROUHET

The epidemiology of infections with ECHO viruses is, to a great extent, the epidemiology of "aseptic meningitis," of acute gastrointestinal syndromes (summer and infantile diarrhea), and of respiratory illnesses. There are also some rather limited observations which deal with paralytic disease. In general, we are concerned with isolated cases whose value lies in the fact that they draw attention to the problem of the pathogenic power of ECHO viruses.

We will describe here, after the general epidemiology of the ECHO viruses, the etiological role of some types in lymphocytic meningitis. Gastrointestinal syndromes are dealt with elsewhere (Part III), as are the respiratory syndromes (Part VI).

HISTORICAL ASPECTS

The ECHO viruses were discovered, by chance and thanks to tissue cultures, during the course of studies on poliomyelitis. In point of fact, they are not pathogenic for laboratory animals, they cannot be grown in fertile eggs, and it is only the cytopathic changes that they produce in tissue cultures that betray their presence. Owing to the fact that their relationship with human disease had not been established, these cytopathic agents, initially recovered from the human digestive tract and then "in search of an illness," were at first designated "orphan" viruses.

Then, in 1955, the term ECHO virus was introduced. This term represents four of the essential characters of these viruses (enteric-cytopathogenic-human-orphan); the National Foundation for Infantile Paralysis set up a committee for their study.[6]

From 1951 onward, such viruses were frequently isolated from infants who were apparently well, but they were also recovered from ill persons suffering from a diversity of diseases. Their numbers increased as virological investigations were made during the course of numerous sporadic and epidemic infections. The degree of their spread among man consequently became evident, together with their biological characteristics and their close relationship with Coxsackie and poliomyelitis viruses.

In 1957, all these viruses were grouped into the same family, that of the enteroviruses (see Chapter 3).

WORLD DISTRIBUTION

ECHO viruses, as well as the other enteroviruses, are frequently recovered from healthy carriers. Nevertheless, Sabin, in 1956, affirmed that ECHO viruses could not be considered part of the normal bacterial flora of the intestine. They reside in the alimentary tract only temporarily and are able to induce transitory infections, particularly in children.

The epidemiology of these viruses has

been clarified, thanks to the study of their clinical manifestations and to large-scale epidemiological investigations carried out in healthy subjects. A low proportion of infections is associated with illness. More frequently, ECHO viruses infect man subclinically and the encounter of a population with the virus is demonstrated by the acquisition of immunity.

Their great similarity to other enteroviruses is shown by the frequent coexistence of polioviruses, Coxsackie viruses, and ECHO viruses in the same population, sometimes in the same individual. Like the polioviruses, the ECHO viruses are probably ubiquitous. Virological and serological investigations of sufficiently wide scope have shown all, or almost all, types of ECHO viruses in healthy populations of the temperate zones. Nevertheless, epidemics also spread in equatorial and tropical zones. Even if these viruses are universally distributed, a regional pathology is found in which certain types are recovered more frequently than others. In addition, in the same region, some types appear one year, then disappear the following year; thus polioviruses, ECHO viruses, or Coxsackie viruses may follow each other. For example, in Minnesota, Coxsackie virus B5 was epidemic in 1956[29] and ECHO virus type 9 in 1957.[22]

SEASONAL DISTRIBUTION

Seasonal variations are due essentially to changes in the conditions of exposure to infection. The appearance of epidemics is, in all likelihood, explained by the presence in the population of a sufficient proportion of persons who are susceptible to infection. Annual variations may be explained, to some extent, by the state of immunity of the population.

The waves of virus spread rise to a peak during the summer and the autumn.

The longitudinal study of 136 healthy preschool children who were followed for 29 months in Charleston, West Virginia, showed that 90 per cent of enteroviruses were recovered during the summer and the autumn.[10] Of these, 44 per cent were ECHO viruses, 39 per cent were Coxsackie viruses, and 19 per cent were polioviruses.

In Phoenix, Arizona, and in Louisiana[8] the incidence of enteroviruses was more uniform among healthy children during the course of the year, but the incidence was always greatest from May to October.

Epidemics of ECHO viruses of types 4, 6, 9, 16, and 18 have been observed during the summer and autumn. However, some epidemics are prolonged later or begin in the autumn and end in the winter. As in the case of poliomyelitis, cases sometimes appear in November and December. An outbreak of ECHO 9 infection affecting seven or eight persons in the same family was reported in Nova Scotia during the months of February and March.[7]

SOCIAL ENVIRONMENT

Other factors being equal, the level of infection is higher in poorer populations and much lower among the rich. It was found that 8.3 per cent of the lower classes are virus carriers, whereas among the classes who benefit from better sanitary conditions, 3.1 per cent are carriers of enteroviruses.[10] During an epidemic of ECHO virus, type 4, 8 per cent of the patients were from residential areas and 28 per cent from semirural areas.[15]

Extensive and well-known studies carried out in several American towns[8, 16, 18] have shown a greater incidence of enterovirus infection (poliovirus, Coxsackie, ECHO) among the Negro than among the white population, and, in the latter, among the very poor.

AGE

The average age at which these infections occur is higher in the upper classes and the morbidity appears greater also. Children harbor viruses more readily than adults.

The incidence of ECHO viruses among healthy subjects in Cincinnati in 1953[23] was 5.2 per cent at one to four years, 2.6 per cent at five to nine years, and 0.2 per cent at 10 to 14 years.

More than 16 per cent of ECHO viruses isolated in Mexico during the months of May and June were from children aged one to four years.[24]

Winkelstein et al. in 1957[32] observed that 47 per cent of children were infected by ECHO 6 virus and 17 per cent of adults.

Goldenberg, in 1959, mentioned that 22 per cent of infections with ECHO 9 virus were in children and 11 per cent were in adults.

Studies of virus spread in nurseries emphasize the prolonged excretion of these viruses in the stools, the simultaneous presence of several types of virus, and the low morbidity rate.

Children provide the main source of infection in familial epidemics but, curiously enough, studies carried out in homes for the aged led to the conclusion that the wide spread of these viruses was due, essentially, to collective living.

In general, adults are resistant because of specific immunity induced by previous infection. The findings of Gelfand[9] illustrate this statement. In 1957, in Ohio, not a single ECHO virus was recovered from young men aged 20 to 30.

Different clinical manifestations do not all necessarily occur in the same age groups. Meningitis predominantly affects the child of four years of age and over.[32] This appears to indicate a susceptibility associated with age. Encephalitic and paralytic forms dominate in the adolescent and in the adult. Exanthemata, on the other hand, are more frequent in early childhood, and gastroenteritis occurs almost exclusively in the unweaned infant.

SEX

In epidemics of aseptic meningitis due to ECHO 6 virus, a higher percentage of male than female patients was observed (five males to one female);[11, 32] similarly, in epidemics due to ECHO 9 virus the ratio was two males to one female.[2, 4] These differences do not indicate a greater biological sensitivity in relation to race or sex. Rather, they represent differing exposures to infection due to those social, economic, and sanitary conditions which facilitate infections with ECHO viruses.

Epidemics of mixed etiology with simultaneous ECHO virus, poliovirus, and Coxsackie virus infections are often found. These are due to the identical epidemiological characteristics of this family of viruses. According to certain authors, ECHO and Coxsackie B virus infections influence the spread of poliovirus infections by a mechanism which, in principle, may be related to interference.

SOURCES OF INFECTION

The apparently exclusive source of infection is the person who excretes virus in his stools or in his oropharyngeal secretions. The pharynx is a poorer source of virus than the feces. The nasal secretions, the mouth, and the saliva are routes of secretion rarely mentioned. ECHO virus 9 was found in the saliva of two patients, mother and daughter, with parotitis. In neither case could infection with mumps virus be proved.

It should be mentioned that similar viruses have been found in the digestive tract of animals (fox, pig), and the presence of neutralizing antibodies has been shown in numerous mammals (cattle, goats, cats, wild rodents). It is difficult to state, however, whether cross-neutralization with animal enteroviruses was not involved. These animal viruses form the counterpart of human ECHO viruses, and it appears that host-specificity occurs.

THE VIRUS IN THE EXTERNAL ENVIRONMENT

The relative resistance of ECHO viruses in the external environment explains why they are found outside the digestive tract of man in those areas which may be contaminated by human excretions (stagnant water, contaminated fruit). Children's hands and the dusty living quarters of children who carry virus are, according to Gelfand, an important source of the virus.

Soiled food and water perhaps play a role in the propagation of the virus among populations with low sanitary standards. In this context, and as an indication of the amount of contamination in sewage water, especially during hot weater, by poliovirus, Coxsackie virus, and ECHO virus, the numerous studies made are extremely instructive.[1, 5, 12, 13, 14, 17, 20]

Natural infection of flies is found,[25] but it has not been demonstrated that this virus can spread and multiply in flies or cockroaches.

METHODS OF TRANSMISSION

The method of transmission of ECHO viruses is not at all clear. It is supposed that this is either direct by way of the respiratory or digestive system, or indirect, by way of the hands, fomites, and soiled foods which infect via the digestive system.

Although the ECHO viruses can cause viremia, great significance is not attached to their transmission by way of hematophagous insects, which has been suggested on the basis of some investigations.[28, 30]

The highly infectious characteristics of certain ECHO virus infections, the prolific spread of viruses in the same family or community or in a crowded urban district, plead in favor of a predominantly direct, man-to-man mode of transmission. The gastro-intestinal system is probably of prime importance in this, although we must not overlook the possibility of aerial diffusion. Children infect each other more easily than adults because of their more intimate relations with each other at play. When an excretor of the virus arrives in a family or in a community, all susceptible persons, children and adults, become infected rapidly, a fact in favor of airborne infection.

The virus is eliminated through the stools, mainly during the first two weeks of infection, but the proportion of virus recoveries decreases during the second week. Nevertheless, excretion may persist for one month or even longer, either continually or intermittently.

PATHOGENESIS

Once the virus has entered the body by way of the respiratory or digestive system, what are the reactions of the host?

Sometimes, very rarely, the virus passes through the intestine, leaving no apparent trace, either clinical or biological, and an ECHO virus is encountered by chance in the feces of an individual who has no antibodies and who does not acquire any antibodies subsequently.

Usually, however, virus infection is subclinical or shows itself through an apparent illness. Infection in both cases results in the development of antibodies.

The spread of ECHO viruses throughout the body appears to be similar to that of other enteroviruses. It takes place in several stages:

(1) In the first stage, the virus multiplies at the level of the pharyngeal mucosa, in the tonsils, in lymph nodes, in the intestine, and in Peyer's patches. During the first months of life, ECHO viruses may provoke gastro-intestinal disorders and diarrhea, as in the case of ECHO 14 and ECHO 18 viruses; following experimental infection, ECHO 11 virus has also been shown to produce similar disturbances in young adults (20 years old).

During the epidemic in Milwaukee, Sabin et al.[26] were able to make a careful study of the fecal excretion of ECHO 9 virus at different stages of the disease. The stools contain virus in greatest numbers before the onset of illness. During the first week, the titer is not greater than 10^2–10^3 TCD_{50} per gram of feces. The titer of fecal virus quickly falls toward the end of the second week, the number of positive stools decreasing from 86 per cent during the first week to 74 per cent during the second week, 37 per cent during the third week, and only 5 per cent toward the fourth week. During the fifth through seventh weeks, ECHO 9 virus is occasionally found in the stools in low titer. Sometimes, the concentration of ECHO 9 virus in the oropharynx is very high ($10^{5.3}$ TCD_{50}). Those patients who excrete virus from the throat during the acute phase do not have a positive nasal swab. A single ill person has yielded virus from a swab taken from the underside of the tongue, but in this case the throat swab contained a large quantity of virus.

(2) The second stage, which begins before the appearance of clinical signs and sometimes persists for several days after their appearance, is the stage of transitory viremia.

During the course of an epidemic due to ECHO 9 virus, Sabin et al.[27] showed that virus was present in the blood of a contact 36 hours before the onset of illness. In one subject out of six studied, viremia persisted 24 hours after the illness began. The concentration of ECHO 9 virus in the blood varies from 8 to 164 TCD_{50} per milliliter. ECHO 16 virus was recovered by Neva and Zuffante[19] two days after the onset of illness. Viremia is also observable in humans infected with ECHO 4 virus. ECHO 11 virus, and ECHO 18 virus and in chimpanzees infected by the oral route with ECHO 9 virus.[33]

(3) Finally, virus flowing through the blood may multiply in different organs. A fresh peak in the titer of virus in the blood precedes its attack on the meninges and on the nervous system. Nevertheless, it is not certain whether the migration of virus along the course of the nerves can be absolutely excluded. As a result of the viremia, tissues and organs are invaded which are far from the place of primary multiplication. There are numerous susceptible organs where virus may multiply and finally produce an inflammatory process.* Most frequently, it is the meninges

---

*In experimental infections of monkeys, it is found, for instance, in the liver, the spleen, the lymph nodes, the bone marrow, and the myocardium.

which are attacked. According to Verlinde et al.,[31] ECHO viruses and especially ECHO 9 virus are more frequently recovered in cases of "aseptic" meningitis than polioviruses or Coxsackie viruses. Virus titers reach $10^{3.8}$ TCD_{50}. ECHO viruses of types 2, 4, 5, 6, 9, 11, 14, 15, 16, 18, and 19 have been recovered from the cerebrospinal fluid, most frequently in the course of epidemics or in sporadic cases of lymphocytic meningitis. The recovery of virus from the blood and from the cerebrospinal fluid[3] demonstrates the etiological role of at least certain types of ECHO virus in clinical manfestations. The meninges and probably the cells of the central nervous system in certain individuals appear to be the places where secondary multiplication occurs. In the course of an epidemic of ECHO 9 virus infection, a fatal case in an infant was reported by Verlinde et al.[31] ECHO 9 virus was recovered from the spinal cord in a titer of 10^5 TDC_{50} per milliliter. Re-examining this case, Pette et al.[21] observed that ECHO 9 virus was associated with poliovirus type II. Nevertheless, the fact that ECHO 9 virus was found in the spinal cord of this infant in higher titer than the poliovirus II shows that ECHO 9 virus is capable of multiplying in the central nervous system of man. Studies carried out since that time, however, show that, in monkeys infected with ECHO 9 virus, a meningeal infiltration can be produced only when this virus is inoculated alone.

THE IMMUNOLOGICAL RESPONSE TO INFECTION

Following infection with ECHO viruses, neutralizing antibodies, which confer immunity, appear in the blood. Neutralizing antibodies of maternal origin are transmitted to the fetus in the same titer as in the mother or in a lower titer. This fact has been confirmed for ECHO viruses of types 1, 2, 8, 11, and 20. Some 90 per cent of subjects at birth are carriers of antibody to ECHO viruses; toward the fifth or sixth month of life these antibodies disappear. Immunity due to latent infection is produced in the same way as in the case of polioviruses in the general population. The incidence of neutralizing antibodies increases progressively in a manner which varies from one place to another according to the type of ECHO virus. The highest incidence is found during adolescence and some-

times even later. Most infants (under two years of age) examined by Gelfand[8] did not possess neutralizing antibodies against ECHO viruses of the types 6, 9, and 14, responsible for epidemics; from six to ten years of age, 65 per cent of children possessed neutralizing antibodies to ECHO viruses of types 6, 9, and 11.

Neutralizing antibodies present in human serum against ECHO 16 virus persist for six years following the end of infection, but during the first year their titer falls by twofold to fourfold. After infections of ECHO 11 virus, neutralizing antibodies disappear rapidly — by the end of three weeks in infants and by the end of seven weeks after experimental infection in adults.

BIBLIOGRAPHY

1. Albano, A., and Bonetti, F.: Isolamento del virus poliomielitico dai liquami di fogna di un centro urbano. Boll. Ist. Sieroterap. Milanese, *36*:468, 1957.
2. Archetti, I., Felici, A., Russi, F., and Fua, C.: Recherches sur la définition étiologique de la méningo névraxite des Marches à l'occasion de l' épidémie estivo-automnale de 1955. Scientia Med. Ital., *5*:317, 1956.
3. Arnold, J. H., and Enders, J. F.: Disease in macacus monkeys inoculated with ECHO viruses. Proc. Soc. Exp. Biol. Med., *101*:513-516, 1959.
4. Baumann, T., Barben, M., Marti, R., Hassler, A., and Krech, U.: Erkankungen durch ECHO-virus Typ 9. Eine epidemiologische, klinische und virologisch-serologische Studie. Schweiz. Med. Wschr., *87*:307, 1957.
5. Bloom, H. H., Mack, W. N., Krueger, B. J., and Mallmann, W. L.: Identification of enteroviruses in sewage. J. Infect. Dis., *105*:61, 1959.
6. Committee on ECHO Viruses: Enteric cytopathogenic human orphan (ECHO) viruses. Science, *122*:117-118, 1955.
7. Faulkner, E. S., MacLeod, A. J., and Van Rooyen, C. E.: Virus meningitis — seven cases in one family. Canad. M.A.J., *77*:439-444, 1957.
8. Gelfand, H. M.: The incidence of certain endemic enteric virus infections in southern Louisiana. Southern Med. J., *52*:819, 1959.
9. Gelfand, H. M.: The occurrence of Coxsackie and ECHO viruses. Progr. Med. Virol., *3*:193, 1961.
10. Honig, E. I., Melnick, J. L., Isacson, P., Parr, R., Myers, I. L., and Walton, M.: An endemiological study of enteric virus infections, poliomyelitis, Coxsackie and orphan (ECHO) viruses isolated from normal children in two socio-economic groups. J. Exp. Med., *103*:247, 1956.
11. Karzon, D. T., Barron, A. L., Winkelstein, W., Jr., and Cohn, S.: Isolation of ECHO virus type 6 during an outbreak of seasonal aseptic meningitis. J.A.M.A., *162*:1298, 1956.
12. Kelly, S.: Enteric virus isolation from sewage. Acta Med. Scand., *159*:63, 1957.

13. Kelly, S., Clark, M. E., and Coleman, M. B.: Demonstration of infectious agents in sewage. Amer. J. Public Health, *45*:1438, 1955.
14. Kelly, S., Winsser, J., and Winkelstein, W., Jr.: Poliomyelitis and other enteric viruses in sewage. Amer. J. Public Health, *47*:72, 1957.
15. Lehan, P. H., Chick, E. W., Doto, J. L., Chin, T. D. Y., Heeren, R. H., and Furculow, M. L.: An epidemic illness associated with a recently recognized enteric virus (ECHO virus type 4). I. Epidemiologic and clinical features. Amer. J. Hyg., *66*:63-75, 1957.
16. Melnick, J. L.: Tissue culture techniques and their application to original isolation, growth and assay of poliomyelitis and orphan viruses. Ann. N.Y. Acad. Sci., *61*:754-772, 1955.
17. Melnick, J. L., Emmons, J., Coffey, J. H., and Schoof, H.: Seasonal distribution of Coxsackie viruses in urban sewage and flies. Amer. J. Hyg., *59*:164-184, 1954.
18. Melnick, J. L., and Ledinko, N.: Social serology: antibody levels in a normal young population during epidemic of poliomyelitis. Amer. J. Hyg., *54*:354, 1951.
19. Neva, F. A., and Zuffante, S. M.: Agents isolated from Boston exanthem disease during 1954 in Pittsburgh. J. Lab. Clin. Med., *50*:712, 1957.
20. Pattyn, S. R., Delville, J. P., and Dresse, A.: Recherche de virus poliomyélitiques et Coxsackie dans les eaux d'égoûts à Elizabethville. Ann. Soc. Belg. Med. Trop., *37*:99, 1957.
21. Pette, H., Maass, G., Valenciano, L., and Mannweiler, K.: Zur Frage der Neuropathogenität von Enteroviren. Experimentelle Untersuchungen zur Neuropathogenität verschiedener Stämme von ECHO-9 Virus. Arch. Ges. Virusforsch., *10*:408, 1961.
22. Prince, J. T., St. Geme, J. W., Jr., and Scherer, W. F.: ECHO-9 virus exanthema. J.A.M.A., *167*:691-696, 1958.
23. Ramos-Alvarez, M., and Sabin, A. B.: Characteristics of poliomyelitis and other viruses recovered in tissue culture from healthy American children. Proc. Soc. Exp. Biol. Med., *87*:655-661, 1954.
24. Ramos-Alvarez, M., and Sabin, A. B.: Intestinal viral flora of healthy children demonstrable by monkey kidney tissue culture. Amer. J. Public Health, *46*:295-296, 1956.
25. Riordan, J. T., Paul, J. R., Yoshioka, I., and Horstmann, D. M.: The detection of poliovirus and other enteric viruses in flies. Results of tests carried out during an oral poliovirus vaccine field trial. Amer. J. Hyg., *74*:123, 1961.
26. Sabin, A. B., Krumbiegel, E. R., and Wigand, R.: ECHO 9 virus disease: Virologically controlled clinical and epidemiologic observations during 1957 epidemic in Milwaukee with notes on concurrent similar diseases associated with Coxsackie and other ECHO viruses. A.M.A. J. Dis. Child., *96*:197-219, 1958.
27. Sabin, A. B., Michaels, R. H., Spigland, I., Pelon, W., Rhim, J. S., and Wehr, R. E.: Community-wide use of oral poliovirus vaccine. Effectiveness of the Cincinnati program. A.M.A. J. Dis. Child., *101*: 546-567, 1961.
28. Schwab, M., Allen, R., and Sulkin, S. E.: The tropical rat mite (Liponyssus bacoti) as an experimental vector of Coxsackie virus. Amer. J. Trop. Med. Hyg., *1*:982, 1952.
29. Syverton, J. T., MacLean, D. M., Martins da Silva, M., Doany, H. B., Cooney, M., Kleinman, H., and Bauer, H.: Outbreak of aseptic meningitis caused by Coxsackie B5 virus; laboratory, clinical and epidemiologic study. J.A.M.A., *164*:2015, 1957.
30. Taylor, R. M., and Hurlbut, H. S.: The isolation of Coxsackie-like viruses from mosquitoes. J. Egypt. Med. Assoc., *36*:489, 1953.
31. Verlinde, J. D., Wilterdink, J. B., and Mouton, R. P.: Presence of two interfering enteroviral agents (ECHO virus type 9 and poliovirus type 2) in the human central nervous system. Arch. Ges. Virusforsch., *10*:399, 1961.
32. Winkelstein, W., Jr., Karzon, D. T., Barron, A. L., and Hayner, N. S.: Epidemiologic observations on an outbreak of aseptic meningtis due to ECHO virus type 6. Amer. J. Public Health, *47*:741, 1957.
33. Yoshioka, I., and Horstmann, D. M.: Viremia in infection due to ECHO virus type 9. New Eng. J. Med., *262*:224, 1960.

16

The Principal Epidemics of Meningitis Due to ECHO and Coxsackie Viruses

By V. DROUHET

ECHO VIRUS

Lymphocytic meningitis may appear in the course of ECHO virus infections. Sometimes cases are sporadic, but the epidemic form seems to be the more frequent.

EPIDEMICS OF LYMPHOCYTIC MENINGITIS DUE TO ECHO VIRUS

The number of cases in any one epidemic may vary from only a few up to hundreds or even thousands. The size of the affected community is relevant, but so also are the methods used to determine the incidence of ECHO virus infections. Clinical infections reflect the epidemiology of subclinical or inapparent infections, and the frequency of the latter in a population determines the existence of clinical manifestations. Surveillance of patients in the hospital and their families gives a very limited notion of the incidence of infection, just as does clinical surveillance without virological investigations.

Provided that the ECHO viruses spread rapidly in the communiy and, that their fecal elimination persists, their dissemination is easy to demonstrate in the laboratory. Clinical phenomena resulting from infection by some of the ECHO viruses are seen during epidemics in which a single type predominates. The incidence of clinical syndromes recognized as being due to ECHO virus infection varies with the type and the strain of

virus; it also relates to the incidence of preexisting immunity.

Epidemics Due to Echo 4. ECHO virus type 4 was initially recovered from the stools of a patient with lymphocytic meningitis who was admitted to a hospital in Connecticut in 1951.[27] Since then, numerous epidemics of "aseptic" meningitis have been described — at Marshalltown, Iowa, and its environs in 1955,[5, 22] in Buffalo in 1956,[17] in Sweden in 1956,[15] in Melbourne, Australia, in 1957,[9] in South Africa,[44] and in Poland.

Clinical manifestations consist, in the main, of an abacterial meningitis, sometimes associated with a minor illness, but without a rash. Thus in the course of the epidemic in Marshalltown, Iowa, 107 cases were reported as aseptic meningitides and 79 cases as minor illnesses. The onset was abrupt, with fever, headache localized to the retrobulbar area, nausea, vomiting, or diarrhea in 70 per cent of patients, sore throat in 40 per cent, and muscular stiffness in 40 per cent. Only 31 per cent of cases were reported in children under 14 years of age; in the same family, multiple infections were described. The incubation period was not accurately determined; in some families, the second case supervened toward the fifth day, but in other cases, it occurred after 21 days. The population of Marshalltown is of 20,000. Observations on 500 individuals from 143 families showed that 16 per cent of the population became infected. Fifty-seven subjects were investigated with regard to the possible fecal excretion of virus. ECHO virus type 4 (in four cases associated with poliovirus) was found in only 21: 16 of 31 individuals with abacterial meningitides, three of 15 individuals with illnesses classified as minor, and two of 11 family associates without clinical symptoms.[5]

In the course of the Swedish epidemic, a maculopapular rash was associated with abacterial meningitis on rare occasions.

Epidemics Due to ECHO 6. This type of ECHO virus is most frequently encountered during the investigation of patients with clinical manifestations.

Of 212 instances in which enteroviruses were recovered in healthy infants by Melnick in 1955,[26] ECHO 6 virus was recovered on only one occasion. In the Cincinnati laboratory it was also recovered only once out of 380 cytopathogenic enteroviruses recovered from healthy infants from Cincinnati and Mexico.[36, 37]

In Washington in 1952,[11] 21 strains of ECHO 6 virus were recovered out of 97 enteroviruses (45 polioviruses, 4 Coxsackie B, 12 Coxsackie A, 29 ECHO, and 17 unidentified viruses) obtained from patients with illnesses described as "nonparalytic poliomyelitis."

Strains of ECHO 6 virus were also recovered in sporadic cases of lymphocytic meningitis in California, Florida, and Massachusetts.[29]

Between 1952 and 1955, a number of epidemics of lymphocytic meningitis broke out in the United States, Sweden, Norway, and Australia. In the 1954 Boston epidemic, of 65 enteroviruses, 40 were ECHO 6. In all these cases, the clinical diagnosis was "nonparalytic poliomyelitis." On the other hand, in 1955, during the severe epidemic of poliovirus type I, ECHO virus type 6 was recovered on only ten occasions in lymphocytic meningitides.[19]

In 1955, ECHO 6 was the predominant type among 69 enteroviruses recovered in Connecticut.[7] These viruses were yielded by 35 patients with illnesses diagnosed as "nonparalytic poliomyelitis."

In New York State, in 1955, ECHO 6 virus produced an epidemic of lymphocytic meningitis. Of 172 cytopathic agents which were recovered in tissue culture from individuals in contact with patients, 90 per cent were ECHO 6.[16, 17]

In a few cases, ECHO 6 virus has been recovered from patients with paralysis.

In 1954, in Sweden, Von Zeipel and Svedmyr[45] found, among 51 enteroviruses, 34 strains of ECHO 6 virus. These isolations came from 130 patients with lymphocytic meningitis.

The presence of a rash was not mentioned in any of the epidemics. In Sweden, however, serological evidence of infection by ECHO 6 virus was observed in one case of erythema exudativa multiforme (Stevens-Johnson syndrome). A febrile illness with or without a rash but without meningeal manifestations in the patient's contacts was described by Karzon et al.[17] and by Kibrick.[19]

Epidemics Due to ECHO 9. ECHO virus type 9 was first recovered from the stools of healthy children during a nonepidemic period in Cincinnati.[36, 37] In 1955, when the virus was designated as ECHO 9, the type strain came from a case of aseptic meningitis in West Virginia. But the prominence of this virus as a cause of large epidemics of aseptic meningitis with rash was not realized until 1956, when hundreds of strains were isolated in Belgium, Holland, England, Germany, and Sweden.[3, 14, 23, 33, 41]

ECHO 9 virus was identified as the predominant type during the Swiss epidemic in 1956. It was then identified in Denmark and in Canada. This virus was responsible for small outbreaks in England in 1954 and 1955 and for larger epidemics in Italy in 1955.[1,2, 6, 10, 20, 38]

In Germany, Hennessen[12] and Brohl et al.[4] described cases of meningitis called "Coxsackie" because the virus was pathogenic for suckling mice.

In 1957, widespread epidemics of ECHO 9 affected tens of thousands of persons in the United States. During the 1957 Milwaukee epidemic, it was established that infection with the virus was limited to families which included sick persons.[39, 40] Among 26 families with 104 individuals (both well and ill persons), 58 strains of ECHO 9 virus were recovered. During the same period, in 107 members of 25 families without any ill member, ECHO 9 virus was recovered on only one occasion.

It was estimated that, for every 300 patients who were infected with ECHO 9 virus, one was hospitalized. In this epidemic, which lasted from the end of June to the end of September, 149 persons were admitted to the hospital, but the outbreak probably affected 40,000 persons. This is 4 per cent of the population, as compared with the 16 per cent in the ECHO 4 epidemic in Marshalltown.

The clinical manifestations of infection with ECHO 9 virus, as demonstrated by virus isolation, are aseptic meningitis, febrile episodes with or without rash, and occasional involvement of the central nervous system.

In the majority of epidemics observed in Europe or the United States, a rash is frequently seen, but in those observed in Italy and Switzerland, no rash was observed; this may be due to differing strains of virus.

In the Milwaukee epidemic, the incidence of rashes decreased with increasing age. Considering only those cases which were confirmed virologically, a rash was observed in the majority of infants under the age of three years, in 44 per cent of those between five and 15 years of age, and in 6 per cent of those above 15 years of age.

In Canada, three patients during the course of the epidemic described by Laforest et al.[20] presented with a petechial rash resembling that seen in meningococcemia; one case (proved by laboratory studies) was described in the Milwaukee epidemic.

In a large family infected by ECHO 9 virus in which four persons presented with a rash at the same time as the exanthem, there appeared a unilateral enanthem consisting of yellowish or grayish-white spots, 1 to 3 mm. in diameter, on the buccal mucosa or tonsillar fauces, or both, in some of the patients.

. Conjunctivitis has been observed in 14 per cent of cases which have been confirmed virologically.

Among patients admitted to a hospital and showing neck stiffness, only 50 per cent of those aged less than ten years and 65 per cent of those aged more than ten years showed an increased cell count in the cerebrospinal fluid at the time of the nuchal rigidity.

Virus is sometimes isolated from the cerebrospinal fluid in cases without any meningeal signs.

Epidemics Due to ECHO 16. This virus was discovered in 1951 in Massachusetts in eight patients admitted to a hospital with a meningeal syndrome[19] and, independently, in seven others who presented with a febrile exanthem.[37]

The cases of "aseptic" meningitis observed in Boston in 1951 were, however, not associated with a rash.

The febrile rash appears in a bizarre fashion, hours or days after the decline of fever and the disappearance of other signs.

In 1954, in the suburbs of Pittsburgh, a small epidemic of 24 cases broke out. The disease was known as the "Boston exanthem" and was caused by the same type of virus as that subsequently designated as ECHO 16 by the Enterovirus Committee in 1957.[30, 32]

In intrafamilial infections, discrete eruptions with little fever as well as febrile illness without rash were observed in the children. Epidemics occurred during the summer, recovery was rapid, and in most cases hospitalization was not necessary. Meningism and rash rarely appeared together.

THE ETIOLOGICAL ROLE OF OTHER TYPES OF ECHO VIRUS IN ASEPTIC MENINGITIS

In addition to the types of ECHO virus that cause epidemics, other types are isolated in sporadic cases of lymphocytic meningitis, most frequently from fecal specimens but also from cerebrospinal fluid. The following types of ECHO virus are at present known to be capable of producing lymphocytic meningitis: 1, 2, 3, 4, 5, 6, 7, 8, 9, 11, 12, 13, 14, 15, 16, 17, 18, 19, 20, 21, 22, 24, 25, 30, 31, and 32.[8, 24, 42, 43]

COXSACKIE VIRUSES

It has been observed for many years in Sweden and in the United States that some cases of aseptic meningitis may occur during epidemics of Bornholm disease or may be associated with pleurodynia. In the 1951 epidemic in Oxford, England, 5 per cent of patients presented with aseptic meningitis at the end of the first week of illness. The incidence of aseptic meningitis in Bornholm disease is greatest in children and they do not show the characteristic symptoms of pleurodynia. Pleurodynia, with or without pericarditis, is more frequent in young adults. The clinical features of these meningitides give rise to some peculiarities when they are seen outside epidemics of pleurodynia, where the two clinical pictures may be found together.[46]

Since the first descriptions by Curnen[48] and Melnick[53] in 1949 which enabled us to relate this meningitis with certainty to a Coxsackie virus infection, observations of Coxsackie B meningitis have multiplied throughout the world. They are most frequently caused by viruses of types B1, 2, 3, 4, and 5. The first case of aseptic meningitis caused by Coxsackie B6 was reported by Hammon in 1960.[50]

The viruses of group A (A7, A9) may

Table 16-1. *Enteroviruses Associated with Lymphocytic Meningitis*

POLIOVIRUS	COXSACKIE				ECHO	
Epidemic and Sporadic cases	*A*		*B*		*Epidemic*	*Sporadic*
	Epidemic	*Sporadic*	*Epidemic*	*Sporadic*		
I, II, III	7, 23	2, 3, 4, 5, 6, 9	1, 2, 3, 4, 5	1, 2, 3, 4, 5, 6	4, 6, 9, 16, 19, 30	1, 2, 3, 4, 5, 6, 7, 8, 9, 11, 12, 13, 14, 15, 16, 17, 18, 19, 20, 21, 22, 24, 25, 30, 31, 32

produce the same picture; more rarely cited are types A2, 3, 4, 5, and 6.[47, 49]

It appears that ECHO viruses are not alone in their ability to produce syndromes which include meningism and a rash, since a number of exanthemata arising in the course of meningitides due to Coxsackie viruses have been described.

The virus has been recovered from feces up to the thirteenth day of illness and, intermittently, even later, and from the throat up to the tenth day. Virus is recovered from the cerebrospinal fluid in 47 per cent of cases, even in the absence of an increase in cells. Virus has been revealed in the urine and in the blood; viremia may be detected five days before the onset of meningeal signs.

Coxsackie meningitis is estimated to be one of the most prevalent of the lymphocytic meningitides, second only to mumps meningitis. Nevertheless the frequency appears to vary with age, geographical situation, and the particular year. Thus, in Connecticut, in successive years, Coxsackie viruses accounted for 35 per cent and then only 6 per cent of lymphocytic meningitides.

The meningeal syndrome always presents in the same way, but the virus type responsible changes from one year to another.

Epidemics due to Coxsackie viruses B4 and B2 followed the epidemic caused by Coxsackie virus B5, at any rate in Minnesota. This epidemic began in July, 1956, and the greatest number of cases occurred in August and September, the last occurring in December. The patients' ages varied between five and nine years. This epidemic was independent of that of paralytic poliomyelitis. Of 113 patients in whom the diagnosis was that of "nonparalytic poliomyelitis," Coxsackie B5 virus was recovered from 61; in 32 of these cases the diagnosis was confirmed by the measurement of antibodies against this virus. Poliovirus was not recovered, and the neutralizing antibody titers against poliovirus remained unaltered in the 42 cases investigated in this regard.

In California, in 1958, of 368 cases of lymphocytic meningitis causing hospitalization in Los Angeles, Lennette[52] showed that 43 per cent were due to Coxsackie B and, of these, 32 per cent were due to Coxsackie B5 which represented the highest percentage by far. These Coxsackie virus infections appeared in July.

In southern Sweden, at Malmö, an industrial town of 200,000 inhabitants, an epidemic of paralytic cases and of aseptic meningitis broke out in August, 1952, and lasted until December. Of the 151 cases, 54 per cent were of lymphocytic meningitis; the morbidity rate was 0.41 per cent. Polioviruses were recovered in 50 per cent of cases and Coxsackie B virus in 12 per cent. Coxsackie B3 virus predominated during the first month of the epidemic in children.[51]

BIBLIOGRAPHY

ECHO VIRUS

1. Archetti, I., Felici, A., Russi, F. and Fua, C.: Recherches sur la définition étiologique de la méningo névraxite des Marches à l'occasion de l'épidémie estivo-automnale de 1955. Scientia Med. Ital., 5:317, 1956.

2. Baumann, T., Barben, M., Marti, R., Hassler, A., and Krech, U.: Erkrankungen durch ECHO-virus Typ 9. Eine epidemiologische, klinische und virologisch-serologische Studie. Schweiz. Med. Wschr. *87*:307, 1957.

3. Boissard, G. P. B., Macrae, A. D., Stokes, J. L., and MacCallum, F. O.: Isolation of viruses related to ECHO virus type 9 from outbreaks of aseptic meningitis. Lancet, *1*:500, 1957.

4. Brohl, I., Helmstaedt, K., Lennartz, H., and Maass, G.: Uber eine Epidemie von Coxsackie Meningitis. Z. Aertzl. Fortbild. (Berlin), *12*:499-505, 1957.

5. Chin, T. D. Y., Beran, G. W., and Wenner, H. A.: An epidemic illness associated with a recenty recognized enteric virus (ECHO virus type 4). II. Recognition and identification of the etiologic agent. Amer. J. Hyg., *66*:76-84, 1957.

6. Dalldorf, G.: The enteroviruses and paralytic disease. In: Viral Infections of Infancy and Childhood. New York, Hoeber Division of Harper & Row, 1960.

7. Davis, D. C., and Melnick, J. L.: Association of ECHO virus type 6 with aseptic meningitis. Proc. Soc. Exp. Biol. Med., *92*:839-843, 1956.

8. Drouhet, V., and Goareguer, H.: Sur le diagnostic virologique et sérologique des infections à entérovirus. Path. Biol., *8*:17-29, 1960.

9. Forbes, J. A.: Meningitis in Melbourne due to ECHO virus 4. I. Clinical aspects. Med. J. Australia, *1*:246, 1958.

10. Godtfredsen, A., and Von Magnus, H.: Isolation of ECHO virus type 9 from cerebrospinal fluids. Danish Med. Bull., *4*:233-236, 1957.

11. Habel, K., Silverberg, R. J., and Shelokov, A.: Isolation of enteric viruses from cases of aseptic meningitis. Ann. N. Y. Acad. Sci., *67*:223-229, 1957.

12. Hennessen, W.: Some features of a new type of virus meningitis. Deutsch. Med. Wschr., *81*:2088-2090, 1956.

13. Hobson, D., Hoskins, J. M., Horner, J., Clarke, A. H., and Wood, F. B.: Clinical, epidemiological and virological aspects of ECHO virus type 9 infection in Sheffield, 1960. Brit. J. Prev. Soc. Med., *16*:84, 1962.

14. Johnsson, T.: A new clinical entity? Lancet, *1*:590, 1957.

15. Johnsson, T., Böttiger, M., and Löfdahl, A.: An outbreak of aseptic meningitis with a rubella-like rash probably caused by ECHO virus type 4. Arch. ges. Virusforsch., *8*:306-317, 1958.

16. Karzon, D. T.: Viruses in search of disease. (Discussion). Ann. N.Y. Acad. Sci. *67*:351-352, 1957.

17. Karzon, D. T., Barron, A. L., Winkelstein, W., Jr., and Cohen, S.: Isolation of ECHO virus type 6 during an outbreak of seasonal aseptic meningitis. J.A.M.A., *162*:1298, 1956.

18. Karzon, D. T., Eckert, G. L., Barron, A. L., Hayner, N. S., and Winkelstein, W., Jr.: Aseptic meningitis epidemic due to ECHO virus 4. Amer. J. Dis. Child., *101*:610, 1961.

19. Kibrick, S., Melendez, L., and Enders, J. F.: Clinical associations of enteric viruses with particular reference to agents exhibiting properties of the ECHO group. Ann. N. Y. Acad. Sci., *67*:311-325, 1957.

20. Laforest, R. A., McNaughton, G. A., Beale, A. J., Clarke, M., Davis, N., Sultanian, I., and Rhodes, A. J.: Outbreak of aseptic meningitis (meningo encephalitis) with rubelliform rash: Toronto 1956. Canad. Med. Assoc. J., *77*:1-4, 1957.

21. Lahelle, O.: Aseptic meningitis caused by ECHO virus. J. Hyg. (Camb.), *55*:475, 1957.

22. Lehan, P. H., Chick, E. W., Doto, J. L., Chin, T. D. Y., Heeren, R. H., and Furculow, M. L.: An epidemic illness associated with a recently recognized enteric virus (ECHO virus type 4). I. Epidemiologic and clinical features. Amer. J. Hyg., *66*:63-75, 1957.

23. MacLean, D. M., and Melnick, J. L.: Association of a mouse pathogenic strain of ECHO virus type 9 with aseptic meningitis. Proc. Soc. Exp. Biol. Med., *44*:656-660, 1957.

24. MacNair Scott, T. F.: Clinical syndromes associated with enterovirus and reovirus infections. Adv. Virus Res., *8*:165-197, 1961.

25. Melnick, J. L.: Advances in the study of the enteroviruses. Progr. Med. Virol., *1*:59, 1958.

26. Melnick, J. L.: Tissue culture techniques and their application to original isolation, growth and assay of poliomyelitis and orphan viruses. Ann. N. Y. Acad. Sci., *61*:754-772, 1955.

27. Melnick, J. L., Emmons, J., Coffey, J. H., and Schoof, H.: Seasonal distribution of Coxsackie viruses in urban sewage and flies. Amer. J. Hyg., *59*:164-184, 1954.

28. Melnick, J. L., and Ledinko, N.: Social serology: antibody levels in a normal young population during an epidemic of poliomyelitis. Amer. J. Hyg., *54*:354, 1951.

29. Meyer, H. M., Jr., Rogers, N. G., Miesse, M. L., and Crawford, I. P.: Aseptic meningitis caused by orphan viruses and other agents. Ann. N. Y. Acad. Sci., *67*:332-337, 1957.

30. Neva, F. A.: A second outbreak of Boston exanthem disease in Pittsburgh during 1954. New England J. Med., *254*:838-843, 1956.

31. Neva, F. A., and Enders, J. F.: Cytopathogenic agents isolated from patients during unusual epidemic exanthem. J. Immunol., *72*:307-314, 1954.

32. Neva, F. A., and Zuffante, S. M.: Agents isolated from Boston exanthem disease during 1954 in Pittsburgh. J. Lab. Clin. Med., *50*:712, 1957.

33. Nihoul, E., and Quersin-Thiry, L.: A new clinical entity? Lancet, *1*:269-270, 1957.

34. Ormsbee, R. A., and Bell, E. J.: ECHO viruses from Idaho and Montana. Amer. J. Public Health, *47*:1405-1413, 1957.

35. Philipson, L.: Experiments in human adults with a recently isolated virus associated with respiratory disease. Arch. ges. Virusforsch., *77*:318-331, 1958.

36. Ramos-Alvarez, M., and Sabin, A. B.: Characteristics of poliomyelitis and other viruses recovered in tissue culture from healthy American children. Proc. Soc. Exp. Biol. Med., *87*:655-661, 1954.

37. Ramos-Alvarez, M., and Sabin, A. B.: Intestinal viral flora of healthy children demonstrable by monkey kidney tissue culture. Amer. J. Public Health, *46*:295-296, 1956.

38. Russi, F., and Fua, C.: L' incidenza dell' accertamento virologico nelle varie forme cliniche della meningo-nevrassite coxsackiosa Marchigiana. Policlinico (Prat.), *63*:1-3, 1956.

39. Sabin, A. B., Krumbiegel, E. R., and Wigand, R.: ECHO 9 virus disease: Virologically controlled clinical and epidemiologic observations during 1957 epidemic in Milwaukee with notes on concurrent similar diseases associated with Coxsackie and other ECHO viruses. A.M.A.J. Dis. Child., *96*:197-219, 1958.

40. Sabin, A. B., Michaels, R. H., Spigland, I., Pelon, W., Rhim, J. S., and Wehr, R. E.: Communitywide use of oral poliovirus vaccine. Effectiveness

of the Cincinnati program. A.M.A.J. Child., *101*: 546-567, 1961.

41. Sauthoff, R., and Mittelstrass, H. B.: Neutralisie-rende Antikörper in Menschlichen Seren gegen ECHO virus typ 9. Klin. Wschr., *35*:311, 1957.

42. Thivolet, J., Gaudin, G., and Terraillon, J.: Petite épidémie familiale dûe au virus ECHO de type 9. Sem. Hop. Paris, *9*:1897, 1961.

43. Wenner, H. A., and Lenahan, M. F.: Propagation of group A Coxsackie viruses in tissue cultures. II. Some interactions between virus and mammalian cells. Yale J. Biol. Med., *34*:421, 1961-1962.

44. Wilsen, A. A. J., and Peisach, H.: A closed epidemic of acute aseptic meningitis caused by ECHO virus type 4. S. African Med. J., *35*:330, 1961.

45. Von Zeipel, G., and Svedmyr, A.: A study of the association of ECHO viruses to aseptic meningitis. Arch. Ges. Virusforsch., *7*:355-368, 1957.

COXSACKIE VIRUSES

46. Bayer, P., and Gear, J.: Virus meningo-encephalitis in South Africa. A study of the cases admitted to the Johannesburg fever hospital. S.Afr.J. Lab. Clin. Med., *6*:22, 1955.

47. Chumakov, M. P., Voroshilova, M. K., Zhevandrova, V. I., Mironova, L. L., Itzelis, F. I., and Robinson, I. A.: Vydelenie i izuchenie IV immunologichest-rogo tipa virus poliomielita (Isolation and invesgi-fation of the IV immunological type of poliomye-litis virus). Probl. Virol., *1*:16-19, 1956.

48. Curnen, E. C., Shaw, E. W., and Melnick, J. L.: Disease resembling nonparalytic poliomyelitis associated with a virus pathogenic for infant mice. J.A.M.A., *141*:894, 1949.

49. Grist, N. R.: Isolation of Coxsackie A7 virus in Scotland. Lancet, *1*:1054-1055, 1960.

50. Hammon, W. D., et al.: Isolation and characterization of prototype viruses ECHO 26, ECHO 27, Coxsackie B6. Proc. Soc. Exp. Biol. Med., *103*: 164, 1960.

51. Johnsson, T.: Occurrence of Coxsackie virus infections in an epidemic of poliomyelitis. Arch. Ges. Virusforsch., *6*:216, 1955.

52. Lennette, E. H., Magoffin, R. L., Schmidt, N. J., and Hollister, A. C.: Viral disease of the central nervous system. Influence of poliomyelitis on etiology. J.A.M.A., *128*:1456, 1959.

53. Melnick, J. L., Shaw, E. W., and Curnen, E. C.: A virus isolated from patients diagnosed as non-paralytic poliomyelitis or aseptic meningitis. Proc. Soc. Exp. Biol. Med., *71*:344, 1949.

54. Syverton, J. T., McLean, D. M., Martins da Silva, M., Doany, H. B., Cooney, M., and Kleinman, H.: Outbreak of aseptic meningitis caused by Cox-sackie B5 virus: Laboratory, clinical, and epide-demiologic study. J.A.M.A., *164*:2015, 1957.

17

Lymphocytic Choriomeningitis

(ARMSTRONG'S DISEASE)

By B. KREIS

In 1934, Armstrong and Lillie[5] isolated an infectious agent from a monkey that induced meningitis in mice with involvement of the choroid plexuses. It was named lympho-cytic choriomeningitis virus (L.C.M.). Soon it was also recovered from uninoculated mice.[21a, 43a] Serological studies carried out by Armstrong and Lillie[5] and direct isolation of the virus[35] have demonstrated its role in human lymphocytic meningitis. This we con-firmed with Lepine et al.[21a] by reproducing the disease by subcutaneous injection of the virus in man. It has also been estab-lished that meningitis is only one of the clinical manifestations of a generalized infectious disease which, in our opinion, should be called "Armstrong's disease."[19, 19a]

Identification of L.C.M. requires tech-niques which few laboratories make a practice of applying. Thus, while viral pathology in general has developed considerably, this infection has remained somewhat neglected, although it initially appeared to be one of the most frequent causes of lymphocytic meningitis. More recently, it has attracted attention again as a typical immunological disease and as an example of latent viral infection. We shall not deal with the immuno-logical aspects, important as they may be, but shall emphasize the more recent methods of diagnosis they have led to. These should increase interest in the disease and make possible a closer approximation of its fre-quency.

CLINICAL MANIFESTATIONS

The best-studied manifestations of Arm-strong's disease are those involving the nervous system. Its most frequent form is that of a mild lymphocytic meningitis.

UNCOMPLICATED MENINGEAL FORM

The onset is sudden, with headaches, nausea or vomiting, fever, and meningeal signs. In half the cases, however, a *pro-dromal febrile form* during the preceding two weeks is reported, with chills, myalgia, signs of rhinopharyngeal infection, or productive cough. These symptoms have usually disappeared by the time meningitis sets in. It is characterized by stiffness of the neck, but contractures are moderate. Even Kernig's sign is sometimes absent. Tendon reflexes are more often diminished than hyperactive, and they often disappear temporarily. A transitory Babinski sign has been reported. There is usually no photophobia and rarely papillary edema. The mental state is usually normal, though some degree of obnubilation or sleepiness may be noted. General signs are usually moderate: the temperature may reach from 39° to 40° C.; the pulse is regular and it is not fast—that is, it is not in keeping with the temperature. There may be a cough or signs of pharyngitis. During this phase, the blood cell count may reveal a mild leukocytosis, with 6000 to 15,000 cells per cubic millimeter. The differential blood cell count remains normal (average among 63 cases studied by Adair et al.[2]: 8400 leukocytes per cubic millimeter, 66 per cent of them polymorphonuclear cells). The sedimentation rate is barely increased.

The study of the *cerebrospinal fluid* remains the most important point: the pressure is normal or slightly increased; the fluid is clear or slightly opalescent; a fibrinous coagulum is infrequent. The crucial indications are given by the cell count. In the first four days cellular reaction is intense. There were more than 1000 cells per milliliter in almost half the cases we studied up to 1948, varying from eight to 3200 cells. The average was 728 cells (0—6050) in the 63 cases studied by Adair et al.[2] but 33 of them had fewer than 600 cells. The cells involved are essentially lymphocytes (95 per cent). Sometimes a certain percentage of polymorphonuclear cells is noted (52 per cent in one of Armstrong's cases), but in our own investigations the causal agent of L.C.M. has never been isolated in a case of meningitis with polymorphonuclear cells. The albumin content is variable, often above 1 gm. per 100 ml. The glucose content is normal, or sometimes low (less than 50 mg. per 100 ml. in 19 of the 72 cases observed by Adair et al.). Colloidal reactions are slightly altered.

Improvement is rapid. As a rule, the clinical meningeal phase lasts less than one week; fever disappears within one or two weeks. It takes much longer for the cytology of the spinal fluid to return to normal; there are still more than 100 cells per milliliter in the third week, and it takes two months or more before the spinal fluid is normal again.

In these uncomplicated meningeal forms, recovery is the rule, without noteworthy sequale. However, more or less persistent stiffness and headaches have been reported, as well as temporary loss of memory or depression, and repeated relapses sometimes occur with reappearance of the virus or even progress of the meningitis toward chronicity. *Complications* are exceptional. Orchitis and parotitis[23] can appear, independently of any action of the mumps virus, and even paraplegia due to spinal arachnoiditis has occurred.

FORMS INVOLVING THE CENTRAL NERVOUS SYSTEM

The clinical picture is more serious when the meningeal involvement is complicated by other central nervous system involvement. Occasionally the disease takes the form of a meningomyelitis: then, in addition to loss of reflexes and a transitory Babinski sign sometimes observed in the forms already mentioned, there are more severe manifestations of medullary involvement: objective sensory disturbances, paresis or paralysis of one limb, and involvement of the lumbar or abdominal muscles. In such cases, L.C.M. may be confused with poliomyelitis.[26] More often meningitis is associated with encephalitis. Of 53 cases of L.C.M. observed over five years by Meyer et al.,[27] there were 38 cases of uncomplicated meningitis and 20 of meningoencephalitis. As a rule, the signs of involvement of the central nervous system are limited to high fever, torpor, ocular or facial paralysis, paralysis of limbs, Babinski's sign, and sensory or sphincteral disorders. These signs disappear more or less rapidly, but occasionally some sequelae remain. Much more seldom, the infection takes the form of true coma with fever, with or without hemiplegia. The course of this form was fatal in about ten cases. In such a neurological form, clinical meningeal signs are often absent. The pleocytosis of the cerebrospinal fluid may be marked (1307 cells per milliliter) or moderate (63 cells). In many cases it was not observed at all, since meningitis is not necessarily present in Armstrong's disease, even when the nervous system is involved.

OTHER NEUROLOGICAL MANIFESTATIONS

If there is no meningeal reaction, Armstrong's disease cannot possibly be suspected. Although some inoculations and systematic tests have given positive results in various forms of neurological involvement (encephalitis, poliomyelitis, or radiculoneuritic syndromes), there is still room for doubt concerning their etiology. Our own investigations gave negative results as concerns the L.C.M. virus in 38 cases representing 18 different neurological diseases.

NON-NEUROLOGICAL FORMS OF ARMSTRONG'S DISEASE

The other known forms of Armstrong's disease will only be mentioned here: they are mainly *febrile* forms resembling typhoid or simple influenza, attended by headache, myalgia, arthralgia, constant leukopenia, and neutropenia, but without clinical or biological meningeal manifestations. Recovery occurs in one to three weeks. Recently Baum et al.[6] reported a laboratory epidemic of ten cases. Exceptionally rare were the forms attended by a *rash,* fatal at times, and others resembling an acute respiratory affection or an atypical pneumonia; still others presented as a hematological disturbance with necrotic tonsilopharyngitis, hemorrhage, leukocytosis, and immature cells. Above all, one should mention the *inapparent* forms, revealed by serological study, which may account for the incidence of positive serological tests among laboratory workers or in some communities.

The clinical aspects of Armstrong's disease would probably prove more varied if it were the rule to search systematically for this agent in all infections of unknown cause.

FORMS INDUCED BY INOCULATION

In 16 cases it was noticed[21a] that the subcutaneous, intramuscular, or intravenous inoculation in man of a virulent emulsion of mouse brain induced, after an incubation lasting 36 hours to three days, a sudden rise in temperature, either alone or accompanied by a slight flu-like condition occasionally presenting signs of bronchitis. Marked leukopenia with granulopenia was observed. Then leukocytosis returned to normal, lymphomonocytosis marking the last phase. Cerebrospinal fluid was normal; the fever abated within a few days but another febrile wave sometimes occurred. It was only some three weeks after inoculation (18 to 20 days) that a further rise of temperature was suddenly observed, with headache, meningeal signs, and cytologic reaction of the cerebrospinal fluid (sometimes more than 800 cells per milliliter). Blood and cerebrospinal fluid were virulent during the acute phase, which permitted successive transfers. As a rule recovery occurred in two or three days. Nonetheless, serious encephalitis occurred in some cases.

On other occasions inoculation caused only a short febrile period, or at the most, a late serological reaction, the cerebrospinal fluid remaining normal during the whole course. Such types of inoculation reaction have been fairly often observed in laboratories where L.C.M. studies are carried out.

PATHOLOGY

In man lesions due to Armstrong's disease are not well known, since the meningeal form is mild. In one case, intense lymphocytic and macrophagic infiltration of the meninges was observed, involving also the ventricular walls and the choroid plexuses, in contrast with the other parts of the brain, which remained unaffected. Death was due to subarachnoid block. Most fatal cases, however, were due to encephalitis or encephalomyelitis, often hemorrhagic, with lymphoplasmocytic infiltration and encephalitis nodules or softening. Meningeal reaction is not constant. In most cases, there is no choroid involvement, as was observed by Armstrong, himself.*

Visceral lesions attending the meningeal involvement are not uncommon, particularly bronchopneumonia foci with mononucleated cells and pleural or pericardial fluid. Visceral lesions are of the same type when there is no meningeal involvement.

EPIDEMIOLOGY

The etiological agent of L.C.M. measures from 40 to 60 mμ as estimated by ultrafiltration. As yet, this virus has not been studied under the electron microscope and it has

---

*That is one of the reasons why it seems inconsistent to continue calling Armstrong's disease in humans "choriomeningitis," since the term is too restrictive.

not been classified, but its characteristics are those of an RNA virus.[32]

Its *geographical distribution* is very wide. It has been found in all parts of the United States (Washington, Texas, Los Angeles), in South America (Brazil, Argentina), from West to East Africa (Morocco, Tunisia, Ethiopia), as well as in Asia (Japan, China). In Europe, its presence has been recorded in Great Britain, Ireland, Italy, Germany, Austria, the Netherlands, Rumania, Bulgaria, Yugoslavia, and the U.S.S.R. In France, it has been identified in Paris, Lyons, and Strasburg.

The most current *reservoir of virus* is the house mouse *(Mus musculus),* But other species of mice (namely, laboratory white mice) are natural hosts of the virus. In the United States, the incidence of the infection in mice between 1942 and 1946 varied from 4 to 21 per cent according to the area.[5, 12] The same observations have been made in Germany.[1] Of 376 mouse nesting places examined, 42 were found to be contaminated; the incidence of these infected foci ranged from 15 to 34 per cent according to the areas. Contact with virus-carrying mice, sometimes even a bite, is found in many clinical histories and is the cause of almost all laboratory infections.

Dogs, farm animals (sheep, goats, calves),[34] monkeys, hamsters, rats, and small wild mammals[9] may be carriers, and they have been considered responsible in some circumstances. The virus might be transmitted by ticks or lice, which have been shown to be infected. Moreover, experimentally the infection has been induced in bedbugs and mosquitoes. These facts have led some authors to classify the L.C.M. agent in the arvovirus group.

In man, the portal of entry of the virus seems to be the upper respiratory tract, as a result of mouse secretions or droppings. No man to man contagion has been demonstrated. One case of transplacental transmission, however, has been reported.[18] Human cases are sporadic or limited to minor outbreaks. They usually occur in late autumn and early winter, when mice and men seek shelter indoors.

FREQUENCY

Since no systematic investigations have been made, it is difficult to estimate the prevalence of Armstrong's disease. In 1948 more than 80 observations were reported in world literature.[19b] Later, studies carried out

on cases of meningeal and nervous infections have shown that whereas sometimes the incidence is nil (Sweden[3, 17]; Switzerland; Finland[31]), in other regions the percentages are more or less high: 3.5 per cent in the United States (1950)[28], 12 per cent in Austria (1952),[8] from 5 to 7.3 per cent in the 325 cases studied by the Virus Reference Laboratory in Great Britain (1953)[33]; 9.4 per cent in Rumania (1956)[38]. In Germany, Scheid et al.[37] observed five cases between 1948 and 1955 and nine others with Ackerman et al.[1] from 1955 to 1964, i.e., 14 cases spread over 16 years.

In France, in 1937,[19a] we reported only one probable case among 29 cases of lymphocytic meningitis studied in Paris and none among 30 neurological disturbances of various types. There were eight cases of L.C.M. among 242 cases of meningitis or of meningoencephalitis studied by Sohier[42] in the Lyons area, i.e., 3.3 per cent. At the same time, there were 26 cases due to the mumps virus (10.7 per cent), eight due to poliovirus (3.3 per cent), two due to Coxsackie virus, and one due to herpes[42]. In Alsace,[20] in 499 presumably viral infections observed over an 18-month period, 211 viruses were isolated: 140 Coxsackie viruses, 55 polioviruses, three adenoviruses, and six L.C.M. viruses (3.3 per cent).

The figures reported by some authors are particularly high. In 150 cases of meningitis, spinal arachnoid encephalitis, and polyradiculoneuritis, Shvarev[40] in the U.S.S.R., isolated the L.C.M. agent twice and obtained 23 postive complement-fixation reactions and 34 positive neutralization tests: L.C.M. was probably the etiological agent in one-fourth of the cases studied. In an investigation carried out in 1939 involving more than 200 specimens of serum taken at random in the United States, 11 per cent showed antibodies neutralizing L.C.M. virus.[46] More recently, Lippi,[24] in Italy, obtained 12.5 per cent positive complement-fixation reactions among the general population.

The most informative study was carried out in the United States[2, 27]: 1567 cases of amicrobial meningitis were observed between 1941 and 1958 in the same military environment and a thorough virological study was undertaken. Tests for L.C.M. consisted of inoculation into mice and guinea pigs as well as tests for complement-fixating and neutralizing antibodies.

Between 1941 and 1946, L.C.M. was demonstrated in 32 cases (8.5 per cent) and presumed in 10 cases (2.7 per cent) out of 374. From 1947 to 1952, L.C.M. was demon-strated in 37 cases (8.1 per cent) and pre-sumed in seven cases (1.6 per cent) out of 480. At the same time, in this series, 12 per cent of the cases were due to mumps virus and 5 per cent to herpes virus; and 7 per cent were due to leptospira. The etiology of 75 per cent of the cases remained undetermined.

From 1953 to 1958, L.C.M. was demon-strated in 57 cases (8.1 per cent) of 713 cases and presumed in 10. At the same time, 12.8 per cent of the cases were caused by mumps and 2.7 per cent by herpes virus, 2.7 per cent by leptospira, and 41 per cent by entero-viruses (21 different viruses), and 27 per cent remained etiologically obscure.

Thus when it was systematically searched for, meningitis due to Armstrong's disease recurred over a period of 17 years with a remarkable frequency and regularity, com-parable to that of mumps meningitis.

Local variations of frequency should not be surprising, however, as the disease appears closely connected with the existence of foci of contaminated mice and with dwelling condi-tions facilitating contact between mouse and man.

DIAGNOSIS

A very small number of clinical mani-festations suggest L.C.M.: a febrile pro-dromal period followed by remission, a pos-sible contact with mice, and a very large number of cells in the cerebrospinal fluid. As in all cases of lymphocytic meningitis, diag-nosis can be established only through the systematic search for the virus.

Two kinds of investigations must be car-ried out: those revealing the presence of the virus through inoculation or culture, and serological studies.

ISOLATION OF THE VIRUS

Material. The patient's *blood* or *serum* is used, since blood and serum are infectious from the beginning of the meningeal phase and sometimes until the fifteenth day of the disease. Cerebrospinal fluid contains less virus and ceases to be infectious earlier, in spite of a persisting cellular reaction. Virus concentration in the *urine* is low, but it may be found there even when it is no longer

present in the blood. *Gargle* fluid is some-times positive. Pathological specimens are inoculated immediately after having been taken or transported in a freezing box, since the titer of the virulent emulsion decreases by 10 to 100 times after one hour at 37° C. or 18 hours at 4° C. However, blood remains infectious for a few days in the freezer of an ordinary refrigerator. The virus is not altered by hemolysis. For necropsy material, the best way is to puncture aseptically the liver or spleen: they contain far more virus than blood (up to 1000 times as much). Brain also may contain more virus than blood, but much less than liver.

Inoculation. White mice and guinea-pigs are used.

INOCULATION OF MICE. The white mouse is the animal of choice. Eight mice aged three to four weeks (newborn mice are not receptive) are inoculated intracerebrally with 0.02 ml. of blood or serum (with or with-out 1000 μg./ml. of penicillin); four other mice are inoculated in the peritoneum. After intracerebral inoculation the typical course is this: after an interval of six to seven days, the mouse suddenly ceases to move in its container and its fur is ruffled. If it is held by the tail, it moves its front and rear legs con-vulsively at a very rapid rate. A *tonic crisis* often occurs: the animal stretches out its hind legs, hunches its back, and moves its front legs convulsively. It dies on the seventh to ninth day, often in this characteristic posi-tion. Part of the brain must be examined histologically; the rest should be kept for possible transfers at +4° C. in phosphated glycerin, or frozen at −70° C. or lyophilized. Deaths within the first three days should not be taken into account, and observation should be stopped after the twelfth day. Some strains, said to be *viscerotropic*, do not regularly kill the mouse after intracerebral injection; when injected intraperitoneally, however, they kill 30 to 70 per cent between the fifth and the fourteenth day after inoculation. Recently in-oculation in the *plantar cushion* of the mouse has been stressed as particularly interesting: it provokes a characteristic local edema seven to eight days later.[36a, b]

Histological study after intracerebral inoculation shows an acute leptomeningitis with round cells prevailing at the base and in the septa, and often, though not always, dif-fuse infiltrations of the choroid plexuses. Moreover, leukocytic infiltration or rare encephalitic nodules can be observed in the nervous tissue of the perivascular layers. In addition, round cell infiltrations are observed in almost all the viscera, in particular the liver, the lungs, the kidney, the pancreas, the heart, the uterus, and even the salivary glands, the testicles, or the ovaries. Such visceral lesions prevail when the brain has not been inoculated, the meninges and choroid usually remaining untouched.[5] Various types of *cellular inclusions* have been described, but they are only occasional.

After intracerebral injection, lesions are as a rule very characteristic. Nevertheless, it is most advisable to authenticate them by fixing *fluorescent antibodies* active on a known L.C.M. virus.[45] Fluorescence is observed in the foci of meningeal infiltrations; it is limited to the cytoplasm of the infected cells, where it forms small perinuclear, intracytoplasmic, or peripheral clumps. Their presence is decisive evidence.

Another test is the search, by ultracentrifugation of the spleen, for a *soluble antigen*[41] which appears in it during the very first days of the infection and which fixes complement in the presence of an experimental anti-L.C.M. serum. Furthermore, the brains of the mice killed by inoculation can be used for successive transfers.

Later evidence can be given by the resistance of mice having survived the intracerebral or intraperitoneal inoculation of the pathological specimen for a month by results of a trial inoculation of a virulent L.C.M. strain.

Thus, inoculation of mice is an excellent method for revealing the virus. A serious cause of error, however, is that the breeding group may naturally be infected with L.C.M. This *natural infection* has two aspects, as very well shown by Traub[43b] as early as 1936 in a remarkable series of works which have been elaborated upon since. If adult mice are infected, the disease is acute; later, antibodies are formed, the virus is eliminated, and the animals become resistant to further infection. Such mice, when inoculated with a virulent pathological specimen, show neither signs nor lesions, and diagnosis of L.C.M. is mistakenly rejected. If on the other hand mice are infected *in utero* or at birth, no antibodies are formed and the animals remain healthy virus carriers all their lives. Like the mice that have formed antibodies, they are completely resistant to inoculation of virulent material. But intracerebral inoculation of

inert matter may cause the virus to circulate, and the mice may show the usual signs of the disease. In such cases, the material injected may be wrongly considered responsible for the disease. Therefore any diagnosis based on inoculation of mice can be completely reliable only if the mice belong to a *selected breeding group,* evidence being provided that the animals are sensitive to the virus and that there is no latent infection.

Inoculation of Guinea Pigs. In order to avoid the aforementioned drawbacks, the standard procedure is to inoculate, in addition to the mice, six guinea-pigs intraperitoneally. These animals are practically always free from natural infection by L.C.M. The dose injected can be 100 times as high as in the mouse (2 ml. of blood), and it does not matter too much if the product injected is not perfectly sterile. The temperature curve must be watched. Typically, in a positive reaction, the temperature remains normal, around 39° C., for four to five days. Then it rises to 40° C. and above and remains high for four to 12 days. Mortality varies according to the strains. If a fever occurs, blood specimens are injected into mice. Two guinea pigs are killed around the tenth day for transfers, search for soluble antigen, and postmortem examination. However, autopsy is not always decisive (there are strictly visceral lesions, with pleuropulmonary foci and histological liver lesions, which can be authenticated by means of fluorescent antibodies). Another test is intradermal inoculation.[36a] The surviving guinea pigs are inoculated a month later with trial injections of a virulent L.C.M. strain. Half of them are inoculated intracerebrally, the others intraperitoneally.

It is pointless to use other species of animals, either sensitive (monkeys, dogs) or liable to inapparent infection (rabbits, hamsters). Inoculation of the *chorioallantoid* membrane of chick embryo is easy, but is not usually followed by typical lesions and does not always lead to the formation of a specific antigen.

Culture. Culture on *cell lines* (FL or, if not available, KB or Hep 2) is of great value, since the difficulties due to latent infection of the animal are thus averted. However, the cytopathogenic effect is often absent. On chick embryo fibroblasts, the mouse virus may induce *plaques* revealing its presence; a specific antiserum inhibits the formation of these plaques.[10] Nevertheless, with some human strains no plaques have been obtained. Here again, identification of the virus in all cultures by means of fluorescent antibodies (Cohen et al.[11]) will probably yield the rational solution to these difficulties.

SEROLOGICAL DIAGNOSIS

No virus should be considered pathogenic if concomitant formation of specific antibodies is not observed. On the other hand, the appearance of such antibodies is in itself enough to make the diagnosis. The various antibodies will be discussed here in their order of appearance.

Fluorescent Antibodies. A culture of L.C.M. virus on monkey or baby hamster kidney cells is placed in contact first with the patient's serum, and then with an anti-human globulin labeled with a fluorescent compound, according to the indirect Coombs' technique. If the serum under study contains an anti-L.C.M. virus antibody, fluorescent clumps appear among the cells.[11]

Antibodies responsible for this reaction are found in the serum very early — sometimes even on the first day of meningeal signs. They reach high titers, around $1/64$ or $1/128$, which persist for at least two to three weeks, and then decrease. These antibodies have been observed in cases when search for the virus and complement-fixation reaction had been negative. Experience with this method of investigation, however, is still very limited.

Complement-Fixing Antibodies. On the other hand, the complement-fixation reaction, developed in 1938[21b, 29] and improved by the use of a soluble antigen extracted from the spleen,[41] has been used extensively. Sixteen patients out of 16 experimentally inoculated exhibited a positive reaction. However, it has seemed at times that the reaction was not very sensitive.[2] At present, it is possible to obtain more specific antigens from cultures on embryonated eggs or on cell lines.[7, 37b]

These antibodies appear two to three weeks after clinical onset. At about the fifth to the sixth weeks they reach a rather low maximum titer (from $1/4$ to $1/64$), which decreases slowly and is nil several months later.

Neutralizing Antibodies. While the fluorescent and complement-fixing antibodies reveal infection, the neutralizing antibodies, which were the first to be known, reflect immunity.

They appear late, from six weeks to two months after onset, but their presence can be shown for six months to five years or more.

These antibodies, when placed in contact with the virus, neutralize its noxious effects. Proving their presence, however, is a rather laborious matter.

The surest test is intracerebral inoculation of mice. It requires a strain of mice of known sensitivity, free from natural infection, and a reference virus the titer of which has been measured repeatedly. Several dilutions of virus are placed in contact (two hours at 37° C.) with the serum under study as well as with a negative normal serum and a positive experimental one. Each mixture is inoculated into six mice, as are also the dilutions of pure virus in another series. The decrease in titer due to the serum under study is calculated on the basis of the mortality rate. One should bear in mind that some sera that are considered "normal" have an inhibitory action.

The neutralization reaction has recently been modified by the use of the property the virus has of causing a local swelling when injected into the *plantar cushion* of mice. Serum containing neutralizing antibodies inhibits this swelling.[16b] The titer is the highest dilution that decreases this swelling by 75 per cent or more as compared to the control sera (sera of normal and immunized rabbits, and normal human serum).[11]

DIFFERENTIAL DIAGNOSIS

L.C.M. virus is not antigenically related to any known virus. Viruses very similar to that of L.C.M. have been observed,[13, 21c, 25, 39] but they usually did not show cross-immunity with L.C.M.

PROPHYLAXIS

Prophylaxis rests on the identification of foci of contaminated mice and on strict precautions in laboratories where the virus is used. Under some epidemiological conditions, it is necessary to search for infection among dogs, rodents, or cattle and for the possible role of ticks or mosquitoes.

The infectious agent resists 0.5 per cent phenol but is inactivated by heat (20° to 58° C.), 0.05 per cent formol, many detergents, and ultraviolet rays. Various experimental *vaccines* have been prepared, but they have not been clinically tested. There remains to be mentioned *interference* phenomena of possible, but as yet entirely undemonstrated, applicability in prophylaxis. Interference is observed between the L.C.M. agent and Rickettsia, as well as various viruses: poliovirus, hamster MM virus, Rauscher's leukemia and guinea pig L2 C leukemia viruses, vesicular stomatitis, and the viruses of eastern equine encephalomyelitis. On the contrary, the action of the rabies virus is enhanced.

TREATMENT

Although in a few cases sulfonamides or aureomycin has apparently brought about improvements, no chemotherapeutic agent is known to have any action on the L.C.M. agent. However, some vegetal extracts recently isolated in China have proved very active in mice.[14] Deficiency in folic acid is an aggravating factor in mice. The results of preventive serotherapy in mice have sometimes been positive, sometimes negative. Serotherapy fails as a curative treatment, probably because of the meningeal barrier.[30]

Thymectomy,[22] administration of antithymocyte serum early in the course of infection,[15b] and various immunodepressive treatments (α-methopterin, guanazole, 500 r irradiation the day before inoculation)[16] protect the mouse against a lethal dose of L.C.M. and inhibit lesions while the virus circulates in the blood.

This has led some authors to infer that the virus itself is harmless (in addition, it is not always cytopathogenic) and that the illness is due only to the phenomena connected with the immunological response.[16] This interpretation may be questioned, since the phenomenon is peculiar to the mouse, and the transplantation of competent cells induces a marked immunological reaction without causing manifestations of the disease.[44] Nevertheless, these observations could suggest the therapeutic trial of *corticosteroids* in large doses.

Such problems should attract renewed attention to the meningitis of Armstrong's disease.

BIBLIOGRAPHY

A list of references appearing prior to 1946 can be found in Kreis, B.: Chorio-méningite lymphocytaire (maladie d'Armstrong). In Levaditi, C., and Lépine, P.: Les ultra-virus des maladies humaines. Paris, Flammarion, 1964, pp. 877-895.

For details of techniques one can consult Sohier, R.: Chorio-méningite lymphocytaire. In: Diagnostic des maladies à virus. Paris, Flammarion, 1964, pp. 877-895; and Virat, J.: La chorio-méningite lymphocytaire. In: Lépine, P.: Virologic humaine. Paris, Masson et Cie, 1964, pp. 447-462.

Among recent reviews one can consult those by Volkert[44] and by Wilsnack, R. E.: Lymphocytic choriomeningitis. Nat. Cancer Inst. Monogr., *20*:77-86, 1966.

1. Ackermann, R., et al.: Uber die Verbreitung des Virus der lymphozytären Choriomeningitis in West Deutschland. Deutsch. Med. Wschr., *89*:325-328, 1964.
2. Adair, C. V., et al.: Aseptic meningitis, a disease of diverse etiology: Clinical and etiologic studies on 854 cases. Ann. Int. Med., *39*:675-704, 1953.
3. Afzelius-Alm, L.: Aseptic encephalomeningitides in Gothenburg, 1932-1950. Acta Med. Scand., *140*, suppl. 263, 1951.
4. Armstrong, C.: Some recent research in the field of neurotropic viruses with especial reference to lymphocytic choriomeningitis and herpes simplex. Milit. Surgeon, *91*:129-146, 1942.
5. Armstrong, C., and Lillie, R. D.: Experimental lymphocytic choriomeningitis of monkeys and mice produced by a virus encountered in studies of the 1933 St. Louis encephalitis epidemic. Public Health Rep., *49*:1019-1027, 1934.
6. Baum, S. G., et al.: Epidemic nonmeningitic lymphocytic-choriomeningitis-virus infection. An outbreak in a population of laboratory personnel. New Eng. J. Med., *274*:934-936, 1966.
7. Benson, L. M., et al.: Cytopathogenicity and plaque formation with lymphocytic choriomeningitis virus. Proc. Soc. Exp. Biol. Med., *103*:623-625, 1960.
8. Bieling, R., et al.: Versuch einer klinischen differential-diagnose der abakteriellen meningitis. Ztschr. Kinderh., *72*:85-112, 1952.
9. Blanc, G., et al.: Les petits mammifères sauvages peuvent-ils être porteurs du virus de la chorioméningite lymphocytaire? Arch. Inst. Pasteur Maroc, *6*:125-130, 1961.
10. Chastel, C.: Technique des plages et de l'inhibition des plages en cultures cellulaires pour l'identification du virus de la chorio-méningite lymphocytaire. Ann. Inst. Pasteur (Paris), *109*:874-886, 1965.
11. Cohen, E. P., et al.: Immunofluorescent detection of antibody to lymphocytic choriomeningitis virus in man. J. Immunol., *96*:777-784, 1966.
12. Dalldorf, G., et al.: Choriomeningitis in apartment harboring infected mice. J.A.M.A., *131*:25, 1946.
13. Durand, P.: Virus filtrant pathogène pour l'homme et les animaux de laboratoire et à affinité méningée et pulmonaire. Arch. Inst. Pasteur Tunis, *29*:179-227, 1940.
14. Furusawa, E., et al.: Antiviral activity of higher plants on lymphocytic choriomeningitis. Infection in vitro and in vivo. Proc. Soc. Exp. Biol. Med., *122*:280-282, 1966.
15a. Haas, V. H., et al. Sparing effect of α-methopterin and guanazole in mice infected with virus of lymphocytic choriomeningitis. Virology, *2*:511, 1956.
15b. Hirsch, M. S., Murphy, F. A. Russe, H. P., and Hicklin, R. D.: Effects of anti-thymocyte serum

20

Epidemic Myalgia (Bornholm Disease): Epidemiology and Clinical Description

By B. GRENIER

Of all the infections due to Coxsackie viruses, epidemic myalgia is certainly the one that has been known the longest by names describing the various territories where the most characteristic epidemics have been observed. Daae[7] and Homann[21] identified it for the first time in Norway, in 1872, as an autonomous contagious disease. Finsen,[12] who as early as 1852 had observed similar cases, gave in his thesis for his doctor's degree in 1874 a more detailed description of "epidemic pleurodynia" as the result of an epidemic that had occurred in Iceland. In 1888, Dabney[8] reported the first epidemic to be described on the new continent in Virginia, under the name of "Devil's grip." In 1933, in a now classic monograph, Sylvest[36] compiled all the observations previously published in Europe under the names of Skien, or Bamle, or Drangedal's disease, and, following an epidemic in Bornholm, a Danish Baltic island, ascribed the name of Bornholm disease.

The viral etiology was not established until September, 1948, by Curnen et al.,[6] who isolated the virus now classified as a Coxsackie B1 from a 14-year old boy, suffering from an illness resembling epidemic myalgia. The study of samples collected in 1947 during a typical outbreak of epidemic myalgia in Massachusetts was pursued by Weller et al.,[39] who identified four new strains of Coxsackie virus B1. Finally, from numerous studies of sporadic cases or epidemics, or even laboratory infections, it was possible to confirm the etiological responsibility of the Coxsackie virus B, types 1 to 6.

EPIDEMIOLOGY

Initially described in the northern European countries and in North America, Bornholm disease has been observed at all latitudes in all races. It generally occurs in *minor epidemics* limited to several families, a district, a village, or an island. After isolated cases have been reported over several weeks or months, the epidemic shows a sudden outburst and dies down just as quickly.[34]

The spread of Coxsackie virus B is generally closely connected with that of the enteroviruses. Both are widespread in the warm subtropical regions, probably in relation with poor sanitary conditions.[13, 16] In the temperate zones, their incidence predominates in the summer-autumn period. Epidemics of Bornholm disease are frequently associated with other epidemic or sporadic manifestations of Coxsackie virus B infections, e.g., acute lymphocytic meningitis, "minor disease," "summer influenza," and, less frequently, acute infantile myocarditis. The clinical manifestation of the viral infection is influenced by age,[24] epidemic myalgia being more frequent in the adult; it is much rarer in children, in whom the infection usually takes the form of an acute lymphocytic meningitis with nonspecific characteristics; acute myocarditis due to Coxsackie virus is almost exclusively limited to the neonatal period.

The spread of the Coxsackie virus, like that of the enteroviruses, depends directly or indirectly on a human source. No other natural reservoir has been discovered. The viruses may be found in the throats and especially in the stools of patients or healthy carriers. Fecal elimination may last for one or two months; hence interhuman contamination can occur either directly, through the air via the pharynx, or more likely indirectly, by the fecal-oral pathway. The Coxsackie viruses have been isolated from sewers, drain water, swimming pools, domestic flies, and cockroaches.[29] These passive factors must play a negligible part in the spread of infection, since a common source of contamination has never been demonstrated.[16, 31]

In the community or in the family, as is the case for other enteroviruses, children are the principal agents for spreading infection.[19, 30, 31] In spite of a brief period of viremia during the first days of the disease, no transmission of the Coxsackie viruses by arthropods has yet been demonstrated.

Despite the fact that the same epidemiological characteristics have been witnessed with regard to all the enteroviruses, it seems that there is an inverse relationship between epidemics of poliomyelitis and those of infections due to Coxsackie virus B, probably for reasons similar to those involved in the *in vitro* interference phenomena that exist between these two groups of viruses. In any one region or period of the year, the incidence of paralytic poliomyelitis and that of infections due to Coxsackie B, especially epidemic myalgias, are inversely proportional.

CLINICAL DESCRIPTION

This disease is known by various *synonyms:* Bornholm disease, epidemic myalgia, epidemic pleurodynia, Devil's grip, epidemic diaphragmatic spasm, epidemic acute dry pleurisy, and epidemic muscular rheumatism.

The *incubation* period lasts two to four days.

The *onset* is usually *sudden.* A violent, abrupt *pain* in the thorax, like the stroke of a dagger, may occur while the patient is at work or at any other activity, or it may suddenly wake the patient from sleep. Less frequently the pain occurs progressively. In 25 per cent of the cases it is preceded by one to ten days of fever, anorexia, malaise, stiffness, and upper respiratory tract infection.

The clinical picture of epidemic myalgia emerges more or less rapidly, dominated by the *pain,* which is usually located in the *lower portion of the thorax,* the upper part of the abdomen, and the region of insertion of the diaphragm, near the costal margin. Most often it is lateral, sometimes anterior or posterior. It may be retrosternal, abdominal, scapular, or dorsal; occasionally it is lumbosacral. The pain is extremely intense and excruciating. It is exacerbated by spontaneous paroxysms, between which it becomes attenuated or even disappears. It is enhanced by respiratory movements (and thus blocks respiration) as well as by coughing, changes in position, and walking; even decubitus is uncomfortable when the pain is retrosternal.[20]

Fever is a constant, ranging from 38 to 40° C., with consequent tachycardia. The general condition is altered; the patient becomes agitated in an attempt to find a painless position. *Hypersudation* is a classic manifestation, although not constant.[20] There is pronounced headache, diffuse, frontal or retro-orbital. Multiple pains in the neck, lumbar region, abdomen, and limbs are often mentioned. Coughing is frequent (20 to 30 per cent of the cases). It is painful and non-productive.[11]

Other symptoms are rarer[11]: nausea and vomiting (10 to 15 per cent of the cases); diarrhea (5 to 7 per cent of the cases); shivering (15 to 20 per cent of the cases); and pharyngeal pain (10 per cent of the cases).

The physical examination of the patient, prostrated with pain, reveals in contrast few objective signs: the hemithorax affected is barely mobile. In the painful area a cutaneous hyperesthesia may render even contact with clothing painful. Palpation is painful: the muscles affected are in contracture. Auscultation sounds are generally normal; often (25 per cent of cases, according to Finn et al.[11]) there is a pleural friction rub localized at the base, sometimes bilateral; it may appear within the first few days or in the second week; sometimes transient, in some patients it may be prolonged for two weeks. On radiological examination the thorax appears normal. Usually there is no meningeal syndrome; occasionally there is moderate polyadenopathy or pharyngitis or both; very infrequently, there is a transitory splenomegaly.[11] The deep and cutaneous reflexes are normal; there is no deficiency in muscular strength.

The routine biological examinations show

no characteristic modifications: the blood count is generally normal, and the erythrocyte sedimentation rate is but slightly altered. The urine is normal.

A few authors have reported the results of a muscle biopsy from the painful area[2, 9] generally taken during surgery[33]; the histology of the painful muscle is usually normal.[33] Brown[2] and Lepine et al.[28] have described inflammation and modifications of the muscle fibers with isolation *in situ* of the Coxsackie virus B. These facts do not seem to have been confirmed subsequently.

The outcome is always spontaneously favorable, but sometimes only after several successive outbreaks at intervals of two to eight days. The site of pain may vary during the illness. Cure of the acute phase is usually obtained in three to ten days, but asthenia, discomfort, and tenderness may persist for several weeks. Relapses have been mentioned to occur from two weeks to several months after the initial attack.[26] It seems that accounts of recurrences have never been published, although the antigenic multiplicity of the viruses that can cause Bornholm disease would, theoretically at least, permit these recurrences.

Epidemic myalgia may assume other clinical forms and become associated with various complications. In young children, pain is more apt to be abdominal. Accompanied by a parietal muscular defense mechanism or even by nausea and vomiting, it may be suggestive of an illness requiring surgery. The abdominal viscera are normal.[33] Rarely the pain has a more ectopic localization: e.g., the neck, lumbar region, or limbs. The pain may be of *moderate* intensity.

Finally, the viral infection may cause other clinical manifestations that occur as *complications* of epidemic myalgia. These are, essentially, meningitis and, more rarely, symptoms of the involvement of the central nervous system, pericarditis, and orchitis.

An acute lymphocytic meningitis may occur several days before the epidemic myalgia or accompany it at the onset or during a recurrence of pyrexia. There is stiffness of the neck; the cerebrospinal fluid is clear and the pressure is increased; the lymphocytic cellular reaction reaches 100 to 300 cells per cubic millimeter; the chemical composition of the fluid is barely modified. In these cases it has been possible to isolate the Coxsackie virus B.[18] This meningeal in-

volvement has no effect on the prognosis of the disease; it ceases spontaneously in eight to ten days.

Sometimes, especially in young children, the myalgia may be moderate and occur in an atypical or variable site: the clinical picture, dominated by meningeal symptoms, may be mistaken for a nonparalytic poliomyelitis. There is never any muscular deficiency in epidemic myalgia.

It should be remembered that epidemics of Bornholm disease are often associated with those of acute aseptic meningitis due to Coxsackie virus B. The incidence of meningitis in patients suffering from epidemic pleurodynia is low, in the neighborhood of 3 to 5 per cent.[5]

Symptoms of an actual neurological affection, such as vertigo, photophobia, convulsions, or delirium, are observed even less frequently.[11]

An acute pericarditis, occurring at the same time as the first outbreak or with a recurrence, may be reflected by retrosternal pain that is more marked by changes in position, by pericardial rub, and by modifications of the electrocardiogram.[18] It is cured spontaneously in four to six days. It is known that the Coxsackie virus B, in children as well as in adults, is able to cause epidemics of acute primary pericarditis.[26]

Acute curable myocarditis and pleuritic exudation have been described.

The occurrence of *orchitis* in the adult has been mentioned by Sylvest[36] and by Warin et al.[38] It is not infrequent (2 to 3 per cent on the average). It affects only the adult; it is a complication that occurs relatively late, usually concurrent with the first or second relapse; the temperature becomes elevated again, sometimes with a renewal of the thoracic myalgias. One testicle becomes enlarged and sensitive, and inflammation often spreads to the epididymis. Spontaneous abatement takes place in three to five days. The second testicle may be affected two to three days after the first. No after-effects have been mentioned, nor any secondary atrophy of the testicles. A Coxsackie virus B5 has been isolated from a testicular biopsy taken during the acute phase of the orchitis.[26]

The possibility of an *acute pancreatitis* may be suggested by the presence of violent transfixing epigastric or left subcostal pain, with marked general involvement and vomiting. This is confirmed by the fact that experimental infection with Coxsackie virus B can cause an acute pancreatitis. Indeed, a significant increase in the serum amylase level has sometimes been noted in these patients apart from any infection with mumps.[30] Certainly a pancreatic involvement by the Coxsackie virus B is quite rare in man even when there is violent epigastric pain.

Finally, epidemic myalgia may sometimes be accompanied by an erythematous or purpuric cutaneous eruption[3, 17] and by arthralgias of the ankles, knees, wrists, or fingers.[11]

CLINICAL DIAGNOSIS

The clinical form of Bornholm disease and the usual conditions under which it occurs nearly always enable one to establish the diagnosis without the assistance of biological examinations. But great care must be taken to eliminate numerous other painful illnesses that are more frequent or more serious than they first appear to be. Depending on the age of the patient and the site of the pain one should consider the possibility of pleurisy, spontaneous pneumothorax, or pneumonia; pulmonary infarction or acute pericarditis; myocardial infarction or an attack of angina (both of which are suggested by the sudden intensity of the pain and by the intensity of the general symptoms, particularly the subsequent asthenia); biliary colic or acute pancreatitis; or, finally, appendicitis (some patients with pleurodynia have even been subjected to unjustified surgery).

VIROLOGICAL DIAGNOSIS

Biological confirmation is indispensable to establish the clinical diagnosis and confirm the viral spread in the surroundings.

All the various antigenic types of Coxsackie virus B, from 1 to 6, may be the cause of Bornholm disease. Other enteroviruses infrequently may be the direct cause of an identical clinical picture: Coxsackie A types 4, 6, and 10, and ECHO types 6, 8, and 9.[26] But epidemic myalgia is the most typical manifestation and the most characteristic of the infections due to Coxsackie virus B.

The virological diagnosis is based on the isolation and identification of the virus and on the simultaneous serological response (cf. Chapter 3B).

TREATMENT OF EPIDEMIC MYALGIA

In the absence of any therapeutic agent active against the enteroviruses, treatment can only be symptomatic and aims essentially at relieving the pain.

Acetylsalicylic acid has little effect and increases hypersudation. The more active analgesics may be used in the severe forms. Cortisone treatment, which experimentally aggravates infections by Coxsackie viruses, is ineffective and would seem to be contraindicated[9] in the case of Bornholm disease, in which the evolution is always benign.

BIBLIOGRAPHY

1. Artenstein, M. S., Cadigan, F. C., Jr., and Buescher, E. L.: Clinical and epidemiological features of Coxsackie Group B virus infections. Ann. Int. Med., *63*:597-603, 1965.
2. Brown, N.: Muscle biopsy and ACTH in Coxsackie virus. New York J. Med., *53*:2994-2996, 1953.
3. Candy, J. P.: Petechiae and fever; Infection with Coxsackie virus group B type 3: Case report. Clin. Pediat., *2*:187-188, 1963.
4. Cramblett, H. G., Moffet, H. L., Black, J. P., Shulenberger, H., Smith, A., and Colonna, C. T.: Coxsackie virus infections: Clinical and laboratory studies. J. Pediat., *64*:406-414, 1964.
5. Curnen, E. D.: The Coxsackie viruses. Pediat. Clin. N. Amer., *7*:903-925, 1960.
6. Curnen, E. D., Shaw, E. W., and Melnick, J. L.: Disease resembling nonparalytic poliomyelitis associated with a virus pathogenic for infant mice. J.A.M.A., *141*:894. 1949.
7. Daae, A.: Epidemi i Drangedal of akut Muskelrheumatisme udbredt ned Smitte. Norsk mag. f. laegevidensk, *2*(n.s.):409-413, 529-542, 1872; cited by Huebner et al.[22]
8. Dabney, W. C.: Account of epidemic resembling Dengue, which occurred in and around Charlottesville and University of Virginia in June 1888. Amer. J. Med. Sci., *96*:488, 1888.
9. Desse, G.: Maladie de Bornholm. Sem. Hop. Paris, *29*:3539-3540, 1953.
10. Felici, A., and Gregorig, B.: Contribution to the study of diseases in Italy caused by Coxsackie B group of viruses: II. Epidemiological, clinical and virological data obtained in the course of a summer outbreak caused by Coxsackie B4 Virus. Arch. Ges. Virusforsch., *9*:317-328, 1959.
11. Finn, J. J., Weller, T. H., and Morgan, H.: Epidemic pleurodynia: Clinical and etiologic studies based on one-hundred and fourteen cases. Ann. Int. Med., *83*:305-321, 1949.
12. Finsen, J.: Iagttagelser angraende Sygdoms-forholdene i Island (Afhandling for den Medicinske Doktorgrad ved Kobenhavns Universitet). Copenhagen, C. A. Reitzels, 1874, pp. 145-151; Cited by Husbener et al.[22]
13. Fox, J. P.: Epidemiological aspects of Coxsackie and Echo virus infections in tropical areas. Amer. J. Public Health, *54*:1134-1142, 1964.

14. Gabinus, O., Gard, S., Johnsson, T. and Pöldre, A.: Studies in the etiology of epidemic pleurodynia (Bornholm disease). I: Clinical and virological observations. Arch. Ges. Virusforsch., *5*:1-13, 1952.

15. Gamble, D. R.: Isolation of Coxsackie viruses from normal children aged 0-5 years. Brit. Med. J., *1*: 16-18, 1962.

16. Gelfand, H. M.: The occurrence in nature of the Coxsackie and Echo viruses. Progr. Med. Virol., *3*:193-244, 1961.

17. Ginevri, A. and Felici, A.: Contribution to the study of diseases in Italy caused by Coxsackie B group of viruses. I. Clinical and virological aspects of an outbreak of Bornholm disease. Arch. Ges. Virusforsch., *9*:310-316, 1959.

18. Gordon, R. B., Lennette, E. H., and Sandrock, R.: The varied clinical manifestations of Coxsackie virus infections. Observations and comments on an outbreak in California. Arch. Int. Med., *103*: 63-75, 1959.

19. Heggie, A. D., et al.: An outbreak of a summer febrile disease caused by Coxsackie B2-virus. Amer. J. Public Health, *50*:1342-1348, 1960.

20. Hervouet, D., Herbouiller, M., Bodic, L. and Orieux J.: Myalgie épidémique. J. Med. Nantes, *5*:159-167, 1965.

21. Homann, C.: Om en i Kargerø Laegedistrikt herskende smitsom Febersygdom. Norsk. mag. f. laegevidensk. 2(n.s.):542-545, 1872, cited by Huebner et al.[22]

22. Huebner, R. J., Risser, J. A., Bell, J. A., Beeman, E. A., Beigelman, P. M., and Strong, J. C.: Epidemic pleurodynia in Texas: A study of 22 cases. New England J. Med., *248*:267-274, 1953.

23. Johnson, R. T., and Bvescher, E. L.: The laboratory in the study of enterovirus epidemics. Amer. J. Public Health, *50*:937-941, 1960.

24. Johnsson, T.: Family infections by Coxsackie viruses. Arch. Ges. Virusforsch., *5*:384-400, 1954.

25. Johnsson, T.: Studies on the etiology of Bornholm disease (epidemic pleurodynia). II. Epidemiological observations. Arch. Ges. Virusforsch., *5*:401, 1954.

26. Kibrick, S.: Current status of Coxsackie and Echo viruses in human disease. Progr. Med. Virol., *6*:27-70, 1964.

27. Kilbourne, E. D.: The Coxsackie viruses and human disease. Amer. J. Med. Sci., *224*:93-102, 1952.

28. Lepine, P., Desse, G., and Sautter, V.: Biopsies musculaires et isolement du virus Coxsackie chez l'homme. Bull. Acad. Nat. Med. (Paris), *136*: 66, 1952.

29. Lerner, A. M., and Finland, M.: Coxsackie viral infections. Arch. Int. Med., *108*:329-334, 1961.

30. Murphy, A. M., and Simmul, R.: Coxsackie B4 virus infections in New-South Wales during 1962. Med. J. Australia, 2:443-445, 1964.

31. Paffenbarger, R. S., Jr., Berg, G., Clarke, N. A., Stevenson, R. E., Pooler, B. G. and Hyde, R. T.: Viruses and illnesses in a boys' summer camp. Amer. J. Hyg., *70*:254-274, 1959.

32. Siegel, W, Spencer, F. J., Smith, D. J., Toman, J. M., Skinner, W. F., and Marx, M. B.: Two new variants of infection with Coxsackie virus group B Type 5 in young children. New England J. Med. *268*:1210-1216, 1963.

33. Sneierson, H.: Pleurodynia (Coxsackie virus infection goup B) and acute abdominal condition in children. Amer. J. Surg., *88*:393-398, 1954.

34. Surjus, A.: Les maladies à virus Coxsackie: étude générale. Sem. Hop. Paris, *10*:1587-1598, 1962.

35. Surjus, A., Lausecker, C., Reeb, E. and Lavillaureix, J.: Les maladies à virus Coxsackie en Alsace. Epidémiologie et gravité au cours des années 1956 à 1961. Sem. Hop. Paris, *11*:149-161, 1963.

36. Sylvest, E.: Epidemic Myalgia: Bornholm disease. London, Oxford University Press, 1934.

37. Walker, S. J., McNaughton, G. A., and McLean, D. M.: Coxsackie B5 virus infections in children: Toronto, 1958. Canad. J. Public Health, *50*:461-467, 1959.

38. Warin, J. F., Davies, J. B. M., Sanders, F. K., and Vizoso, A. D.: Oxford epidemic of Bornholm disease, 1951. Brit. Med. J., *1*:1345-1351, 1957.

39. Weller, T. H., Enders, J. F., Buckingham, M., and Finn, J. J., Jr.: The etiology of epidemic pleurodynia: A study of two viruses isolated from a typical outbreak. J. Immunol., *65*:337, 1950.

PART III

Viral Infections in Which the Predominating Manifestations Affect the Digestive System

21

Virus Infections with Manifestations Predominating in the Digestive Tract Proper

By MARCEL LELONG

A large number of viral infections can be accompanied, notably during the invasive stage, by digestive manifestations which generally form a part of a general infectious syndrome.

We shall consider here only those viral diseases in which manifestations involving the digestive system clearly predominate, the patient being seen first for such symptoms.

From this standpoint, in the present state of our knowledge only two chapters can be clinically individualized: viral stomatitis, pharyngitis, and angina; and viral enterocolitis (or diarrhea).

VIRAL STOMATITIS, PHARYNGITIS, AND ANGINA

In viral stomatitis, pharyngitis, and angina, the clinical manifestations affect the oral cavity and the pharynx. Their appearance is highly suggestive of the viral nature of the disease in question. Such is the case with *measles, rubella, varicella, smallpox, herpes,* and even *influenza*. These diseases are described in special chapters to which the reader is referred.

We shall devote our attention more specially to herpangina, a more recently recognized clinical entity, and to foot-and-mouth disease, a very rare infection in man

but one that has, in some cases, been unquestionably confirmed by laboratory data.

HERPANGINA

History. The term "herpangina" was coined in 1924 by Zahorsky[112] to designate a clinical entity distinct from herpetic angina. The clinical manifestations reminded him of case reports he had published in 1920,[111] but which at the time he had related to herpes. In February of the same year Marfan[85] described and illustrated with nine personal cases a type of angina which he called "pustular angina," which he definitely separated from herpes and considered to be a different disease due to "some unknown virus." These two authors must therefore be given credit for the clinical individualization of the syndrome. Of the two names suggested (both equally poorly chosen), herpangina has been internationally adopted, in spite of the regrettable confusion with herpes that it perpetuates; for this reason it would be preferable to speak of Marfan-Zahorsky's angina, although the publications of these two authors were soon forgotten.

In 1939, Levine et al.[80] revived interest in the question by publishing under the title "Vesicular Pharyngitis and Stomatitis" a report on 186 cases of an epidemic which they had difficulty separating from herpes. In 1941 Breese[36] reported an epidemic of 28 cases of "aphthous pharyngitis" similar to those of Levine et al., the etiology of which had remained unsolved. To Huebner and his co-workers[68, 69, 70] must be given the credit of having shown, by clinical, epidemiological, and virological studies carried out systematically since 1949, the responsibility (which they believed to be specific) of Coxsackie group A viruses. Similar findings have since been obtained in many countries in America, Europe, and Asia. In France, Gerbeaux et al.[55] published in 1960 a clinical and virological study on an epidemic in a hospital, with isolation of a Coxsackie A4 virus.

It should be mentioned, however, that more recently, in 1965, Cherry and Jahn[5] broadened the etiologic spectrum of herpangina by incriminating Coxsackie group B viruses as well as ECHO viruses.

Conditions Under Which Herpangina Occurs. Herpangina is a seasonal disease, occurring mainly in summer; it is most frequent from June to October. It preferentially affects children under age three.

Although sporadic cases exist, reports emphasize its epidemic nature, most epidemics occurring in collectivities such as hospitals, nurseries, and families. When a case occurs in a collectivity, the epidemic is sudden and massive; it rapidly assumes an explosive character. Many epidemics have been reported in the United States, Cuba, Canada, Brazil, Australia, and Japan, as well as in Europe, particularly Sweden and France.

Incubation Period. The incubation period is short; according to Huebner, it does not exceed three to five days.

Clinical Picture. In the typical form of the disease the onset is abrupt and is marked by a rise in temperature that is usually moderate, 38.5° to 39° C. (101.4° to 102.2° F.), but may reach 39° to 40° C. (102.2° to 104.0° F.). Fever lasts two to three days. It may be accompanied by cephalalgia, vomiting, chest or abdominal pains, myalgias, or convulsions.

In two-thirds of the cases dysphagia draws attention to the throat, where the characteristic lesions are found. Against a diffuse erythematous pharyngeal background which is more pronounced along the free border of the palatum molle and on the uvula appear round, hemispherical, or even conical vesicles 1 to 2 mm. in diameter. Encircled by a small red areola, they are grayish white and contain an opalescent fluid. They are not numerous, five or six up to 15 at the most. They are located on the arcus palato-

glossus, on the uvula, more rarely on the tonsils and the posterior wall of the pharynx, and very exceptionally inside the cheeks and on the tongue. They are usually bilateral, irregularly distributed on either side of the median line, isolated and not clustered, never confluent. They may be present on one side only.

The lesions run their course rapidly. In a few hours (48 at the most) they pass from the erythematous to the vesicular stage, the contents of the vesicles being clear at first and then becoming cloudy and opaque (pustules). Rupture of the vesicopustules leaves exulceratio simplex or small, round, grayish ulcerations which heal in a few days after defervescence. There is little or no hypertrophy of the submandibular lymph nodes.

Blood count is normal except when there is a bacterial superinfection.

Atypical forms can be observed: exclusively erythematous forms without any vesicles or ulcerations. There may be acute lymphonodular pharyngitis[19a] with lesions whitish to yellowish in color, solid and not vesicular and surrounded by a zone of erythema, 3 to 6 mm. in diameter. It does not ulcerate even superficially. The most frequent locations of lesions were on the uvula, anterior pillars, and posterior pharynx. There also exist purely febrile forms reduced to solely systemic signs; forms with cutaneous eruptions (erythema, papules, vesicles); forms complicated by diarrhea, parotitis, laryngeal dyspnea, or meningoencephalitis; and asymptomatic forms, i.e., detectable only by serological reactions.

The forms with cutaneous eruptions may be compared with the hand-foot-and-mouth disease described in 1958 by Robinson et al.[17] in connection with an epidemic in a suburb of Toronto, Canada. Epidemics of this disease were subsequently reported by other authors: Magoffin et al. in California (1959); Alsop et al.[2] in Birmingham (1959); and Burtt Richardson and Leibovitz[4] in Tucson, Arizona (1965). All these authors attributed the syndrome to a Coxsackie A group 16 virus.

Clinical Diagnosis. The typical forms offer no difficulties, and thrush, erythematous or erythemopultaceous tonsillitis, varicella, and even herpetic angina are easily eliminated.

Virological Diagnosis. Virological diagnosis is based on the isolation of the virus and on a significant increase in the serum titer of complement-fixing or neutralizing antibodies.

The virus is isolated either from the stools (or a rectal swab) or from a throat swab. The virus is too scarce to be found easily in the throat after the third day of the disease, but it persists longer in the stools, about three weeks and, exceptionally, one to two months. During epidemics the virus can be found in healthy individuals who are in contact with the patients (46 per cent of the contacts, according to Huebner). In summer it can be found in 1.5 to 7.5 per cent of individuals who are healthy or apparently free from disease.

The rise in titer of complement-fixing or neutralizing antibodies reaches a maximum during the month that follows infection; the titer remains elevated for several weeks or even up to three or four months.

The first epidemics that were studied (Huebner,[68, 69, 70] Parrott et al.,[14, 15] Gerbeaux et al.,[55] etc.) showed the part played by Coxsackie A viruses, type 4 being most frequently involved, followed by types 2, 5, 6, 7, 8, 9, 10, 16, and 22, so that the herpangina syndrome apparently could be considered specific of this group of viruses.

But as the number of investigations increased, the "etiologic spectrum" (Cherry and Jahn[5]) of the disease broadened, Coxsackie B viruses being reported, and then ECHO viruses. In 1960 Lerner et al.[10] found Coxsackie B type 3 in two cases. In studying an epidemic of eight cases, Cherry and Jahn[5] found the following viruses: ECHO 9, ECHO 17 (two cases), Coxsackie B4, Coxsackie B1, Coxsackie A9, and Coxsackie A16 (two cases). Many other authors have reported similar findings: Marchessault et al.[12] (Coxsackie B2), Agar et al.[1] (Coxsackie B2), Lerner et al.[10] (Coxsackie B3), Felici and Gregorig[6] (Coxsackie B4), Artenstein et al.[3] (Coxsackie B4 and B5), Glick and Stroud[8] (Coxsackie B3), St. Geme and Prince[19] (Coxsackie B5), Reinhard[16] (Coxsackie B1, B5, A7, and A9 and ECHO 9), Lepow et al.[9] (ECHO 9), Sabin[18] (ECHO 9), and Neva et al.[13] (ECHO 16).

In the hand-foot-and-mouth syndrome — which doubtless is a herpangina with associated cutaneous lesions — the following viruses have been found: Coxsackie A type 4: Magoffin et al.; Coxsackie A type 5: Flewett et al.[7]; Coxsackie A type 16: Burtt Richardson and Leibovitz,[4] Robinson et al.,[17] and Alsop et al.[2]

Treatment. The prognosis of herpangina is excellent, with spontaneous cure within a few days. There is no known specific treatment.

FOOT-AND-MOUTH DISEASE (APHTHOUS FEVER)

Foot-and-mouth disease is an infectious illness caused by a specific virus to which cloven-footed animals are particularly sensitive: horned cattle, goats, sheep, and pigs are susceptible among the domestic animals, as are deer, bison, and antelopes among the wild species.

In receptive animals the disease is contagious and spreads very rapidly in epizootics which may be extremely severe. It is characterized by a generally febrile state and by papular and papulovesicular eruptions on the mucous membranes and the skin which may easily become secondarily infected and cause suppuration. The seat of these eruptions is usually in the mouth and around the nails or the hooves. The mortality rate is usually moderate. Most often the infection in due course attains self-cure; it may cause visceral injuries and a protracted weakening of the affected animal, which has a poor milk yield although it generally recovers. A foot-and-mouth epizootic is always an economic scourge for the area where it occurs. These facts are incontestable in veterinary pathology.

What is the position of aphthous fever in man? What is the relationship between "aphthous stomatitis" or the "aphthae" described in humans and foot-and-mouth disease in animals, particularly cattle? In other words, is the foot-and-mouth virus also pathogenic in man?

For the authorities before 1940 (Lebailly[23] and Nicolle and Bazolet[25]) the question was solved: bovine foot-and-mouth disease was not transmissible to man and aphthous stomatitis was not transmissible to cattle. New facts observed in the necessary critical light, i.e., by experimental research and the diagnostic facilities available to modern virology, make it necessary today to make a little less absolute the affirmations of the past. Although it is true, by and large, that man is but slightly receptive to the foot-and-mouth virus, he may still be affected, as confirmed by the excellent studies carried out in Great Britain.

Epidemiology. Foot-and-mouth disease is a cosmopolitan zoonotic disease. There are seven immunologically distinct virus types, three of which are currently confined to Africa. The infectious particle contains RNA. Serious epizootics generally break out among cattle, and the epidemic wave surges very rapidly. The years 1937-1939 were marked in almost all European countries by severe epizootics among cattle and pigs.

Systematic mass vaccination campaigns have much reduced the extent of epizootics. Virus inactivated with formaldehyde and combined with various adjuvants is used today. Immunity lasts only four to eight months, so that yearly vaccinations that protect against the type that is epizootic are necessary. Prophylaxis by vaccination is not used in some countries such as Great Britain, where a most severe panepizootic exploded fairly recently.

Human receptivity is certainly poor, for, whatever the severity of epizootics, human cases are few and isolated. Human resistance is normally so high that several attempts to infect humans artificially by injecting blister fluid from animals have failed: no lesions were produced and virus could not be recovered from the volunteers' blood at any time after the injections. Foot-and-mouth disease in man raises complex and unsolved pathogenic problems. Armstrong et al.[20] considered the possibility that in some cases preexisting skin disorders have reduced the normally very high human resistance to infection by foot-and-mouth disease virus.

Humans may be contaminated by the content of the vesicles or the saliva of animals, and very rarely by the stools or the urine.

The skin, especially if it is damaged, may become the port of entry for the virus. Infection by oral intake of raw milk from sick animals, or even by the consumption of the meat of slaughtered sick animals, has certainly occurred. Milk infection may be the result of viremia or consequential to infection of the cow's udder. The virus could be preserved for a fairly long time in raw milk left standing at normal temperature. Human contamination may also be caused by soiled household implements. Contamination from man to man has not yet been proved.

Nearly all reported cases have been due to type O virus, though one case due to type C virus has been recorded (Eissner et al.[22]).

Anatomical and Clinical Picture. The disease in humans is quite exceptional in its *apparent clinical and typical form.*

The *lesions* are located in the alimentary tract, although not exclusively; they may also affect the skin and the viscera. To consider only the alimentary tract, the foot-and-mouth virus causes stomatitis both in man and in animals. The lesions are first vesicles, then pustules. They are localized in the epithelium and mucous Malpighian body. Although there are only a few reports of autopsies performed on humans who have died of foot-and-mouth disease, it can be stated that the foot-and-mouth virus produces both in man and in animals aphthous pustules all along the alimentary canal and also involves the respiratory tract, the liver, the kidneys, the spleen, the muscles, and the myocardium (steatosis-necrosis).

The average *incubation period* is from three to eight days; it may last a minimum of two days and a maximum of eighteen days.

The first clinical signs are not very characteristic: general discomfort, weariness, headaches; the mucous membranes feel dry and burning, especially the mouth and throat. Examination shows that the tongue, mouth, and throat are reddish. The temperature rises to 39-40° C., accompanied by tachycardia and arterial hypotension.

The primary *vesicular pustules* appear at the point of inoculation; in the mouth in the case of contamination by raw milk or meat, and on the hands in the case of a farmer who was infected at milking by the lesions on the cow's udder.

It is possible to make a theoretical distinction between a primary phase of inoculation followed by a secondary phase of viremia.

The *aphthae* are more particularly located on the lips, in the mouth, on the tongue, and in the pharynx. Quite often they overflow on the nostrils and the neighboring skin. Generalized erythema has also been noted, predominating on the terminal parts of the members.

The aphthae are vesicles a few millimeters in size, of round or oval shape. They seldom merge. At first they contain a clear serous fluid. This becomes less transparent and is transformed into pus. The vesicles are extremely fragile, and their rupture leaves behind crevices or ulcers blood red at the bottom. These aphthae are very painful and extremely sensitive to all irritants; they cause intense dysphagia accompanied by a burning sensation and abundant salivation. The pain may render any food intake through the mouth impossible. There are no hematological data on these patients. It may be assumed that the red blood cell count is normal or decreased and that leukocytosis exceeds 10,000 to 12,000 only in cases of secondary infection. In the latter cases polymorphonucleosis is increased. Moderate eosinophilia has been noticed during convalescence.

The clinical period of the disease lasts from ten to 15 days. Convalescence is protracted after recovery. Nails have been observed to fall out and new growth takes several months. Convalescence is hampered by difficulties in food intake.

This is the typical form; it is extremely rare. *Varied clinical forms* may be observed. First, there are *complicated forms:* an ataxic-adynamic form, a form with merging and repeated eruptions, a form accompanied by intense glossitis and edema of the glottis, a tracheobronchial or bronchopneumonic form, a gastroenteric form, a hepatic form accompanied by jaundice, a myocardial form, and hemorrhagic forms.

These complications are frequently caused by secondary infections; the risk of a secondary infection is particularly great in a rural environment.

Simple or *attenuated* forms in man are probably much more frequent than realized (an apparently inexplicable fever, aphthae in the mouth, and so on, but inapparent infection seems to be rare. Neutralizing antibodies have been reported in a few laboratory workers exposed over long periods to a high level of infection. But during the Northumberland epizootic, sera were collected from five veterinary officers who had been in contact with infected cattle and from 12 members of the staff of the Animal Virus Research Institute. All samples were negative except that of one staff member (Armstrong et al.[20]).

Diagnosis. There are various methods of diagnosis.

(1) *Isolation of virus by inoculation* of the vesicle content into an animal. This is accomplished by cutaneous scarification of a guinea pig or, even better, a piglet. If the foot-and-mouth virus is involved, the vesicles form within four to five days (Schneider, Magnusson, cited by Mohr[24]). Virus isolation in monolayer cultures of calf thyroid cells was described by Snowdon.[27]

(2) Use of the *complement-fixation test* has been described by Traub and Mohlmann.

The titer obtained may be quite high in man, but the value of this reaction remains debatable.

(3) Use of *neutralization tests.*

(4) Use of *projection tests on guinea pigs.* A small quantity of serum from the suspect patient is injected into two guinea pigs which were previously inoculated with the typical virus. If the reaction is positive the guinea pigs show a complement-fixation reaction (Flaum, Schneider, Magnusson cited by Mohr[24]).

Clinical diagnosis, suspected when vesicular eruption occurs in man during an outbreak of foot-and-mouth disease in cattle, can be accomplished only by laboratory investigations, i.e., isolating virus from vesicular lesions and finding significant titers of specific antibodies.

Indeed, most of the supposed cases of human foot-and-mouth disease are caused by other agents, of which the most important are Coxsackie viruses, usually type A16, occasionally A5 or A10 (see page 000). The lesions caused by these Coxsackie viruses are in some cases so similar to the vesicles of foot-and-mouth disease that the illness is often and misleadingly referred to as "hand-foot-and-mouth disease." This name leads to confusion. Foot-and-mouth disease in man manifests itself by vesicles in the oral mucosa and in the skin of the hands. The lesions caused by Coxsackie viruses are generally more scattered and rarely reach 5 mm. in diameter; they never reach the size (1 to 2 cm. diameter) of lesions on hands infected with foot-and-mouth virus. Isolation of Coxsackie viruses in suckling mice can easily confirm the diagnosis.

In the same way, isolation of herpes virus will confirm the diagnosis of acute herpetic gingivostomatitis. Certain clinical criteria point to herpetic infection: the vesicles are grouped in clusters; they involve the mucocutaneous border line of the lip; they are fairly superficial and almost painless.

Laboratory investigations provide no clue to the diagnosis of nonspecific ulcerations of the oral mucosa often called simply recurrent aphthae; their etiology is unknown. These "aphthae" are small ulcerations which are not very numerous (usually there are only two). They never merge and are strictly localized on the buccogingival mucous membrane. There is no accompanying fever. In women they often appear at the menses. In both male and female patients they often coincide with dental caries and the consumption of "irritating" foods. When these aphthae are numerous the term "aphthous stomatitis is acceptable and is used. This aphthous stomatitis usually has nothing in common with foot-and-mouth disease in cattle.

Of the other diagnostic possibilities, zona has a limited and characteristic topography, and herpangina is also specific. Sometimes the lesions suggest Bazin's hydroa or Fiessinger's syndrome (Stevens-Johnson syndrome).

Prognosis. The prognosis for foot-and-mouth disease in man is generally good, at least in the absence of any secondary complication.

Prophylaxis. Prophylaxis consists primarily in the control of foot-and-mouth disease in animals, particularly cattle. In some countries the veterinary service is responsible for the detection of the animal infection and may call for the necessary police ordinances: slaughter of the infected cattle and isolation of stables. Milk from diseased animals should be consumed only after boiling or pasteurizing. Vaccination of not-yet-infected cattle is certainly to be recommended. Research on a completely satisfactory live attenuated vaccine is still under way.

Treatment. The treatment of infected humans should aim mainly at preventing secondary infections: in this respect, antibiotics and mouth disinfection by rinsing or bathing may be advised (with, for instance, 5 per cent silver nitrate solution or potassium permanganate).

VIRUS DIARRHEAS

The advances in virological techniques during the past few years justify asking whether there are clinically autonomous virus diarrheas, just as there are diarrheas of mycotic, parasitic, or bacterial origin. Many studies have been published on the subject; they are not all equally convincing. Most frequently they deal with epidemics in collectivities, occasionally with sporadic cases, nearly always affecting newborn infants or very young children, more rarely older children, and exceptionally young adults.

In 1949 the possibility of virus diarrheas was raised by the demonstration by Enders et al.[50] of the presence of several types of viruses in the gastrointestinal tract of man.

It should be remembered, however, that the term "enterovirus," though it specifies the level at which the virus was isolated, carries no clinical significance and is far from implying clinical gastrointestinal manifestations; polioviruses, to mention just one example, are involved in gastrointestinal pathology only in exceptional cases.

Do observations and *experiments on animals* furnish any evidence? The existence of virus diarrheas in cats seems to have been proved by Lawrence and Syverton (1939)[76a] and by Hammon and Enders (1939)[64]; in the mouse, by Pappenheimer and Enders (1947),[89] by Pappenheimer and Cheever (1948),[88] and by Cheever and Mueller (1948)[41]; in calves by Baker (1943)[30]; and in piglets by Doyle and Hutchings (1946).[48]

In *man* experimental findings are also suggestive. In 1943 Light and Hodes[81] produced diarrhea in calves by rhinopharyngeal inoculation with a filtrate of feces from newborn infants during an epidemic in nurseries in Baltimore and Washington: 29 passages from one subject to another were carried out successfully; the neutralizing antibodies against the virus were detected both in the infants and in the inoculated calves. The virus could not be isolated either in normal children or in normal calves.

In 1944, by inoculating the cornea of rabbits with a fecal filtrate from infants suffering from diarrhea with stomatitis, Buddingh and Dodd[38] produced conjunctivitis transmissible from one animal to another, and rabbits which ingested suspensions of infected corneas had diarrhea.

In 1947 Gordon et al.[60] reproduced diarrhea with high fever, nausea, and vomiting in human volunteers who had ingested or inhaled filtrates of diarrheic stools, and antibodies were found in the serum of the convalescents.

Pathological histology yielded an interesting observation: in 1947 Pappenheimer and Enders[89] showed the presence of cells with inclusion bodies, and hence a cytopathogenic effect, in the intestinal mucosa of baby mice.

These investigations opened the way to clinical research. In the present state of our knowledge, what *clinical facts* can be correlated with the virological findings?

In this respect it should be noted that the published reports, while containing much virological data, are poor in clinical data.

They use the terms gastroenteritis, enteritis, enterocolitis, and "diarrhea," the latter in most cases being qualified simply by an adjective: "acute" diarrhea (presumably meaning that it lasts only three to four days), "febrile" diarrhea (and therefore accompanied by systemic signs, but not necessarily by severe dehydration), or "epidemic" diarrhea. None of the laboratory tests that a gastroenterologist would demand are mentioned: no accurate description of the stools (only the number of stools is mentioned, and sometimes their watery consistency); no cytological examination of stool smears; no chemical analysis of the stools; no functional explorations or radiological examinations that might reveal involvement of some given segment of the gastrointestinal tract or some specific type of dysfunction. Such a dearth of information makes it impossible for the clinician to identify any characteristic symptoms or syndrome or to establish any consistent correlation between clinical data and a given virus.

The circumstances attending the onset permit definition of only two facts. The first one is relative to the *age* of the patients: they are mostly newborn infants, premature infants, and infants under six months, or under one year. Past the age of one year, cases become rare. Second, outbreaks occur as explosive epidemics with a short incubation period (three to four days); they spread rapidly and are of relatively short duration (five to six weeks). These epidemics occur in centers grouping premature infants, lying-in hospitals, foundling homes, nurseries, hospital wards, large families crowded in small dwellings in the poor and overpopulated sections of large cities, and much less frequently schools or even barracks. Sporadic cases have been reported, as have asymptomatic forms.

Among the enteroviruses that have been incriminated, *poliovirus* types I, II, and III play only a very limited role. Sims Roberts and Thomson[101] have reported epidemics of severe gastroenteritis in the newborn with, in a few cases, encephalitis discovered at autopsy. These facts suggest the possible existence of fulminating forms camouflaged by the picture of acute diarrhea with great dehydration. However, in poliomyelitis, Debré and Thieffry,[46] though they consider that constipation is the rule, admit that in very young children diarrhea may be predominant in the invasion period. Thieffry et al.[104] found diarrhea in 11 per cent of 250 cases of paralytic poliomyelitis in children aged two to 18 months; diarrhea can be profuse, giving rise to a picture of acute dehydration with toxicosis. The existence of purely gastroenteritic forms of poliomyelitis without neurological signs has not been demonstrated.

ECHO viruses have been held responsible for diarrheic episodes having in common their epidemic character and the isolation from the stools of a virus belonging to this group. The types reported vary from one epidemic to another and from one social level to another.

In a study of the Cincinnati epidemic carried out during the summers of 1955 and 1956, Ramos-Alvarez and Sabin[96, 97] reported the following facts: of 253 children under four years of age, 153 had diarrhea, the stools of the remaining 100 being normal. All belonged to the lowest socioeconomic level; they were examined either as private patients or during hospitalization. The viruses most frequently associated with diarrhea were ECHO types 6, 7, and 14.

The same year, in July, 1956, Eichenwald et al.[49] studied an epidemic of diarrhea that broke out in the nursery for premature infants in a New York hospital. Twelve of the 21 infants had mild diarrhea without appreciable impairment of the general condition, and they recovered in three to five days. Four days later the epidemic spread to infants aged eight days to two months in a neighboring ward. None of these children was a virus carrier before admission. An ECHO virus type 18 was isolated in their stools, and at the same time an increase was noted in the specific neutralizing antibodies in their serum. The same virus was found in the stools of two nurses, and the serum of one of them also showed an increased titer of antibodies against ECHO virus type 18.

Lépine et al.[78] described an epidemic occurring in a nursery in July-August, 1959. On July 19 two children aged nine and 14 months, respectively, were suddenly affected by "gastroenteritis" with fever, bloody mucous diarrhea, and signs of dehydration. Two days later a 16-month-old baby presented the same symptoms. The stools of all three children contained an ECHO virus type 14. The same virus was detected in the stools of seven of the 11 ward mates of the patients, and three weeks later in two children in another ward one floor above. Specific antibodies were found in only two of the three patients and in the seven other infected children in the same ward, but at very low titers. Lépine et al. explain that these low titers may be due either to the fact that children of that age have little antibody-producing capacity, or to the low antigenic potency of ECHO virus type 14.

In 1960 Klein et al.[75] reported a small epidemic of gastroenteritis in three adults, two of whom worked together in the same laboratory. The illness, marked by brutal onset with vomiting, abdominal pains, and watery stools, lasted only 24 hours. An ECHO virus type 11 was found in the stools of two of the patients, with the corresponding antibodies in the serum; the serum of the third patient showed a significant increase in antibodies specific for the same virus. Samples from six healthy subjects in contact with the patients were negative.

In Italy, Felici and Archetti[51] described in 1960 an epidemic of diarrhea with fever, vomiting, and catarrhal pharyngitis in 109 children, most of whom were under five years of age. In virological tests on 53 of them, five viruses were isolated (two ECHO type 9, three Coxsackie B type 3). During the same epidemic Grosso and Bergamini[62] tested 15 stool and pharyngeal samples and 17 serum samples from patients hospitalized for diarrhea and found an ECHO virus type 14 in ten of the patients and an ECHO type 9 in seven.

In Italy also, Bergamini and Bonetti[33] described an outbreak in a nursery of acute gastroenteritis that affected six of 13 children aged four to 11 months. Two of the youngest (aged four and six months) died. An ECHO virus type 11 was found in the pharynx and stools of five of the patients; the specific antibody titer of the serum increased (except in the two fatal cases, where a second sample could not be obtained). ECHO virus type 11 was also found in the stools of two normal children living in contact with the patients.

Worms[107] reported three cases of sporadic gastroenteritis in infants aged three, four, and eight months, with mild diarrhea and fever, without dehydration or serious impairment of the general condition, and with rapid progress toward recovery. ECHO viruses types 18, 13, and 21, respectively, were isolated in the stools, and in all three cases the titer of serum antibodies increased significantly.

Some authors have incriminated *Coxsackie viruses* in widely scattered geograph-

ical areas. Group A viruses were accused much more often than those of group B.

In Brazil, in 1952, Travassos[105] isolated a Coxsackie A in nine of 20 children with gastroenteritis. In Finland, in 1955 Pohjanpelto[93] isolated a Coxsackie A (most frequently type 4) in 4.4 per cent of 187 patients with diarrhea. In the United States, in 1955, Parrott[90] isolated four strains of Coxsackie A type 4 in 165 children with diarrhea. In France, in 1964, Marie et al.[86] attributed to a Coxsackie A type 9 an ulcerohemorrhagic enterocolitis in a newborn infant. In 1967, Gerbeaux et al.[56] attributed to a Coxsackie A virus a hospital epidemic of 13 cases. In Hamburg, in 1960, Prenzel and Lennartz[94] examined the stools of 60 children with diarrhea (of whom 66.6 per cent were under two years of age) and in one case found a Coxsackie B type 2 and in another case a Coxsackie B type 4. In each of these cases the virus was accompanied by *E. coli* 0 86, and the authors are quite cautious in their conclusions.

Pelon et al.[92] described an outbreak of diarrhea in Costa Rica which lasted from February, 1963, to September, 1963, in successive outbursts. Twelve communities of equal population (3000 inhabitants each) were studied. Diarrhea was defined as three or more watery stools per 24 hours in children over one year, and six or more watery stools per 24 hours in children under one year. By these criteria, 1811 children under 10 years were retained and 1584 stool specimens were examined in comparison with those of nondiarrheic children. It was found that 75 per cent of the patients with diarrhea were excreting a virus; in 47 per cent of the cases this was a Coxsackie B, most frequently types 4 and 5. In 25 per cent of the cases a virus other than Coxsackie B was found, and when diarrhea lasted more than 24 to 72 hours the percentage of Coxsackie B decreased and the proportion of the other viruses increased.

Among the other virus groups accused of causing diarrhea, the adenoviruses have been thought by some authors to be responsible for summer epidemics of diarrhea, whether or not the gastrointestinal troubles were associated with pharyngoconjunctivitis (Kjellén et al., 1957[74]; Ramos-Alvarez and Sabin, 1958[97]).

Abdominal syndromes with fever, abdominal pains, vomiting, and diarrhea with numerous watery and at times mucous and bloody stools have been attributed to adeno-viruses. In such cases adenoviruses are rela-tively easy to isolate by tissue culture pro-vided the material (stools or rectal swab) is collected early, as soon as possible after the onset of the disease, and promptly brought to the virological laboratory.

Myxovirus influenzae and *myxovirus parainfluenzae* also have been held re-sponsible for gastrointestinal disorders. Need it be recalled that, prior to the era of virologi-cal techniques, standard textbooks described a gastrointestinal form of epidemic influenza?

A difficult problem is the one of *double infections* in which both a virus and an enteropathogenic bacterium are found in the intestine and in the stools. In such cases the virus most frequently found is an ECHO and the associated bacteria are most often a staphylococcus or an *Escherichia coli.*

According to Ramos-Alvarez and Sabin, mild forms seem to be more frequent in children with a virus only, whereas the forms with severe dehydration are more frequent in children with a simultaneous bacterial infection. The incidence of blood in the stools is about the same (17 to 20 per cent of the cases) in those infected with a virus only and with both virus and bacteria.

Brokman et al.[37] believe that in these double infections the virus created the con-ditions favorable for the bacterial pathogenic manifestations. They carried out simultan-eous bacteriological, virological, and serolog-ical tests on 156 children with diarrhea. In 76 they found pathogenic bacteria: *Escher-ichia coli*, shigella, and salmonella. This group was compared with 80 other children in whom no pathogenic bacteria had been found. In children with bacteriologically positive stools the chances of finding an ECHO virus as well were four times greater than in children with stools negative for bacterial pathogens. For the other viruses the authors did not find any significant difference.

In examining the appendices of 642 patients who underwent surgery for acute suppurative appendicitis, Takayoshi[103] (of Kyoto) found a Coxsackie virus in 17 cases and an adenovirus in seven, associated with the pyogenic organisms. He supposed that in these 24 cases the virus was the agent that triggered the attack of appendicitis.

No final conclusions can be drawn from the publications which we have just re-viewed, the list of which is necessarily in-complete. The problem in question is under-

going constant evolution, and our knowledge is as yet only fragmentary. Nevertheless, we can attempt to point out a few guiding principles.

Normally, stools do not contain any viruses. Whereas the intestine harbors a normal bacterial flora that takes part in the physiology of digestion, *the intestine does not contain any viral flora that could be con-sidered normal in this sense.* Furthermore, such a hypothesis would give rise to in-superable objections. As a virus contains only one nucleic acid and no ribosome or mitochondria, it is incapable of synthesizing enzymes, whereas bacteria possess all the genetic and functional equipment required for protein synthesis. It is a well-known fact that these bacterial syntheses are essential for intestinal digestion, and it is impossible to imagine that viruses could fulfill such a function.

Viruses are to be found only transiently in the intestine and stools (as well as in saliva) for periods never exceeding a few weeks. Though viruses are excreted epi-sodically in the stools, anatomical studies have to date revealed specific lesions in the digestive epithelium (other than the mal-pighian epithelium of the mouth and eso-phagus) only in very exceptional cases. As regards enteroviruses (more particularly poliovirus), it has been shown (Bodian[34]) that they multiply in the lymph nodes and cannot be isolated in the gastrointestinal epithelium, in which they do not multiply.

The transient excretion of viruses in the stools is always accompanied by the *appear-ance of specific antibodies, even in the absence of any apparent clinical sign.* How, then, should the exact role of the virus be interpreted when it is associated with clini-cal signs? What can be the explanation of the cases in the same community and during the same epidemic in which different viruses are isolated in different individuals, for instance, an ECHO in some, a Coxsackie in others, and in still others an adenovirus?

To show the direct pathogenic action on the digestive tract of a virus and its power to produce a recognizable autonomous clini-cal symptomatology, *constant concordance is essential* between a homogeneous group of clinical signs and invasion of the intestine by the virus, and such concordance must be present not only from one epidemic to another, but also among the different patients in the same epidemic, as well as in sporadic cases. The mere finding of a virus in the stools, even accompanied by a rise in serum antibodies, is not sufficient. Experimental reproduction of the disease should be obtained.

In the light of our present knowledge, only epidemiological studies, that have yielded homogeneous results and, especially, that were carried out in comparison with valid control groups (of the same age groups and living under the same geographical, climatic, seasonal, and socioeconomic conditions) should be taken into consideration. Such conditions have been fulfilled only exceptionally, and the findings reported are not conclusive. Consider Sommerville's[102] study in Glasgow. It covered a period of one year and included 338 children with diarrhea and 115 controls. The incidence of enterovirus seemed greater in the patients, but the difference was not statistically significant and the author refrains from stating that the viruses had a pathogenic action.

Ramos-Alvarez and Sabin,[96, 97] on the other hand, who studied 97 patients and 100 controls, found ECHO viruses six times as often in the children with gastroenteritis as in the controls. A recent study carried out in Lille by Simon-Lavoine et al.[100] also shows the necessity of caution. It covered 343 children under two years of age, of whom 218 were hospitalized in 1960-1961 for gastroenteritis, and 125 controls who were hospitalized for various reasons exclusive of any intestinal manifestations. The authors noted the predominant part played by enteropathogenic bacteria (37.6 per cent in the patients, 13.4 per cent in the controls). As to the viruses (poliovirus, ECHO, Coxsackie, adenoviruses), they were isolated in 25.8 per cent of the patients and in 31.2 per cent of the controls. Here, again, the difference is not statistically significant.

In brief, pending more complete information, the existence of virus gastroenteritis as an autonomous clinical entity is as yet only hypothetical and a subject for research.

BIBLIOGRAPHY

HERPANGINA

1. Agar, E. A., Felsenstein, W. C., Alexander, E. R., Wymer, M. E., Sabotta, E., and Ashby, V.: An epidemic of illness due to Coxsackie virus Group B type 2. J.A.M.A., *187*:251, 1964.

2. Alsop, J., Flewett, T. H., and Foster, J. R.: Hand-foot-mouth disease in Birmingham in 1959. Brit. Med. J., 2:1708, 1960.

3. Artenstein, M. S., Cadigan, F. C., and Buescher, E. L.: Epidemic Coxsackie virus infection with mixed manifestations. Ann. Int. Med., 60:196, 1964.

4. Burtt Richardson, H., and Leibovitz, A.: Hand, foot and mouth disease in children. J. Pediat., 67:6-12, 1965.

5. Cherry, J. D., and Jahn, C. L.: Hand, foot, and mouth syndrome. Report of six cases due to Coxsackie virus, group A, type 16. Pediatrics, *37*:637-643, 1966.

6. Felici, A., and Gregorig, B.: Contribution to the study of diseases in Italy caused by the Coxsackie B group of viruses. II. Epidemiological, clinical, and virological data obtained in the course of a summer outbreak caused by Coxsackie B 4 virus. Arch. Ges. Virusforsch., *9*: 317, 1959.

7. Flewett, T. H., Warin, R. P., and Clarke, S.: Hand-foot and mouth disease associated with Coxsackie A5 virus. J. Clin. Path., *16*:63, 1963.

8. Glick, S. M., and Stroud, R.: An usual case of Coxsackie B infection. Arch. Int. Med., *109*:297, 1962.

9. Lepow, M. L., Carver, D. H., and Bobbins, F. C.: Clinical and epidemiologic observation on enterovirus infection in a circumscribed community during an epidemic of E.C.H.O. 9 infection. Pediatrics, 26:12, 1960.

10. Lerner, A. M., Klein, J. O., and Finland, M.: Infection with Coxsackie virus group B, type 3 with vesicular eruption: Report of two cases. New Eng. J. Med., 263:1305, 1960.

11. Lerner, A. M., Klein, J. O., Levin, H. S., and Finland, M.: Infections due to Coxsackie virus Group A type 9 in Boston 1959. New Eng. J. Med., 263:1265, 1960.

12. Marchessault, V., Pavilanis, V., Podoski, M. O., and Clode, M.: An epidemic of aseptic meningitis caused by Coxsackie B type 2 virus. Many patients with pharyngitis, crops of small vesicles on the tonsillar pillar and the uvula. Canad. Med. Assoc., J., 85:123, 1961.

13. Neva, F. A., Feemster, R. F. and Gorbach, I. J.: Clinical and epidemiological features of unusual epidemic exanthem. J.A.M.A., *155*:544, 1954.

14. Parrott, R. H., Ross, S., Burke, F. G., and Rice, E. G.: Herpangina: Clinical studies of specific infectious disease. New Eng. J. Med., *245*: 275-280, 1951.

15. Parrott, R. H., et al.: Further observations on herpangina and its relation to the Coxsackie viruses. Clin. Proc. Child. Hosp., 8:118-124, 1952.

16. Reinhard, K. R.: Ecology of enteroviruses in the western Arctic. J.A.M.A., *183*:410, 1963.

17. Robinson, C. R., Doane, F. W., and Rhodes, A. J.: Report of an outbreak of febrile illness with pharyngeal lesions and exanthem: Toronto 1957. Isolation of group A Coxsackie virus. Canad. Med. Assoc. J., 79:615, 1958.

18. Sabin, A. B.: Role of ECHO viruses in human disease. In: Rox, H. M., ed.: Viral infections of infancy and childhood. Symposium No. 19. Section on Microbiology, New York Academy of

Medicine. New York, Hoeber Division, Harper & Row, 1960, pp. 78-100.

19. St. Geme, J. W., and Prince, J. T.: Vesicular pharyngitis associated with Coxsackie virus Group B, type 5. New Eng. J. Med., *265*:1255, 1961.

19a. Steigman, A. J., and Lipton, M. N.: Acute lymphonodular pharyngitis. A newly described condition due to Coxsackie A virus. Arch. Ges. Virusforsch., *13*:143-150, 1963.

FOOT-AND-MOUTH DISEASE

20. Armstrong, R., Davie, J., and Hedger, R. S.: Foot-and-mouth disease in man. Brit. M. J., *1*:529-530, 1967.

21. Drey, A.: Etude clinique de la fièvre aphteuse humaine. Thèse de Lyon, 1920-1921.

22. Eissner, G., Böhm, H. O., and Jülich, E.: Eine Maul-und-Klauenseuche-Infektion beim Menschen. Deutsch. Med. Wschr., *92*:830-832, 1967.

23. Lebailly, C.: La fièvre aphteuse bovine n'est pas transmissible à l'homme; la stomatite aphteuse humaine n'est pas transmissible aux bovins. C.R. Acad. Sci. Paris, *17*:1140, 1921.

24. Mohr, W.: Maul und Klauenseuche. In: Gsell and Mohr: Infektions Krankheiten. Stuttgart, Springer Verlag.

25. Nicolle, C., and Bazolet: L'homme est insensible même sous forme d'infection inapparente à l'inoculation des virus aphteux de types connus. C.R. Acad. Sci. Paris, *197*:374-376, 1933.

26. Roch, M., and Roch, R.: La fièvre aphteuse. In: Lemierre, Lenormant, Pagniez, Savy, Fiessinger, de Gennes, and Ravina, eds.: Traité de médecine. Vol. II. Paris, Masson et cie, 1948, pp. 194-201. This article is an excellent review up to 1948 and contains a detailed bibliography. We have borrowed a great deal from this article.

27. Snowdon, W. A.: Growth of foot-and-mouth disease virus in monolayer cultures of calf thyroid cells. Nature, *210*:1079-1080, 1966.

VIRUS DIARRHEAS

28. Alessandro, G., and Dardanoni, L.: Bacterial and viral etiology of diarrhoeal diseases in infancy. Riv. Ist. Sieroter. Ital., *36*:129-137, 1961.

29. Artenstein, M. S., Cadigan, F. C., Jr., and Buescher, E. L.: Epidemic Coxsackie virus infection with mixed clinical manifestations. Ann. Int. Med., *60*:196, 1964.

30. Baker, J. A.: Filtrable virus causing enteritis and pneumonia in calves. J. Exp. Med., *78*:435, 1943.

31. Barenberg, L. H., Levy, W., and Grand, M. J. H.: An epidemic of infectious diarrhoea in the newborn. J.A.M.A., *106*:1256-1260, 1936.

32. Behbehani, A., and Wenner, H.: Infantile diarrhea: a study of the etiologic role of viruses. Amer. J. Dis. Child., *111*:623-629, 1966.

33. Bergamini, F., and Bonetti, F.: Episodio epidemico di gastro-enterite a cuta da virus E.C.H.O. 11 in un brefôtrofio. Boll. Ist. Sieroter. Milan, *39*:510-515, 1960.

34. Bodian, D.: Viremia, invasiveness, and the influence of injections. Ann. N.Y. Acad. Sci., *61*: 877-882, 1955.

35. Brancato, P., Guillotti, A., and Dardanoni, L.: Diffusione di enterovirus in due diversi gruppi socio-economici della popolazione infantile di Palermo. Riv. Ist. Sieroter. Ital., *37*:630-637, 1962.

36. Breese, B. B.: Aphthous pharyngitis. Amer. J. Dis. Child., *61*:669, 1941.

37. Brokman, H., Imbs, D., Lachowicz, K., Paytsch, F. Z., Truchanowicz, Z., and Wankowicz, R.: Signification des infections concomitantes virales et bactériennes dans les états diarrhéiques. Helv. Paediat. Acta, *20*:592-597, 1965.

38. Buddingh, G. J., and Dodd, K.: Estomatitis y diarrea en los niños causados por un virus hasta ahora desconocido. Pediat. Americas, *5*:83-84, 1947.

39. Celers, J.: Diarrhées à virus. Journées Africaines de Pédiatrie (publication of the Centre International de l' Enfance), pp. 213-216, April, 1960.

40. Celers, J., Drouhet, V., and Gerbeaux, J.: Bull. Inst. Nat. Hyg., *14*:505-522, 1959.

41. Cheever, S. F., and Mueller, J. A.: Epidemic diarrheal disease of suckling mice. III. Effect of strain, letter, and season upon the incidence of disease. J. Exp. Med., *88*:309, 1948.

42. Cherry, J. D., and Jahn, C.: Herpangina: the etiologic spectrum. Pediatrics, *36*:632-634, 1965.

43. Cramblett, H. G., et al.: Coxsackie virus infections. J. Pediat., *64*:406, 1964.

44. Cramblett, H. G., and Siewers, C. M.: The etiology of gastro-enteritis in infants and children with emphasis on the occurrence of simultaneous mixed viral-bacterial infections. Pediatrics, *35*:885-898, 1965.

45. Dalldorf, G.: Coxsackie viruses. Amer. J. Public Health, *40*:1508, 1950.

46. Debré, R., and Thieffry, S.: Encyclopédie médico-chirurgicale: Maladies infectieuses.

47. Dick, G. F., Dick, G. H., and Williams, J. L.: Amer. J. Dis. Child. *35*:955, 1928.

48. Doyle, L. P., and Hutchings, L. M.: Transmissible gastro-enteritis in pigs. J. Amer. Vet. Med. Assoc. *108*:257, 1946.

49. Eichenwald, H. F., Arabio, A., Arky, A. M., and Hartman, A. P.: Epidemic diarrhea in premature and older infants caused by ECHO virus type 18. J.A.M.A., *166*:1563-1566, 1958.

50. Enders, J. F., Weller, T. and Robbins, F. C.: Cultivation of the Lansing strain of poliomyelitis virus in cultures of various human embryonic tissues. Science, *109*:85-89, 1949.

51. Felici, A., and Archetti, I.: Contributo allo studio eziologico della forme diarroïche epidemiche. Boll. Ist. Sieroter. Milan, *39*:485-494, 1960.

52. Felici, A., Archetti, I., Russi, F., Bellochi, C., and Mazzi, F.: Contribution to the study of diseases caused by the Coxsackie 13 groups of viruses in Italy. III: Role of Coxsackie B virus type 3 in summer diarrheal infections in infants and children. Arch. Ges. Virusforsch., *11*:592, 1961.

53. Felici, A., and Gregorig, B.: Contribution to the study of diseases in Italy caused by the Coxsackie B group of viruses. II. Epidemiological, clinical, virological data obtained in the course of a summer outbreak caused by Coxsackie B-4 virus. Arch. Ges. Virusforsch., *9*:317, 1959.

54. Galbraith, N. S.: A survey of enteroviruses and adenoviruses in the feces of normal British children aged 0-4 years. J. Hyg., *63*:441-455, 1965.

55. Gerbeaux, J., Couvreur, J., Hebert-Jouas, J., Virat, J., Maurin, J., and Chany, C.: L'herpangine;

étude clinique, virologique et sérologique d'une épidémie en mileiu hospitalier. Presse Méd., *18:* 675-678, 1960.

56. Gerbeaux, J., et al.: Une épidémie de gastro-entérite associée à un virus Coxsackie A. Journées Parisiennes de Pédiatrie, Oct., 1967.

57. Ginevri, A., and Felici, A.: Contribution to the study of diseases in Italy caused by Coxsackie B group of viruses. I. Clinical and virological aspects of an outbreak of Bornholm disease. Arch. Ges. Virusforsch., *9:*310, 1959.

58. Goldenberg, M. I., and Gudnadottir, M.: Studies on an outbreak of ECHO 9 virus infection in a circumscribed population. Conn. Med. J., *23:* 693-696, 1959.

59. Gordon, I., Ingraham, H. S., and Korns, R. F.: Transmission d'une gastro-entérite à des volontaires humains par administration de filtrats de selles diarrhéiques. J. Exp. Med., *86:*405, 1947.

60. Gordon, I., Ingraham, H. S., and Korns, R. F.: Transmission of epidemic gastroenteritis to human volunteers by oral transmission of fecal filtrates. J. Exp. Med., *86:*409, 1947.

61. Gordon, J. E., and Rubinstein, A. P.: Epidemic diarrhea of the new-born. Amer. J. Med. Sci., *220:*339, 1950.

62. Grosso, E., and Bergamini, F.: Sindrome gastro-intestinale infantile epidemica da enterovirus (E.C.H.O. 14 et 9, polio virus 3). Boll. Ist. Sieroter. Milan, *39:*495-509, 1960.

63. Guardiola-Rotger, A., et al.: Studies on diarrheal diseases. J. Pediat., *65:*81, 1964.

64. Hammon, W. D., and Enders, J. F.: Virus disease of cats, principally characterized by aleucocytosis, enteric lesions and presence of intranuclear inclusions bodies. J. Exp. Med. *69:*327, 1939.

65. Heggie, A. D., Schultz, I., Gutekunst, R. R., Rosenbaum, M., and Miller, L. F.: An outbreak of a summer febrile disease caused by Coxsackie B-2 virus. Amer. J. Public Health, *50:*1342, 1960.

66. Hodds, H. L.: The etiology of infantile diarrhea. Adv. Pediatr., *8:*45-47, 1956.

67. Honig, E. I., et al.: An endemiological study of enteric viruses infection. Poliomyelitis, Coxsackie and ECHO viruses isolated from normal children in two socio-economic groups. J. Exp. Med., *103:*247-262, 1956.

68. Huebner, R. J..: Herpangina. Lecture presented at the Children's Hospital, Cincinnati, Ohio, 1956.

69. Huebner, R. J., Armstrong, G., Beeman, E. A., and Cole, R. M.: Studies of Coxsackie viruses. Preliminary report on occurrence of Coxsackie virus in a southern Maryland community. J.A.M.A., *144:*609-612, 1950.

70. Huebner, R. J., Beeman, E. A., Cole, R. M., Beigelman, P. M., and Bell, J. A.: The importance of Coxsackie viruses in human disease, particularly herpangina and epidemic pleurodynia. New Eng. J. Med., *247:*249-256, 285-289, 1952.

71. Johnson, T.: Family infections by Coxsackie viruses. Arch. Ges. Virusforsch., *5:*384, 1954.

72. Joncas, J., and Pavilanis, V.: Diarrhoea and Vomiting in infancy and childhood: Viral studies. Canad. Med. Assoc. J., *82:*1108-1113, 1960.

73. Jordan, W. S., Jr., Gordon, I., and Dorrance, W. R.: Study of illness in a group of Cleveland families; transmission of acute non-bacterial gastroenteritis

to volunteers: evidence for 2 different etiologic agents. J. Exp. Med., *98:*461, 1953.

74. Kjellén, L., Zetterberg, B., and Svedmyr, A.: An epidemic among Swedish children caused by adenovirus type 3. Acta Paediat. Scand., *46:* 561-568, 1957.

75. Klein, J. O., Lerner, A. M., and Finland, M.: Acute gastroenteritis associated with ECHO virus, Type 11. Amer. J. Med. Sci., *240:*749-753, 1960.

76. Kojima, S., et al.: Studies on causative agent of infectious diarrhea. Records of experiments on human volunteers. Japanese Med. J., *1:*467, 1948.

76a. Lawrence, J. S., and Syverton, J. T.: Spontaneous agranulocytosis in cat. Proc. Soc. Exp. Biol. Med., *38:*914-918, 1938.

77. Leener, L. de: Le problème étiologique de la diarrhée épidémique des nouveau-nés. Arch. Franc. Pediat., *5:*324-329, 1948.

78. Lépine, P., Samaille, J., Maurin, J., Dubois, O., and Carre, M. C.: Isolement du virus E.C.H.O. 14 au cours d'une épidémie de crèche de gastro-entérite. Ann. Inst. Pasteur (Paris), *99:*161-166, 1960.

79. Lépine, P., Samaille, J., Virat, J., Carre, M. C., and Simon-Lavoine, N.: Enquête sur la fréquence et la signification de l'isolement des entérovirus au cours des gastro-entérites infantiles. Arch. Ges. Virusforsch., *13:*201, 1963.

80. Levine, H. D., Hoerr, S. D., and Allenson, J. C.: Vesicular pharyngitis and stomatitis: an unusual epidemic of possible herpetic origin. J.A.M.A., *112:*2020, 1939.

81. Light, J. S., and Hodes, H. L.: Studies on epidemic diarrhea of the newborn: isolation of a filtrable agent causing diarrhea in calves. Amer. J. Public Health, *33:*1451, 1943.

82. Light, J. S., and Hodes, H. L.: Isolation from cases of infantile diarrhea of a filtrable agent causing diarrhea in calves. J. Exp. Med., *90:*113, 1949.

83. Lyon, G. M., and Folsom, T. G.: Epidemic diarrhea of newborn; clinicoepidemic, pathologic and therapeutic aspects. Amer. J. Dis. Chil., *61:*427, 1941.

84. Malherbe, H., Roux, P., and Kahn, E.: The role of enteropathogenic bacteria and viruses in acute diarrheal disorders of infancy and childhood in Johannesburg. II. "Non-specific" gastro-enteritis. S. Afr. Med. J., *37:*259, 1963.

85. Marfan: L'angine pustuleuse. Arch. Med. Enf., *27:* 65-93, 1924.

86. Marie, J., et al.: Entérocolite ulcero-hémorragique chez un nouveau-né avec présence dans l'intestin du virus Coxsackie A-9. Sem. Hôp. Paris, *40:* 275, 1964.

87. McLean, D. M., McNaughton, G. A., and Wyllie, J. C.: Infantile gastroenteritis: further viral investigations. Canad. Med. Assoc. J., *85:*496-497, 1961.

88. Pappenheimer, A. M., and Cheever, S. F.: Epidemic diarrheal disease of suckling mice. IV. Cytoplasmic inclusion bodies in intestinal epithelium in relation to the disease. J. Exp. Med., *88:*317, 1948.

89. Pappenheimer, A. M., and Enders, J. E.: An epidemic diarrheal disease of suckling mice. II. Inclusions in the intestinal epithelial cells. J. Exp. Med., *85:*417, 1947.

90. Parrott, R. H.: The clinical importance of group A

Coxsackie viruses. Ann. N.Y. Acad. Sci., *67*: 230-240, 1957.

91. Parrott, R. H., et al.: Clinical and laboratory differentiation between herpangina and infectious (herpetic) gingivostomatitis. Pediatrics, *14*:122-129, 1954.

92. Pelon, W., et al.: Coxsackie group B virus infection and acute diarrhea occurring among children in Costa Rica. Arch. Dis. Child., *41*:636-641, 1966.

93. Pohjanpelto, P.: Coxsackie group of viruses; epidemiological studies. Ann. Med. Exp. Biol. Fenniae (Suppl. 6), *33*:1-75, 1955.

94. Prenzel, I., and Lennartz, H.: Zür Frage der viralen Enteropathien. Mschr. Kinderheilk., *108*:527-530, 1960.

95. Ramos-Alvarez, M., and Olarte, J.: Diarrheal diseases of children. Amer. J. Dis. Child., *107*:218-231, 1964.

96. Ramos-Alvarez, M., and Sabin, A. B.: Intestinal viral flora of healthy children demonstrable by monkey kidney tissue culture. Amer. J. Public Health, *46*:295, 1956.

97. Ramos-Alvarez, M., and Sabin, A. B.: Enteropathogenic viruses and bacteria; role in summer diarrheal diseases of infancy and early childhood. J.A.M.A., *167*:147-156, 1958.

98. Reitano, G., and Dardanoni, L.: Enterobacteri ed enterovirus in casi di diarrea infantile in Sicilia. Riv. Ist. Sieroter. Ital., *36*:28, 1961.

99. Sanyal, S. K., et al.: Fatal myocarditis in an adolescent caused by Coxsackie virus group B type 4. Pediatrics, *35*:36, 1965.

100. Simon-Lavoine, N., et al.: Enquête sur la fréquence et la signification de l'isolement des bactéries entéropathogènes et des entérovirus au cours des gastro-entérites infantiles. Ann. Inst. Pasteur Lille, *14*:159-181, 1963.

101. Sims Roberts, J. T. C., and Thomson, D.: Poliomyelitis in infancy, especially in the neonatal period. Report of an outbreak. Monthly Bull. Min. Health (London), *12*;152-163, 1953.

102. Sommerville, R. G.: Enteroviruses and diarrhoea in young persons. Lancet, *2*:1347-1349, 1958.

103. Takayoshi, T.: Inapparent virus infection as a trigger of appendicitis. Lancet, *1*:1343-1346, 1965.

104. Thieffry, S., Arthuis, M., and Martin, C.: In: Sixth Symposium de l'Association Européenne contre la Poliomyélite.

105. Travassos, J., et al.: Occurencia de Coxsackie no Rio de Janeiro. II. Isolomento do virus un crianças con disturbio gastro-intestinale. Ann. Microbiol., *2*:83-88, 1952-53.

106. Walker, J. J., et al.: Infantile gastro-enteritis: A search for viral pathogens. Canad. Med. Assoc. J., *83*:1266-1267, 1960.

107. Worms, A. M.: Contribution à l'étude des infections à virus. E.C.H.O. Thèse Nancy, pp. 85-92, 1964.

108. Yamamoto, A., Zennyoji, H., Yanagita, K., and Kato, S.: Research into causative agent of epidemic gastroenteritis which prevailed in Japan in 1948. Japanese Med. J., *1*:379, 1948.

109. Young, V. M., et al.: Studies of infectious agents in infant diarrhea: Bacterial viral and parasitic agents in feces of Puerto Rican children. Amer. J. Trop. Med., *11*:830, 1962.

110. Yow, M., Melnick, J., Blattner, R., and Rasmussen, L.: Enteroviruses in infantile diarrhea. Amer. J. Hyg., *77*:283-292, 1963.

111. Zahorsky, J.: Herpetic sore throat. South. M. J., *13*:871-872, 1920.

112. Zahorsky, J.: Herpangina: A specific infectious disease. Arch. Pediat., *41*:181-184, 1924.

113. Zakstel'skaya, L. Y., et al.: On the etiology of diarrhea with respiratory syndrome in young children. (In Russian.) Vop. Virus., *9*:205, 1964.

114. Zourbas, J., and Drouhet, V.: Etude immuno-épidémiologique de deux collectivités de nourrisons en crèche infectés par des virus poliomyélitiques. Sem. Hôp. Paris, *35*:1356-1362/SP, 1959.

22

Coxsackie Group A Viruses

By P. DUC-GOIRAN and C. CHANY

The Coxsackie A viruses form part of the broader group of viruses known as enteroviruses. They are characterized by their nucleic acid (RNA); their symmetrical cubic structure; the absence of an outer membrane; and an average diameter of 28 mμ.

Most Coxsackie viruses multiply in vitro only in cells of human origin. Some can be detected only by their pathogenicity for newborn mice and hamsters.

They are responsible for a wide variety of clinical syndromes. Their geographic and seasonal distribution is very similar to that of polioviruses and ECHO viruses.

HISTORY

The first strains of Coxsackie A virus were isolated by Dalldorf and Sickles in 1948[10] from two patients with paralytic poliomyelitis. In 1949 Dalldorf suggested calling these isolates Coxsackie virus, after the name of the town where the organism was first isolated.

Various strains of Coxsackie group A virus were isolated during epidemics of herpangina by Huebner et al. in 1951[22] and subsequently by other investigators (Coxsackie viruses A2, 4, 5, 6, 8, and 10).

Other strains of Coxsackie virus (A2, 4, 7, 9, 10) were recovered from patients with aseptic meningitis. Steigman et al.[42] in 1953 and later Chumakov[6a] in 1956 isolated a Coxsackie group A virus from a clinical syndrome suggestive of poliomyelitis. Chumakov proposed designating this virus poliovirus type IV, but it has since been classified by Habel and Loomis[20] as Coxsackie virus A7.

STRUCTURE

Size. Filtration studies using graduated permeable membranes show an average particle diameter of 20 to 29 mμ; electron microscopic measurements give a value of 28 mμ.

Density. Density was determined by ultracentrifuging in sucrose gradient. The sedimentation constant is 150S. In cesium chloride gradient, virus is found principally in a layer corresponding to a density of 1.34.[29]

Crystallization. Coxsackie A10 virus was purified and crystallized by Mattern and du Buy in 1956.[30] They obtained crystals equivalent to 90 to 99 per cent of the infectivity. These values do not differ significantly from those obtained in studies on poliovirus.

Morphological Structure of the Virion. The capsid of the virion presents a cubic symmetry; the number of capsomeres is still unknown. There is no external membrane.

Genetic Material. The genetic material is ribonucleic acid. Table 22-1 (from Mattern[29]) shows the proportions of the various bases in Coxsackie A9 and A10 viruses, the composition of poliovirus (mean values for three strains) being used as reference. Both these viruses contain more guanine and less adenine than poliovirus.

Table 22-1 *Proportions of Various Bases in RNA of Coxsackie A9 and A10**

	A9	A10	POLIOVIRUS	TURNIP YELLOW MOSAIC	
Guanine	1.11	1.13	0.96	0.75	0.69
Adenine	1.08	1.09	1.14	0.92	0.91
Cytosine	0.82	0.84	0.88	1.52	1.53
Uracyl	0.99	0.93	1.01	0.86	0.89

*From Mattern.[29]

PHYSICAL-CHEMICAL PROPERTIES

Effects of Temperature

1. Viruses of this group are stable and can be stored for lengthy periods at $-20°$ C. without a significant loss of infectivity. Similarly, they remain stable at $+4°$ C. for over a year if stored in 50 per cent glycerol or horse serum.

2. When diluted in an aqueous solvent, they are inactivated by heating for 30 minutes at $60°$ C. Higher temperatures are required when the viruses are suspended in milk or cream.

Effect of pH. These viruses retain their infectivity over a pH range of 2.3 to 9.4 for a period of 24 hours, and over a pH range of 4 to 8 for a period of seven days.[37]

Effect of Antiseptics. These viruses, like all enteroviruses, are resistant to ether and to a number of antiseptics such as ethanol and lysol, but are inactivated by N/10 hydrochloric acid and formaldehyde.

MULTIPLICATION OF COXSACKIE VIRUSES IN TISSUE CULTURE

The Different Types of Tissues. Unlike the Coxsackie group B viruses, which grow well on cultures of monkey kidney cells and on most human cell cultures, the group A viruses in general do not multiply in these cells. However, the A11, 13, 15, 18, and 20 strains can be isolated directly by using human cell cultures. Others, however, multiply in cell culture only after adaptation. Strains A1, 4, 5, 6, 19, and 22 can be isolated or maintained only after inoculation of newborn mice. Strains A10 and 14 multiply only in newborn mice (intraperitoneal inoculation).

Multiplication in Organ Culture. Came and Crowell[6] have shown that mouse fetuses inoculated in utero are sensitive to infection by Coxsackie virus A13. Fragments from such an infected fetus continue to shed virus when cultivated in vitro. However, viral adsorption on embryonic tissues cultivated in vitro has not been demonstrated. Hence, it has been postulated that mouse embryo cells isolated from their normal tissue environment lose "receptors" for this virus.[6]

Cytological Lesions. The lesions are the same as those induced by other enteroviruses. The cells become rounded, the nucleus becomes pyknotic, and the cell sheet is destroyed. After fixing and staining, an eosinophilic intracytoplasmic mass is seen in the center of the cell pushing the nucleus toward the periphery.

Sarkar and Ray[38] described an increase in the number of amniotic cells in mitosis after infection by Coxsackie A9 virus. The number of cells in mitosis was seven to 15 per 5000 in a normal culture, and increased to 30 to 75 per 5000 after 24 hours' infection. This effect was inhibited by a specific immune serum.

Buthala[5] observed a variation in the cytopathic effect of Coxsackie A21 and its capacity to produce plaques on cell cultures ("ML" strain isolated from mouse embryo liver) by varying the CO_2 concentration in the surrounding air from 0 to 10 per cent. In the absence of CO_2, microplaques were obtained; with 2 per cent CO_2, 1- to 2-mm. plaques; with 4 to 5 per cent CO_2, the maximal size was 4 to 8 mm., as with 8 per cent. Above 8 per cent, the size of the plaques decreased.

Multiplication of the Virus. On the basis of chemical analysis and the distribution of the various fluorescent antigens within the cell, Mattern and Chi[31] suggested a schematic representation of the succession of events that occur in viral multiplication.

During the first and second hours the virus penetrates the cell and migrates toward the nucleus. The role of the nucleus in the synthesis of viral RNA is not clear. Two hours after infection a considerable rise is noted in the cytoplasmic RNA, followed by the appearance of viral protein.

Guanidine and HBB (α-hydroxybenzyl-2-benzimidazole) inhibit the multiplication of the virus. Guanidine inhibits Coxsackie A7, 11, 13, 16, and 18, and HBB inhibits only Coxsackie A9 and 21.[44] Synergistic action of the two inhibitors on Coxsackie A9 is observed at concentrations which, independently, have no effect.[12]

Length of Cycle. The duration of the cycle is approximately six to seven hours, with a latent period of three and one-half hours.

PATHOGENICITY FOR EXPERIMENTAL ANIMALS

The pathogenicity of these viruses for newborn mice and hamsters is one of the most characteristic biological properties of the Coxsackie viruses. The animal of choice is the newborn mouse, although the virus is also pathogenic for other animals: hamster, gerbil, squirrel, and ferret. The anatomical lesions serve as criteria for the identification of Coxsackie viruses and for their classification as group A or B.

FUNCTIONAL SIGNS OF THE DISEASE

Infected newborn animals present a period of muscular asthenia, followed by a flaccid paralysis of the extremities. Death follows rapidly, and is presumably due to paralysis of the respiratory muscles.

HISTOLOGICAL SIGNS

Histological examination of striated muscles reveals diffuse degenerative lesions which do not, however, extend to the tongue and heart. The diffuse nature of the myositis is an important diagnostic factor which permits distinction of the microörganism from Theiler's virus and the encephalomyocarditis virus, which produce localized lesions. There

is no detectable pathological lesion other than the generalized myositis.

The process begins with a loss of muscle striation, with disappearance first of the H and Z lines and then of the A and I disks, followed by a swelling of the myofibrils[1] and finally by hyaline degeneration. In the necrotic muscle segments there is an accumulation of inorganic phosphates (the increase being due to the blocking of the normal production of energy conveyors), iron, and nucleic acid granules or rods evidencing the internal rearrangement of these molecules. Thirty hours following infection, the sodium/potassium ratio is reversed. A rapid loss of creatinine, potassium, and myoglobin is observed in the paralyzed muscles.[17] The third postinoculation day, when the mice are paralyzed, a loss of glycolytic activity is noted.

FACTORS PERTAINING TO THE MULTIPLICATION OF VIRUSES AND THEIR PATHOGENICITY IN VIVO

The Host. The age of the animal seems to be of prime importance. Four- to five-day-old mice are consistently sensitive to the virus. Mice that are a few days older may survive. Rapid muscle regeneration is observed, but there is a slow resorption of the degenerated muscle, furnishing evidence of the disease a few weeks later. Weaned mice, and even older animals, can be infected and paralyzed only by passaged strains of the virus.

Routes of Inoculation. The route of inoculation does not seem to play an important role in the genesis of the lesions. On the other hand, the sensitivity of the animal to inoculation by the viruses seems to vary according to the route of inoculation. Dalldorf therefore recommended that three groups of mice be employed for primary isolation and that the animals be inoculated intraperitoneally, intracerebrally, and subcutaneously, respectively.[8] Oral administration of the virus gives only variable results.

Role of Hormones. Cortisone increases the sensitivity of the animals. It converts a mild infection in adult mice into a fatal infection. The growth hormone has the opposite effect.

Role of Cold. Boring showed that cold increases the sensitivity of adult mice to infection.[3]

The Nature of the Virus

NEUROPATHOGENIC STRAINS. Coxsackie viruses A7, 14, and 16 occupy a special place among the group A Coxsackie viruses, as they are related to polioviruses by their neuropathogenicity. When inoculated into monkeys and adult cotton rats, they cause lesions of the central nervous system similar to those caused by poliovirus. Coxsackie A7 gives rise to a typical paralysis in the monkey and has also been described under the designation "poliovirus IV." In newborn mice, these strains cause only myositis. In the course of repeated passages on monkey kidney cell cultures Koroleva and Frolova[27] observed a decrease in the neuropathogenic potency which was also accompanied by a decrease in the pathogenicity for rodents.

MYOCARDIOTROPIC STRAINS. Coxsackie virus A9, which causes in newborn mice a generalized myositis which spares the heart, produces a subclinical acute myocarditis in 36 per cent of adult mice (eight months), accompanied only by focal lesions of the skeletal muscles.[13] This myocarditis is evidenced by an increase in the weight of the heart. It is more severe in mice that have been subjected to compulsory exercise.[45]

On the other hand, Koroleva and Frolova found focal necrotic lesions in the myocardium of 20 to 30 per cent of newborn cotton rats inoculated with strains A7, 14, and 16.[27]

STRAINS ADAPTED TO VARIOUS ANIMAL SPECIES. Coxsackie virus A2 causes lesions in the striated muscles of chicken embryos. Coxsackie virus A4 can infect cockroaches, the mites of tropical rats, flies, and wild rabbits. Neutralizing antibodies against Coxsackie A10 have been found in pigs.

SEROLOGICAL STUDIES

NEUTRALIZATION TESTS

1. Twenty-three antigenic types of Coxsackie virus group A have been identified on the basis of cross-neutralization tests. Some strains have antigenic variants; Coxsackie A20, for instance, has four subtypes.

2. Neutralization tests represent the most accurate method of demonstrating a type-specific antibody response. After Coxsackie A infection in man, the neutralizing antibody titer remains elevated for a long time.

COMPLEMENT-FIXATION REACTIONS

1. Coxsackie viruses may also be identified and typed by cross reactions in complement fixation, which yield about the same results as the neutralization methods. The use of this method for typing virus strains isolated from patients is of particular interest. Munch[34] demonstrated the specificity of these complement-fixation reactions with hyperimmune mouse sera. He observed cross reactions between strains A5 and 13, 3 and 8.

2. Tests for complement-fixing antibodies are of more limited value for the diagnosis of Coxsackie group A infections in man. Whereas mouse sera provide highly specific reactions, a considerable antigenic cross reaction is observed with human sera.[2] This heterotypic reaction is also observed in rhesus monkeys, chimpanzees, and guinea pigs. Coxsackie A viruses therefore contain a common group antigen in human sera detectable by complement fixation.

Schmidt et al.[39] separated two antigens from Coxsackie A9 virus by density gradient centrifugation in cesium chloride. One fraction corresponds to the group antigen that fixes complement and is responsible for the heterotypic reaction of human sera, identical with the group precipitating antigen, and another fraction fixes complement with monkey homotypic serum. This second antigen corresponds to the type-specific precipitating antigen.

In man, after the acute stage of infection the titer of complement-fixing antibodies falls rapidly and disappears three to four months after the onset of the disease.

HEMAGGLUTINATION

Coxsackie A7, 20, 21, and 24 preparations contain a hemagglutinin.

1. Williamson and Grist[46] studied the hemagglutinin of Coxsackie A7 virus. It agglutinates chicken erythrocytes but not human group 0 erythrocytes. It is a protein distinct from the infectious particle (incomplete form of the particle). The inhibition of hemagglutination is a simple test for the detection of antibodies against Coxsackie A7.[19]

2. Some strains of Coxsackie A21 agglutinate human group 0 erythrocytes (but not those of guinea pig or monkey origin) at a temperature of $+4°$ C. and an optimal pH of 5.8 to 6.8.

The hemagglutinin appears to be associated with the infectious particle, as the latter is absorbed by human group 0 erythrocytes.

Cultures of human embryonic kidney produce a higher titer of hemagglutinating antigen than malignant cells in continuous culture.[25] Schmidt et al.[41] explain these findings by the presence of inhibitors of hemagglutination. These inhibitors are inactivated by treatment with Genetron 113 fluorocarbon, which furnishes the means of unmasking the presence of hemagglutinin in certain preparations.

EPIDEMIOLOGY

Coxsackie A viruses are widely distributed throughout the world. They have been recovered from the pharynx and the feces of man, in sewage, and even from flies.

IN MAN

Influence of Age. Melnick and Ledinko[33] observed an increase in the level of Coxsackie viral neutralizing antibodies in children, with a peak (85 per cent) at the age of seven to nine years and a second peak between ten and 14 years. There is an increase in complement-fixing antibodies in 65 per cent of children of seven to nine years, and in only 25 per cent between the ages of ten and 14. This is probably related to the rapid disappearance of complement-fixing antibodies after infection.

In contrast to other Coxsackie A viruses, strain A21 is more prevalent in adults. A study by Pereira[35] in Great Britain showed a low rate of infection in young children, and a progressively increasing rate with age. Antibodies are frequently found in young male adults.

Influence of Sanitary Conditions. In areas where sanitary conditions are good, Coxsackie viruses are isolated in the summer and fall, whereas in areas of low socioeconomic status, these viruses are present in the fecal material the year round.

Influence of the Seasons. The traditional enterovirus peak is found in the early fall. A study by Melnick et al. in 6-year-old children showed 42 per cent positive serological reactions in May and 65 per cent in November.

Influence of Climate. Whereas poliovirus is predominant in the temperate zones (presumably owing to a longer period of fecal excretion), in the tropics Coxsackie and ECHO viruses are more endemic. This would appear to be due to the insalubrity of these regions. No characteristic epidemics are reported; infection would seem to appear at a very early age.[14]

Diversity of Serological Types. The diversity of serological types is characteristic of this group of viruses. Numerous types are found in entirely different clinical syndromes, as shown in Table 22-2.

IN SEWAGE

Sewage contains Coxsackie viruses chiefly during the summer and fall. At certain periods, the extensive appearance of new types is noted. Treatment of the sewage inactivates these viruses only partially.

IN FLIES

Melnick et al.[32] isolated Coxsackie viruses from flies but did not observe any multiplication. These insects in no way act as vectors.

ASSOCIATED INFECTIONS

1. During a herpangina epidemic in 1960 at the L. Bernard Hospital at Brevannes (Department of Seine-et-Oise), Gerbeaux et al.[16] showed the simultaneous existence of three epidemics in the same community: (a) a Coxsackie A4 epidemic; (b) an ECHO virus epidemic (isolation of the virus in one patient and elevation of the antibody titer in four of 11 subjects); and (c) a poliomyelitis virus epidemic (increase in complement-fixing antibodies in six cases out of nine confirmed by the neutralization test as being of type I in five cases out of five).

2. A study by Melnick carried out over a period of 29 months on healthy children yielded 213 viral isolations from feces of 1540 children tested: 52 per cent were ECHO viruses, 24 per cent were polioviruses, and 24 per cent were Coxsackie viruses.

RELATIONSHIPS WITH POLIOMYELITIS

The novel interest of the Coxsackie viruses lies mainly in their possible relationships with poliomyelitis, with which they have frequently been associated.

1. In man, the first two strains of Cox-

Table 22-2 *Serological Types of Coxsackie A Virus in Various Clinical Syndromes**

	SEROLOGICAL TYPES
Herpangina	A2, 4, 5, 6, 8, 10, 22 (A4 is most frequently found)
Acute lymphonodular pharyngitis	A10
Aseptic meningitis	A2, 4, 7, 9, 10 (Melnick isolated A10 in CSF)
Paralysis	A7 (Chumakov in Russia; Grist[13] in Scotland:37 cases)
Miscellaneous exanthemas	A4, 9, 16 (isolation of A16 in hand, foot, and mouth disease of children)
Coryza	A21, 24 (A21 responsible for acute respiratory tract diseases is identical with Lennette's Coe virus)
Fatal encephalomyocarditis	A16 isolated in a child from myocardium and other organs by Wright et al.[47]
Pneumonia	A9, 16
Hepatitis	A4, 9
Acute hemolytic syndromes	A4
Fever with lymphadenitis	A5, 6

*Adapted from Dalldorf and Melnick[9] and references 18, 21, 36, 43, and 47.

sackie virus were isolated from children with paralytic poliomyelitis by Dalldorf and Sickles in 1948.[10]

The association of paralytic poliomyelitis with the isolation of Coxsackie virus was reported by Melnick and Ledinko[33] in 1951 during a severe, unusual epidemic at Easton, Pa., and in 1952 by Dalldorf during two small epidemics in New York. In 1953 Steigman et al.[42] isolated a Coxsackie virus from a child with fatal poliomyelitis. In 1956 Chumakov[6a] isolated A7 virus from paralyzed children. Kalter's study in 1958 on a group of patients diagnosed as having poliomyelitis showed that Coxsackie viruses were implicated in 3 per cent of paralytic cases.

In 1960, during a herpangina epidemic, routine tests for associated poliomyelitis infection showed a significant rise in the titer of antibodies against poliomyelitis virus type I (Gerbeaüx et al.[16]).

2. Experimentally, no interference phenomena could be elicited between Coxsackie viruses and poliomyelitis virus in either the monkey or the mouse, nor in cell systems in vitro.

BIBLIOGRAPHY

1. Aumonier, F. J.: Structural changes in the skeletal muscles of suckling mice following infection with a Coxsackie virus of the "A" group. Roy. Microscop. Soc. 72:218-222, 1952.
2. Beeman, E. A., and Huebner, R. J.: Evaluation of serological methods for demonstrating antibody responses to group A Coxsackie (herpangina) viruses. J. Immunol., 68:663-672, 1952.
3. Boring, W. D., Zu Rhein, G. M., and Walker, D. L.: Factors influencing host-virus interactions. II. Alteration of Coxsackie virus infection in adult mice by cold. Proc. Soc. Exp. Biol. Med., 93: 273-277, 1956.
4. Briefs, A., Breese, S. S., Jr., Warren, J., and Huebner, R. J.: Physical properties of two group A Coxsackie (herpangina) viruses when propagated in eggs and mice as determined by ultracentrifugation and electron microscopy. J. Bacteriol., 64:237-246, 1952.
5. Buthala, D. A.: Effect of carbon dioxide concentration on ability of Coxsackie A-21 to form plaques. J. Bacteriol., 86:1356-1358, 1963.

6. Came, P. E., and Crowell, R. L.: Studies of resistance of fetal mouse tissues in culture to Coxsackie group A viruses. Virology, *23*:542-552, 1964.

6a. Chumakov, M. P., Voroshilova, M. K., Zhevandrova, V. I., Mironova, L. L., Itzelis, F. I., and Robinson, I. A.: Vydelenie i izuchenie IV immunologichestrogo tipa virus poliomielita [Isolation and investigation of the IV immunological type of poliomyelitis virus]. Prob. Virol., *1*:16-19, 1956.

7. Committee on Enteroviruses: Classification of human enteroviruses. Virology, *16*:501-504, 1962.

8. Dalldorf, G.: The Coxsackie viruses. In: Poliomyelitis: Papers and Discussions Presented at the Fourth International Poliomyelitis Conference. Philadelphia, J. B. Lippincott, 1958, p. 211.

9. Dalldorf, G., and Melnick, J. L.: Coxsackie Viruses. In Horsfall, F. L., and Tamm, I.: Viral and Rickettsial Infections of Man. Ed. 4. Philadelphia, J. B. Lippincott, 1965, pp. 474-512.

10. Dalldorf, G., and Sickles, G. M.: An unidentified, filtrable agent isolated from the feces of children with paralysis. Science, *108*:61-62, 1948.

11. Dunnebacke, T. H., and Mattern, C. F. T.: A comparison of the growth properties of Coxsackie virus strains A-9 and A-10 with poliovirus strain Mahoney in cultures of primary human amnion cells. J. Immunol., *86*:585-589, 1961.

12. Eggers, H. J., and Tamm, I.: Synergistic effect of 2-(α hydroxybenzyl)-benzimidazole and guanidine on picornavirus reproduction. Nature, *199*:513-514, 1963.

13. Federici, E. F., Lerner, M. A., and Abelmann, W. H.: Observations on the course of Coxsackie A-9 myocarditis in C3H mice. Proc. Soc. Exp. Biol. Med., *112*:672-676, 1963.

14. Fox, J. P.: Epidemiological aspects of Coxsackie and Echo virus infection in tropical areas. Amer. J. Public Health, *54*:1134-1142, 1964.

15. Gear, J. H. S.: Coxsackie virus infections in Southern Africa. Yale J. Biol. Med., *34*:289-303, 1962.

16. Gerbeaux, J., Couvreur, J., Hebert-Jouas, J., Virat, J., Maurin, J., and Chany, C.: L'Herpangine: Etude clinique, virologique et sérologique d'une épidémie en milieu hospitalier. Presse Méd., *68*:675-678, 1960.

17. Gifford, R., and Dalldorf, G.: Creatinine, potassium, and virus content of the muscles following infection with the "Coxsackie virus." Proc. Soc. Exp. Biol. Med., *71*:589-592, 1949.

18. Glasgow, L. A., and Balduzzi, P.: Isolation of Coxsackie virus group A, type 4, from a patient with hemolytic-uremic syndrome. New Eng. J. Med., *273*:754-756, 1965.

19. Grist, N. R.: Further studies of Coxsackie A7 virus infection in the West of Scotland. Lancet, *2*:261-263, 1965.

20. Habel, K., and Loomis, L. N.: Coxsackie A7 virus and the Russian "Poliovirus type 4." Proc. Soc. Exp. Biol. Med., *95*:597-605, 1957.

21. Hinuma, Y., Murai, Y., Fukuda, M., Numazaki, Y., and Ishida, N.: An outbreak of aseptic meningitis associated with Coxsackie B5 and A9 viruses in Northern Japan, 1961: Virological and serological studies. J. Hyg. (Camb.), *62*:159, 1964.

22. Huebner, R. J., Cole, R. M., Beeman, E. A., Bell, J. A., and Peers, J. H.: Herpangina: Etiological studies of a specific infectious disease. J.A.M.A., *145*:268-633, 1951.

23. Johnson, K. M., Bloom, H. H., Mufson, M. A., and Chanock, R. M.: Acute respiratory disease associated with Coxsackie A21 virus infection. I. Incidence in military personnel: Observations in a recruit population. II. Incidence in military personnel: Observations in a nonrecruit population. J.A.M.A., *179*:112-119; 120-125, 1962.

24. Johnson, K. M., Bloom, H. H., Rosen, L., Mufson, M. A., and Chanock, R. M.: Hemagglutination by Coe virus. Virology, *13*:373-374, 1961.

25. Johnson, K. M., and Lang, D. J.: Separation of hemagglutinating and nonhemagglutinating variants of Coxsackie A-21 virus. Proc. Soc. Exp. Biol. Med., *110*:653-657, 1962.

26. Kamitsuka, P. S., Lou, T. Y., Fabiyi, A., and Wenner, H. A.: Preparation and standardization of Coxsackievirus reference antisera. Amer. J. Epidemiol., *81*:283-305, 1965.

27. Koroleva, G. A., and Frolova, M. P.: Investigations on Coxsackie A-7, A-14 and A-16 viruses in tissue culture and in animals. Acta Virol., *8*:532-540, 1964.

28. Lenahan, M. F., and Wenner, H. A.: Propagation of group A Coxsackie viruses in primary human amnion cells. I. Cytopathic changes produced by 5 more serotypes. Proc. Soc. Exp. Biol. Med., *107*:544-546, 1961.

29. Mattern, C. F. T.: Some physical and chemical properties of Coxsackie viruses A-9 and A-10. Virology, *17*:520-532, 1962.

30. Mattern, C. F. T., and duBuy, H. G.: Purification and crystallization of Coxsackie virus. Science, *123*:1037-1038, 1956.

31. Mattern, C. F. T., and Chi, L. L.: Studies on the sites and kinetics of Coxsackie A-9 virus multiplication in the monkey kidney cell. Virology, *18*:257-265, 1962.

32. Melnick, J. L., Emmons, J., Coffey, J. H., and Schoof, H.: Seasonal distribution of Coxsackie viruses in urban sewage and flies. Amer. J. Hyg., *59*:164-184, 1954.

33. Melnick, J. L., and Ledinko, N.: Social serology: antibody levels in a normal young population during an epidemic of poliomyelitis. Amer. J. Hyg., *54*:354-382, 1951.

34. Munch, B. S.: On the specificity of complement fixation tests for typing of Coxsackie virus strains. Acta Path. Microbiol. Scand., *56*:89-104, 1962.

35. Pereira, M. S.: Coe virus properties and prevalence in Great Britain. Lancet, *2*:539-541, 1959.

36. Richardson, H. B., Jr., and Leibovitz, A.: "Hand, foot and mouth disease" in children. J. Pediat., *67*:6-12, 1965.

37. Robinson, L. K.: Effect of heat and pH on strains of Coxsackie virus. Proc. Soc. Exp. Biol. Med., *75*:580-582, 1950.

38. Sarkar, J. K., and Ray, H. N.: Effect of a Coxsackie virus on the mitosis of cultured human amnion cells: A preliminary report. Indian J. Med. Res., *52*:1133-1138, 1964.

39. Schmidt, N. J., Dennis, J., Frommhagen, L. H., and Lennette, E. H.: Serologic reactivity of certain antigens obtained by fractionation of Coxsackie viruses in cesium chloride density gradients. J. Immunol., *90*:654-662, 1963.

40. Schmidt, N. J., Fox, V. L., and Lennette, E. H.: Immunologic identification of Coxsackie A-21 virus with Coe virus. Proc. Soc. Exp. Biol. Med., *107*:63-65, 1961.

41. Schmidt, N. J., Fox, V. L., and Lennette, E. H.: Studies on the hemagglutination of Coe (Coxsackie A-21) virus. J. Immunol., *89*:672-683, 1962.
42. Steigman, A. J., Kokko, U. P., and Silverberg, R. J.: Unusual properties of a virus isolated from the spinal cord of a child with fatal poliomyelitis. Amer. J. Dis. Child., *86*:509-510, 1953.
43. Steigman, A. J., Lipton, M. M., and Braspennickx, H.: Acute lymphonodular pharyngitis: A newly described condition due to Coxsackie A virus. J. Pediat., *61*:331-336, 1962.
44. Tamm, I., and Eggers, H. J.: Differences in the selective virus inhibitory action of 2-(α hydroxy-benzyl)-benzimidazole and guanidine-HC1. Virology, *18*:439-447, 1962.
45. Tilles, J. G., Elson, S. H., Shaka, J. A., Abelmann, W. H., Lerner, A. M., and Finland, M.: Effects of exercise on Coxsackie A9 myocarditis in adult mice. Proc. Soc. Exp. Biol. Med., *117*:777-782, 1964.
46. Williamson, J. D., and Grist, N. R.: Studies on the haemagglutinin present in Coxsackie A-7 virus-infected suckling mouse tissue. J. Gen. Microbiol., *41*:283-291, 1965.
47. Wright, H. T., Landing, B. H., Lennette, E. H., and McAllister, R. H.: Fatal infection in an infant associated with Coxsackie virus group A, type 16. New Eng. J. Med., *268*:1041-1044, 1963.
48. Zalan, E., Kelen, A. E., and Labzoffsky, N. A.: Immunofluorescence studies on Coxsackie group A viruses. Arch. Ges. Virusforsch., *5*:668-680, 1965.

23

Infections and Inflammations of the Salivary Glands, the Pancreas, and the Mesenteric Glands

By F. BRICOUT

Viral infections of the salivary glands are frequent. They are marked by certain particularities: (1) They are infections which may involve clinically only the salivary glands but which can also involve other glands, and even other systems, as is the case with mumps virus. (2) These infections sometimes are latent and sometimes dramatic, as is the case with the cytomegalovirus.

Omitting from this chapter the problem of rabies virus, which was discussed along with encephalitis (see Chapter 10), we shall consider essentially the mumps virus and the cytomegalovirus. It also seems appropriate in this chapter to discuss the viruses responsible for mesenteric adenitis and appendicitis.

MUMPS

CLINICAL ASPECTS

After an 18- to 21-day incubation period, the disease is characterized by the appearance of parotitis, sometimes foreshadowed by several signs which, during an epidemic, orient the diagnosis: slight fever, some malaise, discomfort upon chewing, and acute unilateral or bilateral otalgia.

Parotid enlargement, at first unilateral, becomes bilateral in one to five days. The swelling is firm and painful and obliterates the retromaxillary groove; then, enlarging, it pushes forward the pinna and can give a pear-like appearance to the face. The swelling is accompanied by a moderately febrile state, with fever up to 38° C. in the early stage and headache.

Examination reveals the firm and elastic character of the parotitis. It also reveals the swelling and redness of the orifice of Stensen's duct.

The spontaneous pain, contusive and dull, moderate in children, can be acute in adults. It is localized in front of the auricular canal and radiates toward the ear, more rarely toward the neck. It can hinder mastication and result in a very painful reflexive trismus which alters pronounciation and hampers eating. It is increased or aroused by pressure in the parotid region, particularly at the three points designated by Rilliet and Barthez.

At times other salivary glands become involved, as revealed by the palpable swelling of the submaxillary and sublingual glands.

In the usual form of the disease, results of other clinical examinations are normal.

Besides specific biological examinations, which will be considered in the section on diagnosis, two other elements can aid in confirming the mumps origin of parotitis. (1) The blood count often indicates leukocytopenia or isonormocytosis; and (2) blood amylase titration reveals an increase during the first 15 days of the disease.

The evolution of parotitis is benign; after seven to ten days the swelling begins to subside, and it disappears completely, without sequel, toward the fifteenth day.

However, the mumps virus frequently affects other organs. Its localization can be associated with parotitis or can occur without it. These localizations of infection, which can aggravate the disease, are various. Some are well known.

Involvement of the testis, announced by a sharp rise in temperature with high fever, is characterized by swelling of the bursula testium. Only the testis increases in volume; the epididymis and the ductus deferens remain normal. Orchitis occurs in about 20 per cent of postpubescent patients. This percentage can, however, be higher, reaching 40 per cent (Philip et al.[23]).

The prognosis of orchitis is considered excellent, cure occurring in about two weeks, whether the orchitis is unilateral or bilateral. However, sterility due to bilateral testicular atrophy is not unknown (for further details see Chapter 53).

Central nervous system involvement in its most usual form occurs as "aseptic" meningitis (see Chapter 14). This does not differ either in its symptomatology or in its evolution from other virus-induced meningitis. The lymphocyte level of the spinal fluid is often elevated, reaching 400 to 500 elements per milliliter. As a rule it leaves no sequelae, although a certain degree of asthenia and discrete muscular weakness can persist and prolong convalescence. As a rule, the meningeal involvement is so minor that its only clinical signs are bradycardia and headache. In more than 35 per cent of the cases of simple parotitis, with no clinically evident signs of meningitis, the level of lymphocytes in the cerebrospinal fluid is increased. At the other extreme, more serious complications can occur. Deafness is fortunately very rare, but it is one of the most serious complications of mumps (see Chapter 57).

Involvement of the pancreas is exceptional. It begins suddenly with a rise in temperature, persistent dull epigastric pain, and vomiting. Clinical examination eliminates the possibility of a surgical emergency and reveals scarcely more than tachycardia and pallor. Mumps is easily incriminated in the presence of parotitis or if there is a possibility of contact with the disease. Nonspecific laboratory examinations are of only mediocre value in diagnosis.

The blood amylase level is above normal, although this increase may occur without clinically evident impairment of the pancreas, and there are hyperglycemia and transitory glycosuria. Evolution is favorable as a rule, and residual glycosuria is so exceptional that it has been ascribed to coincidence.

Other sites of localization of the mumps virus, whether or not associated with parotitis, are much rarer. Thus involvements of the prostate, epididymis, ovaries, liver, spleen, thyroid, kidneys, labyrinth, thymus, myocardium, and mammary glands have all been described.

THE MUMPS VIRUS AND PREGNANCY

In agreement with earlier work, Philip et al.[23] noted, during an extensive mumps epidemic in a group of Eskimos, that only 40 per cent of pregnant women contracted mumps as opposed to 62 per cent of nonpregnant women, and that after the epidemic only

65 per cent of the pregnant women had developed homologous antibodies as opposed to 92 per cent of the other women.

This significantly lower antibody level among pregnant women is not explained. Among five women infected during the first trimester of their pregnancy, four abortions occurred, whereas none occurred among 15 women exposed during the second or third trimesters of pregnancy.

As for the 16 children born after the epidemic, no anomaly was observed. This absence of a teratogenic capacity of the mumps virus seems to be well established experimentally. Ferm and Kilham[10] inoculated pregnant hamsters intravenously and established that the mumps virus electively multiplies in the uterine tissues and the placenta, where it was found between the fourth and eighth day of infection. It did not seem to be able to cross the placenta, and no histopathological lesion was seen in the fetal tissues. Similarly these authors did not note an increase in fetal deaths or in congenital malformations.

However, it must be emphasized that several more recent articles have mentioned the possible role of the mumps virus as a cause of endocardial fibroelastosis: Shone et al.[29] and St. Geme et al.[28] incriminated prenatal mumps infection. Comparison of groups of children who had fibroelastosis with control groups showed that 90 per cent of the first group had positive skin tests against the mumps antigen, whereas in the control groups only about 10 per cent had a positive skin test.

In eight of 15 cases with positive skin reaction there was a possibility that the mother had been infected by mumps virus during the first trimester of pregnancy, whereas this was not the case in mothers of the control group. However, of 67 children with fibroelastosis studied by the same authors, only five had homologous antibodies.

This lack of agreement between positive skin reactions to mumps antigens and the presence of serum antibodies was also demonstrated in 16 cases of fibroelastosis studied by Gersony et al.[13] Moreover, the mumps virus could not be isolated from any of the children.

Consequently, a certain number of hypotheses have been suggested: Is this a nonspecific hypersensitivity reaction? A cross reaction due to another virus? An *in utero* infection without a rise in the level of antibodies because of their nonelaboration (Shone et al.[29])? Does it represent absence of antibodies owing to weak antigenic stimulation as a result of the limited multiplication of virus *in utero* (St. Geme et al.[28])? No conclusion has yet been reached.

CLINICAL DIAGNOSIS

Clinical diagnosis of mumps is generally easy when there is a bilateral parotitis and difficult when localization occurs unilaterally in the salivary glands or outside the parotid. It becomes extremely difficult when signs of salivary gland or testicular involvement are absent.

In all atypical forms, in which the symptoms are isolated or in which their chronology in relation to the usual localizations is abnormal, epidemiological and clinical evidence should be seconded by a very complete biological study. This study should not only substantiate arguments in favor of mumps but also provide negative evidence eliminating all other bacterial or viral diseases associated with, or simulating, the same clinical picture.

Even in the presence of a bilateral parotitis, laboratory studies are sometimes indispensable.

Other viruses are capable of provoking parotitis: the virus of Armstrong's disease and the Coxsackie A viruses (see Chapters 17 and 22).

Certain cases of *bacterial parotitis* likewise resemble mumps fairly closely. Parotitis can be observed during infections due to pneumococcus, meningococcus, streptococcus, *Escherichia coli,* and so forth. The etiology is then relatively easily established. But one very particular form is the recurrent infectious parotitis of children (Robert Debré), also called chronic parotitis with recurrent exacerbation. Parotid swelling, sometimes unilateral and sometimes bilateral, appears abruptly within several hours. The parotid is more or less swollen, the gland is firm, and the skin is normal, though occasionally reddened. The region is painful spontaneously, upon chewing and swallowing, and on palpation. One main sign permits differential diagnosis: when slight pressure is applied to the parotid a mucopus oozes from the opening of Stensen's duct, bacteriological examination of which may reveal a pneumococcus or *Streptococcus viridans.*

Unilateral involvement similarly poses

the problem of *salivary lithiasis*. But the repetitive crises of obstruction brought on by feeding, which stop with salivary release, are characteristic, and the salivary calculus is visible on x-ray.

For differential diagnosis of other localizations of mumps we refer the reader to the respective chapters discussing orchitis (Chapter 53) and meningitis (Chapter 14).

CHARACTERISTICS OF THE MUMPS VIRUS

The mumps virus is a member of the group of myxoviruses. These viruses have a certain number of characteristics in common. The virions have a helicoid symmetry, they are of ribonucleic acid nature, and they are enclosed in an envelope.

This viral group has been subdivided and the mumps virus has been classified in the same subgroup as the four serotypes of the parainfluenza myxoviruses, as well as the Newcastle disease virus.

Like the other members of this subgroup, the mumps virus measures about 140 mμ. It develops in the cytoplasm of infected cells. It is a very fragile virus, is inactivated in 20 minutes at 56° C., and is well preserved at −70° C. Ether, formalin, and β-propiolactone destroy the infectivity of the virus while conserving its antigenic capacities (Cantell[7]).

A type-specific hemagglutinin, associated with the surface of the virion, is active with respect to a certain number of erythrocytes such as human, sheep, and guinea-pig red blood cells.

After infection, a soluble antigen stimulates the development of neutralizing and complement-fixing antibodies which are also type-specific.

Like the majority of myxoviruses, the mumps virus can be isolated by inoculation into the amniotic cavity of the chick embryo or into various cell systems cultivated *in vitro* (HeLa and monkey kidney cells). Its multiplication is evidenced by the appearance of multinucleated giant cells in the cytoplasm of which appear eosinophilic inclusions that are readily visible in the optic microscope with hematoxylin-eosin staining. However, techniques of virus isolation are relatively more laborious than the usual serological tests and are generally reserved for particular research: epidemiological studies and diagnosis of an atypical mumps localization, for example.

EPIDEMIOLOGY

Man is the only reservoir of the virus, although anti-mumps-virus antibodies have been shown to be present in the sera of healthy dogs.

Mumps infections occur the world over. Children are particularly sensitive to the infection, which strikes both sexes equally, although in the course of certain epidemiological studies boys between two and six years of age appeared to be more susceptible (Meyer[22]).

Contagion essentially occurs by direct and airborne contact. Indeed, saliva is highly contagious during the six days which preceed parotitis, the excretion of virus generally continuing for another nine days. This virulence of saliva is the same in patients not manifesting parotitis who, as unrecognized carriers of the virus, are a source of massive contamination.

Virus is also eliminated in the urine, which could be a second source of contamination. Testing 110 urine specimens from 21 patients, Utz and Szwed[32] isolated mumps virus in 58 per cent of the cases, a percentage which rises to 80 per cent during the first five days of the disease. This viruria exists until the fifteenth day of the disease.

The length of the period of virus elimination explains the high contagiousness of the disease. During an epidemic in a group of Eskimos, among a population of 561 subjects not having encountered the mumps virus for a great many years, Philip et al.[23] noted that 88 per cent were affected. Sixty-five per cent of them had a clinical case of the disease, the number of cases being greater among school-aged children than among young adults and among boys than among girls. During this epidemic, 23 per cent of the subjects had an inapparent disease, a figure lower than during other epidemics, in which inapparent cases represented a proportion as high as 30 to 40 per cent. The inapparent form of the disease was particularly prevalent in the older age groups.

The absence of reservoirs of the virus other than man and the fact that transmission of infection occurs directly from the person carrying the virus to the healthy subject explains the regional variations in the distribution of the disease. Just as in Alaska Philip et al. observed an epidemic in an almost totally receptive population, so in the Antilles Habel noted that the islanders contracted mumps only when they grouped together in the ports. In most urban populations, mumps is endemic, present all year long though predominating in the winter and spring. Epidemics occur in collectivities of young people with a high proportion of receptive individuals and the possibility of repeated, direct contacts between numerous subjects. These are collectivities of children: orphanages, schools, nurseries, and hospitals for convalescent children. Collectivities of young adults, such as military recruits in all armies have paid a heavy tribute to mumps virus. Military physicians have greatly contributed to our current knowledge of mumps. In these groups, mumps rarely constitutes an explosive epidemic. The morbidity curve rises progressively, reaching a peak in six to 11 weeks, and then declines more rapidly.

According to Meyer et al.[22] who studied the epidemiology of mumps in children in family surroundings, in these circumstances the virus diffuses from the school children who secondarily contaminate receptive subjects in their surroundings. On the other hand, very young children seem to be less susceptible to the disease, perhaps because the diagnosis is not made owing to the greater frequency of subclinical or very discrete infections at this age.

SEROLOGICAL STUDIES

Serological studies essentially consist of the search for and titration of hemagglutination-inhibiting and complement-fixing antibodies. The more laborious search for neutralizing antibodies is much less used.

Mumps infection is followed by a rise in the level of antibodies, beginning about the tenth day and reaching a maximum about the fourth week. The complement-fixing antibodies appear first, whereas the hemagglutination-inhibiting antibodies, which appear more slowly, persist for a longer time.

The level of complement-fixing antibodies reaches a maximum toward the fourth to sixth week after the beginning of infection and then falls rapidly. Consequently, for Philip et al.,[23] titration of these antibodies is of little value in studying the previous diffusion of mumps virus. In the study by Philip et al., 48 per cent of subjects infected had an antibody titer below $\frac{1}{10}$ eight to ten months after parotitis.

The antibody level may be less high in person who had an inapparent infection than in others (Philip et al.). However, these inapparent cases seem to confer an equally solid immunity (Meyer[22]).

Although the mumps virus is clearly an individualized myxovirus, a certain number of studies have shown that there can be serological cross-reactions between it and other members of the subgroup.

Using guinea-pig sera, Cook et al.[8] demonstrated an antigenic relationship between mumps virus and type 1 parainfluenza myxovirus in ten patients with mumps. Hsiung et al.[16] noted a concomitant development of anti-type 2 parainfluenza myxovirus antibodies in five cases of mumps and anti-type 3 parainfluenza myxovirus antibodies in one case. Lennette et al.[21] similarly found a rise in heterologous antibodies, notable with respect to type 1 parainfluenza myxovirus, whether the antibodies were complement-fixing or hemagglutination-inhibiting. This frequency of heterologous reactions increases with the patients' age (21 per cent of patients under five years of age and 80 per cent of these over 20 years of age), an observation which made this author think that anamnestic reactions were involved. In the case of mumps infection of a person who had not previously been infected by another myxovirus, there would be no development of heterologous antibodies. On the other hand, in a person previously infected by myxoviruses, infection with mumps could elicit an anamnestic response due to antigens identical with, or closely related to, those of parainfluenza myxoviruses.

Lastly, Johnson et al.[17] established an antigenic relationship between mumps virus and type 4 parainfluenza myxovirus.

PATHOGENESIS AND ANATOMOPATHOLOGY

It seems that mumps virus can reach the parotid and other salivary glands from the buccal cavity via the salivary ducts.

The existence of viremia has been demonstrated at the onset of disease and explains the diffusion of the virus into many organs, the virus being eliminated in the urine. This viremia has been confirmed experimentally since it is possible to cultivate the virus *in vitro* in leukocytes (Duc Nguyen and Henle[9]). Viral multiplication gives rise to histological modifications. In the salivary gland, it is evidenced by degeneration of the duct cells with a serofibrinous and leukocytic exudate. In the testis, there can be destruction of the seminiferous tubules. In the pancreas, there is generally an interstitial edema and a discrete degeneration of the islets of Langherans.

IMMUNITY

The immunity conferred by clinical or subclinical mumps infection results in a clear-cut resistance to reinfection. Cases of clinical recurrence of mumps parotitis are supposed to be the result of an error in diagnosis. It is, however, possible that inapparent infections occur in immunized subjects.

The newborn child is protected for from six to nine months by passively acquired maternal antibodies.

VIROLOGICAL DIAGNOSIS

In addition to studies of the white cell count and the amylase level, which provide indirect proof of mumps infection, virological examinations are indicated whenever the conditions of appearance or a peculiar symptomatology oblige the clinician to seek biological confirmation of his diagnosis.

Specimens. As soon as the diagnosis of mumps is suggested, particularly in the absence of characteristic parotitis, it is important to take a throat swab, a urine specimen, and a cerebrospinal fluid sample if there are biological signs of meningeal involvement. These specimens should be sent immediately to the laboratory, in dry ice, because of the heat sensitivity of the virus.

At the same time as specimens are taken for the purpose of virus isolation, it is essential to draw from 3 to 5 ml. of the patient's blood. A second sample of serum is sent to the laboratory some two weeks later.

Results. Failure to isolate the virus cannot formally eliminate the possibility of mumps infection, since the virus is fragile and might not have been brought to the laboratory under adequate conditions.

The isolation of the virus should be accompanied by a rise in the level of homologous antibodies in order to affirm viral infection. The increase in antibodies ought to be sharp, that is to say, the antibody level should be four times higher in the serum taken during convalescence than in that obtained during the acute phase of disease.

Serological study of only one serum sample taken during convalescence is of little value, since a high level of antibodies could be due to an infection dating back several weeks or even months. Finally, it should again be mentioned that, after a mumps infection there are serological cross-reactions with parainfluenza myxoviruses.

As to the positiveness of the intradermal reaction to mumps antigens in subjects who have been infected by the virus, it has little diagnostic value since it is only indicative of a previous infection without being more exact. Repetition of this test, moreover, runs the risk of provoking the appearance of antibodies, thereby modifying serological data. However, a positive intradermal reaction has aroused interest in the study of endocardial fibroelastosis.

PROPHYLAXIS AND THERAPY

Several prophylaxis measures have been proposed: (1) The use of gamma globulin of sera from convalescents protects a subject from infection for from two to three weeks. (2) The use of vaccines has also been tried, either an inactivated vaccine with two subcutaneous injections of 1 ml. and a booster injection six to eight months later, or an attenuated vaccine.

In 1968 a committee of experts authorized in the United States the generalized use of mumps live virus vaccine attenuated by culture on the embryonated egg and prepared in cellular cultures of chick embryos.[22a]

A single injection produces a nontransmissible inapparent infection. Over 95 per cent of receptive subjects thus acquire specific antibodies. The titer of these antibodies is slightly inferior to that found after a natural infection and the length of duration of these antibodies has not yet been evaluated beyond two years. It is not excluded that the subjects thus immunized may be susceptible, in an epidemic environment, to infection without clinical manifestations but with a booster effect on the titers of antimumps antibodies.[32a]

It has been proposed by some authors that this vaccine and live attenuated measles vaccine be given together. Simultaneous use of gamma globulins has not seemed to modify the percentage of seroconversions.[15a]

Nonetheless this vaccination cannot, at present, be considered as a routine vaccination and should not in any way hinder the application of vaccination programs whose value has long been recognized. On the other hand, it could have great interest in reducing the incidence of mumps orchitis among adolescents and young adults in collective living conditions. However, the difficulties of evaluating the efficacy of a vaccination under these conditions should be noted in view of the high percentage of inapparent mumps infections.

It is not known what criterion other than prevaccination serological test could detect the young men who ought to be vaccinated. Another unknown is whether, in an epidemic period, a vaccination practiced immediately after an infecting contact would assure an effective protection.

In any event, the contraindications are the same as for all other vaccinations with a live vaccine: treatments with immunodepressive agents, leukemia, lymphoma, or other generalized malignant disease, pregnancy, and acute evolving disease.

As to management, it consists essentially of nonspecific measures such as bed rest and analgesics. Currently, there is no specific therapy.

Corticosteroids have been extolled by some, but there is no certain proof of their effectiveness and it has been ascertained, at least experimentally, that they are noxious in certain viral infections.

INFECTION OF THE SALIVARY GLANDS BY THE CYTOMEGALOVIRUS

CLINICAL ASPECT

Cytomegalovirus infections are very frequent, since it appears that 80 per cent of persons over 35 years of age have homologous serum antibodies. Most often the infection is latent, indicated only by the presence of antibodies. But the clinically evident infection is often manifested as a severe process.

The disease can be congenital, being transmitted *in utero* to the fetus, or acquired, usually during infancy.

Congenital Infection. Since this subject will be discussed in the chapter devoted to neonatal virus diseases (Chapter 61*C*), it suffices to mention here that *in utero* transmission of the virus can cause extremely serious disorders in the newborn, the virus being capable of invading numerous organs.

Involvement of the salivary glands is manifested by the elimination of virus in the saliva, an elimination which can continue for months if the nursing infant survives the infection.

Involvement of the liver is characterized by an intense, often dark green jaundice with hyperbilirubinemia of high level, in relation to the hemolysis. The level of serum transaminases is very high.

Blood disorders other than hemolysis are also manifested—e.g., severe thrombocytopenic purpura. Anemia can accompany erythroblastosis.

Examination reveals a certain number of signs indicative of prenatal infection: prematurity, with an obvious weight deficiency at birth and the possible presence of microcephalia and cerebral calcifications decernible in x-ray films of the head.

Evolution of this infectious syndrome can lead directly to death. Hepatosplenomegaly, pulmonary signs indicative of viral pneumopathy, and the appearance of neurological disorders all confirm a diffusion of the virus that will be fatal to the infant.

If the patient survives, it is often at the price of serious sequelae which are notably of three kinds:

(1) Neurological sequelae, characterized by microcephalia, various paralyses, most often of the diplegic or paraplegic types, and visual disorders with chorioretinitis, optical atrophy, and blindness (Weller and Hanshaw,[33] Hanshaw[14]). Eighty-one per cent of the 42 patients with follow-up by Hanshaw showed neurological sequelae.

(2) Hepatic sequelae which evolve toward cirrhosis. Stern and Tucker[30] described biliary malformations with atresia of the external and intrahepatic bile ducts in connection with a cytomegalovirus infection.

(3) Lastly, psychic sequelae, with mental retardation and behavior disorders which become apparent at school age (Medearis).

Acquired Infection. Acquired infection

is certainly less severe but raises the question especially of its relation to various forms of liver involvement.

It can be at the origin of pulmonary disorders that lack characteristics specific for this virus but suggest a viral pneumopathy, of gastro-intestinal disorders linked to an ulcerative process and manifested by hemorrhages, and, lastly, of blood disorders evolving as acquired hemolytic anemia.

This acquired infection can give rise to a mild clinical picture, but Hanshaw et al.,[15] having isolated a cytomegalovirus from 20 apparently healthy children, discovered that 14 of them had hepatomegaly, five of them had splenomegaly, and, finally, two of them had angiomas. In addition, 17 of the children (six times as many as in the control group) had abnormal liver-function test results.

Thus, the role of cytomegalovirus in the etiology of certain hepatomegalies or liver insufficiencies seemed likely to Hanshaw. However, as seen by this author, the exact relationship between the infection and liver abnormalies was not precisely established: "Although it is clear that infected infants can have chronic obstructive hepatitis which may resemble giant cell hepatitis or biliary atresia, it is not known whether chronic infection can result in chronic hepatitis or cirrhosis in older children and adults. The rarity or absence of inclusions in the liver of congenitally infected infants with known virus in that organ suggests that the pathologist may not be able to make this diagnosis on histologic grounds alone."

Latent Infections. The frequency and importance of latent infections have recently become more evident. They most often become apparent in patients with generalized malignant diseases or with leukemia, or patients who are being treated with immunosuppressive agents. In some cases the infection appeared to develop more easily under such conditions and rapidly brought on death (Cangir and Sullivan[6]), in others, the virus was discovered in the urine and saliva, in the absence of clinical signs of infection (Kanich and Craighead[19]), and, finally, in some cases the infection was discovered at autopsy by culture of kidneys from children with cardiac malformations (Benyesh-Melnick et al.[2]).

Possible Role in Infectious Mononucleosis. It must be stressed that Kääriäinen et al. and Klemola and Kääriäinen[18, 20] mentioned the possible role of cytomegalovirus in the origin of a syndrome resembling infectious mononucleosis.

EPIDEMIOLOGY

Cytomegalovirus infections seem to be extremely frequent, as evidenced by the high incidence of homologous antibodies in the sera of persons over 35 years of age. The infected human being eliminates a large amount of virus in his saliva and urine for periods as long as two years (Rowe et al.[27]) This source of contamination, which might not be noticed in asymptomatic carriers, can be the origin of massive epidemics.

PATHOGENESIS

Diffusion of the virus throughout the infected organism manifests itself by the presence of virus or of cells with characteristic inclusions in a great variety of tissues: kidney, liver, lung, pancreas, and, notably, the salivary glands.

According to Wong and Warner,[34] there are marked differences between what happens in the adult and in the child. In the child, it is above all the salivary glands, kidneys, liver, and lungs which are affected, and accessorily, the pancreas, thyroid, adrenals and brain. On the other hand, in the adult sites of infection, in order of decreasing frequency, are the lungs, adrenals, liver, digestive system, spleen, pancreas, and kidneys. In addition, intranuclear inclusions are found essentially in epithelial cells of children whereas in the adult they are found predominantly in the vascular endothelial cells and macrophages.

These differences, according to Wong and Warner, could be explained by a difference in susceptibility of infantile and adult tissues.

VIROLOGICAL DIAGNOSIS

Since this subject will be covered in the chapter devoted to virus diseases of newborns (Chapter 61C), it will not be discussed here.

INFECTIONS OF THE SALIVARY GLANDS BY COXSACKIE VIRUSES

Coxsackie viruses were incriminated by Howlett in the etiology of a parotitis fairly imilar to that of mumps and characterized by fever, dysphagia, and jugal pain, with tumefaction of the parotid, but with painful buccal ulcerations. The disease lasts between five and 23 days, and group A Coxackie virus has been isolated from the patients' throats. Virological diagnosis of Coxsackie A infections is discussed in the chapter dealing with herpangina (Chapter 22).

THE PROBLEM OF MESENTERIC ADENITIS, INTUSSUSCEPTION, AND APPENDICITIS

The problem is assuredly not one of infection of the gastrointestinal glands, but rather of involvement of the mesenteric lymph nodes and the appendix during virus diseases.

Mesenteric adenitis gives rise to a clinical picture which is in all ways comparable to that of acute appendicitis. The diagnosis changes when surgery reveals large swollen lymph nodes, usually in the ileocecal region, and a normal appendix. This virus-induced mesenteric adenitis can cause intussusception, the role of adenitis as its initiator also being discovered at operation.

In this manner, the role in intussusception of adenoviruses and certain other viruses, notably the enteroviruses, has been pointed out (Bell and Steyn[1]; Gardner,[10, 11, 12]; Potter,[24, 25]). During these syndromes adenoviruses types 1, 2, 3, 5, 6, and 7 and ECHO viruses types 7 and 9 have been isolated either from stools or from mesenteric lymph nodes.

Comparable studies have also permitted isolation of a certain number of viruses, especially adenoviruses, from the stools or mesenteric lymph nodes of children operated on in the course of simple mesenteric adenitis.

Indirect proof of the possible role of adenoviruses in the pathogenesis of intestinal intussusception was given by Potter et al.[25] in a study of the incidence of anti-adenovirus antibodies in sera taken during the acute phase of the disease as compared with that in control cases.

On the other hand, the role of viruses in initiating appendicitis is much less clear. Tobe[31] implicated the Coxsackie B viruses and adenoviruses indirectly. The studies of Bonard,[3] Bonard and Paccaud[4] and Bricout et al.,[5] seem to confirm the possible role of certain viruses (adenoviruses and enteroviruses) in the etiology of acute appendicitis.

For details on the biological diagnosis of adenovirus and enterovirus infections, the reader should consult the chapters on the respiratory manifestations of virus diseases (adenoviruses, Chapter 44C) and on neurological syndromes (ECHO viruses and Coxsackie B viruses, Chapter 3B).

BIBLIOGRAPHY

1. Bell, T. M., and Steyn, J. M.: Viruses in lymph nodes of children with mesenteric adenitis and intussusception. Brit. Med. J., 2:700-702, 1962.
2. Benyesh-Melnick, M., Rosenberg, M., and Watson, B.: Viruses in cell cultures of kidneys of children with congenital heart malformations and other diseases. Proc. Soc. Exp. Biol. Med., 3:452-459, 1964.
3. Bonard, E. C.: Appendicites à virus. Helv. Med. Acta, 30:454-460, 1963.
4. Bonard, E. C., and Paccaud, M. F.: Abdominal adenovirosis and appendicitis. Helv. Med. Acta, 33:164-171, 1966.
5. Bricout, F., Fontaine, J. L., Regnard, J., Baheux, G., Guy-Grand, D., and Morel, M.: La place des virus dans l'étiologie des appendicites aigues de l'enfance. Presse Med., 74:2735-2737, 1966.
6. Cangir, A., and Sullivan, M.: The occurrence of cytomegalovirus infections in childhood leukemia. J.A.M.A. 195:616-622, 1966.
7. Cantell, K.: Mumps virus. Advances Virus Res., 8:123-164, 1962.
8. Cook, M. K., Andrews, B. E., Fox, M. M., Turner, M. C., James, W. D., and Chanock, R. M.: Antigenic relationships among the "newer" myxoviruses (parainfluenza). Amer. J. Hyg., 69:250-264, 1959.
9. Duc Nguyen, H., and Henle, W.: Replication of mumps virus in human leukocyte cultures. J. Bact., 92:258-265, 1966.
10. Ferm, V. H., and Kilham, L.: Mumps virus infection of the pregnant hamster. J. Embryol. Exp. Morph., 11:659-665, 1963.
11. Gardner, P. S.: Adenovirus and intussusception. Brit. Med. J., 2:495-496, 1961.
12. Gardner, P. S., Knox, E. G., Court, S. D. M., and Green, C. A.: Virus infection and intussusception in childhood. Brit. Med. J., 2:697-700, 1962.
13. Gersony, W. M., Katz, S. L., and Nadas, A. S.: Endocardial fibroelastosis and the mumps virus. Pediatrics, 37:430-434, 1966.
14. Hanshaw, J. B.: Congenital and acquired cytomegalovirus infection. Pediat. Clin. N. Amer., 13:279-293, 1966.
15. Hanshaw, J. B., Betts, R. F., Simon, G., and Boynton, R. C.: Acquired cytomegalovirus infection. Association with hepatomegaly and abnormal liver-function tests. New Eng. J. Med., 272:602-609, 1965.
15a. Hilleman, M. R., Buynak, E. B., Weibel, R. E., and Stokes, J. Jr.: Live attenuated mumps-virus vaccine. New. Eng. J. Med., 278:227-232, 1968.
16. Hsiung, G. D., Isacson, P., and Tucker, G.: Studies of parainfluenzas virus II. Yale J. Biol. Med., 35:534-544, 1963.

17. Johnson, K. M., Chanock, R. M., Cook, M. K., and Huebner, R. J.: Studies of a new human hemadsorption virus. I. Isolation, properties and characterization. Amer. J. Hyg., *71*:81-92, 1960.

18. Kääriäinen, L., Paloheimo, J., Klemola, E., Mäkela, T., and Koivuniemi, A.: Cytomegalovirus-mononucleosis. Ann. Med. Exp. Fenn., *44*:297-301, 1966.

19. Kanich, R. E., and Craighead, J. E.: Cytomegalovirus infection and cytomegalic inclusion disease in renal homotransplant recipients. Amer. J. Med., *40*:874-882, 1966.

20. Klemola, E., and Kääriäinen, L.: Cytomegalovirus as a possible cause of disease resembling infectious mononucleosis. Brit. Med. J., *2*:1099-1102, 1965.

21. Lennette, E. H., Jensen, F. W., Guenther, R. W., and Magoffin, R. L.: Serologic responses to parainfluenzae viruses in patients with mumps virus infection. J. Lab. Clin. Med., *61*:780-788, 1963.

22. Meyer, M. B.: An epidemiologic study of mumps: its spread in schools and families. Amer. J. Hyg., *75*:259-281, 1962.

22a. Mumps Vaccine. Recommendations of the P.H.S. Advisory Committee on Immunization Practices. Clin. Pediat., *7*:156, 1968.

23. Philip, R. N., Reinhard, K. R., and Lackman, D. B.: Observations on a mumps epidemic in a "virgin" population. Amer. J. Hyg., *69*:91-111, 1959.

24. Potter, C. W.: Adenovirus infection as an aetiological factor in intussusception of infants and young children. J. Path. Bact., *88*:263-274, 1964.

25. Potter, C. W., Smedden, W. I. H., and Zachary, R. B.: A comparative study of the incidence of adenovirus antibodies in children with intussus-

ception with that in a control group. J. Pediat. *63*:420-427, 1963.

26. Rifkind, D.: Cytomegalovirus infection after renal transplantation. Arch. Int. Med., *116*:554-558, 1965.

27. Rowe, W. P., Hartley, J. W., Cramblett, H. G., and Mastrota, F. M.: Detection of human salivary gland virus in the mouth and urine of children. Amer. J. Hyg., *67*:57-65, 1958.

28. St. Geme, J. W., Noren, G. R., and Adams, P.: Proposed embryopathic relation between mumps virus and primary endocardial fibroelastosis. New Eng. J. Med., *275*:339-347, 1966.

29. Shone, J. D., Armas, S. M., Manning, J. A., and Keith, J. D.: The mumps antigen skin test in endocardial fibroelastosis. Pediatrics, *37*:423-429, 1966.

30. Stern, H., and Tucker, S. M.: Cytomegalovirus infection in the newborn and in early childhood. Lancet, *2*:1268-1271, 1965.

31. Tobe, T.: Inapparent virus infection as a trigger of appendicitis. Lancet, *1*:1343-1346, 1965.

32. Utz, J. P., and Szwed, C. F.: Mumps. III. Comparison of methods for detection of viruria. Proc. Soc. Exp. Biol. Med., *110*:841-844, 1962.

32a. Weibel, R. E., Stokes, J. Jr., Buynak, E. B., Leagus, M. B., and Hilleman, M. R.: Jeryl Lynn strain live attenuated mumps virus vaccine. Durability of immunity following administration. J.A.M.A. *203*:14-18, 1968.

33. Weller, T. H., and Hanshaw, J. B.: Virologic and clinical observations on cytomegalic inclusion disease. New Eng. J. Med., *266*:1233-1244, 1962.

34. Wong, T. W., and Warner, N. E.: Cytomegalic inclusion disease in adults. Arch. Path., *74*:403-422, 1962.

24

Viral Hepatitis

By S. KRUGMAN and R. WARD

In many parts of the world viral hepatitis is considered to be the most important unsolved problem in the field of infectious diseases. In the United States, over 72,000 cases were reported in 1961, the peak year since 1952, the year notification was started. It seems highly likely that at least as many cases were not recognized. Although several

viruses are known to be associated with hepatitis in man (yellow fever, varicella, and infectious mononucleosis* in adults, and herpes simplex, cytomegalovirus, Coxsackie virus, and rubella virus in infants), this chapter is concerned with the agents of *infectiou*

---

*Etiology unknown.

epatitis and *serum hepatitis* and their effect n man. Most authorities believe these agents) be viruses despite the fact that so far they ave defied successful or reproducible propagation in any laboratory test object—experimental animal, egg, or tissue culture. Man eems to be the only susceptible host. Moreover, there is no specific immunological test vailable for the recognition of viral hepatitis. /hen these serious drawbacks are overcome, ıpid advances can be expected in our knowldge of the natural history of viral hepatitis nd how to prevent it.

Infectious hepatitis appears to have lagued mankind for a long time under ıch guises as *catarrhal jaundice, epidemic ıundice,* and *acute yellow atrophy of the ver.* Recently, it has also been called *IH* nd *virus A. hepatitis.* The disease occurs in pidemics and sporadically and is spread by ıtestinal-oral pathways, with intimate human ssociation playing a major role. *Serum epatitis,* known also as *homologous serum ıandice, SH,* and *virus B hepatitis,* is a manade disease artificially transmitted by the ıjection of virus contained in blood, serum, r other blood products, or on contaminated edles, syringes, stylets, and other instruents. Serum hepatitis has been recognized ıring the past quarter of a century with ineasing frequency as a result of the wideread use of blood and its products. The pularity of all sorts of injections—justid and unjustified—adds to the incidence hen these are performed after inadequate erilization of instruments.

FECTIOUS HEPATITIS

LINICAL ASPECTS

Description of Syndrome. Infectious epatitis is a common virus infection which is naracterized by fever, gastrointestinal symp•ms such as nausea, vomiting, and abdominal ıin, and laboratory evidence of liver injury. ıundice, a cardinal sign of the disease, is not esent in all cases. The disease in children commonly anicteric.

Incubation Period. The incubation ıriod may range between 15 and 50 days; it usually about 30 days. The duration may e influenced by such factors as virus strain,)se of infective agent, and presence or abınce of a preicteric phase of the disease.

Certain strains of IH virus have been associated with incubation periods of two to three weeks; with other strains it has been as long as four to six weeks. A decrease in the dose of virus has been followed by a prolongation of the incubation period. On the other hand, neither the source of the virus nor the portal of entry has had an effect on the length of the incubation period; it is essentially the same following oral ingestion or parenteral administration of virus- containing materials.

Clinical Manifestations. The clinical picture in infants and young children is more variable than in adolescents and adults. The classic disease, which is observed more often in the older age group, is characterized by two phases, preicteric and icteric. The preicteric phase usually begins with an abrupt onset of fever, anorexia, nausea, vomiting, and abdominal discomfort. These symptoms may persist for four to eight days before jaundice becomes apparent and the icteric phase begins. In children, the fever and other systemic symptoms subside as the jaundice increases in intensity. In adolescents and adults the anorexia and other gastrointestinal symptoms may be prolonged during the early icteric phase. Dark urine, clay-colored stools, and a tender enlarged liver may precede evidence of icteric sclerae and skin.

The duration of jaundice is variable. In young children it rarely persists for more than one to two weeks. In adults it rarely subsides earlier than three to four weeks. The liver decreases in size and in tenderness after a period of one to two weeks. A transient splenomegaly may be present in some patients.

The disease in infants and children is most commonly anicteric and very mild. In an institutional study of infants under three years of age, only one of 36 infants with hepatitis had obvious jaundice. Asymptomatic, anicteric hepatitis was a common observation in the Willowbrook hepatitis studies.

Laboratory Findings. At the present time there is no specific test for the laboratory detection of hepatitis. Consequently, it is impossible to measure an antibody response to this agent. However, it is not difficult to establish the diagnosis by the use of various nonspecific laboratory tests. During the preicteric period there is evidence of a leukopenia. A small number of atypical lymphocytes may be observed on blood smear. Bile is usually present in the urine shortly before the emergence of jaundice. As indicated in Figure 24-1, the serum glutamic oxalacetic transaminase (SGOT) is the first test of liver function to become abnormal. Thereafter, the thymol turbidity and cephalin flocculation tests become positive just before there is a significant rise in serum bilirubin concentration. The van den Bergh reaction is predominantly direct during the early icteric period; later it becomes biphasic, with an increase in the indirect-reacting fraction.

Assay of serum transaminase activity is the most useful test for the diagnosis of infectious hepatitis. The use of other enzyme determinations, such as phosphohexose isomerase, isocitric dehydrogenase, and leucine aminopeptidase, does not offer any advantage. The two transaminase tests which are employed are the serum aspartic-ketoglutaric (serum glutamic oxaloacetic) transaminase or SGOT and the serum alanine-ketoglutaric (serum glutamic pyruvic) transaminase or SGPT. The SGPT assay may be more specific for liver cell injury because, unlike the SGOT, it is not abnormal in patients with myocardial cell necrosis due to infarction.

The pattern of SGOT activity in children with infectious hepatitis is illustrated in Figure 24-2. The crescendo-like rise in SGOT reaches a peak at about the time of onset of jaundice. The SGOT is abnormal in nearly all patients with infectious hepatitis from one week before to one week after appearance of jaundice. In some cases the SGOT may be abnormal as early as three weeks before icterus appears; it is generally normal by the third or fourth week of jaundice.

De Ritis and his associates[4] have used the ratio of SGOT to SGPT activity as an aid to the laboratory diagnosis of acute viral hepatitis. In normal persons the ratio of SGOT to SGPT was greater than 1.0, the mean value being 1.24. They observed a mean value of 0.64 in patients with viral hepatitis. This inverted ratio was not detected in patients with jaundice due to other causes, such as cirrhosis of the liver, bacterial hepatocholangitis, obstructive jaundice, and

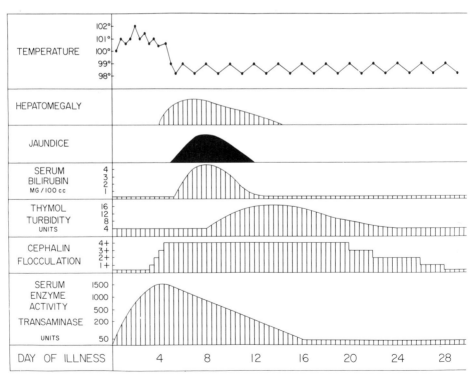

Figure 24-1. Schematic diagram of clinical course of infectious hepatitis; correlation of liver function tests with clinical findings. (From Krugman, S., and Ward, R.: Infectious Diseases of Children. 4th edition. St. Louis, C. V Mosby Co., 1968.)

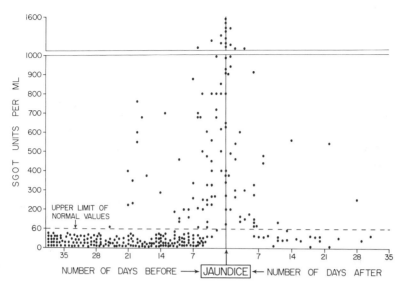

Figure 24-2. Scattergram of serial determinations of serum aspartic-ketoglutaric (serum glutamic oxalacetic) transaminase (SGOT), in 24 children before and after onset of jaundice. (From Giles, J. P., and Krugman, S.: Unpublished studies.)

congestion of the liver due to cardiac decompensation.

Course. The course of infectious hepatitis, especially in children, is usually uneventful and benign. Complications and fatalities are extremely rare. Although the prognosis is generally excellent, there are well-documented reports of fulminating hepatitis with a fatal outcome in children as well as in adults. In these rare situations there may be an abrupt onset of mental confusion, convulsions, coma, intense jaundice, and generalized bleeding in various organs, including the gastrointestinal tract. Occasionally the disease may become progressive or subacute, with subsequent portal hypertension and ascites and possibly death within a year.

Diagnosis and Differential Diagnosis. The diagnosis is usually established by correlating all of the available clinical, epidemiological, and laboratory data. As indicated previously, there is no specific virological or immunological test for the diagnosis of infectious hepatitis.

In the absence of an epidemic it is difficult to establish a diagnosis of either preicteric or anicteric hepatitis. The following diseases may be considered in the differential diagnosis during the acute febrile preicteric period: influenza, salmonellosis, shigellosis, infectious mononucleosis, acute appendicitis, malaria, and dengue. The diagnosis is usually established by detection of the specific causative agent or the results of antibody tests. The diagnosis of appendicitis is confirmed by surgery when it is indicated.

During the icteric phase of the disease the following diseases are considered in the differential diagnosis: serum hepatitis; hemolytic jaundice; obstructive jaundice caused by congenital defects, calculi, or tumors; hepatocellular jaundice caused by chemical poisons and certain drugs; and jaundice associated with a variety of bacterial, viral, and parasitic infections.

SERUM HEPATITIS. This disease may be clinically indistinguishable from infectious hepatitis. The onset is usually more insidious. The abnormal SGOT activity may persist for a longer period; i.e., many months rather than several weeks. The most distinguishing feature is the longer incubation period (50 to 180 days) and the association with parenteral inoculation of blood or blood products.

HEMOLYTIC JAUNDICE. The following differential features are significant; anemia, indirect-reacting van den Bergh, positive Coombs test, and no bile in urine.

OBSTRUCTIVE JAUNDICE. Congenital atresia of the bile ducts may cause extrahepatic or intrahepatic obstructive jaundice. Stones and tumors are rare in children. The clinical course of the illness is the most helpful differential feature.

HEPATOCELLULAR JAUNDICE. A history of ingestion or inhalation of a toxic agent is helpful. Jaundice may be due to the effect of the following drugs on the liver: pyrazinamide, iproniazid, phenothiazine derivatives, gold, cinchophen, methyltestosterone, and arsphenamine.

JAUNDICE ASSOCIATED WITH INFECTIONS. In the neonatal period the most common causes would be bacterial sepsis, congenital syphilis, cytomegalovirus infection, congenital rubella, disseminated herpes simplex virus infection, Coxsackie virus infection, and toxoplasmosis. In older children and adults the following infections should be considered: infectious mononucleosis, yellow fever, spirochetal jaundice (Weils' disease), and amebiasis. The diagnosis of these various infectious diseases is established by culture of the specific causative agent and by a specific serological test.

VIRUS RESPONSIBLE

The past decade has seen an increasing number of reports of the isolation of viruses from patients with infectious hepatitis or serum hepatitis. Although many such candidate viruses have been described in published and unpublished studies, there has been no confirmation of these reports. Some candidate agents have been identified as new types or subtypes of known virus groups such as adenovirus, myxovirus, and reovirus; others have no antigenic relationship with known virus groups. At the present writing none of these candiate viruses can be unequivocally designated the etiological agent of human viral hepatitis. It should be noted, parenthetically, that the classic achievements of Enders and his associates in propagating both poliovirus and measles virus in tissue cultures were promptly reproduced in many other laboratories. So far this has not been the case with candidate hepatitis viruses.

Although a number of viruses have been established as etiological agents of hepatitis in the horse, cow, sheep, dog, mouse, and canary, there is no evidence to indicate that any of these agents is related to viral hepatitis of man. Attempts to transmit the human disease by injecting known icterogenic materials into a wide variety of laboratory animals have yielded negative results. In the case of chimpanzees, there is highly suggestive evidence that transmission may take place in the reverse direction, e.g., from chimpanzee to man: more than 90 cases of infectious hepatitis have occurred among handlers of imported primates, chiefly chimpanzees. Although efforts to induce hepatitis in chimpanzees by giving them human materials have mostly failed, a few suggestive rises in transaminase values have been observed; similar findings in marmosets have recently been mentioned. The reported adaptation of hepatitis virus to the chick embryo has not been confirmed. Despite the enormous efforts on the part of many investigators to adapt hepatitis virus to a laboratory test object, man still appears today to be the only wholly susceptible creature. Most of our knowledge of the properties of hepatitis viruses (IH and SH) and the natural history of the disease has been derived from the use of human volunteers as experimental subjects.

The turning point in our understanding of hepatitis and its probable viral etiology took place about a quarter of a century ago, when the Japanese workers Hiro and Tasaka[15] reported the transmission of hepatitis to children given blood obtained from patients four to five days after onset of the disease. Voegt[29] also reported the successful transfer of infectious hepatitis to man by feeding duodenal contents of a patient with hepatitis. Soon thereafter British investigators described the presence of virus in the blood[1] and in the feces.[19] Several groups of American workers promptly confirmed these findings. Much has been learned about hepatitis despite the severe handicap of using human beings in these and similar studies.

Physical and Chemical Characteristics of Infectious Hepatitis. Although its size has not been measured, IH virus passes ordinary bacteria-retaining filters such as the Seitz; it appears likely to be one of the smaller viruses because its close relative, SH virus, has been measured at 26 mμ or less. IH virus is resistant to various physical and chemical agents; infectivity has been shown to survive 56° C. for 30 minutes, and, in the frozen state, either −18° C. or −70° C. for many years. IH virus resists the action of ether, as well as of chlorine (1 p.p.m.); infectivity is destroyed, however, by coagulation and filtration procedures combined with free residual chlorine concentrations of 1.1 and 0.4 p.p.m.

Distribution of Infectious Hepatitis Virus in Man

VIRUS IN FECES. Since World War II, IH virus has been detected frequently in the stools of patients in the acute stage of the disease. MacCallum and Bradley[19] were the first to demonstrate IH virus in the stools of patients in the preicteric or early icteric phase; this was accomplished by instilling fecal suspensions into the nasopharynx of human volunteers, who acquired infectious hepatitis 27 to 31 days later. Havens et al.[14] promptly confirmed these results. They observed incubation periods of 16 to 34 days after feeding virus and 20 to 31 days after injecting virus subcutaneously or intracutaneously.

More recently the present authors, working with the Willowbrook (WBRK) strain of IH virus, demonstrated it in the feces during the incubation period, approximately two to three weeks before the onset of jaundice (Fig. 24-3). The WBRK virus has also been detected in a pool of feces collected in the first eight days of jaundice, but not thereafter. The question of the persistence of fecal excretion of IH virus is raised repeatedly. The present writers failed to demonstrate WBRK virus in *(a)* the stools of one patient with elevated transaminase values at 32 days and *(b)*, a pool of feces collected from three patients 19 to 33 days after onset of jaundice. Havens[14] described two negative tests for virus in the stools of patients 25 to 29 days after onset of illness. Neefe et al.[24] reported negative results in feces obtained 33 and 43 days after onset (about three weeks after the disappearance of jaundice). On the other hand, Capps et al.[2] reported that IH virus was present in the stools of two infants five and 15 months, respectively, after onset of "chronic hepatitis." These studies were carried out in an orphanage during an epi-

demic of infectious hepatitis among student nurses attributed to the two infants and others like them with "chronic hepatitis." Apparently, the circumstances were such that one could not be certain that these two infants had actually been shedding virus for five and 15 months. In any event, it is obvious that a systematic investigation is required to determine the duration of virus excretion in patients convalescent from infectious hepatitis. The demonstration of the excretion of WBRK strain of IH virus in the stools during the incubation period, two to three weeks before onset of jaundice, suggests that infectious hepatitis, like the enteroviral infections, has an "alimentary tract phase" with multiplication and excretion of virus at a time when clinical manifestations and evidence of liver damages are absent. This finding is of great interest from the public health point of view. It indicates that large amounts of virus may be shed and distributed by ambulatory persons with unrecognized infection.

VIRUS IN THE BLOOD. Viremia has been demonstrated many times during the acute phase of infectious hepatitis. The disease had been produced in volunteers with serum either fed by mouth or injected parenterally; the incubation period of the experimental disease was about the same in each instance. Havens[11] made the important discovery that IH virus injected parenterally into susceptible human beings is excreted in their stools. This finding suggests another difference between infectious hepatitis and serum hepatitis, in that SH virus has not been detected in the feces (Table 24-1). It draws attention to the hazard of cross-infection

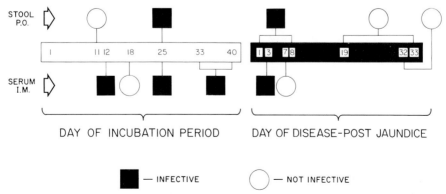

Figure 24-3. Schematic summary of studies of period of infectivity of infectious hepatitis in Willowbrook patients. (Modified from Krugman, S., et al.: New Eng. J. Med., *261*:729, 1959; Amer. J. Med., *32*:717, 1962; and Virology, *24*: 107, 1964.)

Table 24-1. *Comparison of Properties of Infectious Hepatitis and*
Serum Hepatitis Viruses

PROPERTIES	INFECTIOUS HEPATITIS	SERUM HEPATITIS
Size	Unknown; passes Seitz EK filter	About 26 mμ or less
Temperature resistance:		
$\quad$ −15° to − 20° C. (>2 yr.)	Infectivity remains	Infectivity remains
$\quad$ 56° C., ½ hr.	Infectivity remains	Infectivity remains
$\quad$ 60° C., 4 hr.	−	Infectivity remains
$\quad$ 60° C., 10 hr. (albumin)	−	Infectivity destroyed
Resistance to ether	Infectivity remains	Infectivity remains
Resistance to merthiolate 1:2000	−	Infectivity remains
Resistance to chlorine 1 p.p.m.	Infectivity remains	−
Coagulation, settling filtration + chlorine	Infectivity destroyed	−
Virus in stools	+	0
Virus in stools during incubation period	+	0
Virus in blood	+	+
Virus in blood during incubation period	+	+
Virus infective by mouth	+	0
Virus infective parenterally	+	+

resulting from contact with a patient who has acquired hepatitis from blood or plasma transfusion following an incubation period of less than 50 days.

Viremia has also been detected during the incubation period. In 1946 Francis et al.[9] described viremia in a patient three days before onset of symptoms and 13 days before jaundice emerged. Recent studies of the WBRK strain have confirmed and extended this finding: (1) virus was detected in a serum pool formed from patients three to seven days before onset of jaundice; (2) virus was found in a serum pool derived from patients two to three weeks before onset of jaundice (25 days after ingestion of virus) (Fig. 24-3); virus was not detected in a pool of sera from the same patients obtained three to four weeks before onset of jaundice. In another trial, viremia was detected as early as the twelfth day after injection of virus. Although viremia was observed on the third day, it was not found on the seventh day of jaundice. Viremia has also been detected 37 days after feeding virus in a patient who remained completely asymptomatic and in whom the sole abnormality of liver function was a rise in serum transaminase value to 250 units. These results further support the thesis that the most dangerous spreaders

of infectious hepatitis are well persons in whom the presence of virus in blood or stool is not suspected, e.g., those with asymptomatic infection and those in the incubation period.

SEARCH FOR. VIRUS IN NASOPHARYNGEAL SECRETIONS AND IN URINE. Several early investigators reported the possible detection of IH virus in material from the nasopharynx and in the urine. Later, studies by Havens[11] and by Neefe et al.[22a] yielded negative results with these materials. More recently, the studies at Willowbrook have yielded a positive test for virus in urine passed on the first day of jaundice.

EPIDEMIOLOGY

Geographic Distribution. Infectious hepatitis occurs all over the inhabited world. Epidemics have been described in the Scandinavian countries, Iceland, England, Germany, Switzerland, the U.S.S.R., India, Japan, Korea, and the United States. It is endemic in other parts of the world such as the Mediterranean littoral, South and Central America, and other tropical and semitropical areas where its presence is often unsuspected and may be revealed by the advent of susceptible visitors from other countries, as occurs, for example, during military campaigns.

Seasonal Distribution. Infectious hepatitis occurs the year round, but in many countries in the temperate zone there is a seasonal concentration of cases. In the United States the incidence falls to the lowest point each summer, rises during the autumn, reaches a peak during the winter, and declines during the spring months. In Scandinavia the peak occurs in the autumn or early winter months.

Age Distribution. The highest incidence is seen in children under 15 years of age. This is often not appreciated because the disease in children is apt to be so mild as to be overlooked. The relatively immune adult population yields only a few frank cases, and, accordingly, a truly high incidence of hepatitis within a community may be missed. In the Willowbrook State School, an institution for mentally retarded patients where hepatitis has been studied for the past decade, most of the cases occurred in those under 20 years of age. The ratio of icteric to nonicteric hepatitis was about 1:2. The mildness of the infection and often its unsuspected character in infants and young children make them particularly dangerous spreaders of infection. Capps et al.[2] described an epidemic of infectious hepatitis with jaundice in a high proportion of new student nurses caring for infants under three years of age in an orphanage. The source of infection appeared to be endemic hepatitis in the infants, for the most part unrecognized; the evidence for this was supported by the detection of virus in the stools of two of the infants.

Sex Distribution. In general, the sexes seem to be equally susceptible to infectious hepatitis. The incidence has been reported to be higher in girls soon after menarche, and slightly higher for women among parents of the childbearing age. It is possible that these differences can be related to the more intimate contact of mothers and baby-sitters with young children. Ipsen reported a higher morbidity and mortality for chronic hepatitis in postmenopausal Danish women than in men. The reverse seems to be the case in the United States.

Modes of Spread. The evidence points to the intestinal-oral pathways as the most important means of spread of infectious hepatitis. These pathways include the various ways (fingers, flies, sewage, food, water, and so forth) by which virus excreted in the feces of the infected host may reach the mouth of the susceptible person. Support for this concept is derived from (1) trials involving human subjects and (2) epidemiological characteristics.

Trials in Man. Infectious hepatitis virus is shed in large quantities in the feces of persons infected either naturally or artificially. Excretion occurs during the incubation period and in the acute stages of the disease in persons with inapparent hepatitis as well as in those with overt jaundice. The infection has been transmitted experimentally to human beings by feeding infectious hepatitis virus *per os*. Today man appears to be the only established susceptible host and, in all probability, the main source of infection.

EPIDEMIOLOGICAL CHARACTERISTICS

Poor Sanitation. Infectious hepatitis is often endemic or may occur in epidemics in institutions for the mentally retarded, where salmonellosis and shigellosis are also apt to thrive. This is related to the excretory habits of the patients and the impossibility of controlling these conditions in most institutions. Outbreaks of infectious hepatitis have been described in military camps when and where sanitation is defective. Moreover, it is well known that hepatitis emerges in a sizable number of tourists and others following their return from tropical and semitropical countries in which sanitation is poor.

Water-Borne Epidemics. Several explosive water-borne outbreaks have been reported, with summer recreation camps serving as striking examples. In the dramatic epidemic which struck New Delhi during the winter of 1955-1956, jaundice developed in approximately 30,000 people after the city's water supply had been contaminated with raw sewage for a period of one week approximately six weeks before the peak of the epidemic.

Food-Borne Epidemics. Cooks and other persons who handle food while they are in the incubation period or in the early stages of infectious hepatitis, icteric or anicteric, are shedding virus and consequently capable of spreading infection. Outbreaks have been traced to oysters and other shellfish. Other foods have been implicated on other occasions.

The most common mode of spread is most likely through intimate human association such as occurs in households where sanitation may be well above standard. It should be stressed that such "contact infection" includes the intestinal-oral channel and that there are many opportunities for virus excreted in the feces of an infected child— especially if the infection is unrecognized— to reach the mouths of susceptible members of the family.

Although respiratory pathways, droplet infection, and mouth-to-mouth infection have been seriously considered, very little evidence for respiratory spread has been obtained either from trials in human beings or from epidemiological patterns.

Another method of spread of infectious hepatitis, although artificial, is based on the presence of viremia, especially in the incubation period and in cases of unrecognized and anicteric infection. As in serum hepatitis, infection results from blood transfusion or injection of blood products such as plasma or fibrinogen, or from the use of contaminated instruments, syringes, needles, stylets, and so forth. The relatively short incubation period of two to seven weeks in infectious hepatitis may help to distinguish it from serum hepatitis.

PATHOGENESIS

Infection may occur following ingestion of infective material or inoculation of virus-contaminated blood or blood products. The site of initial replication is unknown, but virus is widely disseminated before onset of jaundice. As indicated in Figure 24-3, viremia was detected on the twelfth day of the incubation period, 25 days before jaundice. Evidence of excretion of virus from the intestinal tract was observed on the twenty-fifth day of the incubation period, 18 days before jaundice. In addition, virus was detected in the urine on the first day of jaundice. Virus was not detected in the blood after the third day of jaundice.

One can only speculate about the pathogenesis of infectious hepatitis. The following hypothesis is suggested: Replication of virus occurs first in the cells of the gastrointestinal tract and is followed by a primary viremia. The virus is disseminated to many organs, including the liver and gastrointestinal tract. A secondary viremia may occur one to two weeks before onset of jaundice; at this time constitutional symptoms such as fever, malaise, anorexia, and vomiting may be observed. During this phase, evidence of abnormal serum transaminase activity reflects liver cell damage caused by the virus. Specific anitbody may appear shortly after onset of

jaundice, thereby causing a subsidence of symptoms and an elimination of the virus-carrier state.

It has also been postulated that an autoimmune mechanism may play a role in the pathogenesis of infectious hepatitis, especially the subacute or progressive type of disease. The initial virus infection may cause hepatic necrosis and an antibody response to the byproducts of hepatocellular damage. A subsequent antibody-antigen reaction may play an important role in the continuing hepatic injury.

PATHOLOGICAL ANATOMY

The pathological changes of infectious hepatitis have been studied in both biopsy and necropsy specimens. The liver is usually enlarged. The first microscopic evidence of infection is observed in the appearance of the cells, which become swollen, balloon-like, and irregular in shape. Many cells rapidly undergo lysis and disappear, leaving foci of disturbed architecture. In mild cases, the necrotic foci have a random distribution; larger areas of necrosis are seen in more severe cases. There is a periportal cellular infiltration with a predominance of mononuclear cells and some lymphocytes and plasma cells. In addition, the reticuloendothelial cells are swollen and there is intralobular infiltration. Occasionally, there may be an unusual degree of intralobular bile stasis and a variable amount of necrosis. Later in the course of the disease, regeneration of the liver cells is apparent with complete restoration in two to three months.

The liver is usually small, soft, and reddish brown in color in acute fulminating cases of hepatitis. The capsule is wrinkled. There is histological evidence of massive destruction of the liver cells, but the supporting architectural framework is generally preserved. The sinusoids are congested and the bile ducts are not affected.

In the subacute or progressive type of hepatitis the liver is small; it has a deformed, irregular appearance and the surface is wrinkled and studded with coarse nodules. There is histological evidence of massive cellular destruction as well as irregular areas of formation of new parenchymal cells. The regenerating hyperplastic cells are arranged in an atypical fashion. Extrahepatic manifestations are most often observed in this progressive type of disease. There may be ascites, edema, pleural effusion, and peripheral edema. The regional lymph nodes and spleen may be enlarged. Hemorrahges may be observed in the gastrointestinal tract and elsewhere.

IMMUNITY

One attack of infectious hepatitis with jaundice is usually followed by immunity to a second attack. However, the immunity is not as solid as that conferred by measles, mumps, or rubella. Second attacks have occurred in 5 per cent of more than 1000 cases of hepatitis with jaundice observed at the Willowbrook State School during a ten-year period. Human volunteer studies by Havens[11] revealed protection in adults convalescent from experimental infectious hepatitis when challenged with the same strain of IH virus. Other studies by Neefe et al.[22a] revealed evidence of cross-protection between two separate strains of IH virus.

The most likely explanation for second attacks of hepatitis is the existence of multiple, immunologically distinct types of virus. This phenomenon is observed in enterovirus and adenovirus infections. Other possible causes of second attacks include (1) an overwhelming dose of the infective agent, (2) reactivation of hepatitis virus which may have become latent following the initial infection (3) the presence of an antibody deficiency syndrome, or (4) another virus capable of causing hepatitis. It has been clearly demonstrated that cross immunity does not exist between infectious hepatitis and serum hepatitis.

TREATMENT

No specific drug is available for the treatment of viral hepatitis. Symptomatic therapy includes bed rest and an adequate diet. In children the disease may be so mild that bed rest may be unnecessary; it need not be prolonged beyond the acute phase of the disease.

The child's appetite will determine the type of diet. During the period of anorexia, fluids, including fruit juices, carbonated drinks, and broth, should be offered. If vomiting is severe and persistent, parenteral fluids are indicated. When anorexia subsides, a regular, palatable diet with no restriction of fats should be well tolerated. Corticosteroid therapy is not indicated for the treatment of mild hepatitis.

In mild cases of hepatitis in children, full activity can usually be resumed within two weeks after onset of illness. The decision to return to normal activity is usually determined by the disappearance of jaundice if present, the subsidence of liver tenderness, and the return of normal appetite.

Severe forms of hepatitis with coma, though rare in children, may occur. In such circumstances the treatment should include corticosteroids, withdrawal of protein from the diet, and suppression of intestinal bacterial flora with broad-spectrum antimicrobial agents. The recommended daily dose of prednisone is 20 to 40 mg. The restriction of protein and use of antibiotics are aimed at reducing the formation of ammonia and other toxic materials in the large intestine. Consequently, laxatives and cleansing enemas may also be necessary. Parenteral therapy, including administration of a solution of 10 per cent dextrose, is recommended in the appropriate volume for the size of the patient. Exchange transfusions have been reported to be effective for the treatment of hepatic coma.

PREVENTION

At the present time there is no active immunizing agent available for the prevention of infectious hepatitis. However, there is ample evidence that human immune globulin (gamma globulin) is effective for the prevention or modification of the disease. Gamma globulin administered after exposure may suppress jaundice without preventing infection.

Indications for Gamma Globulin. Gamma globulin is advised for all persons, children as well as adults, who have intimate association with a known case of infectious hepatitis. Intimate contact occurs under conditions which provide opportunity for the transfer of virus-contaminated excreta from person to person. Hepatitis is not spread by the usual causal type of contact on the street, in the church or theater, or in other similar situations; in these circumstances the use of gamma globulin is unnecessary.

SERUM HEPATITIS

Serum hepatitis is a man-made infection caused by the introduction, usually be intravenous injection, of SH virus, which appears to be closely related to infectious hepatitis virus. SH virus is transmitted solely by artificial means, e.g., by injection of blood or blood products or by the use of contaminated syringes, needles, stylets, and other cutting instruments. The disease itself is indistinguishable from infectious hepatitis on the basis of most of the clinical and pathological findings. It is characterized by a longer incubation period than infectious hepatitis and by its apparent lack of communicability.

CLINICAL MANIFESTATIONS

The clinical and pathological features of serum hepatitis are for the most part indistinguishable from those of infectious hepatitis. However, the incubation period is longer, ranging from about 50 to 180 days. This contrasts with the incubation period of infectious hepatitis, which varies from 15 to 50 days. It is said that the onset of serum hepatitis is apt to be insidious and afebrile, while the onset of infectious hepatitis is often abrupt and associated with fever. These reported differences in mode of onset are far from constant and cannot be trusted in differentiating one form of hepatitis from the other. Anicteric hepatitis occurs in both.

The pathological changes, diagnosis, complications, and treatment are identical to those for infectious hepatitis described previously. There are reports suggesting that in serum hepatitis the clinical course may be more severe and the mortality higher than is the case in infectious hepatitis. This apparent difference in prognosis is probably related to the fact that serum hepatitis is seen so frequently in people who are seriously ill, debilitated, or elderly *before* they receive blood or blood products. When a comparison is made of patients of the same age in whom neither cancer nor any other debilitating condition complicates the picture, the outlook is much the same in the two forms of hepatitis.

ETIOLOGY

The properties of serum hepatitis virus suggest that it is closely related to infectious hepatitis virus; the two agents are compared in Table 24-1. Since man is the only established susceptible host for both viruses, research has been severely handicapped by the lack of a practicable laboratory test object.

Physical and Chemical Characteristics. By the method of filtration through collodion membranes, McCollum et al.[20] estimated the size of SH virus to be approximately 26 mμ. It resembles IH virus in its ability to withstand various physical agents. In serum albumin the activity of SH virus survives 60° C. for four hours but is destroyed after ten hours. Its activity is maintained for years in the frozen state and for at least one year in the dried state at room temperature. In serum it survives the action of either merthiolate 1:2000 or tricresol 1:500. Under certain conditions, SH virus is inactivated in serum exposed to ultraviolet light; because the virus has also been shown to withstand ultraviolet light under other conditions, this method cannot be depended on for sterilization.

Viremia. Serum hepatitis has been demonstrated in the blood many times during the acute stage of illness and also during the long incubation period. Neefe et al.[22a] detected virus in the blood 87 days before onset of disease; Paul et al.[25] demonstrated it 60 days before, and Havens,[11] 16 days before the appearance of jaundice. Although early attempts failed to detect viremia during periods of convalescence one to five months after onset of illness, Stokes et al.[27] demonstrated that SH virus may persist in the blood for as long as five years.

All the positive tests cited above were carried out by the parenteral injection of serum or plasma in human volunteers who subsequently developed hepatitis with jaundice. In early limited studies samples of serum or plasma, and even aliquots of known icterogenic serum, when given by mouth, failed to induce hepatitis in the recipients. This observation is in contrast to the positive results which follow the feeding of serum containing IH virus and seems to be another distinctive feature of these two viruses.

Search for Virus in Nasopharynx, Feces, and Urine. Although a limited number of tests for serum hepatitis virus have been done on nasopharyngeal washings, feces, and urine, the results were negative with one possible exception. The exception was reported by Findlay and Martin,[6] who described jaundice in a human volunteer 50 days after intranasal instillation of nasopharyngeal washings obtained from a patient in the acute stage of hepatitis following injection of yellow fever vaccine. This test was performed in a place where infectious hepatitis was endemic, and since we have seen an incubation period of 50 days with the Willowbrook strain of IH virus, the result is difficult to interpret. In summary, there is little or no evidence today for the presence of SH virus in the nasopharynx, feces, or urine. The number of attempts to detect virus in these materials has been limited, however, and when better methods are available, more tests should be carried out.

EPIDEMIOLOGY

The known circumstances under which serum hepatitis occurs are based on the presence of healthy inapparent carriers of SH virus and the demonstration that as little as 0.01 ml. of serum may be infectious. The carrier rate in United States has been estimated by Stokes et al.[27] to vary between 2 and 4 per cent, and the risk to recipients to range from 0.3 to 4.13 per cent. There is reason to believe that a higher carrier rate may be found among professional blood donors. Serum hepatitis virus may be carried in the blood for periods of one to five years. The disease is transmitted to susceptible persons most commonly by blood transfusion; less common sources include blood derivatives such as plasma, convalescent serum, fibrinogen, fibrin foam, and thrombin. During World War II more than 60,000 cases in United States troops followed inoculation of yellow fever vaccine containing human serum. Serum hepatitis has also been transmitted by inadequately sterilized syringes and needles used for injecting insulin, arsphenamine, and other medicaments. Outbreaks have been reported in drug addicts accustomed to unsterilized equipment. The disease may also follow tattooing, withdrawal of blood by venipuncture, or puncture of skin by contaminated stylets for blood counts.

Distribution and Prevalence. Our knowledge of the distribution and prevalence of serum hepatitis is severely handicapped by the lack of clear-cut means of distinguishing it from infectious hepatitis. Consequently, these two forms are generally reported as one disease. To compound this difficulty, IH virus also enjoys a viremic phase during the incubation period and acute phase in both icteric and anicteric or unrecognized cases— circumstances which facilitate transmission by the same channels as those used by SH virus. In support of this concept, prospective studies of post-transfusion hepatitis showed approximately one-third of the cases of jaundice to have incubation periods of two to seven weeks and two-thirds of the cases, eight to 16 weeks.[22]

Serum hepatitis probably exists throughout the world wherever blood transfusions or injections of blood derivatives or of other medications are given. The disease has been reported from the United States, England, Sweden, Russia, and the Middle East. There are indications that the rising incidence of serum hepatitis in the United States is associated with (a) the increasing popularity of injecting blood, blood products, and other materials, and (b) the high incidence of the carrier state (2 to 4 per cent).

Seasonal fluctuation in the incidence of serum hepatitis has not been described. This is consistent with the practice of giving blood transfusions and various other injections at a uniform rate the year round. The factors of *age* and *sex* do not seem to affect susceptibility to serum hepatitis. The predominance in childhood seen in infectious hepatitis does not apply to serum hepatitis, which is said to affect all age groups. In this connection, only six cases of probable serum hepatitis with jaundice were observed at Children's Hospital of Los Angeles during the past eight years. Approximately 33,000 transfusions were given, a rate of approximately 0.2 per thousand. Accordingly, it is our clinical impression that the incidence of serum hepatitis with jaundice in pediatric patients may be appreciably lower than in adults. Although the disease is said to be milder in children, severe cases with high mortality have been reported.

Occupation. Physicians and medical technicians have attack rates for hepatitis higher than those of the general population. In fact, hepatitis is considered to be an "occupational disease" among technicians in blood banks; it is assumed that the cause is SH virus. Drug addicts form another group at greater risk of "syringe hepatitis" for obvious reasons. Tattooed persons represent still another group with higher incidence of serum hepatitis.[17a,28a]

IMMUNITY

Because practical laboratory methods are lacking, our knowledge is scanty concerning the immune response to infection with serum hepatitis virus. Studies with human volunteers carried out by Neefe et al.[22a] showed partial resistance to reinoculation of presumably the same strain of SH virus at intervals ranging from three to 12 months after the first experimentally induced infection. The existence of some degree of protection in the population is suggested by the fact that a large proportion of persons inoculated with SH virus, either as volunteers or as patients receiving blood or blood products known to contain the agent, fail to get the disease. The presence of antibody to SH virus in immune serum globulin is suggested by the early studies of Grossman et al.,[10] confirmed later by Mirick, et al.[22]; these trials indicated that 10 ml. of gamma globulin given on two occasions about one month apart significantly reduced the incidence of post-transfusion hepatitis with jaundice. On the other hand, Drake et al.[5] failed to prevent hepatitis in volunteers injected with mixtures of SH virus and 4 ml. of gamma globulin prepared from persons four months to seven and one-half years after serum hepatitis; nor was hepatitis prevented in volunteers first injected with SH virus and then with 2 ml. of gamma globulin, repeated 40 days later.

The lack of cross immunity between serum hepatitis and infectious hepatitis is unequivocal. Persons who have had a previous attack of serum hepatitis, either naturally or deliberately acquired, are susceptible to infectious hepatitis and vice versa.

CONTROL MEASURES

The transmission of serum hepatitis is accomplished by (1) the extensive use of blood and blood products, (2) the increasing popularity of a wide variety of injections for therapeutic, prophylactic, and other reasons, combined with inadequate methods of sterilization of syringes and needles, and (3) an incidence of 2 to 4 per cent of healthy, inapparent carriers of virus in the general population. The lack of specific laboratory tests for the detection of virus or antibody is a major handicap in attempts to control the disease. Because of the existing difficulties of recognizing the carrier state, the indications for the use of blood or blood derivatives should be carefully weighed against the danger of aggravating the condition of a sick patient by superimposing another disease. Accordingly, the indications for the transfusion of a single unit of blood should be considered with care. It has been shown that the greater the number of donors contributing

to the plasma pool, the greater the risk of its containing virus; therefore, plasma pools should not be used in situations where albumin or stable plasma protein solution are appropriate substitutes. Although the present method of preparing normal serum albumin by heating at 60° C. for 10 hours will inactivate hepatitis viruses without deleterious effect on the albumin, such is not the case with whole blood or its other components. Ultraviolet light has not proved to be a reliable virucidal method. The results of using β-propiolactone in conjunction with radiation of plasma with ultraviolet light are encouraging; similarly, the effect of β-propiolactone alone in whole blood deserves further study.[26a] Storage of liquid plasma at room temperature (27° to 31.6° C.) for six months seems to effect a substantial reduction in the incidence of serum hepatitis; on the other hand, storage of large volumes of plasma presents a variety of problems, including possibility of contamination and denaturation of plasma proteins, which may make this method impracticable.

All equipment* which comes into contact with blood or its derivatives should either be discarded or thoroughly cleaned and then sterilized with heat by boiling in water for 15 minutes, or by autoclaving at 121° C. (15 lb. pressure) for 20 minutes, or by sterilization with dry heat (170° C.) for 30 minutes. The use of disposable needles, syringes, and infusion equipment is strongly recommended to reduce the risk of transmitting hepatitis.

Attempts to control serum hepatitis include screening of blood donors. The following precautions are indicated: Rejection of (1) persons who have received blood or its potentially virus-containing derivatives within a six-month period; (2) persons who have had hepatitis or have been in close contact with a case of hepatitis in the previous six months; (3) narcotic addicts (or suspects); and (4) persons whose blood is suspected to have caused hepatitis in the past.

It is commonly believed that gamma globulin has no effect on serum hepatitis. Although the results of several studies have been conflicting, the early work of Grossman et al.[10] and the more recent work of Mirick et al.[22] indicate that large doses of gamma globulin reduce appreciably the incidence of hepatitis with jaundice which follows trans-

---

*This includes syringes, needles, stylets, surgical and dental instruments, tubing, glassware, and so forth.

fusions in adults. Post-transfusion jaundice includes cases with both long incubation periods (50 to 180 days), or *serum hepatitis,* and short incubation periods (15 to 50 days), or *infectious hepatitis;* in the study reported by Mirick et al.[22] about 30 per cent of the icteric cases fell into the latter group. Gamma globulin seemed to suppress the jaundice associated with both types, but, as in infectious hepatitis, it had no effect on the incidence of anicteric hepatitis. The dose of gamma globulin shown to be effective in reducing the incidence of post-transfusion jaundice is 10 ml. (16 per cent solution) given within one week after transfusion and 10 ml. one month later. From the practical point of view it is impossible to recommend this preventive measure routinely with every transfusion because the available supply of gamma globulin would be rapidly exhausted.

BIBLIOGRAPHY

1. Cameron, J. D. S.: Infective hepatitis. Quart. J. Med., *12*:139, 1943.
2. Capps, R. B., Bennett, A. M., and Stokes, J., Jr.: A prolonged outbreak of infectious hepatitis in nurses due to a group of small children serving as a reservoir of virus. J. Clin. Invest., *29*:802, 1950.
3. Chalmers, T. G., Eckhardt, R. D., Reynolds, W. B., Cigarroa, J. G., Deane, N., Reifenstein, R. W.; Smith, C. W., and Davidson, C. S.: Treatment of acute infectious hepatitis. Controlled studies of the effects of diet, rest and physical reconditioning on the acute course of the disease and on the incidence of relapses and residual abnormalities. J. Clin. Invest., *34*:1163, 1955.
4. DeRitis, F., Coltori, M., and Giusti, G.: An enzyme test for the diagnosis of viral hepatitis. Clin. Chim. Acta, *2*:70, 1957.
5. Drake, M. B., et al.: Failure of convalescent gamma globulin to protect against homologous serum hepatitis. J.A.M.A., *152*:690, 1953.
6. Findlay, G. M., and Martin, N. H.: Jaundice following yellow fever immunization. Lancet, *1*:678, 1943.
7. Findlay, G. M., and Willcox, R. R.: Transmission of infective hepatitis by feces and urine. Lancet, *1*:212, 1945.
8. Fox, J. P., Manso, C., Penna, H. A., and Para, M.: Observations on the occurrence of icterus in Brazil following vaccination against yellow fever. Amer. J. Hyg., *36*:68, 1942.
9. Francis, T., Jr., Frisch, A. W., and Quilligan, J. J., Jr.: Demonstration of infectious hepatitis virus in presymptomatic period after transfer by transfusion. Proc. Soc. Exp. Biol., *61*:276, 1946.
10. Grossman, E. B., Stewart, S. G., and Stokes, J., Jr.: Post-transfusion hepatitis in battle casualties and a study of its prophylaxis by means of human immune serum globulin. J.A.M.A., *129*:991, 1945.
11. Havens, W. P., Jr.: The period of infectivity of patients with homologous serum jaundice and routes of infection in this disease. J. Exp. Med., *83*:441, 1946.
12. Havens, W. P., Jr.: Viral hepatitis: Multiple attacks in a narcotic addict. Ann. Int. Med., *44*:199, 1956.
13. Havens, W. P., Jr., and Paul, J. R.: Prevention of infectious hepatitis with gamma globulin. J.A.M.A., *129*:270, 1945.
14. Havens, W. P., Jr., Ward, R., Drill, V. A., and Paul, J. R.: Experimental production of hepatitis by feeding icterogenic materials. Proc. Soc. Exp. Biol., *57*:206, 1944.
15. Hiro, Y., and Tasaka, S.: Experimental inoculation of epidemic jaundice in children. Acta Paediat. Jap., *47*:975, 1941.
16. Krugman, S., Ward, R., and Giles, J. P.: The natural history of infectious hepatitis. Amer. J. Med., *32*:717, 1962.
17. Krugman, S., Ward, R., Giles, J. P., Bodansky, O., and Jacobs, A. M.: Infectious hepatitis: Detection of virus during the incubation period and in clinically inapparent infection. New Eng. J. Med., *261*:729, 1959.
17a. Kuh, C., and Ward, W. E.: Occupational virus hepatitis; apparent hazard for medical personnel. J.A.M.A. *143*:631, 1950.
18. MacCallum, F. O., and Bauer, D. J.: Homologous serum jaundice: Transmission experiments with human volunteers. Lancet, *1*:622, 1944.
19. MacCallum, F. O., and Bradley, W. H.: Transmission of infective hepatitis to human volunteers: Effect on rheumatoid arthritis. Lancet, *2*:228, 1944.
20. McCollum, R. W., Bech, V., Isacson, P., and Riordan, J. T.: A survey for hemagglutinins in viral hepatitis. Amer. J. Med., *27*:703, 1959.
21. McNalty, A. S.: Acute infectious jaundice and administration of measles serum. Annual report of the chief medical officer of the ministry of health for the year 1937. London, H. M. Stationery Office, 1938.
22. Mirick, G. S., Ward, R., and McCollum, R. W.: The modification of post-transfusion hepatitis by the use of gamma globulin. New Eng. J. Med., *273*:59, 1965.
22a. Neefe, J. R., Gellis, S. S., and Stokes, J., Jr.: Homologous serum hepatitis and infectious (epidemic) hepatitis; studies in volunteers bearing on immunological and other characteristics of etiological agents. Amer. J. Med., *1*:3, 1946.
23. Neefe, J. R., and Stokes, J., Jr.: An epidemic of infectious hepatitis apparently due to a water borne agent. J.A.M.A., *128*:1063, 1945.
24. Neefe, J. R., Stokes, J., Jr., and Reinhold, J. G.: Oral administration to volunteers of feces from patients with homologous serum hepatitis and infectious (epidemic) hepatitis. Amer. J. Med. Sci., *210*:29, 1945.
25. Paul, J. R., Havens, W. P., Jr., Sabin, A. B., and Philip, C. B.: Transmission experiments in serum jaundice and infectious hepatitis. J.A.M.A., *128*:911, 1945.
26. Sherman, I. L., and Eichenwald, H. F.: Viral hepatitis: Descriptive epidemiology based on morbidity and mortality statistics. Ann. Int. Med., *44*:1049, 1956.
26a. Stokes, J., Jr.: The control of viral hepatitis. Amer. J. Med., *32*:729, 1962.
27. Stokes, J., Jr., Berk, J. E., Malamut, L. L., Drake, M. E., Barondess, J. A., Bashe, W. J., Wolman, I. J., Farquhar, J. D., Bevan, B., Drummond, R. J., Maycock, W. d'A., Capps, R. B., and Bennett, A. M.: Carrier state in viral hepatitis. J.A.M.A., *154*:1059, 1954.

28. Stokes, J., Jr., and Neefe, J. R.: Prevention and attenuation of infectious hepatitis by gamma globulin: Preliminary note. J.A.M.A., *127*:144, 1945.

28a. Trumbull, M. L., and Grenier, D. J.: Homologous serum jaundice; occupational hazard to medical personnel. J.A.M.A., *145*:965, 1951.

29. Voegt, H.: Zur Aetiologie der Hepatitis epidemica. Munch. Med. Wschr., *89*:76, 1942.

30. Ward, R., Krugman, S., Giles, J. P., Jacobs, A. M., and Bodansky, O.: Infectious hepatitis: Studies of its natural history and prevention. New Eng. J. Med., *258*:407, 1958.

ADDENDUM

I. Further studies pursued by Krugman, Giles, and Hammond[6], then by Giles and Krugman[3] have shown that two types of "infectious hepatitis" can be distinguished by additional factors. The first type, due to MS-1 virus (closely related to, if not identical with, IH virus) has an incubation period of 31 to 38 days, from date of contamination through the period when serum transaminase level exceeds 100 units. The second type, due to MS-2 virus, in these authors' terminology, is similar to, or identical with, SH virus. It has a much longer incubation period: 41 to 69 days. In both types, the etiological agent is or can be infectious by mouth, as shown by experimentation in human volunteers, and contacts can be more or less readily infected. Convalescents from MS-1 virus infection are immunized against infection by the homologous virus but remain vulnerable to reinfection by MS-2. The same is true for convalescents from MS-2. They remain receptive to infection by MS-1 virus.

The enzymatic and immunological responses to these two types of hepatitis infection likewise differ. MS-1 virus provokes a sudden rise in level of serum transaminases and an equally abrupt fall in the level of these enzymes three to 19 days later. The level of M immunoglobulins (IgM) rises three to four days after the rise in that of the transaminases and returns to normal only five to 35 days later. Results of the thymol turbidity test are consistently abnormal. MS-2 hepatitis is characterized by more gradual but more prolonged rises in transaminase level; the abnormal levels may persist 34 to 200 days after contamination. In contrast, however, IgM level is only slightly modified, and results of the thymol test are often normal.

The first of these types of hepatitis corresponds to the description of infectious hepatitis, the second to that of serum hepatitis.

MS-2 and SH hepatitis differ only by the route of contamination usual in each, i.e., for the first, the buccal portal of entry and the infection of contacts.

II. By what appears to be a geographical accident, an antigen was discovered by Blumberg and his associates[1] in 1963 in the blood of an Australian aborigine. In 1967 the same workers reported that this so-named Australia antigen has a striking association with leukemia, Down's syndrome, and acute viral hepatitis. The relationship of Australia antigen to viral hepatitis is well established.[2] For example, it was revealed in 46 (74 per cent) of patients with serum hepatitis examined by Hirschman et al.[5] in the United States. These patients, who were nearly all in the acute phase of the disease, were the object of weekly blood sampling to follow liver function. Australia antigen became detectable 35 to 120 days after exposure to contaminated blood products; it persisted from one week to three months in 42 patients, and for more than ten months in four patients. (In a different study, persistence of even longer duration was suggested.) Two of 128 healthy chimpanzees and one of 14 healthy gibbons also showed the antigen. The hypothesis has been formulated that monkeys may be contaminated inapparently by man, who thus remains the only known reservoir species.

Australia antigen under the electron microscope seems to be associated with aggregates of small spherical particles approximately 200 Å in diameter. Tubular forms are also found; of similar diameter, they are approximately 3000 Å in length. Cross-striations are frequent.

In a search for Australia antigen in the sera of subjects infected by MS-1 and MS-2, Giles et al.[4] noted that this antigen was never found in association with MS-1, but appeared regularly after infection by MS-2, usually well before the first signs of hepatitis. These authors consider that Australia antigen, SH antigen, and MS-2 antigen are identical.

1. Blumberg, B. S., Alter, H. J., and Visnich, S.: A "new" antigen in leukemia sera. J.A.M.A., *191*:541-546, 1965.

2. Blumberg, B. S., Sutnick, A. I., and London, W. T.: Australia antigen and hepatitis. J.A.M.A., *207*: 1895-1896, 1969.

3. Giles, J. P., and Krugman, S.: Viral hepatitis. Immunoglobulin response during the course of the disease. J.A.M.A., *208*:497-503, 1969.

4. Giles, J. P., McCollum, R. W., Berndtson, L. W., Jr., and Krugman, S.: Viral hepatitis. Relation of Aus-

tralian SH antigen to the Willowbrook; MS-2 strain. New Eng. J. Med., *281*:219-221, 1969.

5. Hirschman, R. J., Shulman, N. R., Barker, L. F., and Smith, K. O.: Virus-like particles in sera of patients with infectious and serum hepatitis. J.A.M.A., *208*:1667-1670, 1969.

6. Krugman, S., Giles, J. P., and Hammond, J.: Infectious hepatitis. Evidence for two distinctive clinical,

epidemiological, and immunological types of infection. J.A.M.A., *200*:365, 1967.

7. Shulman, N. R., and Barker, L. F.: Virus-like antigen, antibody and antigen-antibody complexes in hepatitis measured by complement fixation. Science, *165*:305-306, 1969.

8. Zuckerman, A. J.: Viral hepatitis and the Australia-SH antigen. Nature, *223*:569-572, 1969.

25

Yellow Fever

By R. PANTHIER

INTRODUCTION

DEFINITION

Yellow fever is an acute infectious disease that is endemic-epidemic in certain regions of the intertropical zones of Africa and America. It is highly variable in gravity, ranging from the hyperacute form, fatal within two or three days, to the latent form. The typical cases are characterized by a sudden onset and two-phase development, the two phases being separated by a short remission. The first phase is infectious, without signs of any particular localization; the second is hepatorenal. The causal agent of yellow fever is a filterable virus, an arbovirus of group B (Casals' classification) which is maintained in nature by passage among wild mammals (particularly the monkey) through the agency of wild vector mosquitoes, Aedini, of the genus *Haemagogus* or *Aedes*.

A man who has been contaminated accidentally by a wild mosquito is able to infect urban anthropophilic mosquitoes, in particular *Aedes aegypti*. The passage of the virus through the cycle man-Aedes-man can cause an epidemic of yellow fever the spread of which depends on the density of the vector mosquitoes and the density of the receptive population (i.e., those not immunized against

the disease, either naturally or by vaccination.)

Every case of yellow fever should be reported and subsequently notified to the World Health Organization in Geneva (No. 91 of the nomenclature).

Synonyms: typhus amaril; French: fievre jaune; Spanish: vomite negro, fiebre amarilla; German: Gelbfieber; Portuguese: febre amarella; Italian: febbre gialla.

IMPORTANCE OF YELLOW FEVER IN HUMAN PATHOLOGY

It is difficult to assess the part played by yellow fever among the various serious epidemic diseases that are accompanied by jaundice, and which have been described since the beginning of European penetration in America and tropical Africa. It is nevertheless possible to confirm that this disease has impeded European expansion in these continents. There has been considerable controversy in attempting to establish definitely whether yellow fever originated in America and subsequently contaminated Africa, or whether it was of African origin, since, in Carter's opinion, America was affected by this disease only towards the end of the 17th century. According to this hypothesis, yellow fever spread as far as North America and Europe by means of sea connections, causing brief but deadly epidemics.

The first prophylactic measures following the first epidemiological knowledge, acquired at the beginning of the 20th century, were undeniably effective, but the epidemiological scheme of that period was incomplete. The renewed occurrence of yellow fever in America and Africa in 1927 and 1928 enabled important progress to be made in the knowledge of the disease: it was soon proved that yellow fever in the human being was simply an accident in the cycle maintaining the virus in nature.

Although, in view of this fact, it is no longer possible to envisage the eradication of the virus, at least a more detailed knowledge of the epidemiological chain, the discovery of an efficient vaccine, and severe measures of sanitation control nowadays make it possible to limit the natural outbreaks of infection and sudden epidemics and thus prevent the long-distance spread of the virus. However, it is indispensable, particularly in the areas of receptivity to yellow fever, that all medical practitioners be in a position to establish the diagnosis with all possible speed and accuracy.

CLINICAL STUDY

SYMPTOMATOLOGY

The typical form of yellow fever will first be described as it is usually observed during epidemics. This is practically the only form which the clinician is able to diagnose, confirmation of the diagnosis being of course provided by laboratory tests.

The *incubation* period beteen the time of the infecting bite and the onset of the disease is usually from three to six days (a period of six days is counted for prophylactic purposes); longer incubation periods are possible (Marchoux et al.), but they have mainly been observed in cutaneous contaminations in the laboratory. The incubation period is usually quiescent; occasionally a few vague prodromal symptoms appear a few hours before the onset of fever.

The onset is sudden, often marked by intense shivering of short duration rapidly followed by a rise in temperature to 39° or 40° C. The pulse is rapid (110 to 140) and there is constant headache, usually extremely

intense, producing a sensation of "hammering on the forehead"; it is accompanied by vertigo and generalized muscular pains, and by dorso-thoracolumbar root pain of variable intensity, often sufficiently violent for the patient to have the impression of being "hit by a bar" in the lumbar region.

The usual nausea, although more marked than in the other forms of pyrexia, is often accompanied by vomiting, first alimentary and then bilious.

On examination, the face is congested, the conjunctiva are bloodshot, and the skin is hot and dry; the patient is slightly agitated and anxious; his facies has an "anxious and almost terrified appearance."

The initial period of the disease establishes itself within a few hours.

COURSE OF THE DISEASE

Red Stage. The patient's face gradually takes on the typical aspect of the "yellow fever facies." The bloated face becomes mahogany or wine-colored. This aspect extends over the neck and sometimes even to the upper part of the thorax. Furthermore, a scarlatiniform rash may be observed. The eyes are bright, bloodshot, and sometimes watery; the lips are red and swollen. The saburral tongue is bright red on the edge and at the tip; the buccal mucosa and the gums are also red. There is intense thirst accompanied by total anorexia with fetid breath compared by Marchoux to the sickly odor of butchered meat.

Examination of the abdomen reveals no particular symptom: the abdomen is soft and the liver and spleen are not palpable, but epigastric pressure sometimes provokes intense pain.

The urine, which is dark in color and still sufficient in volume at this stage, does not contain albumin.

This clinical picture remains practically unchanged for two to four days. The headache gradually decreases, the intense congestive condition persists and manifests itself by minor hemorrhages, and in particular epistaxis; small amounts of albumin may appear in the urine. But the temperature, which remains high (between 39° and 40° C.), is often accompanied by a fall in the pulse rate. The pulse rate is rapid at the beginning but slows down from 110 to 80 or from 130 to 90 beats per minute. This dissociation of the pulse and temperature was noted by Faget, who considered it to be a pathognomonic clinical symptom of yellow fever. Faget's sign, which has been described in all the English publications, although it is not constant, remains valid during the "red phase," i.e., the infectious phase of yellow fever.

Remission. At the end of the third day or the beginning of the fourth day, the general symptoms rapidly improve. The headaches disappear, the temperature decreases to approximately 38° C., and the patient often feels better, thus marking the end of the infectious phase. This lull is of short duration, generally of not more than a few hours. The "yellow phase" or the phase of hepatorenal intoxication follows.

Yellow Phase. The temperature rises, but often less than during the first phase. The general symptoms reappear, and the patient is agitated, anxious, then prostrated.

The jaundice, if it has not begun during the remission phase, appears progressively: often barely evident, simply a subicteric appearance of the conjunctiva, with grayish pallor, and it only becomes really intense later on, either immediately before death, or before the convalescent period in case of recovery.

The skin is dry, and, if one presses the thorax with the tip of the finger, "spot signs" appear as described by previous authors: the pale fingerprint, more or less yellow, depending on the intensity of the jaundice, is rapidly replaced by a persistent red mark.

Vomiting recurs and is all the more painful since there is epigastric pain, sometimes of such intensity that the patient is unable to bear the weight of the blankets.

The vomiting is frequent and released by the slightest intake of liquid; the vomitus consists first of mucus and then of gastric juices. Soon afterward it contains digested blood, thus producing the black vomitus or *vomito negro* that is particularly frightening to the patient and persons around him. Sometimes the first black vomit is preceded only by a sharp sensation of hunger (Casanove). In severe cases, the *vomito negro* may be immediately followed by a fatal collapse.

The appearance of the vomitus depends on the quantity of blood digested: it is striated with a few black fragments having sootlike or feathery appearance when the hemorrhage is not abundant, whereas it is completely black, resembling coffee with its grounds, when there is intense gastric hemorrhage.

It is also possible to observe gastrorrhagia of red blood.

Hemorrhages. "Everything is congested at the onset, everything bleeds in the end" (Touatre). The gums, like the whole of the buccal mucosa, are dark red but slightly brighter around the teeth. This mucosa bleeds easily when pressed.

Melena and metrorrhagia may be observed, the latter being frequent among women after menarche, as well as more or less inconstant epistaxis and rare hematuria.

Albuminuria. Generally of sudden onset and rapidly increasing concentration, the albuminuria, which is constant in yellow fever, is, together with the jaundice, one of the basic symptoms of the disease. In the event of recovery, it disappears as rapidly as it appeared. There is a definite correlation between the quantity of albumin found in the urine and the gravity of the disease.

During the "yellow phase" the volume of urine excreted decreases, and often the volume excreted in 24 hours does not exceed 100 ml. Anuria is possible but rare.

Cardiac Involvement. The pulse rate remains dissociated from the fever but the beat becomes weak. The arterial blood pressure is variable. The myocardium is more or less affected, but abnormal electrocardiographic tracings are of no prognostic value. Progressive tachycardia is generally an ominous sign.

Outcome. Death is frequent in the more severe forms, generally occurring from the seventh to the tenth day, with the patient in a state of agitated delirium or coma. Sometimes death follows a black vomit or sudden collapse. Death may be the termination of a uremic coma of extremely rapid evolution, but it may also occur much later on, between the tenth and fifteenth days, or even after a sudden collapse during convalescence (Kirk, 1941[28b]). These later deaths may be more difficult to diagnose, since histological examination of the liver shows altered lesions or lesions undergoing alteration, which are often difficult to interpret. Recovery may occur even after a typical form of the disease characterized by constantly alarming and serious symptoms. The temperature slowly decreases to normal, the urine volume increases, and albuminuria disappears. The jaundice often becomes more pronounced and then slowly disappears. The convalescent stage is long and, at the beginning, is marked by a state of intense fatigue. Complications are exceptional, and the patient remains protected throughout his lifetime against a new attack of yellow fever.

CLINICAL FORMS

Yellow fever, according to this classic description, is easy to diagnose during an epidemic when numerous patients are affected with the same disease. However, even then, not all of the cases are typical or of the same gravity.

According to Symptomatic Prevalence. In the serious forms, certain symptoms may predominate, producing variations of the clinical syndrome described here, rather than separate, distinct forms. In the *hepatic form* the jaundice is very pronounced, the pulse slow, and the liver painful when pressure is exerted; the urinary symptoms are not marked. On the other hand, the *anuric form* is characterized by considerable renal involvement, causing a uremic coma. This may be fatal if the renal involvement occurs early, but the prognosis is more favorable if the anuria occurs later on. The clinical picture of the *hemorrhagic forms* is dominated by the loss of blood. The hemorrhages are either slight but permanent or else massive and rapidly fatal. In the *cardiac forms* the myocardium is affected. The heart beat is faint and rapid, and the arterial blood pressure is low. The slightest movement produces dyspnea, and the patient is syncopal. Recovery may occur, being announced by the return to normal of the pulse and the arterial blood pressure.

In addition, several rather special forms have been described during certain epidemics. An *adrenal syndrome* was observed in one of ten cases during an epidemic in 1927 in Rio de Janeiro. This was a benign syndrome, even though the adynamia, the fall in the arterial blood pressure, and the pronounced bradycardia produced an alarming clinical picture.

Finally, *nervous system involvement,* which is constant throughout yellow fever but usually unobtrusive, may be predominant in certain cases, particularly in alcoholics or during certain epidemics. The predominance of the nervous symptoms was also observed by Kirk[28b] during an epidemic in 1940 in the Nuba Mountain region of the Sudan and subsequently by Berdonneau et al.[11] at the Sudan-Ethiopia border in 1959. The almost purely neuromeningeal symptomatology led to a diagnosis of meningitis with clear fluid of unknown etiology until development of certain symptoms typical of yellow fever — e.g., conjunctival icterus or gastric hemorrhages — incriminated yellow fever.

According to Gravity. The *hyperacute form* is fatal after three days of illness. The exacerbation of the virulence of the yellow fever virus with regard to man during certain epidemics may provoke this rapid and atypical evolution, the only notable symptoms being the hyperpyrexia and pronounced adynamia. A general aspect of this type was observed by Sérié et al.[40] in June, 1961, in Ethiopia, in the province of Wallamo.

In the *abortive forms,* following the remission period, the temperature does not increase and the patient enters into the convalescent stage without going through the "yellow phase."

The *influenza-like* forms are most frequent outside epidemics, but they have always been reported even during epidemics (Nott, 1848). Their frequent occurrence has been proved only quite recently, the fact that the disease is yellow fever being ascertained either by serological conversion or by isolation of the virus (Causey[17b]; Theiler and Casals, 1958[44]). The patient recovers after two or three days of an illness resembling an influenzal infection without pulmonary involvement.

In the asymptomatic forms, the affection passes unnoticed; these forms can be detected only by systematic serological tests. They are nevertheless of great interest, both because the virus can spread without arousing attention and because this unapparent disease produces immunity.

This natural immunization no doubt explains the apparent racial resistance observed among the natives of the zones where yellow fever is endemic, contrasting sharply with the total receptivity of non-vaccinated individuals of any other race who have been transferred from a nonendemic zone to an endemic zone, or who live in a territory free from yellow fever (e.g., Ethiopia, 1961-1962).

CLINICAL LABORATORY TESTS

The principal modifications of the blood, urine, and cerebrospinal fluid are simply noted here, especially those that can be of prognostic value. The data available are insufficient, since yellow fever prevails most often in places which are not easily accessible, and if the patient is hospitalized at all, it is usually in a country hospital with an ill-equipped laboratory.

In the *blood,* a leukopenia is noted that mainly affects the neutrophil polymorphonuclear cells. The blood picture becomes normal again towards the tenth day of illness. The sedimentation rate is accelerated and the blood coagulation time is abnormally long early in the disease, the prolongation of coagulation time being particularly marked in the icteric forms. The prothrombin time, which is usually lowered (65 per cent of normal), is very much lower in the fatal cases (20 per cent). The blood protein level, usually decreased, may fall to less than 5 gm. per liter when the subsequent evolution is fatal. The prognosis is unfavorable if bilirubinemia occurs early and if it is intense, and also if the blood cholesterol level is low and the urea level high.

In the *urine*, the albumin concentration often reaches 5 gm. per liter, but may be massive (up to 40 gm. per liter) in the fatal cases. Albuminuria is constant in yellow fever, but sometimes it is discrete in certain epidemics. When the illness is serious the urinary pH is very low, and the chloride concentration is weak. The concentration of urea in the urine varies with the intensity of the renal involvement: very low in the cases of oliguria, it remains increased in the benign cases or in the icteric or hemorrhagic forms. Bile salts appear at the onset of the jaundice, and bile pigments are observed only during convalescence.

The cerebrospinal fluid is clear, sometimes xanthochromic, and the albumin concentration is always increased (25 to 55 mg.). The pressure of the fluid is raised. The cerebrospinal fluid may contain the virus during the period of viremia.[26]

PROGNOSIS

The prognosis of yellow fever is all the more severe the greater the involvement of the viscera, particularly the liver and kidneys. The death rate is extremely variable depending on the epidemic, ranging from 5 per cent to 90 per cent. Hence, in 1871, during an epidemic in Senegal, 22 of 26 doctors on duty died of yellow fever. In 1961, in Ethiopia, in the province of Goma Gaffa, Sérié

et al.[40] found a single survivor out of 40 inhabitants of a small village following an epidemic wave.

The following features may be considered unfavorable from the viewpoint of prognosis: early jaundice, early and intense albuminuria, marked oliguria, a gradual and considerable increase in the blood urea level, a considerable decrease in proteinemia, a considerable reduction in the prothrombin time, and cardiac disorders. Nevertheless, it should be remembered that even when the clinical picture is serious, the patient may recover: yellow fever is a severe infectious disease of rapid evolution; the extensive anatomical-pathological lesions may be fairly rapidly and completely repaired. On the other hand, in the case of an apparently benign form of yellow fever, death may occur suddenly after a black vomit or even during convalescence, after sudden collapse when the myocardium is impaired.

DIFFERENTIAL DIAGNOSIS

The clinical diagnosis presents various difficulties: although it is easy in the typical forms during an epidemic, it becomes extremely difficult for subacute forms and impossible in most of the atypical forms.

Any person not vaccinated against yellow fever, who lives in an endemic area or has left an endemic area less than six days previously, and who presents an infection of abrupt onset, with headaches, high temperature, generalized pain, and vomiting, must be suspected of having yellow fever. The patient should be isolated and protected from mosquitoes if the latter are possible vectors and if the climatic conditions favor their role.

The responsible physician must contact a competent laboratory that can confirm the diagnosis of yellow fever or of any other tropical infectious or acute parasitic disease, since the differential diagnosis often is difficult to establish by clinical examination alone.

EARLY DIAGNOSIS

At the onset the first disease to be eliminated is malaria. Clinically, the initial symptoms are almost identical: sudden onset, intense generalized aching, headaches, vomiting. The hyperpyrexia is often more severe than in malaria, but this difference alone is not sufficient to orient the diagnosis. The dissociation of pulse rate and temperature (Faget's sign) is more significant but is not constant. The search for the plasmodium of malaria is always necessary, but in the event of primary malarial invasion (particularly in the case of *P. falciparum*) the plasmodium may be extremely rare. Hence the blood smears should be persistently repeated. The presence of numerous parasites would necessitate immediate treatment for malaria, in which case it is rare to observe associated yellow fever, because in yellow fever, the plasmodium, when it is present, is rare in the blood smears. If there are very few parasites, the possibility of yellow fever should be considered and a blood sample should be taken for possible isolation of the virus. The patient should be kept under observation, since the presence of albuminuria is an important factor in favor of the diagnosis of yellow fever.

Hemoglobinuric bilious fever, which is infrequent at present, is usually easy to recognize because of the very early albuminuria and especially the presence of hemoglobin in the urine. Some *arboviruses diseases* are impossible to diagnose without the assistance of a specialized laboratory. *Measles* has sometimes been a cause of error, but is rapidly eliminated by the appearance of Koplik spots. *Relapsing tick fever* is revealed by the presence of spirochetes in the blood; it responds very rapidly to treatment.

DIAGNOSIS DURING THE "YELLOW PHASE"

During the "yellow phase," diagnosis involves the elimination of other possible causes of jaundice. In the case of *epidemic hepatitis* the jaundice occurs only when the temperature has returned to normal. *Malaria* is confirmed, at this stage, by the discovery of plasmodia. *Leptospirosis icterohaemorrhagica*, which is frequently mistaken for yellow fever, is of progressive onset, with a much more severe jaundice; its diagnosis is ensured by the laboratory (isolation of the leptospira and immunological reactions). *Severe yellow atrophy of the liver* and certain *toxic-infectious hepatonephritides* of non-yellow-fever origin are differentiated by the laboratory. Finally, certain cases of *poisoning* (carbon tetrachloride, manioc) are differentiated by anatomopathological examination of the liver when the evolution is fatal.

ANATOMOPATHOLOGY

The macroscopic appearance of the organs of patients who have died of yellow fever varies with the intensity of the jaundice and the degree of involvement of the liver, kidneys, alimentary mucosa, heart, or meninges. However, the microscopic examination of the viscera, and especially the liver, is of greater interest. Since 1930, microscopic examination of sections of the liver sampled by means of a viscerotome (Rickard, 1931) has been performed systematically in South America, in all persons who died within less than 11 days from an illness of undetermined etiology. This measure is part of the inspection program for yellow fever.

The microscopic lesions typically observed in the liver sections have three main characteristics, which may be observed together:

(1) There is a *fatty degeneration* which is constant, essentially consisting of small droplets. The fatty cells are found in the lobules of the liver, close to the healthy cells in the less affected zones. These small droplets observed in the steatosis due to yellow fever contrast with the large droplets in steatosis due to intoxication (e.g., manioc, carbon tetrachloride).

(2) There is a *dissociation of the hepatic lobule* predominant in the middle zone, where the acinous structure has completely disappeared and where necrosis is preponderant. No normal cells remain in this zone. But in the central zone, surrounding the Kiernan's spaces of the central vein, a few normal hepatic cells are always found even when the lesions are extremely severe.

(3) There is a *necrosis of the hepatic cells,* or Councilman's necrosis (1890), which involves particularly the median zone; it is not absolutely specific but is very suggestive of yellow fever.

The affected cells have a nonstainable pyknotic nucleus. They show an eosinophilic hyaline degeneration and Councilman bodies, resulting from this degeneration, which invade the cytoplasm and, on staining with hematoxylin-eosin, take on a salmon-red color. These Councilman bodies do not contain the virus (Hardy, 1963[28a]). The other hepatic lesions are accessory and contingent, i.e., leukocytic infiltration, deposits of bile or blood pigments, sinusoidal congestion. Intranuclear inclusions considered to be specific, described by Torres in the monkey liver and also found by Cowdry in the human liver (Torres-Cowdry granulations), contain protein but not nucleic acid: hence they are not agglomerations of viral particles.[10]

Microscopic examination of the liver enables one to confirm or eliminate a diagnosis of yellow fever only in the typical cases. In other cases there may simply be a suspicion of yellow fever, and these atypical cases risk being interpreted in different ways by different anatomopathologists.[19]

The microscopic lesions of the other organs are less important. In the *kidney* the lesions involve mainly the epithelial cells of the convoluted tubules and the cells lining Bowman's capsule, where necrosis and steatosis are found. The basal layer of the glomeruli is also affected,[8] and the lumen of the tubules is congested with granular debris. These renal lesions are of variable intensity, ranging from a slight degeneration to a severe and extensive nephritis. As in most of the organs, the kidneys also show congestion of the blood vessels and sometimes slight hemorrhage. The adrenals, heart, and brain are affected to varying degrees, with abnormal abundance of lipids in the fasciculi of the adrenals, necrosis of the spongiocytes, fatty degeneration of the myocardial fibers (sometimes even hyaline degeneration), necrosis of the ganglion cells (which would explain the bradycardia), perivascular and cerebral hemorrhages, and even some cellular alterations of the cortex.

Thus, although anatomopathological examination in certain cases permits one to eliminate the diagnosis of yellow fever by revealing another cause of death, and in typical cases it can confirm the clinical diagnosis of yellow fever, in all the other cases it does not alone suffice to establish that the cause of death was yellow fever.

THE YELLOW FEVER VIRUS

In October, 1901, the yellow fever virus became the first human virus to be transmitted experimentally to man after ultrafiltration (Reed and Carrol, 1902). Isolated in 1927 (Stokes, Bauer, and Hudson), it is now included in the group of arboviruses.[17] The virus is thus serologically related to a number of other viruses that have either been known for some time, such as those of tick-borne encephalitis, Japanese type B encephalitis, and St. Louis encephalitis, or

that have been isolated more recently from mosquitoes during epidemiological studies particularly concerned with yellow fever.

Like the other arboviruses the yellow fever virus is small and contains ribonucleic acid, proteins, and lipids; it is sensitive to ether (Andrewes and Horstmann, 1949) and to sodium deoxycholate (Theiler, 1957). Under the electron microscope it appears as a round element of between 38 mμ[12] and 42 mμ (McGavran et al., 1964[30]). It consists of a dense nucleus surrounded by a limiting membrane. The size of 25 to 27 mμ determined previously by physical methods (ultrafiltration and ultracentrifugation) is that of the virus denuded of its limiting membrane.

The prototype strain of yellow fever is the Asibi strain (Stokes, Bauer, and Hudson, 1928), isolated from the monkey *M. sinicus* and, since its isolation, maintained in the laboratory by successive passages in the monkey *M. rhesus*; it has retained its original pantropic nature and virulence for monkey and man. Another strain which was also isolated from *M. rhesus* at Dakar (Mathis, Sellard, and Laigret, 1928) was subsequently inoculated intracerebrally into the mouse (Theiler, 1930) and passed numerous times in this animal, always by the same route. The virulence of this strain became modified, its neurotropism increased, and its pathogenicity considerably decreased with regard to man and monkey. This strain, called the Dakar or French neurotropic strain (or F.N.), is much utilized in the laboratory.

EXPERIMENTAL PATHOGENICITY

The pathogenicity of the Asibi strain for monkeys and of the Dakar strain for mice will be briefly surveyed, after a review of the highly variable susceptibility of other mammals to the yellow fever virus (e.g., the hedgehog, guinea pig, galago) and the multiplication of the virus, with no apparent lesions, in the organism of vector mosquitoes.

The Asibi strain, like most wild strains, causes a severe fatal disease in the monkey, *M. rhesus*. After two to five days' incubation, the animal presents fever and dies toward the fifth day. The viremia is intense. The jaundice is constant but particularly apparent in the viscera. The evolution and lesions caused by the virus closely resemble those in the human hyperacute forms. The monkey's liver contains large amounts of virus remaining virulent even after the animal's death. Manipulation of the infected livers is dangerous to experimental workers. The susceptibility of monkeys other than *M. rhesus* is extremely variable; numerous African monkeys, for example, are almost nonsusceptible to yellow fever virus.

The neutrotropic strain, which causes the death of monkeys inoculated by the intracerebral route and the death by encephalitis of approximately 25 per cent of the monkeys inoculated by other routes, is particularly used to infect mice, which are inoculated intracerebrally. After an incubation period which depends on the dose of virus inoculated (from four to eight days), typical paralysis appears, the hind legs remain extended, and death occurs after one or two days' illness.

Mice one to three days old, as we shall see further on, are just as sensitive to the Asibi strain and other wild strains as to the neurotropic virus: they die of viral encephalitis. All the animals which survive an inoculation of the virus show yellow fever antibodies.

LABORATORY DIAGNOSIS

ISOLATION OF THE VIRUS

Isolation of the virus from the patient's blood or eventually from the cerebrospinal fluid provides the only absolutely unquestionable proof of yellow fever, in the same way that isolation of the virus from ground mosquitoes or from the blood or viscera of animals remains the only conclusive evidence during epidemiological research studies.

Venous blood is taken as early as possible after onset of the disease, and, if it is not possible to inoculate susceptible animals directly from the patient's bedside, then the blood sample should be sent to the laboratory as rapidly as possible.

The animals ordinarily used are newborn mice (one to three days old) of a strain known to be susceptible to the virus. The rhesus monkey, which is extremely susceptible, at least to certain strains of the virus, is too costly, and young mice (three weeks of age) give inconstant results.

One litter of newborn mice is inoculated with pure serum and another litter with serum diluted 1/10. Each animal receives 0.02 ml. intracerebrally and 0.03 ml. intraperitoneally. The litters of mice are inspected twice a day. As soon as one of the animals

shows symptoms of the disease, particularly paralysis or paresis, its brain is removed, finely ground, and inoculated into another litter of mice. If none of the suckling mice of this second inoculated litter show any symptoms of the disease after the seventh day, two or three suckling mice are killed; their finely ground brains are again inoculated into another litter of newborn mice, i.e., "blind passage."

When the isolation is successful, after two or three passages all the suckling mice are paralyzed after a shorter and more constant incubation period. The virus may then be identified.

IDENTIFICATION

The virus is first tested for its sensitivity to ether or to deoxycholate, a reaction common to all the arboviruses. Then, following treatment with Freon or saccharose acetone, an attempt is made to demonstrate the presence of a hemagglutinin in the extract of the infected brain. The hemagglutinin titers with yellow fever virus attain their maximum at a slightly acid pH (approximately 6.4) and at 37° C. The identification procedure is continued by means of serological methods using experimental sera whose specificity and titer have been previously verified.

The diagnosis is oriented toward the probable presence of a group B arbovirus by testing the hemagglutination inhibition provoked by this virus by means of a wide-spectrum serum antiarbovirus B. Subsequently the type is identified by means of a powerful and specific experimental anti-yellow fever serum, which may be derived from horse, rabbit, domestic fowl, or mouse.

The same dilution of experimental serum should inhibit the same number of hemagglutinating units contained both in the antigen obtained from the virus to be identified and in the antigen prepared from the standard reference yellow fever strain.

Identification of the strain is continued by making use of the complement-fixation reaction, performed by cross reactions with increasing dilutions of serum and antigen. The results obtained with the antigen prepared from the strain under observation and with the reference strain are identical. Finally this diagnosis of type is confirmed by determining the neutralization index, which indicates the quantity of virus under identification which is neutralized by the experimental serum, this index being identical, when the neutralization method used is the same, with that obtained with the same serum and with the yellow fever reference strain.

The identification of the yellow fever virus does not usually present any difficulties, since, although this virus is serologically related to the other group B viruses, one can easily obtain experimental sera that are sufficiently specific; furthermore, the different strains of the yellow fever virus are all very similar antigenically. In order to differentiate them serologically, it is necessary to use more specific serological reactions such as study of the absorption of antibodies with regard to homologous or heterologous antigens, a reaction applied to the study of the influenza viruses and adapted by Clarke (1960)[17c] to the study of the arboviruses. Clarke was thus able to demonstrate certain differences between strains of the yellow fever virus isolated in South America, West Africa, and East Africa.

SEROLOGY

It has long been known (Nott, 1848) that an attack of yellow fever confers strong immunity, but the first proof of the presence in convalescent serum of substances capable of conferring passive protection to man was provided by Marchoux, Salimbeni, and Simond (1903). This was substantiated by demonstration of protective anti-yellow-fever antibodies in the serum. The other types of antibodies are complement-fixing antibodies (Frobischer, 1929), precipitating antibodies (Hughes, 1933, who was the first to demonstrate the "soluble antigen"), and hemagglutination-inhibiting antibodies (Casals and Brown, 1954).[17]

We shall not describe here the methods for demonstrating complement-fixing antibodies or hemagglutination-inhibiting antibodies,[18] which are given in Chapter 58. The protective or neutralizing antibodies are demonstrated by the neutralization test performed either in white mice or in cell cultures.

The most current method used is that of Theiler (1930), standardized by a group of W.H.O. experts.[31] The serum protective power is estimated by its capacity to neutralize 100 LD_{50} of the virus (generally, the "French neurotropic" virus), the mixture of the virus and the serum to be tested being inoculated intracerebrally into the mouse. The test results are indicated by the number of mice surviving as compared with the number inoculated, complementary information being provided by the average survival time (Bugher). The results of this test are in agreement with those of the neutralization methods carried out in cell culture (strain 17D and chick embryo cells), the virus titration being performed by the plaque method[28, 37] and the neutralizing power being measured by the inhibition of plaque formation.

The original method for demonstrating precipitating antibodies (Hughes) is not used in practice, i.e., the test for the precipitinogen derived from the serum of a monkey infected with the Asibi strain. However, while this discovery did not find its immediate practical application, it has now aroused renewed interest with regard to immunochemical analysis by precipitation in gelinated media.

The different types of antibodies do not show the same duration or specificity in man. The hemagglutination-inhibiting antibodies persist for a long period, but the complement-fixing antibodies are detectable for only one or two years after the illness. The neutralizing antibodies persist throughout the patient's lifetime after a severe attack of yellow fever. The specificity of the different reactions depends on the patient's state of immunity with regard to the group B arboviruses at the time of onset of the illness.

If yellow fever is the patient's first disease due to a group B arbovirus, then the homologous hemagglutination-inhibiting antibodies are the first to appear, followed by heterologous antibodies for the other arboviruses of the group. The titer of the homologous antibodies remains at least equal to if not higher than that of the heterologous antibodies. The complement-fixing antibodies appear after a variable lapse of time, but the responses are generally specific, the heterologous antibodies appearing only when the homologous titer is extremely high. The neutralizing antibodies are specific, and the heterologous antibodies are of low incidence.

If yellow fever occurs in an individual previously affected by another group B arbovirus, then the serological diagnosis of yellow fever becomes difficult to establish, since the hemagglutination-inhibiting and complement-fixing antibodies appear both rapidly and massively and it is hard to distinguish the specific from the heterologous antibodies. Interpretation of the neutralization test is also made difficult, as an attack of yellow fever always causes formation of neutralizing antibodies and successive attacks by other B arboviruses in the same subject may cause formation of heterologous antibodies capable of neutralizing the yellow fever virus (Smith, 1958;[41] Price et al., 1963[38a]).

Hence, in practice, if one is dealing with an isolated case, to interpret the serological results it is necessary to examine at least two serum samples from the patient, one taken at the onset and another at a later period. If the first sample demonstrates lack of previous infection by any group B arbovirus, the subsequent appearance and rise of the anti-yellow fever antibodies confirms the diagnosis. On the other hand, if antibodies against one or several of the group B arboviruses are found in the first serum sample, the interpretation becomes extremely difficult.

The same problems have occurred during epidemiological investigations. For practical reasons, it is often impossible to obtain two serum samples, one early and one late, from the same patients; this difficulty has been circumvented by taking systematic samples from healthy subjects and from patients or convalescents. From examination of sera from healthy subjects, one can deduce the state of immunity with regard to group B arboviruses of the population before the outbreak of the epidemic. Naturally, only if this basic immunity is low or nil will examination of the sera of patients or convalescents be of full value and easy to interpret.

An epidemic may occur in a population that has been partially vaccinated against yellow fever. In this case the vaccination against yellow fever should be considered as a first infection of an organism by group B arbovirus (Price et al., 1963[38a]); furthermore, the antibody titer found after vaccination varies with the strain used. The titers following vaccination by the Dakar vaccine are intermediary between the high titers observed after an attack of yellow fever and the lower titers observed after vaccination by the 17D vaccine.[13, 35]

Finally, it seems that in certain limited regions (Eritrea) one finds low titers of neutralizing antibodies in the sera of individuals who have never been infected by yellow fever virus. These sera do not contain hemagglutination-inhibiting or complement-fixing antibodies. This anomaly has as yet to be explained.[35]

In short, serological examination can confirm the diagnosis of yellow fever only if the patient has never been previously infected by one of the other group B arboviruses.

EPIDEMIOLOGY

First, an account will be given of the most important stages in the epidemiological studies on yellow fever.

1881: Carlos Findlay was the first to suspect the "Culex mosquito" (*Aedes aegypti*) of transmitting the disease through its bites. Volunteers were infected by *Aedes* which had bitten patients. Findlay was not aware, however, of the extrinsic incubation period of the virus in the mosquito, and consequently the experiments gave variable results.

1900: An American commission (Reed, Caroll, Agramonte, and Lazear) confirmed Findlay's hypothesis during an epidemic in Cuba and established the basis of the epidemiology of yellow fever (urban epidemic form): i.e., the causal agent is a filtrable virulent element, transmitted through the bite of *Aedes aegypti* (only the female bites man). The mosquito is thus infected from the patient's blood, but it becomes infectious only after a certain lapse of time (extrinsic incubation period); in Cuba, this lapse is 12 days. The mosquito remains infectious throughout its lifetime, which may be six months or more. An attack of yellow fever confers immunity. In 1903 these conclusions were confirmed by Marchoux, Simond, and Salimbeni in Rio de Janiero, who also established that the duration of extrinsic incubation varies with temperature. In the case of *Aedes aegypti* it is now known that this incubation period is 12 days at 23° C.; this duration always serves as a basis for the calculation of the average risk of transmission. The incubation period is four days at 37° C., and at 18° C. the mosquito no longer transmits the disease. However, the virus is able to survive at least one month at 8° C., and when the mosquito is replaced at 36° C. it is capable of transmitting the virus after six days. The extrinsic incubation period for other vector mosquitoes is longer (Bates, 1945).

1931: After the virus was isolated in 1927 and the seroprotection test, perfected in

1930, permitted subsequent serological studies, Soper discovered the existence of nonurban yellow fever, transmitted by vectors other than *Aedes aegypti*. Subsequently it was proved that the natural cycle of the yellow fever virus takes place in the tropical and equatorial forest, the virus remaining in the mosquito during the whole of its lifetime. The mosquitoes become infected by biting infected wild animals, especially monkeys and marsupials, during the period of viremia following the bite of an infected mosquito. Hence, the natural cycle is animal-mosquito-animal. Man may accidentally be infected by a wild mosquito or, in some instances, by a domestic mosquito infected by a wild monkey. The passage animal-mosquito-man then takes place. Consequently enzootic and epizootic diseases may provoke sporadic cases if, starting from one infected man, the virus does not spread, or an epidemic if the domestic mosquitoes infected from man in turn bite receptive humans. In the latter case the cycle man-mosquito-man is established: the only one known until 1932, and responsible for the classic epidemics by passage from man to *Aedes aegypti* to man.

The situation is therefore more complex than the early epidemiological observations first led one to suppose, and, although the campaigns for the eradication of *Aedes aegypti* have succeeded in suppressing the urban disease in numerous territories, the virus remains inaccessible in its natural cycle in wild animals and may at any moment provoke serious epidemics.

This brief summary is sufficient to make it evident that different territories are not all exposed to yellow fever to the same extent.

Transmission of the virus may be impossible if there are no vector mosquitoes or if the surrounding temperature is too low for the mosquito to transmit the disease. However, "pseudoepidemics" or sporadic yellow fever may occur (e.g., St. Nazaire, Swansea), if infected vector mosquitoes are imported during the hot season into territories where these mosquitoes are not usually found. The virus is transmitted to every man bitten by the infected mosquitoes, but an epidemic cannot develop.

When the virus is imported either by a patient or by mosquitoes into a territory where vector mosquitoes are present, an epidemic can develop, the gravity of which will depend on several factors: the temperature (which determines the duration of the extrinsic incubation of the virus in the mosquito), the density of the vectors, and the density of the human population receptive to the virus. In temperate zones (e.g., the United States, Spain, Portugal) the epidemics occur during the summer and disappear in the winter. In tropical zones, the epidemic may decrease during the dry season and regain its activity during the following rainy season. Finally, the presence of absence of animals sensitive to the virus determines the temporary or permanent implantation of the virus. In the tropical-equatorial zones of Asia and the Pacific Islands all the conditions necessary for a permanent implantation of yellow fever exist, although until now, these territories have remained free of the disease. The introduction of yellow fever virus into these territories would have disastrous consequences, and therefore the very strict measures of sanitary inspection imposed are completely justified.

Yellow fever is endemoepidemic in the tropical-equatorial zones of America and Africa.

The Americas. In tropical America, *Aedes aegypti* has been eliminated from most of the town centers by eradication campaign undertaken with the aid of the Rockefeller Foundation. This extermination was relatively easy, as the *Aedes aegypti* mosquito recently imported to America is urban and anthropophilic. The area of activity of the virus has thus been considerably reduced: yellow fever has disappeared from the West Indies since 1908, with the exception of a minor epidemic of continental origin occurring in Trinidad in 1954.[22]

In the vast endemic zone of the northern part of South America, the virus is maintained by passages through susceptible animals and vectors. The enzootic disease is thus permanent, often assuming the aspect of a succession of slight epizootic outbreaks. Man is contaminated only accidentally and intervenes relatively little in this epidemiological chain. The whole succesion of events takes place in the forest at a variable height above ground level, very often near the treetops, where the monkeys, marsupials, and mosquitoes are to be found together.

Some of the monkeys are diurnal—e.g., *Ateles* (spider monkeys), *Alouatta* (shrieking monkeys), and *Cebus* (hooded monkeys) while some are nocturnal—e.g., *Aotus*—

sleeping during the day amongst the foliage. As these last are generally susceptible to the virus, they often die of yellow fever, which makes it possible to detect epizootic diseases which proceed over distances from 15 to 200 km. per month. After the passage of an epizootic disease, a new epizootic outbreak is possible only when the forest has become repopulated by young monkeys, offspring of those that survived.

The mosquitoes are of the family Aedinae, either of the genus *Aedes*, particularly *A. leucocelaenus*, or of the genus *Haemagogus* (blue mosquito): *H. spegazzinii, H. capricornii, H. equinus*, and so forth.

Epizootic outbreaks of yellow fever may spread over a wide area, either in the endemic zone (Brazil 1934-1940) or outside this zone (Central America, from the Panama canal to the Mexican frontier 1948-1954). The diagnosis is facilitated by histological examination of the livers of dead monkeys and by isolation of the virus from these organs.[7]

Man may be infected with the virus accidentally, often during the felling of trees, when the mosquitoes descend to ground level. This happened in the epidemic reported by Causey and Maroja.[17a]

Sometimes infected monkeys contaminate rural mosquitoes *(A. scapularis)* in the neighborhood of plantations, i.e., epidemics of borderlands. When the *Haemogogus* swarm, the mosquitoes may invade dwellings and infect the inhabitants.

Each year the yellow fever control organization in the Americas detects cases of yellow fever, very often following systematic histological examination of the liver. In 1964, 105 cases were declared, with 82 deaths, in Peru, Brazil, Bolivia, Columbia, and Venezuela. Obviously the number of cases declared is far less than the actual number of cases occurring. Yellow fever is often pseudo-influenzal or even inapparent in the lower basin of the Amazon (Causey and Maroja[17a]) where 50 per cent of the adult population were shown to possess anti-yellow fever antibodies.

Africa. In Africa, localization of the foci of infection is more difficult than in America, where the foci are fairly easily detected, owing to the fatal simian epizootic outbreaks and the occasional fatal cases among the human population, which are often diagnosed by systematic histological examination. The African monkeys are much less sensitive to yellow fever than the American monkeys; hence the attention of epidemiologists is not drawn by a sudden mortality occurring in colonies of monkeys. Moreover, the population of vast territories has been submitted to a systematic anti-yellow fever vaccination campagin since 1940. Therefore, an active focus of infection may exist in these territories without being detectable by the presence of cases among the human population. Finally, the results of serological surveys performed in these vaccinated populations are falsified by the presence of postvaccinal anti-yellow fever antibodies. Consequently, epidemiological surveys are based on the investigations performed in man, vectors, and wild animals, except in territories where the systematic vaccination undertaken reduces worthwhile investigations to those of the vectors and wild animals.

The serological surveys performed on human sera sampled from a nonvaccinated population demonstrated the presence of antibodies from the 15th degree latitude south to the 15th degree latitude north. The epidemics of yellow fever of any importance in the tropical zone of the northern hemisphere generally occur after the rainy season at the time of massive swarming of the mosquitoes. Endemic yellow fever is mainly observed in the hot, damp, pluvial zone of the Guinean and equatorial forest, where very few clinical cases of human yellow fever are observed, sometimes grouped together in small epidemics. Usually the high level of the anti-yellow-fever antibodies in the population is out of proportion with the small number of clinical cases declared.

During the past few years, epidemics of varying importance have been reported among the nonvaccinated population. In Ghana a few cases of yellow fever occurred in the southern area. In Nigeria, epidemics of varying importance have been observed at the end of the rainy seasons of 1946, 1951, and 1953. The most severe outbreak occurred in 1951 and at the beginning of 1952 in the Eastern provinces (Udi district). In the Congo (Kinshasa), slight epidemics were rapidly overcome in the equatorial provinces (Gemena) and in the Eastern provinces, where, in 1960, Courtois et al.[21] were able to isolate the yellow fever virus for the first time in the Congo.

In Uganda and Kenya, human cases are rare and isolated, despite the presence of natural active foci among monkeys. The most important epidemics were observed in 1940 in the Sudan (Mount Nuba) and in 1960-1962 in southwest Ethiopia, on the border of the endemic zone, particularly south of the Sudan. Taylor et al.[43] called this the "silent zone," suggesting that the maintenance of the virus is based on the compulsory cohabitation of man, vectors, and wild animals in the neighborhood of the water sources in this desert area.

There were over 15,000 cases in the Sudan in 1940, and at least 1500 deaths. In 1959, in the Blue Nile province, a less severe epidemic was observed which extended up to the foot-hills of the Ethiopean plateau.

In southwest Ethiopia, during the later months of 1960, a very serious epidemic broke out which subsequently spread to the north along the Omo river and which was subdued in 1962, after having infected, according to rough estimates, over 100,000 individuals and caused the death of over 10,000. It was the most important epidemic of all those recorded in Africa. One of the factors making this epidemic so severe was probably the absence of antibodies against yellow fever and against the other group B arboviruses among most of the population affected.

In the areas of Africa where mass vaccination campaigns had been undertaken in recent years yellow fever gradually disappeared. These campaigns were reduced or interrupted for several years, since the Dakar vaccine is not entirely free of danger to children and the 17D vaccine has not yet been used for mass vaccination.

In Africa, individuals under 20 years of age represent more than 50 per cent of the total population. If this group is not immunized, an epidemic of yellow fever may occur if the virus is introduced during a period of swarming of the vector mosquitoes. This happened recently east of Dakar, in the region of Diourbel, where a relatively high number of cases of yellow fever were observed among nonvaccinated subjects one to 23 years of age. It was remarkable that none of the children aged less than one year were affected: maternal antibodies had no doubt protected these children against the disease.

THE VECTORS

The vector mosquitoes have been the subject of numerous studies in Africa, particularly in Uganda, where *Aedes africanus* seems responsible for the maintenance of active foci of yellow fever, the mosquito biting the monkeys in the foliage. Sometimes *A. africanus* bites on ground level and becomes responsible for human infections.

The African vectors for humans are mainly *A. aegypti* and *A. simpsoni*. But these mosquitoes are not always anthropophilic. Haddow et al.[26] deduced from this fact the explanation of the surprisingly low number of human cases of yellow fever in Uganda in the zones where the monkeys have been proved to be seriously contaminated by the virus.

In Ethiopia, the vector of the 1960-1962 epidemic was *A. simpsoni,* but *A. africanus* was found to be a carrier of the virus in the forest as soon as the epidemic had reached the forest areas. The part played by other mosquitoes capable of transmitting the virus has not yet been proved. *A vittatus* was suspected to have played an important part in the epidemic of Mount Nuba.

WILD ANIMALS

Monkeys certainly play an important part in the transmission of the virus in nature, but the viremia lasts only three to four days. The mosquitoes infected from these monkeys may, on the other hand, transmit the virus throughout their lifetime. Thus, strictly speaking, there seems to be no reservoir of virus. This cycle certainly plays an important part, but is it unique or are there other animal reservoirs? All the investigations undertaken have so far produced negative results for all animals except the lemurs, especially the galago, and the hedgehog *Ateletrix albiventris,* which are sensitive to inoculation of the yellow fever virus.

To sum up, it is known that in the African forest there still remain foci of yellow fever virus: these foci are not well known and are difficult to inspect and control. The more serious epidemics occur on the edge of the forest, particularly in the Northern Hemisphere, where they may persist at a reduced intensity in the dry season and then set in again after the rainy season, at the swarming period of the mosquitoes. Since the extermination of the vector mosquitoes throughout the areas of Africa involved is impossible, vaccination remains the only practical means of protecting the individual against the disease.

PROPHYLAXIS

The prophylaxis of yellow fever is based, on the one hand, on inspection of the infected areas and then attack against the different links of the epidemiological chain, and on the other, on the protection of man by vaccination. Vaccination serves the dual purpose of protecting the individual and breaking one of the links of the epidemiological chain, since man is an "amplifying host" for the virus.

IN THE ENDEMIC ZONES

Wild Animals. There is no hope of sterilizing the virus reservoirs constituted by wild animals, but in America, and with much more difficulty in Africa, one can detect enzootic and epizootic yellow fever.

Mosquitoes. Although there exists no possibility of destroying all of the sylvatic vectors, it is possible to prevent the spread of an epidemic by massive utilization of insecticides in a limited area. Furthermore, the transit zones for travelers (ports and airports) are freed of mosquitoes and are submitted to a particularly strict inspection with regard to possible vector mosquitoes, principally *Aedes aegypti*.

Man. A properly vaccinated traveler cannot transmit yellow fever. In an endemic zone, the greater the decrease in the number of receptive subjects, the higher the index numbers of vector mosquitoes necessary for an epidemic to spread. Massive vaccination around a focus of yellow fever infection can stop an epidemic.

MEASURES TO BE TAKEN AS SOON AS A CASE OF YELLOW FEVER IS OBSERVED

The patient is isolated under a mosquito net or in a protected room, and suspects or "contacts" who may also have been bitten by an infected mosquito are also isolated.

The case of yellow fever is reported, and an epidemiological investigation is undertaken in order to ascertain the origin and mode of contamination. Massive killing of the possible vector insects (larvae and adults) is undertaken, and the population living in the surrounding region is vaccinated.

In *the event of an epizootic outbreak,* vaccination of the population, before passage of the outbreak to man, prevents an epidemic.

VACCINATION

Two different types of vaccines are used, both consisting of live virus: the 17D and the Dakar vaccine.

The *Dakar vaccine* is prepared from a strain isolated in Dakar in 1927 which was serially propagated in mice by intracerebral administration (Theiler). During the course of the different passages, this strain lost the greatest part of its viscerotropism. It was used for the first attempts at vaccination neutralized by serum from convalescent patients (Sawyer et al., 1931-1932), then attenuated by various methods (Laigret). At present the vaccine prepared with this strain is applied by cutaneous scarification (Peltier et al., 1939).

The vaccine itself consists of a mixture of powder of desiccated brains of mice inoculated with the Dakar virus, at about the 260th passage, together with diatomite.

At the time of use, this powder is placed in suspension in a solution of gum arabic. The Dakar vaccine has principally been used for mass vaccinations in Africa and to combat epidemics in territories that are not easily accessible. It is more stable than the 17D vaccine, not costly, and easy to administer, as well as extremely effective. But although the viscerotropism of this strain has been attenuated after repeated passages in the mouse inoculated intracerebrally, unfortunately its neurotropism has become accentuated.

In approximately 15 per cent of cases febrile reactions have followed vaccination with late neuromeningeal involvement in certain cases, most frequently in children in whom such complications are always more serious than in the adult. Encephalitis also occurs. In most cases it is curable, but it can leave serious sequelae and is occasionally fatal (Costa-Rica, Ghana, Congo, Senegal). Hence, this vaccine should not be used for primary vaccination in children. It is preferable at any age to use it for *revaccination only.*

The *17D vaccine* is a much more attenuated strain, and the reduction in its virulence affects both its neurotropism and its viscerotropism (Theiler and Smith, 1937). It is derived from the pantropic Asibi strain which has undergone numerous passages in embryonic cells of different origins (mouse or domestic fowl). After numerous passages by different methods, the substrain 17D one has been retained for vaccination against yellow fever. The vaccine virus is cultivated in the chick embryo.

The original method of preparation has been modified twice, first by suppression of normal human serum, originally added to facilitate lyophilization and to increase the preservation of the vaccine, since this human serum could, in some instances, contain hepatitis virus (Sawyer et al., 1944), and, secondly, by the production of large batches of primary and secondary seeds so as to avoid repeated passages of this strain of virus, since some substrains have been found to be neurotropic. These seed lots are carefully tested in the monkey *M. rhesus* and stocked at low temperatures (at least −60° C.).

The vaccine consists of a suspension of virulent embryos, centrifuged, lyophilized, rehydrated, and diluted at the time of use. It is inoculated subcutaneously (0.5 ml.).

Reactions are rare (in 2 to 4 per cent of cases) and of slight intensity, usually appearing as a mild febrile syndrome, with mild aching at the worst.

Most countries admit children under one year of age who have not been vaccinated against yellow fever to their territory. This is because nervous system reactions have occasionally followed vaccination in infants; these were, however, benign, curable, and without after-effects.

The 17D vaccine, which contains various proteins of the chick embryo, may cause allergic reactions in sensitive subjects. These reactions may be decreased in number and intensity by performing an intradermal inoculation of the vaccine before the subcutaneous inoculation and by prescribing antihistaminics in the days following the vaccination.

Postvaccinal Immunity. The level of antibodies provoked by the vaccination is higher after vaccination with the Dakar vaccine than with the 17D vaccine. The immunity subsequent to vaccination, whatever the type of vaccine used, is of a high level and durable. This immune state has been proved 2 to 19 years after a single injection of the 17D vaccine.[20, 25, 39] At present a vaccination certificate is considered valid for ten years.

PROTECTION OF TERRITORIES

The protection of countries against pestilential diseases now comes under international health conventions, revised in 1951

by the World Health Organization in the form of an International Health Regulation.

The protection against yellow fever is based on the simple distinction between countries in possible contaminating territories within the endemic zone and territories that may be contaminated and which form the potentially receptive zone.

With a view to reducing as far as possible hindrances to international exchanges, this regulation has been gradually modified, and has become more complex but less strict. The demonstration of the presence of the virus in man or in animals in any one country does not require measures of protection for the whole area of that country, but only for the territory of the infected area. This notion, which appeared in the International Health Regulations of 1957, facilitates international travel without increasing the risks of spreading pestilential diseases. It has, however, not been adopted without reserve by all countries, notably Ceylon, India, Pakistan, South West Africa, and the Union of South Africa, which continue to consider as infected territories the countries included in the endemic zone.

Indeed, thanks to the efficiency of vaccination against yellow fever, the traveler is not only well-immunized against the disease but has free access to all territories without risk of having his voyage interrupted by the quarantine authorities.

TREATMENT

There is at present no specific treatment for yellow fever. A cautious symptomatic treatment should be established to avoid any effort, fatigue, or useless movement for a fragile patient who is always at the mercy of a fatal collapse. The patient should be rehydrated, vomiting should be calmed by bicarbonate preparations, and alkalized water should be given to counteract the fall in the alkali reserve. Aspirin may be used. Laxatives are forbidden; enemas alone should be used to counteract constipation. The cardiovascular analeptics combat the effects of the myocarditis, and total adrenal extracts are advisable in the event of adrenal involvement.

Finally, the treatment consists mainly of minor medical measures to help the patient overcome the different crises of the disease pending the regeneration of the tissues destroyed by the virus.

BIBLIOGRAPHY

STUDIES AND REVIEWS ON YELLOW FEVER CONTAINING NUMEROUS BIBLIOGRAPHIC REFERENCES

1. Bonnel, P. H., and Deutschman, Z.: La fièvre jaune en Afrique au cours des années récentes. Bull. W.H.O., *11*:325-389, 1954.
2. Casals, J., and Reeves, W. C.: The arboviruses. In: Horsfall, F. K., and Tamm, I.: Viral and Rickettsial Infections of Man. Philadelphia, J. B. Lippincott Company, 1965, pp. 580-582.
3. Clarke, D. H., and Casals, J.: Arboviruses: Group B. In: Horsfall, F. K., and Tamm, I.: Viral and Rickettsial Infections of Man. Philadelphia, J. B. Lippincott Company, 1965, pp. 606-658.
4. Demarchi, J., and Bres, P.: Fièvre jaune. In: Encyclopédie Médicochirurgicale. Paris, 1961.
5. Organisation Mondiale de la Santé (World Health Organization): La Vaccination Antiamarile. Série de Monographies No. 30, 1956.
6. Strode, G. K.: Yellow Fever. New York, McGraw-Hill Book Company, 1951.

PRINCIPAL RECENT WORKS

7. Anderson, C. R., and Downs, W. G.: The isolation of yellow fever virus from livers of naturally infected red howler monkeys. Amer. J. Trop. Med., *4*:662-664, 1955.
8. Barbareschi, G.: Glomerulosi toxica in febre gialla. Rev. Biol. Trop., *5*:201-209, 1957.
9. Baruch, E.: Electron microscopic study of spinal cord of mice infected with yellow fever virus. J. Ultrastruct. Res., *9*:209-224, 1963.
10. Bearcroft, W. G. C.: Electron microscope studies on the livers of yellow fever-infected rhesus monkeys. J. Path. Bact., *80*:421-426, 1960.
11. Berdonneau, R. C., Sérié, C., Panthier, R., Hannoun, C., Papaionnou, S. C., and Georgieff, P.: Sur l'épidémie de fièvre jaune de l'année 1959 en Ethiopie (frontiére Soudano-éthiopienne). Bull. Soc. Path. Exot., *54*:276-283, 1961.
12. Bergold, G. H., and Weible, J.: Demonstration of yellow fever virus with the electron microscope. Virology, *17*:554-562, 1962.
13. Bres, P.: La fixation du complément et l'inhibition de l'hemagglutination contre la fièvre jaune par la souche de Dakar. Bull. Soc. Path. Exot., *54*:995-1001, 1961.
14. Bres, P., Lacan, A., Diop, I., Michel, R., Peretti, P., and Vidal, C.: Résultats des campagnes de vaccination antiamarile en République du Sénégal. Bull. Soc. Path. Exot., *55*:1038-1043, 1962.
15. Burton, G. J., Noamesi, G. K., and McRae, T. M.: A survey for the vector of yellow fever in the Damongo Area, Northern Region, Ghana Med. J., *3*:9-15, 1964.
16. Casals, J., and Brown, L. V.: Hemagglutination with certain arthropod-borne viruses. Proc. Soc. Exp. Biol. Med., *83*:170-173, 1953.
17. Casals, J., and Brown, L. V.: Hemagglutination with arthropod-borne viruses. J. Exp. Med., *99*:429-449, 1954.
17a. Causey, O. R., and Maroja, O.: Isolation of yellow fever virus from man and mosquitoes in the Amazon region of Brazil. Amer. J. Trop. Med *8*:368-371, 1959.
17b. Causey, O. R., and Theiler, M.: Virus antibody survey on sera of residents of the Amazon Valley in Brazil. Amer. J. Trop. Med., *7*:36-41, 1958.
17c. Clarke, D. H.: Antigenic analysis of certain group B arthropod-borne viruses by antibody absorption. J. Exp. Med., *111*:21-32, 1960.
18. Clarke, D. H., and Casals, J.: Techniques for hemagglutination and hemagglutination inhibition with arthropod-borne viruses. Amer. J. Trop. Med *7*:561-573, 1958.
19. Courtois, G.: De la spécificité des lésions histologiques dans l'hépatite amarile. Colloque sur la fièvre jaune (5 Sept., 1953). Rapport du Bureau Régional de l'O.M.S. [W.H.O.], Brazzaville, 1954.
20. Courtois, G.: Durée de l'immunité après vaccination antiamarile. Ann. Soc. Belge Med. Trop. *34*:9-12, 1954.
21. Courtois, G., Osterrieth, P., and Blanes Ridaura, G. B.: Isolement du virus de la fièvre jaune au Congo Belge. Ann. Soc. Belge Med. Trop., *40*:29-60, 1960.
22. Downs, W. G., Aitken, T. H. G., and Anderson, C. R.: Activities of Trinidad regional virus laboratory in 1953 and 1954 with special reference to the yellow fever outbreak in Trinidad, B.W.I. Amer. J. Trop. Med., *4*:837-843, 1955.
23. Galindo, P., and de Rodaniche, E.: Surveillance for sylvan yellow fever activity in Panama 1957-1961. Amer. J. Trop. Med., *13*:844-850, 1964.
24. Groot, H., and Ribeiro, R. B.: Neutralizing and haemagglutination-inhibiting antibodies to yellow fever 17 years after vaccination with 17D Vaccine. Bull. W.H.O. *27*:699-707, 1962.
25. Haddow, A. J.: Etat actuel des connaissances concernant la fièvre jaune en Afrique. Ann. Soc. Belge Med. Trop., *38*:271-281, 1958.
26. Haddow, A. J.: Tulloch, J. A., Patel, K. M., Williams, M. C., Woodall, J. P., and Simpson, D. I. H.: Yellow fever in Central Uganda, 1964. Trans. Roy. Soc. Trop. Med. Hyg., *59*:435-458, 1965.
27. Hallauer, C.: Züchtung von Gelbfiebervirus in menschlichen Explanten. Arch. Ges. Virusforsch. *9*:428-441, 1959.
28. Hannoun, C., and Panthier, R.: Application de la méthode des plages en cultures cellulaires à l'étude de vaccin antiamaril 17D. Bull. Soc. Path. Exot., *53*:424-430, 1960.
28a. Hardy, F. M.: The growth of Asibi strain yellow fever virus in tissue cultures. J. Infect. Dis., *113* 1-14, 1963.
28b. Kirk, R.: Epidemic of yellow fever in Nuba Mountains Anglo-Egyptian Sudan. Ann. Trop. Med. *35*:67-112, 1941.
29. Lebrun, A. J.: Jungle yellow fever and its control in Gemena, Belgian Congo. Amer. J. Trop. Med., *12*:398-407, 1963.
30. McGavran, M. H., and White, J. D.: Electron microscopic and immunofluorescent observations on monkey liver and tissue culture cells infected with the Asibi strain of yellow fever virus. Amer. J. Path., *45*:501-517, 1964.

1. Organisation Mondiale de la Santé (World Health Organization): Série de Rapports Techniques No. 136. Comité d'Experts du Vaccin Antiamaril, Premier Rapport, 1957.

2. Organisation Mondiale de la Santé (World Health Organization): Série de Rapports Techniques No. 179. Normes pour les Substances Biologiques: 3. Normes Relatives au Vaccin Antiamaril. Rapport d'un Groupe d'Etude, 1959.

3. Panthier, R.: A propos de quelques cas de réactions nerveuses tardives observées chez des nourrissons après vaccination antiamarile (17D). Bull. Soc. Path. Exot., *49*:477-494, 1956.

4. Panthier, R., and Hannoun, C.: Fièvre jaune ou paludisme; diagnostic d'urgence. Bull. Mem. Soc. Med. Hôp. Paris, *77*:910-913, 1961.

5. Panthier, R., Hannoun, C., and de Looze, L.: Recherche d'anticorps (virus amaril et autres arbovirus) dans des sérums prélevés en Ethiopie de 1954 à 1961. Ann. Inst. Pasteur (Paris), *109*: 204-227, 1965.

6. Porterfield, J. S.: The haemagglutination-inhibition test in the diagnosis of yellow fever in man. Trans. Roy. Soc. Trop. Med. Hyg., *48*:261-266, 1954.

7. Porterfield, J. S.: Plaque production with yellow fever and related arthropod-borne viruses (correspondence). Nature, *183*:1069-1070, 1959.

8. Price, W. H., Lee, R. W., Gunkel, W. F., and O'Leary, W.: The virulence of West-Nile virus and TP 21 virus and their application to a group B arbovirus vaccine. Amer. J. Trop. Med., *10*: 403-422, 1961.

38a. Price, W. H., Parks, J., Ganaway, J., Lee, R., and O'Leary, W.: A sequential immunization procedure against certain group B arboviruses. Amer. J. Trop. Med., *12*:624-638, 1963.

39. Rosenzweig, E. C., Babione, R. W., and Wisseman, C. L., Jr.: Persistence of yellow fever antibodies following vaccination with 17D strain yellow fever vaccine. Amer. J. Trop. Med., *12*:230-235, 1963.

40. Sérié, C.: Andral, L., Lindrec, A., and Neri, P.: Epidémie de fièvre jaune en Ethiopie (1960-1962), Bull. W.H.O., *30*:299-319, 1964.

41. Smith, C. E. G.: The distribution of antibodies to Japanese encephalitis, dengue and yellow fever viruses in five rural communities in Malaya. Trans. Roy. Soc. Trop. Med. Hyg., *52*:237-252, 1958.

42. Spence, L., Downs, W. G., Boyd, C., and Aitken, T. H. G.: Description of human yellow fever cases seen in Trinidad in 1959. West Indian Med. J. *9*:273-277, 1960.

43. Taylor, R. M., Haseeb, M. A., and Work, T. H.: Reconnaissance régionale sur la fièvre jaune au Soudan particulièrement orientée vers les primates. Bull. W.H.O., *12*:711-725, 1955.

44. Theiler, M., and Casals, J.: The serological reactions in yellow fever. Amer. J. Trop. Med., *7*:585-594, 1958.

PART IV

Viral Infections in Which Cutaneous Manifestations Predominate

26

Maculopapular Eruptions: Introduction

By P. MOZZICONACCI AND C. ATTAL

Maculopapular eruptions are a frequent manifestation of viral diseases. We group them into three categories.

The first comprises clinically defined diseases in which the causal virus has been identified. Among them, measles and rubella hold the foremost place. The clinical picture of some other eruptions is less clearly defined although sufficiently individualized to permit a general description. However, the clinical elements alone do not permit easy establishment of the diagnosis.

The second group comprises eruptions, due to various viruses, which present an ill-defined clinical picture. These are exanthems affecting principally very young children. They are attended, more or less, by infectious concomitants; fever, general discomfort, headache, and anorexia. The rash is of various types, most often maculopapular, but occasionally petechial as well, or even of an erythema nodosum type. It may predominate on the trunk or distally. In some cases, the mucosae may be involved. The diagnosis is possible only by demonstrating the virus responsible. But great prudence is required in the interpretation of the virological results.

Discovery of a virus in the course of a clinically ill-defined eruptive fever has no value in itself. Evidence is also required of a rise in the level of antibodies against the virus isolated during the acute phase of the disease, and the presence of another, concomitant viral disease must be eliminated, by thorough virological and serological investigation. The adenoviruses, for example, can persist in latent state in lymphoid tissue, the tonsils in particular, and reëngage in their multiplication cycle when an intercurrent infection occurs. These viral diseases are highly contagious and spread rapidly in collectivities and hospital services. A new infection by a different virus can install itself while the initial pathogenic agent is still present in the organism and thus produce mixed infections. What is true for the adenoviruses is also true for the enteroviruses.

Finally, in a third group, we will consider diverse diseases which present very particular clinical characteristics and generally permit easy diagnosis, but for which it has not been possible to find a specific responsible pathogenic virus.

27

Measles

MEASLES: CLINICAL FEATURES

by C. ATTAL AND P. MOZZICONACCI

Measles is one of the most contagious of the eruptive fevers. Its agent belongs to the myxovirus group, the characteristics of which are now well known. The disease is endemic, with seasonal outbreaks, and occurs the world over. In regions with a high living standard, the prognosis is good, although measles should not be taken lightly because of the serious complications it can involve. In economically ill-favored regions the disease is frequently of extreme severity and still has a very high mortality.

The frequency is such that almost all human beings have had measles at some time. Those who appear to have escaped it perhaps have natural resistance, but it is more probable that they have had an inapparent form of the disease. The near constance of the number of cases from year to year contradicts the hypothesis of a possible genetically transmitted immunity.[60]

CLINICAL DESCRIPTION

Measles is a cyclic disease, always passing through the same phases. We shall first describe the form most common in children.

Incubation Period. This period lasts 10 to 11 days. Its length ordinarily varies little, although in some instances it is longer or is abbreviated to one week.

When the moment of contact with measles is known and the child's temperature is taken regularly during this whole period, a slight rise in temperature, not over 38° C., may be found on the sixth or seventh day; it lasts 24 hours at the most. A few discrete symptoms of upper respiratory infection may be noted concurrently. This in-

cubation period fever is not a constant feature. It is supposedly linked to the first phase of viremia. Partington and Quinton,[51] however, noted considerable variations in the temperature curves in the preeruptive phase; among the 82 patients they studied, some had a moderately high fever that began at the time of contact with measles and lasted four days or more. These authors noted an incubation period fever in 10 per cent of their cases. Then, after an interval of apyrexia, the true fever of invasion installed itself.

Invasion Phase. The usual length of this phase is four days. In certain cases, it is longer and may even stretch out to a week, especially when the incubation phase has been abnormally short. The invasion phase is marked by a series of symptoms so diagnostically characteristic that they enable the physician to predict the appearance of the rash; these are fever and systemic signs, oculonasal catarrh, and pathognomonic enanthem. All these signs increase in intensity up to the outburst of the rash.

1. The *fever* is generally high, exceeding 39° C. (102.2° F.) and often 40° C. (104° F.). It can attain its maximum progressively in four days, up to the time when the rash appears. Sometimes it reaches 40° C. (104° F.) from the first day of the invasion phase and remains level. In the young child, such a brutal rise in temperature may be accompanied by convulsions. The curve may be biphasic: after fever for one or two days, temperature falls to normal and remains so for 24 hours; then it rises again, approximately when the rash bursts out. The fever remains unchanged until the second or third day of the eruption, and then disappears by lysis.

2. The systemic signs are always marked and give the impression of a severe disease characterized by malaise, chills, sweating, prostration and even somnolence,

and occasionally headache and delirium. Pulse rate is accelerated; the urine is highly colored. Blood count reveals a moderate leukopenia affecting mainly the polymorphonuclear cells. The oculonasal catarrh and that of the airways gives a very peculiar and highly significant picture during measles invasion. It disappears with the onset of the eruptive phase.

3. The *conjunctivitis* attracts attention. The eyes are red and weepy. The eyelids and the caruncle are edematous and secrete a small amount of mucus. The patient is photophobic.

4. The *coryza* is first marked by sneezing, then by an abundant nasal discharge that is at first mucous, then mucopurulent, and occasionally even slightly blood-stained, irritating the periphery of the nose and the upper lip. It reaches its maximum at the same time as the eruption, but from the first hours, conjunctivitis and coryza give the face a characteristic aspect: blotched, edematous, and weepy.

5. *Cough,* from the invasion stage on, is never absent. It is dry, incessant, and tiring. It is resistant to the usual treatments. It increases in intensity during the entire period of invasion and persists after the rash has disappeared. It occasionally takes on a rather harsh timbre, owing to laryngitis. Whatever may be its timbre or its intensity, cough should be considered one of the obligatory symptoms of measles and the diagnosis of measles should be rejected if it is absent.

6. *Koplik's spots* confirm the diagnosis of measles. But although they are pathognomonic, they are absent at the onset of the invasion period. They appear only after one or two days of fever, oculonasal catarrh, and cough. The physician often has difficulty in detecting them at their outset. The enanthem described by Koplik in 1896 appears first as small, irregular, bright red spots. They are found on the inner wall of the cheeks facing the second molar teeth. The number is at first limited to two or three elements: small, bluish white, brilliant spots at the center of a reddish areola. This white spot is often so small that it passes unseen if the lighting is insufficient. In very short order, new red spots appear. They are very numerous when the rash appears and then extend over the mucosa of the inner surface of the cheeks and the lips. They become confluent, and the picture is of small grains of sugar strewn over a red background. At this stage, Koplik's spots are evident, but their interest for the diagnosis is diminished since the first cutaneous elements have already appeared. In severe cases of measles, similar elements have been seen on the vulvar mucosa. Koplik's spots begin to disappear on the second day of the rash. The third day, the mucosa is again normal.

7. Even before Koplik's spots appear, a very red aspect or even petechial spotting of the soft palate is almost as constant a feature. It can have a real value for early discovery of contamination.

8. Involvement of the digestive mucosa sometimes manifests itself from the onset of the invasion period by diarrhea, and more rarely by nausea and vomiting. A fugacious scarlatiniform or morbilliform rash may occur before the typical eruption but is rare.

The Rash. The time of onset of the exanthem is remarkably regular, 14 days after contamination. On the average, it appears three to five days after onset of the disease. The eruption is erythematous and maculopapular. Often, an aggravation of the fever, cough, systemic signs, and oculonasal catarrh precedes and accompanies it.

The first macules are situated in the mastoid region, at the roots of the hair. Very rapidly, in a few hours, the eruption invades the upper part of the neck, and on the second day, the face.

It later spreads to the upper extremities and to the trunk, and then to the lower extremities. The areas first involved are those where the rash is the most intense.

The cutaneous elements are red papules that are slightly raised and soft on palpation. Isolated from one another, they are surrounded by areas of healthy skin. They disappear on pressure or stretching of the skin. Their somewhat rounded contours are irregular. On the face, the papules are often confluent, thus forming more or less extensive red plaques, with polycyclic "festooned" edges, but they are always separated by areas of healthy skin.

After two or three days, the rash begins to pale in the areas where it first appeared, but particularly on the face. It changes color, becoming slightly brownish on the fourth day. At this stage, it is no longer effaced by pressure. When the rash has almost disappeared from the face and the upper part of the trunk, it is still visible on the lower extremities. The eruption may be followed, in the areas in which it was most severe, by fine desquamation, often scarcely visible. The skin of the hands and the feet does not desquamate.

At the onset of the eruption, the temperature is always high (40° C.; 104° F.). It remains level during the whole phase of extension, and then returns to normal, as a general rule by lysis, in two or three days, or occasionally less.

When the face is invaded and the fever is at its maximum, the patient is completely prostrated and often somnolent. The eyelids are puffy; the oculonasal catarrh is even more marked than during the invasion period. The cough is incessant. Auscultation of the lungs often reveals no abnormality in uncomplicated measles, but it occasionally reveals bronchial or gurgling coarse rales.

The patient is anorexic. In children under two years of age, diarrhea is frequent. The intense malaise and exhaustion make the patient look miserably ill. But as soon as the rash disappears the child recovers quickly. Only the cough persists several days after temperature has become normal. Convalescence is short.

The total length of acute phase is about six days. The variations depend mostly on the length of the invasion period. The length of the periods of eruption and desquamation is remarkably constant.

Measles, a systemic disease, can involve all organs and provoke lesions of variable importance; some of the lesions are asymptomatic and others are manifested clinically.

1. *Adenopathies* of moderate volume can exist and even involve the whole lymph node system, particularly in severe measles. They may predominate in the occipital, mastoid, or posterior cervical region, as in rubella, but the adenopathies in measles never evolve in the same manner as in rubella.

2. Besides the common respiratory manifestations characteristic of measles, *involvement of the pulmonary parenchyma* is frequent (cf. Chapter 42). During uncomplicated measles, diagnosis of respiratory involvement is possible only by systematic radiography. Abnormal images are found in 60 to 80 per cent of cases. They are of various types. The most frequent consist in hilar widening and an accentuation of the bronchovascular marking. They are entirely nonspecific for measles and resemble the pulmonary images in other viral pneumopathies: starting from the hilus and diverging from there can be seen markings of varying density and thickness, with a more or less precise pattern. The outlines of these images are hazy. They are always bilateral but may be more pronounced on one side than the other. They yield a "butterfly wing" pattern. They are denser in the hilar region and ravel out at the periphery. They appear from the very onset and occasionally persist more than three weeks after disappearance of the clinical manifestations.

Other appearances have been described: intumescence of the peribronchial lymph nodes, linear radiations of inflammatory aspect, micronodular opacities, and pseudomiliary aspect or aspect of scissuritis.

The degree of the radiological anomalies most often contrasts with the discreteness of signs on auscultation.[6, 36, 55] These radiological signs are seen most often in children aged four to five years but they do not differ from those in the adult.

3. The *abdominal manifestations* of measles are ordinarily moderate and limited to a few diffuse pains, and to a not very abundant diarrhea. Mild diarrhea is nonetheless a very frequent symptom, contemporaneous with the invasion period and sometimes with the first day of the eruption.

The abdominal pains are occasionally intense, and are often localized in the right iliac fossa. Certain patients have thus been operated on for appendicitis; in some, the lesions found were those of genuine appendicitis.[32] More often, the lesions are localized in the mesenteric lymph nodes of the ileocecal region. The ileum and the appendix have a congested appearance.

The involvement of the abdominal lymphoid tissue is evidenced only by x-ray examination with barium enema. In 70 per cent of measles patients[21] the radiograph shows intolerance of the last ileal loop with or without permanent spasm and a reticular appearance of the mucosal relief that corresponds to hyperplasia of the follicles. Occasionally, genuine areolar images reveal hypertrophy of Peyer's patches.

The mesenteric ganglia are sometimes voluminous enough to leave their mark on the terminal segment of the small intestine.

All these signs, clinical and radiological, are reversible. They should arouse great prudence in accepting a diagnosis of acute appendicitis in a patient suspected of having measles and call for temporizing whenever possible so as to avert an operation that is at best useless and in some cases highly inopportune.

4. The *neurological complications* of measles are well known. Even in uncomplicated measles, symptoms such as headache, backache, and insomnia or somnolence that may alternate with brief periods of confusion, along with the occurrence of an isolated convulsion, suggest that the central nervous system is not spared.

Electroencephalograms (EEG) recorded in the preeruptive phase have revealed anomalies of short duration: they appear between the fourth day of the incubation period and the eruption and disappear during the eruptive phase. The alterations consist in slowed-down, often irregular, nonspecific activities.[49] They are encountered in 51 per cent of cases of measles.[32a] But there is never a tracing showing spikes or spike-wave complexes, even in children in whom the illness commenced with a convulsion.

The signification of the EEG modifications is uncertain. Some investigators have thought that measles served to reveal anomalies already present but not detected. Others advance the hypothesis of a neurological disturbance due, if not to the virus itself, at least to a "toxic" action secondary to the disease.[49]

5. The *electrocardiogram* is very rarely abnormal. Bengtsson and Berglund[11] found, in 8 among 451 cases of measles, an inversion of T1 and T2 or a flattening out of T. Six of these cases were in adults, and two were in children. The value of this element is open to question despite the possibility of myocarditis during measles.

CLINICAL FORMS

1. In *malignant measles* a group of signs and symptoms appearing from the very onset of the invasion period produces an alarming picture.

The temperature is very high (40° C.—104° F.—or more). From the first, the general physical condition is severely altered. The tongue is dry, the lips are cracked. The livid facies of a child prostrated or in delirium suggests a disease of extreme gravity. Blood pressure is subnormal, and the differential between systolic and diastolic pressure is pinched. The heart sounds are deadened on percussion. The pulse is thready and soft. The urine is emitted rarely, in insufficient amount, and is dark in color. Often the child vomits or has profuse diarrhea. The eruption is pale; it corresponds to "suppressed measles," the gravity of which was emphasized by the writers of earlier periods.

Neurological, hematological, or respiratory signs may predominate. Adynamia with prostration at the limit of coma signifies a severe encephalitic involvement. A cutaneous and mucosal purpura accompanied by hemorrhages and a distressing dyspnea complete the clinical picture (black measles). The patient rapidly becomes cyanotic and is drenched with sweat. Physical examination often reveals extraordinarily few pulmonary signs, at most a few disseminated rales. Occasionally, on the contrary, the physical signs are those of acute pulmonary edema.

These forms are exceptional. Their pathogenesis is not well known. They end in death within a few days.

2. On the other hand, *benign measles* is frequent. In certain cases, each phase of the disease is shortened. Incubation, however, is lengthened. All the symptoms are often attenuated. The fever does not exceed 38° C. (100.4° F.). The oculonasal catarrh may be absent, and the cough is not very distressing. Koplik's spots are present but are not extensive and disappear rapidly. The eruption is not intense and disappears within 24 hours (cf. the description of modified measles in the section on pathogenesis and epidemiology).

3. The variations in the *aspect of the eruption* have occasioned the description of somewhat peculiar clinical forms that are nonetheless easy to recognize within the ensemble of clinical signs. On some occasions, the cutaneous elements are so abundant and confluent that no intervals of healthy skin separate them. Fairly often, in the course of intense measles, the eruption takes on a petechial ecchymotic aspect. A very small hemorrhagic suffusion is at the center of each macule. In such cases, the eruption loses its purely congestive character. Remarkably enough, these types of measles are not, in fact, more serious than the others. More rarely, the physician may note salient highly

colored elements especially on the face (pimple form) or minute blisters filled with clear liquid (miliary sudoral form).

4. Measles is very rare before the sixth month of life in countries with a high living standard. It is then relatively discrete, probably because the infant still retains a certain level of maternal antibodies. Often the incubation period is lengthened and marked by a slight rise in temperature and weight loss. The respiratory signs, the enanthem, and the exanthem are more discrete. But in the slightly older nursling infant, who no longer has any passive protection, measles may be severe. The septic complications that once were almost the rule are less redoubtable today.

5. The same cannot be said of measles in tropical countries. The poor hygiene and the multiple deficiencies from which children in these regions suffer make measles an extremely severe disease. The rapid dehydration of the youngest children and the association with other diseases are responsible for a very high mortality rate.

Respiratory complications are by far the most frequent, often resulting from secondary complications due to various bacteria, but Hendrickse and Sherman,[35a] in a study of fatal forms, observed giant cell interstitial pneumopathy evidencing direct involvement by the measles virus (cf. Chapter 42). Other respiratory complications included empyema, lung abscess, and obstructive laryngitis.

Digestive system involvement is almost as frequent, not merely in the acute phase but also during the convalescent period; diarrhea, anorexia, and vomiting require prolonged medical supervision and parenteral administration of the fluids and electrolytes found requisite by laboratory control tests.

Occasionally, ulcerations of the tongue, of the gums, or of the cheek occur and ultimately produce true gangrene of the mouth, or "noma." The ocular complications are also of particular gravity (cf. p. 327). Encephalitis was noted in 15 of 125 fatal cases, and coma in 25 cases studied by Armengaud and the Dakar workers.[4] The virological studies failed to show any features peculiar to the measles virus.

6. The coincidence of measles with pregnancy and the transmission of the disease to the child have long been known. The first case history dates from 1646 (Fabrice de Hildem). The child was born with a typical eruption. The mother was at the

fourth day of the disease. Since then, numerous other cases have been published (Ledelius, 1685; Vogel and Stark, 1744; Osiander, 1819; Billard, 1828; Caren, 1833; Michaelson, 1836). R Debré and P. Joannon (1926) made a complete study of the question, in connection with some ten cases of congenital measles.

In cases of congenital measles, the lapse of time before appearance of the exanthem is highly variable. The eruption may be evident at birth, when delivery occurs at the moment when the exanthem begins in the mother. But it may also be retarded a few days; the maternal antibodies in these cases may have produced an early seroattenuation and have prolonged the incubation period. The severity of the evolution of congenital measles is variable (cf. Neonatal Virus Infections in Chapter 60).

It is generally considered that measles in the mother never produces malformations in the fetus. Manson, Logan, and Loy[43a] noted seven cases of various malformations in 103 cases of measles supervening in pregnancy but absolute proof of the responsibility of the measles virus was not made. No malformation was seen during the Greenland and the Tahiti epidemics, but the number of abortions and of premature births increased. The measles virus results in death of the fetus when it attacks it in the first weeks of pregnancy (cf. Prenatal Virus Infections in Chapter 60).

7. Measles is considerably more severe in the adult. In certain very isolated regions such as Greenland or Iceland, where epidemics are rare, numerous are the adults without immunity. In the Faeroe Islands, two epidemics broke out within a 65-year interval.[45a] In all these cases, mortality was much higher in adults than in children.

COMPLICATIONS

The complications of measles are due either to the virus itself or to bacterial superinfections, or to both. In all cases, the terrain, the patient's age, and the associated pathology play a preponderant role.

The Respiratory Complications. Before the era of chemotherapy and antibiotics, superinfections were of high frequency and some of them of high gravity. Today they are rarer and less severe; the progress in hospital hygiene plus isolation measures has contributed to their regression, and it has also become possible to determine precisely the role of the measles virus itself in certain localizations.

UPPER RESPIRATORY PATHWAYS. The rhinitis of measles occasionally takes on particular extension and intensity. The purulent nasal discharge erodes the basal periphery of the nose, and the upper lip. The ulcerations crust over. Breathing difficulty results, especially in the young infant. The enanthem may itself become superinfected and provoke a painful stomatitis.

Often, after the eruption, at the time of defervescence or after it, the temperature again rises. The pharynx is covered with mucopus. The tonsils become red and turgescent. Occasionally, a pultaceous coating may be found. Cervical adenopathies are almost always present.

Catarrhal or suppurating *inflammation of the middle ear* are a very frequent consequence of these cases of rhinopharyngitis. They almost always begin at the end of the eruption period. But in some cases, especially in nursling infants, the first sign is a purulent otorrhea. Otitis is particularly feared in children with adenoidism, especially if they have already had attacks of otitis. The superinfecting bacteria are various. In the youngest children, pneumococci and *Hemophilus influenzae* are the most frequently isolated germs. In the older child, staphylococci and streptococci are more often responsible. At present, mastoiditis has become an exceptional complication.

LARYNGITIS. Essentially in children, laryngitis occurs, sometimes at the onset of measles, sometimes at the end of the eruption period.

The early cases of laryngitis are announced by a change in timbre of the voice and of the cough, which become hoarse. Abruptly, the child presents a noisy inspiratory dyspnea with substernal traction and stridor. He is drenched in sweat, becomes agitated, and struggles against suffocation. These cases of stridulent laryngitis in the invasion period or at the onset of the eruptive phase, impressive as they are, usually regress spontaneously. After a half hour or an hour of acute, distressing crisis, respiration becomes easier and the child, exhausted, can fall asleep again. An underlying dyspnea remains, however; it should warn that a renewed attack of suffocation is to be feared the following night.

The late cases of laryngitis linked to bacterial superinfection are much more serious. Alteration of voice and cough is the first sign. Rapidly a permanent dyspnea installs itself with inspiratory traction and stridor progressively accentuated. The child's general physical condition severely deteriorates; he becomes both pale and cyanotic. A picture of this type justifies emergency intubation, or, occasionally, even tracheotomy, for medical means are often inadequate to avert rapid aggravation of the dyspnea. These cases of laryngitis are most often due to streptococci or staphylococci. In certain cases, voice and cough are extinguished, as in true diphtherial laryngitis. Rapid tracheostomy is then obligatory. The secondary prognosis, once redoubtable, today is transformed by antibiotics.

THE PULMONARY AND BRONCHIAL COMPLICATIONS. These are next in order of frequency after the upper respiratory tract infections. Their gravity is extreme. They were once responsible for over 80 per cent of deaths in measles. Occasionally, it is difficult to distinguish clinically between the acute pneumopathies due to the measles virus itself and the bronchopneumonias due to superinfection. Involvement of the lower respiratory pathways by the measles virus is discussed in Chapter 42. We shall describe here the complications due to superinfection.

The late onset, in the midst of full convalescence, of a hyperleukocytosis with polynucleosis and a change in the pulmonary images from those in early x-ray films are elements favorable to the diagnosis of secondary bronchopneumopathy. The secondary infections have a slower evolution and can last several weeks.

Numerous germs can be responsible. The most frequently encountered are pneumococci, hemolytic streptococci, and staphylococci. According to the radiological and anatomical type of these complications, multiple clinical forms have been described.

The Bronchopneumonias. The persistence of the fever at the moment when the eruption pales or reappearance of fever after one or two days of relative apyrexia is often the sign that should arouse attention. The cough that had not disappeared becomes more insistent. At the same time, the first signs of breathing difficulty are noted and they progressively worsen. In a few days, or occasionally even more rapidly, general physical condition deteriorates. The child becomes pale; tongue and lips are dry. He is agitated and anxious. His temperature is above 39° C. (102.2° F.). The heart sounds are deadened, the pulse becomes thready, blood pressure falls, and the differential between systolic and diastolic pressure becomes squeezed.

The cough is then very frequent. The polypnea with flaring of the nasal alae, the cyanosis, and the traction effect in breathing show the involvement of the respiratory system.

Physical examination reveals a mixture of bronchitic rales, coarse subcrepitant rales, bubbling finer rales, and even souffles. All these signs are disseminated in both pulmonary fields without characteristic topography. They are fixed in site in the particular subject.

Radiography shows more or less rounded opacities, variable in number and in size. They are seen in any localization whatever in the pulmonary parenchyma. Polymorphonuclear leukocytosis is always very high.

Before specific treatment became available, the infection often evolved toward a progressive aggravation of the local and the systemic signs and toward the appearance of new foci. Signs of cardiac insufficiency soon appeared. Death usually terminated the process. At present, the prognosis is different in every way. Appropriate antibiotic treatment undertaken from the very onset of signs of bronchopneumonia halts its extension. The disease stops short in a few days. When the treatment is undertaken late, the evolution is much longer. The radiological signs are slow in disappearing. The improvement is slow. But the long-term prognosis is favorable.

Certain bronchopneumonias spontaneously present a prolonged evolution. After an acute onset, all the signs are attenuated. The fever becomes irregular. In the absence of treatment, these subacute bronchopneumonias evolve for several weeks with increasing cachexia. Even when they heal, they occasionally leave severe sequelae, such as chronic bronchitis or bronchial dilatation. Antibiotic treatment causes rapid regression of these subacute forms of bronchopneumonia.

Acute bronchitis. The onset is comparable to that of the bronchopneumonias with fever, cough, and dyspnea with polypnea. Auscultation reveals rhonchi and sibi-

lant diffuse rales with a few scattered foci of mucous rales. Radiography shows the accentuation of the bronchial images that characterizes the measles-involved lung. More or less nodular opacities with ill defined contours do not appear. Signs of upper respiratory infection and hyperleukocytosis always exist; otitis is frequent.

However, despite the severe functional and physical signs, the patient's general physical condition is relatively good. The toxic signs of the bronchopneumonias are lacking.

Acute bronchitis responds with remarkable rapidity to antibiotic treatment and is cured without sequelae.

In certain cases symptoms of a focus of frank pulmonary condensation may appear with tubular breathing and crepitant rales. The unexpected advent of a focus of pneumococcic hepatization is naturally possible. But in most cases the x-ray film shows images of ventilation disturbance: the homogeneous opacity is retractable. Bronchoscopy confirms the cause by showing obstruction of a bronchus by the edema and mucopurulent secretions. Bronchial aspiration sometimes suffices to clear the radiological opacity.

Evolution toward *bullous emphysema* is a relatively frequent possibility in children. More rarely, the rupture of a bubble is the cause of an acute mediastinal emphysema, usually regressive, or of a pneumothorax.

Exceptionally, measles can be complicated by a lung abscess, by scant pleural effusion, or by a purulent pleurisy.

Among the rarer bronchopulmonary complications, a separate place must be given to *capillary bronchitis* (cf. definition in Chapter 42). In fact, it is only one of the elements of the malignant syndrome of measles; it begins at the onset of the invasion period and, from the start, it produces a rapidly fatal hyperacute asphyxia. The temperature reaches and surpasses 41° C. (105.8° F.). The signs of right ventricular insufficiency increase hour by hour. Arterial blood pressure collapses. The dyspnea, often with expiratory predominance, and the incessant cough testify to the participation of the lung in this extremely serious type of measles. The signs on auscultation are variable and occasionally astonish the physician by their discreteness.

The involvement of the pulmonary parenchyma by the virus can produce an interstitial giant cell pneumopathy. The primitive interstitial pneumopathies without eruption are today considered to be a particular form of measles (cf. Chapter 42).

Neurological Complications. Neurological complications are observed, in general, in severe measles. Other than the encephalitides and encephalomyelitides, described in Chapters 6 and 7, isolated lymphocytic meningeal reactions may occur, even without the slightest clinical manifestation. In one case in ten, the number of elements exceeds ten per cubic millimeter. A few cases of neuroretinitis with consequent pigmentation of the retina have also been reported.[10] They are manifest by rapid loss of vision during the acute phase; regeneration is long and often incomplete.

Ocular Complications. Ocular complications are relatively frequent. The conjunctivitis of measles can be superinfected and give rise to purulent discharge that is usually sensitive to local or systemic antibiotic therapy.

Punctiform keratitis of viral origin (Chapter 54) may also be observed, a manifestation ordinarily not very serious and healing spontaneously without sequelae. But bacterial superinfection, still frequent in tropical countries, may, if it is not treated immediately, lead to corneal ulceration and result rapidly in a global suppuration, a frequent cause of blindness.[51a]

Abdominal Complications. The abdominal complications are merely the accentuation of the intestinal lesions so frequent in ordinary, uncomplicated measles. Crises of true appendicitis and acute peritoneal syndromes require surgical intervention, whatever may be the severity of measles in other respects.

Thrombocytopenic Purpura. Thrombocytopenic purpura is exceptional. Digestive hemorrhages, hematurias, or meningeal hemorrhages may result. The thrombocytopenia appears at any time during the evolution. It develops slowly and occasionally takes three months to disappear.[38]

Myocardial Involvement. Myocardial involvement has sometimes been reported. Marinesco[44] noted unquestionable myocardial lesions in six of 28 autopsies in cases of measles. In all six cases, bronchopneumopathy was associated. Histological examination of the myocardium showed lymphohistioplasmacytic infiltrates. Myocarditis is thought to complicate very severe measles,

but it is often difficult to make the clinical or electrocardiographic diagnosis, in a picture of heart failure that may be linked to the pulmonary involvement (cf. Chapter 36).

In one case, Finkel[30] found modifications of ST in the standard deviations and the right precordials with a notable rise in transaminases and acid lactic dehydrogenase.

Postmeasles Nephritis. The cases of postmeasles nephritis reported are probably due to superinfection by a hemolytic streptococcus. It should be pointed out that in the urine of measles patients, epithelial cells with cytoplasmic inclusions[15] or the virus itself[34a] have been found, as well as in a verification of the giant cells in the bladder mucosa. But involvement of the kidney by the virus is not manifested by clinical signs or by histological modifications.

Measles with Tuberculosis. The aggravation of primary or secondary-tertiary tuberculosis by intercurrent measles was once accepted without question. It now seems that this risk was overestimated at a period when no therapeutic agent was available active either on tuberculosis or on the complications of measles.

The negativation of the tuberculin reaction is, however, almost a constant phenomenon. This cutaneous anergy installs itself from the outset of the invasion phase; it lasts one to four weeks after recovery. Are subjects whose cutireaction has become negative more sensitive to Koch's bacillus, as von Pirquet believed? Rather, it would seem that a modification of skin reactivity is in fact involved (Debré, Lesné).

When measles occurs in a preallergic period, in certain cases an aggravated primary infection may be observed. But such aggravation is highly inconstant, and it is impossible to prove the influence of measles on the invasion by tuberculosis.

On the other hand, in a subject with excavated tuberculosis, it is very common to observe a sudden aggravation of the disease after measles. But is this aggravation necessarily due to specific action of the measles virus? Is it not more likely that any intercurrent bronchial or pulmonary disease is susceptible of aggravating a preexistent pulmonary tuberculosis? These risks are in any event diminished when the patient is under antitubercular chemoantibiotic therapy. The Greenland epidemic[8a] showed that the nefarious influence of measles on tuberculosis is not an outdated idea. Mortality was higher in tubercular patients and, moreover, an increase in cases of tuberculosis after the epidemic and a progression of preexistent foci were noted.

Measles with Chronic Respiratory Disease. When measles occurs in a subject with *any chronic respiratory disease,* the latter undergoes a sudden aggravation. Asthma may be worsened by measles, but the aggravation is transitory. In a child with *mucoviscidosis,* measles may produce catastrophic consequences. The respiratory insufficiency is suddenly accentuated and the child may die in a few days. In these subjects prophylaxis by gamma globulins or, better, by vaccination against measles is an absolute necessity.

Measles with Other Eruptive Fevers. The *association of measles with another eruptive fever,* or whooping cough, mumps, or diphtheria, once redoubtable, is no longer so much to be feared. Bastin et al.[8] observed no serious incident among 539 patients who had contracted measles while hospitalized for one of these infectious diseases, nor among 228 measles patients secondarily infected by one or another of the above-mentioned diseases.

Measles with Miscellaneous Other Diseases. The advent of measles in *particular terrains* occasionally gives to measles an atypical clinical aspect and influences, in turn, the primary disease.

1. Thus when measles occurs in a rachitic child, it may be of unusual severity. If the subject already has respiratory disturbances in connection with a "rachitic lung," the extension of a measles pneumopathy may induce a serious respiratory insufficiency.

2. Likewise, the association of measles with malignant hemopathy (acute leukemia, reticulosis) is always of extreme gravity: the giant cell pneumopathy results, in this terrain, in a rapidly fatal aggravation of the original disease.

3. In the tropics, measles is legitimately feared in subjects with kwashiorkor. All the infectious complications of measles are of high frequency. Inversely, measles occasionally reveals a protein deficit, until then approximately compensated, and favors the appearance of clinical signs of kwashiorkor.

4. In the pure nephrosis of childhood, the favorable influence of measles, long reported, is inconstant. In the reactive cases, the proteinuria disappears in a few days and the edema is eliminated. The proteinic-lipidic abnormalities take longer to disappear. But this favorable action is too inconstant and is often temporary. The systematic infection with measles of nephrotic children, which was long in fashion when no efficacious treatment was available, today is abandoned. By what immunochemical intermediary measles may act on childhood nephrosis is unknown.

Measles Virus and Cancer. The hypothesis of a possible cancerigenic action of the virus has been envisaged by certain virologists. The virus is perhaps capable of altering the genetic material of the cell; chromosomic breakage was seen in the leukocytes examined three to eight days after the exanthem (cf. Chapter 61) by Nichols.[47a]

Measles Virus and Subacute Sclerosing Panencephalitis. The role of the measles virus in the genesis of subacute sclerosing panencephalitis (SSPE) and of certain other encephalitides or encephalomyelitides is not yet elucidated (cf. Chapter 19 and Virological Study and Prophylaxis later in this chapter).

It has been maintained that multiple sclerosis could be a late complication of measles. Two lines of argument have been advanced:

1. The cerebral lesions of multiple sclerosis are very similar to those of measles encephalitis. But it is known that these perivenous leukoencephalitides that evolve toward formation of zones of demyelinization are devoid of specificity and that they can be encountered in a number of pathological states.

2. In the cerebrospinal fluid of subjects with multiple sclerosis, there exists a more or less elevated level of antibodies against measles that are lacking in other comparable diseases of the nervous system (Chapter 27).

PROGNOSIS

The case fatality rate due to measles was very high 40 years ago. Since then, the improvement in living standards and the progress in prophylactic methods and hospital hygiene have considerably lowered this mortality rate. For the Claude Bernard Hospital (Paris) the case fatality was 1.2 per cent in 1955[35] and 0.17 per cent from 1959 to 1964.[8] But these figures do not give at all a true picture of mortality from the disease, for the very great majority of cases are not treated in a hospital. Hospitalization is reserved for the cases already complicated or for patients who cannot be cared for at home for socioeconomic reasons. Scarcely over 1 per cent of measles patients are treated in a hospital service.[47] Among 8656 cases of measles followed-up by Bastin et al.,[8] 16 per cent were complicated.

The proportion of complicated forms is notably lower in relation to the total number of cases of measles. From January to the end of April, 1963, an investigation undertaken in England and Wales[47] covered more than 53,000 cases. The total percentage of complications was assessed to be 66.7 per 1000. Their distribution was very unequal in regard to age: 86.2 per 1000 before five months, 83.7 per 1000 from 5 to 11 months, and then a progressive drop according to age that reached 42.8 per 1000 between 10 and 14 years. But, above age 20, the complications were once again as frequent as in the nursling infant (81 per 1000).

The mortality from measles has been evaluated in developed regions at approximately 2 per 100,000 cases. This figure is practically identical for all countries with high standards of hygiene and living. About half the deaths occur in patients with a chronic disease or an infirmity. In relation to the total population, case fatality is estimated to be 0.2 per 100,000 habitants (W.H.O.). In the United States in 1949 it was estimated to be 2.8 per 100,000 before age 4 years, and 0.9 from 5 to 14 years.

These figures contrast with those of tropical countries with underdeveloped hygiene. Case fatality has been estimated to be 550 per 100,000 in Dakar.[4] Measles is a genuine scourge in these regions. It is the number one cause of infant mortality in Dakar (accounting for 24 per cent, an estimate much higher than for tetanus, malaria, and acute meningitides). Comparable figures have been published in Java (25 per cent), in Egypt (28.5 per cent), and in Nigeria (20 to 25 per cent). In hospitals, where the patients can be rehydrated and treated rapidly, the prognosis is hardly better: measles accounted for 17 per cent of deaths in the 725 cases reported by Armengaud.[4]

The respiratory complications were highest in frequency (38.2 per 1000) in Miller's statistics.[47] Otitis followed (25.2 per 1000) and then the neurological complications (3.8 per 1000). Among these last, the frequency of encephalitis or encephalomyelitis was 1 per 1000, and that of convulsions, 1.8 per 1000.

The figures cited by Bastin[8] were slightly different, for they concerned only hospitalized patients. Otitis was the most frequent complication (42 per cent). Respiratory complications represented a total of 25.9 per cent (bronchial and pulmonary complications, 15 and 2 per cent, early stridulent laryngitis, 7.1 per cent, and late laryngitis, 3.3 per cent). Encephalomyelitis occurred in approximately 1.7 per cent. It should be emphasized here that French authors are much more restrictive than certain of their colleagues in the definition of encephalitis (cf. Chapter 7).

From the published results as a whole, it can be concluded that measles has become a relatively benign disease in developed countries but that it remains a serious illness in numerous other regions. Measles is more serious in children aged under 2 years, in overpopulated urban regions, and in children in poor general physical condition or with a chronic disease. The regression of mortality from respiratory complications has considerably improved the prognosis.

Notwithstanding, measles is a tiring disease, from which children often take several weeks to recover completely; occasionally, the complications leave irreversible sequelae, in particular encephalitic.

DIAGNOSIS

In typical forms of measles, the clinical diagnosis presents no particular difficulties.

Invasion Period. In the invasion period, the fever, the cough, and the oculonasal catarrh immediately call to mind the possibility of measles. When the patient is seen on the first day of illness, the presence of an epidemic or of contact with measles and the absence of previous measles are arguments in favor of the diagnosis. Appearance of Koplik's spots removes all doubt. This prodromal phase differs from that of the other eruptive fevers.

RUBELLA. In children, there is no prodrome. The eruption is the first sign of the disease, appearing at the same time as the adenopathies. In the adolescent and the adult the prodrome lasts one to two days with moderate fever. Cough and oculonasal catarrh are absent.

SCARLET FEVER. The fiery red sore

throat suggests the diagnosis; it precedes the eruption by 12 to 24 hours.

EXANTHEMA SUBITUM. The period of fever precedes the eruption by three to four days. The rhinopharyngeal signs are always discrete; they never attain the intensity accompanying measles. Defervescence precedes the eruption.

ENTEROVIRUS INFECTIONS. Boston exanthem, like exanthema subitum, may be preceded by two or three days of fever. The respiratory signs are absent or very moderate. The same is true of other echovirus eruptions and of those due to Coxsackie virus as, in general, fever and eruption appear simultaneously.

MENINGOCOCCEMIA. This infection is manifested by very high fever at the onset, with chills, headaches, and intense malaise. The fever persists; it may present very high spikes with wide oscillations or be of the typhoid type. The eruption appears one to four days after the onset; symptoms of mild upper respiratory infection occasionally appear during the prodrome alone, but the cough and coryza characteristic of measles are lacking.

EPIDEMIC TYPHUS. The eruption is preceded by four to six days of high fever, chills, headache, generalized myalgia, and severe deterioration of general physical condition.

In summary, before Koplik's spots appear, the facial appearance gives a clue. Rarely, in the first 24 hours, are other diagnostic possibilities considered than rhinopharyngitis, bronchitis, or influenza, even when the onset is marked by a crisis of stridulent laryngitis.

Eruption Period. The reddish coloration, the onset on the neck and on the face and the descending extension of the exanthem are fairly peculiar to measles. The rash remains most intense on the face and neck, and more scattered on the limbs.

RUBELLA. The eruption also begins on the face but progresses more rapidly, in one or two days (instead of three days for measles). The cutaneous elements are smaller, more pink than red, and more confluent. They disappear in three days. The areas first involved also pale first. Respiratory signs are lacking.

SCARLET FEVER. The rash starts in the flexion folds and its distribution is rapidly generalized in 24 hours. It is a punctiform, bright red exanthem in large plaques, without intervals of healthy skin. It is intense on the neck and in the flexion folds. The characteristic desquamation predominates on the extremities. The strawberry- or raspberry-red tongue and fiery red throat are essential elements of the clinical diagnosis. The presence of hemolytic streptococci in large numbers, or even in pure culture, in pharyngeal samples confirms the diagnosis. But the practitioner may hesitate to make a diagnosis in certain cases of measles with a confluent miliary distribution in which the hemorrhagic spotting of the soft palate and pillars can suggest the diffuse pharyngeal redness of scarlet fever. The possibility of association of the two diseases must be kept in mind.

EXANTHEMA SUBITUM. The maculopapules may resemble those of measles but usually they are more scattered and more rose than red. They start and remain predominant on the trunk and extend secondarily to the face. At this stage, the fever has disappeared. The eruption pales and disappears in a maximum of two days, sometimes in only a few hours.

ENTEROVIRUS INFECTIONS. The eruption resembles that in rubella or exanthema subitum. The maculopapules do not turn brown and do not desquamate.

ADENOVIRUS INFECTIONS. On the other hand, certain adenovirus infections present a more difficult problem of differential diagnosis when they manifest themselves by both respiratory signs and a morbilliform rash (Chapter 42). The extreme rarity of this association and its advent in the course of adenovirus epidemics that do not produce eruption in other cases make it possible to suspect an etiology that only the laboratory will be able to confirm.

MENINGOCOCCEMIA. The rash is sometimes purpuric, sometimes erythematopapular or erythematovesicular.

EXANTHEMATIC TYPHUS. The eruption is composed of maculopapules and of petechiae that appear on the trunk and spare the face and extremities.

ERYTHEMA INFECTIOSUM. The disease is exempt of fever. The maculopapules are very small and occur only on the extremities or predominate there. The same is true for most *toxic eruptions,* moreover less often morbilliform than scarlatiniform.

A certain number of maculopapular eruptions remain unclassified but none of them presents the clinical aspect and the cyclic evolution of measles. Infectious mononucleosis occasionally presents a morbilliform rash. Acquired toxoplasmosis sometimes manifests itself by a rash at the time of the febrile spike at the onset, but the adenopathies, the chorioretinitis, and the neurological signs occupy the foreground.

The diagnosis is more difficult as concerns measles attenuated by an injection of convalescent serum or of gamma globulins. The rash is then very similar to those of the other viral eruptive fevers. The existence of contact with measles is then the factor determining the clinical diagnosis.

Mild Atypical Forms. For the diagnosis, recourse to laboratory techniques may be required.

The virological diagnosis of measles is described later in this chapter.

Search for multinucleated cells in the saliva and the nasal secretions, or, better, in a smear from the buccal mucosa, is a test that can be made in any laboratory. This giant-cell reaction was first described as early as 1925 by Denton, and in 1931 at the level of the bronchial mucosa in the tonsils by Warthin and by Finkeldey in appendicular foci. It was later found in all lymphatic tissue. After aspiration of the mucus from the posterior nasal region with a sterile polythene tube and preparation of a smear fixed by an alcohol-ether mixture, the smear is colored with methylene blue or Giemsa stain. Two types of giant cells thus become visible:[9]

1. Giant epithelial cells, characteristic of measles, that are comparable to the giant cells of Hecht interstitial pneumopathy and that contain intranuclear eosinophilic granulations;

2. Reticuloendothelial giant cells or Warthin-Finkeldey cells that rarely present intranuclear inclusions. These cells are round and irregularly lobed. The very numerous nuclei (60 or more) are massed in the cell center. Chromatin is scarce and rejected to the periphery.

The cells characterizing measles are slightly different from the giant cells of varicella or herpes, which present less numerous nuclei and a less abundant cytoplasm. They are identical with those in canine distemper. They may be due to fusion of the ciliated cells. But although they are characteristic of measles, and although they are never found in other rhinopharyngeal catarrhs, they are absent in about half the cases of measles. Their absence hence does not authorize the physician to reject the diagnosis.

Presence of abnormal cells in the urine[15] is of short duration and is too inconstant to be utilizable as a routine research measure. These cells may be mononucleated or multinucleated and contain cytoplasmic inclusions.

PATHOLOGY

The lesions of measles are very extensive. The disease is generalized, involving most of the organs, as is shown by the dissemination of Warthin-Finkeldey cells. The latter are visible, from the outset of the invasion phase, in the hyperplastic lymphoid organs. This hyperplasia involves not only the tonsils and adenoids but also the lymph nodes, the appendix, Peyer's patches, the spleen, and the mucosa of the pharynx and bronchi. The conjunctival tissue is infiltrated by mononuclear cells. On the upper respiratory pathways and the bronchi, numerous epithelial cells lose their cilia and their faculty to secrete mucus. The nuclei and the cytoplasm contain eosinophilic inclusions.

Koplik spots are related to inflammatory lesions of the submucosal glands. However, vascular dilatation is not found around the channels of these glands.[54] Associated proliferation of endothelial cells and exudation of serum terminates in formation of a vesicle, then in necrosis of the endothelium. Occasionally, lesions of keratosis and of parakeratosis are noted.

The cutaneous eruption is first marked by the proliferation of the endothelial cells of the superficial layer of the chorion. The serous perivascular exudate reaches the epidermis. Then the epithelial cells vacuolate and necrose, form small vesicles on the corneous layer, and finally desquamate. In places, perivascular red cell infiltrates explain the occasionally hemorrhagic character of the exanthem. In places, lesions of hairs and sebaceous glands may also be observed. At a more advanced stage, perivascular masses of monocytes and lymphocytes may also be detected.

The lesions of the measles-involved lung are, at the onset, bronchial. We have indicated the extension of the lymphoid hyperplasia and of the formation of Warthin-Finkeldey giant multinucleated cells at the level of the bronchial mucosa. These lesions are identical with those described at the level of the alveolar walls by Hecht in interstitial pneumonia, which is known today to be due to the measles virus (cf. Chapter 42).

The same infiltrates of mononuclear giant cells are found in the intestinal submucosa.

The anatomical lesions of encephalitides and encephalomyelitides are described in Chapter 6.

TREATMENT

Treatment of measles should be adapted to each particular case.

Common Uncomplicated Measles of Childhood. No specific treatment active against measles virus exists. The physician should beware of all therapy, useless and inopportune. Nasal or ocular instillations are to be avoided; it is recommended to limit intervention to cleansing the conjunctiva with sterile physiological saline solution and to protect by simple ointments the area around the nose against the irritation due to the coryza. When the conjunctivitis is intense, light should be reduced, but not to total obscurity, and the cornea should be examined to detect any incipient ulceration.

The fever may be combated by small, repeated doses of aspirin. If it exceeds 40° C. (104° F.), cool packings may be necessary.

The cough is the most distressing symptom and the most difficult to combat. In small doses, codeine derivatives or barbiturates can be tried and, prudently (cf. Chapter 42), antihistamine syrups.

The child should remain in bed during all of the febrile and eruptive period. Overheating the room should be avoided and a moist atmosphere should be maintained. Getting up from bed can be authorized in progressive stages after the rash has disappeared. The physician should wait disappearance of cough before giving permission for the child to return to school activity.

Liquid or semiliquid feeding is to be contemplated only during the febrile period or in case of painful stomatitis. As soon as the child feels better, he should be allowed a normal diet.

Antibiotic therapy has no influence on measles virus infection. To prescribe antibiotics systematically with a view toward prevention of complications is futile and can occasionally present distinct disadvantages (possible masking of certain complications such as otitis, and the risk of destroying the bacteriological equilibrium of the upper respiratory pathways).

Although the prognosis of measles in hospitals is not what it was 40 years ago, it is preferable to avoid hospitalization in uncomplicated measles unless the patient cannot be properly cared for at home.

Measles of the Nursling Infant. Measles of the unweaned infant should be considered a serious disease. The fever should be combated if it rises above 39° C. (102.2° F.). Feeding and rehydratation should be adjusted to the fall in body weight. It is prudent to survey the tympanums daily. Systematic use of antibiotics is not recommended. Their use is indicated only when signs of complications appear. But when measles takes on an aspect of particular severity, when the clinical signs of the measles-involved lung are marked, and superinfection is to be feared, it is advisable to administer a broad-spectrum antibiotic (e.g., tetracycline in a dose of 50 mg. per kg. of body weight per day).

Otitis. Otitis due to streptococci and pneumococci, which are the most frequent agents, should be treated by penicillin, tetracycline, or sulfonamides.

Stridulent Laryngitis. Stridulent laryngitis at the onset of measles should be treated by hot compresses around the neck. Corticosteroid therapy is indicated if the dyspnea becomes menacing or if the habitual minor therapeutic means yield no improvements; dexamethasone is injected in a dose of 2 to 4 mg. to be renewed once or twice that day, or, if the infant can drink, 15 to 30 mg. of deltacortisone, according to age and weight. As a rule, it is not useful to pursue this therapy more than 24 or 48 hours.

The late cases of laryngitis are much more resistant. Corticosteroid and antibiotic therapy should be used generously, over a longer period. The gravity of this complication sometimes renders intubation or even tracheotomy obligatory.

Oxygen therapy and humidification of the atmosphere are useful adjuvants. Use of barbiturates is more questionable: although they can lessen angor, they may also induce drowsiness and reduce the capacity to struggle against asphyxia.

The Bronchopneumopathies. (see also Chapter 42)

1. The pneumonias and bronchopneumonias due to superinfection require, first of all, antibiotics or sulfonamides, the choice of which depends on the bacterial agent involved (pneumococcus, staphylococcus, *Hemophilus influenzae,* and streptococci being the germs most often responsible). In case of intense dyspnea, oxygen therapy should be used and digitalin in small daily doses should be initiated without awaiting the first signs of cardiac insufficiency.

2. Measles virus pneumopathies are insensitive to antibiotics. Nonetheless in certain cases the risks of superinfection are such that antibiotics should be employed.

3. Patients with acute bronchiolitis in which the dyspnea is attributable to bronchial spasm should receive, aside from the treatment of all bronchopneumopathies, corticosteroids in sufficient dosage (2 mg. per kg. of body weight per day of deltacortisone) by the systemic route and in aerosols. Theophylline or epinephrine derivatives in nasal inhalations are of dubious usefulness.

Malignant Measles. Malignant measles first of all raises a problem of emergency resuscitation. An intravenous perfusion should be immediately installed in order to assure a sufficient fluid intake (100 to 150 mg. per kg. of body weight per day of physiological glucose and saline solution in equal parts). By the same route antibiotics and corticosteroids are added. The cardiotonics should, in this instance, be prescribed from the onset of the disease. To combat collapse, a transfusion of blood and of plasma and desoxycorticosterone by subcutaneous injection complete the therapeutic schema. But malignant measles often evolves too fast to be brought under control by therapy.

Measles Encephalitis. The treatment of measles encephalitis obeys the same principles. It has been proposed to adjoin to the therapy described in paragraph 6, apart from barbiturates, large doses of gamma globulins. There does not seem to be any significant difference in prognosis after this treatment.[34]

PROPHYLAXIS

1. The isolation of patients is not a measure sufficient to avert the extension of the disease. In the family circle, 90 per cent of subjects without known history of measles contract the disease. In collectivities (nurseries, schools, and so forth), the level varies with the receptivity of the subjects in contact with the disease. Contamination is usually a fact before diagnosis is possible, that is to say, 24 to 48 hours before onset of the invasion period.

Five days before the eruption disappears, the patient is no longer contagious and if only danger to other children were in question, he could return to school.

Isolation of the receptive brothers and sisters is rarely achieved. The attempt never averts extension of the epidemic; it does, on the other hand, needlessly create problems for the family. Subjects are contagious from the eighth day following the infecting contact. If they have received gamma globulins, they should be isolated until the third week, since the incubation period is sometimes prolonged by this measure.

2. Individual preventive measures are much more effective. They should be systematically applied to children under age 2 years, to convalescents from another infectious disease, to children with primary tuberculosis infection or a chronic disease, or simply to subjects with unsatisfactory physical condition. Up to the last few years, prophylaxis depended on convalescent serum or gamma globulins. The problem of vaccination against measles will be treated in a later section of this chapter.

a. Convalescent serum was first tried as a curative measure. Its action proved approximately nonexistent (Charles Nicolle and E. Conseil) (cf. p. 338). In prophylaxis the dose to be injected is 1 ml. by year of age (Robert Debré). If the injection is made before the fifth day following contact with the disease, prevention is total. If it is made from the fifth to the eighth day, the child has discreet measles, with slight fever and slight eruption, of short duration. This attenuated measles confers an immunity that may be as durable as that following ordinary measles. If the injection is made at the onset of the invasion, it cannot hinder the usual evolution of the disease, but the rash does not appear around the point of injection; local inhibition of the eruption alone results, a fact that was long utilized as a mean of specific diagnosis.

b. Gamma globulins are more effective than convalescent serum and have the advantage of containing a much higher antibody level for an equal volume. Prevention or attenuation is assured with a dose of 0.2 to 0.3 ml. per kg. of body weight in intramuscular injection. This dose can be exceeded in any case in which it is deemed necessary. Systematic prevention yields remarkable results. Greenberg obtained 79 per cent of preventions and 19.5 per cent of attenuations; Straus, in 1950,[22] 99.2 per cent of preventions. Debré et al. in 1956[24] had only 1.93 per cent of failures. In an island (St. George) situated in mid-ocean off the Alaskan coast, where measles had not been observed for 21 years, the disease was prevented or attenuated in 92 to 93 per cent of cases.[18]

The results attained are hence excellent, and the injection of gamma globulins is the surest method. Early injection is advised in each case in which prevention of the disease is desired. Children in good health aged over 3 years can benefit from an injection from the sixth to the ninth day after contact with measles. The degree of attenuation is in function of the date of the injection after contact and of the dose administered. Either the prevention is total, averting even an inapparent disease, or an attenuated disease of short duration emerges, that permits an immunization. When the injection is made too late to attenuate measles, a zone free of eruption is often noted round the injection site.

The incidents secondary to the injection are negligible: fairly often erythema at the injection point, and rarely a spike of fever the evening of the day of injection.

The indications are the same as those for convalescent serum. The ease of handling gamma globulins permits extending systematic prevention to hospitals, nurseries, and boarding-in establishments for children.

It should be emphasized that seroattenuation, according to certain authors[34] does not seem to reduce the risks of encephalitis. But the rarity of this complication (less than 1 per 1000) makes it difficult to interpret results.

The length of action of gamma globulins does not extend beyond four weeks. In an epidemic period, the injections must therefore be repeated. But when the child has contacts with measles, he can be immunized definitively by an inapparent disease. Black[13] followed the antibody titer in children who had received gamma globulins. He observed in some of them an astonishing persistence of complement-fixing antibodies up to one year after the injection. The titers were in-

ferior to those observed after ordinary measles or even after attenuated measles. But when the titer of complement-fixing antibodies reaches or is above 1/10, there is a good possibility that the child will remain protected for several years.

3. Prophylaxis by gamma globulins is, notwithstanding, of too short duration and is too costly for it to be used in mass prophylaxis. Measles vaccine, which can be produced on a large scale, is called on in the main to replace it (cf. Virological Study and Prophylaxis, later in this chapter).

BIBLIOGRAPHY

1. Abruzzi, W.: Measles. A serious pediatric disease. J. Pediat., 64:750, 1964.
2. Adams, J. M., Baird, C., and Filloy, L.: Inclusion bodies in measles encephalitis. J.A.M.A., 195:290, 1966.
3. Alexander, E. R., Bansmer, C. A. M., Harris, E. S., Giles, B., and Sparks, M. J.: Measles vaccination in infants (use of killed-live combinations). Amer. J. Dis. Child. 108:470, 1964.
4. Armengaud, M., Louvain, M., Frament, V. and Diop Mar, I.: La mort dans la rougeole en pays tropical. Bull. Soc. Méd. Afr. Noire Langue Franç., 7:197, 1962.
5. Bastin, R.: La rougeole. Rev. Prat., 5:643, 1955.
6. Bastin, R., Morin, H., and Lubetzki, J.: Les complications respiratoires de la rougeole. Rev. Prat., 5:657, 1955.
7. Bastin, R., Cathala, H. P., and Damoiseau, B.: Les complications nerveuses de la rougeole. Rev. Prat., 5:675, 1955.
8. Bastin, R., Verliac, F., and Frottier, J.: La rougeole en milieu hospitalier est aujourd'hui une infection bénigne. Presse Méd., 72:1711, 1964.
8a. Bech, V.: The measles epidemic in Greenland in 1962. (Seminaire Centre International de l'Enfance, Paris, 1964.) Arch. Ges. Virusforsch., 16:53, 1965.
9. Beale, A. J., and Campbell, W.: A rapid cytological method for the diagnosis of measles. J. Clin. Path., 12:335, 1959.
10. Bredossian, R. H.: Neurotinitis following measles. J. Pediat., 46:329, 1955.
11. Bengtsson, E., and Berglund, A.: Electrocardiographic changes in measles. Acta Paediat., 43:426, 1954.
12. Berkovich, S., and Schneck, L.: Ascending paralysis associated with measles. J. Pediat., 64:88, 1964.
13. Black, F. L., and Yannet, H.: Inapparent measles after gamma globulin administration. J.A.M.A., 173:1183, 1960.
14. Bliss, C. I., and Blevins, D. L.: The analysis of seasonal variation in measles. Amer. J. Hyg., 70:328, 1959.
15. Bolande, R. P.: Significance and nature of inclusion-bearing cells in the urine of patients with measles. New Eng. J. Med., 265:919, 1961.
16. Boughton, C. R.: Morbilli in Sydney. A review of

3,601 cases with consideration of morbidity, mortality and measles encephalomyelitis. Med. J. Aust., *2*:859, 1964.

17. Boughton, C. R.: Morbilli in Sydney. II. Neurological sequelae of morbilli. Med. J. Aust., 2:908, 1964.

18. Brody, J. A., and Bridenbaugh, E.: Prophylactic gamma-globulin and live measles vaccine in an island epidemic of measles. Lancet, 2:811, 1964.

19. Cabasso, V. J., Levine, S., Markham, F. S., and Cox, H. R.: Prospects for measles immunization with reference to the relationship between distemper and measles viruses. J. Pediat., *59*:324, 1961.

20. Cathala, F.: Les infections à myxo-virus. Presse Méd., *73*:2483, 1965.

21. Cherigie, E., Tavernier, C., Dupas, J., and Reynal, Les anomalies radiologiques de la région iléocaecale dans la rougeole. Rev. Prat., 5:687, 1955.

22. Coigny, R. L., and Straus, P.: Rôle de la gammaglobuline dans la prévention de la rougeole. Résultats d'une enguête épidémiologique. Presse Méd., *59*:634, 1951.

23. Conference (International) on Measles Immunization, Bethesda, Maryland, 1961. Amer. J. Dis. Child., *103*:395, 1962.

23a. Debré, R., and Joannon, L.: La rougeole: Epidémiologie, Immunologie, Prophylaxie. Paris, Masson et Cie., 1926.

24. Debré, R., and Soulier, J.: Utilisation des gammaglobulines plasmatiques humaines dans la prophylaxie de la rougeole (enquête sur 1259 cas) Presse Méd., *64*:667, 1956.

25. Debré, R.: Vaccinations contre la rougeole. Journées Pédiatriques. Paris, Editions Lanord, 1962, p. 291.

25a. Debré, R.: La prévention de la rougeole par le serum de convalescent (méthode de Charles Nicolle et E. Conseil). Sem. Hôp. Paris, *42*:1875, 1966.

26. De Jong, J. G., and Winkler, K. C.: Survival of measles virus in air. Nature, *201*:1054, 1964.

27. Douglas, J. W. B.: Ability and adjustment of children who have had measles. Brit. Med. J., 2:1301, 1964.

28. Editorial. Epidemiology and prevention of measles and rubella. Lancet, 2:87, 1964.

29. Editorial. Earliest symptoms of measles. Brit. Med. J., 2:687, 1959.

30. Finkel, H. E.: Measles myocarditis. Amer. Heart J., 67:679, 1964.

31. Forbes, J. A.: A current survey of measles in Melbourne including the incidence of measles encephalitis. Med. J. Aust., *1*:170, 1965.

32. Galloway, W. H.: Appendicitis in the course of measles. Brit. Med. J., 2:1412, 1953.

32a. Gibbs, F. A., Gibbs, E. L., Carpenter, P. R., and Spies, H. W.: Encephalographic abnormality in "uncomplicated" childhood diseases. J.A.M.A., *171*:1050-1055, 1959.

33. Gibbs, F. A., Gibbs, E. L., and Rosenthal, I. M.: Electroencephalographic study of children immunized against measles with live attenuated virus vaccine. New Eng. J. Med., *264*:800, 1961.

34. Greenberg, M., Pelliteri, O., and Eisenstein, D.: Measles encephalitis. J. Pediat., *46*:642, 1955.

34a. Gresser, I., and Katz, S. L.: Isolation of measles virus from urine. New Eng. J. Med., *263*:452, 1960.

35. Guran, P.: Epidemiologie, prophylaxie et traitement de la rougeole. Rev. Prat., 5:693, 1955.

35a. Hendrickse, R. G., and Sherman, P.N.: Morbidity and mortality from measles in children seen at University College Hospital, Ibadan. Séminaire, Centre International de l'Enfance, Paris, 1964. Arch. Ges. Virusforsch, *16*:27-34, 1965.

36. Kaplan, M., Fischgrund, A., Blanguernon, R., and Baldino, C.: L'image radiologique pulmonaire au cours de la rougeole non compliquée de l'enfant. Presse Méd., *60*:1428, 1952.

37. Karzon, D. T., Rush, D., and Winkelstein, W., Jr.: Immunization with inactivated measles virus vaccine: effect of booster dose and response to natural challenge. Pediatrics, *36*:40, 1965.

38. Kilic, N.: Hemorrhagic complications of measles. Arch. Pediat. 75:266, 1958.

39. Koprowski, H.: The role of hyperergy in measles encephalitis. Amer. J. Dis. Child., *103*:273, 1962.

40. Krugman, S., and Ward, R.: Infectious Diseases of Children. St. Louis, Mosby, 1964.

40a. Krugman, S., Giles, J. P., Friedman, H. and Stone, S.: Studies on immunity to measles. J. Pediat., *66*:471, 1965.

41. La Boccetta, A. C., and Tornay, A. S.: Measles encephalitis. Amer. J. Dis. Child., *107*:247, 1964.

42. Leading Article. Measles encephalitis. Brit. Med. J., 2:64, 1966.

43. Mande, R., Jammet, M. L., Celers, J., and Boué, A.: A propos de la vaccination contre le rougeole. Résultats des premiers essais de vaccination antimorbilleuse en France avec le vaccin à virus vivant hyperatténué (souche Schwarz). Ann. Pédiat. (Paris), pp. 43-66, 1967.

43a. Manson, M. M., Logan, W. P. D., and Loy, R. M.: Rubella and other virus infections during pregnancy. Report on Public Health and Medical Subjects. No. 101. London, Ministry of Health, Her Majesty's Stationery Office, 1960.

44. Marinesco, G.: Sur la myocardite au cours de la rougeole. Bull. Acad. Nat. Méd. (Paris), *142*:222, 1958.

45. McCarthy, K.: Measles. Brit. Med. Bull., *15*:201, 1959.

46. Medoff, H. S., Hunt, A. R., Karpinski, F. E., Jr., Salitsky, S., Wheeler, J. E., and Hill, D.: Epidemiologic study of inactivated measles vaccine. J.A.M.A., *189*:723, 1964.

47. Miller, D. L.: Frequency of complications of measles, 1963. Report on a national inquiry by the Public Health Laboratory Service in collaboration with the Society of Medical Officers of Health. Brit. Med. J., 2:75, 1964.

47a. Nichols, W. W., and Levan, A.: Measles-associated chromosome breakage. (Séminaire Centre International de l'Enfance, Paris 1964.) Arch. Ges. Virusforsch. 16:168, 1965.

48. La vaccination contre la rougeole. WHO Chron., *18*:87, 1964.

49. Pampiglione, G.: Prodromal phase of measles: some neuro-physiological studies. Brit. Med. J., 2:1296, 1964.

50. Papp, K.: Explication du pathomécanisme de la rougeole. Rev. Immun. 23:97-113, 1959.

51. Partington, M. W., and Quinton, J. F. P.: The preeruptive illness of measles. Arch. Dis. Child. 34:149, 1959.

51a. Quere, M. A., and Rey, M.: Les cécités postrougeoleuses chez l'enfant. Enfant en Milieu Tropical (Dakar and Paris), 23:3, 1965.

52. Reilly, C. M., Stokes, J., Bucynak, E. B., Goloner, H., and Hilleman, M. R.: Living attenuated measles-virus vaccine in early infancy. New Eng. J. Med., *265*:165, 1961.

53. Robbins, F. C.: Measles: clinical features. Amer. J. Dis. Child., *103*:266, 1962.
54. Roberts, G. B. S., and Bain, A. D.: The pathology of measles. J. Path. Bact., *76*:111, 1958.
55. Sédallian, P., Maral, P., de L'Hermuziére, and Traeger, J.: Le poumon dans la rougeole. Pédiatrie, *39*:112, 1950.
56. Tyler, H. R.: Neurological complications of rubeola (measles). Medicine, *36*:147, 1957.
57. van Rooyen, C. E., and Rhodes, A. J.: Virus Diseases of Man. New York, Oxford University Press, 1940.
58. Wallgren, A.: The future of measles vaccination. Acta Paediat., *53*:591, 1964.
59. Watson, G. I.: Serological studies on second attacks of measles and rubella. Lancet, *1*:80, 1965.
60. Wilson, G. S.: Measles as a universal disease. Amer. J. Dis. Child., *103*:219, 1962.

MEASLES: PATHOGENESIS AND EPIDEMIOLOGY

by R. Debré and J. Celers

A universal disease, measles has characteristics so peculiar to it that usually the clinical criteria can be considered valid both in diagnosis and in an epidemiological investigation based on them. Measles has long captivated the interest of minds curious to understand better its transmission and pathogenesis. In our time Enders and his co-workers have brilliantly confirmed facts considered established in the long past on the basis of patient clinical observations. The essential problems of protecting children are now best solved by vaccination; meanwhile new enigmas appear and other questions are raised.

Measles is a viral disease that differs greatly from the other viruses: the *susceptibility* of the human species is extreme, but the adequate *resistance* of the healthy human being toward this aggression is no less striking. G. S. Wilson (of London) remarked, "We have here, therefore, the striking anomaly of a high degree of immunity to death associated with an apparent lack of immunity to attack. In this respect, as in certain others, measles is unique."[33]

Among the other striking aspects is the *solidity of the immunity* (lasting a lifetime) acquired by a single attack of the disease; the natural sensitivity of the human species is such that the receptive subject presents a disease but never becomes a healthy carrier of the virus; in contrast to the untrustworthy protection against other diseases afforded by convalescent serum or gamma globulins from the serum of formerly infected persons the effect against measles is constant, the protection being manifested by different effects according to a very precise chronology related to the time of their administration. Measles is the most striking example, and the most constant, of transplacental transmission of maternal immunity to the infant, this passive immunity remaining effective during the first months of life.

No other disease provokes with equal clarity two singular secondary effects that still lack any satisfactory explanation. These are negativation of the cutaneous reaction to tuberculin, which is a constant phenomenon, and the curative action, which is highly inconstant, produced by measles on the syndrome of lipoid nephrosis of childhood.

In no other viral disease is the influence of socioeconomic conditions on the prognosis as sharply marked. As we shall indicate farther on, the low level of living conditions has determined until now the gravity of measles in countries where part of the population is disfavored (except as concerns measles that is malignant from the onset). Although this phenomenon is capital in the history of measles (we shall return to the point later on) another phenomenon, this one linked to human geography, is striking at present: the contrast between the benignity of measles in the favored countries and the dramatic consequences of measles upon children in the less favored countries. No disease ravages to the same degree as measles the infantile populations of countries where malnutrition is endemic and hygiene poor. In no other viral disease except epidemic influenza do secondary bacterial infections play as important a role as in measles, doubtless owing both to epithelial alterations (in the epithelium of the mouth and the respiratory and the digestive tracts) and to humoral and immunological disturbances.

At present this disease raises still another and different problem: injection of an inactivated measles virus vaccine creates a predisposition to serious clinical symptoms in case of subsequent natural infection. We have had no other example of such a phenomenon until now and its pathogenesis so far remains obscure.

SOURCES OF VIRUS; TRANSMISSION; FIRST MULTIPLICATIONS

The measles virus is a *virus of man*. Outside the human species, the sole natural host now known is the monkey, but this animal is not spontaneously infected under the conditions of its natural habitat; only after capture, contact with human beings ill with measles, and spread of the virus among the animals during collective transport or regroupings, do monkeys become infected.[26] In nature, man constitutes the only source of measles virus propagation.

Contamination takes place by direct *contact between patient and receptive subject*. No human being has been identified as a healthy carrier of measles virus; moreover, indirect contamination has never been rigorously proved. At the most, it has been suggested that, for a few minutes, the physician or nurse passing from a measles patient's room to a contiguous room *might* transport the virus, but proof of this mode of transmission is shaky. Attentive observation long pursued shows that the sick patient is the contaminator and that the transmission takes place chiefly during the invasion period characterized by catarrh of the mucosae of the pathways first involved. The period of the most massive contagiousness, as we know, comes before the eruption; the second day preceding its outbreak can be fixed as the high point when the chances of transmission of measles are at their peak. The length of time of exposure necessary at this point is only a few minutes. The measles patient may be contagious a little before this date (from the onset of catarrh) and a short time thereafter (up to the second or third day of the rash).

During these few days, the patient sneezes and coughs. Moreover, even when he lets out a cry or merely talks, Flügge droplets laden with virus shower about him and, carried by the air, reach and implant themselves in the healthy receptive subject. Virological studies, as will be indicated, confirm this datum that clinical observation had already established.

The spontaneous *penetration* of the receptive subject by the virulent particles has been an object of research work. It has generally been accepted that with the inspired air these particles penetrate the *upper respiratory tract* and implant themselves there. Even before these facts had been proved, physicians considered that development of the virus particles provoked a cellular infection and a pericellular reaction, the virus being transmitted from cell to cell, producing the anatomicoclinical phenomena of viral invasion. The latter phenomena, we know, involve the nasal mucosa, the buccal mucosa (in which Koplik's spots reveal the disease very early), the pharyngeal mucosa, "extending," so to speak, toward the ocular mucosae which are always inflamed from the onset, doubtless also "extending" toward the eustachian tubes and the ears, rapidly reaching the larynx (onset with croup is well known), the trachea, the bronchial epithelium, and even the pulmonary parenchyma. From these multiple involvements arise the signs and symptoms that characterize the period of viral invasion. Likewise the propagation on the digestive mucosa explains the initial diarrhea that is not exceptional in young subjects. The eruption might be considered, as von Pirquet considered it, the translation of a conflict between the virus, disseminated by viremia throughout the body, particularly in the skin, and the antibodies formed by the infected subject. At the moment when the eruption spreads, the catarrhal symptoms increase, attaining a sort of acme that recalls the phenomena of crisis in other infectious diseases (in pneumonia for example) that are considered hyperergic manifestations of a sensitized organism. This acme is followed by a fairly rapid improvement of the general and local phenomena that begins when the antibody level has become sufficient to sterilize the organism, from which event ensue the quickness of recovery and the brevity of convalescence usual in this disease.

In what measure is this schema, established by clinicians, confirmed and completed by virological studies and by experimental trials in man and in the monkey?

First of all, as concerns the natural portal of entry, Karola Papp postulated the hypothesis of a capital role played by the conjunctival mucosa.[28] She demonstrated its unquestionable possibility by infecting receptive subjects by instillation in the conjunctival cul-de-sac of a drop of a measles patient's saliva, then by averting this contamination by the mixing of convalescent serum with the drop of saliva. She even believes that she protected receptive children remaining in contact with patients by having them wear protective goggles. In fact this mode of contamination appears possible, but nothing proves that it plays a role in the natural course of contaminations, and even less that it constitutes the one and only portal. With use of attenuated strains of measles virus, several modes of contamination have been studied, in particular by McCrumb[24] and by Black and Sheridan:[2] conjunctival instillation, nasal instillation, and lastly immediate but more diffuse and doubtless more deep-reaching instillation by aerosols. But the results of experiments utilizing attenuated strains that, as we shall see later, implant themselves less easily than wild strains in the "natural pathways" cannot be transposed to spontaneous measles infection.

It therefore remains highly possible that the salivary droplets and the droplets of mucus secreted by the respiratory pathways penetrate, by the nasal and possibly by the buccal pathways, the upper respiratory tract of receptive subjects and develop there. The diffusion is thus air-borne; the virus's survival outside the human body is very brief and if a draft of air can perhaps carry measles virus a short distance from the patient who emits it, a draft or an exposure to light for several minutes suffices to disinfect a room which a measles patient has inhabited. The presence of the virus detected in the fecal matter and the urine of patients even for several days (up to the fourth day after the eruption[14] has not modified the solidly established concept of direct transmission by the air route. The fragility of the virus (cf. the section on Virological Study and Prophylaxis) explains the impossibility of the virus's survival outside the human body, from which results the absence of indirect hand-borne transmission.

Enders and his collaborators[10] have made a remarkable contribution of exact information concerning all these problems of isolation and culture of the virus. But in justice it should be recalled that Ruckle and Rogers[31] isolated the virus from nasal secretions 48 hours before the rash and 32 hours after its outbreak, thus confirming the early experiments (1911) of Anderson and Goldberger on the infectiousness of buccal and nasal secretions from the sixty-fifth to the hundred and thirteenth hour after the eruption.

DIFFUSION OF THE VIRUS IN THE ORGANISM

The diffusion can be demonstrated by the infectiousness of the different tissues and body fluids for man himself or for the experimental animal, by verification of the virus's presence in tissue culture, and by the lesions it provokes.

The *first experiments on inoculation in man* were made with the desire of obtaining a protection, a "vaccination," by imitating the traditional method of "variolization." These inoculations, accomplished with blood of measles patients at the acute period by Francis Home in Edinburgh in 1758, and then by J. Cook in 1767 with tears of measles patients, experiments renewed with blood by different authors in Great Britain, Italy, and Hungary, by Hectoen in the United States in 1905, by Hirashi and Okamoto in Japan, and by Degkwitz in Germany, have at present only historical interest: that of the history of *measles inoculation*. Obviously they demonstrated that measles virus was present in the patients' blood.

Experimentation in monkeys yielded more precise proof of measles viremia. As early as 1911 Charles Nicolle and E. Conseil (in Debré[8a]) provoked a febrile disease by intraperitoneal inoculation into the monkey (*Macaca rhesus*) of blood of a child with the earliest signs of measles (catarrh and fever) drawn 24 hours before outbreak of the rash. The blood of this monkey permitted contamination in the same manner of two other monkeys and a healthy child. The blood of the second child infected two or three monkeys. This procedure demonstrated precisely for the first time the viremia in measles and its existence before the eruption, as well as the possibility of infecting *Macaca* monkeys. The same year Anderson and Goldberger opened wide this new chapter of experimental pathology. "Thanks to these authors," wrote Charles Nicolle and E. Conseil, "we have learned in a few months: that measles can be inoculated into two species of lower monkeys (*Macaca rhesus* and *M. cynomolgus*); that the virus existed in the patients' blood in the first phase of the eruption; that it disappeared from the blood between the 65th and the 113th hour after the onset of the rash; that the ocular, nasal and pharyngeal secretions were virulent in analogous conditions; lastly, that the specific agent of measles was an invisible, filtrating, fragile microbe, destroyed by heating. The experimental disease of the monkey is translated by a fever of several days' duration, accompanied or not by an eruption of dubious specificity, without tearing eyes, coryza or other symptoms." Nicolle and Conseil completed the fundamental observations of the American authors in other species of monkeys.

These data were to lead the French investigators to attempt *vaccinations in children, under the protection of convalescent serum, by injecting successively the protective serum and then the virulent blood.* With the above data as a starting point, we pursued with Karola Papp and the collaboration of Jean Cros-Decam our trials of active vaccination against measles, demonstrating the possibility of injecting safely into a child a very small dose of blood and of observing in him a slight rise in temperature and a characteristic leukopenia with drop in the percentage of polymorphonuclear leukocytes, a demonstration of the *initial leukopenia.* While we were searching for a purer and richer antigen and drawing on, for the purpose, facts observed in exanthematous typhus by Charles Nicolle, A. Connor, and E. Conseil, we moreover noted that the virus is particularly abundant in the lower layers of the plasma (after collection of blood rendered incoagulable and centrifuged) at the level of the buffy coat.[29] These observations made it seem highly plausible to us that the virus penetrates the polymorphonuclear leukocytes and destroys them by its cytopathogenic power, resulting in the leukopenia in the preeruptive phase in the child which is also regularly produced in the inoculated animal.

More recently, Peebles, and then Gresser and Chany,[15] isolated the virus in vitro from the blood leukocyte fraction and showed that the virus is constantly found there during the first 24 hours that follow the eruption whereas it becomes difficult to isolate after 24 hours, i.e., when circulating antibodies appear. Furthermore, the measles virus can be cultivated in vitro in white cell suspensions, in which it attains infectivity titers comparable to those obtainable in tissue culture.

On the basis of these convergent data, it is entirely reasonable to suppose that measles virus is disseminated in the or-

ganism owing to its multiplication in, and its *transport by, the leukocytes.* It is striking, however, that the white cells are also good producers of interferon and thus capable of inhibiting viral multiplication.[7] Certain mononuclear cells are also considered responsible for the phenomena of delayed hypersensitivity. A more thorough analysis of the hematological phenomena might perhaps solve these problems, by defining the role of the different kinds of leukocytes during the successive phases of the natural infection and of the vaccinal or experimental infection.[5]

The moment at which viremia begins is undetermined, but it seems reasonable to believe, as do S. L. Katz and J. F. Enders,[20] that it intervenes toward the fifth day of the incubation period, i.e., when injection of convalescent serum no longer aborts the infection.

Since isolation of the virus has made great rigor possible in experimental conditions, experiments in the monkey have multiplied. Kraft, Blake, and Trask, Sergiev, and Ryazantseva and Shroit (in Kempe[21] and Mayer[25]) have inoculated cynomolgus monkeys by different routes (intranasal, intravenous, intracerebral, intracisternal, and

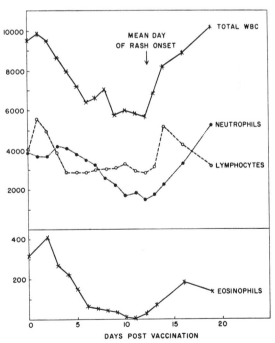

Figure 27-1. Leukocyte counts in vaccinees, median values in 36 subjects. (From Black, F. L.: Measles: its spread from cell to cell and person to person. Canad. J. Public Health, 56:517-520, 1965.)

subcutaneous) and provoked in the animal leukopenia, fever, eruption, and viremia with development of antibodies, reproducing an attenuated measles of sorts, but one typical in this animal.

In the artificially infected monkey, as in man with natural measles, the virus is isolated from the nasal and pharyngeal secretions, from blood, and from urine at the end of the invasion period,[12] but, from the second day following the eruption, the virus ceases to be detectable except in the urine. The diffusion of the virus is easily explained by the viremia and the arrest of this diffusion by the antibodies detectable in the blood. It has been supposed, in accord with the schema established by Fenner for viral ectromelia of the mouse, that there are two phases of viremia; an initial one three days after the inoculation and then, after a viremia-free period of two or three days, a second viremic phase a week after the inoculation. The possibility of two periods of viremia in measles as in ectromelia is a hypothesis that requires confirmation by studies of natural measles in man.

When natural measles virus is inoculated parenterally, the incubation period is shortened to four days, both in man and in the monkey.[10] It is hence possible that, under natural conditions of contamination, an initial phase of viral multiplication leads up to viremia. The most likely site of this phase would be at the level of the upper respiratory pathways, but the possibility of multiplication at the level of the conjunctiva cannot be excluded; the virus has been demonstrated[12] there and, if the second hypothesis proved correct, certain nonbacterial ocular complications would perhaps be explained (cf. Chapter 54).

THE ROLE OF THE MEASLES VIRUS IN THE USUAL SYMPTOMATOLOGY OF MEASLES

Three forms of pathogenic action are attributed to the virus in the genesis of measles: a direct action of the virus on the tissues, a more complex, still ill defined action resulting from both the virus and the organism's defense mechanisms, and, lastly, an action favoring secondary or bacterial infections. The action of the virus on the chromosomes and its possible role in certain chronic diseases of the central nervous system are discussed in other chapters (Chapters 61 and 19).

The direct action of measles virus can logically be considered probable wherever histological examination reveals those multinucleated cells that characterize the multiplication of the virus in tissue culture; the respiratory tract, primarily, is the site where the concordance between the presence of these cells and the clinical symptomatology is the most clear cut (cf. Chapter 42).

The great affinity of natural strains of measles virus for the tissues of the upper respiratory system has, moreover, been emphasized by J. F. Enders, S. L. Katz, and D. N. Medearis[10] in experimental studies comparing virulent and attenuated strains in the monkey. Neither the mode of inoculation (intracerebral or intracisternal injection), nor doubtless the doses of virus, nor the characteristics proper to the animal species make possible the unreserved extrapolation to the human species of the phenomena observed in experiments with the so-called "virulent" strain. Moreover, this is not the end pursued. It is striking, however, to observe the duration and the precociousness of rhinopharyngeal elimination of virus that begins the very day following the inoculation and lasts until the ninth day.

Thus a direct action of the virus might explain in particular the coryza, the cough, certain cases of acute bronchitis, the conjunctivitis, and the interstitial giant cell pneumonia.

On the other hand, neither histological examination of the lesions nor the search for virus in situ makes it possible to incriminate a direct action of the pathogenic agent in producing the enanthem and the exanthem that, for centuries, have permitted clinicians to recognize measles infection.

The hypothesis is advanced that the eruption appearing so regularly 14 days after the contamination (with very few variations plus or minus in the length of this period in natural measles) results from a conflict between the virus and antibodies. Other authors suggest instead the role of a hypothetical antigen derived from the virus.[7] The fact that the eruption breaks out first on the face and descends from head to foot over the rest of the body could encourage the supposition that the cutaneous areas near the regions in which the virus first and most actively developed from the beginning are those first to be sensitized. The hypothesis advanced by von Pirquet is that the exanthem appears where the teguments are best irrigated by the arterial blood and therefore saturated with virus. There is a tendency to accept the hypothesis that the virus, impeded at this moment by the protection of antibodies and their bloodstream diffusion, is localized in the cutaneous capillary endothelia. Without a doubt, by application of a cantharides plaster, Degkwitz and Meyer (in Mayer[25]) isolated the virus from the blister so produced. A reminder as to the effects of convalescent serum on the skin of infected subjects may help the reader at this point to understand the succession of phenomena. The experience we, with P. Joannon (in Debré[8a]), acquired is as follows. Injection of convalescent serum during the first four days of the incubation period halts the blossoming forth of measles; exteriorly at least, nothing betrays that the child has been contaminated. If the injection is made between the fifth and the eighth day of the incubation period, measles appears, but in a modified form, its main features under these circumstances being: prolongation of the incubation period, lessening or suppression of catarrh, attenuation or absence of the eruption, lessened intensity and duration of the febrile period, persistence of excellent general physical condition, absence of anergy to tuberculin, absence of complications, absence of contagion for the surrounding persons, and subsequent presence in the serum of patients who have had this type of measles of detectable immunisins of limited duration (as Karelitz[17] later demonstrated).

When the serum injection is made on the eve of onset of clinical measles or even on the second day preceding it, the disease is absolutely unchanged in its development and not the least attenuated. But on outbreak of the eruption, the zone in which the injection was made is rash-free: around the point where the needle penetrated, the skin is spared, and this area is marked by a white spot surrounded by red macules. Such is the expression of the phenomenon of local inhibition of the rash, which we described with Henri Bonnet and Robert Broca. The cutaneous zone in which the eruption is inhibited is proportionate in extent to the quantity of serum injected and the limits of this zone are sharply delineated. The action of the antibodies against measles has remained local. To borrow Sven Gard's ex-

pression, this phenomenon is one of immuno-inactivation.

The phenomenon of measles eruption remains complex, but that of the cerebral localization is even more so. The clinical, anatomical, and physiopathological characteristics of the cerebral localizations are analyzed in this book in Chapters 6 and 7. Three anatomicoclinical aspects are distinguished that, in order of decreasing frequency, are postinfectious leukoencephalitis of perivenous type, acute encephalopathy, and meningoencephalitis. These three aspects are common to a great number of childhood viral infections and no specific element permits their etiological diagnosis. Despite repeated efforts to track down the measles virus in the cerebrospinal fluid and the brain itself, few investigators have demonstrated its presence in situ. With regard to results positive in this respect, in 1957 Fränkel isolated the measles virus from the cerebrospinal fluid in four cases of measles encephalitis at a time when he could no longer isolate the virus from the blood or the mucosa of the throat. In 1959, Taniguchi (in Mayer[25]) believed he had isolated the virus from blood and cerebrospinal fluid in a case of encephalitis. At present, the hypothesis most often considered remains that of phenomena of indirect reaction comparable to those in experimental allergic encephalitis.

Interferon production, in striking fact, is higher in cell cultures of attenuated virus than of wild virus;[9] this phenomenon had already been observed with the viruses of poliomyelitis and of mumps. As concerns measles virus, the remarkable production of interferon by the attenuated strains is accompanied by a lessening of cytopathogenic effect and viral reproduction in vitro.[20] It will be important to examine in what degree these laboratory data can elucidate human pathology.

MEASLES AND BACTERIAL INFECTIONS; MEASLES AND ASSOCIATED DISEASES

The cases of measles so often complicated and too often fatal that were observed only a few years ago in the favored countries and that are redoubtable today in the disfavored countries present a problem difficult to resolve. What is the part played by the measles virus itself? What is that of secondary bacterial infections? Whatever may be the replies to these questions, the role of the terrain is capital, as is that of the environmental circumstances: the supervention of complications is linked to the nutritional disturbances of childhood, rachitism, insufficiency of protein intake, and various types of malnutrition, on the one hand, and, on the other, to spread of common bacterial pathogens, e.g., streptococci, pneumococci, and pathogenic strains of *Escherichia coli.*

There is no doubt that inflammation of the ear that heals spontaneously at the periods of invasion and of eruption, like early croup, initial capillary bronchitis, and early inflammations of the eyes, may be thought to result from the action of the virus alone; on the other hand, the later bronchopneumopathy, membranous ulceronecrotic laryngitis, suppurative otitis and its local complications are, at least in their majority, caused by microbial aggressions like the pyodermitis or "noma" of the cheek due to anaerobic organisms. To these secondary infections must be added the association, once unexceptional, of various specific diseases, diphtheria for example, to the point that it was advisable to consider this possibility in the presence of all severe cases of laryngitis, or thrush, once so common, or the simultaneous, redoubtable evolution of two childhood diseases: measles and scarlet fever, measles and varicella, measles and whooping cough.

IMMUNOLOGY

Owing to its peculiar immunological characteristics, measles occupies a distinct and separate place in the complex pathology of infection, the importance of which is made obvious by what has been seen recently in African countries.

The immunology of measles indeed merits special attention. We shall emphasize particularly the formation of protective antibodies and their indefinite persistence in the subject after recovery from the disease, their role in prevention, the measles-provoked anergy, in particular toward tuberculin, the shock effect of measles in certain diseases, especially lipoid nephrosis, the modified reactivity to the virus in subjects having received an inactivated measles vaccine, and in what way these different

elements contribute to give to measles a very particular physiognomy.

Before the era of virological and immunological studies, clinicians had shown the receptivity, considered by some of them as absolute, of all mankind to measles, the acquisition of a definitive immunity after even a mild attack, the antibody transmission to the fetus across the placenta of an immunized mother, and the regressive character of this passive immunity in the nursling infant until its disappearance toward the fifth month of life. The progressive character of this disappearance makes possible an attenuated form of measles in the infant still partially, but incompletely, protected by maternal antibodies.

Clinicians opposed measles to diphtheria, for example, in which a spontaneous occult immunization may suffice, whereas active protection against measles is acquired only subsequent to manifest disease. They discussed the exceptional cases of subjects who affirmed that they had never had measles in their life, despite several exposures. Clinicians rejected the hypothesis of an exceptional refractory state, concluding that these cases resulted most probably from mild or unrecognized measles, perhaps from prenatal measles (R. Debré and P. Joannon).[8a] The serological studies now possible will shed light on this particular point.

Since the virus, on the one hand, and the different antibodies, on the other, can be detected, some former suppositions have been confirmed and the facts filled in. We know that antibodies may appear the first or the second day following the eruption, an occurrence explaining the clinical evolution, and attain their highest level at the end of two or three weeks; their level diminishes thereafter during three to six months, but henceforth remains fairly constant for years. The antibodies detected are multiple: those that neutralize the virus, those that inhibit hemagglutination, and those that fix complement. The persistence of these antibodies is not due, as certain studies made in countries in which measles is not endemic appeared to demonstrate, to boosters caused by renewed contacts with the virus.

Thus in 1959, in Tahiti,[4] eight years after the last measles epidemic, the children born since 1951 had no specific antibodies whereas 80 to 100 per cent of subjects born before 1951 had antibodies, at levels comparable to those found in the sera sampled in 1951. It is therefore legitimate to believe that the three types of antibodies against measles (neutralizing, hemagglutination-inhibiting, and complement-fixing) persist at least eight years after the initial infection without change and that this stability is not subordinated to the presence of inapparent infections. The persistence of complement-fixing antibodies without reinfection is emphasized. These antibodies, indeed, are generally considered to be transitory and hence a manifestation of the infection (cf. Introduction, p. 28). The present case marks an exception all the more remarkable for the fact that these very same antibodies have been detected after injection of inactivated measles vaccine into receptive subjects. Their precise significance thus remains to be found.

Is the absence or the rarity of relapses in measles in subjects having had a natural infection linked to the virulence of the agent responsible? In cases of measles attenuated by injection of gamma globulin or by convalescent serum a certain immunity generally follows, the quality and the persistence of which seems comparable to naturally acquired immunity. Notwithstanding, eruptive fevers considered to be measles have been observed, although very rarely, in subjects who several years previously had had a modified case of measles.[17] When these "recurrences" were reported they unfortunately could not be elucidated by serological studies and their real frequency remains undetermined. Doubtless the longitudinal studies pursued with use of modern virological techniques in children vaccinated by attenuated or hyperattenuated strains will give us more precise data in this regard.

One of the points that struck clinicians as soon as the administration of convalescent serum or, occasionally, serum of former measles patients came into use was the small quantity of serum capable of yielding a result valid in prevention of measles. The use of gamma globulins confirmed and defined this action and the variability in effect of the injection of antibodies as a function of the moment of their application. As we indicated earlier, a kind of regressive scale can be established for the activity of antiserum according to the date of its injection. A short time before or a short time after the contamination, the protective action is absolute; it is a form of *seroprophylaxis.* The antiserum in-

jected during the second part of the invasion phase has only a moderating action: "seroattenuation." When it is injected at the onset of the clinical disease, the only action of antiserum is local: *local inhibition of the rash,* becoming evident when the eruption develops amid the other habitual concomitants of the disease. When it is injected later still, i.e., at the end of the invasion period or during the eruptive phase, its action is nil.

Most probably factors other than immunoglobulins are capable of playing a role in human resistance to viral aggression. It was indicated (Introduction, p. 22) that subjects with congenital agammaglobulinemia present measles with a usual evolution and subsequent resistance to reinfection comparable to that of normal subjects. But, when the agammaglobulinemia is associated with lymphocytopenia, measles infection is fatal. These facts throw light on the importance of lymphocytes or of their precursors in the defense of the organism. As concerns this subject, two modes of action have been considered: a nonspecific action consisting in interferon production, and a specific action, the mechanism of which remains a mystery, that is related to the phenomena of delayed hypersensitivity.

As early as 1908 von Pirquet showed the importance of the temporary disappearance of cutaneous reactions to tuberculin in measles; this reaction was reported in 1907 from Vienna by Preisich, who called the phenomenon *anergy.* Anergy in measles has been universally confirmed and has been studied carefully. The child with measles can cease reacting to tuberculin before the eruption, but the anergy attains its acme the day after onset of the eruption. The anergy lasts a week, usually, or exceptionally two, three, or four weeks. In other viral diseases (influenza, varicella), an analogous phenomenon has been detected on occasion, but in no other infectious disease has tuberculin anergy shown both the sharp distinctness and the constancy that it has in measles. Some other phenomena have been related to and compared with von Pirquet's tuberculin anergy: the negativation of the Wassermann reaction (Teisser and Lutenbacher) and of the Widal serum agglutination reaction (Léon Bernard), the adjournment of the vaccinial reaction (Hamburger, Netter, and Gendron), and the decrease in efficacy of antidiphtheria serum.

Another phenomenon that has struck

the clinicians is what can be called—for want of a better term—the "shock-producing" action that measles exerts on different morbid states, especially on eczema of young subjects and on the lipoid nephrosis syndrome. The abruptness of the suspensive effect is unquestionable in certain cases that cannot be ascertained beforehand, for this effect of measles is inconstant. No valid explanation of the effect has been advanced.

Today the action of measles virus on the blood proteins is better known; it is worth mention, for the physician may feel obscurely that a link doubtless exists, on the one hand, between the disturbance in their equilibrium and the phenomena just reported and, on the other, with the susceptibility of measles patients to bacterial superinfections.

Lorenz and Rossipal[23] showed that during the invasion period a fall in serum albumin level is already notable; the lowest point is reached at the moment of the eruption; the level then rises and returns to normal a week after onset of the eruption. The immunoglobulin level falls abruptly at the outset of the eruption, remains low until the fourth day following it, and rises again from that point on. The behavior of the gamma A immunoglobulins (γ_1 A) and of the gamma M immunoglobulins (γ_1 M) is different. The level of the former falls abruptly only after the exanthem but their low level lasts approximately a week, after which the original level is again found. The same is true for the gamma G immunoglobulins, whereas at no time do the gamma M immunoglobulins undergo any appreciable modification (Fig. 27-2). In this connection, should we envisage a parallel, as does J. B. Mayer[25] (of Hamburg, Germany), with the notion established by von Pirquet that tuberculin anergy attains its maximum four days after the onset of the rash? And should not another parallel be drawn with the leukopenia that we have already emphasized?

The last immunological problem that we shall touch on is one that has become known more recently. In 1965 Rauh and Schmidt[30] were struck by atypical cases of measles in children who had received inactivated vaccine and were later exposed to the natural contagion. These children presented occasionally and according to different modalities: petechiae and purpura, urticaria, bullous eruption, peripheral edema, pneumopathy, cephalalgia, abdominal pains, leukocyturia, and also serious systemic signs (prostration, tachypnea) necessitating hospitaliza-

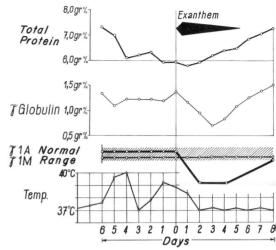

Figure 27-2. Blood protein changes occurring in the course of measles. (From Lorenz, E., and Rossipal, E.: Zur Frage der Resistenzminderung bei Masern. Mschr. Kinderheilk., *113*:161, 1965.)

tion. This description was subsequently completed by that of Nader,[27] and then of Fulginiti et al.[13] and of Lennon and Isacson.[22] This singular clinical picture is perhaps related to observations of early local reactions (48 hours) after the injection of live virus vaccine supervening at the point of injection of this vaccine and characterized by a local inflammatory induration in the subjects who had been previously vaccinated with the inactivated virus.

The details known in regard to this absolutely new phenomenon do not modify its fundamental character. Inactivated measles virus can provoke hypersensitivity to live measles virus. This hypersensitivity can, in the case of local action, be manifested by a reaction similar to the Arthus phenomenon and, as concerns the systemic phenomena, by a very peculiar eruption and by severe disturbances recalling the accidents attributed to allergy or to anaphylaxis by Richet and Portier. No more can be added at present writing, except to call attention to the need for additional knowledge concerning this new immunological feature peculiar to measles and to suggest at least momentary abstention from prophylaxis by inactivated vaccine against measles (cf. Virological Study and Prophylaxis).

Certain forms of measles are also linked to an immunological behavior peculiar to the subject, for example, an incomplete immunization that is responsible for mild measles, measles without eruption, "morbilloid" disease, "modified" measles such as the forms we have described after injections of immunoglobulins. In contrast, the immunological process can fail to establish itself—for reasons that escape us—and in consequence measles then takes on a character of malignity, not so much because of the hemorrhagic character of the eruption (not a sign of gravity as in black smallpox) but because of the exaggeration of all the signs and symptoms from the very onset of the invasion period, with fatal issue shortly after onset of the eruption, with hyperthermia and dyspnea. Occasionally the malignant syndrome occurs in the form popularly known in French as "rougeole rentrée" (essentially, measles without eruption) in which suddenly, after a short incubation, alarming respiratory and nervous system phenomena appear that provoke rapid death without eruption. In large part, immunological deficit is responsible for the high mortality from measles in African countries where malnutrition and its consequences on resistance to infection are so habitual; in certain regions the survival of a young child after measles is considered as "a second birth."

WORLD DISTRIBUTION

The distribution of measles in the world is established in function of three determining factors: the extreme contagiousness of the disease, the exclusive role of man, and of sick man alone, in its spread, and the remarkable efficacy of naturally acquired immunity.

Thus, when a measles epidemic breaks out in a population that has long been sheltered from contamination, more than 99 per cent of subjects contract the disease: such was the case in 1951 in southern Greenland during the first epidemic observed in this territory. If the viral spread cannot be maintained by the renewal of receptive subjects in contact with sick ones, measles disappears until a new epidemic breaks out, sparing the subjects already immunized. The intervals that separate these epidemics diminish with the intensification of means of transport and the greater frequency of human contacts. The first two epidemics described in Greenland were separated by an eight-year interval (1951-1959); the third one, in 1962, had as sole point of departure the arrival by plane from Denmark of one child in the incubation period of measles.[1]

At present, measles rages in an endemic state in most countries in the world and, with rare exceptions, only variations in morbidity rate in function of age, living habits, seasons, and years can be demonstrated.

INCIDENCE IN FUNCTION OF AGE

Study of the prevalence of measles antibodies in different types of population permits an objective estimation of the distribution of measles in function of age.

It shows that, in all the large urban ag-

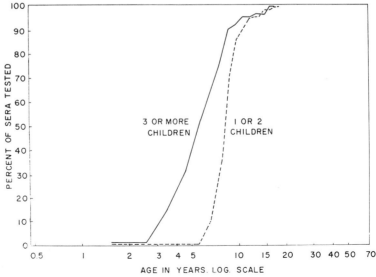

Figure 27-3. Cumulative per cent of positive specimens by age in sera from small and large families in New Haven. (From Black, F. L.: Measles antibody prevalence in diverse populations. Amer. J. Dis. Child., *103*:242-249, 1962.)

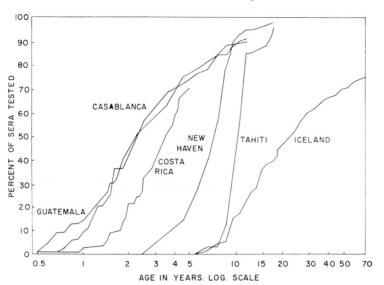

Figure 27-4. Cumulative per cent of sera with measles neutralizing antibodies by age for six geographic areas. (From Black, F. L.: Measles antibody prevalence in diverse populations. Amer. J. Dis. Child., *103*:242-249, 1962.)

glomerations, the quasitotality of subjects have acquired antibodies by age 10. The receptive individuals, capable of transmitting measles on the occasion of their disease, are essentially children under age 10. The adult woman transmits to her infant by the transplacental route antibodies that progressively disappear, protecting the child until the sixth or seventh month. Then, according to the child's contacts with other children, the age of appearance of antibodies consequent to natural infection and the rapidity with which high proportions of antibody-bearing subjects are established vary. Factors such as the number of children in the family and the age at which the child is introduced into collec-

tive life clearly intervene. Thus, in New Haven, Connecticut, if families have an average of one or two children, the acquisition of antibodies begins only with school attendance, i.e., from age five upward, while in families with three or more children 50 per cent of subjects have already had measles before age five. In Costa Rica, the number of children (an average of six per family) is the essential cause to which Black[3] attributes the rapidity of antibody acquisition: 50 per cent of subjects are immunized before age three. In Paris, as in most large French cities, the kindergarten, grouping children from ages three to five years, is an essential factor in the spread of the common diseases

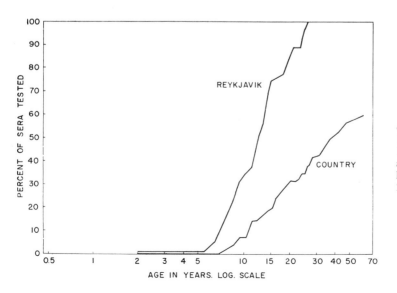

Figure 27-5. Cumulative per cent positive specimens in sera from Reykjavik and from other parts of Iceland. (From Black, F. L.: Measles antibody prevalence in diverse populations. Amer. J. Dis. Child., *103*: 242-249, 1962.)

of childhood, so that at the age of obligatory school attendance 73 per cent of children, according to questioning of the parents, have already had measles.[6]

Inversely, in rural areas where contacts with young children are neither frequent nor renewed, immunity is acquired much later; the study made in Iceland by Black[3] clearly revealed these facts. In the principal city, Reykjavik, antibody acquisition occurs entirely during the schooling period, i.e., between ages 5 and 15 years. In the smaller towns and in the rural zones where population averages approximately one inhabitant per square kilometer, the percentage of antibody bearers progresses much more slowly and the progression continues over almost a lifetime. Such a situation is reminiscent of facts related in France during the 1914-1918 war, which emphasized not only the gravity but also the extreme frequency of measles in young recruits of whom most were of rural origin.[6]

INDICES OF MORBIDITY AND OF MORTALITY

From the time when measles has become endemic and 90 per cent of adults are immunized, the morbidity index should be roughly proportional to the annual live-birth rate in the same population sample. Thus in England and Wales (where an estimated 80 per cent of cases of measles are notified) the morbidity index per 100,000 inhabitants in 1961 was 1650 with, for the same number of inhabitants, 1760 live births.[6]

Nonetheless it is obvious (Table 27-1) that this morbidity incidence undergoes very regular *annual variations* with a rise every two years, particularly intense in 1955 and 1961, as though the years 1954 and 1960 had permitted a renewal of receptive subjects. The annual variations appear less clearly in countries where notification of cases is not as strictly effectuated, or when, as for the United States as a whole, the figures result from disparate data from numerous states in which the climates, the type of dwelling, and the mode of life are highly diverse.

The *seasonal variations* have long been known to physicians and to persons responsible for collectivities of children. Measles appears at the end of winter and early in spring. Probably a great number of factors intervene in these variations. The size of a group of receptive subjects in contact with each other in number sufficient to permit widespread viral diffusion was emphasized by Wilson[33] in connection with London epidemics. Thus, from 1917 to 1939, the morbidity curve showed a spike in winter every year, whereas in 1940 the bombing of the city caused school establishments to be closed and the epidemic did not occur.

But it was also demonstrated[16] that the survival of air-borne measles virus increases when the relative humidity decreases, and, according to the morbidity curves established in England, in London, or in certain subtropical regions, the increase in number of cases parallels the decrease in the relative humidity inside houses.

The intervention of climatic factors hence cannot be neglected; doubtless the

Table 27-1. *Cases of Measles Notified in England and Wales from 1953 to 1962*

YEAR	NUMBER OF CASES NOTIFIED	INDEX OF MORBIDITY PER 100,000 INHABITANTS	NUMBER OF LIVE BIRTHS PER 100,000 INHABITANTS
1953	545,000	1230	1550
1954	147,000	330	1520
1955	694,000	1555	1500
1956	161,000	359	1570
1957	634,000	1407	1610
1958	259,000	572	1640
1959	540,000	1186	1650
1960	159,000	346	1720
1961	764,000	1650	1760
1962	185,000		1800

same is true for phenomena of interference between myxoviruses or for variations in other defense processes, specific or not.

A reminder of the general conditions of mortality from measles can usefully complete the preceding indications.

First of all it should be recalled that in the late nineteenth century, measles, the case fatality of which in Europe was until then less than that due to scarlet fever, to whooping cough, and to diphtheria, little by little conquered the first rank. From the beginning of the twentieth century it caused more deaths than any of these three diseases, this phenomenon being due essentially to a decrease in gravity of scarlet fever and of whooping cough and doubtless at the same time to a decrease in the gravity of diphtheria and to the action of antidiphtheria serum. In France, from 1906 to 1913, measles caused 31,000 deaths—in round numbers—diphtheria 25,000, whooping cough 25,000, and scarlet fever 9800. From 1900 to 1910 in Europe it took approximately a million victims; in the United States, measles provoked more than 100,000 deaths from 1901 to 1920. During this period and in all the countries of Europe and of America considered, measles was, in general, mild in rural areas and in the well-to-do sectors of the large cities, but it hit hard the children of poor families, living in the slums of overpopulated unsanitary neighborhoods. In studying this fact with Pierre Joannon[8] we showed that the case fatality of measles was proportional to the population density and that in the working-class city and suburban areas of the period there was a genuine supermortality from measles due to four causes: the higher frequency of measles infection at an early age; the higher proportion of weakened and ill children; the aggravation of measles by stay in a hospital, and, above all, the gravity of measles in the nursling infant living in an overpopulated hovel. The complications due to the hospital superinfections, then frequent, seemed to us, however, to be at the origin of only a fifth or a sixth of fatal cases. The relationship with overpopulation still seems capital to us; we denounced the slum dwelling or the hovel as the principal cause. Certainly, to the life of the small child in a hovel are added different inevitable faults and defects in hygiene and an extreme facility of spread of various pyogenic bacteria. In any event, it is instructive to recall this situation in the past in the countries

where today an improvement in living standards and in public health has changed the situation that was once disastrous. The average annual death rate from measles in France passed from some 4000 in the first half of the twentieth century to some one hundred from 1960 to 1965. Today it is in the tropical and subtropical countries that measles is one of the most important causes of infant mortality. Measles kills malnourished, debilitated, sick children, children with digestive disturbances, in tropical countries now as it did in the past in the slums of the large European cities. There too, children are protected in large numbers against measles by vaccination, but it should be remarked that in the course of infancy they nonetheless succumb. It must hence be seen whether, after the success of vaccination campaigns, the mortality in young children for the entire year and for the year following has marked a valid decrease.

BIBLIOGRAPHY

1. Bech, V.: The measles epidemic in Greenland in 1962. Arch. Ges. Virusforsch., *16*:53-56, 1965.
2. Black, F. L., and Sheridan, S. R.: Studies on an attenuated measles-virus vaccine. Administration of vaccine by several routes. New Eng. J. Med., *263*:165-169, 1960.
3. Black, F. L.: Measles antibody prevalence in diverse populations. Amer. J. Dis. Child., *103*:242-249, 1962.
4. Black, F. L., and Rosen, L.: Patterns of measles antibodies in residents of Tahiti and their stability in the absence of re-exposure. J. Immun., *88*:725-731, 1962.
5. Black, F. L.: Measles: its spread from cell to cell and person to person. Canad. J. Public Health, *56*:517-520, 1965.
6. Celers, J.: Problèmes de Santé Publique posés par la rougeole dans les pays favorisés. (Séminaire du Centre International de l'Enfance, 17 juin 1964.) Arch. Ges. Virusforsch., *16*:5-18, 1965.
7. Chany, C.: Physio-pathologie de la rougeole. Arch. Ges. Virusforsch., *16*:129-137, 1965.
8. Debré, R., and Joannon, P.: La Rougeole. Epidémiologie, Immunologie, Prophylaxie. Paris, Masson, 1926.
8a. Debré, R.: La prévention de la rougeole par le sérum de convalescents (Méthode de Charles Nicolle et E. Conseil). Sem. Hôp. Paris, *42*:1875-1878, 1966.
9. De Maeyer, E., and Enders, J. F.: Growth characteristics, interferon production and plaque formation with different lines of Edmonston measles virus. Arch. Ges. Virusforsch., *16*:151-160, 1965.
10. Enders, J. F., Katz, S. L., and Medearis, D. N., Jr.: Recent advances in knowledge of measles virus. In: Pollard, M. (ed.): Perspectives in Virology. New York, Wiley, 1959, pp. 103-120.

1. Enders, J. F.: A consideration of the mechanisms of resistance to viral infection based on recent studies of the agents of measles and poliomyelitis. Trans. Coll. Physicians Phila., *28*:68-79, 1960.

2. Enders, J. F.: Measles virus. Historical review, isolation, and behavior in various systems. Amer. J. Dis. Child., *103*:282-287, 1962.

3. Fulginiti, V. A., Eller, J. L., Downie, A. W., and Kempe, G. H.: Altered reactivity to measles virus. J.A.M.A., *202*:1075-1080, 1967.

4. Gresser, I., and Katz, S. L.: Isolation of measles virus from urine. New Eng. J. Med., *263*:452-454, 1960.

5. Gresser, I., and Chany, C.: Isolation of measles virus from the washed leucocytic fraction of blood. Proc. Soc. Exp. Biol. Med., *113*:695-698, 1963.

6. Jong, J. G. de: The survival of measles virus in air, in relation to the epidemiology of measles. Arch. Ges. Virusforsch., *16*:97-102, 1965.

7. Karelitz, S.: Does modified measles result in lasting immunity? J. Pediat., *36*:697-703, 1950.

8. Karelitz, S.: Measles vaccine and immunity. J. Indian Pediat. Soc., *1*:403-411, 1962.

9. Katz, S. L., Medearis, D. N., and Enders J. F.: Experiences with a live attenuated measles virus. A.M.A. J. Dis. Child., *96*:430-431, 1958.

20. Katz, S. L., and Enders, J. F.: Measles virus. In: Horsfall, F. L., and Tamm, I. (eds.): Viral and Rickettsial Infections of Man. 4th ed. Philadelphia, Lippincott, 1965, pp. 784-804.

21. Kempe, C. H., and Fulginiti, V. A.: The pathogenesis of measles virus infection. Arch. Ges. Virusforsch., *16*:103-129, 1965.

22. Lennon, R. G., and Isacson, P.: Delayed dermal hypersensitivity following killed measles vaccine. J. Pediat., *71*:525-529, 1967.

23. Lorenz, E., and Rossipal, E.: Zur Frage der Resistenzminderung bei Masern. Mschr. Kinderheilk., *113*:161, 1965.

24. McCrumb, F. R., Jr., Kress, S., Saunders, E., Snyder, M. J., and Schluederberg, A. E.: Studies with live attenuated measles-virus vaccine. I. Clinical and immunologic responses in institutionalized children. Amer. J. Dis. Child., *101*:701-707, 1961.

25. Mayer, J. B.: Masern (Morbilli). In: Gsell, O., and Mohr, W. (eds.): Infektions Krankheiten. Berlin, 1967, pp. 455-519.

26. Meyer, H. M., Jr., et al.: Ecology of measles in monkeys. Amer. J. Dis. Child., *103*:307-313, 1962.

27. Nader Ph. R., Horwitz, M. S., and Rousseau, J.: Atypical exanthem following exposure to natural measles: eleven cases in children previously inoculated with killed vaccine. J. Pediat., *72*:22-28, 1968.

28. Papp, K., Molitor, I., and Ory, I.: Expériences prouvant que la voie d'infection de la rougeole est la contamination de la muqueuse conjonctivale. Rev. Immun., *20*:27-36, 1956.

29. Papp, K.: Explication du pathomécanisme de la rougeole. Rev. Immun. (Paris), *23*:97-113, 1959.

30. Rauh, L. W., and Schmidt, R.: Measles immunization with killed virus vaccine. Amer. J. Dis. Child., *109*:232, 1965.

31. Ruckle, G., and Rogers, K. D.: Studies with measles virus. II. Isolation of virus and immunologic studies in persons who have had the natural disease. J. Immun., *78*:341-355, 1957.

32. Sergiev, P. G., Ryazantseva, N. E., and Shroit, I. G.: The dynamics of pathological processes in experimental measles in monkeys. Acta Virol. *4*:265-273, 1960.

33. Wilson, G. S.: Measles as a universal disease. Amer. J. Dis. Child., *103*:219-223, 1962.

MEASLES: VIROLOGICAL STUDY AND PROPHYLAXIS

by A. BOUÉ

We owe to the work of J. F. Enders and his co-workers that, from 1954[8] on, techniques for isolating measles virus became available, as did serological techniques of basic importance to progress in understanding the multiple aspects of measles infection. The basic contributions of Enders and his group were destined, moreover, to permit the development of an attenuated strain of virus[6] that is at the origin of most of the live-virus vaccines against measles utilized today.

THE MEASLES VIRUS

The Virus

STRUCTURE. Measles virus is comprised of ribonucleic acid with helical symmetry, within an envelope. Its aspect under the electron microscope has been thoroughly studied, by Waterson et al.[23] in particular; the virus particles, which are roughly spherical, have a diameter between 1200 and 2500 Å, measurement confirming those made by filtration or ultracentrifugation that yielded a diameter of 1400 A.

The virus includes a long nucleocapsid constituted of ribonucleic acid surrounded by units of proteinic structure disposed in a helical pattern, the diameter of the nucleocapsid being 170 Å. This nucleocapsid is contained in a thick envelope of approximately 100 Å with numerous short projections at its surface (Fig. 27-6). The electron microscope preparations often show viral particles with the envelope split open so that long filaments escape from the nucleocapsid. Examination of virus-infected cells revealed that the inclusions were comprised of masses of these elements of the nucleocapsid.

It is tempting to localize the different

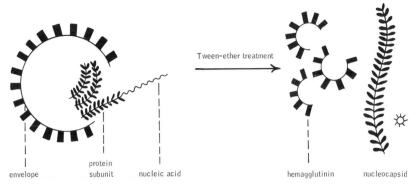

envelope   protein   nucleic acid   hemagglutinin   nucleocapsid
                  subunit

Figure 27-6. Schematic representation of the constituent elements of measles virus.

viral antigens on the elements of the virion: complement-fixing activity is found on the nucleocapsid, but on the envelope, as well. The various constituents of the hemagglutinating activity of the virus are those that have been subjected to the most thorough studies, for, apart from the utilization of this antigen in serological reactions, it was thought possible to prepare, from the starting point of this hemagglutinin, a purified inactivated vaccine devoid of the other viral elements; the research studies on this vaccine are still under way. The hemagglutinin is situated on the viral envelope and is constituted of large and of small particles; they can be separated from the nucleocapsid by Tween-ether treatment.

OTHER PROPERTIES. Measles virus is very sensitive to heat; it is rapidly destroyed at 37° C. and at 20° C. It should preferably be stored at −70° C. Its tolerance to variations in pH is fairly considerable. As noted earlier, it is ether-sensitive.

All these characteristics show that measles virus belongs to the myxovirus group. Waterson[22] divided this group into two subgroups: measles virus figures in the subgroup of large myxoviruses with *Myxovirus parainfluenzae,* mumps virus, and Newcastle disease virus.

Isolation of the Virus. *Cell cultures* represent the sole practical method of isolating the virus.

THE VIRUS'S CYTOPATHOGENIC EFFECT. Described by Enders and Peebles, the lesions produced by measles on cells in culture comprise:

syncytia, giant cells resulting from the fusions of cells that may comprise numerous (more than 100) nuclei, each closely packed against the other (cf. Fig. 2 in the color plate);

spindle cells, so-called because they retract and give an etiolated appearance to the middle of the cellular layer (cf. Fig. 2 in the color plate).

cytoplasmic and nuclear inclusions (cf. Fig. 2 in the color plate):

The nuclear inclusions are eosinophilic and are Feulgen-negative; they spare the nucleolus and are not accompanied by margination of the chromatin; they appear so late that they are rarely noted. The cytoplasmic inclusions are eosinophilic and are found in the syncytia and in the isolated cells; they may be limited in size and fairly dense, or, occasionally, of considerable size, and diffuse (cf. Fig. 2 in the color plate).

The nature, the amount, and the time periods before appearance of the different lesions provoked by the virus differ according to the cellular system used and to the degree of adaptation of the virus strain to these cells.

Numerous cellular systems permit multiplication of measles virus, either immediately or after adaptation. Primary cultures of human or simian renal cells or of human amniotic cells are the most suitable. Measles virus also multiplies in established human cell lines (e.g., Hep 2) or established simian lines (e.g., BSC 1) and on primary dog kidney cells. It can be adapted to other cellular systems, in particular to chick embryo fibroblasts; this adaptation permitted the development of the attenuated strains utilized in vaccines (Edmonston strain).

LABORATORY ANIMALS. The monkey is particularly sensitive to measles; it presents a discrete disease similar to attenuated measles in man.

Approximately a week after intravenous inoculation, a general malaise is apparent and is followed two days later by a maculopapular rash; increase in temperature is slight. This picture is seen only with use of freshly isolated strains; after several passages of these same strains on cell cultures their inoculation provokes a completely inapparent infection.

The major difficulty is to procure receptive animals: the conditions of captivity and of transport of these animals in regions in which measles is endemic in human communities, plus the monkeys' extreme receptivity, mean that almost all the animals, contaminated between their capture and their arrival in laboratories, are already protected by antibodies. These facts explain the irregularity of the results observed at the time of the first attempts to inoculate measles virus into these animals.

Measles virus can also be adapted to the newborn mouse and to the newborn hamster.

SAMPLES

Pharyngeal Samples. The virus is present at the throat level during the days preceding the eruption and immediately after onset of eruption.

The samples should be collected by swabbing the throat with a moistened cotton tab rolled round a wooden stick; the tab is plunged into 1 to 2 ml. of Hank's solution with antibiotics. The sample must be maintained and transported at a temperature far below freezing and the earlier it is utilized to inoculate cell cultures, the better the results will be (ideally, the procedure should be carried out at the patient's bedside).

Blood. The virus is present in the blood immediately before, and at onset of the eruption, until antibodies appear some 48 hours after outburst of the rash.

A good technique is isolation of the virus from the patient's leukocytes by the method proposed by Gresser and Chany:[11] a leukocyte suspension is inoculated onto sensitive cells.

The possibilities of isolating the virus from the urine and from the conjunctival exudate have been reported.

Whatever the method or the material, isolating measles virus is not easy; hope of positive results is limited to a very short period; 48 hours after onset of the eruption, the chances can be considered approximately nil. Moreover, in the first passage, the virus-produced lesions are slow to appear, few in number and discrete; a practiced eye is required to detect them. But, most especially, the quality of the cellular system is an essential element; particularly if, as is recommended, monkey kidney cells are utilized, the known frequency of latent viruses in these cells, some of them provoking formation of giant cells that could be confounded with the lesions produced by measles virus, creates a problem. Hence use of several control tubes is requisite to guarantee the quality of the cells.

Identification of the Virus. Given the difficulties of isolation and the sources of error possible, it is absolutely indispensable to identify the virus even when the aspect of the cellular lesions is suggestive.

The simplest procedure is to perform this identification with use of a specific immune serum by a seroneutralization test.

DETECTION OF THE VIRUS BY IMMUNOFLUORESCENCE OR ELECTRON MICROSCOPY. Among the samples to be effectuated for isolation of the virus, we have not discussed postmortem organ samples.

Except for the isolation by J. F. Enders of measles virus in fatal cases of giant cell pneumopathy,[7] most attempts made under these conditions have failed, in particular in cases of postinfectious encephalitis.

But detection of viral antigens by immunofluorescence may prove to be a method of great interest. This method has been utilized especially in brain sections, and we shall see farther on an application of this technique. The method demands the utmost care and skill, and its results must be interpreted with the utmost prudence.

Electron microscopy makes possible observation of elements of the nucleocapsid within the cells, but this aspect is not specific for measles virus and evidences only the presence of a myxovirus.

SEROLOGICAL METHODS. Three serological techniques are available: seroneutralization in cell culture, complement fixation, and hemagglutination inhibition.

Seroneutralization can be carried out in any of numerous cellular systems. The preferable one is a system to which the virus strains utilized have been adapted and in which characteristic lesions appear rapidly, so as to facilitate reading of the test results.

For the complement-fixation test the Kolmer technique should be used; the antigen can be prepared in cell lines.

Hemagglutination inhibition is the most sensitive technique and is preferable to the others. To increase its sensitivity and precision, use of Tween-ether-treated anti-

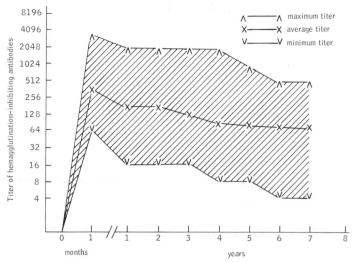

Figure 27-7. Evolution of antibodies against measles in 46 children over a seven-year period. (Adapted from Berman, P. H., and Krugman, S.: Correlation of measles and subacute sclerosing panencephalitis. Neurology, *18*: 91, 1968.)

gens employed according to the Norrby technique[16] is to be recommended.

The evolution of the three types of antibodies is remarkably parallel: they appear as early as the second day following the eruption and attain their maximum titer two to four weeks thereafter (with the hemagglutination technique, the levels are between 1:128 and 1:2048). Antibody levels decrease during the first year (by about one half), and then remain stationary or undergo a slight fall during the following years (Fig. 27-7).

The same pattern being followed by all three types of antibodies, the lifelong persistence of complement-fixing antibodies against measles is striking since it is most unusual in virology; the hypotheses advanced to explain this anomaly of the complement-fixing antibodies lack the support of any scientific proof.

Despite this remarkable relative stability of the antibody level, studies on vaccination have revealed that a booster effect could be observed: after injection of live attenuated vaccine into children already possessing antibodies at a low level (1:4 to 1:16), rise in the antibody level was ascertained (Boué, Katz, and Krugman in separate personal observations) but when the antibody level is originally higher, this booster effect is not observed.

The diagnosis of infection by measles virus must be based on the rise in antibody level between samples, the first being taken at the onset of the illness, and the second, two or three weeks later.

The presence of antibodies, whatever the method used for their detection, is an absolute sign of immunity.

Relationships between Measles Virus and Other Viruses Responsible for Disease in Animals: Distemper Virus and Rinderpest Virus. As early as 1945, Pinkerton[17] noticed the similarity of the anatomical lesions in measles pneumopathy to those in distemper pneumopathy; more recently, giant cells like those due to measles virus were observed in cattle with rinderpest.[18]

The kinship between these three viruses is manifest.

The lesions in cell cultures are absolutely identical, and Shishido[21] adapted these three viruses to the same monkey cell line (Vero); on these cells he observed the same lesions with the three viruses. Under the electron microscope, the aspect of the three viruses is identical. Immunological relationships exist between these three viruses: for example, a young puppy is protected against distemper by inoculation of measles virus or of rinderpest virus. In man, after measles, the blood can be shown to contain not only antibodies against measles but also antibodies against distemper. Nonetheless, the attempts to vaccinate man against measles with a vaccine against distemper result in antibodies detectable against distemper alone and in no antibodies against measles.

Hence an antigenic community between these viruses is unquestionable, but it is only partial; the question can be raised as to whether other viruses as yet unknown do not also have antigenic relationships with these three viruses.

The facts mentioned make difficult the interpretation of research tending to demonstrate the presence or the role of measles virus on the basis of exclusively immunological arguments.

Measles Virus and Subacute Sclerosing Panencephalitis. One of the most recent aspects of research on measles concerns the role that the virus might have in the etiology of subacute sclerosing panencephalitis.

In 1962 Adams and Imagawa[1] noted that in subjects with multiple sclerosis the level of antibodies against measles is higher than the average level in a comparable normal population; moreover, these antibodies can be detected in the cerebrospinal fluid whereas they are not found there in normal subjects. But research investigations have been oriented mainly toward subacute sclerosing panencephalitis; numerous case reports[4] have confirmed the first observations in this regard published by Connolly[5] in 1967.

1. In children with encephalitis, the level of antibodies against measles virus detected by complement fixation, by hemagglutination inhibition, or by immunofluorescence[14] is significantly higher than in normal children. The level of these antibodies during the evolution of the disease may be subject to great increases or decreases even when the children had had measles several years earlier. Thus Berman and Krugman[2] reported antibody titers evolving between 1:16,000 and 1:1000 seven years after the eruption, figures much higher than those found by these authors in normal children (Fig. 27-7).

2. These antibodies can be detected in the cerebrospinal fluid, in which they may also attain fairly high levels.

3. The examinations of histological sections of the brain from necropsy specimens have made it possible to detect measles antigens by the techniques of direct and of indirect immunofluorescence. The cellular localization of the antigens revealed by the fluorescence corresponds to that of the inclusions.

4. The examinations made with the electron microscope have shown, in the nuclear inclusions, structures very comparable to elements of the nucleocapsid of viruses belonging to the group of the large myxoviruses. These observations, first made by Bouteille et al.,[3] have been confirmed by different other authors.

Rustigian[19] obtained experimentally cell lines chronically carrying measles virus antigens and in which detection of the virus in its infectious form proved impossible.

Research by the Wistar Institute shed new light on the problem: Katz et al.[13] seemed to have succeeded in transmitting subacute sclerosing encephalitis to the ferret. The fact that the ferret is a receptive animal strongly confirms that a myxovirus is involved, but these authors believe that it is not measles virus.

Recently several research workers have established cell cultures from necropsy samples. With the help of certain culture techniques, they have obtained the reappearance of the virus in its infectious form: the virus is that of measles.

Today a whole group of arguments leads to the conclusion that measles virus is associated with subacute sclerosing panencephalitis. An important question remains to be answered: what is the role of measles virus in the disease?

VACCINATION AGAINST MEASLES

The Vaccines. Research efforts developed in two directions: toward the selection of strains of attenuated viruses enabling preparation of live vaccines, and toward the preparation of inactivated vaccines.[12, 20]

The Attenuated Live Vaccines. The first strain of attenuated virus was to emerge from the laboratory of J. Enders:[6] starting from the Edmonston strain from the first isolate achieved by this group of workers, they achieved a progressive attenuation by successive passages on different cell systems (human renal cells and human amniotic cells) and especially by adaptation to, and numerous passages on, chick embryo cells. This first attenuated vaccine, tested experimentally from 1958 on, yielded an excellent degree of immunity, but the reactions remained frequent and more or less severe, necessitating the injection of gamma globulins in association with the vaccine.

From the starting point of this Edmonston strain attenuated by Enders or from that of other viral strains, numerous investigators obtained strains of virus further attenuated than Enders' initial vaccine (hyperattenuated strains of Schwarz, Beckenham, Belgrade, Leningrad, Moraten, for example).

INACTIVATED VACCINES. In parallel, research work developed that led to preparation of inactivated vaccines. Two pathways of research were followed:

1. Preparation of vaccines inactivated according to the classic procedures used for other viral vaccines (inactivation by formaldehyde, for example); various improvements have made it possible to obtain vaccines of satisfactory antigenic potency:

2. Preparation of vaccines constituted by the purified viral *hemagglutinin* after Tween-ether treatment of the virus according to Norrby's technique.[16]

But the occurrence of reactions attributed to phenomena of delayed hypersensitivity that are still ill elucidated caused these vaccines to be abandoned. In the children vaccinated with the inactivated vaccines, two types of incidents were observed: (1) severe local reactions (erythema, edema, vesicular or hemorrhagic lesions, adenopathies) on ulterior injection several months or several years later of live vaccine for the purpose of reinforcing immunity;[10] and (2) generalized systemic reactions[9] of occasionally striking amplitude (acute febrile syndrome, pneumonia, atypical eruption commencing on the feet and mounting from there over the whole body) when these children were exposed to the virus during measles epidemics supervening several years after the injection of the inactivated vaccine.

Research on the preparation of purified hemagglutinin vaccines continues, but several years' observation is required to make it possible to certify that these vaccines do not provoke the same phenomena of delayed hypersensitivity.

On the basis of the data at our disposal today, vaccination can be considered applicable in practice only with live hyperattenuated virus vaccines.

The Vaccination. Vaccination comprises a single subcutaneous injection. The presence of transferred maternal antibodies is an obstacle to multiplication of the virus, and for maximum success, this vaccination is recommended only in those over age 10 months.

The reactions due to injection of hyperattenuated virus vaccine are very slight: mainly rise in temperature occurring about a

week after the injection, of short duration (one to two days, average), rarely exceeding 39.5° C. (103.1° F.); higher fever occurs in 5 to 15 per cent of vaccinated subjects without any other systemic sign; a very discrete and fugitive exanthem may be observed in 2 to 5 per cent of cases. On the other hand, when vaccinations are effectuated in closed collectivities, the incidents may be more frequent; they might be linked to more or less latent intercurrent infections aggravated or revealed by the vaccination; but, even in these cases, the reactions have never presented a serious character.[20]

A very detailed study of neurological disturbances occurring in the month following the vaccination was made in the United States.[15] The conclusion of this report was that the number of cases reported was inferior to that of encephalitic manifestations of unknown origin observed in a nonvaccinated population of children during an equivalent period.

It can therefore be stated with certitude that the vaccination produces only minor clinical incidents and that the use on a massive scale of this vaccination in certain populations, that of the United States for example, confirms the benign character of these reactions.

Quality and Duration of the Immunity. Estimated by antibody titration, the conversion rate is above 95 per cent in measles-receptive children. After a slight fall of antibody level during the first year following vaccination (as in the natural disease), the antibody level remains stable in the years following (the length of observation is now eight years for the hyperattenuated vaccines).

Epidemiological studies have shown that

Table 27-2. *Number of Cases of Measles Registered in the United States Since 1957**

1957	487,000	
1958	763,000	
1959	406,000	
1960	441,000	
1961	424,000	
1962	481,000	Doses of vaccine utilized
1963	385,000	3,180,000
1964	458,000	3,820,000
1965	262,000	6,000,000
1966	204,000	8,000,000
1967	62,000	—
1968	22,500	—

*Established according to documents of the United States Public Health Service.

the vaccinated children were resistant to the disease several years after vaccination.

In countries in which the entire population of children has been vaccinated, measles disappears; this is particularly striking in the United States (Table 27-2).

Indications for the Vaccination

SYSTEMATIC VACCINATION OF CHILDREN. With live vaccine against measles, can mass vaccination be envisaged, as for vaccination against poliomyelitis, that would tend—if not to eradicate the disease, which seems utopic—at least to make cases of measles rare?

In countries with a high living standard this is what is being attempted and we see in Table 27-2 the results recorded. Although in such countries measles no longer presents the gravity that it had up to the beginning of the century, it still has encephalitic complications. But such systematic vaccination is recommended for socioeconomic reasons since the child's illness—apart from what it costs—leads to the mother's being housebound for one or two weeks and to loss of her time from work.

But it is above all in the countries where measles is an important cause of mortality in children that this systematic vaccination should be developed (for example, in Latin American countries and in Africa). Vaccination campaigns have already been carried out in some of these countries. But several difficulties have arisen: (1) The material organization of mass vaccination necessitates qualified personnel: the vaccine is lyophilized and, once reconstituted, it is very fragile and should be injected immediately. Collective vaccination with jet gun (Dermojet or similar apparatus) has been successful when all the material was handled by practiced teams, but has yielded an unpredictable percentage of failures when carried out by a local personnel of low competence. The almost endemic character of measles in these regions and the high sensitivity of very small children, between 6 and 18 months old, requires vaccination at an early age. After spectacular results of the first mass campaigns, their spacing out owing to an excessively slow rotation of the vaccination teams has permitted epidemic outbreaks among the young children not yet vaccinated.

Although the introduction of vaccination against measles represents a considerable step forward in the fight against infantile mortality, great rigor in its application is requisite to its success.

VACCINATION OF CERTAIN CATEGORIES OF CHILDREN. In the countries that may not adopt systematic vaccination against measles in the near future, the most important indications of this vaccination are:

1. Certain conditions in children that make measles a serious risk. For example, asthmatics, patients with respiratory insufficiencies, patients with cardiac disease, and children with mucoviscidosis or with congenital adrenal hyperplasia should be vaccinated (vaccination with the hyperattenuated live vaccine is very well tolerated by such children).

2. COLLECTIVITIES. It would be desirable to apply this vaccination in all collectivities of children, in which measles epidemics can be serious, disorganize the operation of the institution, and hence encourage prevention by gamma globulins which even apart from its costliness, provides only transitory immunity.

3. EPIDEMIC PERIODS. Owing to the introduction of the attenuated virus by the subcutaneous route, the cycle of the virus vaccine in the organism is shortened from three to five days in comparison with the normal cycle of the wild virus in the natural disease. This "grace period" can be utilized for prevention of the disease after contact with a source of infection. All the trials effectuated in collectivities of very young children have confirmed the value of this protection, and the injection of live vaccine should now replace the injection of gamma globulins in all the cases in which total prevention of the disease should be sought.

Contraindications. These are the contraindications common to all live vaccines: leukemia and generalized malignant syndromes, treatments with corticosteroids, and pregnancy.

BIBLIOGRAPHY

1. Adams, J. M., and Imagawa, D. T.: Measles antibodies in multiple sclerosis. Proc. Soc. Exp. Biol. Med., *111*:562, 1962.
2. Berman, P. H., and Krugman, S.: Correlation of measles and subacute sclerosing panencephalitis. Neurology, *18*:91, 1968.
3. Bouteille, M., Fontaine, C., Vedrenne, C., and Delarue, J.: Sur un cas d'encéphalite subaiguë à inclusions. Etude anatomoclinique et ultrastructurale. Rev. Neurol., *113*:454, 1965.
4. Conference on measles virus and subacute sclerosing panencephalitis. Neurology, Vol. 18, part 2, 1968.
5. Connolly, J. H., Allen, I. V., Hurwitz, L. J., and

Millar, J. M. D.: Measles virus antibody and antigen in subacute sclerosing panencephalitis. Lancet, *1*:542, 1967.

6. Enders, J. F., Katz, S. L., Milovanovic, M. V., and Holloway, A.: Studies on an attenuated measles virus vaccine. 1. Development and preparation of the vaccine: technics for assay of effects of vaccination. New Eng. J. Med., *263*:153, 1960.

7. Enders, J. F., McCarthy, K., Mitus, A., and Cheatham, W. J.: Isolation of measles virus at autopsy in cases of giant-cell pneumonia without rash. New Eng. J. Med., *261*:875, 1959.

8. Enders, J. F., and Peebles, T. C.: Propagation in tissue cultures of cytopathogenic agents from patients with measles. Proc. Soc. Exp. Biol. Med., *86*:277, 1954.

9. Fulginiti, V. A., Arthur, J. M., Pearlman, D. S., and Kempe, C. H.: Altered reactivity to measles virus. Amer. J. Dis. Child., *115*:671, 1968.

10. Fulginiti, V. A., Eller, J. J., Downie, A. W., and Kempe, C. H.: Altered reactivity to measles virus. J.A.M.A., *202*:1075, 1967.

11. Gresser, I., and Chany, C.: Isolation of measles virus from washed leucocytic fraction of blood. Prqc. Soc. Exp. Biol. Med., *113*:695, 1963.

11a. Hillman, M. R., Buynak, E. B., Weibel, R. E., Stokes, J., Jr., Whitman, J. E., Jr., and Leagus, M. B.: Development and evaluation of the Moraten measles virus vaccine. J.A.M.A., *206*:587-590, 1968.

12. International Conference on Measles Immunization. Amer. J. Dis. Child., March, 1962.

13. Katz, M., Rorke, L. B., Masland, W. S., Koprowski, H., and Tucker, S. H.: Transmission of an encephalitogenic agent from patients with subacute sclerosing panencephalitis to ferrets. Meeting of the American Pediatric Society, March, 1968.

14. Lennette, E. H., Magoffin, R. L., and Freeman, J. M.: Immunologic evidence of measles virus as an etiologic agent in subacute sclerosing panencephalitis. Neurology, *18*:21, 1968.

15. National Communicable Disease Center, Measles surveillance. Report No. 6. 17 April, 1967. U.S. Dept of Health Education and Welfare.

16. Norrby, E.: Hemagglutination by measles virus. Arch. Ges. Virusforsch., *12*:153, 1962.

17. Pinkerton, H., Smiley, W. L., and Anderson, W. A. D.: Giant cell pneumonia with inclusions, a lesion common to Hecht's disease, distemper and measles. Amer. J. Path., *21*:1, 1945.

18. de Rudder, J.: La rougeole. In: Lépine, P.: Techniques de laboratoire en virologie humaine. Paris, Masson, 1964.

19. Rustigian, R.: Persistent infection of cells in culture by measles virus. J. Bact. *92*:1792, 1804, 1966.

20. Séminaire sur l'épidémiologie et la prévention de la rougeole. (Centre international de l'enfance, Paris, 1964.) Arch. Ges. Virusforsch., vol. 16, 1965.

21. Shishido, A., Yamanouchi, K., Hikita, M., Sato, T., Fukuda, A., and Kobune, F.: Development of a cell culture system susceptible to measles, canine distemper and rinderpest viruses. Arch. Ges. Virusforsch., *22*:364, 1967.

22. Waterson, A. P.: Two kinds of myxovirus, Nature, *193*:1163, 1962.

23. Waterson, A. P.: Measles virus. Arch. Ges. Virusforsch., *16*:57, 1965.

RUBELLA: CLINICAL FEATURES
by C. ATTAL AND P. MOZZICONACCI

Rubella is an acute infectious disease, characterized by a maculopapular rash, adenomegalies, and a general syndrome, all of them discrete. For a long time the only problem was to distinguish between rubella and measles in diagnosis. Since 1941, when Gregg first described congenital malformations following a rubella epidemic, this disease has attracted considerable attention. Its teratogenic action has become the subject of extensive research.

It proved possible to transmit the disease to monkeys (Hess, 1914; Habel, 1942) and to children (Hiro and Tasaka, 1938). The virus, however, was not successfully cultured until recently (Weller and Neva[72]; Parkman, 1962). In 1964, an epidemic spread on a broad front over practically the whole of the United States. It led to new progress in the study of rubella and the description of new clinical involvements. The epidemic also gave rise to a statistical, virological, and im- munological study that has shed entirely new light on the pathology of this disease.

CLINICAL DESCRIPTION

TYPICAL FORM

In its typical form, rubella is comparatively easy to identify.

Incubation. Its incubation is asymptomatic. The average incubation period is 16 to 18 days (Krugman[30a]) or 17 days (Bradford). Extremes may vary from 14 to 21 days.

Invasion. Invasion by the disease in the young child is not heralded by any clinical symptoms. The rash is the first sign of the illness. A brief invasion period is rather frequently noted in adolescents and adults, rarely lasting any longer than a few hours or a day. It is marked by moderate fever, slight headache, loss of appetite, and a vague, general feeling of discomfort. A slight catarrh of the upper respiratory tract (Krugman[30a]) or a conjunctival irritation has been observed in some cases. Physical examination may reveal a micropolyadenopathy even at this stage.

Less frequently, a discrete enanthema may be found, composed of minute red spots, and localized on the palate (Forchheimer's sign). These spots are by no means characteristic and may be observed in numerous virus infections. All these signs vanish as soon as the rash appears, or last no longer than 24 hours.

Active Stage. The active stage is marked primarily by a rash, which is, moreover, quite frequently the first symptom of the disease.

THE RASH. The rash always starts on the cheeks, which acquire a bright red coloring, either evenly or in stripes. It then spreads to the neck, arms, trunk, and legs. This process is completed within 24 hours and is much faster than in measles. Occasionally, the rash may be generalized right from the onset. The palms of the hands, the soles of the feet, and the scalp remain unaffected.

The rash is made up of tiny pinhead-sized maculopapules. Alternatively, they may be slightly elongated, 2 to 3 mm. in diameter. They are separated by intervals of healthy skin, but they may join here and there, presenting a scarlatina-like aspect.

The maculae are smaller than in measles, and, most important, they are a shade paler, more pink than red.

The rash lasts a maximum of three days. Most often it begins to fade after 24 hours. The face clears up first, then the trunk.

If the rash is intense it may be followed by faint desquamation. The latter is discrete in the majority of cases. It may remain localized on the face and trunk and appear as a faint diffuse redness, dotted with small darker spots.

The rash is not accompanied by pruritus or by a feeling of warmth.

ADENOPATHIES. Adenopathies are almost a constant finding. They have been noted even in the forms of the disease with a faint and evanescent rash, as well as in those where the rash is altogether absent. They should in themselves determine the diagnosis in times of epidemic, or when contagion is known to exist. They sometimes precede the rash by a week, as in the experimental observations by Krugman.[30a] Adenopathies appear predominantly at the back of the neck, along the sternocleidomastoid and in the mastoidal and suboccipital regions, but the submaxillary, axillary, epitrochlean, and inguinal lymph nodes may also be affected.

The swelling of lymph nodes is especially noticeable on the first day of the rash; the nodes never become very big and do not exceed the size of a hazelnut. On rare occasions they are a little sensitive. The skin covering them remains normal. The swelling continues for two or three weeks, sometimes even longer.

Adenopathies are not pathognomonic of rubella. Other virus diseases may be accompanied by lymph node involvement of the same type (measles, infectious mononucleosis, various rashes caused by adenoviruses). Their frequency and importance in rubella are, however, such that, by themselves, they sometimes suggest the diagnosis.

SPLENOMEGALY. A discrete splenomegaly may be noted sometimes at the onset of the rash. Its frequency is variable. Raybaud[51] found it in 53.8 per cent of his cases.

MODIFICATIONS IN THE BLOOD COUNT. The frequency of blood modifications has been diversely assessed. Blood plasmacytosis, which may attain 15 to 20 per cent of the white count, is not constant. Bernard found from 5 to 10 per cent plasmacytes in 92 per cent of his patients, de L'Hermuzière[34] found them in 50 per cent of his cases, and Raybaud[51] in only 21 per cent. However, American and Australian authors do not appear to attach any particular importance to this fact, and often do not even mention it in their descriptions.

Plasmacytosis is usually present at the beginning of the rash, but probably disappears shortly afterward. Hillenbrand[21] thinks, however, that it continues for a fortnight and may last several months. Raybaud[51] has noted an increase in the number of monocytes more frequently than plasmacytosis. The leukocyte count is generally reduced. However, the blood picture may also remain normal.

There is no parallel between the severity of the disease, the extent and intensity of the rash or the adenomegalies, and modifications in the blood count.

ABATEMENT. The rash disappears in a day or two. The temperature goes back to normal within 24 hours.

ATYPICAL FORMS

Occasionally, the rubella rash becomes diffuse and intense, resembling that of scarlet fever.

Much more frequent and interesting,

however, are the attenuated or inapparent forms of the disease. In such cases, only if the existence of contact is known can a diagnosis be made, and only the isolation of the virus or an increase in the level of antibodies will confirm the diagnosis.

The number of cases of rubella in which there is no rash is difficult to determine. Very often, there is an absence of fever and general discomfort. The clinical expression of the disease is limited to a slight swelling of the occipital or mastoidal lymph nodes, and the patient goes about his business as usual. Therefore, only by a systematic search for the virus and the antibodies can the disease be detected. Brody et al.,[11] Horstmann et al.,[22a] and Sever et al.[59] consider that every second or third case of rubella remains inapparent, whereas Buescher[12] has observed six cases of rubella without rash for every full-blown one. The attention that these cases attract is due to the fact that they can both disseminate the disease and cause malformations in the fetus. It is unfortunately impossible to detect these cases with certainty without the assistance of a highly specialized laboratory. Blood counts, repeated either daily or every second day, sometimes permit identification of either a transient plasmacytosis or a leukopenia with inversion of the blood count. We have seen, however, that modifications in the blood count were not a constant feature. An experimental investigation carried out by Krugman et al.[30a] confirmed the very real occurrence of rubella without rash: of 12 subjects inoculated with the blood and pharyngeal secretions of affected subjects, two had an inapparent disease.

COMPLICATIONS

Complications of rubella are infrequent, and they are observed mainly during widespread epidemics. Superimposed bacterial infections, as occur during measles, have not been observed. Complications are caused either by the direct attack of the virus on normally healthy tissues or organs, or by antigen-antibody conflicts.

Impairments of the Central Nervous System. These may take different aspects:

(1) Encephalitis and meningoencephalitis are much less frequent than in measles and are observed in only one case out of 6000. (See Chapter 9.)

(2) Pure meningeal forms, myelitis and polyradiculoneuritis, have also been described.

Thrombocytopenic Purpura. This is an infrequent complication. Its onset occurs from the second to the eighth day following the outbreak of the rash; this period may even occasionally last until the twelfth day. Its beginning is violent: simultaneously with rising temperature, there appear petechiae, ecchymoses, bleeding from nose and gums, and sometimes hematuria or gastrointestinal hemorrhages. The platelet count falls below 50,000. Sometimes, as in an observation by Svenningsen,[66] the thrombocytes disappear altogether. A slight anemia of the hemolytic type has been concurrently noted in certain cases.

The evolution is ordinarily favorable (23 of 25 cases collected by Wallace[71]). The purpura is rarely complicated by cerebral hemorrhage, and, should this occur, it does so mostly at the onset. In the great majority of cases, cure occurs within two weeks. There have been cases, however, in which thrombocytopenia has persisted for two months. Incidentally, the clinical signs disappear before the hematological modifications.

It is seldom possible to reveal the presence of antiplatelet antibodies (one case in eight, according to Svenningsen[66]). The direct action of the rubella virus on megakaryocytes has not been proved, and the mechanism of this thrombocytopenia remains a mystery.

It is probable that a certain number of cases of so-called idiopathic thrombocytopenic purpura are caused by the rubella virus. Lusher and Zuelzer[39] detected the latter in 15 of 152 patients with purpura.

Arthritis and Synovitis. These are more frequent than was first thought. They occur mainly in female adults and adolescents. In a series of 74 cases of rubella in adults, Fry et al.[17] noted arthritis in approximately 15 per cent in women and 6 per cent in men). However, the same frequency ratio has not been found by all authors who investigated it.

Rubella rheumatism complicates severe cases of rubella. Its onset most frequently occurs toward the second day of the illness, at the time when the rash is beginning to fade (Krugman[30a]). It may, however, precede the fading of the rash, or set in after a longer delay (from the sixth day before, to the fourth day after the rash, according to Chambers and Bywaters[13]). One or more articulations are affected, and almost always the metacarpophalangeal articulations, wrists, and knees. The other joints may also be involved.

Fever, more or less severe pains, swelling, and even articular effusion point to acute articular rheumatism or to rheumatoid arthritis.

The sedimentation rate is accelerated, sometimes moderately. Blood plasmacytosis is variable. Leukopenia is more frequent. The Waaler-Rose test as well as the latex and C-reactive protein tests were negative in the cases observed by Chambers and Bywaters[13] and in those noted by Kantor and Tanner.[27] The latex test was positive in nine cases out of ten according to Johnson and Hall[26] (but these authors also obtained positive tests in the course of two out of seven cases of rubella without arthritis).

Puncture of the synovium yields viscous fluid with a high albumin content, but of nonspecific cytology.[13]

The evolution usually takes a favorable course within some ten days, but it may drag out a full month. No signs of rheumatoid arthritis were detected after two to five years in a series of patients with rubella arthritis (Kantor and Tanner[27]). Arthralgia may, however, persist in certain cases (Lee).

From time to time, rubella may acquire a specific articular tropism, as was the case during an epidemic in Houston (Phillips et al.[48]), where a whole series of patients suffered from severe arthritis subsequent to a rash, which was diagnosed by the detection of viruses and antibodies.

Exceptional Involvements. *Involvement of the myocardium* has been observed with systematic electrocardiograms (Bianchi[6]) during the course of a rubella arthritis. Inversion of the T-waves in the precordial derivations from V_1 to V_4 lasted three weeks, without clinical signs. Quite as exceptionally, a *Stevens-Johnson syndrome* has been described after a case of rubella (Fruehan[16]).

DIAGNOSIS

A clinical diagnosis of rubella is frequently considered in the case of a slightly febrile maculopapular rash that starts with the face, spreads to the trunk, and disappears within one to three days, accompanied almost always by occipital and rear cervical adenopathies and, occasionally, by splenomegaly and blood plasmacytosis.

The characteristics which distinguish rubella from measles and scarlet fever were specified by clinicians a long time ago.

Yet a differentiation of rubella from measles is not always easy. Discrete measles or attenuated measles, e.g., by an injection of gamma globulins, can be misleading. More pronounced adenopathies, especially occipital ones, are in favor of rubella; in favor of measles are oculonasal catarrh and, primarily at the onset of the rash, Koplik's sign. Inversely, rubella may simulate measles. In this case, the absence of respiratory symptoms, cough, conjunctivitis, and high fever permits discarding a diagnosis of measles.

Some severe cases of rubella are suggestive of scarlet fever. However, the skin is not hot and dry, conveying to the touch the rugged feel of grain leather, and the signs are not accentuated in the skin folds. The adenopathy is not merely subangulomaxillary, but also rear cervical and primarily occipital. Finally, the absence of sore throat, tongue modifications, and hemolytic streptococci in the pharyngeal swab will preclude an error.

In fact, the most frequent source of diagnostic errors lies in the varied types of rash caused by numerous viruses which have been identified fairly recently.

Today it is often impossible, except during epidemics, to link up a maculopapular rash with a specific virus. Viruses such as ECHO 16, which was responsible for the "Boston exanthem," or ECHO 9 and 4, may cause exanthems which, owing to their nature and coloring, their seat, and their transience, have been justifiably called rubella-like. It proved possible after identification to attribute a South African "rubella" epidemic to an ECHO virus: hence the neologisms "rubecho" or "echobella" (Phillips et al.[48]).

Adenoviruses were isolated during the course of other exanthems resembling measles or scarlet fever: type 3 (Neva and Enders), type 7 (Dascomb, Sohier), and, more rarely, types 4, 1, or 2.

Viruses of the Coxsackie group more frequently cause vesicular rashes. In certain cases, however, they may cause a rubella-type rash. This also applies to myxoviruses (Pierson) and to reoviruses.

Other fevers accompanied by a rash, such as *exanthema subitum*, may also be mistaken for rubella. Habitually, in these cases, the maculopapules are bigger, less numerous, and located predominantly on the trunk.

Finally, any toxic rash may take on the same aspect. Furthermore, there is very often a risk that this type of rash will be attributed to rubella, in the absence of virological or immunological evidence to the contrary. The apprehension that this diagnosis may cause in the family of a pregnant woman can be allayed only by laboratory examinations.

CONGENITAL RUBELLA

The involvements of congenital rubella are well known today (see also Chapter 61). A great number of studies have been devoted to them since the first descriptions by Gregg (1941) after an Australian epidemic. This work has recently been rounded off, thanks to the isolation and the culture of the virus and to new immunological methods, knowledge utilized in a remarkable series of studies undertaken by American authors during the vast epidemic in the United States in 1963 and 1964. It thus proved possible to describe a syndrome of congenital rubella, distinct in its clinical symptoms from rubella malformations, with which it is frequently associated.

The risk of malformation in a child whose mother acquired rubella during the first weeks of her pregnancy has not always been accurately appreciated. In the years following the publications of Australian authors, and until 1958, the proof of maternal rubella was provided exclusively by questioning the parents. This is the reason for the extraordinarily high figures of the first investigations. Swan et al.[67] considered that 80 to 90 per cent of rubellas occurring in the first quarter of the pregnancy generated embryopathies. An investigation carried out in France by Lamy and Seror arrived at the same conclusions: when rubella occurred between the first and seventh weeks, 95 per cent of the newborn showed malformations (86 per cent, including the eighth week); from the ninth to the twentieth week, the risk still amounted to 20 per cent.

More recent investigations have lessened the pessimism aroused by these authors. Indeed, when it became possible to follow patients and suspects by a systematic search for the virus and the titer of antibodies, it was established that embryopathies were not at all a quasimandatory consequence of rubella. This is one of the most interesting lessons drawn from the study of the 1963-1964 American epidemic.

It has been confirmed that the risk of embryopathies was proportionately higher when rubella occurred earlier in the pregnancy and that during the fourth month this risk decreased drastically, disappearing after this date.

According to different authors and statistics, the number of malformations encountered varies from 10 to 30 per cent. Manson et al.[41] assessed them at 15.6 per cent if the mother had rubella during her first month, 19.7 per cent in the second month, 13 per cent in the third month, and 4.2 per cent in the fourth month. Lundström[36] arrived at lower figures: for the first four months, respectively: 11.1 per cent, 11.5 per cent, 7.9 per cent, and 1.4 per cent. The same author indicated, as a comparison, the global figures of 14 previous investigations, spread between 1946 and 1961, and bearing on the same pregnancy periods; the percentages published were, respectively: 54.8 per cent, 31.4 per cent, 7.1 per cent, and 5.7 per cent. Skinner[63] and Plotkin et al.[50] concluded that there was a 20 per cent global frequency of malformations. Sever et al.[60] arrived at a figure of 10 per cent. Horstmann et al.[22] found eight cases of malformations for 21 mothers who had been ill with confirmed rubella, or 38 per cent. It is not unlikely that certain fluctuations depend on the virulence of the responsible agent and the environment.

All these studies prove that the frequency of embryopathies is less high than originally feared. On the other hand, women who have come into contact with a rubella patient during the first quarter of their pregnancy have, without showing any symptoms of the disease themselves, two and one-half times more malformed children than control subjects (Sever et al.[60]). Cases of inapparent rubella seem, therefore, able to cause embryopathies.

From the clinical point of view, a distinction should be made between congenital malformations as such, and manifestations and complications of the rubella syndrome in the newborn.

CONGENITAL MALFORMATIONS

Fetal Death. The death of the fetus is a well-known possibility subsequent to rubella of the mother. The frequency of spontaneous abortions is, according to Ingalls,[23] in the vicinity of 10 per cent. A study of 826 women affected by a virus during their pregnancy (Siegel et al.[62]), concludes that the percentage is 20.4. Among the viruses causing abortion, rubella takes second place, after mumps (27.3 per cent) and before epidemic hepatitis (16.7 per cent) and measles (15.8

per cent). Among control subjects without a virus disease, the number of interrupted pregnancies amounted to 13 per cent.

Premature Delivery. Premature delivery is a comparatively frequent occurrence. Moreover, practically all babies who have reached full term have both an inadequate weight and height at birth. Their average weight is 2.3 to 2.4 kg., and weight at birth below 2 kg. is not infrequent. The number of stillbirths is relatively high (two cases of 54 in Sever's series).

Malformations. The most frequently observed malformations are as follows:

OCULAR MALFORMATIONS. Among the ocular malformations, first place is taken by cataract—central and subtotal at birth, more often bilateral. It is frequently accompanied by microphthalmia. Its surgical correction is difficult and almost always incomplete. (See Chapter 56.)

Other ocular anomalies are possible, such as transient clouding of the cornea, glaucoma, floating bodies in the anterior chamber, buphthalmia, and atrophy of the iris.

Impairment of the retina is often masked by the cataract. An isolated chorioretinitis may sometimes be observed, with pepper and salt change around the macula or the papilla.

CARDIAC MALFORMATIONS. These have been encountered in 30 to 70 per cent of all cases in observations by different authors. Persistence of the ductus arteriosus is the most common malformation. Cases of interauricular or interventricular communication have been reported, as well as Fallot's tetralogy, aortic or pulmonary stenosis, coarctation of the aorta, Eisenmenger's complex, and transposition of the great vessels.

Among a total of 426 cardiac malformations, Stuckly was able to prove that rubella had been the cause of 44. It is, moreover, probable that this figure errs on the conservative side.

DEAFNESS. Total or partial deafness is extremely frequent (see Chapter 61). It is often belatedly recognized when the child attains school age. This may explain the very considerable discrepancies among the reports of the observers. Furthermore, when deafness is an isolated phenomenon, it is not always easy to prove its origin in rubella.

The physiopathology of the deafness is not fully known. Some physicians think that it is caused by a hemorrhage of the middle ear. Others think in terms of central lesions. Still others refer to the lysis of basal cochlear membrane cells (see Chapter 57).

INVOLVEMENT OF THE NERVOUS SYSTEM. Impairment of the nervous system is expressed by microcephalia and mental retardation. Its frequency is not known and probably varies from one epidemic to another. Among the pupils in an institution for retarded children, Skinner[63] determined only 0.9 per cent of rubella encephalopathies. However, even in cases in which the nervous system does not appear to be impaired, slowness at school has been observed (Lundström[37]). Sheridan,[61] on the other hand, when examining children between eight and 11 years of age, found them to be normally intelligent.

DENTAL MALFORMATIONS. Anomalies of the teeth have been carefully studied by Lundström.[38] Cutting of the first tooth is retarded. Later, the number of teeth is below normal (at 14 months it is 8.6 instead of 9.9). Characteristically one or several incisors are missing. Anomalies of shape can also be observed (pointed teeth). Damage to enamel is infrequent.

RETARDED GROWTH. This has frequently been noted among these children.

MULTIPLE MALFORMATIONS. Multiple malformations, affecting practically every organ system (except the urinary system), have been reported during rubella epidemics: meningocele, cryptorchidism, intestinal atresia, syndactyly, and hypospadias. However, it has not always been possible to ascertain the origin.

HISTOLOGICAL FINDINGS. The histological features of fetuses after the interruption of pregnancy have shown the extreme diffusion and the high frequency of microscopic anomalies (68 per cent of the fetuses examined by Tondury and Smith[69]), present even in cases in which the fetus did not display gross malformations. Tondury and Smith noted cellular and necrotic lesions without inflammatory reaction. These foci of cellular lesions were found in the chorionic epithelium, in the endothelial lining of vessels, in the myocardium, in muscles, and, particularly often, in the crystalline lens, the inner ear, and teeth. For all cases of rubella that occurred before the eleventh week, the authors found evidence of cardiac lesions in 53 per cent of the cases, the crystalline lens in 45 per cent, muscles in 18 per cent and the inner ear in eleven per cent. The affected cells display a pyknotic nucleus and a cytoplasmic swelling, occasionally with eosinophilic inclusions and vacuoles. The frequency of placenta lesions shows convincingly that this is the port of entry for the infection. Alford et al.[1] detected the virus in the placenta in 61 per cent of their cases, whereas only 30 per cent of the fetuses were virus carriers.

THE RUBELLA SYNDROME IN THE NEWBORN

This syndrome was studied during the American epidemic.

The research by Alford et al.,[1] made it known that the virus could be cultured from the placenta, the amniotic fluid, and all fetal tissues a long time after rubella, when the mother had voluntarily interrupted her pregnancy. Later on, systematic throat swabs, urine and blood samples, bone marrow, and rectal secretions cultured on the cells of green monkeys provided evidence of the virus in the newborn, i.e., several months after contamination by rubella (Rudolph et al.[55]; Plotkin et al.[50]). The virus can continue to exist and be cultured even several months after birth (Alford et al.[1]; Cooper et al.[14]).

The number of virus carriers decreases with age. During the first month of life, Phillips et al.[49] found positive throat cultures in 32 per cent of the children whose mothers had had rubella. At the third month of life only 15 per cent were virus carriers. Some of these children had malformations. Others were apparently unaffected. Horstmann et al.[22] found in children affected by the neonatal rubella syndrome that 82 per cent were virus carriers at birth, 70 per cent at the age of one month, 50 per cent at three months, and 8 to 18 per cent from the sixth to the ninth months of life.

Neutralizing antibodies are demonstrable in the blood of these children. The titer remains high in children with congenital rubella, whereas it decreases in healthy subjects. It would seem that the production of antibodies begins in utero.

At the outset, 19S immunoglobulins are developed. Then, 7S immunoglobulins are produced after the third month; 7S immunoglobulins of maternal origin and 19S immunoglobulins of fetal origin are concurrently found in newborn infants.

This remarkable chronicity of rubella acquired in utero may explain the multiplicity of malformations.

The continued presence of the virus in the newborn is the cause of the neonatal rubella syndrome, the clinical symptoms of which are extremely varied.

Thrombocytopenic Purpura. Thrombocytopenic purpura is very frequent: 40 per cent of all newborns in the series of Plotkin et al.[50] and 70 per cent in that of Cooper et al.[14] If the patients of Horstmann et al.,[22] Korones et al.,[29, 30] and Rudolph et al.[56] are added to those of these two authors, the average is 58.7 per cent. If a decrease in the platelet count below 140,000, without purpura, is included, the percentage is 65.3 (Heggie[18]).

The clinical and hematological picture does not differ from that of an acute idiopathic purpura. Cutaneous hemorrhages and hemorrhages of mucous membranes do not display any specific features. Cerebromeningeal hemorrhages may be observed at the onset. The platelet count is usually below 60,000. The megakaryocyte count in the bone marrow is reduced. In some cases there is an associated hemolytic anemia with reticulocytosis and, occasionally, erythroblastemia. Cure occurs within an average of four weeks.

Hepatosplenomegaly. A more or less pronounced hepatosplenomegaly is noted in 75 per cent of the cases. A certain number of cases of neonatal hepatitis may be due to rubella (Stern and Williams[65] and Alagille[1a]).

Myocardial Necrosis. Apart from the previously described cardiac malformations, seven patients with myocardial necrosis were found in a series of 22 cases (Korones et al.[30]).

Bone Lesions. In approximately 36 per cent of the cases (Heggie[18]), the rubella syndrome of the newborn is accompanied by bone lesions. These lesions are metaphyseal, diffuse, and sometimes painful decalcifications. The mechanism is not clear. They are likened to calcification disorders caused by general infection, as in congenital syphilis. Seen through the microscope, the bones are infiltrated by monocytic cells (Korones[29]).

Rudolph et al.[55] think these lesions should rather be connected with a general nutritional disorder, and that they differ from those that are observed during smallpox, vaccinia, inguinal lymphogranulomatosis, or cytomegalic inclusion disease (Sacrez).

Widening of the anterior fontanelle is

frequently noted in these patients (Rudolph et al.[55]).

Pulmonary Disorders. Although pulmonary malformations as such are exceptional in rubella embryopathies, pneumonia was noted in six cases out of 17 (Korones[29]). They were interstitial pneumonias with monocytic infiltration.

Adenomegalies. Adenomegalies have been observed in 32 per cent of the cases (Cooper et al.[14]). Sometimes, in addition, a maculopapular rash completely reproduces rubella.

Neurological Impairment. Impairment of the nervous system is not constant. Korones[29] observed cellularity of the cerebrospinal fluid in three cases and an increase in the protein content in seven. Lindquist et al.[35] observed some discrete neurological impairment in 25 per cent of their patients (bulging of the anterior fontanelle, irritability). Monif and Sever[45] succeeded in isolating the virus in the cerebrospinal fluid and brain of 27 newborn infants who showed clinical signs and symptoms of rubella.

It is probable that this list of manifestations of rubella is not exhaustive. The digestive tract and the gonads may also be invaded by the virus.

Contagion. All these newborn virus carriers are capable of transmitting rubella to nurses, physicians, and the other children in the ward.

TREATMENT AND PROPHYLAXIS

Treatment of rubella in children does not raise any special problems. The benign nature of the disease and its infrequent complications warrant therapeutic abstention. Small doses of aspirin will suffice for the forms of the disease involving fever or arthritis. It is even unnecessary to prescribe bed rest.

Treatment of thrombocytopenic purpura consists primarily in transfusions of fresh blood. Corticosteroid therapy has been added by nearly all authors; it is continued for a month as a safeguard against a relapse. Its effectiveness has been questioned (Lusher and Zuelzer[39]). Svenningsen[66] has used ε-aminocaproic acid, which does not affect the platelet count but which is supposed to exercise a beneficial influence on hemorrhages of the mucous membranes; the dosage is 1 gm. a day per 10 kg. of weight.

Prevention of the disease in pregnant women raises serious problems which have not yet been solved satisfactorily (see the next section).

Surgical treatment of malformations can be appropriate in certain cases. Treatment of the neonatal rubella syndrome may involve corticosteroid therapy, especially in the case of thrombocytopenic purpura or hepatitis. However, the risk of accentuating bone lesions makes caution necessary. Corticosteroids should be prescribed only in the absence of a tendency to spontaneous improvement.

BIBLIOGRAPHY

1. Alford, C. A., Neva, F., and Weller, T. H.: Virologic and serologic studies on human products of conception after maternal rubella. New Eng. J. Med.,
1a. Alagille, D., Habib, E.-C., Gautier, M., Boué, A., and Kocher, S.: L'hépatite de la rubéole néonatale. Arch. Franç. Pédiat., *25*:393-414, 1968.
2. Altman, R.: Rubella virus: Recent advances in its isolation. Clin. Pediat., *2*:433-438, 1963.
3. Babbott, F. L., Jr., Rodenberger, B. M., and Ingalls, T. H.: Rubella. Morbidity in a schoolboy population, 1935-1959, and a comparison with measles, mumps and chicken-pox. J.A.M.A., *178*:542-546, 1961.
4. Banatvala, J. E., Horstmann, D. M., Payne, M. C., and Gluck, L.: Rubella syndrome and thrombocytopenic purpura in newborn infants. New Eng. J. Med., *273*:474-478, 1965.
5. Bernheim, M., and Gilly, R.: La rubéole. Rev. Prat., *10*:1803-1812, 1960.
6. Bianchi, G. N.: Myocarditis in rubella: A case report. Med. J. Aust. *2*:754-755, 1964.
7. Blattner, R. J.: Experimental rubella in human subjects. J. Pediat., *39*:785-787, 1951.
8. Blattner, R. J.: The etiology of rubella. J. Pediat., *62*:147-149, 1963.
9. Blattner, R. J.: Congential rubella: Persistent infection of the brain and liver. J. Pediat., *68*:997-999, 1966.
10. Blomquist, B., Lundstrom, R., and Thoren, C.: Passive immunization against rubella in pregnancy. A follow-up study. Acta Paediat., *49*:653-654, 1960.
11. Brody, J. A., Sever, J. L., McAlister, R., Schiff, G. M., and Cutting, R.: Rubella epidemic on St. Paul Island in the Pribilofs, 1963. I. Epidemiologic, clinical and serologic findings. J.A.M.A., *191*:619-626, 1965.
12. Buescher, E. L.: Behavior of rubella virus in adult populations. Arch. Ges. Virusforsch., *16*:470-476, 1965.
13. Chambers, R. J., and Bywaters, E. G. L.: Rubella synovitis. Ann. Rheum. Dis., *22*:263-268, 1963.
14. Cooper, L. Z., Green, R. H., Krugman, S., Giles, J. P., and Mirick, G. S.: Neonatal thrombocytopenic purpura and other manifestations of rubella contracted in utero. Amer. J. Dis. Child., *110*:416-427, 1965.
15. Dudgeon, J. A., Butler, N. R., and Plotkin, S. A.:

Further serological studies on the rubella syndrome. Brit. Med. J., *2*:155, 1964.

16. Fruehan, A. E.: Erythema multiforme exudativum and arthritis following infection with rubella. New York J. Med., *63*:859-863, 1963.

17. Fry, J., Dillane, J. B., and Fry, L.: Rubella 1962. Brit. Med. J., *2*:833-834, 1962.

18. Heggie, A. D.: Rubella: Current concepts in epidemiology and teratology. Pediat. Clin. N. Amer., *13*:251-266, 1966.

19. Heggie, A. D., and Weir, W. C.: Isolation of rubella virus from a mother and fetus. Pediatrics, *34*: 278-280, 1964.

20. Heggie, A. D., and Weir, W. C.: Rubella in naval recruits: A virologic study. New Eng. J. Med., *271*:231, 1964.

21. Hillenbrand, F. K. M.: Rubella in a remote community. Lancet, *2*:64-66, 1956.

22. Horstmann, D. M., Banatvala, J. E., Riordan, J. T., Payne, M. C., Whittemore, R., Opton, E. M., Florey, C. du V.: Maternal rubella and the rubella syndrome in infants. Amer. J. Dis. Child., *110*: 408-415, 1965.

22a. Horstmann, D. M., Riordan, J. T., Ohtawara, M., and Niederman, J. C.: A natural epidemic of rubella in a closed population. Arch. Ges. Virusforsch., *16*:483-487, 1965.

23. Ingalls, T. H.: German measles and german measles in pregnancy. Amer. J. Dis. Child., *93*:555-558, 1957.

24. Ingalls, T. H., Babbott, F. L., Hampson, K. W., and Gordon, J. E.: Rubella: Its epidemiology and teratology. Amer. J. Med. Sci., *239*:363-383, 1960.

25. Jammet, M. L.: L'embryopathie rubéolique. Rev. Prat., *8*:3649-3658, 1958.

26. Johnson, R. E., and Hall, A. P.: Rubella arthritis: Report of cases studied by latex test. New Eng. J. Med., *258*:743-745, 1958.

27. Kantor, T. G., and Tanner, M.: Rubella arthritis and rheumatoid arthritis. Arthritis Rheum., *5*:378-383, 1962.

28. Kibrick, S.: Rubella and rubelliform rash. Bact. Rev., *28*:452-457, 1964.

29. Korones, S. B.: Congenital rubella syndrome: New clinical aspects with recovery of virus from affected infants. J. Pediat., *67*:166-181, 1965.

30. Korones, S. B., Ainger, L. E., Monif, G. R. G., Roane, J., Sever, J. L., and Fuste, F.: Congenital rubella syndrome: Studies of 22 infants. Myocardial damage and other new clinical aspects. Amer. J. Dis. Child., *110*:434, 1965.

30a. Krugman, S.: Rubella: Clinical and epidemiological aspects. Arch. Ges. Virusforsch., *16*:477-482, 1965.

31. Krugman, S.: Rubella: New light on an old disease. J. Pediat., *67*:159-161, 1965.

32. Krugman, S., and Ward, R.: Rubella. Demonstration of neutralizing antibody in gamma-globulin and re-evaluation of the rubella problem. New Eng. J. Med., *259*:16-19, 1958.

33. Krugman, S., Ward, R., and Jacobs, K. G.: Studies on rubella immunization; demonstration of rubella without rash. J.A.M.A., *151*:285-288, 1953.

34. L'Hermuzière, J. de: Splénomégalie et rubéole. Pédiatrie, *15*:165-169, 1960.

35. Lindquist, J. M., Plotkin, S. A., Shaw, L., Gilden, R. V., and Williams, M. L.: Congenital rubella syndrome as a systemic infection. Studies of affected infants born in Philadelphia, U.S.A. Brit. Med. J., *2*:1401-1406, 1965.

36. Lundstrom, R.: Rubella during pregnancy. A follow-up study of children after an epidemic of rubella in Sweden, 1951, with additional investigations on prophylaxis and treatment of maternal rubella. Acta Paediat., *51*(suppl. 133):5-110, 1962.

37. Lundstrom, R., and Ahnsjo, S.: Mental development following maternal rubella. A follow-up study of children born in 1951-1952. Acta Paediat., *51*(suppl. 135):153-159, 1962.

38. Lundstrom, R., Lysell, L., and Berghagen, N.: Dental development in children following maternal rubella. Acta Paediat., *51*:155-160, 1962.

39. Lusher, J. M., and Zuelzer, W. W.: Idiopathic thrombocytopenic purpura in childhood. J. Pediat., *68*: 971-979, 1966.

40. McCracken, J. S.: Rubella in the newborn. Brit. Med. J., *2*:420-423, 1963.

41. Manson, M. M., Logan, W. D. P., and Loy, R. M.: Rubella and other virus infections during pregnancy. Reports on Public Health and Medical Subjects. No. 101. London, Ministry of Health, 1960.

42. Mellman, W. J., Plotkin, S. A., Morhead, P. S., and Hartnett, E. M.: Rubella infection of human leukocytes. Chromosomal and viral studies. Amer. J. Dis. Child., *110*:473-476, 1965.

43. Meyer, H. M., Jr., Parkman, P. D., and Panos, T. C.: Attenuated rubella virus. II. Production of an experimental live-virus vaccine and clinical trial. New Eng. J. Med., *275*:575-580, 1966.

44. Monif, G. R. G., Avery, G. B., Korones, S. B., and Sever, J. L.: Post mortem isolation of rubella virus from three children with rubella-syndrome defects. Lancet, *1*:723-724, 1965.

45. Monif, G. R. G., and Sever, J. L.: Chronic infection of the central nervous system with rubella virus. Neurology, *16*:111-112, 1966.

46. New rubella syndrome. Brit. Med. J., *2*:1382-1383, 1965.

47. Parkman, P. D., Meyer, H. M., Jr., Kirschstein, R. L., and Hopps, H. E.: Attenuated rubella virus. I. Development and laboratory characterization. New Eng. J. Med., *275*:569-574, 1966.

48. Phillips, C. A., Behbehani, A. M., Johnson, L. W., and Melnick, J. L.: Isolation of rubella virus. An epidemic characterized by rash and arthritis. J.A.M.A., *191*:615-618, 1965.

49. Phillips, C. A., Melnick, J. L., Yow, M. D., Bayatpour, M., and Burkhardt, M.: Persistence of virus in infants with congenital rubella and in normal infants with a history of maternal rubella. J.A.M.A., *193*:1027-1029, 1965.

50. Plotkin, S. A., Oski, F. A., Karnett, E. M., Hervada, A. R., Friedman, S., and Gowing, G.: Some recently recognized manifestations of the rubella syndrome. J. Pediat., *67*:182-191, 1965.

51. Raybaud, A.: Hématologie leucocytaire dans la rubéole. Marseille Med., *103*:224-226, 1966.

52. Reiss, J. S., and Pryles, C. V.: Thrombocytopenia in congenital rubella. New Eng. J. Med., *275*: 264, 1966.

53. Report by the Epidemic Observation Unit of the College of General Practitioners. The infectiousness of rubella. Brit. Med. J., *2*:419-420, 1963.

54. Rubella virus isolation. Public Health Rep., *78*: 149, 1963.

55. Rudolph, A. J., Singleton, E. B., Rosenberg, H. S., Singer, D. B., and Phillips, C. A.: Osseous manifestations of the congenital rubella syndrome. Amer. J. Dis. Child., *110*:428-433, 1965.

56. Rudolph, A. J., Yow, M. D., Phillips, C. A., Desmond, M. M., Blattner, R. J., and Melnick,

J. L.: Transplacental rubella infection in newly born infants. J.A.M.A., *191*:843-845, 1965.

57. Schiff, G. M., Smith, H. D., Dignan, P. St. J., and Sever, J. L.: Rubella: Studies on the natural disease. Amer. J. Dis. Child., *110*:366-369, 1965.

58. Selzer, G.: Virus isolation, inclusion bodies and chromosomes in a rubella-infected human embryo. Lancet, *2*:336-337, 1963.

59. Sever, J. L., Brody, J. A., Schiff, G. M., McAlister, R., and Cutting, R.: Rubella epidemic on St. Paul Island in the Pribilofs, 1963. II. Clinical and laboratory findings for the intensive study population. J.A.M.A., *191*:624-626, 1965.

60. Sever, J. L., Nelson, K. B., and Gilkeson, M. R.: Rubella epidemic, 1964; effect on 6000 pregnancies. Amer. J. Dis. Child., *110*:395-407, 1965.

61. Sheridan, M. D.: Final report of a prospective study of children whose mothers had rubella in early pregnancy. Brit. Med. J., *2*:536-539, 1964.

62. Siegel, M., Fuerst, H. T., and Peress, N. S.: Comparative fetal mortality in maternal virus diseases. A prospective study on rubella, measles, mumps, chickenpox and hepatitis. New Eng. J. Med., *274*:768-771, 1966.

63. Skinner, C. W., Jr.: The rubella problem. Amer. J. Dis. Child., *101*:78-86, 1961.

64. Stark, G.: Rubella retinopathy. An account of six cases. Arch. Dis. Child., *41*:420-423, 1966.

65. Stern, H., and Williams, B. M.: Isolation of rubella virus in a case of neonatal giant-cell hepatitis. Lancet, *1*:283-295, 1966.

66. Svenningsen, N. W.: Thrombocytopenia after rubella (report of two cases). Acta Paediat. Scand., *54*: 97-100, 1965.

67. Swan, C., Tostevin, A. L., and Black, G. H. B.: Final observation on congenital defects in infants following infectious diseases during pregnancy with reference to rubella. Med. J. Aust., *2*:889, 1946.

68. Tartakow, I. J.: The teratogenicity of maternal rubella. J. Pediat., *66*:380-391, 1965.

69. Tondury, G., and Smith, D. W.: Fetal rubella pathology. J. Pediat., *68*:867-879, 1966.

70. Valenti, C.: Cytogenic analysis of abortuses following maternal rubella. Amer. J. Obstet. Gynec., *91*:1141, 1965.

71. Wallace, S. J.: Thrombocytopenic purpura after rubella. Lancet, *1*:139-141, 1963.

72. Weller, T. H., and Neva, F. A.: Propagation in tissue cultures of cytopathic agents from patients with rubella-like illness. Proc. Soc. Exp. Biol. Med., *111*:215-225, 1962.

RUBELLA: VIROLOGY, EPIDEMIOLOGY, PROPHYLAXIS

by A. Boué

CHARACTERISTICS OF RUBELLA VIRUS

Not until 1962 was the rubella virus isolated in tissue cultures. This was accomplished by two groups of American investigators, Weller and Neva in Boston[35] and Parkman et al. in Washington.[23] Knowledge of this virus hence remains limited.[22]

This is a fairly large virus: various estimates based on filtration or electron microscopy attribute to it a size between 100 and 300 mμ. Its density is low, 1.07 gm. per cubic centimeter. Its infectivity is destroyed by ether; it is highly sensitive to heat and to low pH; it is rapidly inactivated at 56° C. and even at 37° C. It is probably an RNA virus. Its different characteristics bring to mind a virus of the paramyxovirus group. A complement-fixing antigen has been demonstrated,[31] and Stewart et al.[33] showed that rubella virus agglutinates blood cells of one-day-old chicks.

VIROLOGICAL AND SEROLOGICAL TECHNIQUES

Laboratory Techniques

Collection of Specimens. The rubella virus is isolated mainly from the throat and nose. These specimens should be taken at the onset of the eruption or, at the latest, within the week following the eruption. The swabs are placed in the liquids usually used in virological research (e.g., Hank's solution) and must be frozen immediately, for the virus is fragile; transfer must also be done in frozen medium.

It is also desirable to take a stool sample. Although rubella virus is rarely isolated from stools, it is sometimes possible to isolate enteroviruses, which are responsible in some instances for rubella-like eruptions. As in all viral infections, a blood sample should be taken at the earliest possible moment and also at a later time (approximately one month). The serum should be decanted rapidly and frozen.

Isolation and Demonstration of Rubella Virus in Tissue Cultures. Different cell systems are susceptible to rubella virus; the action of the virus on these systems permits classifying them into two categories.

1. The first category consists of cell systems in which multiplication of the virus is not accompanied by detectable cellular lesions, but provokes an interference phenomenon that renders this tissue culture insensitive to the inoculation, some days later (ten days in general), of a second virus normally cytopathogenic for the same cell system. This property of rubella virus was demonstrated by Parkman et al. in kidney cells of green monkeys;[24] it was also observed in monkey cell

lines (LLC-MK 2, for example[34]). The viruses used for the interference are either ECHO 11 or Coxsackie A9. On human cells, amniotic cells, and diploid cell strains, the presence of rubella virus can also be detected by interference with Sindbis virus.[3,21]

2. The second category consists of cell systems in which multiplication of rubella virus determines more or less evident cytological lesions. These lesions were observed by Weller and Neva[35] in cultures of human amniotic cells, but are slow to appear (more then three weeks) and require cell cultures that can be maintained in excellent condition. Rubella virus produces lesions in other cellular systems, above all in strains established from rabbit tissues, the RK 13 cell line[17] in particular. But appearance of lesions requires highly precise culture conditions not always easy to reproduce in different laboratories. Moreover, precise titrations are difficult.

In practice, for isolation of the virus, it is best to utilize primary cultures of green monkey kidney cells. Ten days after inoculation of the infected material, 100 TCID^{50} of ECHO 11 virus is added to each tube. Three days later, the tubes are examined. If the cellular layer remains intact, there is interference. Thus the presence of rubella virus should be suspected. But this isolation often requires one or several blind passages,[6] the virus titer obtained during the first passage being insufficient to determine interference. Thus a positive result for isolation of rubella virus can be expected only in two weeks in the exceptionally favorable cases (sensitive cells available, virus produces interference on first passage); usually the procedure will require at least three weeks, after which the virus will have to be identified by a specific antiserum. Unfortunately, in many countries it is difficult to have these cells regularly available in a laboratory. Isolation of the virus is possible in other cellular systems, either in LLC-MK 2 cells, by use of the same procedure as with primary cultures of monkey kidney cells, or in RK 13 cells, in which the virus produces lesions. Systematic blind passages are also required if the results on first passage are negative or doubtful.

Thus it is clear that isolation of the rubella virus is not yet possible in every virology laboratory, since the required cell systems are not currently available in all such laboratories.

The Serological Techniques. Until recently, the same problems that arise for tissue culture also arose for serological techniques. Neutralizing antibodies can be titrated in the different cell systems enumerated above, but the techniques concerned are difficult and slow, and only laboratories doing these tests regularly can be expected to obtain reproducible results. The determination of complement-fixing antibodies requires the preparation of a specific antigen that is difficult to prepare and expensive.

During the autumn of 1966, however, Stewart et al.[33] succeeded in demonstrating the hemagglutinating property of rubella virus and, at the same time, developed a technique for demonstrating hemagglutination-inhibiting antibodies. Rubella virus cultivated in hamster cells (BHK 21 cell line) permits the preparation of an antigen which agglutinates one-day-old chick red blood cells and goose red blood cells. Titration of hemagglutination-inhibiting antibodies is then possible after treatment to rid the sera of the nonspecific inhibitors normally present.

This technique transforms the serological study of rubella and makes it possible to determine precisely, in a few hours, the state of immunity to the infection.

VIROLOGICAL AND SEROLOGICAL STUDY OF THE RUBELLA INFECTION

Since the isolation of the virus it has been possible to undertake detailed studies in the course of experimental infections.[9] The results have been confirmed by laboratory examinations made in the course of the spontaneous disease and, in particular, during epidemics in children's institutions.[12]

Systematic search for the virus has established with precision its presence in the blood, throat, stools, and urine (the studies of Green et al.[9] — Fig. 27-8 — of Schiff et al.,[29] and of Plotkin et al.[27]).

In natural rubella, the virus is found at the level of the throat a week before the eruption, and it is regularly present in the throat during the six days that precede the rash. Schiff et al. showed that, at this time, the titer of the virus in the throat increases progressively, reaching its maximum when the rash appears.

The virus can still be isolated regularly at the throat level during the week that follows the rash; only exceptionally has it been

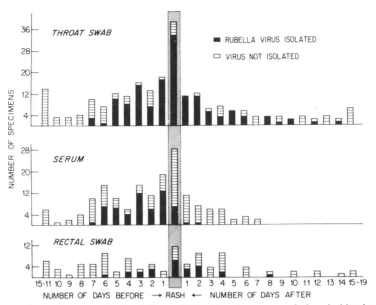

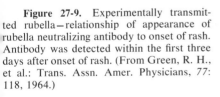

Figure 27-8. Experimentally transmitted rubella—relationship of presence of virus in blood and pharynx to time of appearance of rash. Virus was detected in serum six days before to two days after onset of rash; it was detected in the pharynx seven days before to 14 days after onset of rash. (From Green, R. H., et al.: Trans. Assn. Amer. Physicians, *77*:118, 1964.)

Figure 27-9. Experimentally transmitted rubella—relationship of appearance of rubella neutralizing antibody to onset of rash. Antibody was detected within the first three days after onset of rash. (From Green, R. H., et al.: Trans. Assn. Amer. Physicians, *77*: 118, 1964.)

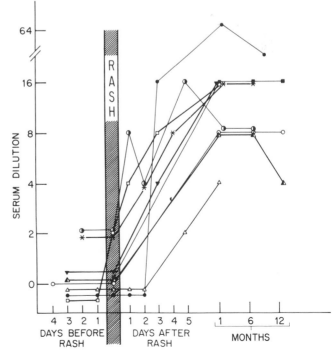

isolated more than two weeks after the rash. Thus virus elimination takes place at the throat level for about two weeks. This long period of contagiousness, and especially its onset well before the eruption, shows the difficulties of effective prophylaxis among pregnant women.

The virus may be isolated from the stools during nearly the same period, but the chances of isolating the virus from stool specimens are much poorer; for this reason, it is preferable to search for the virus in specimens from the throat and nose.

The viremia shows a completely different picture. Isolation of the virus from the blood is frequently possible during the week preceding the eruption but becomes exceptional from the very day the eruption appears. The same is true for the urine, which is thus inappropriate for use in attempts to isolate the virus.

This picture of viral localization is in good accord with results of serological studies (Fig. 27-9); antibodies start to appear from the time of the eruption, which corresponds to the disappearance of the virus from the blood. Nondetectable before the eruption, neutralizing antibodies can be demonstrated from the second or third day after it, their titer reaching a maximum a month afterward. This high level is maintained for six to 12 months, the level diminishing thereafter; the antibodies will, in likelihood, persist at lower levels for the patient's lifetime.

The complement-fixing antibodies also appear shortly after the eruption; their level diminishes progressively, but there seem to be great variations in the persistence of these antibodies, which hence cannot represent a good test of recent infection.

The hemagglutination-inhibiting antibodies seem to evolve similarly to the neutralizing antibodies and are thus also an evidence of immunity.

EPIDEMIOLOGY

ANNUAL AND SEASONAL VARIATIONS

It is not easy to establish a precise picture of the epidemiological characteristics of

Table 27-3. *Rubella in Copenhagen, 1936-1964*

Year	Total No. of Cases	Women Aged 15 to 64 No.	%
1936	1661	247	14.8
1937	189	21	11.1
1938	379	8	2.1
1939	381	12	3.1
1940	2001	366	18.2
1941	9104	1987	21.8
1942	628	29	4.6
1943	643	14	2.1
1944	827	60	7.2
1945	5455	1184	21.7
1946	1739	205	11.7
1947	838	28	3.3
1948	940	38	4.0
1949	1086	44	4.0
1950	1231	45	3.6
1951	1090	19	1.7
1952	970	33	3.4
1953	2634	150	5.6
1954	3922	282	7.1
1955	5246	411	7.8
1956	1130	32	2.8
1957	1296	24	1.8
1958	754	11	1.4
1959	920	37	4.0
1960	1773	117	6.6
1961	648	21	3.2
1962	970	34	3.5
1963	960	58	6.0
1964	3470	317	9.1

ubella. Numerous cases never come to the attention of a doctor, errors in diagnosis are frequent, and cases are declared only exceptionally. These facts make a statistical study difficult.

It would certainly seem that, in Europe, rubella is endemic, with epidemic outbreaks occurring from time to time. This is demonstrated in Table 27-3, which shows the cases of rubella declared in Copenhagen from 1936 to 1964. Likewise, the declarations received by the state of Massachusetts since 1917 show, besides a moderate endemicity, a fairly regular recrudescence of rubella approximately every seven years.[13]

Much better established is the seasonal factor; rubella is a springtime disease. During the last 50 years longitudinal studies made in the United States have shown clearly this annual recrudescence between April and June. Even more precise is the study of the last epidemic in the United States, in which, for the first time, virological study left no doubt concerning the diagnosis.

During the winter and spring of 1964, a considerable epidemic of rubella started in the Atlantic states of the United States, rapidly spreading toward the midwest and the south. The majority of cases were observed from March through June. This epidemic ceased in July, 1964, just as it was reaching the Pacific coast, but it recommenced on the West coast during the winter, attaining its maximum in the spring of 1965, then dis-

appearing during the summer (see Figure 27-10, drawn from the separate graphs published by the Communicable Diseases Center.[28]

These data again show that rubella appears essentially at the end of winter and especially during the spring, whereas summer is very unfavorable to transmission of the virus despite the existence of an abundant source of contamination and a large number of susceptible subjects. These observations were again confirmed by the study of epidemics in the southern hemisphere (New Zealand[16] and the Falkland Islands[11], where epidemics occur during the austral spring, i.e., toward September and October.

The seasonal character is an important element in diagnosis, since many of the rubella-like eruptive diseases of viral origin are due to enteroviruses, and their incidence is higher in summer and in the autumn.

AGE

It seems that rubella generally occurs at a later age than the other common viral diseases of childhood (measles, mumps, chickenpox), but attempts at an estimation, most of them based on questioning of patients, are extremely difficult to interpret. Fry et al.[7] observed during the English epidemic of 1962 the following distribution by age group: 4 per cent of patients under one year, 11 per cent between one and four years, 40 per cent

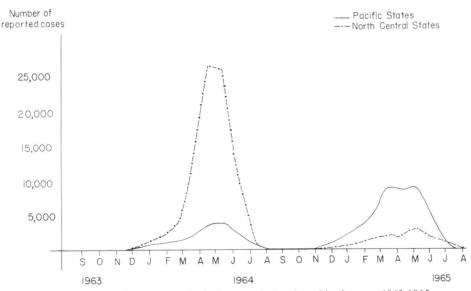

Figure 27-10. Monthly report of rubella cases during the epidemic years 1963-1965.

from five to nine years, 22 per cent from ten to 14 years, and 8 per cent from 15 to 19 years.

The serological studies made during 1963 in Canada[8] and the United States,[32] although oriented toward women aged 15 to 40 years, yielded the figures shown in Table 27-4.

In France, serological surveys undertaken in 1966 and 1967 showed that a high percentage of young women were immune; 90 to 95 per cent of women aged 18 to 30 had antibodies against rubella.

These serological studies confirm the accepted belief that rubella is above all a disease of school-aged children but that a proportion of persons attain adulthood without protection. This proportion can reach alarming size, as was noted by Sever et al.[30] in Hawaii in 1965, where 60 per cent of young women lacked antibodies against rubella.

This phenomenon has been explained by the fact that rubella is less contagious than measles, for example. In the recent epidemics, however, virological studies showed that almost all receptive subjects were infected when they were placed in contact with a patient, although the infection sometimes was inapparent.

The contagiousness is particularly clear in collectivities of school-aged children and in the armed services, where the high proportion of recruits lacking antibodies at the time of their induction results in frequent small epidemics. Thus, in the United States Navy, 33 per cent of recruits of urban origin and 27 per cent of recruits of rural origin lack neutralizing antibodies for rubella and 5 per cent of recruits have clinical rubella in the weeks following their induction.[20]

MODE OF CONTAGION

In view of the constant and prolonged presence of the virus at the throat level in children with rubella, air-borne contamination is most likely. Before the isolation of the virus, the disease was transmitted to volunteers by swabbing the pharynx with pharyngeal secretions taken from patients on the first day of the eruption.

The disease can also be transmitted experimentally by injection of patient's serum up to a dilution of 10^{-3}. This method yields 100 per cent success. The adenopathies appear from the fifth to the eleventh day following the inoculation, with a maximum on the eighth day. The eruption commences about a week later, up to three weeks after the injection.

More recently experimental infections were transmitted by intranasal spray of a suspension of rubella virus grown on tissue cultures; all susceptible children developed a typical rubella.[19]

Recent observations of congenital rubella, which are studied in the preceding section have shown that the newborn eliminate the virus in the throat during the first weeks of life. Infections have thus been observed among the personnel caring for these infants. These highly important observations explain the persistence of the virus between epidemic outbreaks, since the virus eliminated by these children after their birth had been transmitted to them *in utero* several months previously.

Table 27-4. *Percentage of Females in Various Age Groups Showing Immunity Against Rubella: Canada and the United States**

AGE, YR.	SUBJECTS HAVING ANTIBODIES AGAINST RUBELLA VIRUS, %
Canada	
1 - 4	19
5 - 9	27
10 - 14	60
15 - 19	70
20 - 24	80
United States	
14 - 19	75
20 - 25	80

*Based on data from Givan et al.[8] and Sever et al.[32]

INAPPARENT INFECTION, OR RUBELLA WITHOUT RASH

The existence of rubella without rash was demonstrated in 1953 by Krugman et al.[15] during experimental rubella infections in children. Subsequently, virological studies made during epidemics permitted confirmation and more precise knowledge of the incidence of these cases of rubella without eruption. Horstmann et al.,[12] during an epidemic in an institution for children aged 12 to 18 years, determined serologically that there were approximately as many rubella infections with eruption as without. Similar figures were contributed by Brody et al.[4] in a study in the Pribilof Islands (Bering Straits). It appears from his study (see Fig. 27-11) that

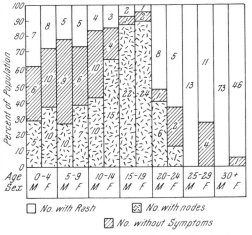

Figure 27-11. Appearance of rash and nodes by age nd sex during rubella outbreak, Pribilof Islands, 1963. From Brody, J. A., et al.: Arch. Ges. Virusforsch., *16*: 88, 1965.)

patients under 15 years of age, less than alf of rubella infections are accompanied y eruption, whereas among those from 15 o 20 years, 90 per cent develop an eruption. Attempts to evaluate the proportion of cases hat occur without rash in adults have yielded ighly divergent results. Brody's observations (see Fig. 27-11) and those of Buescher[5] n American recruits indicate one case with ruption for six to 30 inapparent infections. These results were verified in the laboratory n the basis of virus isolation and serological eactions.

One can attempt to evaluate the importance of rubella without eruption by reviewing he histories of mothers who have given birth o children with congenital rubella. In a study nvolving only infants for whom the diagnosis ad been confirmed by isolation of the virus, 0 per cent of the mothers had no history of ubella with clinical manifestations.

MMUNITY

Without virus isolation, the uncertainties nvolved in all retrospective diagnoses render mpossible any valid study of the immunity conferred by rubella infection; the serological nvestigation done by Sever et al.[32] makes vident the difficulties of diagnosis based on questioning subjects. Among the women leclaring that they had had rubella, 85.2 per cent had antibodies against rubella virus; mong those declaring they had not had ubella, 81.2 per cent had antibodies.

Recent follow-up studies in patients with virologically confirmed rubella all seem to show the solidity of immunity demonstrated by the presence of neutralizing antibodies.

Not a single case of rubella detected either clinically or by a systematic search for the virus has been observed in subjects with neutralizing antibodies at the time of contagion, whether during spontaneous epidemics[12] or subsequent to experimental infections.[29] Moreover, titrations before exposure to contagion or inoculation of the virus and several weeks thereafter did not show modification of the antibody titer.

Thus it is clear that neutralizing antibodies present at the time of exposure are protective against rubella. It would be crucial to know whether the antibodies appearing subsequent to a disease contracted during childhood always persist through adulthood or, at least among women, through the period of fecundity.

PROPHYLAXIS

Because rubella in children is so benign, whereas the risk of malformations consequent to rubella during the first trimester of pregnancy is high, preventive measures ought to attempt primarily to avert the contamination of pregnant women. It has even been suggested that the whole female population ought to contract the disease in childhood; however, because of the epidemiological characteristics of the virus attempts to create "rubella camps" or other conditions favorable to contamination are not regularly successful. Furthermore, the risk of extension of contagion is very high.

The application of preventive measures and, even more, the evaluation of their efficacy, come up against numerous difficulties.

In order to protect pregnant women from the contagion, the contagious subjects must be known, but, as we have already seen, detection of the real sources of contagion is difficult (in view of the inapparent forms of rubella, enterovirus eruptions simulating rubella, and so forth). This is why it is impossible to give any weight to replies to questioning of the pregnant woman as to her history. In the application of preventive measures every woman of childbearing age should be considered as receptive.

Perfection of the serodiagnosis of rubella by means of the hemagglutination-inhibition reaction and the prospect of soon having at our disposal a vaccine constitute the elements permitting a real prophylaxis.

What Preventive Measures Can Be Envisaged?

1. General Measures of Hygiene and of Public Health. Serodiagnosis of rubella makes possible an exact determination of a woman's state of immunity to the disease. It is of great importance to plan the systematic application of this serodiagnosis in those groups of young women who, because of their profession, are particularly exposed: teachers and kindergarten and hospital personnel. The serodiagnosis of rubella made among those who are already working in the professions mentioned will show that practically all these women are immune (99 per cent was ascertained for the personnel of Paris nurseries); made at the time when young women enter these professions, it will detect exactly those who are receptive.

Serodiagnosis could be practiced regularly at the pre-marital examination.

Should an epidemic occur in the school or hospital, all the receptive young women should be evacuated to a safe distance. As soon as pregnancy is suspected in a woman without antibodies, it ought to be possible immediately to accord her leave of absence, and a biological diagnosis to confirm pregnancy should then be made.

2. Specific Prophylactic Measures. Since an efficacious vaccination is not yet at hand, it is necessary to consider the only prophylactic methods at present available.

Numerous studies have attempted to evaluate the protection provided by administration of gamma globulins. The results show wide variations due to the diverse methods of evaluating protection and to the difficulties encountered when there are no biological criteria for scientific study of the problem. The general impression from all these studies is not very favorable.

We have already indicated some of the features of rubella that create difficulties in the use of gamma globulins for prophylaxis. Since the disease is contagious for several days before the rash appears, and since inapparent forms are so common, contact with the disease is often unrecognized or recognized too late for effective treatment. Thus the injection of gamma globulins is often made after the viremia has already developed which will transport the virus to the embryo (viremia begins a week before the rash). Often the only result of this injection is suppression of the rash; the rubella infection develops notwithstanding, but in an inapparent form.

Experimental studies[10] have shown that the injection of gamma globulins prior to experimental inoculation of the virus prevents the infection, but that this same injection made even very shortly after the experimental inoculation often fails to prevent viremia.

Nonetheless, according to certain investigations it seems that, injected early and in large doses, gamma globulins have diminished the incidence of malformations. It is with this modest hope — and for want of something better — that use of gamma globulins is still recommended. The physician unfortunately is almost always ignorant as to whether the woman has previously had a rubella which would have conferred natural immunity. It would be important to be able to practice systematic serological examinations (in the framework of the premarital examination for example) that would reveal immunity or lack of it in these women and thus avoid during an epidemic, both the untimely use of gamma globulins and the distress of the mother.

The only genuine prophylactic solution is vaccination. The first research works showed the weak antigenic power of the virus and the difficulties of obtaining viral suspensions of high titer: conditions indispensable for preparation of an effective inactivated vaccine.

Thus efforts have been directed toward perfecting a live virus vaccine. The development of live vaccines against poliomyelitis and measles has shown that such live vaccines are attainable.

Parkman and Meyer and their colleagues[18, 19, 25] were the first to propose a live vaccine against rubella. After 77 passages in green monkey kidney cells they obtained an attenuated strain of rubella virus which produces in children an infection followed by appearance of antibodies, without any clinical reaction; above all, this strain of virus seems to have lost all capacity to propagate from one vaccinated subject to another. A few limited trials in collectivities of children have confirmed this absence of contamination of others by the vaccinated children.[19] This property is absolutely esential, for pregnant women must not be contaminated by vaccinated children, even though it also seems that this attenuated virus has lost the property of affecting the tissues of the embryo.

More recently, other investigators (Hilleman, Prinzie, Plotkin) have also perfected strains of attenuated virus that could be utilized as a vaccine.

The work in progress should, in short order, permit selection of the best attenuated strains and will define the modalities of the vaccination; either systematic vaccination of all children to halt the spread of the virus and also protect pregnant women, or vaccination of young girls toward the age of 13 years and of women without antibodies against rubella who are not pregnant.

Now that the chronic and evolving aspect of rubella infection in the embryo and fetus is known, it might be possible to attempt to limit or even arrest this infection and thus to safeguard certain organs that the virus reaches late.

During intrauterine life, the total lack of action of maternal antibodies excludes all hope for the action of gamma globulins, but the development of synthetic antiviral agents or the possible action of interferon in the equilibrium between the virus and the host cell might offer therapeutic solutions.

After birth, the treatment of certain late-appearing lesions of congenital rubella (deafness, retinopathy, mental retardation) might be more effective. Dudgeon suggested the treatment from birth onward of children in whom the diagnosis of congenital rubella has been made by laboratory examinations. In this case, early and prolonged treatment with gamma globulins could be envisaged.

BIBLIOGRAPHY

1. Boué, A.: Le sérodiagnostic de la rubéole. Bull. Acad. Nat. Med., *151*:266, 1967.
2. Boué, A., Nicolas, A., and Lang, R.: La réaction d'inhibition de l'hémagglutination pour la sérologie de la rubéole. Ann. Inst. Pasteur, *114*:317, 1968.
3. Boué, A., Plotkin, S. A., and Boué, J. G.: Action du virus de la rubéole sur différents systèmes de cultures de cellules embryonnaires humaines. Arch. Ges. Virusforsch., *16*:443, 1965.
4. Brody, J. A., Sever, J. L., McAlister, R., Schiff, G. M., and Cutting, R.: Rubella epidemic on St. Paul Island in the Pribilofs, 1963. 1. Epidemiological, clinical and serological findings. Arch. Ges. Virusforsch., *16*:488, 1965.
5. Buescher, E. L.: Behavior of rubella virus in adult populations. Arch. Ges. Virusforsch., *16*:470, 1965.
6. Burnett, J. W., and Alford, C. A.: Comparative effectiveness of two cultures techniques for isolation of rubella virus. Proc. Soc. Exp. Biol. Med., *120*:569, 1965.
7. Fry, J., Dillane, J. B., and Fry, L., Rubella 1962. Brit. Med. J., *2*:833, 1962.
8. Givan, K. F., Rozee, K. R., and Rhodes, A. J.: Incidence of rubella antibodies in female subjects. Canad. Med. Assoc. J., *92*:126, 1965.
9. Green, R. H., Balsamo, M. R., Giles, J. P., Krugman, S., and Mirick, G. S.: Rubella: Studies on its etiology, epidemiology, clinical course and prevention. Trans. Assoc. Amer. Physicians, *77*:118, 1964.
10. Green, R. H., Balsamo, M. R., Giles, J. P., Krugman, S., and Mirick, G. S.: Experimental studies with rubella: Evaluation of gamma globulin for prophylaxis. Arch. Ges. Virusforsch., *16*:513, 1965.
11. Hillenbrand, F. K. M.: Rubella in a remote community. Lancet, *2*:64, 1956.
12. Horstmann, D. M., Riordan, J. T., Ohtawara, M., and Niederman, J. C.: A natural epidemic of rubella in a closed population. Arch. Ges. Virusforsch., *16*:483, 1965.
13. Ingalls, T. H., Babbott, F. L., Jr., Hampson, K. W., and Gordon, J. E.: Rubella: its epidemiology and teratology. Amer. J. Med. Sci., *239*:369, 1960.
14. Krugman, S.: Rubella: clinical and epidemiological aspects. Arch. Ges. Virusforsch., *16*:477, 1965.
15. Krugman, S., Ward, R., Jacobs, K. G., and Lazar, M.: Studies on rubella immunization. I. Demonstration of rubella without rash. J.A.M.A., *151*:285, 1953.
16. Liggins, G. C., and Phillips, L. I.: Rubella embryopathy, an interim report on a New Zealand epidemic. Brit. Med. J., *1*:711, 1963.
17. McCarthy, K., Taylor-Robinson, C. H., and Pillinger, S. E.: Isolation of rubella virus from cases in Britain. Lancet, *2*:593, 1963.
18. Meyer, H. M., Jr., Parkman, P. D., and Panos, T. C.: Clinical trial of an experimental live, attenuated rubella virus vaccine. New Eng. J. Med., *275*:575, 1966.
19. Meyer, H. M., Jr., Parkman, P. D., and Panos, T. C.: Clinical experience with natural and attenuated virus infections (in press).
20. Miller, L. F.: Rubella in naval recruits. Meeting of Ad Hoc Committee on Rubella Virus Vaccines, National Institutes of Health, February 26, 1964.
21. Neva, F. A., and Weller, T. H.: Rubella interferon and factors influencing the indirect neutralization test for rubella antibody. J. Immunol., *93*:466, 1964.
22. Parkman, P. D.: Biological characteristics of rubella virus. Arch. Ges. Virusforsch., *16*:401, 1965.
23. Parkman, P. D., Buescher, E. L., and Artenstein, M. S.: Recovery of rubella virus from army recruits. Proc. Soc. Exp. Biol. Med., *111*:225, 1962.
24. Parkman, P. D., Buescher, E. L., Artenstein, M. S., McCown, J. M., Mundon, F. K., and Druzd, A. D.: Studies of rubella. 1. Properties of the virus. J. Immunol., *93*:595, 1964.
25. Parkman, P. D., Meyer, H. M., Korschstein, R. L., and Hopps, H. E.: Development and characterization of a live attenuated rubella virus. New Eng. J. Med., *275*:569, 1960.
26. Parkman, P. D., Mundon, F. K., McCown, J. M.,

and Buescher, E. L.: Studies of rubella. 2. Neutralization of the virus. J. Immunol., *93*:608, 1964.

27. Plotkin, S. A., Cornfeld, D., and Ingalls, T. H.: Studies of immunization with living rubella virus. Amer. J. Dis. Child., *110*:381, 1965.

28. Rubella. Communicable Disease Center Morbidity and Mortality Weekly Report: 1964-13-93, 1965-14-138, 1965-14-354.

29. Schiff, G. M., Sever, J. L., and Huebner, R. J.: Clinical and laboratory findings of experimental infection with rubella virus. Clin. Res., *11*:296, 1963.

30. Sever, J. L., Fabiyi, A., McCullen, P., Chu, P. T., Weiss, W., and Gilkeson, M. R.: Rubella antibody among pregnant women in Hawaii. Amer. J. Obstet. Gynec., *92*:1006, 1965.

31. Sever, J. L., Huebner, R. J., Castellano, G. A., Sarma, P. D., Fabiyi, A., Schiff, G. M., and Cusu-

mano, C. L.: Rubella complement fixation test Science, *148*:385, 1965.

32. Sever, J. L., Schiff, G. M., and Huebner, R. J.: Frequency of rubella antibody among pregnant women and other human and animal populations. Obstet Gynec., *23*:153, 1964.

33. Stewart, G. L., Parkman, P. D., Hopps, H. E. Douglas, R. D., Hamilton, J. P., and Meyer, H. Jr.: Rubella virus hemagglutination-inhibition test New Eng. J. Med., *276*:554, 1967.

34. Veronelli, J. A., Maassab, H. F., and Hennessy A. V.: Isolation in tissue culture of an interfering agent from patients with rubella. Proc. Soc. Exp. Biol. Med., *111*:472, 1962.

35. Weller, T. H., and Neva, F. A.: Propagation in tissue culture of cytopathic agents from patients with rubella-like illness. Proc. Soc. Exp. Biol. Med. *111*:215, 1962.

MORE RECENTLY IDENTIFIED ERUPTIVE FEVERS

by P. Mozziconacci, C. Attal, and V. Drouhet

ERUPTIONS DUE TO ECHO VIRUS

ECHO Virus 16: Boston Exanthem

During the summer of 1951, there occurred in the Boston area an epidemic disease characterized in some patients by a rash, and in others by aseptic meningitis. A cytopathogenic infectious agent was isolated from stools, pharynx, and blood. Neva and colleagues,[29,30] who studied this epidemic, observed another in 1954 in Pittsburgh, although it was less widespread.[28] They demonstrated that the virus was the same.[31] Later studies confirmed the serological relationship of these different strains, of which one is the prototype of ECHO 16.

Circumstances of Appearance. The disease affects both children and adults. It manifests itself after an incubation period of four to five days.

Clinical Description. The disease begins with a few functional and systemic manifestations which precede the eruption: fever, pharyngeal pain, headache, shivering, myalgias, and ocular burning sensation. All these symptoms are marked, particularly in adults. In the form associated with a rash, the fever lasts only a day or two. In the meningeal forms the fever lasts longer, but meningeal involvement is never associated with eruption; ECHO 16 virus produces either meningitis or exanthem, and the association of the two has not been reported to our knowledge. It is not rare for the eruption to appear after the fall in temperature. The rash is macular or maculopapular, of salmon-pink color, made up of small elements (1 to 2 mm.), usually thin-spread, occasionally abundant or even confluent. It appears above all on the face, chest, and back but may extend to the extremities, the palms of the hands, and the soles of the feet. An enanthem composed of red spots or yellowish-white erosions sometimes occurs on the pharyngeal mucosa, the gums, and the inner surface of the cheeks. In the exanthemic form, the cerebrospinal fluid is normal. The number of leukocytes in the peripheral blood is normal. The virus can be found in the stools, the throat, and possibly in the blood, where it was isolated on one occasion. In the convalescent period, neutralizing or complement-fixing antibodies are found. They persist several years. The course is benign; no serious case has been reported.

Contagiousness is high, and it is not unusual for all the children in one family to be affected, as well as one or both parents.

THE MENINGOERUPTIVE SYNDROMES

During numerous summer epidemics, observers have often described the association of a morbilliform eruption with a meningeal syndrome. The meningoeruptive syndrome linked to infections by ECHO viruses 9, 4, and 6 represents one of the most interesting and the most characteristic among the clinical manifestations of ECHO virus infections.

ECHO 9 Virus. Since 1955, the date

of the first epidemic observed in Italy, a series of summer epidemics of aseptic meningitis has been described, frequently associated with a morbilliform rash, occurring in different European countries, in Canada, and in the United States, and linked to a virus of ECHO 9 type. In 1957, a particularly widespread epidemic was reported first in England and Scotland, thereafter spreading to numerous countries of Western Europe (Belgium, the Netherlands, Denmark, Germany, Switzerland, and Italy), extending to Iceland, Canada, and parts of the United States, and finally reaching Australia.[8, 11, 15, 23, 32, 35, 37, 38]

The association of an erythema with meningitis is not constant but is frequently observed and seems fairly particular to this type of virus.

CIRCUMSTANCES OF APPEARANCE. The disease affects both children and adults. Its incubation period is three to five days, possibly longer.

CLINICAL DESCRIPTION. The gravity of the invasion period varies according to the epidemics and the patient's age. In the adult, onset is often brutal, accompanied by frontal and retroörbital cephalgia, photophobia, attacks of nausea and of vertigo, and stiffness of the nape of the neck. In the young child, the onset is often marked by abdominal pains, with attacks of nausea and vomiting, but generally without diarrhea.

The rash has been present in all the epidemics described except two. It generally appears one or two days after the onset of the disease. It affects the face, the trunk, the extension zones of the arms and legs, the palms of the hands, and the soles of the feet. Usually it appears first on the face and the trunk, where it predominates; occasionally it remains limited; if not, it extends to the rest of the body only in the following six to 12 hours.

The rash is generally maculopapular, composed of elements 1 to 3 mm. in diameter, rose-colored or brown, and may be accompanied by petechiae or ecchymoses resembling the cutaneous lesions in meningococcemia.

The evolution may occur in two or three outbursts marked by recrudescence of fever and eruption.

An enanthem may appear in the form of white or grayish spots on the buccal mucosa facing the molars; vesicles or small ulcerations may also appear on the tongue.

CLINICAL FORMS. The disease takes four forms: (1) meningitis without eruption; (2) eruption without meningitis, apparently at least; (3) meningitis with eruption; or (4) a purely febrile form of "summer influenza."

EPIDEMIOLOGY. Numerous epidemics have been reported since 1955, and it seems probable that numerous cases of meningo-encephalitis with rubella-like eruption described in earlier years were related to this disease.

Diffusion of the infection is rapid within population groups, from one group to another, and even from country to country. The disease affects equally newborns, older children, and adults, and it spreads massively. The epidemic in the Milwaukee area in 1957 affected over 40,000 subjects among an estimated population of 900,000.

ECHO 4 Virus. The meningoeruptive syndrome due to ECHO 4 virus is much less frequent. The infection manifests itself most often in the form of a lymphocytic meningitis or as a minor illness of very short duration. In the Melbourne epidemic,[7] eruption was noted only in rare cases (two of 263). However, in the Swedish epidemic, rubella-like exanthem was present in most cases, eight of 13[11]; Karzon et al., in 1961,[13] encountered eruption in only three cases of 82. Rather often, a few vesicular elements appear in the eruption.

ECHO 4 virus was isolated from the liquid of vesicular lesions and from the blood during an epidemic in Germany.[27] It was also found in food believed to have played a role in causing the infection.

In the ECHO 4 infections in Iowa[17] and those of South Africa[10,26,39] no rash was noted.

ECHO 6 Virus. ECHO 6 virus is most often the cause of meningitis; in a few cases, the illness is accompanied by exanthem with generalized maculopapular lesions affecting even the palms of the hands and the soles of the feet[35] or by cutaneous lesions of the erythema exudativum multiforme or polymorphous erythema type.[40]

Erythematous buccal lesions have also been reported in children living in an environment in which ECHO 6 infections were rife.[35]

Other ECHO Virus Types. An epidemic due to ECHO 2 virus, occurring in an orphanage, was characterized by respiratory signs with rash. The eruption was most often associated with ECHO type 2 virus, which was isolated in five of 15 children from the stools and once from the throat.[33]

Finally, it is worth mentioning a curious epidemic that occurred in Germany in 1958;

Table 27-5. *Eruptions Due to ECHO Viruses*

ECHO VIRUS TYPE	CLINICAL ASPECT	REFERENCES
16	Boston exanthem Exanthema subitum-like	Neva et al.[28, 29, 30, 31] Lerner et al.[18]
4, 6, 9, 14, 16, 18	Meningoeruptive syndrome: fever, meningitis, maculopapular exanthem, petechiae, various erythemas	Nihoul and Quersin-Thiry,[32] Verlinde and Wilterdink,[38] Johnsson et al.,[11] Sabin et al.,[35] Forbes,[7] Karzon et al.,[12, 13] Godtfredsen and von Magnus,[8] Tyrrel et al.,[37] Laforest et al.,[15] MacLean and Melnick[23]
4, 9, 11	Vesicular erythema	Munk and Nasemann[27]
6	Maculopapular exanthem Polymorphous erythema	Von Zeipel and Svedmyr[40]
2, 7	Eruption and respiratory syndrome Macular eruption and paralysis	Rendtorff et al.[33] Lerner et al.,[18] MacAllister,[22] Steigman et al.[36]
14	Erythema Febrile exanthem	Fleurette et al.[5]
1, 3, 11, 19	Erythema	MacAllister,[22] Cramblett et al.[1]
5, 12	Vesicular and bullous lesions	Enders-Ruckle et al.[3]

the patients presented vesicular or even bullous lesions. Throat-washings and stool specimens permitted isolation of ECHO viruses of types 5 and 12, but the increase in titer of homologous antibodies was slight.[3]

In the absence of any epidemic, ECHO viruses 4, 6, 9, 14, 16, and 18 have been isolated from sporadic cases of meningo-eruptive syndrome. In addition, ECHO 2 virus was cited by Lerner et al.[18] and by MacAllister.[22] Steigman et al.[36] isolated it from the central nervous system in a fatal case in a child who had presented paralyses and a macular eruption on the abdomen and thorax.

Erythema was noted in a child infected by an ECHO 14 virus,[35] a virus that usually causes acute meningitis or summer diarrhea in children. In France, Fleurette et al. in 1962[5] isolated this type from the stools in two cases of exanthem and demonstrated the appearance of homologous antibodies. ECHO 1 virus was cited in MacAllister's studies in 1960.[22]

Table 27-5 gives a list of eruptions due to ECHO viruses.

ERUPTIONS ASSOCIATED WITH COXSACKIE VIRUSES

COXSACKIE VIRUSES OF GROUP A

Coxsackie A Type 9 Virus. Coxsackie A9 virus has been isolated[2,14] in patients presenting a febrile infectious state with erythematous or sometimes vesicular pharyngitis accompanied by maculopapular cutaneous lesions and even petechiae or vesicles. The eruption, often followed by adenopathy, is epidemic and occurs mainly in the summer. The infection has at times provoked meningitis.[9] It is, above all, interesting to note that, in the Boston epidemic, in the 15 patients affected by Coxsackie A9 virus who were seen by Lerner et al.,[20] the virus was isolated from the throat, the stools, the cerebrospinal fluid, and, for the first time, from the blood in five patients. Antibodies neutralizing Coxsackie A9 virus were present in all cases, and their increase was demonstrated in nine cases. The vesicular lesions accompany pulmonary involvements, whereas they are not observed in patients presenting meningitis in whom maculopapular lesions or petechiae may occur, possibly giving rise to errors of interpretation and, in particular, suggesting a meningococcosis. In certain cases the rash, of exclusively maculopapular form, is accompanied by an infectious state with pharyngitis, rhinorrhea, and meningeal reaction.

In a 16-month-old child presenting exanthem with pulmonary signs who died in a convulsive state, without meningeal reaction, the virus was isolated from the liver and the lung.

Coxsackie A Type 16 Virus. Several epidemics linked to this serological type have been described, the first in Toronto during the summer of 1957. Sometimes the term "hand, foot, and mouth disease" has been applied to the eruptions observed on these occasions, with the risk of confusion between Coxsackie A16 virus and the viruses of animal aphthous fever (foot and mouth disease).

The disease manifests itself, after three to six days' incubation, by a febrile period of three to five days, followed by an exanthem. In the mouth, the exanthem is made up of vesicular and ulcerous lesions affecting not only the oropharynx, as in herpangina, but also the buccal mucosa, the tongue, and the gingivolabial groove. The lesions commence with a macula, which is then surmounted by an oval vesicle 1 to 3 mm. in diameter, which may unite with neighboring vesicles to form a large ulcer.

On the body the exanthem is maculopapular and vesicular, most often affecting the hands and the feet, and occasionally also the limbs and the trunk; it is not a very abundant rash, often consisting of only two or three vesicles, but evolving by successive outbursts, the vesicles being situated most often on the dorsal surface of the fingers and toes and on the lateral borders of the feet, more rarely on the palms or the soles, where they form deep lesions having the aspect of grains of rice. The eruption lasts two or three

Table 27-6. *Eruptions Due to Coxsackie Viruses*

COXSACKIE VIRUS TYPE	CLINICAL ASPECT	REFERENCES
A9	Maculopapular, petechial, vesicular exanthem and vesicular erythematous pharyngitis	Dubin and Horstmann,[2] Kilbourne and Goldfield[14]
	Exanthem and pulmonary syndrome	Lerner et al.[20]
	Exanthem and meningeal reaction	Habel et al.[9]
A16	Exanthem and vesicular stomatitis (buccal mucosa and tongue) Maculopapular, vesicular exanthem	Robinson and Rhodes,[34] Magoffin et al.,[25] Lerner et al.[18]
A2, A4, A5	Maculopapular erythema Vesicular erythema and herpangina	MacNair Scott,[24] Flewett et al.[6]
A23	Exanthem and aseptic meningitis	Lamy et al.[16] (one case)
B1	Febrile erythema	Lycke et al.[21]
B2	Febrile erythema	Lamy et al.[16]
B3, B5	Vesicular eruption	Lerner et al.[19]
B4	Febrile maculopapular exanthem	Felici et al.[4]
B5	Exanthema subitum-like and vesicular pharyngitis	Lerner et al.[18]

days. It is occasionally accompanied by con-junctivitis, cough, abdominal pains, diarrhea, and headache.

Other Coxsackie Group Viruses. Types A2, A4, A5, and A23 can in certain cases be responsible for a maculopapular erythema.

THE COXSACKIE GROUP B VIRUSES

Infections accompanied by exanthems due to Coxsackie group B types 1, 2, 3, 4 and 5 have been described. *Coxsackie B1* has caused infectious states accompanied by a cutaneous erythema, as described by Lycke et al.[21]

Coxsackie B3 provokes summer epi-demics of infections with vesicular eruptions. Lerner[19] reported the cases of two infants aged nine and six months. The first presented an infectious state with torpor, dyspnea, generalized adenopathies, and a vesicular eruption initially considered to be due to chickenpox. The eruption involved the trunk, the abdomen, the shoulders, the fingers, and the legs. In the second case there were fever and sore throat with small ulcerations and vesicular lesions on the arms and hands, as well as adenopathies. The virus was isolated from the vesicle fluid. In other cases, the virus has been isolated from throat washings or stools, and in certain cases proof of the role of the virus is given by the rise in neu-tralizing antibody titer.

In the course of an epidemic of 70 cases in an Italian village, Felici et al.[4] observed an infection characterized by fever, headache, diarrhea, and in 11 per cent of cases, an exan-them consisting of maculopapular elements on the face and thorax and presenting a morbilliform aspect in certain cases. Forty-one per cent of the ill children had a rash, and 27.5 per cent of the adolescents; few rashes were reported among adults. Rashes were thus heavily predominant in children. *Cox-sackie B4 virus* was isolated from throat washings and stools, and a significant rise in antibody titer was detected in a certain number of patients.

The existence of vesicular pharyngitis with infection by *Coxsackie B5 virus*[18] and the observation of oropharyngeal lesions different from those of herpangina and pro-ducing the picture of "hand, foot, and mouth syndrome" show clearly that herpangina is not characteristic of Coxsackie group A infections.

It is important for the clinician to know these different pictures for the differential diagnosis with polymorphous erythema, Stevens-Johnson disease, or even chickenpox.

Lamy et al.[16] conducted a two-year study (1959-1961) at the medical genetics clinic in Paris. Among the 62 cases they saw in which a virus was isolated, an eruptive disease due to Coxsackie B viruses (B2 and B4) was found in four cases, and cutaneous exanthem associated with Coxsackie A23 was found in two cases, in one of which there was also an "aseptic" meningitis.

Table 27-6 gives a list of eruptions due to Coxsackie viruses.

BIBLIOGRAPHY

1. Cramblett, H. G., Moffet, H. L., Middleton, G. K. Jr., Black, J. P., Shulenberger, H., and Yongue, A.: ECHO 19 virus infections. Clinical and laboratory studies. Arch. Int. Med., *110*:574-579, 1962.
2. Dubin, L., and Horstmann, D. M.: Epidemiology of aseptic meningitis and related nonspecific diseases in Connecticut, 1957: Virological and clinical studies. Yale J. Biol. Med., *30*:429-441, 1958.
3. Enders-Ruckle, G., Heite, H. J., and Siegert, R.: Klinische und virologische Studie über das akute epidemische Exanthem, sog. bläschenkrankheit I. Besprechung der Krankheitsfälle und der zuge-hörigen Isolierungsversuche. II. Mitteilung. Identifizierung der zytopathogenen Agentien und serologisches Verhatten der Pattenten. München Med. Wschr., *101*:490, 1213, 1959.
4. Felici, A., Archetti, I., Russi, F., Bellochi, C., and Mazzi, F.: Contributo alla studio delle malattie da virus Coxsackie. Manifestazione epidemics ad impronta diarreica causata da un virus Coxsackie type B3. Rendic. Ist. Sup. Sanit., *23*:695, 1960.
5. Fleurette, J., Sohier, R., and Chardonnet, Y.: Les exanthémes dùs à des virus chez l'enfant. Rev. Hyg. Med. Soc., *10*:355, 1962.
6. Flewett, T., Warin, R. P., and Clarke, S. K. R.: Hand, foot and mouth disease associated with Coxsackie A5 virus. J. Clin. Path., *16*:53-55, 1963.
7. Forbes, J. A.: Meningitis in Melbourne due to ECHO virus 4. I. Clinical aspects. Med. J. Australia, *1*:246, 1958.
8. Godtfredsen, A., and Magnus, H. von: Isolation of ECHO virus type 9 from cerebrospinal fluids. Danish Med. Bull., *4*:233-236, 1957.
9. Habel, K., Silverberg, R. J., and Shelokov, A.: Iso-lation of enteric virus from cases of aseptic meningitis. Ann. N.Y. Acad. Sci., *67*:223-229, 1957.
10. Howarth, W. H., et al.: A closed epidemic of acute aseptic meningitis caused by ECHO virus type 4. II. Laboratory studies. S. Afr. Med. J., *35*:333-335, 1961.
11. Johnsson, T., Bottiger, M., and Lofdahl, A.: An out-break of aseptic meningitis with a rubella-like rash probably caused by ECHO virus type 4. Arch. Ges. Virusforsch., *8*:306-317, 1958.
12. Karzon, D. T., Barron, A. L., Winkelstein, W. J.,

and Cohen, S.: Isolation of ECHO virus type 6 during an outbreak of seasonal aseptic meningitis. J.A.M.A., *162*:1298, 1956.

3. Karzon, D. T., Eckert, G. L., Barron, A. L., Hayner, N. S., and Winkelstein, W. J.: Aseptic meningitis epidemic due to ECHO virus 4. Amer. J. Dis. Child., *101*:610, 1961.

4. Kilbourne, E. D., and Goldfield, M.: Coxsackie viruses and "virus-like" diseases of the adult. A three-year study in a contagious disease hospital. Amer. J. Med., *21*:175, 1956.

5. Laforest, R. A., McNaughton, G. A., Beale, A. J., Clarke, M., Davis, N., Sultamian, I., and Rhodes, A. J.: Outbreak of aseptic meningitis (meningoencephalitis) with rubelliform rash: Toronto, 1956. Canad. Med. Assoc. J., *77*:1-4, 1957.

6. Lamy, M., Jammet, M. L., Ajjan, N., Nezelof, C., and Bonnisol, C.: Les infections à virus dans un service de pédiatrie. Arch. Ges. Virusforsch., *13*:24, 1963.

7. Lehan, P. H., et al.: An epidemic illness associated with a recently recognized enteric virus (ECHO virus type 4). I. Epidemiologic and clinical features. Amer. J. Hyg., *66*:63-75, 1957.

8. Lerner, A. M., Klein, J. O., Cherry, J. D., and Finland, M.: New viral exanthems. New Eng. J. Med., *269*:678-685, 736-740, 1963.

9. Lerner, A. M., Klein, J. O., and Finland, M.: Infection with Coxsackie virus group B type 3 with vesicular eruption; report of two cases. New Eng. J. Med., *263*:1305, 1960.

10. Lerner, A. M., Klein, J. O., Levin, S. H., and Finland, M.: Infections due to Coxsackie virus group A type 9 in Boston, 1959, with special reference to exanthema and pneumonia. New Eng. J. Med., *263*:1265, 1960.

11. Lycke, E., Hultgardth, A., and Redin, B.: Coxsackie B1 virus and febrile illness with rash. Lancet, *1*: 1097, 1959.

12. MacAllister, R. M.: ECHO virus infections. Pediat. Clin. N. Amer., *7*:927, 1960.

13. MacLean, D. M., and Melnick, J. L.: Association of a mouse pathogenic strain of ECHO virus type 9 with aseptic meningitis. Proc. Soc. Exp. Biol. Med., *44*:656-660, 1957.

14. MacNair Scott, T. F.: Clinical syndromes associated with enterovirus and reovirus infections. Adv. Virus Res., *8*:165-197, 1961.

15. Magoffin, R. L., Jackson, E. W., and Lennette, E. H.: Vesicular stomatitis and exanthem: syndrome associated with Coxsackie virus group A type 16. J.A.M.A., *175*:441, 1961.

16. Malherbe, H., Harwin, R., and Smith, A. H.: An outbreak of aseptic meningitis associated with ECHO virus type 4. S. Afr. Med. J., *31*:1261-1264, 1957.

27. Munk, K. K., and Nasemann, T.: Untersuchungen über die Ätiologie der in Süddentschland beobachteten Fälle des variablen infektiosen exanthems isolierung eines ECHO virus. Klin. Wschr., *37*:371, 1959.

28. Neva, F. A.: A second outbreak of Boston exanthem disease in Pittsburgh during 1954. New Eng. J. Med., *254*:838-843, 1956.

29. Neva, F. A., and Enders, J. F.: Cytopathogenic agents isolated from patients during an unusual epidemic exanthem. J. Immunol., *72*:307-314, 1954.

30. Neva, F. A., Feemster, R. F., and Gorbach, I. J.: Clinical and epidemiologic features of an unusual epidemic exanthem. J.A.M.A., *155*:544-548, 1954.

31. Neva, F. A., and Zuffante, S. M.: Agents isolated from Boston exanthem disease during 1954 in Pittsburgh. J. Lab. Clin. Med., *50*:712, 1957.

32. Nihoul, E., and Quersin-Thiry, L.: A new clinical entity? Lancet, *1*:269-270, 1957.

33. Rendtorff, R. C., Walker, L. C., Hale, B. D., Billheimer, G. J., Jr., and Roberts, A. M.: An epidemic of ECHO virus 2 infections in an orphanage nursery. Amer. J. Hyg., *79*:64-73, 1964.

34. Robinson, C. R., and Rhodes, A. J.: Vesicular exanthem and stomatitis. Report of an epidemic due to Coxsackie virus group A type 16. New Eng. J. Med., *265*:1104, 1961.

35. Sabin, A. B., Krumbiegel, E. R., and Wigand, R.: ECHO 9 virus disease: virologically controlled clinical and epidemiologic observations during 1957 epidemic in Milwaukee with notes on concurrent similar diseases associated with Coxsackie and other ECHO viruses. J. Dis. Child., *96*:197-219, 1958.

36. Steigman, A. J., Kokko, U. P., and Silverberg, R. J.: Unusual properties of a virus isolated from the spinal cord of a child with fatal poliomyelitis. A.M.A. J. Dis. Child., *86*:509, 1953.

37. Tyrrell, D. A. J., Lane, R. R., and Snell, B.: Further studies of an epidemic of exanthem associated with aseptic meningitis. Quart. J. Med., *27*:323, 1958.

38. Verlinde, J. D., and Wilterdink, J. B.: Neuropathogenicity of non polio enteroviruses with special reference to ECHO 9 virus. Folia Psychiat. Neerl., *61*:670, 1958.

39. Wilsen, A. A. J., Peisach, H., and Howarth, W. H.: A closed epidemic of acute aseptic meningitis caused by ECHO virus type 4. I. Epidemiological and clinical studies. S. Afr. Med. J., *35*:330-333, 1961.

40. Von Zeipel, G., and Svedmyr, A.: A study of the association of ECHO viruses to aseptic meningitis. Arch. Ges. Virusforsch., *7*:355-368, 1957.

LABORATORY DIAGNOSIS OF VIRUSES ASSOCIATED WITH EXANTHEMS

by V. DROUHET

Virus Associated with Exanthems	VIROLOGICAL DIAGNOSIS									SEROLOGICAL DIAGNOSIS						
	SPECIMENS					INOCULATIONS				SERUM SAMPLES (Days After Onset)			TESTS			
						New-born Mice	Tissue Cultures									
							Primary		Cell Line							
	Throat	Feces	Skin Lesions	Blood	CSF	New-born Mice	Monkey Kidney	Miscella-neous	Cell Line	1st	2nd	3rd	C.F.	H.I.	Hemad.	Neu
Polioviruses I, III	+	+		±	±	+	+	amnion	+ HeLa, KB etc.	5 to 15	10 to 40	30	+			+
ECHO Viruses																
16	+	+		+	+	+	+	amnion						±		+
4, 6, 9, 14, 16, 18	+	+	type 4 (vesicles)	+	+	+	+	amnion						type 6	types 6, 18	+
1, 11, 3, 19	+	+	type 11 (vesicles)	±		+	+	amnion							type 11	
5, 12	+	+		±		+	+	amnion							type 12	
2, 7	+	+		±		+	+	amnion								
Coxsackie Viruses A																
A9	+ (vesicles)	+		+	+	+ IM	+	amnion					+			+
A16, A5	+ (vesicles)	+	+ (vesicles)	+		+ IM							+			
A2, A4	+ (vesicles)	+		+		+ IM			A4 HeLa				+			
A11, A21, A23		+		+		+ IM							+			
Coxsackie Viruses B																
B3, B5	+ (vesicles)	+	type 5 (vesicles)	+	+	+ IC	+	±	±					+		+
B1, B2, B4		+		+	+	+ IC	+	±	±					type B1		+
Adenoviruses																
3	+	+				±		amnion	+	3	7 to 10		+	+		+
4	+	+				±		amnion	+				+	+		+
7	+	+				±		amnion	+				+	+.		+
1, 2	+	+				±		amnion	+				+	+		+
unidentified	+	+				±		amnion	+				+	+		+
Reoviruses																
1, 2	+	+				+		human kidney	HeLa	10 to 15			+	+		±
Parainfluenzae Myxoviruses																
3	+					+				7 to 10			+	+	+	+
Respiratory Syncytial Viruses	+	+				+			Hep. 2 KB, HeLa	3 7	20	50	+			
Infectious Mononucleosis										Heterophil antibody test						

*CSF = Cerebrospinal fluid; C.F. = complement-fixing antibodies; H.I. = hemagglutination-inhibition test; Hemad. = hemadsorption; Neut. = neutralizing antibodies; IM = intramuscular; IC = intracerebral.

28

Clinically Ill-Defined Eruptions
Due to Various Viruses

By P. MOZZICONACCI, C. ATTAL, AND V. DROUHET

POLIOVIRUSES

Polioviruses have often been isolated from the stools of subjects with an eruption, but their pathogenic role has not always been demonstrated serologically. It is more likely that, in the course of an exanthemic infection, an inapparent infection by polioviruses plays only an accompanying role. Ferola et al.[6] observed in Naples in 1961, in the course of a poliomyelitis type I epidemic, five cases of febrile exanthem in which they isolated poliovirus type I and demonstrated a significant level of homologous antibodies. Fourrier et al.[8] published two case reports of exanthem in children aged two and one-half years during a small poliomyelitis epidemic in Lille. The presence of poliovirus type III in the stools and the increase in antibody titer were contemporaneous with the clinical manifestations and confirmed the existence of the infection.

ADENOVIRUSES

The adenoviruses, like the enteroviruses, can circulate in human collectivities, especially among young people, in hospital wards, in nurseries, and in military barracks, where conditions are favorable to their spread. The excretion of adenovirus by children in closed residential institutions was studied by Gardner et al.[10] over a period of a year. Types 1 to 7 were found in stools. Adenovirus type 5 was isolated from no less than 50 per cent of the children, and some of them excreted adenovirus type 5 for periods of three to six months. As a rule, these infections remained inapparent. Therefore, great prudence is required in interpreting the etiologic role of adenoviruses, which can be found in the stools several weeks or even months after the infection.

In most cases described in the literature, the laboratory diagnosis was based on isolation of the virus and demonstration of antibodies in the patient's blood. Adenoviruses of types 3, 4, and 7 are the most often cited.

In 1954, Neva and Enders[19] noted, in association with adenovirus type 3, a maculopapular eruption in the course of an infectious state with fever, coryza, sore throat, and adenopathy, recovery occurring after two to three days.

In 1957, Fukumi et al.[9] isolated from a throat washing a type 3 adenovirus, and also found a significant increase in neutralizing antibodies, in a 3-year-old child hospitalized for febrile pharyngoconjunctivitis, accompanied by a morbilliform maculopapular erythema of the face and then the trunk and limbs. The rash disappeared in five days but left a slight pigmentation.

In 1958, Munro-Ashman et al.[18] isolated a type 3 adenovirus in the course of a pharyngitis with scarlatiniform erythema.

Type 7 was isolated by Dascomb and Hilleman[5] in 1956 in United States Army recruits presenting an infectious state with rhinopharyngitis, tracheitis, adenopathy, occasionally digestive disturbances, and, in 429 of these patients, a fairly intense erythema of the neck and thorax. This illness lasted one to two days. The serological reactions proved the infection to be due to adenovirus type 7.

Sohier et al.,[22] in 1957, studying an influenza-like epidemic among young military recruits, isolated type 7. In one patient they noted a rubella-like erythema. The etiology was confirmed by the significant increase in complement-fixing antibodies.

In 1961, Gutekunst and Heggie[11] described in United States Navy recruits 122 cases of rubella-type infections with fever, rhinopharyngotracheitis, conjunctivitis, and postauricular, mastoidal, and cervical adenopathy. The isolation of adenovirus type 4 or 7, with an increase in antibodies, proved the etiology in 43 cases.

Barr et al.[1] in 1958 drew attention to infections by adenoviruses of types 3 and 7 in children having scarlet fever or rubella; the adenoviruses were found in the stools several weeks, and even two months, after the infection.

Chany et al.[4] in 1957 reported on five cases of fleeting maculopapular rash among 27 cases of adenovirus pneumonia.

In 1959 Breton et al.[3] proved serologically the role of adenoviruses in determining acute infectious states in children aged 18 months to four years; the infection was accompanied by oculonasal catarrh, pharyngitis, fever, and a morbilliform rash on the face and chest, disappearing in three to seven days.

In 1960 Laurensich et al.,[14] in a study of adenovirus infections, found 47 infections without exanthem and seven with morbilliform exanthem.

In another study, Fleurette et al.[7] in 1962 reported on four cases of exanthems due to viruses in children. Adenoviruses types 1, 2, and 3 were isolated from stools and throat, and their role was proved by a rise in the level of homologous antibodies.

MYXOVIRUSES

A small epidemic of exanthems due to myxoviruses was described by Pierson et al. in 1963.[20] It affected infants, aged three to 16 months, hospitalized from November 16 to November 24, 1961, for various illnesses. The child who appeared to have contaminated the others entered the service for an exanthem accompanied by discrete respiratory manifestations and slight adenopathy. Exanthem was the only symptom presented by the four infants contaminated.

Parainfluenza virus 3 was isolated from throat specimens. Rectal swabbings gave negative results. Serological study demonstrated the appearance of antibodies in three cases and the existence of a high level of antibodies in the serum at a late date in one case.

While in the epidemic described by Pierson et al. exanthem was the major constant sign and even, in some cases, the sole symptom, cutaneous manifestations were rarely observed by Lippi et al.,[16] who in 1962 reported only three morbilliform rashes among 75 cases of myxovirus infection.

REOVIRUSES

At present, most of the symptoms imputable to enterovirus infections are fairly well known, but the role of reoviruses is still ill defined. Lerner et al.[15] made a study of the possible relationships of reovirus type 2 with cutaneous exanthems. In the course of systematic investigations, they demonstrated the increase in titer of antireovirus 2 in seven infants, of whom six presented cutaneous manifestations (five maculopapular eruptions and one vesicular eruption), but reovirus type 2 could be isolated in only three cases.

The relative frequency with which these viruses can be isolated in healthy subjects should indicate the need for extreme prudence in the interpretation of virological results obtained in the course of an infectious syndrome of only slight specificity. The case report by Turpin et al.[23] of a polymorphous erythema in a four-and-one-half-month-old infant after prescription of phenobarbital, with isolation of a type 1 reovirus and progressive increase in level of serum antibodies, illustrates the difficulty of establishing a link between a particular viral infection and the concomitant symptoms. The viral infection definitely occurred, but the virus was isolated not from the cutaneous lesions but from the stools; moreover, the fact that it was isolated well after appearance of the clinical signs leaves room for the possibility of a hospital contamination.

The studies of reovirus infections show the frequency of latent infections and the rarity of cutaneous manifestations.

OTHER VIRUSES

Among the other viruses that can provoke eruptions should be cited the *arboviruses*. These eruptions are described in relation to each type involved (see Chapter 58).

The *respiratory syncytial virus* can also provoke eruptions. In 15 respiratory infections shown serologically to be due to the respiratory syncytial virus, Moss et al.[17] twice observed erythematous eruptions, involving the face in one case and the trunk in the other. Berkovich and Kibrick[2] observed in a two-year-old child the association of croup with an eruption that seemed very probably also linked to the presence of respiratory syncytial virus, since an epidemiological investigation (virological and bacteriological) in the child and surrounding persons failed

Table 28-1. *Viruses Associated with Clinically Ill-Defined Eruptions*

VIRUS	TYPE	CLINICAL ASPECT	REFERENCES
Polioviruses	I	Febrile exanthem	Ferola et al.[6]
	III	Exanthema subitum-like	Fourrier et al.[8]
Adenoviruses	3	Maculopapular eruption, fever, sore throat, adenopathy	Neva and Enders,[19] Barr et al.[1]
		Pharyngoconjunctivitis, maculopapular morbilliform erythema	Fukumi et al.[9]
		Scarlatiniform erythema, pharyngitis	Munro-Ashman et al.,[18] Fleurette et al.[7]
	4	Rubella-like erythema, rhinopharyngoconjunctivitis	Gutekunst and Heggie[11]
	7	Influenza-like syndrome, rubella-like erythema	Dascomb and Hilleman,[5] Sohier et al.,[22] Gutekunst and Heggie[11]
	1, 2	Exanthema subitum Exanthem	Jansson et al.,[13] Fleurette et al.[7]
	Not typed	Morbilliform rash, pharyngitis, oculonasal catarrh	Chany et al.,[4] Breton et al.,[3] Laurensich et al.[14]
Myxoviruses Parainfluenzae	3	Exanthem, respiratory syndrome, adenopathy	Lippi et al.,[16] Pierson et al.[20]
Reoviruses	1	Polymorphous erythema	Turpin et al.[23]
	2	Vesicular maculopapular rash	Lerner et al.[15]
Respiratory syncytial virus		Respiratory syndrome, nonspecific erythema	Moss et al.[17]
		Pharyngitis, maculopapular erythema	Berkovich and Kibrick[2]
Infectious mononucleosis		Pseudodiphtheritic form, morbilliform rash	Sohier[21]
Arboviruses		Various exanthems	See Chapter 58

to reveal other germs capable of explaining the exanthem. The erythema appeared on the fourth day of the disease, affecting the shoulders and chest, and diffused the fifth day over the entire trunk and the anterior surface of the arms, assuming a maculopapular aspect; a few perianal lesions were noted. The eruption disappeared 12 hours later, at the same time as the fever.

INFECTIOUS MONONUCLEOSIS

Even though the pathogenic agent of infectious mononucleosis has not been isolated, it seems proper to include the subject in this chapter, the infection being well defined and most probably provoked by a virus.

Eruptions are not rare in this disease. Certain authors estimate that they occur in 10 or 15 per cent of cases. All types have been described: scarlatiniform, morbilliform, rubella-like, or even papulovesicular, nodular, or urticarial.

Particular interest is attached to the rubella-like exanthem which is occasionally associated with infectious mononucleosis, especially in children, and which can lead to an erroneous diagnosis of rubella. Hematological examination and the Paul-Bunnell test are sometimes indispensable to establish the differential diagnosis.

BIBLIOGRAPHY

1. Barr, J., Kjellen, L., and Svedmyr, A.: Hospital outbreak of adenovirus type 3 infection. Acta Paediat., *47*:365, 1958.
2. Berkovich, S., and Kibrick, S.: Exanthem associated with respiratory syncytial virus infection. J. Pediat., *65*:368-370, 1964.
3. Breton, A., Voisin, C., Gaudier, B., and Martin, G.: Réactions sérologiques positives vis-à-vis des adénovirus et érythèmes morbilliformes. Sem. Hôp. Paris, *35*:1083, 1959.
4. Chany, C., Lépine, P., Lelong, M., Le-Tan-Vinh, Stagé, P., and Virat, J.: Severe and fatal pneumonia in infants and young children associated with adenovirus infections. Amer. J. Hyg., *67*:367-378, 1958.
5. Dascomb, H. E., and Hilleman, M. R.: Clinical and laboratory studies in patients with respiratory disease caused by adenoviruses (RI-APC-ARD agents). Amer. J. Med., *21*:161, 1956.

6. Ferola, R., Morrone, G., and Nuziata, B.: Contributo alla conoscenza degli esantemi da poliovirus. Pediatria (Napoli), *5*:949, 1962.
7. Fleurette, J., Sohier, R., and Chardonnet, Y.: Les exanthèmes dûs à des virus chez l'enfant. Rev. Hyg. Med. Soc., *10*:355, 1962.
8. Fourrier, A., Hollinghausen, J., Bossuyt, J., and Samaille, J.: Un novel exanthème viral rappelant l'exathème subit dans deux cas d'infection par le poliovirus III. Lille Med., *11*:6-12, 1966.
9. Fukumi, H., Nishikawa, F., Nakamura, K., Watanabe, T., and Kitayama, T.: Further studies of the cases associated with adenoviruses. Jap. J. Med. Sci. Biol., *10*:407, 1957.
10. Gardner, P. S., Wright, A. E., and Hale, J. H.: Faecal excretion of adenovirus in a closed community. Brit. Med. J., *2*:424-426, 1961.
11. Gutekunst, R. R., and Heggie, A. D.: Viremia and viruria in adenovirus infections. Detection in patients with rubella or rubelliform illness. New Eng. J. Med., *26*:374-378, 1961.
12. Hummeler, K., Kirk, D., and Ostapiak, M.: Aseptic meningitis caused by Coxsackie virus with isolation of virus from cerebrospinal fluid. J.A.M.A., *156*:676, 1954.
13. Jansson, E., Wager, O., Forssell, P., and Halonen, H.: An exanthema subitum-like rash in patients with adenovirus infection. Ann. Paediat. Fenn., *7*:3, 1961.
14. Laurensich, A., Bassanetti, F., and Giovannelli, G.: La clinica delle adenovirosi. G. Mal. Infett., *12*:857, 1960.
15. Lerner, A., Cherry, J., Klein, J., and Finland, M.: Infection with reoviruses. New Eng. J. Med., *267*:947, 1962.
16. Lippi, M., Benedetto, A., Fontana, G., Frugoni, G., and Sebastiana, A.: Epidémie due au virus parainfluenzae type 3 (hemadsorption type I) dans une collectivité infantile en Italie. Ann. Inst. Pasteur (Paris), *102*:567-579, 1962.
17. Moss, P. D., Adams, M. O., and Tobin, J. O.: Serological studies with respiratory syncytial virus. Lancet, *1*:298, 1963.
18. Munro-Ashman, D., Gardner, P. S., Taylor, C. E. D., and MacDonald, J. C.: Acute pharyngitis associated with adenovirus type 3 infection. Lancet, *2*:121, 1958.
19. Neva, F. A., and Enders, J. F.: Isolation of a cytopathogenic agent from an infant with a disease in certain aspects resembling roseola infantum. J. Immunol., *72*:315-321, 1954.
20. Pierson, M., De Lavergne, E., Gilgenkrantz, S., and Worms, A. M.: Aspect clinique et épidémiologique de quelques cas d'infections à myxovirus parainfluenzae III (EA 102). Arch. Ges. Virusforsch., *13*:257-264, 1963.
21. Sohier, R.: Etiologie et pathogénie de la mononucléose infectieuse. Rapport du III Congrès de Pathologie Infectieuse, Bucarest, 1962.
22. Sohier, R., Bensimon, P., Chardonnet, Y., Challut, F., and Freydier, J.: Une épidémie d'infection à adenovirus. Rev. Hyg. Med. Soc., *5*:423, 1957.
23. Turpin, R., et al.: Erythème polymorphe et infection à réovirus. Ann. Pediat., *12*:36, 1965.

29

Clinically Defined Eruptive Fevers Whose Viral Origin Has Not Been Demonstrated

By P. MOZZICONACCI AND C. ATTAL

The diseases described here have a definite clinical autonomy, but proof of their viral nature has not yet been established.

EXANTHEMA SUBITUM OR ROSEOLA INFANTUM

Exanthema subitum is sometimes called the "sixth disease," following scarlet fever, measles, rubella, a fourth disease, Filatow and Duke's disease, whose very existence seems debatable, and epidemic megalerythema. It is one of the most frequent eruptive fevers of infancy, but although it was described over 50 years ago by Zahorsky, its etiology is still not known.

Circumstances of Appearance. Exanthema subitum is a disease of infants: 90 to 95 per cent of cases occur in children under the age of two years, and a diagnosis of roseola infantum after this age has every chance of being erroneous. Furthermore, if the very great probability of mild cases passing unnoticed is taken into consideration, it is probable that the disease is more or less obligatory during the first two years of life.[5]

The incubation period varies from five to 15 days, with an average of 12 days.

Clinical Description. The usual form is very benign. It begins with a sudden increase in temperature, to 39° C. on the average. The fever persists approximately three days, sometimes continuously, sometimes with remissions; then the fever falls abruptly and the rash appears. Granulocytopenia is usually observed and it confirms the diagnosis.

The fever, usually high, is generally well supported; occasionally a slight anorexia, vomiting once or several times, a slight diarrhea, or moderate agitation may be observed. A convulsive crisis may mark the temperature rise.

Examination reveals few notable signs. One-third of the infants have a slight pharyngitis, a few have a slight tonsillar exudate. Occasionally, minor adenopathies are encountered, some disseminated, others localized to the cervical or occipital regions. The spleen may be palpable. A slight meningeal-type stiffness may be observed.

Hematological examination is rarely undertaken at this point. The blood count is not yet typical, showing a decrease in the leukocyte count, with a relative increase in granulocytes.

The fever usually lasts three days, and then the temperature suddenly falls. The rash appears in the 24 hours following the fall in temperature. The eruption affects principally the nape of the neck and the trunk; often it is more marked at the level of the

385

back and spares the face; it rarely affects the limbs, and then is reduced to a few dispersed elements at the level of the thighs and the arms.

It is composed of macular elements 2 to 4 mm. in diameter, pale rose-colored, recalling the eruption in rubella. Its intensity is, moreover, highly variable; it may be slight, made up of disseminated elements and separated by spaces of healthy skin, or it may be dense and confluent.

The eruption is evanescent, lasting only one day or often only a few hours; it can even appear during the night and disappear the next morning. It never appears in recurrent outbursts. It involves neither desquamation nor persistent discoloration of the skin. There is no enanthem.

Finally, after the fever falls the general condition is excellent, and recovery occurs in the usual forms without sequelae.

Hematological examination during the eruptive period shows a highly characteristic pattern: a clearly marked granulocytopenia with decreased leukocytes (3000 to 7000) and a low level of polymorphonuclear cells (8 to 30 percent). Even when leukopenia does not exist, the level of polymorphonuclear cells is, in general, greatly decreased. The lymphomonocytosis, relative or absolute, which accompanies it is not accompanied by the appearance of hyperbasophilic pseudoplasmocytic elements analogous to those encountered in rubella or other viral diseases. The leukocytopenia, usually short-lived, occasionally persists two or three weeks.[5]

Clinical Forms. One of the characteristics of exanthema subitum is the relative frequency of nervous system manifestations accompanying it. Thus the convulsions at its onset may recur, the meningeal signs may be accompanied by discrete alterations in the cerebrospinal fluid, and, finally, an encephalitic form can exist. In this last, the initial state of agitation gives place to progressive torpor, a picture which may be completed by the appearance of a hemiplegia or monoplegia with Babinski's sign. A certain number of reports of this form are found in the literature.[3,4] The evolution is always toward rapid recession, although occasionally there are convulsive sequelae.

The cell count of the cerebrospinal fluid, even in these forms, is generally normal or very slightly altered. In the study that Joseph et al.[3] devoted to the nervous forms of exanthema subitum, two patients with encephalitis showed altered electroencephalographic tracings with localized anomalies related to the hemiplegia.

Diagnosis. Exanthema subitum must be differentiated from rubella. It must, however, be noted that the notion of contagion has never occurred with exanthema subitum, whereas it is frequently found in rubella, and that the leukocyte picture in rubella is very different, because it includes hyperbasophilic plasmocytic elements. The other diagnostic error arises from the fact that during the febrile phase medicines are often administered that can cause cutaneous eruptions and granulocytopenia. It is probable, as emphasized by Monnet and Fleurette,[5] that many eruptions in infants reported as reactions to drugs are, in reality, manifestations of exanthema subitum. The problems of differentiation from eruptions due to adenoviruses or ECHO viruses, are related rather to etiology: however, it is to be noted that illnesses linked to adenoviruses are often accompanied by conjunctivitis or involvement of the upper respiratory tract, which is lacking in exanthema subitum.

Pathology. No histological findings have been reported.

Epidemiology. The disease affects infants almost exclusively. The fact that older children are spared suggests that many infants affected by unexplained fever have, in fact, had an incomplete form of roseola infantum and that they thus have acquired immunity. In the first six months of life, the illness is exceptional, probably owing to transplacental passive immunity.

Exanthema subitum is apparently only very slightly contagious. The disease never affects more than one child in the same family, and its transmission in hospital wards is not to be feared, since epidemics are rare. A few have been reported, however, particularly in maternity hospitals. In fact, the mode of transmission remains undetermined.

ERYTHEMA INFECTIOSUM OR EPIDEMIC MEGALERYTHEMA

The autonomy of the "fifth disease" has often been contested. It is true that, when it occurs in the form of sporadic cases, it is difficult to recognize and probably often remains unrecognized. But when it assumes the aspect of a major epidemic, it appears as a clearly defined disease whose individuality is indisputable. Such major epidemics have been reported by German and Italian authors, to whom we owe the description of the disease; epidemics have also occurred in the United States and France.

Circumstances of Appearance. The disease generally affects children of school age. Its incubation period is estimated to be five to ten days with a mean of eight days. The disease generally begins with a rash on the face at the very start; it is, however, occasionally preceded by two or three days of symptoms: fever, rarely above 38° C., slight digestive disturbances, anorexia, vomiting, diarrhea, abdominal pains, and moderate impairment of general physical condition.

Clinical Description. The rash appears first on the face. Boulard and Pierre[1] described it perfectly. At the onset small red spots appear that are slightly papular, smaller than a lentil, and disappear on pressure; they swell rapidly in a few hours, giving to the skin a homogeneous, bright red aspect. The rash affects the cheeks but halts suddenly at the nasolabial groove, leaving untouched the base and the dorsal surface of the nose, the chin, the eyelids, and, generally, the forehead. Occasionally a few isolated elements are found at the base of the nose, on the chin, on the lateral surface of the neck, or behind the ears. The facial erythema takes the form of butterfly wings. The erythematous zone is smooth to the touch, but tight-drawn and hot. This facial erythema persists two to three days and then pales, but it may reappear transiently during the days following.

During a second phase the eruption involves the limbs, where it propagates centripetally. On the upper limbs, the eruption begins on the external surface of the arms, more rarely at the shoulder, then involves the forearm, predominating on its posterolateral surface, and the back of the hand, sparing the palm.

The rash on the forearms may be almost the sole manifestation of the disease: it begins on the posterior surface and mounts the lateral surface, particularly on the external side, leaving the elbow fold untouched. It extends at its periphery in an areolar manner, while small clear surfaces of irregular contour form at its center, growing and coalescing in a "geographic map" pattern. These clear zones with bright red border are very characteristic in aspect.

The lower limbs are affected almost simultaneously, especially the anterolateral surface of the thighs and the buttocks; the legs are less involved. The soles of the feet are untouched. Occasionally there are disseminated elements on the thorax. The abdomen is never involved. Small lymphadenopathies, in particular epitrochlear, often exist. The rash lasts one or two weeks. Its regression is not regular: several successive erythematous outbursts occur. The eruption is never followed by pigmentation or desquamation.

In general, there is no enanthem. However, Grimmer and Joseph[2] reported the possible presence of dark red spots on the gums, the soft palate, and the pharynx. The possibility has also been reported of vesicular or erosive lesions of the buccal cavity and also of the genital regions.

After the onset the systemic signs are minimal: the temperature is normal or subnormal and there is no asthenia.

The white cell count often shows slight lymphocytosis and often there is a marked eosinophilia.

Recovery is rapid and total, without complications or sequelae.

Pathology. The cutaneous lesions present a few distinctive histological features. The epidermic cells are edematous and infiltrated by histiocytes. The endothelium of the superficial vessels is swollen. Mononuclear cells have infiltrated around arterioles, venules, and capillaries.

Epidemiology. The disease generally affects children between the ages of five and 15 years, but infants are affected occasionally. Girls are affected more often than boys.

The occurrence of successive cases in schools or in members of the same family demonstrates the contagiousness of the disease, but its mode of transmission is poorly known, and during epidemics the cases are often scattered. It seems probable that very mild cases, without eruption or with discrete eruption, play a role in transmission of the disease. This epidemic form seems to be characterized by a high risk of infection within families and slow propagation by extrafamilial contacts; in this respect, the disease more resembles affections linked to enteroviruses than those due to respiratory viruses, such as influenza.

ECTODERMOSIS EROSIVA PLURIORIFICIALIS

Ectodermosis erosiva pluriorificialis, also called Stevens-Johnson or Rendu-Fiessinger disease, associates involvement of the mucosae, cutaneous eruption, and an infectious syndrome that is sometimes very intense. Stomatitis and conjunctivitis, however, constitute the dominant element in this clinical picture.

The very unity of this syndrome is not established with certainty. Certain forms are accompanied by a very severe effect on the general physical condition and can be fatal. In benign forms recovery takes place in two weeks on the average.

Whereas a viral etiology for exanthema subitum is probable, as shown by transmission of the disease to the monkey from patients' serum, and whereas it is probable that a nonidentified virus is responsible for epidemic megalerythema, the viral etiology of ectodermosis pluriorificialis is far from being proved.

BIBLIOGRAPHY

1. Boulard, P., and Pierre, R.: Le mégalérythème épidémique. A propos d'une grande épidémie régionale. Sem. Hôp. Paris, *29*:4059-4064, 1953.
2. Grimmer, H., and Joseph, A.: An epidemic of infectious erythema in Germany. A.M.A. Arch. Derm., *80*:283-285, 1959.
3. Joseph, R., Ribierre, M., Job, J. C., and Gabilan, J.: Les complications nerveuses de l'exanthème subit. Sem. Hôp. Paris, *34*:546, 1958.
4. Kaplan, M., Bijaoui, G., Kramarz, P., and Van Houtte, N.: Les manifestations neurologiques de l'exanthème subit. Etude de 20 observations. Ann. Pediat. (Paris), *11*:428-440, 1964.
5. Monnet, P., and Fleurette, J.: La 6ème maladie ou exanthème subit. Ann. Pediat. (Paris), *10*:190-195, 1963.

30

Varicella-Herpes Zoster Infections

CHICKENPOX (VARICELLA): CLINICAL FEATURES

by C. Attal and P. Mozziconacci

Chickenpox is a benign, highly contagious disease caused by herpes zoster-varicella virus (see page 402). It is characterized by a vesicular eruption with successive brief crops occurring at short intervals, ending in a crust-forming stage. It mainly attacks children aged two to ten, with a peak between four and eight years, but can also be observed in infants or newborn children or in adults; in these cases the systemic and cutaneous manifestations are more severe.

The immunity induced by varicella is strong and lasting. Recurrences have not been confirmed to date by laboratory investigations. Varicella rarely occurs before the third month of life, a fact which suggests that antibodies are transmitted by the mother. However, it is less rare than measles at that age, possibly because the transplacental passage of antibodies is not so constant or because the protection of the newborn child by antibodies is not always effective.[31]

Both sexes are equally susceptible, and all races are receptive.

Chickenpox is worldwide in distribution. It occurs in all seasons, predominantly in winter (March), at least in temperate climates.

Like all eruptive fevers, it is more frequent in the large urban centers. Epidemics do not occur as regularly as with measles, but a slight recrudescence can be noted every two or three years, related to the increase in receptive subjects.

Varicella is one of the most highly contagious diseases. It is transmitted from patient to patient by direct contact, probably via the respiratory route. However, the possibility of transmission by a healthy carrier, within a limited area and for a very short time, is not excluded (Ross).

The duration of the contagious phase is variable (see Varicella-Herpes Zoster: Virological Features.

PATHOLOGY

The lesions of varicella are identical to those of herpes simplex or herpes zoster. The vesicles are intraepidermic. The vesicle fluid is produced by the lysis and the liquefaction of stratum mucosum cells. In the first stage the cells degenerate, fill up with water, and detach themselves one from the other; they are often enormous. Many of them contain eosinophilic intranuclear inclusions, with a clear halo and a peripheral circle of chromatin.

When the fluid becomes cloudy, it is invaded by polymorphonuclear leukocytes. The crust which is formed afterwards is first adherent to the deep layer but later is easy to detach. On the mucous membrane, there is no crust. When the vesicle disrupts, it leaves a superficial ulceration which heals very quickly.

In the very rare fatal cases of varicella, the lesions observed at autopsy are widespread. Many organs are found to be involved: esophagus, liver, pancreas, kidney, ureter, bladder, uterus, adrenal glands. Foci of necrosis and acidophilic inclusion cells have been observed there.

On histological study, the lung shows scattered lesions of interstitial pneumopathy and many nodular hemorrhagic areas. The latter consist of exudates which contain fibrin, blood red cells, and many mononuclear cells, some of them containing intranuclear inclusion bodies. Macroscopically, rounded red areas, 2 to 4 mm. in diameter, are sometimes observed. But in other cases, no anomaly is noted. Microscopic examination alone permits the detection of the foci of peribronchial necrosis, the fibrinoleukocytic exudates, and the intranuclear inclusions, which are the three characteristic elements of these cases of varicella pneumopathy.

CLINICAL FEATURES

Incubation. The incubation of varicella is not apparent. It lasts 14 to 16 days, the extreme limits being ten to 20 days. In children, the *invasion* period lasts only a few hours, 24 at the utmost. It is characterized by a moderate fever and a discrete malaise. Often the systemic manifestations and the eruption start at the same time.

In the adolescent and in the adult, the invasion period is sometimes longer. Fever, headache, and malaise are generally more marked and may precede the eruption by two or three days.

Eruption. The eruption, sometimes preceded by a brief scarlatiniform rash, is characterized by its aspect and the rapidity of its progression. At first some macular elements appear; they become slightly papular, 2 to 4 mm. in diameter, pinkish, congestive. A few lesions disappear after this stage, but most of them become covered with superficial vesicles surrounded by a very thin red areola. Their content is clear and their surface is distended. The vesicle is then like a dewdrop, 3 or 4 mm. in diameter, round or oval in shape. The following day, the vesicle fluid becomes turbid and the vesicle quickly deflates, then dries and crusts.

This crust, which is darkish, drops off within a week on the average (extreme limits; five to 20 days).

At this stage, pruritus frequently occurs. The total evolution of each element is brief and the succession macula-papule-vesicle-crust may last only six to eight hours and sometimes ends two or three days later.

The elements appear on various parts of the body, but mainly on the trunk (centripetal distribution). The face and the scalp are always involved. In the mild cases, only a few scattered vesicles are observed there. On the limbs, the vesicles are more numerous on the proximal parts.

The exanthem develops in successive crops, on an average three or four crops within three or four days, which accounts for the presence, at the same site, of elements of different age. On the whole, they have all reached the crust-forming stage within six to eight days. With each crop, the temperature rises; moreover, the fever reflects the intensity of the eruption. In some cases, the eruption is very discrete and there are no more than about 10 or 20 vesicles, which evolve in a single crop. On the other hand, in some cases the crops are more numerous and the cutaneous elements, which are countless, spread on the face, the scalp, and the limbs, but are invariably predominant on the trunk.

After the crusts fall off there remain small unpigmented areas, but there is no scar, except in case of superinfection.

Mucosae are often involved, in particular the buccal mucosa. The elements are mainly located on the palate or on the anterior pillars. It is difficult to observe the vesicle because it disrupts very early and is replaced by an ulceration, 2 to 4 mm. in diameter, rounded, white, surrounded by a red areola, very superficial and rarely painful. The same elements may be present on the palpebral conjunctiva, where they are very painful, on the vulval mucosa, and even on the pharynx and the larynx.

The systemic manifestations vary, like the fever, according to the intensity of the eruption. They consist of headache, malaise, and anorexia. When all the elements have reached the crust stage, these manifestations have all disappeared.

CLINICAL FORMS

Since chickenpox is remarkably benign and has such a characteristic symptomatology, it generally raises few problems for the physician. Occasionally, however, it takes on misleading aspects: its evolution, especially in some patients, may be redoubtable.

Unusual Aspects of the Eruption. In some cases, the vesicles, widely spread, form large polycyclic bubbles, over 1 cm. in diameter. The eruption consists either of these bubble elements alone or of both vesicles and bubbles. The benign prognosis is that of a common varicella, but such eruptions may suggest a pemphigus or even a vesicular prurigo.

In other cases, some vesicles are filled with hemorrhagic fluid or there is a thin ecchymotic edge at the base of the cutaneous element. In the absence of extensive ecchymosis and of important systemic manifestations or other hemorrhagic manifestations, the possibility of dangerous hemorrhagic varicella can be rejected.

Hemorrhagic Varicella. Hemorrhagic varicella is very rare and extremely serious. It is characterized by high fever, severe constitutional symptoms, and generalized hemorrhage, in the vesicles and also in the form of petechiae, ecchymoses, even epistaxis and hematemesis. It is often fatal. In some cases it is related to depression of the patient's immunological defenses.

This is what happens when chickenpox occurs during a hemopathy, in particular acute or chronic leukemia treated with certain antimitotic drugs such as methotrexate. In recent years, the extension of corticosteroid treatments has created a new type of extremely serious hemorrhagic varicella which is often fatal.

It always occurs in patients who have been under treatment for some time. Its severity does not depend upon the original disease which necessitated the treatment (rheumatic fever, asthma, collagen disease); it seems related above all to the comparative adrenal insufficiency of those subjects. If the steroid therapy is stopped or even if the doses are only lowered, the clinical picture becomes worse. This accounts for the recommendation that corticosteroid treatment be continued during the entire course of the disease, or, better, that the dosage be increased slightly.[22] However, these complications should not be regarded as constant. Falliers and Ellis[21] did not observe any case of aggravated varicella among their patients with asthma undergoing prolonged hormone therapy, possibly because the doses used were lower.

Varicella in the Newborn Child. In the newborn child, chickenpox is often benign. Sometimes, however, the lesions are widely disseminated. The general state is seriously impaired and the child may die. Postmortem examination reveals lesions in all viscera (metastatic varicella).

Usually, the newborn infant is infected by his mother at the moment of delivery and the disease starts after an incubation period of normal length. In some cases, however, placental transmission may occur (see page 402). Such cases of congenital varicella, with an incubation period of less than ten days,[19] can be very severe and accompanied by multiple visceral localizations. They also can be absolutely benign (O'Neil[30]). However, the mortality of congenital varicella is 21 per cent (Newman).

Varicella in the Adult. In the adult, varicella can be much more severe than in the child. The prodrome is longer, the fever is higher, the headache and the malaise are more intense. The eruption is more profuse and complications are more frequent. The severity as well as the rarity of these forms of varicella in adults accounts for the frequent difficulty in distinguishing it from smallpox. Such cases are an absolute indication for epidemiological and virological investigations (see page 402).

COMPLICATIONS

The rarity of complications other than cutaneous superinfection should be emphasized.

Cutaneous superinfection can cause either pyodermitis or impetigo. They remain localized and produce scars.

Until antibacterial chemotherapy came into use, such superinfections were the source of severe disseminations: bacterial pneumopathy, septicemia, osteomyelitis. This type of complication is no longer observed in the developed countries. These superinfections are probably related to the cases of varicella nephritis described by earlier authors. In all probability, they were cases of glomerulonephritis subsequent to superinfection of the skin by group A hemolytic streptococci. However, since the varicella virus spreads throughout all the organs, its possible role in causing nephritis cannot be ruled out entirely.

Certain localizations of the vesicles may cause local complications: for example, shedding of the crusts on the nasal mucosa may provoke an epistaxis which is sometimes considerable. More severe is dyspnea due to the extension of the laryngeal eruption; acute inspiratory dyspnea accompanied by intense respiratory traction may require a tracheotomy in severe cases.

Other complications are common to many viral diseases and are the consequence of unusual localizations or of the extension to tissues not usually involved.

Cases of thrombocytopenic purpura have been observed occasionally. They do not differ from those described in other eruptive fevers such as German measles or measles. Their prognosis, as a rule, is favorable.[23] In other cases, the picture of purpura fulminans has been reported.[8]

Still rarer is gangrenous varicella. The few observations published concern children whose varicella had seemed to progress normally until the eighth day. Then, suddenly, large necrotic areas appeared on the skin, along with a hemorrhagic syndrome caused by afibrinogenemia. The prognosis is most unfavorable.[13, 24]

Varicella pneumopathy is less exceptional than had been thought. It is more frequent in adults than in children (see Chapter 42).

Lesions of hepatitis have occasionally been discovered at autopsy in these cases of varicella pneumopathy, although there had been no clinical manifestations other than a subicterus.

The neurological complications (encephalitis, myelitis, polyneuritis) are discussed in Chapter 9.

Ocular complications other than conjunctivitis due to local vesicles have been described. Sometimes ulcerous keratitis, central or marginal, may be the cause of corneal opacity. However, as a rule, it is transient and benign. Uveitis is rarer. Retrobulbar optic neuritis and edematous papillitis have also been reported. Involvement of the optic nerve, as well as of the motor nerves, seldom occurs alone. As a rule, it is one of the elements of chickenpox encephalitis.[7]

A few cases of varicella orchitis have been reported.

Some observations of hypoglycemia with convulsions have also been reported.[6] Their significance is not clear. In Krugman's opinion salicylate therapy, rather than varicella itself, was responsible.

DIFFERENTIAL DIAGNOSIS

The differential diagnosis is, as a rule, easy.

OTHER CUTANEOUS ERUPTIONS

Some of the most common cutaneous affections have at times led to diagnostic errors, but usually these errors were soon corrected.

Strophulus Infantum. The cutaneous element of strophulus infantum is different from that of varicella: it is, above all, a papule, and if, fairly often, there is a central vesicle, it is like a needle-point but never like a "dewdrop." Moreover, the strophulus eruption never involves the scalp but is sometimes located on the palms of the hands. Buccal lesions never occur. The papules are grouped in clumps of eight to ten elements and are never scattered all over the body. They never have the characteristic centripetal disposition. Fever and malaise are not observed. The evolution is longer. Each element remains unchanged for several days, even for one or two weeks. Pruritus, however, provokes lesions due to scratching that often undergo secondary infection. Infected strophulus may, then, look like a superinfected varicella vesicle.

Some cases of vesicular strophulus have a different aspect: they consist of some elements, vesicular at the onset, without papule. These bubbles are usually much larger than varicella vesicles (1 cm. in diameter). No crust covers them and they persist a long time without alteration.

Impetigo. The cutaneous lesion of impetigo is vesicular at the onset. Very soon the fluid seems purulent and a crust is formed. Impetigo exclusively involves the uncovered parts of the body, with a marked predilection for the lips and the surface around the nose. It does not progress through successive crops. Adenopathy in the involved zone frequently occurs.

Scabies or Insect Bites. These cannot be mistaken for varicella since their site is characteristic and their course prolonged.

SMALLPOX. Smallpox is not a frequently suggested diagnosis in most European or North American countries. Nevertheless, persistent endemic centers in Central and South America, in Africa, and in Southeast Asia, the insufficient guarantees of the international certificates of vaccination, and the speed of air transport which makes possible the travel of patients in the incubation period, require physicians to be vigilant. The elements of the differential diagnosis are well known for the characteristic forms. The prodromal period of variola lasts at least

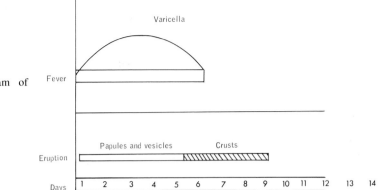

Figure 30-1. Schematic diagram of the clinical evolution of varicella.

three days. It is characterized by a high fever, malaise, headache, and severe constitutional symptoms.

The eruption, at first papular, as in varicella (but in smallpox the papules are larger), progresses much more slowly: the succession papule-vesicle-pustule-crust occurs over five to six days, not a few hours. Each element is deeper in the skin. This evolution is not manifested by crops scattered all over the body; in any one anatomical area, the elements are all of the same age.

The systemic signs remain marked during the whole course. The lesions are predominant on the face and on the hands and feet.

Smallpox may, however, present more deceptive aspects, with discrete systemic signs and a moderate eruption. The fact of recent successful smallpox vaccination, which must be verified by the presence of a scar, is a valuable argument against variola. However, when the vaccination is not recent variola may present a particularly deceptive aspect. Therefore, when a possible contamination is suspected, when atypical varicella occurs

during a smallpox epidemic, or when the patient is an adult, the highly specialized laboratory should be called on without hesitation and, within a few days, it will provide the indispensable differential diagnosis (see pages 402 and 421).

RICKETTSIALPOX

In rickettsialpox, the generalized papulovesicular eruption follows a primary escharotic lesion located anywhere on the body surface and an influenza-like syndrome lasting a few days. Moreover, the vesicles, smaller than those of varicella, top an indurated papula. A specific complement-fixation test permits the diagnosis. The vector agent, *Rickettsia akari*, is transmitted to man by the bite of the mouse louse.

COXSACKIE A 16

In the course of some Coxsackie A 16 virus epidemics, vesicular eruptions have been mistaken for varicella. These eruptions

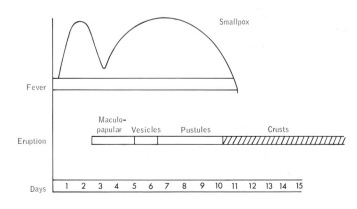

Figure 30-2. Schematic diagram of the clinical evolution of smallpox.

are, however, rarely strictly vesicular. Many maculopapular elements are also present, predominantly at the extremities. These eruptions are always accompanied by characteristic lesions in the mouth and on the tongue. They progress in a single crop (see Chapter 27).

HERPES ZOSTER

Lastly, we shall consider the very particular problem of the differential diagnosis with herpes zoster. Those two diseases have the same etiological agent but usually occur under completely different conditions (see page 402). Moreover, the zoster eruption is not very similar to that of varicella. It is unilateral and is located along the nerve endings; its vesicles are small, bright, and confluent on an erythematous plaque; it is accompanied by pain, which does not exist in varicella; adenopathy is constant and the scars are pigmented or achromic. However, extremely rare cases have been reported in which the two diseases occurred simultaneously. As a rule, the onset is that of herpes zoster, followed by a generalized eruption.

Most of these diagnoses lead to controversy only in atypical varicella. Almost invariably, varicella is recognized at first sight. The associated papulovesicular eruption is characteristic enough, with its mild general signs and moderate fever, its rapid succession through macula, papule, vesicle, crust, progressing in several successive crops; it has a centripetal distribution but covers the scalp and leaves shallow small white ulcers on the buccal mucosa. The usual laboratory tests are of no help. The blood count is generally normal; however, marked leukocytosis may be found in cases of superinfection of the cutaneous lesions or of varicella pneumopathy. The virological investigations, which can be made in highly specialized laboratories, can be considered only for systematic studies, although they are sometimes imperative to differentiate chickenpox from smallpox.

TREATMENT

The treatment of uncomplicated chickenpox is merely symptomatic. To date, the antiviral substances have not yielded any appreciable results. Various preparations have been tried, in particular xenalamine[12] and ABOB[14] (see page 402).

Low doses of aspirin can be prescribed for high fever or marked systemic signs. Pruritus may be attenuated by local application of 1 per cent mentholated talc. The effect of antihistaminic drugs per os is not very convincing. Antihistaminic creams must be absolutely forbidden, for they often cause dermatitis. However, a very old treatment remains valid: xylol, which is administered at a dose of 60 to 120 drops per day, in three intakes, in a small quantity of milk (the mixture must be taken immediately). It attenuates pruritus and accelerates the evolution of the cutaneous elements.

It is important, especially with children, to cut the nails closely and to observe hygienic precautions strictly, both to limit the scratching and to avoid superinfection. When the vesicles are the site of bacterial superinfection (as a rule by *Staphylococcus aureus*) a local treatment is usually sufficient (application of a 2 per cent eosin solution in 60° alcohol).

In serious cases, the treatment of pulmonary localizations may be difficult. Antibotics have no action on the virus; however, they must be prescribed to avert secondary bacterial infections (see Chapter 42).

Although steroid therapy has been suggested in the treatment of virus pneumopathy, it is questionable in this case. It should be borne in mind that cases of varicella have been fatal when they occurred in the course of steroid treatment. It has not been proved that such treatment undertaken after the onset of the disease entails the same risks, but it is not certain either that hormonal treatment has a favorable influence upon varicella pneumopathy, and, since there is room for doubt, it is more reasonable not to undertake such therapy.

The same remarks apply to the use of steroid drugs during encephalitis. A great risk is certainly not involved, but the profit is uncertain. Rehydration, barbiturates in case of convulsions, and assisted respiration whenever necessary are the steps to be taken.

PREVENTION

Varicella prevention should be resorted to only in the newborn, in patients under steroid treatment, or in those suffering from malignant hemopathy. Ross considers that injection of gamma globulins in a dose of 0.15 mg. per kilogram of body weight might attenuate the disease, but the results are inconsistent (see page 402).

With normal children, practically no precaution is useful. Isolation of the patients, which in France legally lasts 15 days, has never succeeded in limiting the spread of the disease. Isolation of brothers and sisters assumed to be in the incubation period is difficult to obtain, and these children are contagious 24 hours before the onset of the disease.

BIBLIOGRAPHY

1. Appelbaum, E., Rachelson, M. H., and Dolgopol, V. B.: Varicella encephalitis. Amer. J. Med., *15*: 223-230, 1953.
2. Aula, P.: Chromosomes and viral infections. Lancet, *1*:720-721, 1964.
3. Bastin, R., Binard, C., and Phav-Sany: Les manifestations pulmonaires au cours de la varicelle. Presse Med., *71*:1873-1875, 1963.
4. Bernheim, M.: Maladies à virus et hormonothérapie. Arch. Franc. Pediat., *16*:240-250, 1959.
5. Blair, A. W., Jamieson, W. M., and Smith, G. H.: Complications and death in chickenpox. Brit. Med. J., 2:981-983, 1964.
6. Blattner, R. J.: Serious complications of varicella, including fatalities. J. Pediat., *50*:515-518, 1957.
7. Bonamour, G., and Gaillot: Les complications oculaires de la varicelle. J. Med. Lyon, *40*:663-669, 1959.
8. Bouhasin, J. D.: Purpura fulminans. Pediatrics, *34*: 264-270, 1964.
9. Canby, J. P., and Blakely, L.: Bullous chickenpox (varicella bullosa). Clin. Pediat., *2*:13-15, 1963.
10. Carstairs, L. S., and Emond, R. D. T.: Chicken-pox virus pneumonia. Proc. Roy. Soc. Med., *56*:267-270, 1963.
11. Charles, R. H. G.: Post varicella polyneuritis. Brit. Med. J., *1*:908, 1965.
12. Colomb, D.: Xenalamine dans le traitement des dermatoses virales du groupe herpès-zona. Bull. Soc. Franc. Dermat., *68*:14, 1961.
13. Crocker, A. M., and Middelkamp, J. N.: Varicella gangrenosa. J. Pediat., *54*:104-108, 1959.
14. Curwen, M. P., Emond, R. T. D., and MacKendrick, G. D. W.: Controlled trial of ABOB in measles, chicken-pox and mumps. Brit. Med. J., *1*:236-237, 1963.
15. Editorial: Fatal chicken-pox. Brit. Med. J., *2*:954-955, 1965.
16. Editorial: Varicella encephalitis. Lancet, *2*:821-822, 1953.
17. Editorial: Complications of chicken-pox. Lancet, *2*:839, 1957.
18. Editorial: Orchitis as a complication of chicken-pox. Brit. Med. J., *1*:1203-1204, 1953.
19. Ehrlich, R. M., Turner, J. A. P., and Clarke, M.: Neo-natal varicella. A case report with isolation of the virus. J. Pediat., *53*:139-147, 1958.
20. Eisenklam, E. J.: Primary varicella pneumonia in a three-year-old girl. J. Pediat., *69*:452-454, 1966.
21. Falliers, C. J., and Ellis, E. F.: Corticosteroids and varicella. Six years experience in an asthmatic population. Arch. Dis. Child., *40*:593-594, 1965.
22. Gerbeaux, J., Couvreur, J., Baculard-Beauchef, A., and Jay, J. P.: Maladies infectieuses sous corticothérapie au long cours (194 observations dont 102 varicelles). Sem. Hop. Paris, *39*:61-75, 1963.
23. Giraud, P., Orsini, A., Pinsard, N., and Pieron, H.: Purpura thrombopénique post-varicelleux. Pediatrie, *19*:861-864, 1964.
24. Grenier, A., and Marlat, J. M.: Syndrome hémorragique par afibrinogénémie au cours d'une varicelle. Arch. Franc. Pediat., *21*:207-211, 1964.
25. Knyvett, A. F.: Complicated chicken-pox. Med. J. Aust., *2*:91-93, 1957.
26. Krugman, S.: Varicella and herpes virus infection. Pediat. Clin. N. Amer., *7*:881-902, 1960.
27. Krugman, S., and Ward, R.: Infectious Diseases in Children. 3rd ed. St. Louis, C. V. Mosby Company, 1964.
28. Leonardi, G., Zulian, G., and Ghio, T.: Effect of a new antiviral substance (xenalamine) in chickenpox. Lancet, *2*:718-719, 1961.
29. Nakao, T.: Primary varicella pneumonia. Tohoku J. Exp. Med., *72*:249-252, 1960.
30. O'Neil, R. R.: Congenital varicella. Amer. J. Dis. Child., *104*:391-392, 1962.
31. Readett, M. D., and McGibbon, C.: Neo-natal varicella. Lancet, *1*:644-645, 1961.
32. Rotem, G. E.: Complications of chickenpox. Brit. Med. J., *1*:944-947, 1961.
33. Rotem, G. E.: Primary chickenpox pneumonia. Israel Med. J. *20*:226, 1961.
34. Seigerman, H., and Zonis, M. H.: Varicella bullosa, a case report. J. Pediat., *62*:302-304, 1963.
35. Tan, D. Y., Kaufman, S. A., and Levene, G.: Primary chickenpox pneumonia. Amer. J. Roentgen., *76*:527-532, 1956.
36. Vic-Dupont, and Vachon, F.: La varicelle. Rev. Prat., *16*:1159-1165, 1956.
37. Weber, D. M., and Pellechia, J. A.: Varicella pneumonia: study of prevalence in adult men. J.A.M.A., *192*:572-573, 1965.
38. Weinstein, L., and Meade, R. H.: Respiratory manifestations of chicken-pox. Arch. Int. Med., *98*: 91-99, 1956.
39. White, H. H.: Varicella myelopathy. New Eng. J. Med., *226*:772-773, 1962.
40. Wouthard, M. E.: Roentgen findings in chickenpox pneumonia. Amer. J. Roentgen., *76*:533-539, 1956.

HERPES ZOSTER: CLINICAL FEATURES

by C. ATTAL AND P. MOZZICONACCI

Herpes zoster holds a special place among the infectious diseases. Although it is now established that the responsible virus is that of varicella, the natural history of the disease is not well known. The interpretation of clinical, anatomical, and virological facts is partly hypothetical.

As a rule, the clinical aspect of the zoster rash is characteristic enough to be recognized immediately. Its segmentary distribution, emphasized by Bright as early as 1831, is not observed in any other infection. Herpes zoster is always a benign disease. Even though painful sequelae occur in some cases, it is never fatal alone.

The cutaneous localization of the virus may be considered secondary, although it comes first in the clinical picture: the neurological lesion is the most important element.

ETIOLOGY

Although it is generally easy to establish the clinical diagnosis, the occurrence of zoster is unforeseeable and does not obey any known rules of transmission of viral diseases. Zoster rarely attacks children. Its incidence increases with age and is highest after 50 years of age. Zoster is not an epidemic disease. With certain exceptions, the cases observed are sporadic, and there is no seasonal recrudescence.

The influence of the subject's general health has long been known. Zoster occurs more often in tired persons or in those with an infection, a metabolic disease, or neoplasia or leukemia. In some cases, it may appear as the consequence of intoxication (lead, especially arsenic, carbon monoxide, and also sulfonamides and bismuth), of trauma, of corticosteroid therapy,[17] of a neurological lesion of the cord (tabes, tumor, myelitis), or even of sunburn. These secondary cases of zoster are located on the metameric area of the myelopathy or on that of the trauma. Cases of reflex zoster have been described, during pleuropneumopathies or after hepatic or nephritic colic. They are located in the area of the affected organ. The relationship between primary zoster and so-called secondary zoster was the object of much discussion until

the unity of the disease and of the agent was definitely established.

It is difficult to determine the incidence of zoster, since many forms are very mild and medical aid is not sought. In the outpatient department of a hospital, the cases of zoster represent hardly 1 per cent of the patients. A survey of 1000 families showed a much higher incidence, about 15 per cent.[19]

PATHOLOGY

1. The skin lesions are no different from those of varicella and herpes simplex. During the first stage of the rash, some cells of the malpighian layer proliferate. This results in formation of giant multinucleated cells. At the same time, others undergo ballooning degeneration. The vesicle, at first unilocular, becomes bigger. The content seems to press on the walls, which are made of balloon cells. Finally a multilocular cavity is achieved. Its tegmen is made of the corneal layer of the epidermis and it rests on the malpighian layer. Its content is serofibrinous, but there are some polymorphonuclear cells. The vesicular fluid may turn purulent and an inflammatory dermal reaction may occur all around; the dermis becomes infiltrated with polymorphonuclear cells and lymphocytes.

The cells with intranuclear inclusions are not a constant finding. These inclusions, at first basophilic, turn acidophilic in the older lesions; they are colored red by Giemsa's stain and green by Pappenheim's stain. They are visible mainly in the cells that have undergone ballooning degeneration but may appear around the vesicle and in the conjunctive tissue. They are identical to those observed in herpes simplex.

Sometimes, small granular inclusions are seen in the nucleus and the cytoplasm of some epithelial cells.

2. Lesions in the spinal ganglia were first observed by von Barens-Prung in 1862. Head and Campbell studied them with great care in 1900.

The spinal ganglion involved is infiltrated with mononuclear leukocytes. It is scattered with hemorrhagic areas which are sometimes large enough to destroy it almost completely. On healing, a secondary gliosis is observed. The afferent peripheral nerve is congestive and infiltrated with round cells. The nerve fibers which end in the impaired ganglion cells degenerate. Degeneration can also occur in the efferent posterior root, with secondary sclerosis.

Even in the cases of uncomplicated zoster, the neurological lesions are not limited to ganglia and to the sensory nerves. They reach the posterior horn of the cord, which is infiltrated with mononuclear cells. Head and Campbell wrote that zoster was actually acute posterior poliomyelitis. Sometimes, even the bulb and the pons are invaded (Wohlwill).

The myelitis, which remains unilateral, may also spread to the anterior horn (Denny-Brown).

Finally in the areas of ganglionic, radicular, and medullar involvement, lesions of leptomeningitis are almost invariably observed (Goodbody and Cheatham). Whatever the site of the zoster, rachidian or cranial, the lesions are the same.

CLINICAL FEATURES

If it is assumed that herpes zoster is due to the reactivation of a virus which has been latent for many years, it is clear that discussion of the length of the incubation period is meaningless. Zoster is characterized by an erythematous and vesiculous eruption with a very special topography; signs of involvement of the nervous system; local adenopathy; and systemic signs of varying severity.

1. At the onset, the signs are usually neurological (68 per cent of the cases). There is a sensation of prickling along an intercostal nerve. Sometimes the pain remains moderate, and it may disappear after a few days. But it may also persist during the rash and even after, for a longer or shorter period. The pain varies greatly in intensity and in type from one patient to another. The onset is either sudden or more progressive; sometimes the pain rapidly becomes more and more intense and may be unbearable, neuralgia-like or more often burnlike. It is either intermittent or constant. The area most often involved is that of dorsal ganglia (intercostal zoster). In some cases, limited areas of hypoesthesia or of anesthesia can be observed at the very onset. Occasionally the anesthetic area is clear-cut and large. This is called syndrome of painful anesthesia.

Vasomotor disturbances are almost constant; sweating is suppressed (André Thomas).

As a rule, painful phenomena appear four to five days before the cutaneous signs, but may last ten to 15 days. Sometimes they are even the only symptom of the disease; in such cases the eruption does not occur or is limited to a few maculae, without vesicles (zoster without rash). On the other hand in some cases the pain is very discrete, especially in children; abnormal sensations, more unpleasant than painful, may be felt.

At that stage, lymphadenopathy develops in the corresponding area (Bartholomew's sign).

2. The most characteristic feature is the localization of the rash. It is nearly always unilateral (bilateral zoster represents only 0.5 per cent of the cases). It is present all along the endings of the intercostal sensory nerves. The rash starts proximally and spreads distally along the nerve. It almost never spreads beyond the median line. Occasionally, one or two aberrant elements can be noted on the opposite side. The metameric involvement is greater or lesser. Most often, a single rachidian ganglion and a single area are involved. Sometimes, the eruption covers a wider band, corresponding to two neighboring ganglia. Much more rarely, two separate areas are affected.

The first erythematous plaques or papulae are oval, 1 to 2 cm. long and 1 cm. wide, and irregularly outlined. Their axis has the same direction as the nerve. They are located at three points: near the spine, in the axillary area, and near the sternum. Within the next 12 to 24 hours, small, white, bright vesicles appear, more or less numerous. On the third day, the vesicular fluid, previously clear, turns turbid. The eruption becomes pustule-like. At this stage, the subjacent erythema starts disappearing. Some aberrant vesicles are frequently seen besides the plaques.

A week later, the pustulae are dry and covered with crusts, which drop off within two or three weeks. The affected skin may remain pigmented or, on the contrary, achromic, and sometimes a small area of hypoesthesia or of anesthesia is noted.

The severity of the eruption varies greatly. In mild cases, it remains maculo-papular, without vesicles; it decreases and disappears within a week. The total duration of the eruption depends very much on the time of appearance of the vesicles: when they come out in 24 hours, they disappear between the tenth and the sixteenth days, but when they do not become visible until the seventh day, they do not disappear until the fifth week.

In severe cases, the plaques may be confluent and the vesicles may have a gangrenous aspect. Healing occurs only many weeks later.

In most cases, there are six to ten plaques with intervals of healthy skin, but the eruption may be limited to one single element.

3. Systemic signs are usually less marked. There is no fever, or the temperature does not exceed 38° C. Headache, general malaise, and stiff neck are sometimes noticed. In adults, these symptoms are encountered only in 5.8 per cent of the cases of zoster.[6] They are assumed to be more frequent in children. Firm and painful swelling of axillary lymph nodes is a constant feature.

The laboratory tests are of little avail for the diagnosis. The blood count is normal or reveals a slight increase in leukocytes, with moderate polymorphonucleosis.

The cerebrospinal fluid often shows a slight lymphocytic reaction and an increase in protein level (in 50 to 70 per cent of the cases), but the mere fact that the cerebrospinal fluid is normal does not prove that the disease is not zoster.

On the whole, the disease lasts from ten to 30 days.

As a rule, there are no sequelae after the cure, but occasionally (12 per cent of the cases), and mainly in aged people, pain is persistent and permanent and unforeseeable recrudescences may occur. Such pain is often a severe trial to the patient and eventually impairs his physical and moral resistance.

CLINICAL FORMS

As already described, the rash may be limited to a single plaque of erythema or to a single cluster of vesicles.

Sometimes, however, it is more serious, with a hemorrhagic or even gangrenous or extended eruption. At its worst, it may become generalized. In addition, the zoster eruption itself may be followed by an outbreak of varicella vesicles scattered all over the body. Generalized zoster often appears as a severe disease, very febrile, attended by polymorphonuclear hyperleukocytosis. Com-

plications, mainly pulmonary and neurological, are very frequent in such cases.

The general physical condition of the patient may affect, to a degree, the aspect and the course of the disease.

1. In children, zoster is less serious than in adults. The eruption and lymphadenopathy are no different, but the general symptoms are absent; pain is absent or very slight and transient. Post-zoster pain is never seen. The total duration of the disease is shorter: of patients with zoster up to age 20, 94 per cent recover in seven to 14 days, whereas of patients aged 40 to 59, only 49 per cent recover within two weeks.

2. Zoster in newborn children or in infants is very rare. When it does occur it is not easily accounted for. In patients who have not previously had varicella, the transplacental route is considered responsible for the transmission of the virus, as well as for an antibody level sufficient to control its spread. A case of zoster in an infant age 30 hours which involved the inferior maxilla has been reported.[1] According to generally held opinion, the disease in infants is benign and recovery is rapid, without sequelae.

3. A particular problem is the high incidence of zoster during malignant diseases: leukemia, Hodgkin's disease, lymphosarcoma, carcinoma. Estimates of this incidence vary according to the authors, the type of disease, the patient's age, and, probably, the duration of observation. In a study of 70 cases of lymphoid leukemia[5] the incidence was as high as 15.7 per cent. It ranges around 3 per cent in children with Hodgkin's disease, a particularly high incidence for that age.[12]

It is in such cases that serious hemorrhagic, generalized, and even fatal forms of zoster are most often encountered. However, this association is not constant and less severe forms of zoster often occur.

Various factors are assumed to be the cause of the incidence and the relative seriousness of zoster in malignant diseases: inhibition of the defense mechanisms, aggravation by therapy (corticosteroid therapy, radiotherapy, alcoylant agents), local irritation in spinal ganglia (tumoral or leukemic infiltration, compression, radiotherapy). In this respect, it is relevant to mention that accidental or surgical traumas involving spinal roots or nerves play a well-known triggering role.

According to its *topography,* zoster often has a special aspect. Zoster located in the upper thorax may be associated with an eruption on the internal side of the arm. Zoster involving the limbs has a characteristic radicular topography; the cutaneous elements are no different from those of intercostal zoster. Zoster of the sacral roots causes eruptions on the buttocks or the perineum. The pain felt in the genital organs may suggest a urinary disease.

In patients over 40 years of age, thoracic or lumbar zoster represents 65.4 per cent of the cases, ophthalmic zoster 20 per cent, and zoster of the maxillary and mandibular nerves 1.3 per cent each. Zoster of the cranial nerves is much less frequent under the age of 20; in such patients intercostal zoster is observed in 89 per cent of the cases and zoster of the cranial nerves is the second most frequent form.

Cranial zoster is more severe than others; it is usually associated with sympathetic disturbances and paralysis. In some cases, the mucosae are involved.

Zoster of the ophthalmic branch of the trigeminus nerve is the most severe form (see also Chapter 54).

The preëruptive pains are very intense; they are located on the forehead, the orbit, and the eyeball; the systemic symptoms are more marked than in other types of zoster, with fever, shivering, and often signs of meningeal irritation.

The eruption is preceded by edema of the eyelid. Most often it involves only one branch of the ophthalmic nerve. When it is the frontal branch, the eruption spreads fanlike from the upper eyelid to the scalp.

When the lacrimal branch is involved, the eruption affects the temporomalar area and the external half of the upper eyelid. Weeping resulting from the lacrimal gland involvement is also noted.

Involvement of the nasociliary branch is characterized by an eruption on the internal angle of the eye, the conjunctiva, and the root of the nose. It is associated with a unilateral coryza and above all with a corneal anesthesia, and the physician must be aware of the risk of local complications.

As a matter of fact, often the infratrochlear branch alone (root of the nose, internal angle of the upper eyelid) or the anterior ethmoidal branch (lobule and mucosa of the nose) is electively affected.

The submaxillary and preauricular lymphatic glands always become enlarged and painful. A meningeal reaction, clinical and biological, is constant.

The course of ophthalmic zoster is often identical to that of intercostal zoster in that cure occurs within three to five weeks. But more frequently than with other localizations, neurological complications lead to a poor prognosis.

The post-zoster pain is, in this case, often severe: extremely intense, permanent, and often attended by painful vasomotor disturbances. Cutaneous anesthesia is frequent. No therapy is effective against these pains, which may last for several years, if not for the patient's lifetime.

The corneal involvement may be superficial (scratchlike keratitis) or more extended (interstitial keratitis revealed by biomicroscopic examination). These lesions eventually heal but with painful leukomas.

Neuroparalytic keratitis, more serious but exceptional, may later develop on an anesthetic cornea. It results in an extended leukoma and occasionally causes a purulent degeneration of the eye. Only tarsorrhaphy, made early, can stop this evolution. Sometimes, too, an iritis may induce posterior synechias.

Paralyses of the third cranial pair, often partial, are not infrequent, yielding paralysis of the oculomotor nerve, raising the eyelid, paralytic mydriasis, Argyll-Robertson's sign. More rarely, the fourth or the sixth pair is involved, and still less frequently a Claude Bernard-Horner's syndrome occurs.

Zoster of the maxillary nerve is characterized by an eruption on half of the soft palate, on the anterior pillar, and on the uvula.

Zoster of the mandibular nerve is characterized by an eruption on the tongue, the gums, and the lower lip.

Zoster of the facial nerve (Ramsay-Hunt's syndrome) or zoster of the geniculate ganglion affects the Wrisberg's nervus intermedius and starts with unilateral auricular pain, followed by an eruption on the external ear and occasionally on the tongue. A peripheral facial paralysis is often the first symptom, which may be due either to a compression of the trunk of the seventh nerve, caused by edema of the geniculate ganglion or by a direct lesion of the nucleus. Sometimes, the involvement of the eighth pair is characterized by hypoacusis or by cochleovestibular disturbances (vertigo).

Zoster of the glossopharyngeal or of the

vagus nerve is noted occasionally; the eruption covers the oral or the pharyngeal mucosa, and may spread over the vocal cords.

COMPLICATIONS

1. As already mentioned, a discrete meningeal reaction frequently occurs in noncomplicated zoster. In some cases, the eruption is associated with an acute lymphocytic meningitis which is the most important element of the clinical picture: fever, stiffness, vomiting, rachialgias, and headache are unusually accentuated. Changes in the cerebrospinal fluid are more marked. Zoster meningitis leaves no sequelae.

2. As indicated, the incidence of paralysis is high in zoster of the cranial nerves. Partial peripheral paralysis may also be observed in spinal zoster: mild flaccid paralysis with absent or decreased tendon reflexes, with a radicular topography superimposable on that of the eruption. Such cases of paralysis are more easily detected in the limbs or the abdominal muscles, but they are also often associated with intercostal zoster.

More unusual localizations have been reported: hemidiaphragmatic paralysis during zoster involving C3 and C4, syndrome of the cauda equina.

Very few cases of peripheral paralysis located far from the eruption have been reported.

In the limbs, vasomotor disturbances may also be noted in the involved area; in such cases the pilomotor reflex is absent.

All these complications clear up spontaneously, without sequelae, at the same time as the zoster.

3. In some cases, more serious neurological complications have been described: leukoencephalitis, encephalopathy, myelitis, Guillain-Barré type polyradiculoneuritis (see Chapter 5).

4. Zoster pneumopathy occurs in some cases.

In intercostal zoster, pleural sounds may be heard, sometimes with thoracic pain occuring in rhythm with respiratory motions; the pain is different from the usual superficial type. The respiratory symptoms are rarely more marked than cough and rhonchi. Bronchial vesicles have even been seen on bronchoscopy (Andrews).

A few cases of real pneumopathy have been mentioned, resembling those observed in varicella. The most important elements are the functional signs, fever, hyperleukocytosis, and polymorphonucleosis. The physical signs are not very marked. Radiographic examination shows nodular, miliary or segmental opacities, which may persist a fairly long time.[21] These pneumopathies are usually encountered in cases of generalized zoster.

5. Other complications are exceptional, such as endocarditis or arthritis of the small joints in zoster of the limbs.[20] Epigastric, urinary, or precordial pain of anginal type have also been mentioned.

6. The most frequent complications of zoster are the persistent neuralgias occurring in 9.7 per cent of the cases.[6] They are rare in patients under the age of 40, but their incidence increases with age. They are particularly dangerous in subjects over 60. They are very serious because of their intensity and their resistance to all treatments.

7. Skin atrophy, retractions of aponeuroses and muscles in cases of limb zoster, and some cases of arthropathy with osteoporosis should also be mentioned.

DIAGNOSIS

In the usual forms, zoster cannot be mistaken for any other eruptive disease, although in some rare cases of herpes simplex the topography may be pseudoradicular. However, the absence of pain, of a prodromal phase, and of erythematous plaques prior to vesiculation aid in diagnosis. Laboratory tests are usually unnecessary. Since the pathology of herpes zoster and herpes simplex is similar, virological investigation may be necessary (see later in this chapter).

The other vesicular eruptions never show the typical distribution of zoster. The association of varicella and zoster may be a matter at issue. Such cases are caused by generalized zoster in which the typical elements precede the dissemination of the vesicles.

Insect bites may have a bandlike distribution, but their elements are different from those of zoster in that they are smaller, and there are no multiple vesicles and no pain.

Neither impetigo nor pemphigus affects the same areas; it is impossible to mistake them for zoster.

Finally, mucous localizations (zoster of

he geniculated ganglion) may be mistaken or stomatitis, but stomatitis never has the unilateral topography of zoster.

TREATMENT

Local. No irritating or dermitis-inducing drugs should be applied. It is advisable to use neutral products: talcum powder, dry dressing, or a 2 per cent eosin solution in 90° alcohol. MacCallum recommends 5-iodo-2-deoxyuridine; its local action upon viruses is assumed to be satisfactory.

In the cases of ophthalmic zoster, rigorous asepsis of the cornea is imperative; antiseptic solutions or antibiotics (Aureomycin) must be used. However, the use of hydrocortisone drops is not generally accepted. Atropine collyrium must be used in case of iridocyclitis. Finally, for lasting corneal anesthesia tarsorraphy is indicated.

Systemic. Many treatments have been attempted: emetine (40 mg. every other day), griseofulvin, and lysozyme. The results have been inconstant and not very convincing. Antibiotics (Aureomycin, spiramycin, Terramycin) sometimes seem to have a favorable effect. It seems that corticosteroids entail more side-effects than advantages. As a matter of fact, since there is no effective antiviral treatment, there is no etiological therapy.

Pain. As for the treatment of pain, numerous approaches have all failed. The usual antalgic drugs are invariably ineffective: vitamins B_1 and B_{12} at high doses, ganglioplegic drugs, as well as chlorpromazine and imipramine. A new antiepileptic, 5-carbamoyl-5*H*-dibenzo(*b, f*)azepine (Tegretol) is effective for primary neuralgia of the trigeminal nerve but not for post-zoster pain.

Physiotherapy (ultraviolet rays, infrared rays, ionization) does not have a constant effect. Radiotherapy at anti-inflammatory doses directed to the spinal ganglia sometimes diminishes pain, provided it is begun at the very onset of the disease.

Painful Sequelae. Treatment of the painful sequelae is equally disappointing. Because of their chronicity and their severity, surgery is sometimes attempted. Posterior rhizotomy and retrogasserian neurotomy proved useless. Chordotomy and prefrontal lobotomy are too serious operations to be widely used. Attempts at cutaneous denervations seem more effective. Quite often, however, for the elderly patient in poor general condition the only solution is the use of opiates and dextromoramide (Palfium).

BIBLIOGRAPHY

1. Adkisson, M. A.: Herpes zoster in a newborn premature infant. J. Pediat., *66*:956, 1965.
2. Appelbaum, E., Kreps, S. I., and Sunshine, A.: Herpes zoster encephalitis. Amer. J. Med., *32*: 25, 1962.
3. Bacon, G. E., Oliver, W. J., and Shapiro, B. A.: Factors contributing to severity of herpes zoster in children. J. Pediat., *67*:768, 1965.
4. Boudin, G., and Labet, G.: Zona et Herpes secondaires. Rev. Prat., *11*:2317, 1961.
5. Bousser, J., Christol, D., and Groubermann, S.: Les lymphadénies, terrain d'élection pour certains virus ectodermoneurotropes. Le virus varicellozonateux en particulier. Sem. Hop. Paris, *35*: 2572, 1959.
6. Burgoon, C. F., and Burgoon, J. S.: The natural history of herpes zoster. J.A.M.A., *164*:265, 1957.
7. Downie, A. W.: Chickenpox and zoster. Brit. Med. Bull., *15*:197, 1959.
8. Forest, A., and Jeglot, A.: Zona ophtalmique. Rev. Prat., *11*:2287, 1961.
9. Fourrier, A., and Bonte, C.: Lille Med., *10*:40, 1965.
10. Herbeuval, R., Remy, M., and Pierson, M.: Les pneumopathies zostériennes. J. Franc. Méd. Chir. Thorac., *4*:466, 1950.
11. Hope-Simpson, R. E.: The nature of herpes zoster: A long term study and a new hypothesis. Proc. Roy. Soc. Med., *58*:9, 1965.
12. Keidan, S. E., and Mainwaring, D.: Association of herpes zoster with leukemia and lymphoma in children. Clin. Pediat., *4*:13, 1965.
13. Kissel, P., and Dureux, J. B.: Formes cliniques et complications du zona. Rev. Prat., *11*:2275, 1961.
14. McAlpine, D., Kuroiwa, Y., Toyokura, Y., and Araki, S.: Acute demyelinating disease complicating herpes zoster. J. Neurol. Neurosurg. Psychiat., *22*:120, 1959.
15. Pek, S., and Gikas, P. W.: Pneumonia due to herpes zoster. Ann. Int. Med., *62*:350, 1965.
16. Pestel, M.: Le zona: Thérapeutique quotidienne. Presse. Med., *69*:347, 1961.
17. Rado, J. P., Tako, J., Geder, L., and Jeney, E.: Herpes zoster house epidemics in steroid treated patients. Arch. Int. Med., *116*:329, 1965.
18. Rose, F. C., Brett, E. M., and Burston, J.: Zoster encephalomyelitis. Arch. Neurol., *11*:155, 1964.
19. Scott, T. F. M., Coriell, L., Blank, H., and Burgoon, C. F.: Some comments on herpetic infection in children with special emphasis on unusual clinical manifestations. J. Pediat., *41*:835, 1952.
20. Van Rooyen, C. E., and Rhodes, A. J.: Virus Diseases in Man. New York, Thomas Nelson, 1948.
21. Wilson, F. W., and Natlock, T. B.: Herpes zoster pneumonitis: case report. Dis. Chest, *40*:74, 1961.

VARICELLA-HERPES ZOSTER: VIROLOGICAL FEATURES

by R. NETTER

The concept that the varicella and herpes zoster viruses are identical was suggested by von Bokay and A. Netter. This has been shown to be true during recent years, thanks to the isolation by Weller of the responsible viruses in tissue culture and subsequent studies of their properties. The varicella-zoster (V-Z) virus belongs to the same family as herpes simplex and cytomegalic inclusion viruses. It is icosahedral, measures 180 mμ in diameter, and is protected by an envelope. It contains DNA and at first develops in the nucleus of the infected cells, where it determines the formation of a nuclear inclusion, then in the cytoplasm. Its multiplication is hampered by halogenated deoxyuridines, which alter thymidine, indispensable to its synthesis. The techniques of virus culture are not yet sensitive enough to make possible a deep study of the physicochemical factors likely to alter the wild virus.

According to the system of cell culture used the virus is intracellular or extracellular. The virus in cell cultures is much more sensitive to cold than that contained in the vesicles; slight variations of medium composition are likely to alter it.*

DIAGNOSIS OF VARICELLA AND HERPES ZOSTER

Although the diagnosis can usually be made without laboratory tests because the clinical criteria are explicit enough, for some atypical forms laboratory tests are useful or even necessary. However, one should bear in mind that such tests are often time consuming and require techniques or reagents which are not available to all laboratories. Whenever there are sound reasons to suspect smallpox, further precautions must be taken in order to avoid any risk of contamination by the samples (see page 421).

TAKING OF SAMPLES

The mode of taking the samples varies according to the stage of the disease and the test to be made.

_____

*For those who are interested by these problems, more comprehensive bibliographies can be found in references 58 and 60.

Vesicles

ELECTRON MICROSCOPY. This examination is quite justifiable for some cases of very difficult differential diagnosis with smallpox. A little vesicular fluid is put on a slide or the bottom of a small tube, and the placement of the infectious material is carefully indicated on the external face of the glass.

SMEARS. The inside of a vesicle is scratched and the fluid is spread by means of another slide; the slide is quickly dried as if it were a blood smear.

VIRUS ISOLATION. The patient must go to the laboratory or the technician must come to the patient's room to take the sample and inoculate it immediately. The vesicles are superficially cleaned with normal saline solution, then they are pricked with a tuberculin syringe or a thin Pasteur pipette. The small amount of fluid taken is then scattered over cell cultures previously deprived of their nutrient medium: human diploid cells, human thyroid cells, amniotic cells, or even simian renal cells (more currently used in laboratories, but also less sensitive).

Whenever it is impossible to seed the vesicular fluid immediately, it must be diluted in a little sterilized skim milk and preserved in a sealed ampule at a temperature as low as possible ($-70°$ C.). Another technique, equally satisfactory, is to dilute the fluid of three or four vesicles in 0.3 ml. of skim milk and to lyophilize immediately.

The herpes zoster vesicles are larger and contain more virus than the varicella vesicles. Three or four days after the vesiculation has started, the chances of success are more limited because of the decrease in infectious particles and the possibility of superinfection, generally by staphylococcus. At the crust stage, there is practically no chance of isolating the virus.

Crusts. Crusts are collected by scratching or with forceps, then put into a small tube which is capped. These crusts, ground up in the laboratory, yield an antigen which can be used for complement-fixation and immunoprecipitation reactions. Both tests are possible only with a sufficient amount of crusts.

Blood. The blood is taken without an anticoagulant. Neutralizing, precipitating or complement-fixing antibodies are looked for in the sera.

Cerebrospinal Fluid. A meningeal reaction rarely occurs in the course of varicella whereas a lymphocytic reaction is usually observed during the first week in patients *ith herpes zoster. This may range between* *)* and 200 lymphocytes per cubic milliliter.

Gold and Robbins[7] even reported the *olation* of virus from the cerebrospinal fluid *a* a patient with herpes zoster.

Postmortem Examinations. Postmortem *pecimens* are taken either for histological *xamination* or for virus isolation. According *o* the purpose, the samples are put in a suit-*ble* fixative or immediately carried to the *boratory* for inoculation.

The V-Z virus may be isolated from var-*ous* organs, in particular the kidney, eight *ours* after death[5]; explant cultures[12] or inoc-*lation* of ground up fragments on tissue *ultures* can be used.

ESULTS AND INTERPRETATION

Electron Microscopy. Such an examina-*on* requires only a few hours. It permits the *uick* classification of the virus; but diagnosis *f* a V-Z infection cannot be made because *ne* virus cannot be differentiated from the *erpes* virus, which also belongs to the same *mily.*

Staining of Smears. These techniques *re* quick, but they must be carried out and *nterpreted* only by highly qualified tech-*icians.*

The low number of viral corpuscles *evealed* by Gutstein's stain suggests vari-*ella.*

The presence of Tzanck's multinucleate *iant* cells may be a source of error, as was the *ase* in South Africa during a smallpox epi-*emic* reported by Heydenreich.[33]

The detection of V-Z antigen by the im-*munofluorescence* technique requires great *rudence* because the poor state of the cells *nay* give rise to nonspecific staining.

Histological Examination. About one *veek* is required to fix, include, cut, and *tain* the various fragments. The intranuclear *nclusions* are particularly sought for in the *pidermal* cells, the esophageal mucosa, and *ne* bile ducts; they are more rarely found in *ne* muscular cells or the endothelial cells of *ne* capillary blood vessels. The liver and *pleen* are the sites of micronodular necro-*is;* the adrenal glands are hemorrhagic. Ex-*mination* of the lungs reveals an acute alveo-*itis* with intranuclear inclusions and multiple *nicroscopic* necrotic foci.[39, 51]

The nuclear inclusions observed in the *istological* preparations of organs are not *athognomonic* of varicella, but only of the *nerpes* virus family.

Immunoprecipitation in Agar Medium. This rapid and specific method, which can be applied during all stages of the disease, in-cluding the crust stage, permits a diagnosis in four or five hours.

According to the circumstances, the iden-tification will concern the antigen of the crusts or the precipitating antibodies of the serum. In the first case, a known precipitating serum must be available; in the second case, a con-trol varicella antigen is necessary.

Only a positive result is valid. The sera of patients recovering from varicella never contain sufficient antibodies to cause pre-cipitation, while sera of some patients re-covering from herpes zoster are likely to attain that critical level.

Isolation of Virus in Cell Culture. This technique is always time consuming. As a rule, the first cytopathogenic lesions appear from the fourth to the seventh day; some-times they appear still later, after the third week. Theoretically, microscopic examina-tion by the fluorescent antibody technique a few days earlier might be of some avail; however, since it is generally not possible to inoculate a large number of tubes at the beg-inning, it is difficult to waste tubes which are not numerous for an uncertain result. The aspect of the cytopathogenic lesions after staining and the fact that the virus grows slowly on particular cells are in favor of vari-cella. To confirm the diagnosis, one to five more days are necessary to permit an im-munofluorescence reaction on cells, a sero-neutralization reaction against a known zoster serum, or a complement-fixation test with the cell culture itself as antigen.

Complement-Fixation Test. This is the easiest reaction to carry out if a stock of anti-gen is available in the laboratory.

A recent study by Gold and Godek[6] revealed that in 71 cases out of 72, the reac-tion was positive after one week in varicella. Five of ten patients with zoster showed a titer of antibodies higher than $1/4$ as early as the fourth day. High titers, which, accord-ing to the technique used, varied from $1/64$ to $1/520$, persisted for a few months, then gradually decreased so that, after one year, less than 25 per cent of the subjects had detectable antibodies. This was true for pa-tients with varicella or zoster.

It is of interest to note that a second exposure to varicella does not cause an in-crease in antibodies.

The specificity of the reaction does not

seem absolute, and two recent publications question it. The sera of patients with herpes simplex reacted 12 times out of 49 in the presence of varicella antigen.[36]

On the other hand, according to Ross et al.,[56] the sera of ten out of 19 patients with varicella and five out of 19 with zoster reacted in the presence of herpes antigen. Thus the complement-fixation reaction does not permit a diagnosis of encephalitis, except with precise analysis. It is a useful reaction to detect the acute cases but does not indicate the individual's protection.

Neutralization Test. A V-Z virus strain must be available in the laboratory. The results are not very precise, since it is not possible to make limit dilutions with either the virus or the serum; finally, what is calculated is the percentage reduction in number of plaques as compared with those in non-neutralized control tubes or flasks. According to Taylor-Robinson (cited by Sohier and Netter[58]), the serum of a patient recovering from herpes zoster shows a percentage of reduction ranging between 60 and 90 per cent, whereas that of a normal adult is approximately between 10 and 30 per cent. Recently Schmidt et al.[57] suggested distributing the various serum dilutions on the surface of smears of V-Z virus-infected cells; the union of V-Z virus with homologous antibodies in patients' sera is detected by the indirect fluorescent antibody staining technique with the use of fluorescein-labeled anti-human immune globulins prepared in rabbits. This process gives results which are superimposable on those yielded by the complement-fixation test, and the titers diminish in the same way during the months following the disease. It still is not known whether this process permits measurement of the antibodies responsible for immunity.

EPIDEMIOLOGY OF VARICELLA AND HERPES ZOSTER

VARICELLA

Although varicella occurs all over the world, it has always been difficult to obtain a clear picture of the epidemiological problems owing to the fact that the disease is usually benign. It is seldom compulsory to report the disease, and thus it is difficult to estimate the number of cases occurring at home; the number of patients hospitalized is not an exact reflection of what happen in the whole of the population. Finally techniques of virus isolation and serologica diagnosis, although recently improved, ar still confined to a limited number of special ized laboratories.

This paucity of information accounts fo the interest of the survey made by Gordon[2] in which he analyses the statistics for the stat of Massachusetts, where, since 1907, it ha been compulsory to report cases of varicella

Morbidity. In Massachusetts, varicell incidence has increased: for each 100,000 in habitants, there were 70 cases in 1910 an 286 in 1961. However, the curve is not linea and shows peaks, usually every two or thre years.

Sex. As had already been suspected by many authors, sex does not seem to have any influence, since the 159,512 cases observec between 1952 and 1961 were distributed fairly equally between boys (52 per cent) an girls (48 per cent).

Age. In insular territories or in closed communities, fresh epidemic outbreaks may occur, even now, attacking children and adults indiscriminately. It is then difficult for the physician to differentiate the disease from variola, and he cannot make the diagnosis without laboratory tests. We recently had the opportunity of studying several such epidemics, one of them in a mental hospital in Guadeloupe.

In the Western Hemisphere, cases of varicella in adults, if not exceptional, are infrequent because, owing to increasing urbanization, contacts among individuals are frequent at an early age. In England, at the beginning of the century, 16.7 per cent of patients with varicella were over 18 years; in Massachusetts, between 1952 and 1961, only 2.6 per cent were over 15 years. In Massachusetts, between 1942 and 1951, 84 per cent of the children with varicella were younger than ten years; during the following ten years, between 1952 and 1961, this proportion reached 90.5 percent. The greatest number of cases occur in children between five and nine years of age, with a peak at six years, when children start school (Table 30-1).

Varicella in the Pregnant Woman and the Newborn Child. Varicella is always more severe in the adult than the child, and gravidity is an additional aggravating factor. In Pearson's statistical study[51] based on 70,000 postmortem examinations, only one woman

Table 30-1. *Varicella in Relation to Age in Children Under Ten: Massachusetts, 1942-1952 (Total Reported Cases, 171,419)**

AGE	%
< 1	2.8
1	4.1
2	5.8
3	6.6
4	7.8
5	12.7
6	18.6
7	13.0
8	8.0
9	4.7
Total	84.1

*From Gordon.[28]

Thus it is clear that, in the highly urbanized regions, varicella attacks children from their earliest youth and protects them from a second attack when they are adults; as for the pregnant woman, since her disease is usually very remote, she transmits only a weak and transitory immunity, which accounts for the possible occurrence of neonatal varicella.

was found to have died of varicella. Pearson recorded 16 cases of varicella among 46,000 pregnant women; only three of the 16 delivered prematurely. In other statistics mentioned by the author, the proportion is 25 per cent. The transmission of varicella to the fetus is far from constant; on the basis of clinical arguments only, the proportion of newborn children with varicella less than ten days after birth was five of 16 in Pearson's series, four of 14 for Abler,[1] and two of seven for Newman.[48]

The question whether varicella may cause congenital anomalies was studied by Dumont[17] in a prospective investigation bearing on 224 women, half of whom had contracted an infection during the first three months. The percentage of congenital malformations observed was 1.8 per cent, while the usual rate ranges between 2 and 3 per cent. Thus, this study yielded no evidence that varicella has a teratogenous action.

Seasonal Occurrence. The study of 75,284 cases observed from 1956 to 1961 in Massachusetts reveals a minimum in September and a maximum in March. Winter and spring are the most propitious seasons (Fig. 30-3). On the other hand, zoster has no seasonal prevalence; moreover, the infectious mechanism is totally different, as we shall see.

Mortality. When varicella occurs in a region which has been untouched for many years, it may cause real ravages. In 1935, in the former French Equatorial Africa, Millous (mentioned by Gordon[28]) observed an epidemic of 1919 cases; 370 persons died (19 per cent). The population had been well vaccinated against smallpox and a diagnosis of variola was definitely eliminated.

It must be admitted that such epidemics are becoming rarer owing to the numerous international exchanges of the present time. Maretić and Cooray[43] found that varicella, without attaining the case fatality rate above, is more serious in tropical regions (0.58 per cent mortality); most often it attacks adults, who often have pneumonic, nervous, hemorrhagic, or bacterial complications. The average annual mortality due to varicella per 100,000 inhabitants in Massachusetts between 1910 and 1959 was estimated by Gordon[28] to be 0.12. Table 30-2 clearly shows the relation between the patient's age and the seriousness of the disease.

According to Newman,[48] the mortality rate is much higher for neonatal varicella; in his own series of 38 cases it was 21 per cent. These statistics must be interpreted with some reservations. Although it is probable that the disease is more serious during the first year of life, it is not certain that the mortality is so high. Since neither autopsies nor

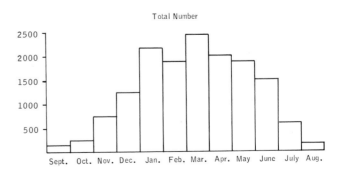

Figure 30-3. Number of cases of varicella observed in Massachusetts between September 1, 1956, and August 31, 1961. (From Gordon.[28])

Table 30-2. *Mortality, by Age, Due to Varicella in Massachusetts Between 1942 and 1952**

AGE, YR.	NO. CASES OF VARICELLA	NO. OF DEATHS	RATE PER 10,000
<1	4,856	18	37
1	7,130	6	8
2	10,009	1	1
3	11,291	3	2.7
4	13,408	4	2.9
5 to 9	97,807	7	0.7
10 to 14	14,429	0	0
15 and up	6,260	5	7
unknown	6,229	0	0
Total	171,419	44	2.5

*From Gordon.[28]

virological tests were made, it is possible that at least some of the deaths were due to other causes.

Reservoir of Virus. For a long time the absence of a sensitive laboratory animal and of apparent lesions after inoculation into embryonated eggs hampered the study of varicella. The sensitivity of the monkey was also questioned; however, it is possible that this resistance is only the consequence of an early infection, as is the case with measles. Henschelé (mentioned by Gordon[28]) thinks that he observed, in a zoo, three anthropoids with varicella at a time when varicella was raging in the town. Because of the absence of serological or virological studies proving the possible existence of an urban or sylvan animal reservoir, we have to admit that, for the time being, man is the sole known reservoir.

Varicella is transmitted from child to child. The possible existence of healthy carriers of varicella is mentioned in our discussion of congenital varicella. As we shall see farther on, there is the possibility of a latent infection by the varicella virus which, without any manifestations, remains quiescent in the nervous ganglia for a few years and appears as herpes zoster.

Thus in an island such as Iceland, when it was almost completely isolated, varicella recurred regularly, whereas, measles, mumps, and rubella completely disappeared after the whole population had been attacked, until the virus was again introduced into the island.

Mode of Transmission

DIRECT ROUTE. *Air Route.* Our methods of virus culture are not yet sensitive enough to make such a study possible; how-

ever, the epidemics, as observed in children's wards, spread so quickly that we are inclined to believe that airborne transmission occurs. It is possible that the lesions of the buccal mucosa and the upper respiratory tracts are responsible.

Blood Route. Blood-borne transmission is possible, and Beckeman (mentioned by Gordon[28]) reported a case of varicella occurring after a transfusion. If this observation has remained exceptional, it is undoubtedly because varicella is so unusual in adults.

Transplacental Route. Varicella is considered congenital only if the eruption occurs less than ten days after delivery; after that, varicella is usually called neonatal. Thirty-eight observations published before 1965 have been collected by Newman.[48] Earlier reports mentioned by Gordon[28] describe cases of varicella appearing a few days after birth even though the mother did not exhibit any eruption and had not been in the presence of persons with varicella. A further observation by Eichenwald, reported by Newman, confirmed those facts.

Three mechanisms have been suggested: passage of the virus through intact chorionic villi; passage of the virus through altered chorionic villi; and infection of the fetus through the cutaneous or respiratory route by contaminated amniotic fluid. At present no decision concerning the mechanism is possible; Pearson[51] examined, with negative results, nine placentas of women with varicella who had given birth to apparently healthy children. Pearson mentioned only one published report which described multiple necrotic foci.

INDIRECT ROUTE. The indirect spread of virus can be asserted only on epidemiological ground. Laporte[37] considers the fact that it is so difficult to stop the disease from spreading in a hospital ward as evidence of possible infection through a third person or by means of material or toys used in common.

Duration of Incubation. Kundratitz and Brunsgard (cited by Gordon[28]) inoculated vesicular fluid into children and estimated that the incubation was between seven and 14 days; however, this experiment was carried out under conditions too far from reality to be perfectly exact. By studying hospital epidemics following accidental introduction into the service on a known date of a child or of a nurse with the virus, Gordon and Meader, and then Evans (cited by Gordon[28]) furnished proof that the incubation ranges beween ten and 20 days, with the peak from the hirteenth until the seventeenth days.

Varicella acquired from a patient with oster has a similar incubation period.

In congenital varicella, there is usually a ortnight between the mother's varicella and hat of the baby (six to 15 days) (Table 30-3).

Period of Contagion. It has long been nown that the disease is most infectious arly in its course. In 1929, Gordon and Meader (cited by Gordon[28]) published observations on four patients with varicella vho, on the eighth day after the eruption, iid not transmit the disease to their conacts (21 children, all receptive). Modern irology further confirmed this by recommending that virus isolations be made from resh vesicles, if possible more recent than hree days. Bearing in mind these arguments nd the mildness of the disease, there is no ound reason to isolate patients for a long time.

A patient may be contagious before the ruption. Gordon and Meader (cited by jordon[28]) described a case in which the atient left the hospital the day before the ash emerged; in spite of all precautions, variella appeared in the ward after the usual inubation period. Similar cases of contagion ne to four days before the first symptoms vere also reported by Evans (mentioned by jordon[28]). The presence of enanthema on the uccal or nasopharyngeal mucosa before the utaneous rash is probably responsible for he early contagiousness.[37]

Contagiousness and Receptivity. In spite f the high contagiousness of the virus and the great receptivity of human subjects, it has never been observed that 100 per cent of the sensitive individuals in contact with one varicella patient contract the disease. Gordon, on the basis of his own observations and those of Kling, Rabinoff, and Simpson estimated that the proportion of sensitive individuals contracting varicella after a first contact ranges between 61 and 75 per cent.[28] These figures are only an average because, in young children, the proportion may reach 81 per cent; after a second contact, only 0.6 per cent of individuals remain unaffected. In adults, there is a striking discrepancy between the 30 per cent who claim never to have had varicella and the very small proportion of clinical cases after exposure. No doubt there are many attenuated or inapparent forms inducing a certain resistance. The results of a limited serological investigation carried out in children were favorable to this hypothesis.[46]

As we see it, most of the epidemiological problems concerning varicella are based on clinical considerations; unfortunately, because of the difficulties of virus culture and the mildness of the disease, research workers do not undertake further investigations.

HERPES ZOSTER

Although the viruses of varicella and herpes zoster are identical, the two infections differ from one another in certain points. It is difficult to obtain a precise idea of the epidemiology of herpes zoster because it is not

Table 30-3. *Incubation Period of Congenital Varicella*

	DAYS ELAPSED	
REFERENCE	Mother's Varicella to Confinement	Confinement to Child's Varicella
Ehrlich and Turner, 1958[19]	2	7
Freud, 1958[22]	8	2
Librach, 1959[40]	10	4
Bertram, 1961[6]	14	1
Hanauer, 1961[30]	1	7
O'Neil, 1962[50]	5	8
Laramée, 1963[38]	6	7
Neustadt, 1963[47]	14	1
Abler, 1964[1]	5	9
Baldasseroni and Ulivelli, 1964[3]	"some days"	5
Pearson, 1964[51]	10	5
Pearson, 1964[51]	3	8
Pearson, 1964[51]	5	10
Pearson, 1964[51]	1	5
Newman, 1965[48]	1	9

compulsory to declare the disease. However, the recent review by Hope-Simpson[34] and various other publications make some statistics available which, although confined to a particular region of England, are extremely valuable.

Morbidity. The average annual incidence was 3.4 per 1000 in the series of Hope-Simpson,[34] who over 16 years observed 192 cases of zoster in Cirencester, a British town of 3500 inhabitants; this rate is slightly lower than that (4.5 per 1000) reported in the Scottish statistics compiled by MacGregor[42] over a seven-year period. Zoster is thus far from rare, since the rates reported are fairly close to and even higher than for varicella; as a matter of fact, although varicella induces immunity so strong as to make recurrence exceptional, this is not the case with herpes zoster. In Hope-Simpson's series, eight of the 192 cases represented second attacks and one case was the third attack. Calculating the incidence per 1000 per year, it appears that the 2.9 rate observed by Gordon[28] for varicella is not very far from the rate for zoster, which ranges between 3.4 and 4.8.

Sex. Although it is frequently said that men are more often attacked by this disease than women, Hope-Simpson[34] found that the annual rate per 1000 was 3.6 for men and 3.2 for women; similarly, the statistics of MacGregor[42] and Burgoon et al.[10] do not show significant differences in favor of either sex.

Age. It is well known that herpes zoster generally occurs after the age of 20 whereas varicella usually occurs much earlier.[10] However, this rule is far from absolute; varicella does occur in adults and may even be difficult to differentiate from variola; conversely, zoster in children is not rare. In Hope-Simpson's series, six of 192 cases of herpes zoster occurred in children younger than ten years. Table 30-4 shows the age distribution of zoster in Hope-Simpson's series.

The age group from birth to nine years, for which the morbidity for herpes zoster is lowest, is precisely the age group attacked by varicella. The more remote is childhood, the greater is the risk of herpes zoster. Age also affects the evolution of herpes zoster: in those under 20 years, neither ophthalmic herpes zoster nor post-zoster neuralgia is observed, since recovery from the disease is usually complete within 15 days.[10]

Influence of Season. While varicella is definitely a seasonal infection, this is not the case with herpes zoster. The statistics of Hope-Simpson and MacGregor both show insignificant monthly variations, which is not surprising since the disease is sporadic and nonepidemic.

Mortality. We could not find any information concerning the mortality due to herpes zoster; we therefore must say that the risk is limited, death usually being caused by an intercurrent agent.

Virus Reservoir. Man is his own reservoir of virus. According to the prevailing hypotheses, herpes zoster represents the reappearance of a virus that was introduced into the organism during varicella and then remained there in latent form (see section on mechanisms of infection).

Mode of Transmission

Air Route. This route can be rejected because an epidemic of herpes zoster has

Table 30-4. *Occurrence of Herpes Zoster in Relation to Age; Rate per 1000 Inhabitants per Year. Cirencester, England, 1947-1962**

Age, Yr.	Population	Cases of Zoster	Rate per 1000 Inhabitants per Year
0 - 9	510	6	0.74
10-19	455	10	1.38
20-29	412	17	2.58
30-39	491	18	2.29
40-49	492	23	2.92
50-59	454	37	5.09
60-69	350	38	6.79
70-79	263	27	6.42
80-89	99	16	10.10
90-99	8	–	–
Total	3534	192	3.39

*From Hope-Simpson.[34]

ever been observed. Nor is zoster connected with varicella epidemics, for no statistical parallel is noted between recrudescences of varicella and zoster. In fact, in Hope-Simpson's statistics, the opposite fact is reported three times out of four, as if contact with a patient with varicella conferred a certain protection against zoster. Moreover, among the 1287 persons who had domestic contact with patients with varicella, no cases of zoster were reported; this is important because the contagiousness of varicella is very great.

Transplacental Route. The hypothesis that the mother infected while pregnant may transmit the disease to her child is not new, and Lomer (mentioned by Hope-Simpson[34]) in 1889 reported the case of a four-day-old child with herpes zoster of the penis which had delayed circumcision. Investigation showed that the mother had been in close contact with a patient with zoster during the third month of pregnancy. By 1952, about 10 cases of neonatal herpes zoster had been reported; in one of them, well studied by Feldman, the mother remembered that she had had herpes zoster about the time of conception (reported by Hope-Simpson[34]).

Several more or less recent publications mention the possibility of congenital malformations in children whose mother was infected while pregnant. Until a statistical investigation is undertaken, it will be difficult to know whether there is a causal relationship or merely an unfortunate coincidence.

Incubation. Accuracy is not easy as concerns the incubation of herpes zoster, which varicella has always preceded. Elderly people may vaguely remember the varicella they had in early childhood. Some incubations are counted in decades; some are short in the six children observed by Frischknecht[23] the interval varied between five months and a little over seven years).

Contagious Material and Contagiousness. The V-Z virus is very abundant in the zoster vesicles before they dry; in spite of this, zoster is but slightly contagious, either because the mucous lesions responsible for respiratory infections are rare, or because the number of lesions and the fact that they are usually on parts of the body that are covered with clothing do not promote dissemination.

Epidemic Herpes Zoster. Unlike varicella, which is very contagious, zoster occurs out sporadically. In Hope-Simpson's series,[34] there were no cases of zoster among the 318 persons having had domestic contact with patients suffering from the disease, in spite of the great risk of infection. On the other hand, in a hospital environment Aubertin observed several grouped cases suggesting an epidemic; this may have been the result of the patients' original diseases or of the treatments they were undergoing.

VARICELLA SPREADING FROM HERPES ZOSTER

After von Bokay had emphasized the closeness of the relations between cases of varicella and those of herpes zoster, A. Netter and A. Urbain noted, on the basis of over 100 cases, that varicella habitually preceded herpes zoster and the secondary occurrence of cases of varicella in the surrounding persons, and that the incubation period of varicella was the same as in the usual condition of contagion.

The transmission of varicella to children by means of herpes zoster virus was achieved by Kundratitz (mentioned by Hope-Simpson[34]) and by Brunsgard (mentioned by Gordon[28]) in 1932.

In 1946, Peterson and Black (mentioned by Gordon[28]) noted that in the Shetland Islands varicella epidemics developed after exposure to herpes zoster just as they did after exposure to varicella. During a five-year period investigations carried out by the British Medical Research Council recorded the occurrence in boys' boarding-schools of 20 epidemics of varicella derived from zoster (mentioned by Burgoon et al.[10]).

MECHANISM OF THE VARICELLA-HERPES ZOSTER INFECTION

Two features concerning the pathogenesis of varicella and herpes zoster have been known for almost a century: the diseases are related to one another, and, in herpes zoster, the sensory ganglia are involved. The links that unite the two diseases are unquestionably proved by epidemiology and virology.

The neurological involvement in herpes zoster is confirmed by clinical studies; indeed, the distribution of the lesions fairly closely corresponds to the area distribution of one or several sensory ganglia.

Hope-Simpson,[34] on the basis of his own observations and those of Head and Campbell, clearly showed the prevalence, in cases of herpes zoster affecting the trunk, of lesions located in the dermatomes related to D3 to L2 ganglia, as well as to those of the fifth cranial nerve; however, there is no appreciable difference between the attack rates for the right and the left sides. In view of the centripetal disposition of the varicella lesions, one is struck by the fact that the same zones are the most common sites of eruption in both varicella and herpes zoster.

Histological studies[61] reveal hemorrhagic and necrotic acute inflammation of the sensory ganglia and nerves; even the sensory neurons are involved.

Irreversible lesions of the cord and of the brain are the cause of paralysis or encephalitis, although van Bogaert considers the latter to be allergic in origin. The involvement of the sympathetic system accounts for the painful phenomena and the vasomotor reactions. We shall not describe here all the well-known lesions which caused zoster to be called neuroganglioradiculomyelitis.

HYPOTHESES CONCERNING THE MECHANISM OF VARICELLA-HERPES ZOSTER INFECTION

Varicella. Although there is no proof of the mode of infection, it is generally believed that, in view of the high contagiousness of varicella, the virus is introduced into the organism through the respiratory tract. The lengthy incubation suggests that the virus starts multiplying and that, owing to a brief viremia allows the virus to reach the cells of the reticuloendothelial system where it again multiplies; a second viremia, which has not yet been proved, is thought to disseminate the virus to almost all organs in malignant varicella, and more especially at the level of the cutaneous and mucous areas in the usual forms; this viremia is thought to occur in successive waves that are accompanied by systemic signs (malaise, fever) and cause the outburst of crops of cutaneous lesions at various stages.

Spreading from all the involved areas, the virus is supposed to reach the sensory ganglia by following the nerves; this was demonstrated by Johnson,[35] who used fluorescent antibody staining to study herpes simplex infection in suckling mice inoculated by the parenteral route. The virus then is assumed to remain in the nervous cells in a latent state, perhaps as a provirus or as a complete virus; there it is insulated and pro-

tected from the effects of the neutraliz[ing] serum antibodies, the titer of which, at th[is] stage, is sufficient. As yet, however, no o[ne] has succeeded in demonstrating the presen[ce] of the virus in human ganglia, either by vir[us] isolation or by immunofluorescent stainin[g].

Herpes Zoster. For some years, t[he] provirus is confined to the ganglia, and a[ny] issue out of the ganglion is immediate[ly] stopped by the serum antibodies. Periodical[ly] contacts with patients with varicella te[m]porarily increase an unsteady level of an[ti]bodies, which accounts for the low inciden[ce] of herpes zoster during varicella outbreak[s]. Years later, the titer of antibodies declin[es] below the critical value, and the virus ca[n] again multiply in the dorsal root ganglion cells, where it causes an intense inflammatio[n]. Then it returns to the skin, following the ner[ve] and causing neuritis, neuralgia, and vesicul[o] pustular lesions. Hope-Simpson believes th[at] this mechanism of temporary storage of t[he] virus for tens of years accounts for the recu[r]rence of varicella in certain insular popula[tions] tions among which the number of birth[s] would seem insufficient to maintain regular[ly] a virus as fragile as that of varicella.

It is assumed that generalized herpe[s] zoster results from severe viremia concomi[t]ant with the progress of the virus along th[e] nerves even before elaboration of new ant[i]bodies has intervened.

Factors Predisposing to or Aggravatin[g] Varicella. Periodically reports appear d[e]scribing an increased rash after sunburn or drug injection.

LYMPHOID LEUKEMIA. The aggrava[t]ing effect of lymphoid leukemia has probabl[y] been exaggerated. As early as 1953 Bierma[n] et al.[7] showed that, in three patients wit[h] varicella and leukosis who had not undergon[e] any treatment during the incubation or th[e] eruption, the evolution was normal; in tw[o] cases they even observed a spectacular hema[to]togical remission, the number of leukocyte[s] decreasing from 200,000 to 40,000 withi[n] two days. Bodey et al.[8] report that 12 leu[?] kemic patients recovered from varicella whil[e] they were undergoing various treatment[s] methotrexate, 6-mercaptopurine, and cort[i] costeroids. Eight of them were in total remis[?] sion, two were in partial remission, and tw[o] were in full relapse when varicella occurred[.] The disease seemed more severe in thos[e] being treated with steroids: three of the si[x] had a pneumopathy. Of six patients no[w] being treated with corticosteroids, one, wh[o]

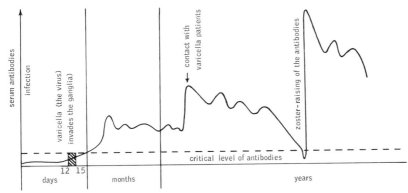

Figure 30-4. Diagram of the suggested nature of herpes zoster (according to Hope-Simpson[34]).

as in full relapse of leukemia, had a pneu-opathy which predated the varicella. According to Bodey the tendency to publish ily serious cases has led to overestimation the risk of varicella in the course of leu-emia.

CORTICOSTEROIDS. Josserand (cited by ordon[28]) and many others have insisted the aggravating effect on varicella of opping corticosteroid treatment. In par-cular, they observed that the eruption be-omes hemorrhagic or pemphigoid and that eumopathy and pericarditis occur more equently.[7, 16, 20, 32, 39]

Since steroids are used for the treatment patients with rheumatic fever or leukosis, rousseau's aphorism "never has a physician en a patient die of varicella" is not true. erbeaux et al.,[24] who collected reports by authors prior to 1963 of 102 cases of vari-lla occurring in patients under steroid ther-by, note that about one-third died.

The study of 274 cases of varicella oc-urring during steroid therapy gathered by alliers and Ellis,[21] corroborates these data d shows that the accidents occur only with tients who already have an immunological fect or whose steroid therapy has been opped; thus since 1958, 231 patients had en treated without incident (p. 391).

ECZEMA. Unlike vaccinia, for which zema is an aggravating factor, varicella veloped normally in two young patients scribed by Nonclercq and Levy[49]; in one the two, the eczema even was attenuated ring the varicella eruption.

Factors Predisposing to or Precipitating erpes Zoster. It has long been known that ad, arsenic, chronic or acute infections, and syphilis can provoke the appearance of zoster. Earlier physicians also suspected trauma to have an influence. In Hope-Simpson's statistics there are only two examples of a causative agent: one case occurred after a horsefly bite, the other 15 days after one leg had been wounded. Frischkneckt[23] several times noted that contusions of the head and of the spine were at the origin of cases of infantile herpes zoster.

HEMOPATHY. The negative influence of hemopathy has long been known. Bousser et al.[9] surveyed the subject as early as 1959. By combining their observations and those found in several recent reviews, it is possible to form a clearer idea of the problem.

Frequency of Herpes Zoster. Wright and Winer,[62] in a study involving 55,279 patients admitted to a medicosurgical center over five years, found that only 0.22 per cent of patients without cancer suffered from herpes zoster. Burgoon et al.[10] found a 2 per cent rate. On the other hand, a much higher frequency of herpes zoster is observed in patients with Hodgkin's disease (8 per cent for Sokal and Firat[59], 9 per cent for Wright and Winer,[62] 8.1 per cent for Bichel and Thorling,[6a] 4.6 per cent for Heine,[31] 4.16 per cent for Craver and Haagensen [cited by Bousser et al.[9]]). An increase of the same magnitude is also found in patients with lymphosarcoma (7 per cent for Craver and Haagensen [mentioned by Bousser et al.[9]]), or chronic lymphoid leukemia (15 per cent for Bousser et al.[9] and 10 per cent for Heine[31]).

Spread of Lesions. While generalized herpes zoster is comparatively rare and usually occurs only in subjects over 50, it is particularly frequent in certain patients, whatever their age. The zoster was generalized in 43 per cent of the patients with lymphomatosis or leukemia seen by Merselis et al.;[45] in 33 per cent of the patients with Hodgkin's disease seen by Dayan (mentioned by Sokal and Firat[59]); and in 27 per cent of the 49 patients with Hodgkin's disease seen by Sokal and Firat.[59]

Sokal and Firat, having studied 49 cases of herpes zoster among 800 patients with Hodgkin's disease, concluded that generalized zoster occurs mainly in patients at stage III of the disease, i.e., when the lesions are disseminated. The prognosis is, thus, particularly pessimistic, and any case of generalized herpes zoster should lead one to seek a hemopathy.

Protracted Evolution. Nuclear inclusions are observed in the cutaneous lesions for a long time. Furthermore, herpes zoster leaves necrosis and scars.

Role of Treatments for Hemopathies. The anergy of patients with Hodgkin's disease is well known and suffices, according to Sokal and Firat, to account for their deficient immunological defense against zoster: there is a close connection between the severity of the disease and the generalization of herpes zoster, and it is not surprising that in these very ill patients a multiplicity of therapies have been tried.

Moreover, the doses administered to the patient of x-rays, cytostatic agents, or corticosteroids are quite a bit lower than those which would be required to inhibit the immunological defenses.[59] In particular, the steroid agents do not seem to have increased or aggravated the cases.[59]

Radiotherapy seemed to "localize" a subsequent zoster eruption in 20 to 40 per cent of the cases. But Sokal and Firat suppose that when radiotherapy was prescribed it was precisely because this area contained a tumor which could reactivate the virus of the ganglia or of the nerve roots nor far from it. Administration of gamma globulins was beneficial only in a few cases of zoster, although the doses were high (80 to 150 ml.). Because of the risk to patients with tumors or blood diseases, it is imperative to take every precaution to avert contact with zoster or varicella. Merselis et al.[45] even suggest stopping the treatments in the presence of risk alone that the patient has been exposed.

Organ Transplant. The incidence of zoster is increased after organ transplant. Rifkind[54] published observations on six cases

of zoster among 73 young patients receivi㎜ renal transplant. Splenectomy, thymectom㎜ azathioprine, or corticosteroids did not see㎜ responsible. On the other hand, local x-irradi㎜ tions did seem important, and Rifkind o㎜ served six cases of zoster among 34 irradiat㎜ patients; four of these cases appeared fro㎜ six to 23 days after the irradiation.

Moreover, complement-fixing antibodi㎜ belonging to the 7S gamma globulin grou㎜ appeared at the usual time and level.

This confirms the opinion that, in hem㎜ pathy, it is the disease itself and not the im㎜ muno-suppressive therapy which is respo㎜ sible for the weakness of antibody respons㎜

PROPHYLAXIS AND TREATMENT OF VARICELLA AND HERPES ZOSTER

VARICELLA

Prophylaxis

ISOLATION AND QUARANTINE. T㎜ *Patient.* It is absolutely ineffective to isola㎜ the patient, since contagion quite often occu㎜ prior to the eruption; after the eruption, ㎜ is infectious only until the fifth day; it is ther㎜ fore unnecessary to insist upon the usual 2㎜ days.

Contacts. People who have been i㎜ contact with varicella patients should be ke㎜ at home only if they exhibit fever indicati㎜ the onset of varicella.

Patients Undergoing Steroid Therap㎜ These patients should be isolated in order ㎜ prevent if possible their contracting varicell㎜

DISINFECTION. The virus is so fragi㎜ that there is little chance for it to surviv㎜ until the disease is over. American attempt㎜ (reported by Gordon[28]) to sterilize the atmo㎜ phere in schools or in hospital rooms b㎜ means of ultraviolet rays were reported t㎜ have led to a lower rate of morbidity; how㎜ ever, when the same experiment was carrie㎜ out in the country it was without avail becaus㎜ the contagion occurred out of school, in th㎜ bus conveying the children.

VACCINATION. Vaccination against var㎜ cella, tried about 25 years ago, is of onl㎜ historical interest. *At present, there is n㎜ vaccine against varicella.*

SEROTHERAPY. Convalescent serum o㎜ specific gamma globulins contain more anti㎜ bodies than the serum taken over a year afte㎜ the disease. The available quantity of specifi㎜

rum would not be sufficient to forestall an
ɔidemic; in any case, *the efficacy of sero-
•erapy is questionable* if one considers the
iscrepancies among the results obtained by
arious authors (mentioned by Gordon[28]).
hus Funkhauser deemed it useful, Schaeffer
nd Toomy considered it ineffective, and
rimble noted only a weak action in two chil-
ren out of four. Ross[54] treated 242 children
ithin the three days following a contact.
ʻhose who received 0.1 ml. immunoglobulin
er pound of body weight exhibited only
ɔpproximately one-third as many vesicles as
ontrol subjects, while the children receiving
,6 ml. per pound of body weight exhibited
nly one-eighth as many. The fever was
lightly lower than in control subjects.

ANTIVIRAL THERAPY. *Xenalamine.*
ʻhis aldehyde, the full name of which is
-[(α-ethoxy-p-phenylphenacyl)amino] ben-
ɔic acid, was preventively used by Calonghi[11]
ı 28 children; at a dosage of 1 gm. per day,
his drug is well tolerated but ineffective.

ABOB (Virustat). ABOB, or chlorhy-
rate N′,N′-anhydrobis(β-hydroxyethyl)bi-
uanide, has been used preventively as well
s curatively; its effect upon varicella is
ncertain.[14, 44]

SEARCH FOR CONTACTS. The mildness
f the disease makes a search for contacts
nnecessary. On the other hand, *whenever
ariola is suspected, it is compulsory.* This
•ractice is thus extremely desirable in all
ases of varicella in adults; some health au-
horities also seek the contacts of young variella patients at the outbreak of the epidemic
•nly, as long as the diagnosis of variola has not
•een definitely rejected.

Treatment. Varicella is not a serious
lisease and, as a rule, is cured by itself. Even
he encephalitic complications are among the
nost benign ones. Specific immune globulins
ıre reserved for the treatment of the com-
•licated forms or of very young patients,
ılthough their efficacy has not been proved.

No definite evidence of any activity of
he antiviral therapies has yet been given.

Patients Undergoing Steroid Therapy. In
•atients who are already undergoing cortico-
teroid treatment, the interruption of this
herapy may have dramatic consequences.
ʻhe patient cannot resist a serious infectious
lisease; it is therefore necessary to go on with
ınd to increase steroid therapy, administering
ıgain the maximal doses used at the beginning
f they had been lowered or stopped.

In case of emergency, hydrocortisone

hemisuccinate by the intravenous route can
be truly lifesaving. Of course, immune globulins and antibiotics are very useful comple-
ments.

As for the cases of encephalitis (1 in 1000
cases of varicella) Bastin et al.[4] do not advise
administration of steroids, since varicella
encephalitis is generally cured spontaneously
and totally in a few weeks. Gerbeaux et al.[25]
report a case of encephalitis occurring in
the course of steroid therapy. Such cases also
require prudence, and cortisone must be administered only if the patient is already undergoing such treatment or if, because of the
serious state of the patient's condition, it is
the only solution left.

HERPES ZOSTER

Treatment of Herpes Zoster. Most often
zoster is cured in two to four weeks without
complications. Ophthalmic complications
and residual and obstinate pains in aged patients call for treatments the variety of which
reveals the limit of their activity.

CHEMOTHERAPY. *Xenalamine.* This
drug was administered by Colomb[13] at a dose
of 1.5 mg. per day; in reality, only the fever
and the eruption were improved in 50 per cent
of the cases, and the pains persisted.

5-Iodo-2′-deoxyuridine. This drug, in a
0.1 per cent solution, was locally applied
every other hour by MacCallum et al.[41] In two
cases, the lesions dried well in three days;
in the other four cases, the results were
slower and the pains persisted.

ABOB. Duperrat,[18] compiling his results and those of various authors, reports
the results obtained with 150 patients treated
with 800 mg. per day for one week. In 75 per
cent of the cases, the evolution of zoster
seemed shorter and the pains stopped in most
cases within 48 hours. However, this action
was obvious only when the patients were
treated at the onset, as soon as the diagnosis
had been made.

SPECIFIC THERAPEUTICS. *Immunoglobulins.* Use of the serum of patients re-
covering from zoster was recommended by
Tzanck. At present, some authors assert that
they are fairly successful in administering 5
ml. of 16.5 per cent immunoglobulins, once
or twice a day, until the pains have disappeared and the lesions have dried. Others
regard the action of globulins as rather irregular. Nonetheless, their use is perfectly
justified with severe cases or with patients

undergoing anti-inflammatory therapy which tends to lower the production of antibodies (e.g., for cancer or malignant hemopathies).

ANTI-INFLAMMATORY THERAPIES. *X-Rays*. A prospective study recently carried out by Rhys-Lewis[53] in 409 patients with herpes zoster revealed that radiation is of very little use in treating the ganglionic roots. It is thus pointless to discuss further this expensive therapy, the results of which are very uncertain.

Emetine. Use of this drug was suggested to a physician who had observed an improvement of zoster in patients he was treating with emetine. Griveaud and Achard[29] report on 160 cases of herpes zoster treated with a dose of 40 to 60 mg. every other day for a total of three to seven subcutaneous injections; ophthalmic zoster is more resistant and requires one injection every day. Although the results seemed favorable for the cases treated early, emetine was of little use in treating post-zoster pain.

The Corticosteroids. Corticosteroids have been used with a certain prudence since the accidents that have been observed with their use during varicella. The cases of herpes zoster occurring in the course of corticosteroid treatment are different from the usual ones in that they are often painless and their evolution is mild. Moreover, when the corticosteroids are stopped, zoster is not aggravated, contrary to what happens with varicella.[25] Pestel[52] thinks that short corticosteroid treatments (3 or 4 days) have an appreciable action if administered at the preeruptive or at the eruptive stage of the disease, and some effect upon the late painful phenomena. The dosage recommended for triamcinolone is 16 mg. in four doses for the first two days, 12 mg. in three doses for the next two days, and 8 mg. in two doses for the next three days.

In a 71-year-old patient treated by Elliot[20] with prednisone the pains disappeared within three and a half days instead of the three and a half weeks for the control subjects. The doses administered were 60 mg. of prednisone per day for seven days, 30 mg. of prednisone per day for the next seven days, and then 15 mg. of prednisone per day for seven days.

While a mild eruption does not require corticosteroid treatment, this therapy may be resorted to for the obstinate forms; in any case, there is no reason to fear that herpes zoster may occur in patients given corticosteroids.

BIBLIOGRAPHY

1. Abler, C.: Neonatal varicella (occurrence in bab born of infected mothers). Amer. J. Dis. Chil *107*:492-494, 1964.
2. Aubertin, M. E.: Epidémie de zona. J. Med. B deaux, *140*:440, 1963.
3. Baldasseroni, G., and Ulivelli, A.: La varicella periodo neonatale e nel primo mese di vita. R Clin. Pediat., *74*:46-51, 1964.
4. Bastin, R., Verliac, F., Maugey, F., and Christop P.: Les encéphalites des maladies éruptives. Ar Franç. Pediat., *21*:1073, 1964.
5. Benyesh-Melnick, M., Rosenberg, H. S., and Watso B.: Viruses in cell cultures of kidneys of childr with congenital heart malformations and oth diseases. Proc. Soc. Exp. Biol. Med., *117*:45 459, 1964.
6. Bertram, A.: Neonatal varicella. Lancet, *1*:891, 196
6a. Bichel, J., and Thorling, K.: Herpes zoster Hodgkin's disease. Danish Med. Bull., *14*:68-7 1967.
7. Bierman, H. R., Crile, D. M., Dod, K. S., Kell K. H., Petrakis, N. L., White, L. P., and Shimki M. B.: Remissions in leukemia of childhood follo ing acute infectious disease. Cancer, *6*:591-59 1953.
8. Bodey, G., MacKelvey, E., and Karon, M.: Chicke pox in leukemic patients, factors in prognosi Pediatrics, *34*:562-564, 1964.
9. Bousser, J., Christol, D., and Groubermann, S.: L lymphadénies, terrain d'élection pour certai virus ectodermo-neurotropes (varicello-zonateu en particulier). Sem. Hôp. Paris, *35*:2572, 1959.
10. Burgoon, C. J., Burgoon, J. S., and Baldridge, G. D Natural history of herpes zoster. J.A.M.A., *16* 265-269, 1957.
11. Calonghi, F.: Essai de xenalamine dans la proph laxie de la varicelle. G. Mal. Infett., *162*:141-14 1964.
12. Cheatham, W. J., Weller, T. H., Dolan, T. F., an Dower, J. C.: Varicella: report of 2 fatal cases wi necropsy, virus isolation and serologic studie Amer. J. Path., *32*:1015, 1956.
13. Colomb, D.: Xenalamine dans le traitement de dermatoses virales du groupe herpès zona. Bu Soc. Franç. Derm. Syph., *69*:828-829, 1962.
14. Curwen, M. P., Emond, R. T. D., and McKendric G. D. W.: Controlled trial of A.B.O.B. in measle chicken-pox and mumps. Brit. Med. J., *1*:23 237, 1963.
15. Degos, R., Lortat-Jacob, E., and Veron, P.: Var celle hémorragique au cours d'une leucose lym phoide traitée par corticoides. Bull. Soc. Fran Dermat. Syph., *68*:14-15, 1961.
16. Domart, A., Hazard, J., Labram, C., Husson, R and Portos, J. L.: Varicelle hémorragique ave pneumopathie chez un adulte traité par la delta cortisone pour leucose aiguë. Presse Méd., *72* 235-236, 1964.
17. Dumont, M.: Viroses inapparentes et malformation foetales. Presse Méd., *68*:1087, 1960.
18. Duperrat, B.: Le virustat en dermatologie. Sem Hôp. Paris, *39*:686-691, 1963.
19. Ehrlich, R., and Turner, J.: Neonatal varicella. Pediat., *53*:139, 1958.
20. Elliott, F. A.: Treatment of herpes zoster with hig doses of prednisone. Lancet, *2*:610-611, 1964.
21. Falliers, C. J., and Ellis, E. F.: Corticosteroids an

varicella. Six years' experience in asthmatic population. Arch. Dis. Child., *40*:593-598, 1965.

22. Freud, P.: Congenital varicella. Amer. J. Dis. Child., *96*:730, 1958.

23. Frischknecht, W.: Zur Pathogenese des Herpes zoster. Helv. Paediat. Acta, *20*:222-226, 1965.

24. Gerbeaux, J., Couvreur, J., Baculard-Beauchef, A., and Joly, J. B.: Maladies infectieuses sous corticothérapie au long cours (194 observations dont 102 varicelles). Sem. Hôp. Paris, *39*:61-74, 1963.

25. Gerbeaux, J., Couvreur, J., and Tron, P.: Sur un cas d'encéphalite de la varicelle survenu au cours d'une corticothérapie chez un enfant. Arch. Franc. Pediat., *20*:1165-1171, 1963.

26. Gold, E., and Godek, G.: Complement fixation studies with varicella-zoster antigen. J. Immunol., *95*:692-695, 1965.

27. Gold, E., and Robbins, F. C.: Isolation of herpes zoster from spinal fluid of a patient. Virology, *6*: 293, 1958.

28. Gordon, J. E.: Chickenpox: An epidemiological review. Amer. J. Med. Sci., *244*:362-389, 1962.

29. Griveaud, E., and Achard, J.: L'émétine dans le traitement du zona. Sem. Hôp. Paris, *35*:872-875, 1959.

30. Hanauer, L.: Neonatal varicella. Lancet, *1*:891, 1961.

31. Heine, K. M.: Zoster in leukosis and lymphogranuloma. Munch. Med. Wschr., *21*:1038-1041, 1965.

32. Helmly, R. B., Smith, J. O., and Eisen, B.: Chickenpox with pneumonia. J.A.M.A., *186*:870, 1963.

33. Heydenreich, J. S. S.: An outbreak of smallpox in an urban area. S. Afr. Med. J., *39*:463-466, 1965.

34. Hope-Simpson, R. E.: Nature of herpes zoster. A long term study and a new hypothesis. Proc. Roy. Soc. Med., *58*:9-20, 1965.

35. Johnson, R. T.: Pathogenesis of herpes virus encephalitis. J. Exp. Med., *119*:343-356, 1964.

36. Kapsenberg, J. G.: Possible antigenic relationship between varicella zoster virus and herpes simplex virus. Arch. Ges. Virusforsch., *15*:67-73, 1964.

37. Laporte, A.: La varicelle. In: Traité de Médecine. Vol. 1. Paris, Masson et Cie, 1948, pp. 714-722.

38. Laramée, B.: A propos d'un cas de varicelle maligne congénitale. Un. Med. Canada, *92*:543-545, 1963.

39. Le Tan Vinh, Canlorbe, P., Gentil, C., and Lelong, M.: Varicelle maligne pluriviscérale. Sem. Hôp. Paris, *33*:3989, 1957.

40. Librach, I. M.: Congenital chickenpox. Postgrad. Med. J., *35*:575-577, 1959.

41. MacCallum, D. I., Johnston, E. N., and Raju, B. H.: 5 Iodo-2'-deoxyuridine in the treatment of herpes zoster. Brit. J. Derm., *76*:459-462, 1964.

42. MacGregor, R. M.: Herpes zoster, chickenpox and cancer in general practice. Brit. Med. J., *1*:84-87, 1957.

43. Maretic, Z., and Cooray, M. P. M.: Comparisons between chickenpox in a tropical and a European country. J. Trop. Med. Hyg., *66*:311-315, 1963.

44. Menut, G., Dieu, J. C., and Adenis-Lamarre, F.: Les échecs d'une chimiothérapie anti-virale (ABOB) au cours d'une épidémie de varicelle. Arch. Franç. Pediat., *21*:859-869, 1964.

45. Merselis, J. G., Jr., Kaye, D., and Hook, E. W.: Disseminated herpes zoster. Report of 17 cases. Arch. Int. Med., *113*:679-686, 1964.

46. Netter, R.: Etude sur le virus de la varicelle. Path. Biol. (Paris), *12*:467-471, 1964.

46a. Netter, A., and Urbain, A.: Le virus varicello-zonateux. Ann. Inst. Pasteur, *46*:17-26, 1931.

47. Neustadt, A.: Congenital varicella. Amer. J. Dis. Child., *106*:96, 1963.

48. Newman, C. G. H.: Perinatal varicella. Lancet, *2*: 1159-1161, 1965.

49. Nonclercq, E., and Levy, G.: Contagiosité de la vaccine et de la varicelle au contact d'eczémateux. Bull. Soc. Franç. Derm. Syph., *64*:729-730, 1957.

50. O'Neil, R. R.: Congenital varicella. Amer. J. Dis. Child., *104*:391-392, 1962.

51. Pearson, H. E.: Parturition varicella-zoster. Obstet. Gynec., *23*:21-27, 1964.

52. Pestel, M.: Le zona. Presse Med., *69*:347-348, 1961.

53. Rhys-Lewis, R. D. S.: Radiotherapy in herpes zoster. Lancet, *2*:102-104, 1965.

54. Rifkind, D.: The activation of varicella-zoster virus infection by immunosuppressive therapy. J. Lab. Clin. Med., *68*:463-474, 1966.

55. Ross, A.: Modification of chickenpox in family contacts by administration of gamma globulin. New Eng. J. Med., *267*:369-375, 1962.

56. Ross, C. A. C., Subak Sharpe, J. H., and Ferry, P.: Antigenic relationship of varicella-zoster and herpes simplex. Lancet, *2*:708-711, 1965.

57. Schmidt, N. J., Lennette, E. H., Woodie, J. D., and Ho, H. H.: Immunofluorescent staining in the laboratory diagnosis of varicella-zoster virus infection. J. Lab. Clin. Med., *66*:403-412, 1965.

58. Sohier, R., and Netter, R.: Varicella, zona. In: Traité de Diagnostic des Maladies à Virus. Paris, Flammarion, 1964.

59. Sokal, J. E., and Firat, D.: Varicella-zoster in Hodgkin's disease. Amer. J. Med., *39*:452-463, 1965.

60. Weller, T. H.: Varicella, herpes zoster virus. In: Lennette, E. H., and Schmidt, N. J.: Diagnostic Procedures for Viral and Rickettsial Disease. New York, American Public Health Association, 1964.

61. Wohlwill, F.: Le zona. In: Levaditi, C., and Lepine, P.: Les Ultravirus des Maladies Humaines. Paris, Masson et Cie, 1948.

62. Wright, E. T., and Winer, L. H.: Herpes zoster and malignancy. Arch. Derm., *84*:242-244, 1961.

31

Smallpox

SMALLPOX: CLINICAL ASPECTS, DIAGNOSIS, AND TREATMENT*

F. DEKKING

Smallpox usually is acquired by the respiratory route, but infection can take place by inoculation of the skin or mucous membranes, accidentally or intentionally.

INCUBATION

The incubation period has a remarkably uniform length of 12 to 13 days, and variations are rare. It can be shorter (six to nine days), mostly after inoculation or intrauterine infection. It can be longer, 16 and even 21 days having been described. This lengthening might be caused by the fact that the dose of infective virus was very small or that the infection was caused by a mixture of virus and antibody such as crusts may contain, or after an unsuccessful attempt at passive immunization. After infection the virus multiplies locally and in the regional lymphoid tissue. Then, after 24 to 48 hours a first, transient viremia is postulated by which the reticuloendothelial system of liver, spleen, and bone marrow is infected. There the virus multiplies until the end of the incubation period, when the second viremia causes the first symptoms of the disease. This viremia in the ordinary forms lasts about two days, but in the severe forms it continues unabated until the death of the patient.

---

*For figures, see color plate.

INITIAL STAGE

The disease begins with a vague syndrome consisting of fever, headache, pain in the lumbar region, and vomiting. The fever can be slight or very high, and the other symptoms very severe, without prognostic significance. The patient may be clear-headed or delirious. Children may have convulsions. A dry cough, coryza, and conjunctivitis not unlike the prodromal stage of measles may be present. Sometimes there may be an initial petechial ("swimming trunk") rash in the groins.

This initial phase lasts two to three days (longer in the fatal cases). At the end of this period the temperature drops to normal and there is a marked amelioration in the patient's condition, followed by the eruption of the rash.

ERUPTIVE STAGE

The ordinary smallpox eruption is characterized by the aspects of its elements and by their distribution.

THE ELEMENT OF THE ERUPTION

The element starts as a macule the size of a pinhead. It is level with the skin, but may already feel like a tough, submerged papule, into which it quickly develops by growing. The emerged papule still lies deep in the skin and feels like a very hard, rubbery bead. If scratched with a needle for diagnostic purposes its tip will always contain a little fluid (the beginning of vesiculation), which

416

distinguishes it from most other papules, especially those of secondary syphilis. The maculopapular stage takes two days, when the vesicle develops inside the papular lesion. Right from the start the vesicle is deep-seated like the papule and multilocular: when opened, only part of its fluid may come out. The wall of the vesicle is tough and thick, the fluid pearly or slightly turbid. The vesicle slowly grows to a maximum diameter of 4 to 5 mm. It is circular, and may show a central umbilication. It is surrounded by a sharply defined, narrow erythematous zone. After two days the vesicle becomes pustular, and in the course of four days this pustule may grow to its maximum size of 8 to 10 mm. Then it dries out and a crust is formed which usually falls off around the fourteenth day of the eruption. The time schedule of about eight days from macule to crust is fairly rigid; it may be shortened in the modified form to three to four days. This development is very rarely lengthened; eruptions lasting for several weeks certainly are not smallpox. The development of the eruptive element compares very well with the course of the vaccinial lesion after primary vaccination; and an accelerated course is similarly seen in the presence of a partial immunity, as after revaccination.

DISTRIBUTION OF THE RASH

The peculiar distribution of the smallpox rash is governed by Rickett's law: the rash will be denser in those spots where the blood circulation in the skin is stimulated by movement, temperature changes, pressure, friction, or trauma. Thus the rash will be densest on exposed parts—face and hands—and on extensor surfaces. Hollows and shallows escape at the expense of ridges and prominences. There will be more lesions on the moving limbs than on the less mobile trunk, more on the back of the trunk than in front, more on the thorax than on the abdomen, and orbita and axilla may be spared altogether. Why this law holds for smallpox and not for chickenpox (although in that disease local irritation of the skin will also cause a denser eruption in the irritated area) is one of the many riddles of this disease.

The eruption occurs not only on the skin but also on the mucous membranes, sometimes even preceding the skin eruption. Smallpox lesions usually can be found in the mouth, on the hard palate, and on the tongue; sometimes the larynx may be affected. The rectal mucosa also can show lesions which at times can be quite extensive. Sometimes, in the modified form, there may be many lesions in the mouth with very few or no eruptive elements on the skin. Epidemiologically such patients may be very dangerous.

The first macules appear on the face and the upper part of the trunk, then slowly spread to the extremities and the lower part of the body. This spreading may take 24 to 36 hours, and the facial elements remain further along in development throughout the course of the disease. Thus scabbing may start in the face while pustulation is not yet completed on the skin of the lower extremities. In any individual anatomical area, however, all the eruptive elements are in the same stage of development, in contrast to chickenpox, in which newer crops may be found in the same areas as older elements.

CLINICAL FORMS OF SMALLPOX

Smallpox can manifest itself in various clinical forms, from very mild to extremely severe. Dixon[1] classified these forms partly according to the clinical aspects, and partly according to the distribution of the lesions, with a result which is not logically satisfying. I prefer the classification given by Rao[2] based on the observation and treatment of more than 20,000 smallpox patients in the Infectious Diseases Hospital at Madras, probably the most extensive single personal experience of the disease in modern times. In this classification, four basic groups are distinguished, according to the character of the eruption: hemorrhagic, flat, ordinary, and modified. In group 1 a distinction is made between early and late hemorrhagic smallpox; groups 2, 3, and 4 are subdivided, according to the distribution of the lesions, into confluent, semiconfluent, and discrete. In group 4, the modified form, the eruption may be lacking altogether, so a fourth variant is distinguished: variola sine eruptione. This classification has the didactic advantage that it stresses the relative unimportance of the distribution and number of the lesions: the ordinary confluent form has a better prognosis than the flat discrete one with far fewer eruptive elements.

HEMORRHAGIC FORMS

These are characterized by bleeding in the skin and from all the hollow viscera, and by their almost invariably fatal course. In Madras this form was seen in about 2.5 per cent of all smallpox patients.

The Early Hemorrhagic Form. The early hemorrhagic form stands quite apart from the other clinical manifestations of smallpox. The initial period is extended for several days and characterized by very severe headache and backache, restlessness, prostration with unimpaired consciousness, and awareness of the fatal end. Bleeding precedes the rash, which seldom has time to erupt, as most patients die on about the sixth day. In these patients the coagulation mechanism is severely disturbed: there is thrombocytopenia, a decrease in prothrombin and proconvertin, and a marked decrease in accelerator globulin (factor V), and a circulating antithrombin is found. The blood, until the last day, contains such a high titer of virus that it can be used as a precipitating antigen in the gel diffusion test. In the serum of an exceptional patient who survived until the tenth day no neutralizing antibodies could be found, while these are present in the ordinary form on about the fifth day. It looks as if all the patient's defenses are overrun by an enormous and continuous production of virus. This form is invariably fatal. It is more frequent in adults than in children and in females than in males. In Rao's series about two-thirds of the female patients were pregnant, while of all smallpox patients only three per cent were pregnant. It does not spare the vaccinated.

The Late Hemorrhagic Form. In the late hemorrhagic form the initial period is slightly extended, the rash develops to the papulovesicular stage, and then hemorrhages occur in the lesions and the viscera. The mortality is 95 to 100 per cent, death occurring on the fifth to eighth day. In the blood only thrombocytopenia is found.

THE FLAT FORM

In this form also the patients are severely ill in the initial period, which may last three to four days. The eruption of the rash generally is not accompanied by a fall in temperature. The maturation of the elements is very slow, and true round vesicles do not develop. The lesions, although they contain a little fluid and are sometimes blood-stained, stay flat. In the confluent forms large blebs may form, and when the patient is moved or handled the skin may strip off over large areas, leaving a raw oozing surface. Mortality is 95 per cent in the unvaccinated, and 70 per cent in vaccinated patients. The discrete form, although less severe, still carries a mortality of 85 per cent in the unvaccinated.

THE ORDINARY FORM

The initial period lasts two to three days, and then the eruption develops as described. The temperature at this stage is normal or only slightly elevated, and the patient does not feel very ill. On the fifth day of the eruption, with pustulation, there is a secondary rise in temperature: this is the fever of suppuration, which may last until the ninth or tenth day. This fever, which can be suppressed only partially by antibiotics, may also be caused by the resorption of toxic products from the skin lesions. At this stage the patient may become irrational and even delirious. The mortality is about 28 per cent in the unvaccinated, and 2 per cent in the vaccinated, mostly in those with the confluent forms.

MODIFIED FORM

The initial period has a normal length of two to three days. There is always fever, and the clinical picture may be either very mild or severe. The eruption may show an accelerated course, with scabbing already starting on the tenth day of the disease. The modified form is not always linked with vaccinial immunity; among the unvaccinated patients in Madras about three per cent showed this clinical variety of smallpox. The modified confluent form is very rare, about 0.1 per cent of all cases, and occurs only in the vaccinated. The modified form carries no mortality.

It should be stressed that in this form the eruption may lack almost all of the characters typical of smallpox. The distribution may be erratic, even localized, and asymmetrical. I have seen a patient with a typical zoster-like distribution of the rash, consisting of about 50 vesicles, from which variola virus was isolated. The eruptive elements may be very small, irregular in outline, superficial, and in different stages of maturation.

In the extreme variety of the modified form, variola sine eruptione, the rash is lacking completely, and the diagnosis is suspected only because of the contact with a smallpox patient, the typical incubation period, and the initial phase which may show the complete

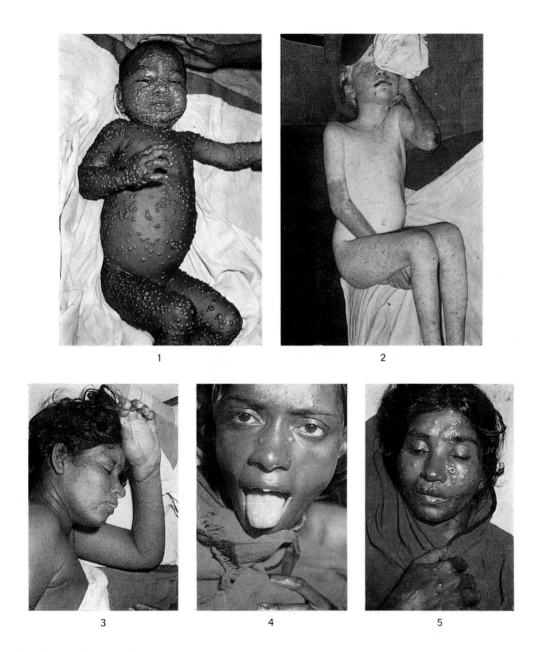

See Chapter 31, page 416.

Figure 31-1. Ordinary discrete, typical distribution. Day 6.

Figure 31-2. Hemorrhagic smallpox in an albino Indian girl. Day 6. Death on day 7.

Figure 31-3. Flat form of smallpox in a pregnant woman. Day. 5. Note enormous bullae on hand. Spontaneous abortion day 6. Death day 7.

Figure 31-4. Very mild variola with multiple lesions in the mouth. This form is highly contagious.

Figure 31-5. Mild smallpox in a partially immune patient. Atypical lesions, in different stages of development.

smallpox syndrome. The diagnosis can be confirmed by serological methods. These patients sometimes have lesions in the mouth whose variola character can be confirmed by virus isolation: for that reason they may be contagious.

COMPLICATIONS

Complications in smallpox are relatively rare. Secondary infection of the skin lesions with abscesses and boils can occur in the malnourished or under poor hygienic conditions. Conjunctivitis, rarely with keratitis, is seen in the eruptive stage in about 5 per cent of the patients and has a fairly good prognosis. Conjunctivitis from which no virus can be isolated can also occur during convalescence, with keratitis leading to corneal ulceration and loss of the eye. It is seen in the malnourished and might be caused by vitamin A deficiency. Osteomyelitis, probably caused by the virus, and secondary arthritis are rare. Encephalomyelitis, common in other exanthematous diseases, is a fairly rare complication. Orchitis is sometimes seen. Bronchopneumonia probably is not viral in origin, but caused by bacterial superinfection. Respiratory symptoms in the modified forms are considered by some to be of an allergic origin.

VARIOLA MINOR: ALASTRIM

All the clinical forms described, including the severe early hemorrhagic form, can also be seen in variola minor, but the severe forms are exceedingly rare. The diagnosis of variola minor can thus never be made in the individual patient: it can only be made at the end of an epidemic by taking the mortality into consideration, or by laboratory examination of the causative virus. The over-all mortality of variola major is 25 to 30 per cent, of variola minor less than 1 per cent.

DIFFERENTIAL DIAGNOSIS

As a rule the differential diagnosis with the ordinary forms of smallpox will not pose many problems, if it is remembered that the rash is general and symmetrical, that the elements are uniform in character, and that their size seldom exceeds 10 mm. In the initial stage diagnosis is impossible, but the lumbar pain is rarely as severe in other feverish conditions as it is in smallpox. In the macular stage, differentiation will be necessary with other acute exanthematous fevers, and especially with measles if coryza and conjunctivitis were present in the initial stage. Here again the distribution can help, and also the feeling of the rash: the macules in measles are superficial, slightly elevated, and velvety to the touch, and tend to be much larger than in smallpox. In the papular stage differentiation from secondary syphilis may be a problem, but the luetic papules as a rule contain no fluid. The early hemorrhagic form is almost impossible to recognize when smallpox is not suspected. The peculiar blood picture, with its preponderance of lymphoid elements and many immature forms, often suggests acute leukemia: this is the most frequent false diagnosis of this form in Western Europe. The characteristic symptoms of the initial stage may be of help in such cases. Sometimes malignant measles is suspected, and sometimes typhus, dengue, or other hemorrhagic fevers. Some patients in whom hematemesis and melena are the only symptoms may be brought to surgical departments with the diagnosis of a bleeding ulcer. It is the modified form, however, which causes most difficulties, and if only a few eruptive elements are present and the intial fever has been so slight as to pass unnoticed, clinical diagnosis is impossible and only virus isolation may bring the answer. Because the modified forms are mostly mistaken for chickenpox, points in the differential diagnosis of the two conditions are listed in Table 31-1. It must be stressed that chickenpox in an adult traveler, returning from an area in which smallpox may be prevalent, should always be diagnosed as smallpox until disproved by laboratory investigation.

THERAPY

There is no specific therapy for smallpox. As detectable antibodies can already be found in the serum on the second day of the rash, specific immunoglobulin is of no value and should not be given.

N-Methylisatin-β-thiosemicarbazone (Marboran), an antiviral substance, will prevent the outbreak of smallpox if given during the incubation period up until, as far

Table 31-1. *Differential Diagnosis of Variola and Varicella**

CLINICAL FEATURE	VARIOLA (SMALLPOX)	VARICELLA (CHICKENPOX)
Fever	Precedes eruption by 2-3 days; no fever at outbreak of eruption, temperature rises again after about 7 days	*Starts with eruption;* reaches climax 2-3 days later. If, in exceptional cases, there is an initial fever, it is never severe, and there is no headache, low back pain, or vomiting
Rash Distribution	Mostly on face and hands, less on trunk. See text	Mostly on trunk, less on face and hands
Character of lesions	Papules: *deep and hard*	Papules: *superficial and soft*
	Vesicles: *deep,* thick wall, fluid pearly or turbid. Mostly multilocular	Vesicles: *superficial,* thin wall, fluid clear. Unilocular
	Shape: round, surrounded by narrow circular areola	Shape: irregular, areola oval and directed along "splitting" lines of the skin
Evolution of lesions	In one area all in the same stage. Maturation from macule to scab takes ± 10 days	In one area all different stages can be found. Maturation takes 36-48 hours
	Crusts remain fixed for several days, leave scar	Crusts fall off quickly, leave no scar

*The italicized criteria are the only reliable ones to distinguish modified discrete smallpox, with but a few lesions, from chickenpox. In such cases, however, only the virology laboratory can give the final diagnosis.

is known now, the ninth day of that period. If given during the eruptive phase of smallpox it will not modify the course of the disease. A related compound has been tested early in the initial period, and, although this proved to be inactive, a trial with Marboran in the first days of the initial period might still be worthwhile.

Given the exceptional disorders in the early hemorrhagic form, with its lack of immunological defense and its thrombocytopenia and allied clotting disorders, a trial should be made in such condemned patients of massive exchange transfusions with fresh whole blood of recently vaccinated donors or from those convalesing from recent smallpox. The patient will then be provided not only with blood platelets and neutralizing antibodies, but also with immunologically competent lymphocytes.

In the ordinary forms it is necessary to give broad-spectrum antibiotics or penicillin from day six to 14 of the disease as a prophylactic measure against bacterial complications. Antibiotics are useless in the severe, quickly lethal forms, and unnecessary in the modified forms.

Patients with the confluent or semicon-

fluent forms may suffer from dehydration after about the tenth day of the disease, either from impaired fluid intake caused by the difficulty of swallowing or from fluid loss through the skin lesions. If possible they should be treated like burn patients, with control of the electrolyte balance. If intravenous fluid therapy is impossible because of the skin condition, sternal puncture might be tried or the fluids might be given by nasal intubation.

The application of oily lotions to the skin in the scabbing stage is pleasant to the patient and may speed the detachment of the scabs. The firmly embedded scabs in the sole of the foot and the palm of the hand should be taken out with the aid of scissors: this will speed the discharge of the patient by about a week.

BIBLIOGRAPHY

1. Dixon, C. W.: Smallpox. London, Churchill, 1962.
2. Rao, A. R.: Some epidemiological and clinical features of smallpox and its diagnosis. Bull. Ind. Soc. Malaria, *3*:96, 1966.
3. Ricketts, T. F., and Byles, J. B.: The Diagnosis of Smallpox. London, Cassall & Co., Ltd., 1908.
4. Smallpox Eradication. WHO Technical Report Series, No. 393, p. 12.

SMALLPOX: VIROLOGY, EPIDEMIOLOGY, AND PROPHYLAXIS

by R. NETTER

VIRUS RESPONSIBLE

DEFINITION

Viruses of the poxvirus group such as the variola and vaccinia viruses are big and brick-shaped, about 230 mμ wide and 295 mμ long, with a swollen nucleoid and two characteristic lateral bodies. They are fairly resistant to exterior agents owing to an envelope.

They are comprised of deoxyribonucleic acid (DNA); they develop in the cytoplasm of the infected cells, forming inclusion bodies. The nucleotid can be selectively altered by ultraviolet rays and the nitrogen mustards, and the enveloping protein by urea or heat.

Some substances, such as the halogenated deoxyuridines and the thiosemicarbazone compounds, inhibit the virus by their action on thymidine, which is indispensable to DNA synthesis.

PROPERTIES

In practice, the heat resistance of these viruses increases the dryer they are; when freeze-dried, they resist even 100° C. for several hours. Ultraviolet rays have an effect on contact. Phenol (1 per cent) has only a moderate influence. Ether resistance is a property of the group. The action of iodized compounds is not trustworthy since they have an influence only in protein-free media. Oxidizing agents such as sodium hypochlorite or permanganate are efficacious. *Cresyl* and *formalin* are the very basis of disinfection whenever either flaming or autoclaving cannot be used; crusts are more difficult to sterilize than dusts.

LABORATORY DIAGNOSIS OF SMALLPOX

In most cases, the clinical diagnosis of smallpox is enough, provided it is established. However, because of the heavy responsibility which is laid upon him, the practitioner tries to have both clear-cut and doubtful cases confirmed by the laboratory. Of course, any error is prejudicial in either direction, but better too much affirmation than not enough. Moreover, the practitioner should not think that the mere fact that he has asked for laboratory tests relieves him of the responsibility for the usual sanitary steps. It is easy to assert that a laboratory result is positive, but it is much more difficult and time-consuming to affirm that a sample is free of virus. In order to obtain a result as soon as possible and to avoid any risk of contamination, it is recommended that one use only laboratories that specialize in this type of test, whose staff members are regularly vaccinated, and where inoculation material is available at any time.

SAMPLES (Table 31-2)

The more abundant the sample, the quicker the laboratory's answer.

Cutaneous Samples. During the *maculopapular stage,* scraping specimens are sent.

During the *vesicular stage,* the lesions are cleaned with normal saline solution and the vesicular fluid is taken by suction. The whole capillary tube is sent, or only its content, in a small screw flask, itself placed in a metal tube as a safety measure.

Smears can be utilized for immunofluoresence tests only if they are suitably fixed, with anhydrous calcium chloride-dehydrated acetone cooled to −20° C.

During the *pustular stage,* the pus is taken; smears are unreliable because the cell fragments are a cause of error.

During the *crusting stage,* several crusts are detached by means of a vaccinostyle, scalpel, or forceps, and are put in a small flask. The infectious material can be used either to reveal an antigen rapidly or to cultivate the virus.

Blood. The tubes used for the blood should not contain any anticoagulant.

BLOOD COUNT AND THE HEMOGRAM. Leukopenia invariably occurs in the serious cases of smallpox[15]; it is only transitory in the mild forms and then becomes a leukocytosis. During the last epidemic in Bradford, England, a general practitioner was able to warn the responsible authorities; he based his diagnosis on granulopenia and the comparative increase in mononuclear cells. Thus, although such a result is not pathognomonic of smallpox, in a febrile patient exhibiting a more or

Table 31-2. *Laboratory Tests Generally Used to Diagnose Smallpox*

	MATERIAL TO SEND	VIRUS DETECTION			
		ELECTRON MICROSCOPY	SEROLOGIC METHOD	EGG CULTURE OR CELL CULTURE	ANTIBODY DETECTION
Maculopapular stage	Cutaneous scraping specimen	+		+	
Vesiculopustular stage	Vesiculopustular fluid	+	+	+	
Crusting stage	Crusts	+	+	+	
Retrospective diagnosis or noneruptive forms	Serum				+
Time required for the test (hr.)		$^{1}/_{2}$-2	2-24	24-12	24
Can differentiate vaccinia from variola		no	no	yes	no
Can differentiate herpes-varicella from vaccinia-variola		yes	yes	yes	yes

less typical eruption and dying within a few days it is suspicious enough to justify further investigations.

VIRUS CULTURE. The interest of virus culture is mainly theoretical. MacCallum et al.[37] recovered the virus one day prior to and one day after the eruption in two patients out of seven. Downie et al.[19] have shown that a considerable and persistent viremia after the third day was, as a rule, characteristic of the fatal cases. The blood must be inoculated for culture rapidly, since under refrigeration it quickly loses its infectious capacity.

TITRATION OF SERUM ANTIBODIES. This is required only for a retrospective diagnosis of smallpox, when all traces of lesion have disappeared, or for noneruptive febrile illnesses.

Urine. The search for the variola virus in urine has only a theoretical interest. Downie et al.[21] found it in half their patients with smallpox but in the absence of catheterization exterior contamination could not be excluded.

Saliva. The variola virus is present in the saliva when there exist buccal enanthematous lesions,[22, 37] i.e., when the cutaneous lesions are well developed. MacCallum et al.[37] found the virus on the second or third day after the eruption in two patients out of ten. The patient gargles with 5 ml. of 10 per cent peptone water which also contains 300 units of penicillin and 300 mg. of streptomycin per milliliter.

Dispatching the Samples. The safety of those who will be handling the samples must always be kept in mind. The double-box system is imperative. Only the flasks or the inside metal box can come near the patient. Then, they are painted over with an antiseptic solution and the whole thing is packed in the second box, outside the contaminated area. Inside, a slip is included which states the type of investigations required and the following information: name and age of the patient, name of the physician or public health body, date of the disease onset, date of the last antivariolic vaccination, whether there was known exposure to smallpox or varicella, and whether the patient has recently been in an area where smallpox is endemic.

Refrigeration is unnecessary during transportation. The parcel must be sent the fastest way possible, and the specialized laboratory must be notified immediately by telephone or cable.

RESULTS AND INTERPRETATION

We classify the laboratory tests according to the rapidity of their results.

Quick Orientation Diagnosis

ELECTRON MICROSCOPY. Electron microscopy can be utilized only with vesiculo-pustular fluids; it provides an orientation diagnosis within a few hours, classifying the virus in the poxvirus group (variola, vaccinia, cowpox) or the herpesvirus group (herpes, varicella-zoster).

IMMUNOFLUORESCENCE. This is a quick method for detecting the antigen. Avakian et al.,[2] as well as Kirsch and Kissling,[33] have adopted the direct method, whereas Murray[45] prefers the indirect technique. Either way, great prudence is required because a badly fixed smear may cause serious errors.

AGAR IMMUNOPRECIPITATION. The minimum sample required for agar immuno-precipitation is a large crust; the amount of vesicular fluid available is usually insufficient for this easy reaction, which is as rapid as the preceding ones. In the fulminating and extremely serious forms, the concentration of soluble antigen in the patient's blood is sometimes sufficient for a positive precipitation reaction with rabbit hyperimmune serum; only a diagnosis for the viral group orientation is theoretically possible.

COMPLEMENT-FIXATION REACTION. This reaction is occasionally the key to a differential diagnosis of varicella. At the vesicular stage, the reaction may not be very sensitive,[29] nor is it very specific when there is no suitable control. In any case, it is a group reaction which does not differentiate vaccinia from variola.

A negative result is significant only if there is a sufficient dose of antigen. For this reaction, Downie et al.[19] sometimes used the patient's serum as antigen; the prognosis was pessimistic when there was a positive reaction, since in all such cases death occurred rapidly.

MICROSCOPIC EXAMINATION OF STAINED SMEARS. Downie, of Liverpool, remains faithful to this technique. The greatest prudence is imperative especially if it is used from the pustular stage on, when many artifacts distort the interpretation. In a recent unfortunate experience a diagnosis of varicella, supposedly confirmed by the presence of Tzanck's cells, considerably delayed the diagnosis of smallpox.[29]

MODERATELY RAPID DIFFERENTIAL DIAGNOSIS BETWEEN SMALLPOX AND VACCINIA. Inoculations into embryonated eggs make it possible to distinguish, within three days, vaccinia and variola or cowpox viruses; if there is a small amount of virus in the specimen, a further passage is sometimes necessary to isolate it. In cell culture, the lesions induced by the variola virus are different from those caused by the vaccinia or even the herpes virus. Since the cytopathogenic action of variola is evident as early as the third day, the virus cannot be mistaken for that of varicella, which requires at least one week to produce cytopathogenic lesions. Before the third day, it is possible to detect a hemadsorbent antigen by adding chick red blood cells after 24 hours of culture; immuno-fluorescence[11, 26, 34] may permit diagnosis within six hours if the specimens are highly infected[26] and plentiful. As a matter of fact, the cases that are difficult for the clinician to diagnose are equally difficult for the laboratory staff because they receive only very small specimens. Should the sample be kept at room temperature there is no chance of isolating the varicella virus. Whereas the latter disappears rapidly from the cutaneous lesions and cannot be recovered at the crusting stage, that of variola persists for a very long time, although its infectiousness decreases.

Late Diagnosis: Distinction Between Variola Major and Minor.

The diagnosis is based on the difference in mortality in chick embryos inoculated with a high dose of virus (Helbert's test),[28] or on the difference in percentage of lesions observed either on the chorioallantois of the embryonated egg[23] or on cell cultures[46] incubated at various temperatures. Downie et al.[17] and Rossi,[49] using these tests, unquestionably established the diagnosis of alastrim (variola minor); the smallpox epidemic in Tanganyika[6] may have been caused by an intermediary virus, a little less thermosensitive than the real strains of variola minor.

SEROLOGICAL TESTS

Serological tests are used to establish a diagnosis for the noneruptive or only slightly

eruptive febrile illnesses or for the posteruptive period. In cases of fulminating
variola, when death occurs at the very onset
of the disease, antibodies generally have no
time to appear.

Immunoprecipitation. The sera of subjects vaccinated against smallpox never
precipitate in the presence of ground vaccinia virus-infected chorioallantoic membrane.

However, some serious forms of smallpox induce a level of antibodies sufficient for
this reaction to be positive.

Complement-Fixation Reaction.[18, 39] The
titers obtained vary with the method used.
In nonvaccinated subjects with smallpox the
results are invariably positive from the
eighth to the tenth day, the titer reaching 1/80.
In subjects with smallpox who were vaccinated in the past, the titers are higher and
the antibodies appear earlier. However, in
about 50 per cent of the subjects who have
been vaccinated against smallpox, antibodies
appear between the seventeenth and the
twenty-third day and disappear within six
months; they may appear again after revaccination.

In doubtful cases, high levels or increasing levels of antibody are required to establish the diagnosis. A positive reaction in a
subject suspected of having smallpox who has
not been vaccinated for one year is of great
value.

Hemagglutination Inhibition Test. In
nonvaccinated subjects with smallpox,
hemagglutination-inhibiting antibodies appear
between the third and the fifth day and are
always present on the seventh day;[18] in subjects with smallpox who were vaccinated in
the past, titers are higher and antibodies
appear earlier.

One should bear in mind that hemagglutination-inhibiting antibodies reach titers
of 1/800 after vaccination and persist at low
titers of about 1/40 long afterward.

In case of doubt, high levels or increasing levels of antibodies are required for
diagnosis.

Seroneutralization Test. The search for
neutralizing antibodies on embryonated egg
chorioallantoic membrane or cell culture is
always time consuming. In nonvaccinated patients with variola, these antibodies are always
present on the sixth day of disease. Their titer
is higher than after just one vaccination but
is as high as during generalized vaccinia

(1/10,000 and up). In patients with smallpox
who were vaccinated in the past, antibodies
appear as early as the second day. In fatal
cases, the reaction is often negative. Antibodies persist at low rates of 1/2 to 1/64 long
after smallpox vaccination, whereas the titer
one month after vaccination is usually 1/120
to 1/330.

EPIDEMIOLOGY

The speed of air transport has greatly
increased the risk of infection: it brings into a
receptive country subjects incubating variola
who show no signs of disease when they arrive, whereas during voyages in the past the
disease would have broken out on board ship.

Unfortunately, the vaccination certificate
required from international travelers is not an
absolute guarantee, first, because the result
of revaccination is not checked, second, because the passenger is permitted to leave
immediately after revaccination, even
though he might be incubating variola, and,
third, because many false certificates are
made out by unscrupulous physicians.

During the smallpox epidemic in Paris,
in 1948, Boyer and Roussel[8] noted three
flagrant examples: the first patient had obtained a false certificate for an international
trip; the second had obtained a false certificate with a view to an examination; and the
third, fearing a reaction to the vaccine,
wiped it away.

MORBIDITY

Figure 31-1 shows the incidence of
variola in Africa, America, and Asia during
the past ten years. Since 1958, the incidence
of smallpox has decreased owing to mass
vaccination campaigns in the most infected
areas. These are Asia (with India, Indonesia,
and Pakistan the largest reservoir of smallpox), then Africa, and Central and South
America. Europe is not represented in Figure
31-6 because the number of cases of smallpox is always very small. In 1963, however,
five imported cases caused 124 secondary
cases (98 in Poland, 26 in Sweden, no
secondary cases in Hungary, Switzerland,
and Germany).

Table 31-3 shows the smallpox rates in
the countries declaring more than 500 cases
in 1964. It is to be noted that the incidence

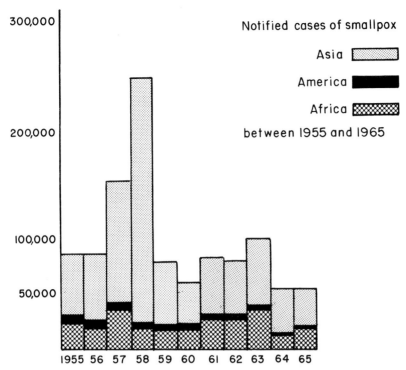

Figure 31-1. Notified cases of smallpox between 1955 and 1965.

per 100,000 inhabitants is higher in Africa than in Asia. Probably this only reflects the inadequacy of the vaccination campaigns in Africa as compared to Asia because of the more scattered population.

Sex. During some epidemics, such as that in Paris in 1942, it was noted that the incidence was higher in women than in men. Of the 61 typical cases of variola studied by Boyer and Roussel,[8] 36 occurred in women and only 12 in men; the others were in children. This difference is accounted for by the fact that the men had been revaccinated not only during military service but also during World Wars I and II.

Age. The age at which vaccination takes place affects the morbidity. As a result of a letdown in vaccination campaigns during the war, most patients in the variola epidemic in Paris in 1947[8] were younger than five years in age.

Table 31-3. *Smallpox Incidence per 100,000 Inhabitants in Countries Declaring More Than 500 Cases in 1964*

	COUNTRY	NO. OF CASES	INCIDENCE PER 100,000 IN- HABITANTS
Africa	Congo	2,324	15
	Dahomey	703	34
	Malawi	712	24
	Nigeria	1,454	3.9
	Swaziland	517	194
	Tanganyika	1,461	19
	Ouganda	523	7
	Zambia	2,209	90
America	Brazil	1,791	2
Asia	India	32,480	7
	Indonesia	1,745	1.8*
	Pakistan	896	0.9

*Approximate figure.

Among vaccinated subjects, children under ten years are rarely attacked because of their recently acquired immunity, whereas age groups over 30 are far from being spared.

Blood Group. In order to account for the unequal distribution of the blood groups over the world, it has been suggested that variola may have been more lethal to those in blood group A, whereas plague was more lethal to those belonging to group O. The recent investigation of Downie et al.[20] clearly shows that, in 337 hospitalized patients, the incidence and the seriousness of variola had no connection at all with any blood group.

Seasonal Behavior. There are no recent statistics showing a seasonal incidence in variola. Therefore, in temperate zones, the sanitary authorities must be vigilant at all times.

Mortality

At least 9000 persons died of smallpox in 1964. Table 31-4 shows the world-wide mortality and morbitity rates, based on notifications made to the World Health Organization (Epidemiological Reports).

The mortality is highest in Asia, ranging from 25 to 30 per cent and up, whereas it is only about 10 per cent in Africa or Europe. In Asia, the form is always variola major; in South America, where mortality is lower than 0.1 per cent, it is a type of variola minor.[15]

Effectiveness of Vaccination. From the statistical study of the epidemics which took place in England in 1927 and 1958, Dixon[15] has recorded the following figures: For patients under 20 years of age, the mortality was 0 per cent for those who had been vaccinated as children and 33 per cent for those who had not been vaccinated. The corresponding figures for patients over 20 years of age were 20 per cent and 54 per cent. In India, the difference is not always so spectacular in people under 20; this fact seems to be without connection with the vaccine, and we cannot account for it. Nevertheless it is obvious that mortality has decreased owing to vaccination.

Age. Sensitivity is more marked at both extremes of life. In aged subjects this is probably the result of intercurrent diseases or remoteness of vaccination. Pregnancy is undoubtedly an aggravating factor.

Virus Reservoir

The existence of an animal reservoir of variola virus has never been proved. Accordingly, a patient is almost always at the origin of an epidemic. Therefore, it is important to identify the primary case as soon as possible in order to prevent secondary or tertiary cases.

The Patient. Smallpox is not contagious during the incubation period, but it may become contagious after the hyperthermic

Table 31-4. *Morbidity and Mortality of Variola, 1960-1965*

Continent	1960	1961	1962	1963	1964*	1965*
Africa						
Cases	15,851	24,025	24,188	16,735	12,417	16,590
Deaths	1,017	1,798	2,423	1,669	819	1,428
America						
Cases	3,090	1,939	3,029	6,431	2,230	1,072
Deaths	–	–	–	16	–	–
Asia						
Cases	39,221	53,549	46,374	76,271	35,329	31,088
Deaths	9,639	13,081	12,287	22,858	9,285	8,643
Europe						
Cases	47	24	137	129	–	1
Deaths	–	4	27	11	–	–
Total						
Cases	58,209	79,537	73,728	99,566	49,976	48,750
Deaths	10,656	14,883	14,737	24,554	9,304	10,071

*Incomplete figures.

viremic phase. The cutaneous lesions, including crusts, are rich in virus. The disease is less contagious in its late stage.

The enanthematous lesions are equally virulent. One hundred fifty specimens out of 309 (48.5 per cent) obtained by buccal washings with peptone solution were positive; the optimal time for isolation was between the third and the ninth day after the onset of the eruption. Seventeen forms in which exanthemata were absent or very mild did not yield any positive results, although the examinations were repeated;[22] such forms are known to be only slightly contagious.

All the organs of a patient with smallpox are contagious. Therefore the greatest care is required during autopsy.

Bedding and Clothes. The bedding and clothes of the patient and the hospital staff are infected with virus; thus laundrymen, particularly those who inhale dust when unwrapping the linen, have often been infected. Patients were also infected by doctors and nurses at a time when it was not the rule to change hospital clothing after contact with a suspect patient. Downie, Dumbell, and MacCallum detected amounts of virus, occasionally considerable, in the dust of patients' rooms.

Hair of Domestic Animals. This route has often been considered the link between several cases of variola, but its existence has not been proved.

Cotton. The experiments carried out by MacCallum and MacDonald, mentioned by Dixon,[15] show that variola crusts artificially introduced into raw cotton are infectious for more than one year at room temperature, especially if the humidity is low. According to Dixon, the fact that smallpox often infects workers in the cotton industry is not adequate evidence that cotton is the source because such factories are in towns where most of the population works in the cotton industry, and these towns are harbors where ships and crews arrive from areas infected with variola. The same could be said of supposed contamination by imported wool.

Ambient Air. Infection of the ambient air has been held responsible when no other cause could be found. This hypothesis has been supported by MacCallum,[38] who tested the survival of the vaccinia virus in aerosol at various temperatures and relative humidities. After 23 hours at 11° C. and 50 per cent humidity, 59 per cent of the virus was still viable.

MODE OF TRANSMISSION

Direct Route. This is the usual route and it explains the occurrence of many secondary and tertiary cases; a very brief contact, for instance just passing through a room, is enough if the patient is in the period of maximal infectiousness.

AIR ROUTE. This was the route usually used for variolations in China: ground smallpox crusts taken at a late stage of the disease were blown through the nostrils by means of a brass tube. Downie et al.[21] attempted to isolate the virus by placing uncovered Petri dishes for 10 to 15 minutes near the patient's mouth while the patient was talking; they also used an exhaust-bubbling apparatus. They were able to isolate far less virus than when the dusts went back into the atmosphere owing to motion or handling of clothes and bedding.

This mode of contamination is undoubtedly more usual than one reported by Boyer and Roussel:[8] during the variola epidemic in Paris in 1942, the infection was transmitted to the upper floor of a hospital because of a defective hot-air vent common to both wards.

There are not many observations that really prove that the few cases of variola which occur near isolation hospitals are caused by inhaling air and not by contact with a person with variola at a subclinical stage.

CUTANEOUS ROUTE. The Greco-Turkish variolation method involved the cutaneous route. Cases of contamination from wounds incurred in the autopsy room are well known. During the epidemic in Vannes, in 1955, Le Bourdelles[35] observed two children with pulpal paronychia due to smallpox; a technician had taken blood for hemograms immediately after drawing blood from a patient seriously ill with smallpox. The aggravating role of various cutaneous affections is alleged, although there is no positive evidence for this.

DIGESTIVE ROUTE. In India, variolation used to be carried out through the digestive route. In practice, alimentary transmission does not seem to play an important role.

TRANSPLACENTAL ROUTE. When smallpox occurs at the beginning of pregnancy, miscarriage is likely. At the end of pregnancy, the fetus may be infected. Marsden (mentioned by Dixon[15]) described 34 women who became infected in late pregnancy.

Only 17 of the infants became infected in utero; the incubation period between the appearance of the mother's rash and that of the child lasted only nine to 12 days, i.e., a little less than the usual incubation period.

The transplacental route should be regarded as certain if the eruption starts less than ten days after birth.

Indirect Route. Transmission by the indirect route is proved by epidemiological considerations. Inhaled virus may remain viable for 24 hours on the rhinopharyngeal mucosa of healthy carriers. Moreover, there are many instances in which contamination could have occurred only through healthy carriers or through contaminated clothes, bedding or other objects; therefore, those most often attacked are laundrymen, wardrobe dealers, hotel maids, or the hospital staff taking care of the laundry and handling bedding.

CONTAGIOUSNESS

Incubation. The disease is not contagious for at least the first ten days of incubation. Therefore, contacts from this time are usually permitted to circulate freely. The patient starts to be dangerous when viremia develops, which is revealed by pyrexia.

Onset of the Eruption. At its onset, the rash is not very dangerous, as proved by two recent observations mentioned by Boyer and Roussel:[8] the first is the case of a medical student who, in 1947, 17 days after he had been contaminated in the hospital, traveled by subway to a specialist's consulting room; at this time he already had a rash. He sent his wife to the country before going to the hospital by ambulance. In spite of all these imprudences, no secondary cases occurred. The other case is that of a Pakistani who, in 1961, stopped in Rome and then in Paris, where he spent the whole afternoon in the transit room at Orly airport. However, his rash, although beginning, was obvious enough that passengers kept away from him on the plane. In spite of all the possible contacts between this patient and passengers or crew, no secondary cases were detected in either Italy or France. It was not until he arrived in England that the patient, who subsequently died, caused an epidemic.

Differences in Contagiousness of the Various Forms. The study carried out by Boyer and Roussel[8] during the Paris epidemic of 1942 shows that, in two hospital wards, the patients' receptivity was only about 30 per cent; after one smallpox patient was introduced, 14 patients out of 40 and 18 out of 78 exhibited more or less severe forms of variola.

It is difficult to guess what the smallpox incidence would be without any immunization at all, because all the contacts are usually vaccinated. However, Dixon[15] thinks that, with variola major, at least 50 per cent of the subjects would contract the disease, and with variola minor, only 20 per cent.

The fulminating forms are less contagious than the serious ones because the patient dies before the virus can be eliminated. The mild or noneruptive influenza-like forms are not very dangerous either, for the period of virus elimination is probably very short.

The intermediate forms are contagious for at least five to six days. Contaminations may occur up to 45 days later, but no doubt they are infrequent even though the virus is still present in the crusts. In observations of very prolonged incubation periods, one can never be sure that the contamination was not indirect, due to virus remaining on some objects after the patient left.

INFECTIOUS MECHANISM

VARIOLA INOCULATA

Inoculation can occur accidentally in the laboratory, the autopsy room, or the funeral parlor. When variolation was a common procedure against variola, inoculation was voluntary.

Dixon,[15] referring to earlier publications, noted that the incubation period after inoculation is short, since the vesicle appears on the fifth day and the progress is rapid, everything being back to normal within three weeks.

The fact that the incubation period is short may be due to the amount of virus inoculated, to its greater ability to develop in the skin, or to its direct passage in the lymphatics or in the blood.

Actually, these experiments do not exactly reflect the facts, for a point of cutaneous inoculation is never found in the usual forms of variola. Moreover, the amount of virus inoculated is much greater than in the natural infection. Finally, the crust virus is not very dangerous, since the mortality was only 1 per cent with cutaneous or respiratory variolations, whereas it exceeds 30 per cent with variola major. Wheelock[52] thinks that the interferon he was able to reveal in the vaccinia crusts may be responsible for the phenomenon.

CONGENITAL SMALLPOX

Congenital smallpox results from actual inoculation of the virus into the fetus by the blood route. The incubation period is two to three days shorter than in the usual forms; this is probably because the virus is transmitted before the appearance of the mother's cutaneous lesions.

COMMON SMALLPOX

Introduction of the Virus. All epidemiologists agree that respiratory contamination occurs. Only a few infectious units are required; MacCallum[38] succeeded in infecting, by aerosol, three rabbits out of three with only 4 infectious units of vaccinia virus, a virus that probably behaves exactly like variola.

However, it has never been possible to show primary pulmonary lesions due to the variola virus. Although theoretically the contaminated subject could immediately transmit the virus which has just reached his respiratory mucosa, there is no epidemiological evidence that the virus multiplies there, since there is no risk of contagion during the incubation period.

THE NONERUPTIVE FORMS. Since the disease is benign and does not cause death, no virological or histopathological information can be obtained. It is not contagious and its existence is revealed mainly by radiological examinations. Since these influenza-like forms usually occur in vaccinated subjects, Dixon[15] does not exclude an allergic origin, at least in the forms with brief incubation.

Incubation. Once the virus is in the organism, it cannot be recovered until the stage of viremia, which is marked by fever and which precedes the eruption. In other words, it cannot be recovered during the incubation period, which lasts an average of 12 days.

By analogy with the work carried out by Fenner[24] on ectromelia in mice, by Bedson and Duckworth[5] on rabbit pox, and by Hahon and Wilson[27] on experimental variola in the monkey, the following cycle can be assumed: (1) the virus infects the lung, and the cervical and tracheobronchial lymphatic ganglia; (2) a first, brief viremia carries the virus into the spleen and the liver, where it multiplies rapidly in the cells of the reticuloendothelial system[6, 27, 48] but produces no macroscopic lesions.

Mims,[44] using the immunofluorescence method, observed that 90 per cent of the vaccinia virus injected intravenously is rapidly localized in the Kupffer's cells of the liver and go further only if the strains are virulent. Earlier observations by Councilman, mentioned by Downie,[16] that hepatic sinusoids disappear in fatal forms, might be evidence of this intense multiplication within the Kupffer cells.

Viremia. Fairly frequently, MacCallum[37] and Downie et al.[19] isolated the virus from blood drawn during the first two days of the eruption. This second viremia phase, more intense and longer than the first, corresponds to the hyperthermic phase. In serious forms, it persists for several days, whereas in benign forms it may not exceed a few hours. It spreads the virus through the whole body.

Histopathology of the Cutaneous Lesions. The dermal capillaries are dilated and surrounded with mononucleated cells. The epithelial cells of the malpighian layer are distended; they may or may not contain viral cytoplasmic inclusions. The fluid collects between the degenerated cells and forms a vesicle. Then the mononuclear and the polymorphonuclear cells go from the capillaries to the impaired epithelial layers and the vesicle turns into a pustule.

In malignant forms, the destructive process causes little reaction from the host, whereas in benign forms the reaction is intense and superficial.

Immune Phenomena. Neutralizing antibodies soon appear in the serum and limit the viremia. Since the incubation period lasts about 12 days and, in subjects vaccinated for the first time, neutralizing antibodies appear around the eleventh day, it is easy to see why vaccination on the day of the contact is of some avail. Revaccination or infection with the variola virus in a vaccinated subject very rapidly induces a further increase in antibodies which inhibits the viremia and neutralizes the virus.

The virus that is already intracellular

and that is therefore insensitive to antibodies continues to grow in the cutaneous lesions until further mechanisms such as interferon check its multiplication.[52]

The longer the period between contact and vaccination—that is, the shorter the period between vaccination and the appearance of the rash—the more unlikely it is that a vesiculopustule will be induced by vaccination. Such failures are accounted for only by a refractory state of the skin because, at that stage, antibodies are either not present or present at a low level.

A Few Remarks. Many problems remain to be solved. For instance, the vaccinia and variola viruses are very similar, yet one of them causes a localized and only slightly contagious disease, while the other causes a generalized highly contagious disease. Interferon is found very early in the vaccinia virus-induced lesions. However, such an observation has never been made with variola, whose virus may provoke the production of less interferon.

One may also wonder why the incubation period is so long in congenital vaccinia and so short in congenital variola—whether this is because variola has a greater tendency to terminate the pregnancy than vaccinia, and if so, why.

PROPHYLAXIS

PROPHYLAXIS DURING NONEPIDEMIC PERIODS

In countries where variola is not endemic, prophylaxis is essentially based on protection of the individual by vaccination and on measures to prevent patients with variola from entering the country.

Antivariolic Vaccines

STRAINS. The history of the vaccinia strains used all over the world is usually not well known. Jenner's cowpox strain, transmitted from arm to arm, even during smallpox epidemics, was lost several times. The strain presently used by the Lister Institute, London, was obtained from a soldier with smallpox during the 1870 war. The strain of the Vaccinia Institute of Paris is derived from Naples cowpox and was cowpox-enriched early in this century. The strains, originally different, were later maintained on various animals. At present, they are different in that experimentally they are more or less neuro-

tropic or have more or less tendency to cross over the epithelial barrier and to develop in the mesoderma; they have in common the capacity to protect against variola.

THE VARIOUS VACCINES. *Glycerinated Fresh Vaccine.* In temperate regions, the glycerinated fresh vaccine is undoubtedly the most convenient. At $-30°$ C., it can be maintained for over 15 months. At room temperature, its activity starts to diminish during the very first week.

Freeze-Dried Vaccine. In France, the first freeze-dried vaccine was prepared by Camus and d'Arsonval as early as 1914, Such a preparation is of great help in tropical countries, since it remains very well preserved: the vaccine retains its original efficacy for years at $+4°$ C., for months at $45°$ C., and even for one hour at $100°$ C. Once the vaccine is again in solution, it is absolutely comparable to fresh vaccine.

Egg Vaccine. The advantage of such a vaccine is that it is free of bacteria. However, it has not been demonstrated that the number of cases of postvaccinial encephalitis is smaller than that following use of the usual vaccines. Therefore, the vaccine prepared on egg has never been unanimously accepted and is used only in Texas (since 1939) and in Sweden.

Tissue Culture Vaccine. Of course, this preparation is attractive owing to its bacteriological sterility. But it is expensive, an important consideration with regard to mass vaccinations. Moreover, it has not yet proved its worth in countries where variola is endemic, and it is not certain whether the neutralizing antibodies this vaccine induces really reflect a refractory state with regard to variola. Investigation of this problem is in full progress.

Attenuated or Inactivated Vaccines. It has never been proved on a sufficient scale that the use of attenuated or inactivated vaccines prevents the complication of encephalitis. Furthermore, it has been unanimously accepted until now that they are not effective against smallpox. Exception could be made in the case of vaccines partially inactivated by formalin or merely diluted vaccines, but the percentage of cases in which the vaccine causes a vesiculopustular reaction is too low.

Any generalized use of such vaccines would be disastrous to smallpox prophylaxis, first, because they do not necessarily protect against encephalitis, and, second, because physicians or health agencies might be lulled into neglecting to follow up this injection with that of a classic vaccine, the only one that reliably confers immunity.

Combined Vaccines. It is most advisable to use combined vaccines in developing countries where various severe diseases are endemic and where difficult transport hampers mass vaccination campaigns. In the former French territories of equatorial Africa, the vaccinia virus and the anti-yellow fever vaccine were often used jointly. More recently, the vaccinia virus has been given with BCG,[36] with the live antimeasles vaccine,[42] or even with the measles vaccine plus yellow fever vaccine.[41]

VACCINATION TECHNIQUE. The vaccine is introduced into the skin by making one scarification with a vaccinostyle, by pressing the cutting edge of a Hagedorn's needle repeatedly, or by making multiple punctures at one time, according to Krawitz's technique.

Intradermal Jet Inoculation. The advantage of this process is that it is rapid and requires a smaller and more precise amount of vaccine.[43] Very good seroconversion is obtained for the hemagglutination-inhibiting antibodies, even when there is no local reaction;[42] several vaccines can be used jointly. Users should nonetheless be on their guard against the aerosols emitted by the functioning apparatus.

ADVANTAGES OF VACCINATION AND A FEW POINTS TOO OFTEN UNKNOWN. Figure 31-2, a diagram from an early publication by Camus,[10] is very significant. The enormous difference in morbidity and mortality during the 1870-1871 war and World War I, i.e., before the smallpox vaccination law and after, is further shown in Table 31-5.

The usual vaccination processes protect an individual against a serious attack only if he has developed a vesicle or, better, a pustule. Table 31-6 clearly shows the relation of earlier vaccination to mortality and recovery in 17 aged women in a home for the aged. Their vaccination scars dated back 60 to 80 years.

In India, during an epidemic which in 1961-1962 killed 144 of 440 patients, De[14] observed only 14 per cent of confluent forms in the vaccinated subjects, but 56 per cent in the nonvaccinated patients. Among the vaccinated subjects showing one or two scars, 34 per cent caught the disease and 13 per cent died, whereas in those having three or four scars the morbidity was only 26 per cent and the mortality 8.5 per cent.

In a recent WHO (OMS) publication[12] it is estimated that the risk of an attenuated form of variola after an adequate first vaccination, as compared to that in nonvaccinated subjects, is 1/1000 during the first year, 1/200 for three years, 1/8 for 10 years, and 1/2 20 years after the vaccination.

Whenever the protective power of a vaccine is found insufficient, the date and results of the last vaccination must be referred to.

Vaccination should not be a mere ad-

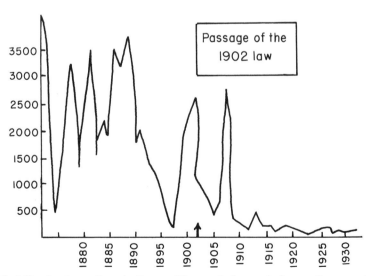

Figure 31-2. Mortality due to smallpox in France, 30 years before and after smallpox vaccination became compulsory. (From Camus: Ball. Acad. Nat. Med. (Paris), *110*:207-216, 1933.)

Table 31-5. *Effect of Vaccination on Smallpox in the French Army During Two Wars*

	DURATION	SOLDIERS	CASES OF VARIOLA	DEATHS
1870-1871 war	6 months	600,000	125,000	23,740
World War I	4 years	8,000,000	12	1

*From Camus.[10]

ministrative formality. Although WHO deemed it convenient to mention, in the international vaccination book, only the date of revaccination, it is imperative that the subject be informed of the results and their possible interpretation and consequences.

Too often the term "revaccination" is used to refer to subjects who have no primary vaccination scars.

Repeated negative reactions do not mean protection; Dixon[15] reported cases in which nurses caught smallpox soon after they showed negative reactions.

The effect of vaccination does not last forever; the immunity must be maintained by revaccination every ten years in countries where smallpox is not endemic, every three years in travelers to countries where there is a risk of variola, and every year during an epidemic or in subjects who may at any moment be in contact with a variola patient.

Physicians, the entire hospital staff, however employed, and other personnel such as ambulance men are in particular danger; during the recent epidemics in Western countries, 20 per cent of the cases occurred in the medical or the hospital administrative staff: five benign cases of 33 during the Paris epidemic in 1947,[8] 17 of 94 during the epidemic in Brittany in 1955,[35] and 24 of 79 cases during the Polish epidemic in 1963. This confirms the observations by Smith et al.[49a] who found that, of 7500 hospital staff members, 35 per cent had not been revaccinated for 15 years.

Public Health Measures. Any clinical or *even suspected* case must be isolated immediately and the local person responsible to the public health authorities must be notified by telephone. As long as the diagnosis is not certain, the patient may be kept at home or sent to the hospital by ambulance, which must be carefully disinfected afterward. In any case, all the patient's close contacts must be revaccinated.

PORT AND AIRPORT CONTROL. In Article 83 of the International Sanitary Regulations, revised August 1, 1963, it is stipulated that a valid certificate of smallpox vaccination may be required by any administration of the port of call. If, during the past 14 days, the person in question has been traveling in an infected country and has not been *successfully* vaccinated or revaccinated, the sanitary authorities may require vaccination control or, according to the circumstances, isolation for 14 days from the last possible smallpox contact.

MEASURES DURING EPIDEMICS

Any hesitation may be fatal; rapid but efficient steps should be taken. Several recent publications[13, 40] have clearly outlined the necessary measures. Here are some substantial extracts:

The Patient. If the diagnosis is certain, the patient must be isolated in a hospital or, in exceptional cases, at home.

The old saw, "burn all but the patient," is now somewhat moderated; only the patient's belongings and bedding must be sterilized, as well as the ambulance and the laundry where his linen was washed.

Frequently an epidemic originates not from the first case observed, but from a second or even a third case. The point is thus to recover this primary case in which the atypical

Table 31-6. *Relation of Vaccination in the Distant Past to Smallpox in a Group of 17 Aged Women*

	NUMBER OF SCARS FROM EARLIER VACCINATION				
	0	1	2	3	4
Death	6	1	2	1	1
Recovery				1	5

*From Stanley-Banks.[50]

form of the disease led to an incorrect diagnosis (scarlet fever, varicella, leukemia) but which may possibly have contaminated other patients than those under examination. In adults, a diagnosis of varicella should be accepted only after variola has been ruled out by laboratory tests. Since the incubation period is not dangerous, a possible contact is looked for during the 12 days preceding the febrile peak in the patient recognized.

Contacts. It is most important to detect contacts, both to protect them before smallpox can occur and to protect society by cutting as soon as possible the links in the epidemic chain.

GROUP 1: KNOWN AND PROBABLE CONTACTS. This group is made up of members of the family, colleagues, or any person in contact with the patient after the febrile peak, and those having entered the patient's room before the final disinfection: physician, ambulance men, staff who carried the patient's things, laundrymen, hotel maids, worker repairing something in the patient's room, postman, and priest or undertakers in fatal cases.

All of them must be vaccinated or revaccinated *immediately* by a two-incision scarification. The vaccination result is recorded on the third day.

All these persons must be observed for 16 days from the last contact. Their temperatures should be taken daily and, from the eighth day, the physician must examine the whole surface of their body.

If these conditions are met, moving about is not prohibited. However, some physicians have contacts isolated from the tenth through the sixteenth day.

Specific immunoglobulins are recommended, at a dose of 0.2 to 0.3 ml. per kilogram body weight, for those who were not vaccinated within 24 hours after contact.

During the 1955 epidemic in France, Le Bourdelles[35] reported that, of 64 patients treated in this way, 40 did not contract smallpox, 12 had a benign form, and 11 a non-eruptive one; only one death was recorded.

An inquiry was carried out in Madras, under the auspices of WHO, on two groups of contact individuals;[31] there was about the same number of immune subjects in each group. Only five cases of smallpox occurred in the group of 326 contacts having received specific immunoglobulin (1 gm. in adults and 0.5 gm. in children), whereas there were 21

cases of variola in the group of 379 controls. Thus, there was about a 70 per cent reduction of the risk.

Since immunoglobulins are expensive, this therapy should be reserved for the subjects most in danger or for those in whom vaccination is contraindicated (persons with leukemia or active eczema).

GROUP 2: INDIRECT OR POSSIBLE CONTACTS. This group includes travelers in the same plane or ship as a patient, guests at the patient's home who were not in direct contact with him or his clothing, and colleagues working in the same place as the patient but not side by side with him. *They must be revaccinated* and the result examined three days later; in case of fever within the 16 following days, it is advisable to call a doctor.

GROUP 3: REMOTE OR DOUBTFUL CONTACTS. Members of this group are the most difficult to detect, since contact occurred in public: train, bus, football match, cinema, theater. The sanitary authorities establish an order of preference in emergency and recommend revaccination according to the circumstances.

Mass vaccination campaigns are ordered only if nothing else can check the epidemic. Usually, fear of smallpox is enough to induce people to be vaccinated on their own.

Disinfection. The disinfection processes have not changed much. They are, in decreasing order of preference: fire, steam disinfection, and chemicals (cresyl, formalin). Formalin is more active against dusts than against crusts; moreover, it must be left in place long enough to act. Oxidizing agents such as sodium hypochlorite or potassium permanganate are more efficacious than the iodized compounds, which have little activity in the presence of protein.

Special care should be taken to disinfect the ambulance (inside, and outside door handles) and to assure that the ambulance men change their clothes after disinfection of the vehicle.

Corpses. All those who have handled the corpse must be duly vaccinated or revaccinated, and the result should be examined. The shroud is impregnated with disinfectant, as is the stuffing of the coffin. Plastic bags with cotton-stoppered tubes to permit fermentation gas to escape are recommended because it is easy to paint the outside of the bag with antiseptic solutions.

Table 31-7. *Results of Preventive Trials with Marboran**

India[4]	1126 revaccinated	78 cases of smallpox (12 deaths)
	1100 revaccinated + Marboran	3 cases of smallpox (mild)
South Africa[25]	570 revaccinated	0 cases of smallpox
	43 revaccinated + Marboran	4 cases of smallpox (1 death)
Brazil[51]	219 never vaccinated	38 cases of alastrim
	267 first vaccination after contact	42 cases of alastrim
	187 never vaccinated + Marboran	7 cases of alastrim
	215 first vaccination after contact + Marboran	8 cases of alastrim

*Subjects treated between the first and ninth days after contact.

However, it is difficult to know whether these measures to disinfect the corpse are efficacious. As a matter of fact, as emphasized by Dixon,[15] death usually occurs around the eleventh day, at a time when the contacts coming to the funeral are already contagious.

International Measures. The following measures must be taken by the national health authorities: (1) WHO and the neighboring countries are notified by telegram of the existence of a smallpox epidemic. (2) Special measures are taken concerning ships, cars, and planes coming from infected regions, according to the international sanitary laws.[30] (3) Stricter control of travelers' vaccinations is undertaken; report of the result and revaccination can be made obligatory.

Outlook for Chemoprophylaxis. We wish to be somewhat optimistic on this subject, in view of the paper published by Bauer et al.[3] on the preventive action of N-methylisatin-β-thiosemicarbazone (metisazone, Marboran, 33T57) on the infant mouse inoculated with variola.

Therapeutic trials on humans by Pickford Marsden[47] and Benn[7] in 1962 were not successful. Ker[32] administered 1 gm. of Marboran every six hours in a subject who had formerly been vaccinated but who was suffering from variola, febrile, and showing petechial forms. This treatment resulted in a fall in temperature within 24 hours but did not inhibit the formation of a few generalized papular lesions which, it is true, evolved rapidly. In the therapeutic trial by Rao et al.[47a] there were no differences in the mortality rates for 629 treated patients and 601 controls.

Three *preventive trials* carried out in Asia, Africa, and South America gave the results shown in Table 31-7. The discrepancies noted may have been due to a failure of absorption of the drug due to its conditioning or to an excess of absorption causing nausea and vomiting of the product in 16 to 26 per cent of the subjects treated.

Although the beginnings of this chemical preventive therapy are promising, it would be desirable to find a posology or a related compound that does not have the drawbacks mentioned.

At present there is no possibility of substituting chemotherapy for vaccination. As the old maxim says, "Prevention is better than cure;" fortunately, vaccination makes prevention possible.

BIBLIOGRAPHY

1. Arendzikowski, B., Kocrelska, W., and Przestalska, H.: Epidemic smallpox in Wroclain in 1963. Cited in Bull. Hyg. (Camb.), *39:*1246, 1964.
2. Avakian, A. A., Altshtein, A. D., Kirillova, P. M., and Bykovskii, A.: [Technique of direct fluorescence applied to diagnosis of variola.] Vop. Virus., *6:*196, 1961. Russian.
3. Bauer, D. J., Dumbell, K. R., Fox-Hulme, P., and Sadler, P. W.: The chemotherapy of variola major infection. Bull. WHO, *26:*727-732, 1962.
4. Bauer, D. J., St. Vincent, L., Kempe, C. H., and Downie, A. W.: Prophylactic treatment of smallpox contacts with N-methylisatin-β-thiosemicarbazone (compound 33T57, Marboran). Lancet, *2:* 494-496, 1963.
5. Bedson, H. S., and Duckworth, M. J.: Rabbit pox: an experimental study of the pathways of infection in rabbits. J. Path. Bact., *85:*1-20, 1963.

6. Bedson, H. S., Dumbell, K. R., and Thomas, W. R. G.: Variola in Tanganyika. Lancet, *2*:1085-1088, 1963.

7. Benn, E. C.: Smallpox in Bradford, 1962. Proc. Roy. Soc. Med., *56*:343, 1963.

8. Boyer, J., and Roussel, A.: Epidémiologie et prophylaxie de la variole. Monographie No. 25. Institut National d'Hygiène, 1962.

9. Bradley, W. H.: Smallpox in England and Wales. Proc. Roy. Soc. Med., *56*:335-338, 1963.

10. Camus, L.: Trente ans de fonctionnement de l' Institut Supérieur de Vaccine. Bull. Acad. Nat. Med. (Paris), *110*:207-216, 1933.

11. Carter, G. B.: Rapid detection, titration and differentiation of variola and vaccinia viruses by a fluorescent antibody coverslip cell monolayer system. Virology, *25*:659-661, 1965.

12. Chron. OMS: La Variole: Lutte et prophylaxie. Chron. OMS, *18*:443-448, 1964.

13. Comité OMS d'Experts de la Variole: Rapport technique No. 283. Genève, 1964, pp. 1-41.

14. De, S. K.: Investigation of an outbreak of smallpox in a police station area within Basirhat sub-division of West Bengal. J. Indian Med. Assoc., *42*: 374-380, 1964.

15. Dixon, C. W.: Smallpox. London, J. & A. Churchill Ltd., 1962.

16. Downie, A. W.: Infection and immunity in smallpox. Lancet, *1*:419-422, 1951.

17. Downie, A. W., Dumbell, K. R., Ayroza-Galvao, P. A., and Zatz, I.: Alastrim in Brazil. Acta Leidensia, *32*:75-79, 1963.

18. Downie, A. W., and MacCarthy, M.: Antibody response in smallpox. J. Hyg. (Camb.), *56*:479-487, 1958.

19. Downie, A. W., MacCarthy, K., MacDonald, A., MacCallum, F. O., and Macrae, A. D.: Virus and virus antigen in the blood of smallpox patients. Lancet, *2*:164, 1953.

20. Downie, A. W. Meiklejohn, G., St. Vincent, L., Rao, A. R., Sundara Babu, B. V., and Kempe, C. H.: Smallpox frequency and severity in relation to ABO blood groups. Bull. WHO, *33*:623-625, 1965.

21. Downie, A. W., Meiklejohn, G., St. Vincent, L., Rao, A. R., Sundara Babu, B. V., and Kempe, C. H.: Recovery of smallpox virus from patients and their environment in a smallpox hospital. Bull. WHO, *33*:615-622, 1965.

22. Downie, A. W., St. Vincent, L., Meiklejohn, G., Ratnakannan, N. R., Rao, A. R., Krishnan, G. N. V., and Kempe, C. H.: Virus content of mouth washings in the acute phase of smallpox. Bull. WHO, *25*:49-53, 1961.

23. Dumbell, K. R., Bedson, H. S., and Rossier, E.: The laboratory differentiation between variola major and variola minor. Bull. WHO, *25*:73-78, 1961.

24. Fenner, F.: The pathogenesis of the acute exanthems; interpretation based on experimental investigations with mouse-pox (infectious ectromelia of mice). Lancet, *2*:915-920, 1948; Clinical features and pathogenesis of mouse-pox (infectious ectromelia of mice). J. Path. Bact., *10*:529-552, 1948.

25. Ferguson, D. L.: Some observations on the role of methisazone (Marboran) in the prophylaxis of smallpox in a rural area. S. Afr. Med. J., *38*:868-869, 1964.

26. Gurvich, E. B., and Roihel, V. M.: Use of fluorescent antibody technique in the detection and differential diagnosis of smallpox. Acta Virol. (Praha), *9*:165-171, 1965.

27. Hahon, N., and Wilson, B. J.: Pathogenesis of variola in Macaca irus monkeys. Amer. J. Hyg., *71*:69 1960.

28. Helbert, D.: Smallpox and alastrim: use of chick embryo to distinguish between variola major and variola minor. Lancet, *1*:1012-1014, 1957.

29. Heydenreich, J. S. S.: An outbreak of smallpox in an urban area. S. Afr. Med. J., *39*:463-466, 1965.

30. International Sanitary Regulations, WHO Regulations No. 2, Technical Report No. 41. Geneva, 1951.

31. Kempe, C. H., Bowles, C., Meiklejohn, G., Berge, T. O., St. Vincent, L., Sundara Babu, B. V., Govindarajan, S., Ratnakannan, N. R., Downie, A. W., and Murthy, V. R.: The use of vaccinia hyperimmune gamma-globulin in the prophylaxis of smallpox. Bull. WHO, *25*:41-48, 1961.

32. Ker, F. L.: Smallpox treated with compound 33T57. Brit. Med. J., *2*:734, 1962.

33. Kirsh, D., and Kissling, R.: Use of immunofluorescence in the rapid presumptive diagnosis of variola. Bull. WHO, *29*:126-128, 1963.

34. Kratchko, A., Netter, R., and Thivolet, J.: Méthode rapide de recherche de virus vaccinal par mise en culture sur cellules et identification par immunofluorescence directe. Ann. Inst. Pasteur (Paris), *107*:184-191, 1964.

35. Le Bourdelles, B.: Données actuelles sur l'épidémiologie et la prophylaxie de la variole. Rev. Hyg. Med. Soc., *4*:13-40, 1956.

36. Lin, H. T.: Study of effect of simultaneous vaccination with BCG and smallpox vaccine in newborn infants. Bull. WHO, *33*:321-326, 1965.

37. MacCallum, F. O., MacPherson, C. A., and Johnstone, D. F.: Laboratory investigation of smallpox patients with special reference to infectivity in the early stage. Lancet, *2*:514-517, 1950.

38. MacCallum, F. O.: Airborne spread of smallpox. In: Symposium internationale sur la vaccination antivariolique. Paris, Mérieux, 1963.

39. MacCarthy, K., Downie, A. W., and Bradley, W. H.: Antibody response following vaccination. J. Hyg. (Camb.), *56*:466, 1958.

40. Memorandum on the Control of Outbreaks of Smallpox. London, H. M. Stationery Office, 1964, pp. 1-27.

41. Meyer, H. M., Hostetler, D. D., Bernheim, B. C., Rogers, N. G., Lambin, P., Chassary, A., Labusquiere, R., and Smadel, J. E.: Response of Volta children to jet inoculation of combined live measles, smallpox and yellow fever vaccine. Bull. WHO, *30*:783-794, 1964.

42. Meyer, H. M., Bernheim, B. C., and Rogers, N. G.: Titration of live measles and smallpox vaccines by jet inoculation of susceptible children. Proc. Soc. Exp. Biol. Med. *118*:53-57, 1965.

43. Millar, J. D., and Roberto, R. R.: Vacunación intradérmica contra la viruele pov inyección a presión. Bol. Ofic. Sanit. Panamer., *57*:537-547, 1964.

44. Mims, C.: An analysis of the toxicity for mice of influenza virus. Brit. J. Exp. Path., *41*:593, 1960.

45. Murray, H. G. S.: Diagnosis of smallpox by immunofluorescence. Lancet, *1*:847-848, 1963.

46. Netter, R.: Discussion de la communication de MM. Kirn, Braunwald et Scherrer. Ann. Inst. Pasteur (Paris), *108*:339-340, 1965.

47. Pickford Marsden, J.: Case of malignant smallpox treated with compound 33T57. Brit. Med. J., *2*:524, 1962.

47a. Rao, A. R., MacFadzean, J. A., and Kamalakshi, K.: An isothiazole thiosemicarbazone in the treatment of variola major in man. Lancet, *1*:1068-1072, 1966.

48. Roberts, J. A.: Histopathogenesis of mousepox. Brit. J. Exp. Path., *44*:465-471, 1963.

49. Briceno Rossi, A. L.: Las diferencias del virus de alastrim. Bol. Ofic. Sanit. Panamer., *54*:419-424, 1963.

49a. Smith, J. W., Seidl, L. G., and Johnson, J. E.: Small-

pox vaccination in hospital personnel. J.A.M.A., *197*:309-314, 1966.

50. Stanley-Banks, H.: Smallpox in England and Wales. Proc. Roy. Soc. Med., *56*:345, 1963.

51. do Vale, L. A. R., de Melo, P. R., and de Salles Gomes, L. F.: Methisazone in prevention of variola minor among contacts. Lancet, *2*:976, 1965.

52. Wheelock E. F.: Interferon in dermal crusts of human vaccinia virus vaccinations. Possible explanation of relative benignity of variolation smallpox. Proc. Soc. Exp. Biol. Med., *117*:650-653, 1964.

32

Vaccinia

By R. NETTER

Unlike the other diseases studied in this book, vaccinia is an artificial disease, generally benign and provoked by man for prophylactic vaccination against smallpox.

CLINICAL ASPECTS

The appearance and development of the vaccinial lesion varies according to whether the subject is being vaccinated for the first time or has been vaccinated previously.

PRIMARY VACCINATION

Three or four days following inoculation of the vaccine a maculopapule appears which from the fifth day becomes separated into two distinct regions, a central vesicular region and a surrounding inflammatory region that is somewhat red. The vesicle gradually becomes depressed and is transformed into an umbilicated pustule with a raised irregular edge, very typical on the ninth day. Frequently at this stage one can observe lymphangitic trails toward the neighboring lymph nodes, bouts of fever of up to 39° C., and hyperleukocytosis with mononucleosis. About the twelfth day, the peripheral inflammation regresses and the pustule becomes brown in color, dries up, and produces a scab which falls off at about the third week, leaving a permanent scar; this scar has its importance since it is the indelible stigma of the success of the vaccination.

Among infants vaccinated before the age of three to six months, the vaccinal reaction is sometimes minimal or negative as a result of the persistence of the antibodies of maternal origin, particularly if the mother has been revaccinated shortly before pregnancy.

REVACCINATION

Early reaction may be observed in individuals who have been vaccinated against smallpox recently or frequently: a pruriginous papule is observed the same day, reaches its acme within 24 hours, and disappears two days later. This reaction does not necessarily involve immunity; it may be provoked by an inactivated vaccine, out of date or completely lacking in activity. If vaccination is not repeated, the medical practitioner cannot guarantee that the subject is protected against smallpox. Dixon[24] cites the case of young nurses revaccinated six times without success who died of smallpox during the Glasgow epidemic in 1950.

The *accelerated reaction* is that usually observed when a certain amount of time has elapsed since the previous vaccination. The papule appears much earlier and the vesicle is not always transformed into a pustule; the inflammatory reaction reaches its maximum on about the sixth day; the general symptoms are more discrete than during the primary vaccination. Depending on the interval since the last vaccination, the subsequent development resembles that of the primary vaccination or that of the early reaction. There exists no definite rule with regard to this interval; some individuals react as if to a primary vaccination less than one year after a valid primary vaccination, whereas others produce accelerated reactions more than 15 years after a first vaccination.

Lack of any reaction whatsoever is often the consequence of a faulty vaccination technique or a faulty vaccine. Only rarely does it indicate solid immunity; one can only presume this explanation if one is sure of the technique and of the vaccine and if one has attempted two further vaccinations eight and 15 days later.

COMPLICATIONS

The vaccinia virus artificially introduced in man usually produces no more than a moderate reaction; but it can in some instances cause complications.

CUTANEOUS COMPLICATIONS

The cutaneous complications of smallpox vaccination vary in gravity; those really deserving to be called "generalized vaccinia" are most uncommon.

Benign Rashes. Benign rashes are morbilliform or scarlatiniform and appear two to 14 days after vaccination; their evolution is rapid and does not exceed two to four days.

It is usually not possible to demonstrate the presence of the vaccinia virus in the vesicular lesions.

During a period of epidemic the diagnosis of an allergic origin is retained only after the diagnosis of smallpox has been ruled out. These rashes react fairly well to antihistamines. In Glasgow in 1942, as in Edinburgh in 1944,[18] these rashes appeared in one-fourth of the 5000 persons vaccinated.

Vaccination of Traumatic Origin and Autoinoculation. In these cases, contamination is always of external origin and the lesions are few in number.

Vaccinial paronychia is fairly common. The case reported by Witham[97] is much less so: a boxer recently vaccinated soiled his glove in replacing the dressing covering his lesion; then, with a direct blow to the jaw, he inoculated his opponent—a fact that was discovered two days later.

Autoinoculations are usually located on the face, the virus being transported by the hands and inoculated by scratching with the nails; it is not infrequent to observe a secondary lesion only, the vaccination having been completely wiped off the site of the primary inoculation. Depending on the date of the autoinoculation, the evolution of the secondary lesion is identical to or shorter than that of the primary lesion.

The lesions may also be spread by contiguity following scratching, if woolen clothing covers the vaccinial lesion, or by soaking in soiled diapers of infants if the vaccination has been performed in the thigh or buttocks for esthetic purposes.

Eczema Vaccinatum. This eruption is either varicelliform, according to the first description made by Kaposi in 1895, or more frequently it is varioliform, according to that of Juliusberg. It is situated in the region of a recent or former patch of eczema; a distal eruption may appear simultaneously or subsequently. Attempts at isolation have revealed a variety of bacteria (staphylococcus, diphtheria bacillus), herpes virus, or vaccinia virus; hence English authors have drawn a distinction between eczema vaccinatum and eczema herpeticum in Kaposi's disease.

ROLE OF ECZEMA. It is somewhat reassuring to know that only 25 per cent of patients with eczema show vaccinial complications. All types of eczema can give rise to eczema vaccinatum, but Copeman's statistics[19] show a definite preponderance of atopic eczemas (80 per cent) that had started in infancy and were more or less connected to other allergic manifestations. It is not only the current eczemas that run the risk of eczema vaccinatum: two-thirds of the cases of eczema vaccinatum occur in persons who had previously had eczema.

In a case described by Jeune et al.,[44] the primary vaccination of a ten-month-old child who had been free of eczema since the age of six months provoked a new outbreak 21 days later, followed 15 days later by diffuse vaccinial lesions. In this child, with hypoproteinemia, the disease was fatal.

ROLE OF VACCINATION. In primary vaccinations, the risk of eczema vaccinatum is of the order of from one in 20,000 according to Copeman[19] to one in 250,000 according to Conybeare,[18] both of whom based their results on over a million vaccinations. Among revaccinated subjects the risk is minimal: none in 1,250,000 to one in 3,250,000.[18, 19]

The risk is by no means negligible among nonvaccinated subjects who have contact with a classmate, or hospital patient, or member of the family who has recently been vaccinated[19, 83]; two cases of eczema vaccinatum out of three enter into this category, and the affection in such cases is even more serious.[24]

MORTALITY RATE. The overall mortality rate for eczema vaccinatum is only 6 per cent; 75 per cent of these fatal cases occur in children under five years of age.[19] According to Conybeare[18] the mortality is 50 per cent in children less than one year of age.

TREATMENT. Antibiotics, if the patient has not become sensitized to them, will prevent secondary infection.

Specific gamma globulins (0.6 ml. per kilogram of body weight) are administered prophylactically to subjects who are not already contaminated, or up to the seventh day after vaccination if required to reduce the vaccinial reaction and block a possible viremia. Used therapeutically they are capable of curing a large number of patients.

Corticoids should not be given because of the risk of the eruption spreading.

Marboran (methisazone; CT 57), sometimes combined with other treatments, has been considered useful by various authors. Bauer[3] reviewed 22 cases treated with various doses: there were 12 favorable results (six of them in children less than two years of age); six other results were doubtful (one death); in four other cases the drug had no effect (three deaths). These results can be improved by administering a full dose of 200 mg. per kilogram, then 400 mg. per kilo-

gram divided into several doses per day over two days. The addition of gamma globulins is not necessary. A new favorable case has since been published.[1]

Chronic Progressive Gangrenous or Ulcerative Vaccinia. The original vaccinial lesion, instead of regressing after the tenth day, continues to proliferate on the surface for several months and spreads in depth, causing such damage that it is sometimes necessary to perform skin grafts[40, 49] or even amputations. Pustular lesions at a distance often suggest the diagnosis of generalized vaccinia, as in the case described by Sedallian et al.[78] in which viremia persisted for more than one month and the patient died of toxemia. Conditions of hypogammaglobulinemia or agammaglobulinemia, either of congenital origin[33, 95] or related to the development of leukemia or Hodgkin's disease[21, 22] or to their treatment by x-rays or cortisone,[72] have been suspected to be at the origin of this redoubtable complication. However, Gitlin and Good, according to Ultman,[90] observed primary vaccinations and revaccinations which evolved classically in hypogammaglobulinemic subjects.

In the report by O'Connell et al.[71] the gamma globulin level was normal and that of the neutralizing antibodies or those inhibiting hemagglutination was even quite adequate (IHA 1/1000, N.A. 1/32 to 1/447).

Ehrengut[26] also observed ulcerative vaccinial lesions in subjects sensitized by an injection of inactivated smallpox vaccine.

INCIDENCE AND MORTALITY OF ULCERATIVE VACCINIA. With primary vaccination the risk is one in 475,000; for children it is even higher, according to Conybeare.[18] Following revaccination Conybeare did not find a single case among more than one million persons vaccinated. The mortality is alarming: seven patients out of eight die whatever the treatment.

TREATMENT. The transfusion of blood from a hyperimmune donor[17, 95] or gamma globulins is not very certain: three of four of Conybeare's patients died, whereas four of five of Sussman and Grossman's[83] patients were cured.

The transfusion of fetal liver or spleen tissues,[17] the intramuscular injection of washed leukocytes,[71] and lymph node grafts[49] have given variable results.

Ehrengut[26] successfully desensitized ten subjects by means of repeated injections of small doses of inactivated vaccine in the neighborhood of the lesion.

Interferon was found to be ineffective in one case described by Connolly et al.[17]

Bauer[3] reviewed the cases of ten patients treated with Marboran (methisazone; CT 57).[17, 21, 22, 33, 40, 95] Five patients were cured, and these results could have been improved by administering first a loading dose of 200 mg. per kilogram and then 400 mg. divided into several doses over two days. Combination with gamma globulins is also useful.

Generalized Vaccinia. If one discards autoinoculations, eczema vaccinatum, progressive vaccinia, and benign rashes in which the vaccinia virus has not been isolated, there remain but few cases that can truly be called generalized vaccinia.

During the massive vaccination campaign in 1947 in New York, only seven cases were observed among 5 million persons vaccinated, i.e., one case for 710,000 persons vaccinated.

Generalized vaccinia presents a serious problem of diagnosis during an epidemic of smallpox.[11] The onset is sudden, accompanied by a fever and chills; then the eruption appears suddenly and literally pits the whole body. The disastrous role played by chronic leukemia has been demonstrated by Kempe:[49] of 62 cases of generalized vaccinia which he collected before 1960, three showed the presence of chronic myeloid leukemia as well; from 1960 to 1964 he observed seven additional patients all affected with chronic leukemia, but two of them did not show hypogammaglobulinemia (cited by Ultmann[90]).

Scabies may favor a generalization of the vaccinial lesions.[83]

TREATMENT OF GENERALIZED VACCINIA. Specific gammaglobulins administered in massive doses have a good effect;[49] an improvement is observed in one day and a cure obtained in eight days. Cocchi and Ulivelli[15] use locally applied 5-iodo-2'-deoxyuridine, although other authors question its efficacy.[6]

POSTVACCINIAL ENCEPHALITIS

This complication, which occurs as an after-effect of smallpox vaccination, has given rise to much discussion, even with regard to the name, since it may be applied to complications occurring after almost any vaccina-

tion; for this reason de Vries[93] suggested the name "postvaccinial" concerning the observations made after smallpox vaccination.

The incidence of this complication is extremely variable, depending on the country or even the province within the country; in certain countries such as Holland and Austria the rate is higher than in others.

The same variability is observed with regard to time. In France, where the usual incidence is one per 100,000 vaccinated, the morbidity attained a level of one per 298 in Alsace in a region where, according to Rohmer et al.,[76] in 1947 there was an outbreak of lymphocytic meningitis and encephalitis of undetermined origin.

It does not seem, either, that the incidence of this complication is proportional to the number of persons vaccinated, since, in 1955, when mass vaccinations were performed in relation to the epidemic in Vannes, France, cases reported were fewer than in the previous years.

Clinical Criteria. The clinical criteria adopted by medical practitioners to identify postvaccinial encephalitis are extremely variable; Spillane and Wells[81] classified their 39 observations of nervous complications into the following categories: I. encephalomyelitis; II. encephalopathy; III. meningism; IV. epilepsy; V. multiple sclerosis; VI. polyneuritis; VII. brachial neuritis; VIII. myasthenia. Only 14 cases out of the 39 reported belonged to the first two categories.

Histological Criteria. Before two years of age the toxic edematous encephalopathic form is the type most commonly observed; evolution is rapid, often terminating in sudden death. After two years of age the microglial form with demyelination of the perivenous leukoencephalitis type is the form most frequently observed.

In fact, neither of these two types of lesions is truly specific for postvaccinial en-

Table 32-1. *Declared Cases of Postvaccinial Encephalitis in France from 1950 to 1955*

YEAR	1950	1951	1952	1953	1954	1955
Number of cases declared	136	156	142	129	140	118*

*This was a year in which a mass vaccination campaign was carried out.

Table 32-2. *Comparison of the Incidence of Diseases of the Central Nervous System Following Primary Vaccination and Revaccination**

| | | REVACCINATION | |
	PRIMARY VACCINATION	WITHIN 15 YR.	AFTER 15 YR.
Number vaccinated	3,820,369	235,682	1,004,962
Diseases of the CNS	56	0	8
Rate per 100,000	1.46	0	0.79
Deaths	19	0	8
Rate per one million	4.97	0	2.98

*From Conybeare.[18]

cephalitis, and the glial form in particular may also be observed in other cases of posteruptive encephalitis.

Virological Criteria. Modern virology is as yet unable to provide definite proof one way or the other.[68] In view of this uncertainty one should be cautious in interpreting statistics, some of which are based on an insufficient number of vaccinated subjects and others of which only take into account the cases of encephalitis that have been reported.

From the British statistics compiled by Conybeare[18] (Table 32-2) it appears that the risk is less with revaccination, especially if the time elapsed since the primary vaccination is not too long.

Table 32-3 shows the incidence in Great Britain in terms of age. It appears that, contrary to general opinion, the first year of life is not the most favorable period for primary vaccination. This is probably due to the fact that vaccination is not compulsory in Great Britain, and hence few mothers transmit a basic immunity to their infants.

Treatment. Sussman and Grossman[83] were able to cure four cases of encephalitis out of five by means of gamma globulins.

The reader interested in further details on the problem of nervous complications following smallpox vaccination can refer to Chapter 9, as well as to works by Dixon,[24] de Vries,[93] and Lhermitte.[55]

OCULAR COMPLICATIONS

Two important sets of statistics exist, but they are insufficient to indicate the risk of ocular complications following vaccination. Sedan et al.[79] observed 19 cases after 800,000 vaccinations performed in Marseilles in 1952. Greenberg, quoted by Sudarsky,[82] observed none after the 5 million vaccinations performed in New York in 1947. The cases observed resulted either from autoinoculations by splashing the vaccine while breaking the ampule or by contamination through the use, for example, of soiled towels.

Clinical Aspect.[28, 79, 82] Vaccinia essentially affects the eyelid, the conjunctiva, or the cornea. Infection of the eyelid is the most frequent and generally precedes the other two.

Table 32-3. *Incidence, in Relation to Age, of Diseases of the Central Nervous System Following Primary Vaccination in Great Britain**

	UNDER 1 YEAR	1 YEAR	2-4 YEARS	5-14 YEARS	15 YEARS AND OVER
Number vaccinated	2,661,448	298,918	188,134	264,316	407,513
Diseases of the CNS (rate per 100,000)	39 (1.46)	1 (0.33)	2 (1.06)	8 (3.02)	6 (1.47)
Deaths (rate per one million)	16 (6.01)	1 (0.03)	1 (5.31)	0 (0)	1 (2.45)

*From Conybeare.[18]

The pustules are smaller and more ulcerous, and edema dominates the picture.

Vaccinial keratitis is the most dangerous because of the irreversible lesions it is liable to produce (perforation, albugo, glaucoma, hypopyon), but fortunately it represents only 10 to 30 per cent of the ocular forms.[79, 82, 83] Sudarsky[82] in 1957, found reports of only two cases in different publications. The laboratory is then responsible for establishing a differential diagnosis by isolating a staphylococcus, a herpes virus, a vaccinia virus, or even a smallpox virus during a period of epidemic. It should also be noted that previous lesions of the eye (e.g., blepharitis, eczema, chronic conjunctivitis) may exacerbate the infection.

Treatment. The administration of antibiotics prevents secondary ocular infection.

Specific gamma globulin,[39, 49] administered by intramuscular injection at a dose of 0.6 ml. per kilogram of weight (with a maximum dose of 10 ml. for children and 20 ml. for adults), reinforces immunity. In serious cases two drops of gamma globulin are instilled every hour during the day and every two hours during the night.

Interesting results have been obtained with 5-iodo-2'-deoxyuridine even at the stage of ulcer of the cornea, in rabbits that were treated every two hours for two days.[48]

A favorable evolution has been reported by Goldman[38] in a patient without keratitis who was given 10 ml. of gamma globulin intramuscularly, instillations of 0.1 per cent iododeoxyuridine every hour during the day and every two hours during the night, and applications of chloramphenicol ointment three times a day.

Steroids should be used only with great caution and even then only in the later stages, when one is sure that there are no longer any infectious viruses.

Interferon[45] can produce improvements in one to four days in patients already suffering from opacities or even ulcerations; it must be administered every half hour.

For further details on these problems the reader should refer to Chapter 54.

CARDIAC COMPLICATIONS OF VACCINATION

Cardiac involvement by a certain number of viruses is now sufficiently well known for one to suppose that the vaccinial virus is not an exception to the general rule. The only statistics that are of any real value are those of Dolgopol et al.,[25] who observed only one case in New York among 5 million vaccinated in 1947. If it is possible that the vaccination can be made responsible either directly or indirectly, formal proof has, however, not been provided in the case published by Dolgopol, nor in the cases described in Table 32-4.

The risk of "cardiac complications" is therefore fairly slim when one considers the enormous number of vaccinations performed throughout the world; moreover, comparison should be made with a nonvaccinated population. It could certainly be reduced if one avoided vaccinating elderly people who had previous heart conditions such as infarction.

Certain authors such as Finlay-Jones[32] are of the opinion that the delay in appearance of the lesions of six to 19 days could indicate an allergic manifestation, a hypothesis supported by the presence of eosinophilic cells in the infiltrates.

Study of the serological reactions can be of no help whatsoever, since all of the patients have been vaccinated; only isolation of the virus in the actual site of the damage or during a later viremia could provide arguments of any weight, but it should be added that to date these proofs are lacking.

COMPLICATIONS IN PREGNANCY

Smallpox vaccination presents no particular danger to pregnant women any more than it does to nonpregnant women.

In two sets of statistics out of the five available, the *incidence of abortion* was clearly increased when the vaccination was performed during the first three months of pregnancy; later on vaccination had no influence (see Table 32-5).

Rates of *prematurity or perinatal deaths* are not modified by smallpox vaccination (see Table 32-5).

It is interesting to note that none of the fetuses or stillborn showed clinical stigmata of vaccinial infection. Furthermore, Bienarz and Dobrowski examined 23 fetuses from vaccinated mothers and were unable to isolate vaccinia virus (cited by Lemoine and Lafontaine[54]).

Smallpox vaccination does not increase the risk of congenital malformation, no matter what the stage of pregnancy when it is performed (see Table 32-6).

Table 32-4. *Summary of 26 Observations of Cardiac Complications Occurring as the Result of Smallpox Vaccination*

Author	Patient's Age (Yr.)	Primary or Revaccination	History	Incubation (Days)	Symptoms	Outcome (Cure or Death)
Dolgopol et al.[25]	34	?	?	9	Myocarditis	D
Lagerlof	20		?		Myocarditis	C
(cited by	21		?		Myocarditis	C
Bengtsson and	22		?		Myocarditis	C
Lundstrom[5])						
Mathieu[64]	57	R	Diabetes, Infarction	6	Infarction	D
	53	R	Infarction	10	Algidity	D
	56	R	Infarction	7-10	Anteroseptal ischemia	C
	63	P	0	7	Anteroseptal ischemia	D
	58	?	Infarction	7-10	Shock, infarction	D
	58	R	0	7	Posterolateral ischemia	C
	64	P	0	13	Murmur, infarction	C
	83	?	0	7	Infarction	D
Dalgaard[20]	22	P(probable)	0	10	Pericarditis +myocarditis	D
Majdalani[61]	13 months	nonvaccinated	Eczema	?	Eczema vaccinatum +myocarditis	C
Bengtsson and Lundstrom[5]	19	P	Eczema	7	Eczema vaccinatum +arrhythmia	C
	16	nonvaccinated	Eczema	14	Eczema vaccinatum +tachycardia	C
Cangemi[14]	56	P	0	14	Pericarditis	C
Caldera et al.[13]	11 months	P	0	12	Heart failure	D
	8 months	P	0	19	Pericarditis	C
MacAdam and and Whitaker[58]	49	P	0	13	Pain + abnormal E.C.G.	C
	57	R	0	13	Brachial pain + pericardial rub	C
	37	P	0	3	Abnormal E.C.G.	C
Mant[62]	48	R	?	11	Myocarditis, sudden death	D
Finlay-Jones[32]	39	P	?	11	Myocarditis	D
Conybeare[18]	?	R	?	8	Coronary thrombosis	D
Van der Noorda[91]	19	P	0	15	Myocarditis	D

Table 32-5. *Prematurity, Abortion, Stillbirths, or Perinatal Mortality in Women Vaccinated During Pregnancy*

		No. of Women	Time of Vaccination	Premature No.	%	Abortion %	Perinatal Mortality %
Bellows et al.[4] (New York)	Vaccinated	153	Before 4½ months			3.2	
	Nonvaccinated	62				3.2	
Greenberg* (New York)	Vaccinated	4172	1st trimester	343	8.2		
	Nonvaccinated	2186		185	8.5		
MacArthur[59] (Glasgow)	Vaccinated	6720	1st trimester			24.0	
		69	2nd trimester			3.0	
		67	3rd trimester			2.0	
Bienarz and Dabrowski* (Poland)	Vaccinated	1270	1st trimester			24-30	
	Nonvaccinated	3515				12.0	
Abramowitz* (South Africa)	Vaccinated	510	Late				3.5
	Nonvaccinated	201					3.0
Liebschuetz[56] (London)	Vaccinated	157	Before 5 months			5.1	1.9
	Nonvaccinated	1657				4.5	1.2
Bourke and Whitty[8] (Ireland)	Vaccinated	114	1st trimester			0.9	2.6
	Nonvaccinated	453				0.9	1.3

*Quoted by Lemoine and Lafontaine.[54]

Transmission of vaccinia to the fetus remains exceptional, since until the present it has been possible to collect only 12 observations (see Table 32-7). It has been observed following both primary vaccination and revaccination or even in the absence of vaccination.[96] The evolution is slow, since the interval between vaccination and expulsion of a fetus or infant showing all the stigmata of vaccinia has been from four to 12 weeks.

Several of the fetuses were alive or macerated on expulsion; five premature infants died rapidly. All of the observations described insist on the generalization of the macular, vesicular, and pustular cutaneous lesions, which are grayish in color, circular, and often confluent. The postmortem and histopathological examinations performed by Entwistle et al.,[29] Naidoo and Hirsch,[66] and Lycke et al.[57] also showed an internal generalization appearing in the form of small necrosis-like nodules of the size of a grain of rice in the kidney, the liver, the lungs, and especially the placenta.

The virus has often been isolated in numerous organs,[29, 57, 66, 87, 96] including the placenta.[66, 96]

OSTEOARTICULAR COMPLICATIONS

The incidence of this complication is certainly extremely low. We found a few observations in recent publications.

Elliott's case[27] concerns a five-month-old baby who showed pseudo-paralysis with swelling of the elbow a fortnight after vaccina-

Table 32-6. *Congenital Malformations in Infants Whose Mothers Were Vaccinated During Pregnancy*

		NO. OF MOTHERS STUDIED	MALFORMATIONS No	%
Bellows et al.[4]	Vaccinated	571	16	2.8
	Nonvaccinated	173	4	2.3
Greenberg*	Vaccinated (1st trimester)	4172	68	1.63
	Nonvaccinated	2186	30	1.37
Abramowitz*	Vaccinated (after 3 months)	510	8	1.5
	Nonvaccinated	201	3	1.5
Liebschuetz[56]	Vaccinated (before 5 months)	157	3	1.9
	Nonvaccinated	1657	22	1.3
Bourke and Whitty	Vaccinated (1st trimester)	114	3	2.6
	Nonvaccinated	453	3	0.7

*Quoted by Lemoine and Lafontaine.[54]

Table 32-7. *Neonatal Vaccinia*

AUTHOR	VACCINIAL REACTION	STAGE OF GESTATION AT TIME OF VACCINATION	INTERVAL BETWEEN VACCINATION AND EXPULSION
Lynch†		5th month	4 weeks
MacDonald and MacArthur†	P	3rd month	11 weeks
Wielenga[96]	N	18th-19th week	8 weeks
Kropholler†	P	15th week	7 weeks
Entwistle et al.[29]	P	19th week	5 weeks
Tucker and Sibson[87]	P	13th week	9 weeks
Hood and MacKinnon[42]	P	7th week	3 months
Killpack†	R	12th week	1 month
Naidoo[66]	P	22nd-24th week	8 weeks
Lycke et al.[57]	P	23rd week	5 weeks
Tondury and Foukas[86]	R	52nd day	12 weeks
Tondury and Foukas[86]	P	3rd week	65 days

*P = primary vaccination, R = revaccination, N = nonvaccinated.
†Quoted by Lemoine and Lafontaine.[54]

tion in the same arm. The author observed, on x-ray examination, bone destruction with periosteal reaction and subsequent deformation of the bone during the following days. No attempt was made to isolate the virus, hence the diagnosis was based on supposition.

Sewall's case which in reality hid a bony sequestrum (cited by Elliott[27]) is similar: two weeks after vaccination a swelling appeared on the anterior portion of the radius. A biopsy taken from the radius made it possible to isolate the virus.

The observation by Cochran et al.[16] is just as demonstrative: 70 days after vaccination a child showed the presence of periosteal scapular, mandibular, and costal lesions which persisted for a period of one year. There was nothing that could distinguish the disorder from cortical hyperostosis, and only the viral proof provided the key to the diagnosis of this scapular lesion. Treatment with gamma globulins for a period of 103 days finally counteracted this tenacious infection.

In the last case observed by Silby et al.[80] arthritis of the knee appeared ten days after vaccination; vaccinia virus was isolated after puncture.

RENAL COMPLICATIONS

No statistics are available which indicate the extent of renal complications. Schafer[77] presented 21 cases published up until 1964 of acute glomerulonephritis which appeared in vaccinated subjects most of whom had previously been in good health. All except one of the vaccinations were primary. The patients' ages varied from one to 36 years. The clinical symptoms appeared four to 25 days after vaccination, mainly within seven to 12 days, which suggest an allergic cause. In only three caues of 20 were there antecedents of eczema, angina, or hay fever. It would be advisable to perform virological isolations in order to be sure that these somewhat rare complications are not simply coincidental. Lamache et al.[53] describe the reactivation of a scarlatinal nephritis that had occurred in infancy in a man 31 years of age, with albuminuria, azotemia of 0.42 per 1000, hematuria and edema of the face which persisted for a week.

CANCER AND LEUKEMIA

Vaccination is contraindicated in these diseases; it risks provoking massive vaccinial reactions, or a new outbreak of cancer or leukemia.[9]

Melanoma. Marmelzat et al.[63] reported six cases in which malignant melanomas appeared on scars five to 35 years after vaccination. Taking into account the millions of vaccinations performed throughout the world, and assuming that these cases were not simple coincidences, the proportion is very small. On the other hand, Burdick and Hawk[10] mention a personal case, and several others, of melanomas treated in situ by means of smallpox vaccine.

TUBERCULOSIS

Various authors[53, 85, 92] observed reactivations in formerly tubercular patients; these consisted of pleurisy, meningitis, polyarthritis, and tuberculids which appeared seven to 15 days following vaccination.

VARIOUS COMPLICATIONS

Asthma, urticaria,[43] psoriasis, and varicose ulcers are sometimes reactivated. The consequences are not serious if the subject has not been sensitized with calf serum.

New outbursts of multiple sclerosis and epilepsy may also follow vaccination.

THE VIRUS

The main characteristics of the vaccinia virus have been described in the section on the variola virus, which it resembles. Indeed, the vaccinia virus is essentially differentiated from the variola virus by the culture processes on the chorioallantois of the chick embryo and by the general aspect of the lesions in cell cultures (see page 421).

ANTIVIRAL MEDICAMENTS

5-Iodo-2'-deoxyuridine was originally synthesized and studied as an antineoplastic agent; it interferes with the utilization of thymidine necessary to the cell and also during multiplication of the virus. Because of the risk of genetic mutation, it is generally administered only locally as an antiviral agent.

N-Methylisatin-β-Thiosemicarbazone (methisazone, Marboran, CT 57). This compound was derived from the discovery by Domagk of the antitubercular action of the thiosemicarbazones and by Hamre in 1950 of their antivaccinial effect. The first clinical or prophylactic tests date back to 1960. In weak doses the product acts only on the thymidine used in viral synthesis but not on the nucleic acid of the host. It affects only the intracellular virus and does not have an antiseptic action.

SAMPLING, REACTIONS, AND INTERPRETATION OF THE RESULTS

SEARCH FOR THE VIRUS

Cutaneous Lesions: Vesicular Stage. After cleaning with physiological saline solution the vesicular fluid is drawn up by means of a hypodermic syringe or a capillary tube. If it is to be transported, the capillary tubes are placed in a sterile flask, or else the liquid, with rinsings (the minimum amount of isotonic buffer solution or physiological saline), is projected into a small tube or well-stoppered flask.

Pustular Stage. If the serous fluid is difficult to sample by suction, then a vaccinostyle or a small scalpel is used.

Scab Stage. Several scabs are detached by means of a Hagedorn needle, small scalpel, vaccinostyle, or forceps and placed in a small flask.

Autopsy. In the case of generalized vaccinia or progressive necrotic vaccination, nearly all of the organs are virulent.

Urine. After the urinary meatus has been cleaned, 50 ml. of urine is collected.

Serological Examinations. The blood is sampled without heparin or sodium citrate solution, as at high concentrations they hinder seroneutralization or inhibition of hemagglutination reactions. An electrophoresis can be requested in order to determine the level of gamma globulins.

Dispatching the Samples. The vaccinia virus is very resistant and does not require refrigeration for transport when it is in appreciable quantities, as in cutaneous samples; as for the other samples destined for isolation of the virus, in view of the fact that they usually contain only a small quantity of virus, it is advisable to transport them at low temperature. If the result is required urgently then it is always wise to contact the laboratory by telephone.

Naturally, a detailed case history should be included, mentioning the date of vaccination and the result, the possibility of contagion by variola or varicella, as well as any other information on the complications that have justified the sending of a sample for examination, and the treatment administered.

THE REACTIONS

In function of the emergency of the diagnosis and the size of the sample, it is generally possible to obtain a guiding diagnosis within 24 hours and a nearly certain one in three days.

The reader who is interested in these techniques and in the bibliography will find descriptions in two recent treatises in English[50] and French.[69]

The Electron Microscope. This type of examination is requested only in extremely urgent cases when smallpox is suspected. It is easily practicable only at the vesicular stage, and within an hour it is possible to classify the virus in the pox family (i.e. variola, vaccinia, cowpox) or in the herpes group (i.e., herpes, varicella-zoster).

Immunoprecipitation. The amount of scab sent as a sample should be sufficient. The result can be obtained within a few hours but, as in the case of the electron microscope, it is possible only to classify the virus in the pox or herpes family. The immunoprecipitation reaction performed by using the sera of the vaccinated subjects as antigen or antibody is always negative in the absence of complications.

Culture of the Virus. *On the chorioallantoic membrane of the embryonated egg* the result requires a minimum of three days, provided the laboratory has embryonated eggs 10 to 12 days old at its disposal, and laboratories responsible for confirming the diagnosis of smallpox are sure to have them.

In cell culture it requires three days on an average, but it is often possible to confirm the diagnosis earlier by means of hemadsorption by chick red blood cells or by techniques using immunofluorescence.

When the virus is only present in small amounts, as in the case of blood samples, urine, or the organs, several passages are sometimes necessary, which causes a delay of approximately three weeks.

Antibody Titration

THE COMPLEMENT-FIXATION REACTION. The production of an antigen for identification purposes from the scabs is feasible only if the sample is sufficient in amount and is not anticomplementary. On the other hand, testing the patient's serum for complement-fixing antibodies is technically easier, since the laboratory possesses a standardized antigen.

SERONEUTRALIZATION. This method is far more delicate to perform than the complement-fixation reaction, whether in the embryonated egg or in cell culture. The latter method may be less sensitive than the former[7]; it consists in determining the highest dilution of serum which neutralizes 50 per cent of the pathogenicity. There is no exact relationship between the level of neutralizing antibodies and the degree of protection: hence, after injection of a vaccine that has been inactivated by formalin or ultraviolet rays, neutralizing antibodies appear that are insufficient to prevent the development of a vaccinial pustule after reinoculation of a live vaccine.

INHIBITION OF HEMAGGLUTINATION. The antibodies inhibiting hemagglutination are more often sought because of the simplicity of the technique, provided sensitive chick red blood cells are available. The antibodies are a sign of viral multiplication within the organism, and the totally inactivated vaccines do not cause the formation of these antibodies. No doubt the formalin-treated vaccines that cause formation of these antibodies after injection are not totally inactivated. The specificity of the reaction has been debated during recent years; in patients suffering from coronary artery disease Neff (cited by Netter[69]) noted a higher proportion of positive inhibition tests than in normal subjects, no doubt because of the presence of a nonspecific lipid factor. In the cerebrospinal fluid of vaccinated or nonvaccinated subjects with a high protein concentration, it is also possible to observe positive non-specific tests of hemagglutination inhibition.

INTERPRETATION OF THE RESULTS

In the Absence of Complications

ISOLATION OF THE VIRUS. The virus is present in the vaccinial lesion at all stages, although in variable proportions. Measured as number of plaque-forming units per gram, the proportions are as follows: fifth day, 4 million; 7th day, 23 million; 9th day, 16 million; 12th day, 400,000.

Proof of viremia or of the excretion of the virus in the urine is very difficult to establish.

A positive viral isolation test at a distance from the point of inoculation is a substantial argument if one can be certain that the virus has not been merely transported mechanically from the vaccinial inoculation lesion.

SEROLOGICAL REACTIONS. *The Complement-Fixation Reaction.* After primary vaccination, approximately 50 per cent of the vaccinees may have titers in the order of 1/10 after the thirteenth day and for six months at the most.[60]

After revaccination, a rise in the level of these antibodies may occur, but no statistics are available that indicate the extent.

The Seroneutralization Reaction. After primary vaccination, the antibodies appear after the tenth day; they increase up to the end of the third week to a titer of approximately 1/300, are maintained at this level for some time, and then regress slightly and subsequently persist for a very long time.

After revaccination, the increase in the antibodies is apparent from the seventh day,[60] but the level which confers protection has not been defined.

The Hemagglutination-Inhibition Reaction.[7, 60] After primary vaccination, the antibodies appear after the tenth day; they may reach a level of 1/320 within several weeks, regress, and then persist at low levels of 1/4 to 1/32 for several years.

Revaccination causes a moderate increase in these antibodies, but a correlation between the antibody level inhibiting hemagglutination and any protective capacity has not yet been demonstrated.[70]

In the Presence of Complications

ECZEMA VACCINATUM. In eczema vaccinatum the virus has been isolated from the urine by Gresser (quoted by Netter[69]). There is a delay in appearance of the antibodies. In the five cases of Kempe[49] neutralizing antibodies were undetectable at the time of death.

PROGRESSIVE VACCINIA. Persistence of the virus is noted in the region of the lesions for several months together with the spread of the virus to the regions of the brain, kidneys, and adjacent lymph nodes.[33]

One patient only, in contrast to the 18 others discussed by Kempe,[49] showed no antibodies at the beginning of the treatment. Two patients with normal amounts of gamma globulins lacked vaccinial antibodies. In one case[71] progressive vaccinia continued to evolve despite an appreciable level of antibodies.

SEVERE GENERALIZED VACCINIA AND MULTIPLE CUTANEOUS VACCINIAL LESIONS. The virus is isolated fairly easily from the blood from the twelfth to seventeenth day. In one of Kempe's[49] untreated cases the viremia was still demonstrable after six months. The supernatant of the urine after centrifugation contains cultivable virus.[7] There is also a delay in the appearance of the antibodies, which enables the viremia to be prolonged.

BENIGN RASH. It is difficult to demonstrate the presence of the vaccinia virus in or near the lesions, which are, furthermore, evanescent.

POSTVACCINIAL ENCEPHALITIS. The serological reactions of vaccinia are usually the common ones: an attempt may be made to search for vaccinia virus in the blood; samples should also be taken of the secretions from the throat and stools in an attempt to demonstrate the presence of another virus. In case of death a postmortem examination should be performed and detailed investigations made of numerous organs.

NEONATAL VACCINIA. The vaccinia virus is easily isolated not only from the cutaneous lesions but also from numerous viscera. The serological tests that have been performed in normal newborn infants show that their level of antibodies is approximately the same as, or slightly higher than, that of the mother.[49] Newborn infants suffering from neonatal vaccinia generally die rapidly after birth and no information is available in the literature as to their serological reactions, the investigation of which might prove extremely interesting.

OSTEOARTICULAR VACCINIA. The virus may be isolated from the lesion itself.[16, 80]

EPIDEMIOLOGY

Unlike smallpox, which is extremely contagious, vaccinia has only meager ability to spread, in a population vaccinated or not. Hence, epidemics of vaccinia are unknown; at the most, accidental contaminations occur here and there by autoinoculation or heteroinoculations. Two-thirds of the cases of eczema vaccinatum occur in nonvaccinated children who have simply had contact with a vaccinated child.

To study the complications it is necessary not only to isolate the vaccinia virus but also to estimate the risk in terms of the number of vaccinated subjects; one should further specify whether one is dealing with a primary vaccination or revaccination, and the result observed.

When the virus is not isolated, the procedure is to compare the incidence of the suspected complications in two similar groups, one vaccinated and the other not. When isolated observations are published, some doubt remains and no definite conclusions can be established.

MECHANISM OF INFECTION

There is no doubt that the *cutaneous route of entry* is that of typical vaccinations, autoinoculations, or heteroinoculations of traumatic origin. It is less certain that this is the route in the case of eczema vaccinatum in nonvaccinated subjects or in the case reported by Sussman and Grossman[83] of a nonvaccinated father who was undergoing treatment for a burn of the forearm and who became contaminated while transporting the football equipment of his recently vaccinated son. Indeed, in the rabbit inoculated intravenously with vaccinia virus, it is easy to localize the infection in a cutaneous region by previously creating irritation by epilation or scarification.

Entry via *the respiratory tract* is probable in the case described by Wielenga et al.[96]: a nonvaccinated pregnant mother who herself had not shown any cutaneous reaction was infected by contact with her recently vaccinated son and subsequently contaminated her fetus; the fetus, with vaccinia contamination virologically proved, could have contracted the disease only via the blood. The virus multiplies locally, as demonstrated by Plotz in the experiments cited by Gastinel and Fasquelle[36]; fragments of rabbit skin were taken for several hours at variable distances from the point of inoculation. After the fourth day the virus was found only in the lesion itself.

The Ganglionic Stage. The regional lymph node enlargement which accompanies the pustule on about the eighth day is well known to clinicians. Svet-Moldavskaya,[84] in rats inoculated subcutaneously in the foot, demonstrated the presence of the virus in the popliteal nodes for 96 to 120 hours and in the inguinal and peritoneal nodes for only 48 hours. Siegert isolated the vaccinia virus from the lymph nodes of a certain number of patients suffering from postvaccinial encephalitis (cited by Blattner et al.[7]).

Viremia. When vaccination is not followed by any complications viremia is difficult to demonstrate. Blattner et al.[7] noted failure to isolate the virus in any of seven subjects after primary vaccination. No doubt the very unobstrusive and transitory nature of this viremia, which occurs at about the seventh day, accounts for these failures.

When there are complications, viremia is easier to detect. Blattner et al.[7] proved viremia in two children suffering from eczema vaccinatum, as did Siegert (cited by Blattner et al.[7]) in a certain number of subjects suffering from postvaccinial encephalitis.

The virus is carried by the leukocytes in man[7] and also in animals[2, 37, 84]: hence the necessity, when attempting culture, of eliminating the serum, which could contain antibodies. Whereas the virus disappears from the region of the inguinal or retroperitoneal lymph nodes within two months, it persists in the region of the axillary nodes and the spleen for a maximum of one week.

It has been suggested that the neutralizing antibodies act by limiting the duration of the viremia. However, they are far from essential for cure of the initial lesion: chick embryos incapable of producing antibodies can survive vaccinia or variola infection (Baron and Isaacs, cited by Friedman et al.[35]); guinea pigs irradiated with x-rays in an attempt to block the formation of antibodies (Friedman and Baron, cited by Friedman et al.[35]) recovered from the vaccinial lesion just as quickly as nontreated animals.

In hypogammaglobulinemic human subjects (Baron et al., cited by Kempe[49]) and in 33 agammaglobulinemic children (quoted by Kempe[49]) vaccination took place normally despite the paucity or even the absence of specific antibodies.

In spite of the considerable importance of the antibodies, as demonstrated by the results of numerous treatments with specific gamma globulins, no doubt there exist certain other defensive mechanisms.

Cutaneous Hypersensitivity. In a subject undergoing primary vaccination with fresh vaccine, the reinoculation of live vaccinia three to six days later provokes an accelerated reaction; whereas killed vaccinia causes the appearance of an early reaction. After the fifteenth day there is no difference between the results of reinoculations of live or killed vaccinia, which both provoke the early appearance of a papule. The cutaneous hypersensitivity thus causes a local blocking of infection.

Levaditi and Sanchis Bayarri (cited by Gastinel and Fasquelle[36]) showed that it was easy to dissociate the two phenomena: indeed, the repeated injection of killed vaccinia gives rise to production of an "allergy" attested by the accelerated evolution of the reinoculation lesion, but not of immunity, as a live vaccine nevertheless gives rise to a pustule. Flick and Pincus[34] demonstrated the generalization of vaccinia infection when the "allergic" phenomena are suppressed. They rendered rabbits immunotolerant by inoculating a strong dose of inactivated virus at birth. When they were reinoculated later on, this time with a live vaccinia virus, most of the animals died from generalized infection. The fact that the survivors of this test showed no "allergic" reaction or detectable antibodies suggests that survival resulted from another mechanism. Ehrengut[26] is also of the opinion that an anomaly in the "allergic" responses is responsible for several complications of vaccination; the hypoallergy of generalized vaccinia might be stimulated by inactivated vaccine, whereas the hyperergia of ulcerative necrotic vaccinia regresses under the influence of a desensitizing treatment consisting basically of small doses of inactivated vaccine.

Interferon. The existence of a neutralizing factor in the dermal vaccinial lesions at the time when the serum antibodies have yet to be formed was demonstrated as early as 1939 by Vieuchange and Galli and confirmed by Hartley in 1940 (cited by Gastinel and Fasquelle.[36]). Further proof was provided by Friedman et al.[35] in guinea pigs whose immunological defenses were blocked by methotrexate and x-rays.

Interferon was found in the vaccinial lesions in human subjects, where it no doubt limits viral multiplication[94]; it has also been demonstrated in white blood cells,[37] a possible explanation as to why vaccinia virus does not multiply.

Petralli et al.[74] suggest that the presence of interferon in the blood explains why only 20 per cent of smallpox vaccinations "take" in children vaccinated nine to 15 days previously with a live measles vaccine.

Since virologists know that vaccinia in cell culture passes from cell to cell without being affected by the antibodies of the surrounding medium, a substance that would act on the intracellular virus is of primary importance. It is probably thanks to interferon that chick embryos which are unable to produce antibodies manage to survive vaccinia infection. It is also by means of interferon that agammaglobulinemic human subjects are able to recover from vaccinial prophylaxis. Interferon of leukocytic origin probably was what enabled Kempe[49] to arrest the development of progressive vaccinia by several injections of leukocytes from vaccinated individuals around the edge of the lesion.

Other nonspecific factors, such as the temperature factor, also intervene in blocking infection; Kirn et al.[51] showed that rabbits in which pyrexia was prevented by antipyretic agents had more severe infections than the controls.

Hence the usual limitation of the vaccinial reaction is the result of the simultaneous action of several factors. A certain number of factors still remain unknown concerning the maintenance of immunity: would it consist, as Olitzky and Long first supposed in 1929 (quoted by Gastinel and Fasquelle[36]), of an immunity against infection that is maintained by the persistence of the virus in the human body? As far as the problem of the prolonged development of intrauterine vaccinia is concerned, could this be explained by an accidental phenomenon of immunotolerance, a defect in the production of interferon, or an unusual retention of the maternal antibodies by the placental filter?

PROPHYLAXIS AND TREATMENT

As concerns a vaccination, questions of prophylaxis and treatment seem shocking, the disease being not in fact an accidental illness but a benign illness that has been voluntarily transmitted in order to protect the individual against attack by redoubtable variola infection. Prophylaxis concerns complications, which are, after all, fairly rare.

Nonvaccination. This would certainly be the best form of prophylaxis, but as long as smallpox remains endemic in certain countries, this would be risky except perhaps in countries having a highly developed health organization. Regular vaccinations would then be performed only among the medical or hospital personnel who run the risk of being in contact with variola patients before the health authorities are informed of the introduction of smallpox into the territory, and the remainder of the population would be vaccinated only in case of emergency.

Early Vaccination and Regular Revaccination. Most of the incidents reported occurred at primary vaccination or very late revaccination performed over 15 years after the first vaccination. It is easy when smallpox has disappeared from a country to state that the number of postvaccinial complications exceeds that of the actual cases of smallpox; it would be vexatious, to say the least, to be constrained by events to regret this judgment the next day.

In countries where vaccination is compulsory the maternal immunity transmitted to the child results in the vaccinial reactions being less marked if the vaccination is performed before one year of age. Moreover, not long ago vaccinations were performed in the maternity wards, and it was precisely because of the weak reactions and the necessity of beginning again several times that this practice was abandoned. In countries where vaccination is not compulsory it is no doubt preferable to wait until the second year, when the child is better able to defend himself in general. Revaccinations are performed in many countries every five to ten years up to the time of military service.

Mechanical Protection. A dressing which is sufficiently wide for the adhesive portion not to provoke irritation and sufficiently aerated for it not to cause maceration, should avoid many autoinoculations or heteroinoculations.

The persons performing the vaccinations as well as the producers of the vaccine are advised to wear glasses so as to avoid ocular contaminations.

Contraindications. In a nonepidemic period it would be wise, even if the risk is slight, to postpone vaccination in a certain number of cases. Such conditions include:

1. malignant affections: cancer and leukoses;

2. acute or subacute infectious diseases (tuberculosis);

3. eczema, pyodermatitis, varicose ulcers, and burns: for this class of disease

vaccination in the neighborhood of the lesion can be dangerous;

4. hypogammaglobulinemia or agammaglobulinemia: this condition should be suspected if the child suffers from repeated infections;

5. pregnancy;

6. diabetes: the risk is twofold, i.e., exacerbation of the local reaction and ketosis;

7. diseases of the nervous system: epilepsy, encephalopathies and sequelae of encephalitis, hemiplegias, and multiple sclerosis; vaccination should be delayed (if possible) even in regions where epidemics or neurotropic virus diseases occur;

8. active heart diseases;

9. corticosteroid treatment, although there is no formal proof that it causes difficulties in man;

10. serious allergic conditions and acute nephritis.

Finally, the association of live vaccines should be avoided such as BCG, smallpox vaccine, yellow fever vaccine, and measles vaccine, except when the difficulties of transport or the importance of the epidemics justify them. This attitude is strictly preventive, as it has yet to be proved that the association increases the risk of complications.

Vaccination before two years of age and revaccination regularly every five years provides without risk an effective protection.

Prevention of Complications of Late Vaccinations against Smallpox in the Child or Adult. Although the origin of postvaccinial encephalitis is still somewhat mysterious, it seems logical to attempt to reduce this risk by decreasing the vaccinial reaction.

Vaccines prepared in eggs or cell culture offer the advantage of greater sterility in their preparation. Nevertheless, as emphasized by Fenje,[31] neurological complications have also followed administration of these vaccines, which tends to prove that the absence of contaminating substances does not settle the problem. The Rivers' strain cultured on the chorioallantoic membrane of chick embryo produces fewer local and general reactions after vaccination. It also forms a good protection against complications of revaccination with the classical type of vaccine.[23] A strain derived from the Rivers strain has even been used successfully and without incident by Kempe[50a] in eczematous children.

Less virulent vaccines may be obtained

by different means: by aging until about or past their date limit; by simple dilution,[30] by partial attenuation with formaldehyde, or even by limitation of the length of scarification or the number of scratches. It should be mentioned that the survey made by Polak et al.[75] on 1968 soldiers of the Dutch army concluded that the variations in the activity of the vaccines used bore no relationship to the incidence and gravity of the vaccinial reactions.

Totally inactivated vaccines are delicate to prepare if it is necessary to destroy their virulence without diminishing their antigenicity. Ramon's anavirus treated with formaldehyde has been studied by Herrlich.[41] Various forms of vaccines inactivated by irradiation with gamma or ultraviolet rays or by photosensitization have been studied since 1945 by Levinson and Milzer, by Habel and Sockride, and by a team of research workers of the Lister Institute.[46, 47, 88]

No formal proof has yet been provided as to the efficaciousness of any of these vaccines in preventing postvaccinial encephalitis. Koch[52] even reported a case of postvaccinial encephalitis that was not prevented by this prevaccination, and Ehrengut[26] described a progressive generalized vaccinia subsequent to the sensitization provoked by the first inactivated vaccine.

Furthermore, it is certain that none of these vaccines have sufficient activity to counteract smallpox. Thus any generalized use would give a false impression of security both against the complications and against smallpox in the event, as could well happen, that the population would not seek a second injection of the classic vaccine, reputed to be dangerous.

The injection of specific gamma globulins (0.1 ml. per kilogram of body weight) in an attempt to decrease the reactions or complications, as suggested by Nanning,[67] has only a limited effect and is available only for certain individuals because of the cost and the limited stocks available of this product.

Treatment. The specific treatment (gamma globulins and chemotherapy) has been given separately for each complication of vaccinia.

BIBLIOGRAPHY

1. Adels, B. R., and Oppe, T. E.: Treatment of eczema vaccinatum with N-methylisatin-β-thiosemicarbazone. Lancet, *1*:18-19, 1966.

2. Baratawidjaja, R. K., Morrissey, L. P., and Labzoffsky, N. A.: Demonstration of vaccinia, lymphocytic choriomeningitis and rabies viruses in the leukocytes of experimentally infected animals. Arch. Ges. Virusforsch., *27*:273, 1965.

3. Bauer, D. J.: Clinical experience with the antiviral drug Marboran. Ann. N. Y. Acad. Sci., *130*: 110-117, 1965.

4. Bellows, M. T., Hyman, M. E., and Merrit, K. K.: Effect of smallpox vaccination on the outcome of pregnancy. Public Health Rep., *64*:319, 1949.

5. Bengtsson, E., and Lundström, R.: Post-vaccinial myocarditis. Cardiologia (Basel), *30*:1-8, 1957.

6. Bjornberg, A., Hellgren, L., and Seeberg, G.: Treatment of cutaneous vaccinia with iodoxuridine. A double-blind investigation. Arch. Derm. (Chicago), *90*:581-582, 1964.

7. Blattner, R. J., Norman, J. O., Heys, F. M., and Aksu, I.: Antibody response to cutaneous inoculation with vaccinia virus: viremia and viruria in vaccinated children. J. Pediat., *64*:839-852, 1964.

8. Bourke, G. J., and Whitty, R. J.: Smallpox vaccination in pregnancy. Brit. Med. J., *1*:1544-1546, 1964.

9. Bousser, J., Christol, D., and Quichaud, J.: Accidents locaux et généraux de la vaccination jennerienne chez les leucosiques. Presse Med., *63*: 1797-1798, 1955.

10. Burdick, K. H., and Hawk, W. A.: Vitiligo in a case of vaccinia virus-treated melanoma. Cancer, *17*: 708-712, 1964.

11. Bureau, Y., Barriere, H., and Bruneau, Y.: Les accidents cutanés de la vaccination antivariolique. Sem. Hôp., Paris, *75*:4053-4058, 1955.

12. Calabresi, P., MacCallum, R. W., and Welch, A. D.: Suppression of infection resulting from DNA virus (vaccinia) by systemic administration of 5-iodo-2'-deoxyuridine. Nature, *197*:767-769, 1963.

13. Caldera, R., Sarrut, S., Mallet, R., and Rossier, A.: Existe-t-il des complications cardiaques de la vaccine? Sem. Hôp. Paris, *37*:1281-1284, 1961.

14. Cangemi, V. F.: Acute pericarditis after smallpox vaccination. New Eng. J. Med., *258*:1257, 1958.

15. Cocchi, P., and Ulivelli, A.: Vaccino generalizzato trattato con 5-iodo-2'-desossiuridina. Riv. Clin. Pediat., *73*:1-9, 1964.

16. Cochran, W., Connolly, J. H., and Thompson, I. D.: Bone involvement after vaccination against smallpox. Brit. Med. J., *2*:285, 1963.

17. Connolly, J. H., Dick, G. W., Field, C. M. B.: Fatal case of progressive vaccinia. Brit. Med. J., *1*: 1315, 1962.

18. Conybeare, E. T.: Illness attributed to smallpox vaccination during 1951-1960. II. Illness reported as affecting the central nervous system. III. Fatal illness reported as associated with vaccination. Monthly Bull. Minist. Health (London), *23*:126-133, 150-159, 182-186, 1964.

19. Copeman, P. W. M., and Wallace, H.: Eczema vaccinatum. Brit. Med. J., *2*:906-908, 1964.

20. Dalgaard, J. B.: Fatal myocarditis following smallpox vaccination. Amer. Heart J., *54*:156, 1957.

21. Daly, J., and Jackson, E.: Vaccinia gangrenosa treated with N-methylisatin-β-thiosemicarbazone. Brit. Med. J., *2*:1300, 1962.

22. Davidson, E., and Hayhoe, F. G. J.: Vaccination and leukaemia. Brit. Med. J., *1*:790, 1962.

23. Dekking, F., and Van der Noorda, J.: In: Symposium internationale sur la vaccination antivariolique. Paris, Mérieux, 1963, pp. 263-268.

24. Dixon, C. W.: Smallpox. London, J. & A. Churchill Ltd., 1960.

25. Dolgopol, V. B., Greenberg, M., and Aronoff, R.: Encephalitis following smallpox vaccination. Arch. Neurol. Psych., *73*:216, 1955.

26. Ehrengut, W.: Allergie vaccinale, vaccines generalisées et vaccines ulcéreuses. Presse Méd., *72*: 1957-1958, 1964.

27. Elliott, W. D.: Vaccinial osteomyelitis. Lancet, *2*: 1053-1055, 1959.

28. Ellis, P. P., and Winograd, L. A.: Ocular vaccinia. Arch. Ophthal. (Chicago), *68*:600-609, 1962.

29. Entwistle, D. M., Bray, P. T., and Laurence, K. M.: Prenatal infection with vaccinia virus. Brit. Med. J., *2*:238-239, 1962.

30. Espmark, J. A.: Smallpox vaccination studies with serial dilutions of vaccine. II. Statistical evaluation of quantal response data. Acta Path. Microbiol. Scand., *63*:116-126, 1965.

31. Fenje, P.: Advances in the immunoprophylaxis of smallpox. Canad. J. Public Health, *55*:346-352, 1964.

32. Finlay-Jones, L. R.: Fatal myocarditis after vaccination against smallpox. New Eng. J. Med., *270*: 41-42, 1964.

33. Flewett, T. H., and Ker, F. L.: Case of vaccinia necrosum (or progressive vaccinia), with severe hypogammaglobulinemia, treated with N-methyl isatin beta-thiosemicarbazone (33T57). J. Clin. Path., *16*:271-276, 1963.

34. Flick, J. A., and Pincus, W. B.: Inhibition of the lesions of primary vaccinia and of delayed hypersensitivity through immunological tolerance in rabbits. J. Exp. Med., *117*:633-646, 1963.

35. Friedman, R. M., Baron, S., Buckler, C. E., and Steinmuller, R. I.: Role of antibody, delayed hypersensitivity and interferon production in recovery of guinea pigs from primary infection with vaccinia virus. J. Exp. Med., *116*:347, 1962.

36. Gastinel, P., and Fasquelle, R.: Virus vaccinal. In: Levaditi, C., and Lepine, P.: Les ultravirus des maladies humaines. Paris, Maloine, 1948.

37. Glasgow, L. A.: Leukocytes and interferon in the host response to viral infections. I. Mouse leukocytes and leukocyte-produced interferon in vaccinia virus infection in vitro. J. Exp. Med., *121*: 1001-1018, 1965.

38. Goldman, A.: Ocular vaccinia. Med. J. Aust., *2*: 921-922, 1963.

39. Gould, E. L., Havener, W. H., and Andrew, J. M.: Vaccinia lid infection. Amer. J. Ophthal., *56*: 830-832, 1963.

40. Hansson, O., and Vahlquist, B.: Vaccinia gangrenosa and compound 33T57. Lancet, *2*:687, 1963.

41. Herrlich, A.: Uber vakzine antigen. Munchen. Med. Wschr., *101*:12, 1959.

42. Hood, C. K., and MacKinnon, G. E.: Prenatal vaccinia. Amer. J. Obstet. Gynec., *85*:238-240, 1963.

43. Jacquelin, A.: Dangers de la vaccination antivariolique. Sem. Hôp. Paris, *56*:2911-2916, 1963.

44. Jeune, M., Sohier, R., Carron, R., and Challut, F.: Vaccine tardivement généralisée et développée sur eczéma apparu postérieurement à la vaccination. Presse Med., *63*:962, 1955.

45. Jones, H. B. R., Galbraith, J. E. K., and Hussaini, M. K. A.: Vaccinial keratitis treated with interferon. Lancet, *1*:875-878, 1962.

46. Kaplan, C.: Antigenicity of gamma irradiated vaccinia virus. J. Hyg. (Camb.), *4*:391-398, 1960.

47. Kaplan, C., Benson, P. F., and Butler, N. R.: Immunogenicity of ultraviolet irradiated noninfectious vaccinia virus vaccine in infants and young children. Lancet, *1*:573-574, 1965.

48. Kaufman, H. E., Nesburn, A. B., and Maloney, E. D.: Cure of vaccinia infection by 5-iodo-2′-deoxyuridine. Virology, *18*:567-569, 1962.

49. Kempe, C. H.: Studies on smallpox and complications of smallpox vaccination. Pediatrics, *26*: 176-189, 1960.

50. Kempe, C. H.: In: Diagnostic Procedures for Viral and Rickettsial Diseases. H. Lennette and N. J. Schmidt. New York, American Public Health Association, 1964.

50a. Kempe, C. H.: Smallpox vaccination of eczema patients with attenuated live vaccinia virus. Yale J. Biol. Med., *41*:1-11, 1968.

51. Kirn, A., Dammron, A., Braunwald, J., and Wurtz, R.: Relation entre la fièvre et la survie des lapins infectés avec le virus vaccinal. C. R. Acad. Sci. (Paris), *261*:1923-1925, 1965.

52. Koch, F.: Encephalitis postvaccinalis und Varimpfung mit Vakzine Antigen Herrlich. Deutsch. Med. Wschr., *88*:1937-1940, 1963.

53. Lamache, A., Bourel, M., Richier, J. L., Dauleux, L., and Lenoir, P.: Les lendemains de la vaccination jennérienne. Sem. Hôp. Paris, *32*:1962-1970, 1956.

54. Lemoine, P. E., and Lafontaine, A.: Vaccination antivariolique et grossesse. Arch. Belg. Med. Soc., *5*:295-309, 1964.

55. Lhermitte, F.: Les Leucoencéphalites. Paris, Flammarion, 1950.

56. Liebeschuetz, H. J.: The effects of vaccination in pregnancy on the foetus. J. Obstet. Gynaec. Brit. Comm. *71*:132-134, 1964.

57. Lycke, E., Ahren, C., Stenborg, R., Bernler, G., and Spitz, S.: A case of intra-uterine vaccinia. Acta Path. Microbiol. Scand., *57*:287-294, 1963.

58. MacAdam, D. B., and Whitaker, W.: Cardiac complications after vaccination for smallpox. Brit. Med. J., *2*:1099-1100, 1962.

59. MacArthur, P.: Congenital vaccinia and vaccinia gravidarum. Lancet, *2*:1104-1106, 1952.

60. MacCarthy, K., Downie, A. W., and Bradley, W. H.: Antibody response following vaccination. J. Hyg. (Camb.), *56*:466, 1958.

61. Majdalani, E.: Complications vaccinales observées au cours du mois de janvier, 1957. Rev. Med. Moyen Orient, *14*:334, 1957.

62. Mant, A. K.: Mort subite due à une myocardite focale suivant une vaccination contre la variole. Ann. Méd. Lég. (Paris), *43*:49-52, 1963.

63. Marmelzat, W. L., Hirsch, P., and Martel, S.: Malignant melanomas in smallpox vaccination scars. Arch. Derm. (Chicago), *89*:823-826, 1964.

64. Mathieu, L., et al.: Vaccination antivariolique et thrombose coronarionne aigüe. Arch. Mal. Coeur, *48*:802-806, 1955; and cited in Lyon, E.: Probleme der cardiovasculären Komplikationen nach Pockenschutzimpfung. Med. Klin., *52*:1947-1949, 1957.

65. Mims, C.: An analysis of the toxicity for mice of influenza virus. II. Intravenous toxicity. Brit. J. Exp. Path., *41*:593, 1960.

66. Naidoo, P., and Hirsch, H.: Prenatal vaccinia. Lancet, *1*:196-197, 1963.

67. Nanning, W.: Prophylactic effect of antivaccinia gamma globulin against postvaccinial encephalitis. Bull. WHO, *27*:317-324, 1962.

68. Netter, R.: Les encéphalites post vaccinales, le point de vue du virologiste. Arch. Franç. Pédiat., *21*:606-612, 1964.

69. Netter, R.: In: Sohier, R.: Diagnostic des maladies à virus. Paris, Flammarion, 1964.

70. Nyerges, G., Losonczy, G., Erdos, L., and Petrass, G.: Significance of haemagglutination inhibiting antibodies in the evaluation of vaccinial reactions. Acta Microbiol. Acad. Sci. Hung., *11*:139-145, 1964.

71. O'Connell, C. J., Karzon, D. T., Barron, A. L., Plant, M. E., and Vilayat, M. A.: Progressive vaccinia with normal antibodies. A case possibly due to deficient cellular immunity. Ann. Intern. Med., *60*:282-290, 1964.

72. Olansky, S., Smith, J. G., Jr., Hansen-Pruss, O. C. E.: Fatal vaccinia associated with cortisone therapy. J.A.M.A., *162*:887, 1956.

73. Ortel, S.: Haemagglutination inhibiting antibody against vaccinia virus in the population and after revaccination. Z. Hyg. Infektionskr., *150*:300-307, 1965.

74. Petralli, J. K., Merigan, T. C., and Wilbur, J. R.: Action of endogenous interferon against vaccinia infection of children. Lancet, *2*:401, 1965.

75. Polak, M. F., Beunders, B. J. W., Van der Werff, A. R.: A comparative study of clinical reaction observed after application of several smallpox vaccines in primary vaccination of young adults. Bull. WHO, *29*:311-322, 1963.

76. Rohmer, P., Sacrez, R., and Rohmer, J. A.: A propos de cinq cas d'encéphalite vaccinale. Bull. Acad. Med. Paris, *131*:60-64, 1947.

77. Schäfer, K. H.: Nierenerkrankungen nach Erstimpfung gegen Pocken. Mschr. Kinderheilk., *111*: 361, 1963.

78. Sédallian, P., Badon, A., Fayolle, J., and Rouchon, J.: Vaccine généralisée mortelle avec virémie et agammaglobulinémie. Presse Méd., *65*:319-321, 1957.

79. Sedan, J., Ourgaud, A. G., and Guillot, P.: Les accidents oculaires d'origine vaccinale observés dans le département des Bouches-du-Rhône au cours de l'épidémie variolique de l'hiver 1952. Ann. Oculist. (Paris), *186*:34-61, 1953.

80. Silby, H. M., Farber, R., O'Connell, C. J., Ascher, J., and Martini, E.: Acute monarticular arthritis after vaccination. Ann. Intern. Med., *62*:347-350, 1965.

81. Spillane, J. D., and Wells, C. E. C.: The neurology of Jennerian vaccination. Brain, *87*:1-44, 1964.

82. Sudarsky, R. D.: Postvaccinial disciform keratitis. Amer. J. Ophthal., *44*:810, 1957.

83. Sussman, S., and Grossman, M.: Complications of smallpox vaccination. Effects of vaccinia immune globulin therapy. J. Pediat., *67*:1168-1173, 1965.

84. Svet-Moldavskaya, I. A.: Dynamics of antibody production and of the plasmocytic reaction on immunization with vaccinia virus. Nature (London), *206*:963, 1965.

85. Tapie, J., Monnier, J., Le Tallec, Y., and Delande, A.: Coexistence de pleurésie sérofibrineuse et de vaccine. Rev. Tuberc., *21*:1401, 1957.

86. Tondury, G., and Foukas, M.: Danger pour le foetus humain de la vaccination antivariolique au cours de la grossesse. Path. Microbiol. (Basel), *27*:602-623, 1964.
87. Tucker, S. E., and Sibson, D. E.: Foetal complication of vaccination in pregnancy. Brit. Med. J. *2*:237-238, 1962.
88. Turner, G. S., and Kaplan, C.: Observations on photodynamic inactivation of vaccinia virus and its effects on immunogenicity. J. Hyg. (Camb.), *63*:395-409, 1965.
89. Turner, W., Bauer, W., and Smith, N.: Eczema vaccinatum treated with N-methylisatin. Brit. Med. J., *1*:1317, 1962.
90. Ultmann, J. E.: Generalized vaccinia in a patient with chronic lymphocytic leukemia and hypogammaglobulinemia. Ann. Intern. Med., *64*:728-732, 1964.
91. Van der Noorda, J.: Primary Vaccination of Adults with an Attenuated Strain of Vaccinia Virus.

Doctoral thesis. University of Amsterdam. 1964.
92. Véran, P., et al.: Vaccination antivariolique suivie de choc et d'une pleurésie de substitution developpée dans un ancien pneumothorax. Bull. Soc. Med. Hôp. Paris, *71*:670-676, 1955.
93. de Vries, E.: Postvaccinial perivenous encephalitis. New York, American Elsevier Publishing Company, 1959.
94. Wheelock, E. F.: Interferon in dermal crusts of human vaccinia virus vaccinations. Possible explanation of relative benignity of variolation smallpox. Proc. Soc. Exp. Biol. Med., *117*:650-653, 1964.
95. White, C. M.: Vaccinia gangrenosa due to hypogammaglobulinemia. Lancet, *1*:969, 1963.
96. Wielenga, G., Van Tongeren, H. A. E., Fergusson, A. H., and Rijssel, T. G.: Prenatal infection with vaccinia virus. Lancet, *1*:258-260, 1961.
97. Witham, K. M.: A case of traumatic vaccinia. Lancet, *2*:202, 1962.

33

Cowpox and Paravaccinia

By J. CELERS

Among the human poxvirus infections, certain infections common to man and farm animals (cattle and sheep) deserve mention both for their historical role and for their peculiar epidemiological characteristics. We shall study cowpox first; milker's nodules or pseudocowpox and the contagious pustular dermatitis of sheep or orf* belong to another subgroup, i.e., paravaccinia.

COWPOX

Known well before the end of the eighteenth century, cowpox was described by Edward Jenner who recognized its immunizing properties against smallpox and showed that farm workers accidentally in-

fected during their work later resisted smallpox, whether the latter appeared in epidemic form or had been voluntarily injected during sessions of "variolation." From cowpox transmitted from arm to arm by Jenner, to the numerous strains of vaccinia now utilized in production of vaccine in different countries, it is not always easy to retrace what was the pathway (cf. Chapter 32), but both vaccinia and cowpox immunize against smallpox, and cowpox must be clearly distinguished from a disease with which it was long confounded: milker's nodules, which results in no immunity to either smallpox or cowpox.

Clinical Aspects. *An incubation period* of two or three days, without the least local or systemic sign, separates the moment of inoculation from the clinical onset.

When the lesions appear, they are located most often on the hands, in particular

---

*"Orf" is probably derived from the Old-English word "hreof" = rough, knotty.

between the thumb and the index finger, less often on the forearm, the face, and the buccal mucosa. At first one or several papules appear that progressively increase in size and vesiculate on the fourth or fifth day. Toward the seventh to eighth day, at the moment when the vesicles are extremely voluminous, they are often filled with a bloody liquid. The evolution is fairly similar to that of Jennerian vaccination, but with more intense systemic and local signs.

Considerable *edema* develops round the vesicles, and *lymphangitis* and *lymphadenia* appear. The *adenopathy,* in connection with hand lesions, is both epitrochlear and axillary, the latter often being more striking than for an initial Jennerian vaccination in the deltoid region. The lesion is *painful,* fever of 38.8° C. (101.6° F.) is frequent; the patient is prostrated.

Resorption is long; the scab falls off only toward the twenty-fifth day, and an indelible scar remains with, especially when the scar is on the face, a retraction exactly comparable to that left by Jennerian vaccination.

Cowpox is habitually considered to be a benign illness, but Dixon[1] in his treatise considers that generalizations of the infection are possible in suckling infants with eczema and cites a case reported by Jansen of fatal encephalitis.

Cowpox immunizes against vaccinia and vice versa; like vaccinia, it does not confer a definitive immunity. Two attacks of cowpox have been observed at several years' interval, and extremely severe forms have been noted five or six years after a successful Jennerian vaccination.

Diagnosis. The clinical diagnosis of cowpox in man is founded on the circumstances of its appearance, the site of the lesions, their evolution, and their aspect. The disease affects the personnel of farms and of dairies, but also appears in quarterers of animal carcasses, butchers, and veterinarians, whose profession leads to the examining, caring for, palpating, milking, killing, or cutting up of cattle. The intensity of the local and the systemic signs distinguishes cowpox from milker's nodule. The site of the lesions, the bluish hue of the areola, the frequently bloody character of the vesicular fluid are all elements permitting exclusion of a vaccinial etiology of the lesion.

The vesicular fluid contains a virus that can be identified in the laboratory as having all the characteristics of the cowpox virus or of that of vaccinia, from which it can be differentiated in vitro only by the aspect of the pustules obtained after inoculation of the chorioallantoic membrane. Antibodies neutralizing these two viruses appear from the eighth to the tenth day.

Epidemiology and Pathology. Cowpox virus is thus entirely comparable with vaccinia virus, which probably was derived from it. Both of them, under the electron microscope, appear similar to that of variola, and the serological reactions are identical (cf. Chapter 32).

It is generally accepted that cowpox is more virulent for man than vaccinia and that, inversely, vaccinia is more virulent for cattle than cowpox. But as concerns both types of virus, each has more or less virulent strains.

Dixon[1] supposes that just as vaccinia is probably a product obtained by man from the starting point of cowpox, cowpox is probably the product of the spontaneous adaptation to cattle of another virus, itself derived more or less directly from smallpox. Whatever the facts may be in this regard, cowpox and vaccinia have identical animal hosts, and epizootics of cowpox in cattle (including horses) from recently vaccinated human beings have been described.

Cowpox can involve a rather large number of domestic animals and, in particular, draft horses. Man is most often infected from the lesions on the udders and teats of cows. In the animal the disease is mild and does not much reduce milk productions, and farmers do not notify it. Thus, most often, the lesions of human cowpox lead the veterinarian to examine the herd. Cowpox is evidenced by several vesicles that evolve toward pustulation and then form a crust. The lesions remain localized on the udders and teats, and the manipulations necessary to milking occasion both the infection in man and the spread of the disease to the whole herd.

Epizootics have been described in England and Wales at a variable rhythm. From 1944 to 1950, Downie[2] examined material collected in ten epizootic outbreaks. Cases were also reported by F. Dekking in Holland, by Leroy[6] in France, in Poland, in Germany, and in North America, but the real incidence of the disease in animals and in man is unknown.

Treatment and Prophylaxis. Treatment of the usual forms is of the simplest: dry bandage to avert bacterial superinfection or transmission of the disease. Only in the presence of a secondary bacterial infection should the appropriate antibiotic therapy be applied. Generalized cowpox of an eczematous suckling baby can be treated with immunoglobulins specific for vaccinia.

It is important to diagnose early human cowpox so as to avert accidental transmission to other subjects, in particular to those with eczema. The diagnosis of human cowpox also permits measures to avert spread of the disease to the rest of the herd and vaccination or revaccination against smallpox of the farm workers. The rareness of epidemics in France is probably due to the high degree of protection conferred by obligatory vaccination against smallpox.

PARAVACCINIA

The viruses of the paravaccinia subgroup cause in man a disease that, according to the conditions in which it appears, is called either milker's nodule or pseudocowpox, either contagious pustular dermatitis of sheep or orf.

Clinical Aspect. After a four to eight day *incubation period,* the lesions appear and evolve with a slowness peculiar to them. Usually the lesion is single, occasionally there are two, three, or four elements.

Their *site* is most often on the fingers and the hand, but localizations on the arm, the face, the neck, and even the lower limbs have been reported.

Different aspects have been described.[3] Usually the disease first presents as violet-red papules or nodules that reach 5 to 15 mm. in diameter and are sometimes topped by a small white blister. Ulceration is the rule. The lesions can also take the form of granulomas in which ulceration occurs with proliferation of grayish epidermal tissue. Despite their vesicular appearance, it is often difficult to extract a liquid.

The most striking fact is that these lesions are *painless* even though resembling acute inflammatory lesions. Lymphangitis and lymphadenitis have been reported but, in comparison with the lymphadenopathies in human cowpox, they seem rare. There are usually no systemic disturbances. In only one case in 19 described by Leavell et al.[5] did chills and fever occur.

The lesions persist about five to eight weeks and are resorbed spontaneously. A single attack seems to confer a durable immunity against reinfection, but there is no cross-immunity either with cowpox or with vaccinia.

Diagnosis. The clinical diagnosis of paravaccinia in man is founded on the epidemiological context and the site and aspect of the lesions. Unlike cowpox and vaccinia, the disease rarely produces systemic manifestations; unlike the lesions in the first two diseases, those of paravaccinia rarely vesiculate; lymphangitis is rare, and no indelible scar remains. The name attributed to the infection depends on the animal which was the probable source of infection. The result is that orf or contagious papular dermatitis of sheep is diagnosed in shepherds, wool shearers, veterinarians, butchers, or even in cooks, while milker's nodule, although it can be found in veterinarians, is observed more specifically in the keepers of herds of cattle even when the cows are mechanically milked.

Epidemiology. Milker's nodule arises from a viral infection of the cow's teat producing small papulovesicular lesions evolving chronically, with rather frequent recurrences. These lesions differ from those of cowpox, with which they were long confounded, from which fact arises the name of pseudocowpox also given to this zoonosis. It should moreover be noted that repeated trauma provoked by milking modifies the aspect of the lesions, which become less easy to recognize. This lesion is probably very frequent in cattle; it has been described especially in Norway, the United States, New Zealand, and Great Britain.[8] Bovine papular stomatitis described in the United States is now thought to be due to a virus related to the other paravaccinia virus, if not identical with it, and produces in man lesions clinically identical with those of milker's nodule and, like them, appearing on the hands and forearms of agricultural workers.[3]

Orf, or contagious pustular dermatitis of sheep, produces buccal lesions in this animal, most often in ewes and especially in the lamb, in which they can be a transitory hindrance to feeding and growth. Recovery, without complications, occurs in about four weeks, but the epizootic can spread to the whole herd and evolve over a period of several months, causing death only when superinfection has occurred.[5]

The relationships between these three animal infections are obscure, but in man all of them produce the same lesions. Moreover, Lauder et al. (cited in the British Medical Journal editorial[3]) demonstrated that the bovine virus of milker's nodule inoculated into the gums and lips of lambs can produce lesions impossible to distinguish from those of orf.

Virology. The paravaccinial viruses share a common general aspect: oval or cylindrical shape, dimensions (160 to 280 mμ), and, under the electron microscope, the same characteristic picture in which the appearance of criss-cross surface banding represents the rolling back upon itself of a tube 80 to 90 Å in diameter, as in a skein of wool.[8-10] They are DNA viruses, as are all the poxviruses. The virus of milker's nodule and that of orf have the same cultural characteristics[8] and can be isolated from crusts or cutaneous biopsies in primary cultures of bovine testicular cells, in human amniotic cells, or in those of monkey kidney. Their multiplication is nonetheless very slow and is hindered by fungal or bacterial superinfection. Nagington[8] considers examination under the electron microscope to be the surest and the most rapid method of identifying them.

Treatment. The spontaneous evolution is toward healing, and only bacterial or mycotic superinfections necessitate the therapy then appropriate.

BIBLIOGRAPHY

1. Dixon, C. W.: Cowpox. *In*:Smallpox. Churchill Ltd., London, 1962, pp. 160-169.
2. Downie, A. W.: Jenner's cowpox inoculation. Brit. Med. J., 2:251-256, 1951.
3. Editorial, Brit. Med. J., 2:308-309, 1967.
4. Friedman-Kien, A. E., Rowe, W. P., and Banfield, W. G.: Milker's nodules: isolation of a poxvirus from a human case. Science, *140*:1335-1336, 1963.
5. Leavell, U. W., McNamara, M. J., Muelling, R., Talbert, W. M., Rucker, R. C., and Dalton, A. J.: Orf; report of 19 human cases with clinical and pathological observations. J.A.M.A., *204*:657-664. 1968.
6. Leroy, D., Bizais, J., Richier-Chevrel, M. E., and Richier, J. L.: Une épidémie humaine de cowpox en Bretagne. Bull. Acad. Nat. Méd. (Paris), *136*: 546-549, 1952.
7. Moscovici, C., Cohen, E. P., Sanders, J., and Delong, S. S.: Isolation of a viral agent from pseudocowpox disease. Science, *141*:915-916, 1963.
8. Nagington, J., Tee, G. H., and Smith, J. S.: Milker's nodule virus infections in Dorset and their similarity to orf. Nature (Lond.), *208*:505-507, 1965.
9. Nagington, J., Plowright, W., and Horne, R. W.: The morphology of bovine papular stomatitis virus. Virology, 2:361-364, 1967.
10. Peters, D., Müller, G., and Buttner, D.: The fine structure of paravaccinia viruses. Virology, *23*: 609-611, 1964.

34

Herpes

By N. NEIMANN, E. DE LAVERGNE, and D. OLIVE

INTRODUCTION AND HISTORICAL ACCOUNT

Derived from the Greek word ερπης, "scurf," or perhaps from the verb ερπω, "I crawl," the term herpes originally denoted all vesicular lesions of the skin. It was subsequently agreed that it should apply to an autonomous disease whose manifestations were far from being merely cutaneous. In 1913, Gruter was the first to succeed in inoculating the cornea of the rabbit with scrapings from a corneal herpetic lesion from a human being. Identification of the cutaneous and corneal herpes was then confirmed by Levaditi and Harvier, who demonstrated the ultrafiltrable nature of the causative agent. By means of the phenomenon of neuroprobasia these same authors were able to explain the affinity of herpes virus for the nervous tissues, first suggested by Doerr and Vöchting in 1920.

From 1930 onward more and more precise data were acquired on the different modes of herpetic infection. It was possible to distinguish between the clinical manifestations of primary herpetic infection and recurrent herpes. With regard to the anatomical-pathological aspect, Unna, Loewenstein, Lipschutz, and Levaditi described the specific nuclear inclusions of herpetic infection.

Recent technical progress has made it possible to identify the virus by its isolation in cell culture and by establishing proof of specific antibodies.

Herpes simplex hominis is classified among the viruses containing deoxyribonucleic acid (DNA). It possesses a capsid showing cubic symmetry and consisting of 162 capsomeres, and is surrounded by a lipoprotein outer wall.

It belongs to the group of herpes viruses of 100 to 200 mμ in size and which produce intranuclear inclusions of Cowdry's type A in culture, just as they do in the cells of infected subjects.

The first part of this chapter is devoted to the clinical study of primary and secondary manifestations of herpes.

The different means of laboratory diagnosis will then be considered. The epidemiology and pathogenesis are studied in a third section, and finally treatment and prophylaxis will be discussed.

CLINICAL MANIFESTATIONS

Infection of a receptive organism by herpes virus remains clinically inapparent in 90 per cent of the cases, being reflected simply by the appearance of specific antibodies. In 10 per cent of the cases it gives rise to variable clinical patterns depending on age, general state of health, and the portal of entry, i.e., *primary herpetic infection.* Secondarily, the

virus, which remains in the tissues in a latent condition, is able to recover its virulence and shows its presence by producing, usually, well-defined lesions i.e., *recurrent herpes.*

The characteristics of primary herpes — its occurrence in young subjects, the multiplicity of its clinical manifestations, its tendency to affect the viscera, and the very serious prognosis of some of its forms — contrast point by point with those of recurrent herpes, which usually occurs in older children or adults, is localized exclusively in the skin or mucous membranes, spares the viscera, and always has a favorable prognosis.

PRIMARY HERPETIC INFECTION

Herpes in the Newborn. The development of herpes in the newborn is extremely dangerous. It presents two distinct clinical patterns, herpetic septicemia and meningoencephalitis.

HERPETIC SEPTICEMIA IN THE NEWBORN. Since the first-published case, reported by Hass in 1935, 42 cases have been described in the world literature. Herpetic septicemia usually affects a child of low birth weight, a premature infant, or a twin, who is contaminated during or immediately after the confinement, either by its mother or by a person in its surroundings who is a carrier of a patent herpetic infection, or often of a latent one.

After four to ten days of inapparent incubation, the patient suddenly manifests anorexia, hyperpyrexia or hypothermia, and a rapid deterioration of the general condition.

At the acme the clinical manifestations are numerous.

Lesions of the skin and mucous membranes are not a constant finding, but they are extremely valuable for diagnosis. The skin may be the seat of characteristic groups of vesicles filled with transparent fluid and which occur in variable zones. Often the cutaneous lesions are not very striking, e.g., macules, papules, ulcerations, or scabby lesions. Lesions of the same type may occur in the region of the conjunctiva or mucous membranes of the mouth, larynx, and nose.

Hepatic lesions are a constant finding, with hepatomegaly, obstructive jaundice, gastric hemorrhages, and purpura occurring singly or together. Size of the spleen also is increased.

Cardiopulmonary disorders occur, consisting of dyspnea, cyanosis, and a blurred effect in the x-ray picture of the thorax.

Neurological disorders consist of somnolence and convulsions.

Digestive disorders are manifested by vomiting and diarrhea.

A *severe infectious syndrome* is seen, consisting of toxic facies, hyperpyrexia or hypothermia, and loss of weight.

Subsequent development produces death within five to ten days.

The biological examinations (blood count, blood culture, Bordet-Wassermann test) are of little assistance; they simply enable one to discard the diagnosis of bacterial septicemia or neonatal syphilis.

It is much more difficult to distinguish the other types of neonatal hepatitis from hepatitis due to virus A or B, congenital toxoplasmosis, and especially diseases due to cytomegalic inclusions, whose symptomatology is very similar.

Only histological examination and isolation of the virus in the samples taken before or after death permit a definite diagnosis of the disease.

MENINGOENCEPHALITIS. Although it is much more rare, meningoencephalitis occurs under the same conditions as generalized herpes. The neurological symptoms predominate. They occur after the cutaneomucous lesions or at the onset. Depending on the case, the meningeal syndrome or encephalitic symptoms predominate. Involvement of the other systems is less severe, and there is no hepatic insufficiency. Development is not always fatal, but sequelae, such as chorioretinitis and mental retardation, are common.

It should be mentioned that neonatal infection by herpes virus is not always this dramatic: it is possible to observe purely cutaneous lesions (Wilson, Mitchell, Lamy, Neimann, Bach) without any visceral disorder in newborn infants who nevertheless lack antibodies.

Herpes Simplex Hepatitis and Generalized Herpes Diseases in the Infant. Since the first observations by Zuelzer and Stulberg in 1952, 30 other cases have been recorded in infants nine to 25 months old, in a poor general state of health or who were affected by a debilitating illness. These mostly concern Africans affected with kwashiorkor (MacKenzie; Armengaud).

The illness begins with cutaneous symptoms, particularly stomatitis. At the acme of the disease, the symptoms of hepatic involvement predominate, i.e., jaundice, hepatomegaly, and a hemorrhagic syndrome.

The general state of health is greatly altered, and temperature is always above normal. The gastric, cardiopulmonary, and neurological disorders are not constant. Subsequent development is nearly always fatal in eight to 15 days, the clinical pattern being that of collapse, coma, and profuse hemorrhage.

In Tolentino's case, in which recovery occurred, the diagnosis resulted from the histological examination of a fragment of liver sampled by punch biopsy. Consequently, it may be that hepatic involvement during the common or curable forms of primary herpetic infection is more frequent than is supposed.

Cutaneous and Mucous Membrane Forms. At the level of the skin and mucous membranes herpes virus produces a vesicular eruption that evolves in three stages (Fournier): the preeruptive stage with erythema and marked subjective signs (burning, itching, prickling, or tingling sensations), the stage of vesicular eruption, then that of scab formation, which gives place to a transitory red or pigmented macula.

In the various localizations, the eruption lasts an average of a week or two and is accompanied by a moderate, tender adenopathy.

Cutaneous herpes occurs habitually on the face, most commonly about the nostrils or the lips, more rarely on the chin, ears and cheeks (Fig. 34-1).

The following forms suggest even more the possibility of a primary infection:

TRAUMATIC HERPES (Findlay; MacNair Scott). Cutaneous burns and wounds may serve as a portal of entry for the virus, particularly in subjects who lack antibodies. Vesicles appear around the wound, and the temperature rises moderately. Recovery is complete in eight to ten days.

HERPETIC PARONYCHIA (Stern; Chancellor[15]). The infection, which has been described among hospital nurses who did not possess serum antibodies, appears in the form of a pyogenic paronychia. The presence of vesicles should be a guide to diagnosis and thus avert a contraindicated incision.

KAPOSI-JULIUSBERG'S DISEASE OR "VARICELLIFORMIS ERUPTION" OR "PUSTULOSIS VARIOLIFORMIS ACUTA" (Fig. 34-2). The eruption in this case is pustular; it occurs

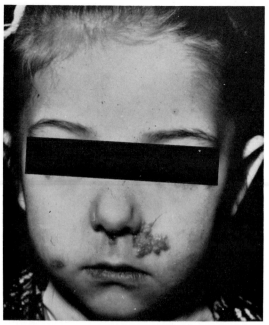

Figure 34-1. Grouped outbursts of herpes vesicles on the face.

mostly in young subjects with pre-existent lesions of the constitutional eczema type. In the areas involved earlier, but also in the previously healthy areas of skin, there appear vesicles rapidly becoming pustules that rest on an edematous and painful plaque. There is a deterioration in the general condition and a high temperature. Previously, development was always fatal, but the disease can now be cured except in the event of complications such as extension of the herpetic infection and especially staphylococcal superinfection of the cutaneous lesions. Proof of the herpetic etiology of the disease is provided by taking cutaneous samples. The vaccinial virus and herpes virus are both responsible in approximately 45 per cent of the cases (Barton, Seidenberg, Jackson, Ruchmann).

NASAL HERPES. Ruchmann and Dodd have described an acute febrile rhinitis with eruption of vesicles around the nostrils, ulcerous lesions of the nasal mucous membrane, and isolation of the virus from the nasal mucus.

BUCCAL HERPES. Buccal herpes assumes two clinical aspects: acute gingivostomatitis, which is the most common form of primary infection in children, and herpetic tonsillitis, which is much rarer and mainly observed in adults.

Herpetic Gingivostomatitis. First described by Dodd et al. in 1938, it occurs mainly in children one to three years of age, and less frequently in adults. The onset is progressive, marked by a rise in temperature, anorexia, dysphagia, and a buccal erythema.

At the acme, the tongue, the gums, the internal face of the cheeks, and the pharynx, which are swollen and painful, are studded with lesions that are above all erosive rather than frankly ulcerated. The pustular vesicle stage is transitory and most often passes unnoticed. Submental and submaxillary adenopathies are always present. The lesions may spread to the periphery of the lips or even beyond, affecting other mucous membranes (conjunctivitis). The temperature is always high, and dysphagia is intense and considerably impedes feeding. The pulmonary and gastric symptoms are not constant. Cure occurs in eight to 16 days. The herpes virus is isolated from throat samples in nearly all of the cases. In all of the cases of gingivostomatitis which we have had occasion to observe it has been possible to isolate the herpetic virus from the lesions of the mucous membrane and observe a significant increase in the serum antibodies. However, it should be mentioned that certain infections due to Coxsackie virus A16 may cause aphthous

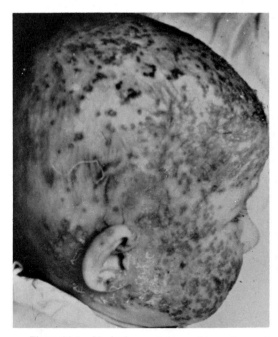

Figure 34-2. Vesicular, pustular, scabby and necrotic lesions in Kaposi's disease.

stomatitis, with exanthema and vesicles of the extremities. Cases of this general type have been reported by Richardson during an epidemic affecting 21 children.

Herpetic Tonsillitis. This occurs in the form of groups of vesicles on an erythematous base, situated in the region of the soft palate and tonsils to the exclusion of the tongue and the mucous membrane of the cheeks and gums. Fever is high. Recovery occurs within a week. Virological and bacteriological examinations make it possible to exclude the possibility of a bacterial origin and particularly Vincent's angina, as well as other types of viral pharyngitis such as herpangina due to Coxsackie A virus and to certain Coxsackie B viruses (Parrott).

GENITAL HERPES. The genital localizations in women usually give rise to extensive and particularly painful lesions; the Mauriac form (neuralgic herpes) has the additional components of rectal and vesical tenesmus and sphincteric spasms.

The very ephemeral vesicular stage is followed by confluent ulcerations often covered by a grayish yellow pseudomembrane and extending to the whole area surrounding the vulvar orifice and occasionally as far as the anus.

Inguinal adenopathy is always present and is tender; fever is usual, and there even occur in severe cases (Ravaut and Darré) cellular reactions in the cerebrospinal fluid.

The multiplicity of the ulcerations, their site, and their frequent superinfection explain the slowness with which cicatrization takes place.

In men, in contrast to women, genital herpes provokes discrete lesions, usually on the penis and the prepuce; the vesicles, few in number, are grouped together, open quickly and thus form erosions with polycyclic contours letting exude a clear serosity: herpes "weeps" (Leloir).

Other localizations, although rare, are possible, for example in the ureter, the fossa navicularis, where they are revealed by an abacterial ureteritis.

In both sexes, genital herpes recurs frequently and can, in even the most benign cases, represent a portal of entry for venereal infection.

OCULAR HERPES. We shall not stress the isolated and benign affections of the eyelids or conjunctiva. Herpetic keratoconjunctivitis is far more serious and more frequent.

It occurs in the child or young adult either alone or accompanying another herpetic lesion. Different aspects are described, especially superficial punctate keratitis (Braley), dendritic ulcer of the cornea, disciform keratitis, and marginal herpetic ulcers (cf. Chapter 54).

The evolution is variable; scars (leukoma) are frequent; complications (e.g., superinfection, iridocyclitis), which are enhanced by corticosteroids, may render the prognosis discouraging. The possibility of recurrences persists.

Herpetic Encephalitis and Meningoencephalitis. The affinity of the herpes virus for the central nervous system was proved experimentally by Doerr and Vöchting in 1920, but the role of herpes in human neurological affections was more difficult to establish, particularly after the confusion arising from Levaditi's hypothesis, according to which Von Economo's encephalitis could be attributed to herpes.

At present, numerous observations have been made in which affection of the central nervous system by herpes has been proved by isolation of the virus from the cerebrospinal fluid or from the brain, by the presence of specific histological lesions, and by serological data (Smith, Armstrong, Afzelius-Alm, Ross, Bernheim, Thieffry) (cf. Chapter 6).

The actual frequency of herpetic neurological infections is difficult to establish. Afzelius-Alm attributes 7 per cent of the cases of severe lymphocytic meningitis to herpes. Adair reduces this incidence to 5.3 per cent; Sohier and Bussiere isolated the herpes virus in only one case out of 377 cases of meningitis or encephalitis.

These disorders always consisted of primary infections affecting children or young adults.

Involvement of the central nervous system may be primary; the entry is then nasopharyngeal. In some instances it is secondary to an initial extracerebral localization; e.g., stomatitis or genital or cutaneous herpes occurs eight to ten days prior to the neurological disorders. The mode of propagation of the virus to the central nervous system is debatable: its advance along a peripheral nerve by neuroprobasia (Levaditi, Goodpasture) may explain certain cases.

The hypothesis of a viremia is probable, but it has rarely been verified. The lymphatic vessels of the pharynx may also serve as a pathway for spread of the virus. It should be noted that not all strains show a tropism for the nervous system and that the virulence of each strain certainly plays a determining factor in the development of cerebral lesions.

As a rule, the onset is progressive, marked by an infectious syndrome and variable neurological symptoms, including headaches, jacksonian attacks, and language defects.

The usual clinical pattern is that of an acute meningoencephalitis: disorders of consciousness and tonicity, convulsions, paralysis, diffuse cerebral disorders shown by the electroencephalogram, stiff neck, with hypercytosis and increased albumin content of the cerebrospinal fluid.

Sometimes there is an isolated lymphocytic meningitis and, more rarely, an encephalitis without any meningeal reaction.

These neurological symptoms are associated with an infectious syndrome or, in some cases, with a cutaneous or mucous herpes, which provides a useful guide for diagnosis.

The disease is often fatal, with a clinical pattern of coma and vegetative disorders, but some forms are regressive. Sequelae occur mainly in adults and are psychic, psychomotor, purely motor, or epileptic.

Diagnosis is based on the isolation of the virus from the mucocutaneous lesions and from the cerebrospinal fluid, where its presence is temporary and in which it survives with great difficulty. Very often the diagnosis can be established only after death by means of histological and virological examinations of the brain. Some authors were able to isolate the virus from a fragment of the brain sampled by biopsy.

Serological proof of recent herpetic infection should always be considered in terms of virological and histological criteria.

Recurrent Herpes

Although specific antibodies appear during primary infection, herpes virus may remain in a latent condition in the tissues and reassert itself when some stress or hormonal modification occurs; it then gives rise to various manifestations that are usually benign, but troublesome because of their repetition and the functional disorders they produce. The recurrences often involve the same cutaneous region or mucous membrane.

In addition to the genital and peribuccal localizations that are by far the most frequent, there also occur, occasionally, recurrent forms of herpes on the cheeks, the buttocks, the fingers and the hands.

Atypical incomplete forms reduced to localized itching sensations (Gougerot) may alternate with a vesicular eruption.

Many women are affected with *recurrent genital herpes*, often connected with the menstrual cycle.

Recurrent ocular herpes is not infrequent. Its manifestations are sometimes in the form of benign lesions: blepharitis, palpebral herpes; or serious lesions: e.g., dendritic keratitis, which may leave sequelae. Ocular herpes is the disease for which keratoplasty is most justified.

LABORATORY DIAGNOSIS

It is easy to relate herpes virus to the presence of cutaneous vesicles of common aspect and development, but this is not so for the other manifestations, where the etiological diagnosis is based above all on the biological criteria.

Histological examination serves as a guide for diagnosis by identifying typical lesions in the skin, mucous membranes, and organs sampled on postmortem examination. *Virology* is able to establish the etiology by isolation and identification of the virus. *Serological data* are indispensable to confirm the primary or recurrent nature of the herpetic infection.

Histology

The fragments sampled by biopsy in the region of the mucocutaneous lesions, by punch biopsy of the liver and brain, or during postmortem examination, are fixed and stained by the current techniques.

Mucocutaneous Lesions. Unna's vesicle is not specific, since it is also observed in chickenpox and herpes zoster.

Hollowed out in the rete mucosum, its inner wall consists of epithelial cells that have undergone so-called ballooning degeneration; the stroma is infiltrated with inflammatory cells.

The structure of the vesicle is identical at the level of the mucous membranes. The cellular lesions are the same in all the infected cells, both in vivo and in vitro, by inoculation of an egg embryo or in cell culture. On the edge of the lesions of the tissues, the chromatin of certain nuclei is compressed in masses toward the periphery (margination of the chromatin), whereas a single or multiple homogenous acidophilic inclusion (Feulgen) occupies the center of the nucleus; it is separated from the chromatin by a transparent halo. This aspect is that of the type A inclusions described by Cowdry. The cytoplasm remains intact up to the death of the cell.

Visceral and Nervous Lesions

MACROSCOPIC EXAMINATION. The presence of small necrotic nodules on the surface and in the parenchyma of certain organs is fairly characteristic. In the case of generalized herpes these lesions are always found in the liver and adrenals and are frequent in the lungs and kidneys. In the case of meningo-encephalitis the brain and meninges appear congested; foci of softening may be seen on histological section.

HISTOLOGICAL EXAMINATION. There are two types of lesions: nodular zones of acidophilic necrosis of the "coagulation necrosis" type, and acidophilic intranuclear inclusions in certain cells situated on the edge of these zones.

In the liver the patches of necrosis are of variable size; they may invade several lobules and render the parenchyma hardly recognizable. The same occurs in the adrenals, where only the cortex is affected, as well as in the spleen, kidneys, lungs, alimentary mucosa (particularly the esophagus), lymph nodes, and bone marrow.

In the brain the lesions are characteristic. They are predominant in the rhinencephalic, temporal, and insular cortices. They show acidophilic nuclear inclusions in the nerve and glial cells with foci of necrosis, hemorrhage, and inflammatory phenomena. In

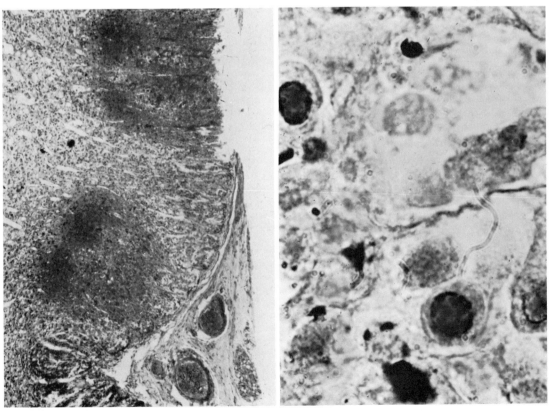

Fig. 34-3.   **Fig. 34-4.**

Figure 34-3.   Foci of acidophilic necrosis in the adrenal cortex. (× 100.)

Figure 34-4.   Dissociation of the hepatic parenchyma. Margination of the chromatin. Eosinophil nuclear inclusion body. Numerous granules of hemosiderin. (× 500.)

short, in all of the affected tissues one finds foci of hemorrhagic necrosis where it is possible to identify cells with inclusions of type A Cowdry.

However, these lesions are not specific; other viruses of the herpes group, such as the varicella-zoster virus, induce similar alterations. Lesions due to cytomegalic inclusion body disease may be distinguished by the giant type (20 to 35 μ) of infected epithelial cells, the "owl's eye" appearance of the nuclear inclusions, and the presence of small cytoplasmic inclusions.

ISOLATION AND IDENTIFICATION OF THE HERPETIC VIRUS

Sampling. The samples are taken early, between the first and fourth day of the illness, and should be inoculated either immediately or after passage through a transport medium (Hank's solution to which antibiotics have been added or Lepine's buffer glycerine solution). One thus avoids the risk of superinfection or alteration of the virus.

The virus is fragile. It is sensitive to heat and is destroyed by 24 hours at 37° C. and by three days at 22° to 37° C. It resists cold better, which permits its prolonged preservation: eight to 15 days at +4° C. and several months at −20° C. Its instability at an acid pH should also be mentioned.

Herpes virus can easily be isolated from the fluid of cutaneous or mucous vesicles, from scrapings of ulcerations, and from throat samples or saliva (but one should be wary of healthy carriers). Isolation from the cerebrospinal fluid is difficult, since the virus is present only briefly. The stools are not, except in the opinion of Buddingh, a good place to seek the virus. The virus may also be present in the blood or serum (Ruchmann, Pugh, Bird), but the viremia is short lived and does not exceed 24 to 48 hours. The virus can be found in fragments of organs sampled less than six hours after death; these may be inoculated after crushing.

Methods of Isolation. Herpes virus was originally isolated by inoculation into animals, and then by inoculation onto the chorioallantois of chick embryos. At present the best method is cell culture.

ISOLATION IN CELL CULTURE. *Sensitive Cultures.* All cell strains can be used. Those most often used are shown in Table 34-1.

Table 34-1. *Cell Systems Most Often Used for Culture of Herpes Virus*

Primary cultures
    Animal origin
        Monkey kidney
        Rabbit kidney
        Cat kidney
        Chick embryo tissues
        Sheep embryo tissues

    Human origin
        Thyroid
        Amnion
        Kidney

Cell strains

    Of cancerous origin
        Hela
        KB
        Hep$_2$

    L (mouse fibroblasts)
    FL (amniotic origin)

Diploid human cells

Cystopathogenic Effect. Examination of the fresh sample. The cellular lesions are identical whatever the type of culture used. Twelve to 16 hours after inoculation, foci of rounded refractive cells appear, well separated from each other. Toward the forty-eighth hour the lesions are more extended, and the cells show a characteristic appearance, like bunches of grapes. The culture degenerates in three to five days. Certain strains give rise to the formation of multinucleated giant cells as a result of the disappearance of the cell membranes. Gray, MacNair Scott, and Hoggan and Roizman classified the herpes strains into two types according to the cytopathic effect observed. Certain authors are of the opinion that these syncytia are related to well-defined antigenic structures. Others believe that they are induced by various external factors (e.g., type of culture, dose of inoculum, temperature).

Examination after fixation and staining. The use of tubes containing cover slips makes it possible to identify the lesions after fixing and staining with hemalum or hematoxylin-eosin. They are essentially nuclear: the nucleolus disappears, and the chromatin is compressed into dense masses against the nuclear membrane. The eosinophilic inclusion body appears in the center, separated from the border by a transparent halo, and Feulgen negative.

This inclusion body does not contain the virus, as has been demonstrated by Lebrun, using immunofluorescence, and by Morgan, using the electron microscope. It represents the trace of the passage of the virus, which has already left the cell when the inclusion appears.

The effect of herpes on mitoses has been studied by Stoker and Newton and by Wildy. Mitoses are gradually reduced in number until after 24 hours they are nonexistent. Recent studies have been devoted to the action of herpes on the chromosomes (Stich and Hsu, Hampar and Ellison, Mazzone and Yerganian and Tanzer, Bernard). In vitro, 24 hours after inoculation, herpes causes a considerable amount of breaking up of the chromosomes. This is responsible for the death of the cell. It is possible that these lesions are the cause of certain abortions or malformations but proof has not been furnished.

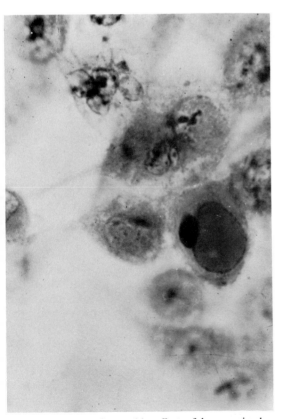

Figure 34-5. Cytopathic effect of herpes simplex virus cultured on human thyroid cells. Margination of the chromatin and eosinophil nuclear inclusion body. ($\times$ 500.)

Study with the electron microscope (Wildy, Russell, Horn). The electron microscope has made it possible to identify the cellular lesions and to study the structure of the virus particles and their multiplication cycle. The virus particles are seen initially in the nucleus and then in the cytoplasm, showing their three parts: the central nucleus or nucleoid, consisting of DNA, which is the carrier of genetic information, and the icosahedral capsid together with the lipoprotein outer wall.

ISOLATION IN THE CHICK EMBRYO. This method, which was devised in 1931 by Goodpasture, Woodruff, and Buddingh, was frequently used at one time but has now been superseded by the cell culture method. It can also serve in the preparation of antigens for the complement-fixation reaction. The inoculation is made in the chorioallantois of chick embryos 11 to 13 days old (Beveridge; Burnet). In 48 to 72 hours, after one or several passages, a marked thickening of the inoculated area is observed and pustules 0.5 to 2 mm. in diameter appear, the centers of which are opaque and sometimes necrotic. They vary in number according to the quantity and virulence of the virus, and thus titration is possible according to the number of pustules obtained (Burnet's pock-counting method).

It is sometimes difficult to distinguish the herpes lesions from those produced by the vaccinia virus, but the presence of nuclear inclusions will remove any doubts. It should be remembered that the varicella-zoster virus does not develop in the embryonated egg.

INOCULATION INTO ANIMALS. This was the first method of isolation of herpes virus (Grüter), and it is still used nowadays to confirm a diagnosis that has been established by cell culture or to estimate the efficaciousness of certain therapies in vivo.

The rabbit is the best animal for this purpose. It is mostly inoculated by scarification of the cornea. Two or three days afterward a herpetic keratoconjunctivitis is observed which evolves either toward healing within 15 days or else to local or systemic complications. The systemic complications are of the encephalitic type, with convulsions, coma, and alterations of the electroencephalogram occurring between the eighth and tenth days. These have recently been studied in detail by Tamalet. Histological examination shows the presence of typical lesions in the region of the eye or the encephalon, on Ammon's horn.

The rabbit can also be inoculated intracerebrally, cutaneously, intravenously, or via the viscera. Involvement of the central nervous system depends on the virulence of the strain (weak and strong strains according to Levaditi), the dose inoculated, and the treatment undergone (aggravating role of cortisone).

In the *guinea pig,* which is less sensitive than the rabbit, the virus may be introduced by cornea scarification (keratitis), intracerebral inoculation (encephalitis, found irregularly), or intradermal inoculation (vesicular eruption).

Newborn mice die as a result of septicemia following intraperitoneal inoculation (Kilbourne and Horsfall).

Adult mice, after intracerebral, peritoneal, or intravenous inoculation, die of encephalitis.

Identification of the Virus. Isolation of the virus should always be followed by its identification. The means include the seroprotection tests in animals, neutralization and complement fixation, performed by means of specific antisera prepared by immunization of the animals. Even more interesting is the direct or indirect fluorescent antibody technique devised by Coons; this was applied to herpes by Biegeleisen. It makes possible simultaneous isolation and identification of the virus by placing the pathological specimen in contact with antiherpes antibodies labeled with fluorescein. In this way a fluorescent antigen-antibody complex is obtained.

SEROLOGY

Antigenic Structure. According to the data advanced by Artzet, Hayward, and Schneweis, herpes virus possesses three types of antigen: an antigen V, linked to the virus particle, which fixes the complement and is resistant to heat and ultraviolet rays; an antigen N, which is soluble, neutralizing, extremely thermolabile, but resistant to ultraviolet rays; and an antigen S, which is soluble and which fixes complement, its sensitivity to heat being intermediate between that of antigens V and N.

At present it is thought that the various viral strains do not have a single common antigenic structure. Schneweis was able to differentiate two serological types, differing in their cytopathic effect (the production or

not of giant cells), in the size of the plaques produced, and possibly in their pathogenicity with regard to animals and man.

The antigenic capacity of herpes virus is reflected by the appearance of specific antibodies in all the infected subjects, as demonstrated by neutralization reactions, complement fixation, and skin tests. The first two tests are performed with two blood samples, the first taken within the first four days of illness, the other 15 to 20 days later. It should be emphasized that herpes simplex hominis virus shows certain antigenic, clinical, and epidemiological similarities to Sabin's virus B of the monkey (Herpes simiae). But the antigenic properties of the former differ from those of the other viruses of the herpes group.

Neutralization Reaction

PRINCIPLE. The neutralization reaction consists in determining the presence of antibodies neutralizing the lesions produced by a herpes virus of known infectious titer in the animal, in the embryonated egg, and especially in cell cultures. The latter method is the simplest and most rapid.

The serum to be tested is inactivated for 30 minutes in a water bath at $56°$ C. The virus which serves as antigen is diluted in such a way that the addition of an equal volume of serum brings the final dilution up to LTD_{50}. Increasing dilutions of serum are placed in contact with the virus for two hours at $37°$ C. ("virus constant, serum variable" method), and are then inoculated into cell cultures. The serum titer of neutralizing antibodies corresponds to the highest dilution that completely prevents the appearance of the cytopathogenic effect.

INTERPRETATION OF RESULTS. In the case of a primary herpetic infection the neutralizing antibodies appear between the fourth and eighth days of the illness. The level gradually increases to a maximum at about the beginning of the third week. It lies between $1/32$ and $1/256$. This level is maintained for three to four weeks, then it steadily decreases to a certain lower limit, varying according to the individual, but generally above $1/8$. The persistence of these antibodies does not prevent recurrences, but they are rendered benign. Attacks of recurrent herpes occur in subjects possessing variable but relatively low amounts of antibodies, this level being increased barely or not at all following the new attacks. Moreover,

Andrewes and Wheeler showed that herpes virus multiplies within the cells despite the presence of gamma globulins or specific neutralizing antibodies in the serum.

Complement-Fixation Reaction

PRINCIPLE. Because of the difficulties encountered in the preparation of antigens, this reaction has only recently been applied to the diagnosis of herpes. At the moment, extracts of the chorioallantois and especially the allantoic and amniotic fluids of infected eggs are being used. Comparable results have been obtained by Hayward, Gajdusek, Coriell, and Sohier. The antibodies are estimated according to Kolmer's technique, by making increasing dilutions from $1/8$ to $1/512$ of the patient's serum.

INTERPRETATION OF RESULTS. The complement-fixing antibodies appear in the second week of development of primary herpetic infections. The level subsequently increases and attains a maximum ($1/64$ to $1/128$) in three to four weeks. Then it gradually decreases to a fairly constant level.

Comparative Value of Tests for Neutralizing Antibodies and Complement-Fixing Antibodies. All primary herpetic infections become apparent by the presence of two different types of antibodies that evolve in a comparable manner (Nathalie, Gajdusek, Holzer, and ourselves). However, the level of the complement-fixing antibodies is often lower than that of the neutralizing antibodies. Serological proof of a primary infection can be made as well by one reaction as by the other.

Similarly, in systematic tests for antibodies against herpes made in a given population, the results from the two methods were entirely comparable.

SKIN TEST

The hypersensitivity of the skin to extracts of chick embryo infected by herpes virus was observed for the first time by Nagler in 1944. From 0.01 to 0.05 ml. of antigen is administered by intracutaneous inoculation. The reaction is positive when a round papule of over 0.5 cm. in diameter appears within 18 to 24 hours. The antibodies responsible for this reaction appear at the same time as those studied previously.

However, this reaction is not as reliable and is not often used in current practice.

EPIDEMIOLOGY AND PATHOGENICITY

The cycle of herpetic infection is determined by a certain number of humoral and clinical phenomena.

As far as the clinical aspect is concerned, the primary infection often is not observed. MacNair Scott estimated the number of clinically evident infections to be between 1 and 10 per cent, and these were mostly represented by cases of acute gingivostomatitis in infants or young children (Dodd). Sometimes there are recurrences of the this infection or subsequent secondary herpetic disease. In conjunction with this clinical cycle there is a humoral cycle which is characterized by the appearance and persistence of specific antibodies. Hence, most adults possess these antibodies: 63 per cent according to Scott, 80 per cent according to Hayward, 73.9 per cent in our experience, and 90 per cent according to Buddingh. The percentage of subjects infected shows a definite increase under unsanitary living conditions (Coetze; Burnet; Armengaud).

RESERVOIR OF VIRUSES

The ubiquity of the virus should be stressed, but the reservoir of this virus seems to be man alone – sometimes patients with a patent infection, or convalescents (who may harbor the virus for 15 to 40 days), or healthy carriers (Buddingh).

AGE AT WHICH PRIMARY INFECTION OCCURS

The age at which primary infection usually occurs can be deduced from study of the distribution of antibodies according to age (Scott, Buddingh, Anderson and Hamilton, and ourselves).

The newborn infant possesses antibodies of maternal origin, transmitted via the placenta. The level gradually decreases up to the age of six months. Few children are protected from six months to two years of age (less than 5 per cent according to Scott). From three to 14 years of age, the percentage rises and reaches that observed for adults.

The period of loss of the maternal antibodies corresponds to the maximum incidence of primary infections; that is, between six and 24 months of age.

CIRCUMSTANCES OF CONTAMINATION

Apart from direct contamination by a subject suffering from a skin lesion, the principle agents of infection are the saliva and the stools (Buddingh, Scott). The portal of entry is variable, frequently nasopharyngeal, but also cutaneous, genital, ocular, or gastric. Certain factors favor infection in the child: frequent contacts with the family, lesions of the mucous membranes of the mouth (dental eruptions) or of the skin. In this regard the part played by eczema in the occurrence of Kaposi's disease should be mentioned, as well as the frequent localizations in the region of wounds and sores.

Certain factors aggravate primary herpes infection: e.g., extremely young age, intercurrent diseases, bacterial superinfections, hypogammaglobulinemia or agammaglobulinemia, and cortisone treatment.

CONTAGIOUSNESS

Since herpes is an endemic disease, the infection may give rise to minor epidemics among groups of receptive subjects. Since such epidemics have occurred in family groups, hospitals, and institutions, it has been possible to study them from the clinical, virological, and serological point of view. The risk of infection in collectivities is high: according to Anderson, 100 per cent of the children in an Australian orphanage were infected before two years of age, 50 per cent of the infections being apparent clinically. Hale[27] found 77 per cent affected in a group of orphans 11 to 35 months old.

In a collectivity of children underdeveloped owing to various constitutional or acquired diseases, we observed an epidemic of primary herpetic infection which affected 12 girls, two and a half to five years of age, living in the same ward. The incubation period lasted five days on an average. Six children had an initial febrile herpetic tonsillitis for three to four days; then, after a latent period and apyrexia lasting three to seven days, gingivostomatitis followed. In five cases it consisted of a vesicular tonsillitis and in one only did the stomatitis occur immediately. In ten of the 12 cases the etiology was ascertained by isolation of herpes virus from throat samples or from the vesicles.

Among these 12 children, no neutralizing or complement-fixing antibodies were found in blood sampled at the onset of the illness or between the two clinical manifestations. A positive reaction was always found on the twentieth day of illness.

The peculiarities of this epidemic consisted in the number of children infected, in its clinical development in two stages (not previously mentioned in any publications), and finally in the reliability and correlation of the laboratory tests.

DURATION OF THE INCUBATION PERIOD

The incubation period is not well defined, since the contamination, usually by a healthy carrier, often passes unnoticed. During different epidemics, it has been established at two to 12 days, one week on an average.

PATHOGENESIS OF HERPES DISEASE IN NEWBORN INFANTS

The rare occurrence of herpes in the newborn and its serious and spectacular manifestations and evolution give it its individuality.

Source of Infection. This has been established in approximately half the cases. Very often it is the mother, who has an outbreak of genital, buccal, or cutaneous herpes at the time of confinement. Sometimes the child is contaminated by family or medical personnel.

Circumstances of Contamination. Contamination may occur at the time of confinement if the mother has an outbreak of genital herpes or in the first few days of life, by direct or indirect contact (saliva) with a virus carrier.

Transplacental contamination is possible. An in utero infection should be incriminated in the case reported by Mitchell in a newborn infant whose cutaneous herpes was recognized an hour after birth. This is also substantiated by the observations of Witzleben, who was the first to show the presence of necrotic foci together with nuclear inclusion bodies in the placental villi.

Virological studies performed in gravid rabbits by Biegeleisen and Scott have demonstrated viremia following infection of the mother and the subsequent infection of the fetus via the placenta.

Portal of Entry. The entry may be nasopharyngeal, cutaneous, conjunctival, or genital.

Generalization of the Infection. The infection becomes generalized via the blood. Demonstrated experimentally by Slavin and Berry, the viremia of the newborn infant seems to be confirmed by the presence of specific lesions of the vascular endothelia described by Zuelzer and Felder.

Susceptibility of the Newborn. It is generally agreed that immunological factors play the principal role. Most newborn infants possess antibodies of maternal origin. Their protective action has been proved experimentally in the newborn mouse: infected intranasally, it is protected by the administration of immune serum. Furthermore, its natural immunity seems to be diminished once it has been weaned (Berry and Slavin). Generally, herpetic disease of the newborn is observed only in the absence of a passive immunity of maternal origin. This would explain the particular susceptibility of the premature infant, who is not so well immunized because of the late passage of antibodies during pregnancy. The disease can, however, occur in newborn infants who possess antibodies. On the other hand, benign neonatal herpes has been known to occur even in the absence of antibodies.

The possibility of infection despite the presence of antibodies confirms the observations made by Wildy and Wheeler in vitro and would explain the failure of treatment by gamma globulins. No doubt *factors of predisposition* are involved.

The immaturity of the tissues of the newborn, especially the premature infant, seems to increase the susceptibility to infection. Anderson obtained generalized lesions in very young chick embryos, whereas after the eighteenth or nineteenth day the lesions remained localized.

Intercurrent diseases may play a part in promoting infection. Becker, Armengaud, and MacKenzie have described severe infections in undernourished African children; the same would hold in the case of *bacterial superinfections* with *Pseudomonas pyocyanea* (Pugh), staphylococcus (Ericson), meningococcus (Finberg), colibacillus (Langvad), or fungi (Möbius).

Colebatch stresses the part played by *factors affecting the mother:* e.g., obstetrical shock (Bird), diseases occurring in the last trimester of pregnancy.

MacCallum is of the opinion that generalization of infection occurs when the dose of virus is massive as compared to the amount of fetal antibodies.

Teratogenic Role. If herpes simplex is able to infect the fetus transplacentally at the end of pregnancy, then a point in question is whether it can be held responsible for certain abortions and particularly certain congenital malformations when an infection has occurred at the beginning of pregnancy. No information is available as far as the human being is concerned. The most accurate research work has been carried out by Ferm and Low on the gravid hamster. Intravenous injection between the first and eighth days of gestation was not followed by either abortion or malformations, despite the presence of histological lesions in the placenta and in the adrenals and liver of the mother. If herpes is inoculated into the fetus itself, it dies in utero within 24 to 48 hours, and the virus is found in its tissues.

Finally, it should be mentioned that research concerning the effect of herpes virus on the chromosome system of the cell is at present under way.

PATHOGENESIS OF RECURRENT HERPES

Recurrence occurs under various circumstances: the time interval of the recurrences is variable and sometimes curiously periodic.

Outbreak of herpes may be incidental to certain generalized *infections:* e.g., by pneumococci, meningococci, influenza virus, spirochetes, the rickettsiae of typhus.

Certain cases of herpes are favored by *foci of local infection:* e.g., dental alveolus, nasopharyngitis, otitis, genital infection.

Humoral shocks caused by injections of medicaments or vaccinations are sometimes to blame.

Recurrent herpes may occur after accidental or surgical *trauma:* e.g., lumbar punctures, spinal anesthesia, operation on the gasserian ganglion, dental treatment.

Certain physiological phenomena seem to release the outbreaks. The frequency of herpes associated with menstruation and with gestation is well known. Coitus can also be held responsible, as can any emotion; hence, Hellig and Noff have provoked pyschogenic herpes under hypnosis.

Secondary herpes often occurs during *malignant hemopathies and neoplasia* which compress or infiltrate the spinal ganglia or roots.

The pathogenesis of recurrent herpes is obscure. The animals inoculated acquire complete immunity. In man, the disease occurs in spite of the presence of serum antibodies, which simply attenuate the manifestations, the benign character of which contrasts with the extensive nature and sometimes dangerous evolution of the primary infection. During the course of human infection, cellular immunity appears to play an important part, but it is difficult to assess. The results of the first vaccination tests seem to confirm the importance of skin allergies in the determination of recurrences (Hénocq, Lépine, de Rudder).

TREATMENT

TREATMENT OF PRIMARY INFECTION

Herpes of the Newborn. The possibilities of treatment are somewhat limited. Antibiotics are ineffective. The use of gamma globulins at first raised some hope, but so far has never prevented death. Only products that are rich in herpes antibodies should be used. They should be injected early; otherwise the virus, once it is fixed in the cell, escapes the action. The dose should be strong: 10 cu. mm. per kilogram per day, three days running (Felder).

The *prophylactic* action of the gamma globulins seems more plausible. Their use is recommended to try to protect a newborn infant who has been in contact with a subject suffering from herpes.

Witzleben performed a cesarean section in a pregnant woman affected with genital herpes. Nevertheless, the child was born infected. Consequently one is confined to purely symptomatic treatment: maintenance of water and electrolyte balance, transfusions of fresh blood and plasma, and administration of vitamin K_1.

The situation is the same with regard to the treatment of herpetic hepatitis in the infant.

However, some recent work suggests the possibility of employing IDU (cf. Introduction: Specific Therapy) *by perfusion* in certain serious forms of herpes for which we have had no effective treatment: generalized neonatal herpes (Partridge) and encephalitis (Bellanti).

Mucocutaneous and Ocular Herpes. Various local treatments have been recommended. *For the skin,* inert powders have been used as well as dyes, antiseptics, and dabbing with a 1 per cent solution of silver nitrate.

Antibiotic ointments and lotions are used in the event of bacterial superinfection, usually in Kaposi's disease. The local or general use of corticosteroids is useless and even harmful.

Cicatrization of the mucous lesions is facilitated by the application of antiseptic solutions, e.g., methylene blue. *For the eye,* many treatments have been used, ranging from the venom of the bee to x-rays! Before the era of antiviral substances, abrasion of the infected tissues was performed by means of cytoplasmic poisons (e.g., iodine, silver nitrate, phenol, alcohol) or proteolytic enzymes (chymotrypsin) or by curettage followed by dabbing with iodized alcohol or permanganate. Here again, the use of corticosteroids locally should be proscribed.

A new phase in the treatment of viral infections began in 1960 with the production of *antiviral substances.* Despite initial enthusiasm, a certain number have already been discarded. This is the case with xenalamine and ABOB or Virustat, but not with 5-iodo-2′-deoxyuridine (IDU), the use of which has transformed the prognosis of cutaneous and particularly ocular herpes.

IDU is an analogue of thymidine, from which it differs only in the substitution of an I for a CH_3 radical in position 5. It acts as antimetabolite, being substituted for thymidine during the synthesis of DNA. It also inhibits the enzymes necessary for the use of thymidine in the synthesis of DNA. These properties explain its effect on viruses consisting of deoxyribonucleic acid: IDU governs the formation of "fraudulent" DNA and hence of incomplete viral particles that no longer have the ability to infect (Smith, Siminoff, Roizmann, de Lavergne). Experiments on animals were performed with success by Kaufmann: IDU prevented the occurrence of herpetic keratitis in the rabbit or attenuated its development and prevented cerebral complications.

In man, IDU has been used with success in numerous cases of *cutaneous herpes.* A 0.1 per cent or 0.5 per cent solution of IDU is dabbed on every two hours. Evolution of the lesions is considerably shortened (48 hours), and the pruritus disappears at the beginning of the treatment.

Mucous herpes, particularly of the

mouth, is less accessible for this treatment: the solution is swept away by the saliva and cannot remain in contact with the infected cells. For this reason IDU is ineffective in the treatment of gingivostomatitis.

IDU finds its main application in the treatment of *herpetic keratitis;* instillations of a collyrium containing 0.1 per cent IDU or applications of IDU gel are renewed every two hours. The functional symptoms rapidly recede, the evolution is shortened, complications are rarer, and numerous keratoplasties are thus avoided.

Because of its possible interference in the metabolism of the cell (possible risk of cancerization), the use of IDU is, in general, local; however, as we mentioned earlier, it has been used by the systemic route in certain serious forms of primary herpes. Its action is temporary. It has no effect on recurrences of herpes. Furthermore, research studies in vitro seem to indicate that certain strains may become resistant. We have had occasion to reproduce this phenomenon in cell culture, after Dubbs and Kitt.

TREATMENT OF RECURRENT HERPES; VACCINATION

So far no medicament has prevented recurrences; hence the advantage of a treatment that would make use of immunological mechanisms.

The first attempts at specific prevention by means of a vaccine were made by Fournier and Levaditi (1928); Urbain and Schaeffer (1929), Bedson (1931), and Burnet and Lush (1939): these authors used an antigen prepared from the brain of the mouse or rabbit.

Antivariola vaccination, based on the erroneous belief that there is an antigenic relationship between herpes and vaccinia virus, had its passing fashion; it was used by Kubelka and Wassermanova[39] in 1959 in secondary ocular herpes.

Even more interesting are the attempts at desensitization with regard to herpes antigen by repeated autoinoculations of the fluid from the vesicles from the patient himself (Macher, Goldman). Jawetz obtained 50 per cent favorable results in this way.

In 1958, Biberstein and Jessner prepared an antigen from rabbit brain, inactivated by heat, which produced active skin tests in 24 out of 28 cases of recurrent herpes. In 1960, Söltz-Szöts obtained good results by vaccinating with purified anti-

gen S: he believed that recurrences are preceded by a fall in anti-S antibodies. In 1960, Chu and Warren succeeded in immunizing mice with a vaccine obtained from cell culture of rabbit kidney, inactivated by formalin. In 1961, Anderson and Kilbourne prepared a vaccine with a strain cultured on chick embryo cells and inactivated by means of ultraviolet rays.

In France, Lepine and de Rudder published extremely encouraging, though somewhat limited, results obtained with an inactivated antiherpes vaccine prepared in cell culture of sheep fetus kidney and inactivated by means of ultraviolet rays. This strain lost its virulence with regard to the rabbit and the mouse. Its cytopathic effect passed from the type of "microplaques" to the "syncytial" type. A toxicological and pharmacological study showed that it had completely lost all toxicity. This vaccine protected the rabbits against a lethal dose of virus and caused them to acquire two different types of antibodies. The mice were protected against 1000 LD_{50}, but the level of their antibodies did not exceed $1/16$.

This vaccination finds its application in all manifestations of herpes in man. It acts on both the outbreak and recurrences, and the results do not depend on the length of the illness, its periodicity or its localization, the age and sex of the patient, or previous treatment.

The first results have proved encouraging. In cases of mucocutaneous herpes the lesions healed in less than 48 hours, and recurrences were avoided or less frequent in 38 cases out of 50 (Degos) and in 18 cases out of 20 (Henocq and Touraine). The best results were obtained in menstrual herpes.

In ocular herpes, Pouliquen obtained 12 improvements in 20 cases treated. Recurrences were less frequent and, especially, much attenuated. The action of IDU is thought to be enhanced by this vaccine.

The method of treatment should take into account the possibility of local reaction at the point of injection and especially the danger of reactivating the lesions. Consequently, Pouliquen and de Rudder, in the case of ocular herpes, advise alternating intradermal and subcutaneous injections and gradually increasing the doses administered. They inject, every four days, 0.1 ml. of a 1/100 solution, then a 1/10 solution, and finally the pure vaccine.

To treat cutaneous herpes, Henocq

injected subcutaneously 1 ml. of the vaccine immediately after performing a skin test on the patient by an intradermal injection of 0.1 ml. of the pure solution.

Weekly injections are given for at least six weeks and continued until the recurrences disappear. It seems that the vaccine does not cause an increase in the circulating antibodies (Henocq and Lepine). It would seem to intervene at the cellular level by a mechanism as yet obscure.

BIBLIOGRAPHY

A more complete bibliography up to 1964 can be found in: Olive, D.: Thèse. Nancy, Imprimerie G. Thomas, 1964.

1. Antonova, N. I.: Virological and serological investigation of acute aphthous stomatitis in children. Acta Virologo., *4*:383-391, 1960.
2. Armengaud, M.: Note préliminaire à l'étude de la primo-infection herpétique de l'enfant africain (à propos de 244 observations). Bull. Soc. Méd. Afr. Noire Lang. Franç., *8*:358-375, 1963.
3. Bach, C., Schaefer, P., and Babinet, B.: Primo-infection herpétique bénigne chez un nouveau-né. Ann. Pédiat. (Paris), *13*:57-60, 1966.
4. Baden, E.: La gingivo-stomatite herpétique chez le jeune adulte. Rev. Franc. Odontostomat., *3*:75-91, 1956.
5. Baylet, R. J.: Valeur et limite de la réaction de déviation du complément dans le diagnostic de la maladie herpétique de primo-infection. Bull. Soc. Méd. Afr. Noire Lang. Franc., *8*:422-425, 1963.
6. Becker, W., Naude, W. D., and Kipps, A.: Virus studies in disseminated herpes simplex infections. Association with malnutrition in children. S. Afr. Med. J., *37*:74-76, 1963.
7. Bedson, S. P.: Immunisation with killed herpes
7a. Bellanti, J. A., Guin, C. H., Grassi, R. M., and Olson, L. C.: Herpes simplex encephalitis: brain biopsy and treatment with 5-iodo-2'-deoxyuridine. J. Pediat., *72*:266-275, 1968.
8. Biberstein, H., and Jessner, M.: Experiences with herpin in recurrent herpes simplex, together with a review and analysis of the literature on the use of C.N.S. substances as a virus antigen carrier. Dermatologica (Basel), *117*:267, 1958.
9. Biegeleisen, J. Z., Scott, L. V., and Lewis, V.: Rapid diagnosis of herpes simplex virus infections with fluorescent antibody. Science, *129*:640-641, 1959.
10. Bird, T., Ennis, J. E., Wort, A. J., and Gardner, P. S.: Disseminated herpes simplex in newborn infants. J. Clin. Path., *16*:423-431, 1963.
11. Blattner, R. J.: Latent virus infection: recurrent herpes simplex. J. Pediat., *59*:784-786, 1961.
12. Bloedhorn, H.: Herpes-simplex-Enzephalitis des Erwachsenen mit tödlichen Ausgang D. Mediz. Wochschr., *87*:1247-1249, 1962.
13. Brégeat, P.: La 5-iodo-2'-désoxyuridine (I.D.U.) dans le traitement de l'herpès de la cornée. Etude expérimentale et clinique. Arch. Ophtal. (Paris), *23*:433-440, 1963.

14. MacCallum, F. O., Potter, J. M., and Edwards, D. H.: Early diagnosis of herpes simplex encephalitis by brain biopsy. Lancet, *2*:332-334, 1964.
15. Chancellor, A. H. R.: Herpes simplex of the fingers. Med. J. Aust., *1*:517-518, 1961.
16. Chu, L. W., and Warren, G. H.: Pathogenicity and immunogenicity of herpes simplex virus strains propagated in rabbit kidney tissue. Proc. Soc. Exp. Biol. Med., *105*:396, 1960.
17. Coetzee, J. N.: Epidemiology of herpes simplex in Pretoria Bantu population. S. Afr. J. Lab. Clin. Med., *1*:52-56, 1955.
18. Cogan, D. G.: Herpes simplex retinopathy in an infant. Arch. Ophthal. (Chicago), *72*:641-645, 1964.
19. Corwin, M. E.: A double blind study of the effect 5-iodo-2'-deoxyuridine on experimental herpes simplex keratitis. Amer. J. Ophthal., *55*:225-229, 1963.
20. Degos, R., and Touraine, R.: Traitement de l'herpès récidivant par un vaccin spécifique. Bull. Soc. Franc. Derm. Syph., *71*:161-166, 1964.
21. Dodge, P., and Cure, C.: Acute encephalitis with intranuclear cellular inclusions. A nonfatal case of probable herpetic etiology diagnosed by biopsy. New Eng. J. Med., *255*:849-853, 1956.
22. Eilard, U., and Hellgren, L.: Herpes simplex. A statistical and clinical investigation based on 669 patients. Dermatologica (Basel), *130*:101-106, 1965.
23. Ferm, V. H., and Low, R. J.: Herpes simplex virus infection in the pregnant hamster. J. Path. Bact. *89*:295-300, 1965.
24. Fisher, A. A.: Herpes simplex of a hand (due to contact with sibling who had herpetic gingivostomatitis). A.M.A. Arch. Derm. (Chicago). *80*:598-599, 1959.
25. Garcia, A. G.: Fatal infection in chicken-pox and alastrim with histopathologic study of the placenta. Pediatrics, *32*:895, 1963.
26. Goldman, L.: Reactions of autoinoculation for recurrent herpes simplex. Arch. Derm. (Chicago), *84*:1025-1026, 1961.
27. Hale, B. D.: Epidemic herpetic stomatitis in an orphanage nursery. J.A.M.A., *183*:1068-1072, 1963.
28. Hampar, B., and Ellison, S. A.: Chromosomal aberrations induced by an animal virus. Nature (London), *192*:145-147, 1961.
29. Havener, W. H., and Wachtel, J.: IDU therapy of herpetic keratitis. Amer. J. Ophthal., *55*:234-237, 1963.
30. Hénocq, E., Rudder, J. de, Maurin, J., and Lépine, P.: Etude clinique et allergologique des herpès récidivants à l'aide d'un nouveau vaccin antiherpétique. Rev. Franç. Allerg., *4*:196, 1964.
31. Hogan, M. J., Kimura, S. J., and Thygeson, P.: Pathology of herpes simplex kerato-iritis. Amer. J. Ophthal., *57*:551-564, 1964.
32. Jack, I., and Perry, J. W.: Herpes simplex infection in the new-born. Med. J. Aust., *2*:640, 1959.
33. Johnson, R. T.: The pathogenesis of herpes virus encephalitis. I. Virus pathways to the nervous system of suckling mice demonstrated by fluorescent antibody staining. J. Exp. Med., *119*:343-356, 1964.
34. Jorgensen, G.: Herpes gestationis with habitual death of the foetus. Nord. Med., *50*:1551, 1953.

35. Juel-Jensen, B. E., and MacCallum, F. O.: Herpes simplex lesions of face treated with iodoxuridine applied by spray gun: results of a double blind controlled trial. Brit. Med. J., *1*:901-903, 1965.

36. Kaufman, H. E.: Chemotherapy of virus disease. Chemotherapia (Basel), 7:1-16, 1963.

37. Kaufman, H. E., Martola, E. L., and Dohlman, C. H.: Herpes simplex treatment with IDU and corticosteroids. Arch. Ophthal. (Chicago), *69*:468-472, 1963.

38. Kern, A. B., and Schiff, B. L.: Vaccine therapy in recurrent herpes simplex. Arch. Derm., *89*:844-845, 1964.

39. Kubelka, V., and Wassermanova, V.: Antiherpetic vaccine in ophthalmology. Cesk. Oftal., *15*:1, 1959.

40. Kusano, N.: Herpetic hepatitis, with special reference to its transition to giant cell hepatitis. Acta Path. Jap., *10*:549-564, 1960.

41. Laibson, P. R., Sery, T. W., and Leopold, I. H.: The treatment of herpetic keratitis with 5-iodo-2'-deoxyuridine (IDU). Arch. Ophthal. (Chicago), *70*:52-58, 1963.

42. Lamy, M., Jammet, M. L., Ajjan, M. N., and Bonissol, C.: L'herpès de première invasion (la gingivostomatite herpétique de l'enfant). Presse Med., *72*:1045-1046, 1964.

43. Langvad, A., and Voigt, J.: Herpes generalisata infantum: a review and report of a new case. Danish. Med. Bull., *10*:153-158, 1963.

44. Lavergne, E. de, Olive, D., and LeMoyne, M. T.: Action de l' I.D.U. sur quelques virus à A.D.N. en cultures cellulaires. Rev. Immun. (Paris), *29*:241-266, 1965.

45. Lelong, M., Simon-Lavoine, N., Dubois, O., and Samaille, J.: Etude des réactions sérologiques au cours des gingivo-stomatites herpétiques de l' enfant. Rev. Immun. (Paris), *27*:291-300, 1963.

46. Lépine, P., and Rudder, J. de: Aspects cliniques et immunologiques du traitement de l'herpès récurrent par un vaccin inactivé. Rev. Méd. (Paris), 1061-1070, 1964.

47. Lépine, P., Rudder, J. de Maurin, J., and Hénocq, E.: Essai de thérapeutique de l'herpès récidivant par un vaccin préparé en culture cellulaire et inactivé par les rayons ultra-violets. I. Préparation du vaccin et essais d'immunisation sur l' animal. II. Essais cliniques. Sem. Hop. Paris, *40*:1471-1480, 1964.

48. Macher, E.: Zur Behandlung des chromisch-rezidivierenden Herpes simplex. Z. Haut. Geschlechskr., *23*:18, 1957.

49. Martins, A. N., Kempe, L. G., and Hayes, G. J.: Acute haemorrhagic leucoencephalitis (Hurst) with a concurrent primary herpes simplex infection. J. Neurol. Neurosurg. Psychiat., *27*:493-501, 1964.

50. Maxwell, E.: Treatment of herpes keratitis with 5-iodo-2-deoxyuridine (IDU). A clinical evaluation of 1500 cases. Amer. J. Ophthal., *56*:571-573, 1963.

51. Möbius, G., and Möbius, M.: Zur pathologie der generalisierten Herpes simplex-virus-infektion des Neugeborenen. Monat. Kinderheilk., *111*:246-252, 1963.

52. Moses, H. L., and Cheatham, W. J.: The frequency and significance of human herpetic esophagitis. An autopsy study. Lab. Invest. *12*:663-669, 1963.

53. Neimann, N., Pierson, M., Lavergne, E. de, Gilgenkrantz, S., and Olive, D.: La primo-infection herpétique. Etude clinique et biologique. Arch. Franc. Pediat., *21*:273-295, 1964.

54. Offret, G., Payrau, P., Rudder, J. de, Pouliquen, Y., Faure, J. P., and Cuq, G.: De l'application du vaccin inactivé dans le kératite herpétique. Arch. Ophtal. (Paris), *25*:287-300, 1965.

54a. Partridge, J. W., and Millis, R. R.: Systemic herpes simplex infection in a newborn treated with intravenous idoxuridine. Arch. Dis. Childh., *43*:377-381, 1968.

55. Pettit, T. H., Kimura, S. J., and Peters, K.: The fluorescent antibody technique in diagnosis of herpes simplex keratitis. Arch. Ophthal. (Chicago), *72*:86-98, 1964.

56. Platt, H.: The local and generalized forms of experimental herpes simplex infection in guinea-pigs. Brit. J. Exp. Path., *45*:300, 1964.

57. Plummer, G.: Serological comparison of the herpes viruses. Brit. J. Exp. Path., *45*:135-141, 1964.

58. Rey, M.: Essais de chimiothérapie antivirale dans la primo-infection herpétique de l'enfant africain. Bull. Soc. Méd. Afr. Noire Lang. Franç., *9*:446-451, 1964.

59. Richardson, H. B., and Leibovitz, A.: "Hand, foot and mouth disease" in children. An epidemic associated with coxsackie virus A$_{16}$. J. Pediat., *67*: 6-12, 1965.

60. Russell, W. C., Watson, D. H., and Wildy, P.: Preliminary chemical studies on herpes virus. Biochem. J., *87*:26-27, 1963.

61. Scott, T. F. M., and Tokumaru, I.: Herpes virus hominis (virus of herpes simplex). Bact. Rev., *28*: 458-471, 1964.

62. Simon, G.: Psychosis and recurrent herpes simplex. New Eng. J. Med., *271*:1070, 1964.

63. Smith, K. O., and Dukes, C. D.: Effects of 5-iodo-2'-desoxyuridine (IDU) on herpes virus synthesis and survival in infected cells. J. Immun., *92*:550-554, 1964.

64. Söltz-Szöts, J.: Neu Methode einer spezifischeu Vaccination bei rezidivieren dem Herpes simplex. Hautarzt, *11*:465, 1960.

65. Szögi, S., and Berge, I.: Hepatoadrenal necrosis in newborn infants due to herpes simplex virus infection. Patol. Avd. Cenc-Las. Boros-opusc. Med. (Stockholm), *9*:344-348, 1964.

66. Tamalet, J., Toga, M., Delmon, J., Regis, H., Duc, P., and Dubois, D.: L'encéphalite herpétique expérimentale du lapin. Corrélations électrocliniques et anatomiques dans 13 cas. Rev. Neurol. (Paris), *108*:865-885, 1963.

67. Tanzer, J.: Alterations chromosomiques observées dans des cellules de rein de singe infectées in vitro par le virus de l'herpès. Ann. Inst. Pasteur. (Paris), *107*:366-373, 1964.

68. Uchida, Y., and Kimura, S. J.: Fluorescent antibody localization of herpes simplex virus in the conjunctiva. Arch. Ophthal. (Chicago), *73*:413-419, 1965.

69. Vigier, P.: Remarques sur le traitement de l'herpès récidivant par la vaccination antivariolique. Bull. Soc. Franc. Derm. Syph., *71*:556, 1964.

70. Watson, D. H., and Wildy, P.: Some serological properties of herpes virus particles studied with the electron microscope. Virology, *21*:100-111, 1963.

71. White, J. G.: Fulminating infection with herpes-

simplex virus in premature and newborn infants. New Eng. J. Med., *269*:455-460, 1963.

72. Witzleban, C. L., and Driscoll, S. G.: Possible transplacental transmission of herpes simplex infection. Pediatrics, *36*:192-199, 1965.

73. Wright, H. T., Miller, A.: Fatal infection in a newborn infant due to herpes simplex virus. Report of a case diagnosed before death. J. Pediat., *67*: 130-132, 1965.

ADDENDUM

In 1962 Schneweis demonstrated the presence of two serologically distinct types (see p. 466). Other workers, especially Dowdle and Nahmias,[1] were able to throw more light on the distinction made earlier. In addition to their serological differences, the two herpes viruses can be distinguished by physicochemical characteristics: sensitivity to heat, sensitivity to these viruses of chorioallantoic membrane and of cell cultures, and, most striking, differences in pathogenicity for man.

Type 1 virus, the more frequent, is found in all sites above the belt: especially in lesions of the face (skin and mucosae), including ocular lesions.

Type 2 virus is associated with lesions below the belt, genital herpes in particular. Recent investigation shows that a type 2 virus is found in most cases of neonatal herpes and seems to be responsible for congenital malformations and abortions.

By the kinetics of seroneutralization, the types of circulating antibodies can be determined. This technique has revealed that 80 per cent of women with cancer of the uterus have antibody against herpes virus type 2; this antibody is found in only 10 to 20 per cent of adult women.

South et al.[2] reported the case of a premature infant born with lesions of type 2 herpes virus. The child showed microcephaly, microphthalmia, and retinal dysplasia. This case probably represented a fetopathy by intrauterine herpetic infection.

1. Nahmias, A., and Dowdle, W. R.: Antigenic and biologic differences in herpes virus hominis. Progress in Medical Virology, *10*:110, 1968.

2. South, A., Tompkins, W. A. F., Morris, C. R., and Rawls, W. C.: Congenital malformation of the central nervous system associated with genital type (T.2) herpes virus. J. Pediat., *75*:13-18, 1969.

35

Warts and Molluscum Contagiosum

By J. HEWITT and F. HAGUENAU

Warts and molluscum contagiosum are small cutaneous tumors that are frequently mentioned together because of a series of common features. In both cases, the tumors are benign; they are often multiple and may regress spontaneously. They affect mainly children and they are induced by viruses.

In both cases, the viruses are not detectable in the basal layer, which is the initial seat of hyperplastic proliferation; they are, however, apparent in the more superficial layers of the skin. Their appearance is linked to cellular lysis.

Despite these common traits, the viruses responsible for these two lesions could not be more different, either in their structure or in their mode of development in the epidermal cells.

The molluscum contagiosum virus is voluminous and belongs to the *Poxviridae* family, whereas the wart virus is small and belongs to the *Papillomaviridae* family. The cycle of the former virus can be completely followed in the cytoplasm, while that of the latter occurs only in the nucleus. In addition, the mechanism by which hyperplasia is induced appears to be entirely different in these two diseases.

For all these reasons, each of them will be considered separately.

VERRUCA (WART)

Verrucae are benign hyperkeratosic proliferations of the epidermis growing on hyperplastic papillary shafts. They are contagious and of viral origin. This definition excludes from this category various benign wart-like, though nonviral, proliferations, in particular the seborrheic wart (or verruca senilis).

Despite their banality, the verrucae as a whole represent a highly challenging type of affection to research workers. Not only is it well established now that they are due to a virus, many experiments of autoinoculation having succeeded but spectacular work performed with the electron microscope has shown that the virus belongs to the *Papillonaviridae* family, some members of which are either highly oncogenic in various animal species (for instance polyoma in mice) or may become so (for instance SV40 in hamsters).

Finally, the other known papilloma viruses (in the rabbit, deer, calf, etc.) induce tumors that may become malignant (Shope papilloma in the rabbit) or "transform" cells in vitro (bovine papilloma).

We are thus dealing with a human growth which, although it never evolves toward cancer, is induced by a virus of a type similar to cancer-inducing viruses in other species.

In this respect it is perhaps of interest to mention here the still discussed kinship between *epidermodysplasia verruciformis* of Lewandowski-Lutz and verruca plana. The former consists of small flat papules with a singular resemblance to verruca plana, but the lesions are often purplish red and generalized and tend to undergo malignant transformation (spinous cell carcinoma). Electron microscopy has revealed the presence of wart-like viruses.[8] However, malignancy here is thought by many authors to result from the genetic make-up of patients.

A virus of the same group has also been shown to be present in the brain of patients with progressive multiple leukoencephalopathy, a disease strikingly associated with other malignancies in the same individual.[9]

In addition to the stimulating problems just mentioned, the clinical behaviour of warts also raises questions of the greatest interest. On the one hand, these are tumors which regress spontaneously in a great number of cases (30 per cent); on the other hand, one often observes the disappearance of all tumors (daughter tumors) following treatment of only one. Finally, the fact that regression can often be obtained by autosuggestion, a phenomenon which is used with therapeutic success, escapes explanation for the moment.

SYMPTOMATOLOGY

There are two clinical types of warts: verruca vulgaris, with its numerous varieties, and verruca plana. They are very frequent in children.

Verruca Vulgaris. Verruca vulgaris corresponds typically to the general definition of warts.

Warts show their most characteristic aspect on the fingers and hands, where they take root preferentially, either isolated or in groups (Fig. 35-1). They appear as little epidermal tumors one or several millimeters in diameter, being well defined and rounded or oval. Sometimes they are larger or polycyclic owing to confluence of several warts or to growth by budding. Yellowish or grayish, firm, dry, rough to the touch, they can be bristly. Painless, they become painful by fissuration when they are voluminous or traumatized or secondarily infected.

Evolution begins with a very small papule (pinhead size) which is skin colored and visible only under skimming light. Such secondary outcroppings, a source of recurrence, should be sought. After attaining several

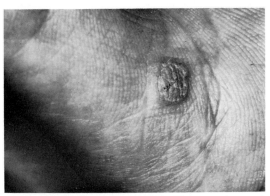

Figure 35-1. Verruca vulgaris. Macroscopic aspect.

millimeters in size, warts often remain stable for several months, or years. Finally, they can disappear spontaneously, sometimes all existing warts suddenly disappearing at the same time. On the other hand, sometimes after a long period of stability, an explosive evolution may occur during which warts grow and multiply at the same time.

The site at which warts appear determines their characteristics:

Warts *around the nails* take root in the periunguinal furrow, where they are mistaken for simple hyperkeratoses until they overlap the adjacent skin and take on a typical aspect.

Subunguinal warts heave up the nail and are painful.

Verrucae plantaris, which are very common, especially in adults, take on a variety of aspects. Their most consistent feature is acute pain upon pressure and walking, often a revealing symptom since verrucae plantaris are usually located at the weight-bearing points. Because of the pressure to which they are subjected and the thickness of the cornified layer covering them, verrucae plantaris do not form salient warty tumors but grow in depth. In their most typical form they constitute, in the center of a thickened cornified layer, a depressed, rounded or oval area with a grayish surface that is rough or frankly warty (Fig. 35-2). The rounded limit of the central wart is marked by a precise, characteristic groove.

Small verrucae of the sole of the foot may be very difficult to diagnose. At times only a minute white circle is present, which may be mistaken for the vestiges of dysidrosis vesicles: the fact that the inferior surface of the circle is slightly lower than the epidermal plane allows identification.

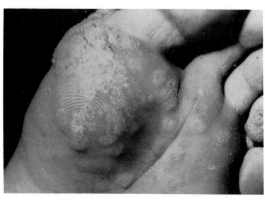

Figure 35-2. Verruca plantaris. Macroscopic aspect.

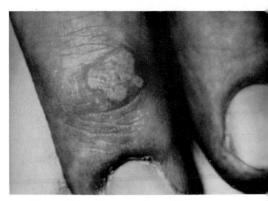

Figure 35-3. Verruca plana. Macroscopic aspect.

At other times there is no depression, rather there is a small hard encased mass, often embedded in a callosity.

All callosities which become painful should be suspected of harboring a wart. Sometimes the wart can be made out as a translucid pseudocyst in the center of the callosity. Sometimes the wart remains invisible and is manifested only by acute pain upon pressure at a calloused point: it can be discovered only by successively exfoliating the epidermal layers, and it appears as a profoundly inserted rounded white mass.

In contrast, confluent plantar warts ("in sheets," "in mosaic") form relatively painless keratotic surfaces which often go unrecognized or are mistaken for mycosis or psoriasis.

Pedicular, digitiform, or *filiform* warts are seen primarily on the face (eyelids, chin) and on the neck.

Among warts must be included *condyloma accuminata (venereal vegetation)* which develops on the supple, humid skin of the external genitalia and the perianal region and on the vulvar and vaginal or anal mucosa. Its appearance differs greatly depending on the location. The most characteristic is the "cockscomb," a sort of pediculated papilloma, red and flattened, the borders of which bristle with fine keratotic projections. Sometimes these growths are confluent (cauliflower excrescences); these can become infected and suppurate, particularly during pregnancy. On the neighboring skin they spread as simple nonkeratotic warts. On the internal mucosa they are difficult to recognize, appearing either as pink translucent papillomas, recognizable by their bristling surface, or as minute pale protrusions.

Verrucae plana. These so-called juve

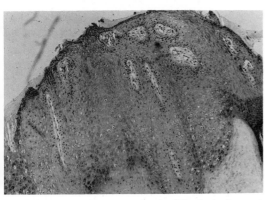

Figure 35-4. Verruca vulgaris. Histological aspect. × 300.

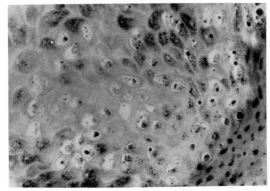

Figure 35-5. Verruca vulgaris. Histological aspect: detail on an area where cytological lesions are easily observed. × 1200.

nile warts are frequent in children and young girls. They differ from verruca vulgaris in that their surface is not papillomatous but smooth and barely protruding. Always multiple, of 1 to 5 mm. in diameter, with rounded or polygonal edges, and appearing preferentially on the face, the back of the hands, the forearms, or the legs, they often form linear striations due to post-trauma inoculation and may be confluent. Of normal skin color or grayish, they are hardly visible and are recognized by their shiny surface when illuminated from certain angles. Their evolution is unpredictable, and after having persisted several years, they may suddenly disappear spontaneously.

HISTOLOGY

Verruca vulgaris is a papilloma with acanthosis and hyperkeratosis.

Toward the deep layers of the skin, the elongated and regular epidermal buddings converge toward the central area but do not go beyond the level of the basement membrane of the normal skin. The dermal papillae, which are very elongated, rise from the deep central regions toward the surface, diverging as they go. Under the hyperkeratotic cornified layer, the epidermis covering the papillae has a thickened granulosum layer, whose cells are often vacuolated and contain large, unequal patches of keratohyaline and sometimes dyskeratotic cells.

Verruca plantaris is the variety for which histological diagnosis is most evident. The acanthotic and papillomatous proliferation which deeply indents the dermoepidermal junction early contains cells with clear cytoplasm which tend to isolate themselves from the others (dyskeratosis) on passing through the granulosa. This thickened layer is the site of marked cellular abnormalities: cytoplasmic and nuclear vacuolization, mounds

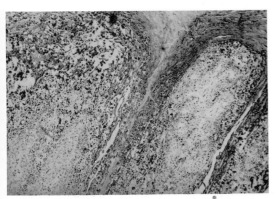

Figure 35-6. Verruca plantaris. Histological aspect. × 300.

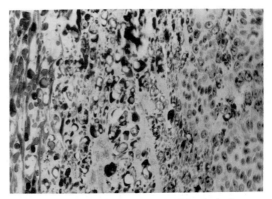

Figure 35-7. Verruca plantaris. Histological aspect. × 1280.

of keratohyaline, pools of eosinophilic hyaline substance.

Inversely, *verruca filiformis,* a simple projection of the skin made up of a dermal papilla covered by a layer of epithelium, shows few cytological abnormalities and can be mistaken for a banal inflammatory papilloma.

As for *verruca plana,* a simple epidermal thickening, it usually shows inequalities in the distribution of keratohyaline, and its cornified layer exhibits a "wickerwork" appearance.

EXPERIMENTAL RESEARCH

There is good evidence that warts are transmitted from one person to another both directly by contact with wart tissue and indirectly by contact with virus-contaminated objects. Several successful transmission experiments in man have been reported.[7]

Experiments involving transmission to species other than man are less convincing. Likewise, the recent results reported on replication of the agent in tissue culture still need confirmation.

Data concerning the immunology of warts are relatively scarce. Complement-fixing antibodies have been detected in approximately 50 per cent of patients. No "tumor antigen" has been demonstrated as yet; viral antigen is evidenced by immunofluorescent methods in the nuclei of the granular layers and the lower portion of the cornified layer of the epithelium. This is in accordance with the findings of electron microscopy.

ELECTRON MICROSCOPY

Two types of observations have been made. They concern, on the one hand, development of the virus inside tumor cells, and on the other, the structure of the viruses examined after extraction. In the first case,[1] no virus particles were found in the basal layers of verrucal growths under the electron microscope, although this is the layer where cell proliferation takes place. But the virus appears progressively as cells migrate to the surface and while they undergo the differentiation that will lead finally to keratinization and cell necrosis. The first indications of virus formation are found in the nuclei of the cells of the stratum spinosum, while in the stratum granulosum masses of clustered viruses are

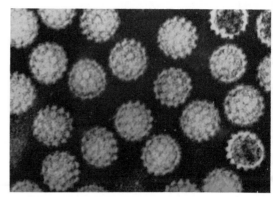

Figure 35-8. Wart virus examined under the electron microscope with the negative contrast technique. × 300,000. (Electron micrograph courtesy of Dr. Howatson.)

observed and correspond to the inclusion bodies visible with fluorescein-conjugated antisera. In the most superficial layers, in which all cellular structures become unrecognizable, these closely packed aggregates of viruses are surrounded by keratinous debris.

Because of the high virus content (7.3 × 10^9) of some warts (the amount varies greatly from wart to wart), extraction and examination of purified preparations with the negative-contrast technique is easy. Their characteristic structure has thus been revealed.[4, 5, 6]

The viruses are spherical particles measuring 52 to 55 mμ in diameter and possessing an outer capsid composed of morphological units (capsomeres) arranged with cubical symmetry (Fig. 35-8). The number of capsomeres, which may be calculated from their arrangements in relation to one another, has been the object of much debate, some authors holding the correct number to be 42, others 92, others still 72 (see details and references in Rowson and Mahy[7]). The last possibility now seems to be the one which is most generally accepted.

Inside the capsid is double-stranded deoxyribonucleic acid (DNA) (5.3 × 10^6 m.w.), the linear, circular, and helical configuration of which has been beautifully shown with the electron microscope.[3]

TREATMENT

Verruca Vulgaris. Because of the mode of transmission of warts, there is advantage in acting as quickly as possible in order to prevent spread.

A first attempt can be made with a

systemic treatment which often works: tincture of *Thuja occidentalis* (50 to 80 drops), magnesium oxide (0.2 to 1 gram per day), and magnesium chloride (1.2 grams per day).

The part played by suggestion in the cures thus obtained is doubtless important, especially in the case of verruca plana juvenilis. Disappearance of verrucae can be obtained with *suggestion* alone.[7]

In general, however, treatment will consist in destroying the warts by *physical methods.*

Warts on the fingers and hands can easily be eliminated under local anesthesia with 1 per cent Xylocaine (not 2 per cent, which may cause necrosis), by *galvanocauterization,* or, better, by *electrocoagulation* with prior or secondary curettage. If electrocoagulation is not possible, the Aurégan technique (ablation with a curette followed by filling the resulting cavity with powdered potassium permanganate) yields good results.

One or two treatment sessions with dry ice or liquid nitrogen can also give good results, particularly if the warts are not widespread.

Periunguinal or subunguinal warts are much more difficult to treat: liquid nitrogen is effective but painful. In exceptional cases, ablation of the nail is necessary.

Radiotherapy (dose of 1200 r very lightly filtered) is remarkably successful but requires the maximum of precautions. Its use is shunned by numerous authors, because of the serious radiodermitis it may cause, the effective doses being situated at the limit of the risk of x-ray dermitis.

The best treatment is *cryocauterization* with liquid nitrogen. If the warts are few, superficial electrodesiccation suffices.

Verrucae Plana Juvenilis. Since these warts are located mainly on the face and are usually numerous, it is especially necessary to avoid scarring.

Systemic treatments, such as humoral shock by vaccine injections or by autohemotransfusion, can be very effective, probably acting through suggestion. Carteaud also advises dabbing with the following solution:

Lactic acid	10 gm.
Acetic acid	10 gm.
Precipitated sulfur	20 gm.
Glycerin	40 gm.

Verrucae Plantaris. Chemical cauterization or systemic therapy may be effective,

inasmuch as simple suggestion can result in the disappearance of verrucae plantaris, though less often than for verruca vulgaris. But this type of wart most often requires a small operation under local anesthesia with one per cent Xylocaine. The simplest and most effective procedure is, after removing the cornified layer, to scoop out the wart with a *curette* and to *galvanocauterize* or *electrocoagulate* the sides and the bottom of the wound.

Scarification requires three to five weeks; the sooner the patient gets up after the operation, the longer it takes. Two or more days of immobilization are often necessary.

MOLLUSCUM CONTAGIOSUM

Molluscum contagiosum is a benign tumor of the skin, contagious, self-containing, and due to a poxvirus. Typically, it appears as small epithelial tumors with such characteristic appearance that the diagnosis is usually immediate.

From a theoretical point of view, mulluscum contagiosum, like warts, is a particularly interesting disease in that it is caused by a *virus* and it induces *in man a tumoral lesion.* In this respect it is of importance to those cancerologists interested in the possible viral origin of cancer.

However, in man, molluscum contagiosum tumors are always benign and often regress spontaneously. The mechanism of the hyperplastic cell reaction almost certainly differs from that involved in other virus-induced tumors (warts included), for it has been shown that when poxviruses replicate in an infected cell, cellular DNA synthesis is inhibited and cell multiplication ceases (for references, see review by Joklik[14]).

In spite of these remarks it must be recalled that in animals benign tumors due to a pox-like virus also occur (e.g., Shope fibroma in the rabbit; fibromas in deer, hare, and squirrel; Yaba tumor in the rhesus monkey). In the case of Shope fibroma of rabbits malignant evolution of the tumors may be induced by acting on the immunological defenses of the host (cortisone treatment of rabbits, injection of Shope fibroma virus into newborn rabbits) (see Kato et al., 1966).

As for the virus causing the Yaba tumor in the rhesus monkey, it is of interest to note that it is transmissible to man, in whom it induces small histicytomas which regress spontaneously.[12]

Thus from an experimental point of view molluscum contagiosum represents an example of a hyperplastic cell response to a virus in humans, and its study is of theoretical significance in spite of the fact that its characteristics make it, at least for the present, a wholly unique entity.

EPIDEMIOLOGY

Ever since the first clinical description it has been apparent that molluscum contagiosum is infectious and that spread can occur through direct contact, especially when lesions are at the eruptive stage. Intradermal inoculation was achieved by various authors.[17]

True epidemics do occur: Overfield and Brody[16] have recently reported 13 cases among 46 members of eight families in Anchorage, Alaska. No defective hygienic conditions could account for this. All patients were, as is most often the case with this disease, children, their ages ranging from 10 months to 13 years. Duration of the disease ranged from two weeks in the mild cases to 18 months in the more severe attacks. Recurrence occurred in eight of the 13 cases.

Antibody response is usually difficult to elicit, although the level of antibodies detectable by complement fixation was studied in some patients. Early spontaneous regressions have been observed and may be taken as indication of the existence of an immunological response. However, the course of the disease is lengthy, and serological studies are of little help in diagnosis.

DIAGNOSIS

A diagnosis of mulluscum contagiosum must be considered when there are small scattered, rarely single, tumors occurring preferentially on the face (in particular on the eyelids and forehead) and on the genital, anal, and cervical areas, though all cutaneous regions can be affected.

The diagnosis will rest essentially on the characteristic aspect of each cutaneous tumor: small, hemispheric, umbilicated, and hard. The adult element of molluscum contagiosum is in fact a prominent *hemispheric,* well-delimited tumor, varying in volume from 1 mm. in diameter to about the size of a pea (Fig. 35-9). It is pale, rosy-white or milky or more rarely yellowish. Its surface is smooth and shiny except at its summit, where the

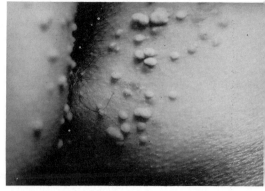

Figure 35-9. Molluscum contagiosum. Macroscopic aspect.

characteristic central *umbilication* appears. Often on small tumors this depression is reduced to a simple dull white, flattened area which the physician must know how to look for.

The consistency of the tumor is smooth and firm. It resists finger pressure, and on firm squeezing it emits a small hard crumbly plug from the central umbilication which, examined under the light microscope, is seen to consist of cornified cells and refringent, ovoid corpuscles, the classic "molluscum corpuscles."

The small immature tumors, the size of the head of a pin, are much more difficult to diagnose, for they lack the umbilication. Diagnosis will be based on their regional topography and dissemination and on their resistence to pressure with the finger.

Secondary inflammation of molluscum contagiosum can cause pruritis, reddening, and formation of a scab. This complication is particularly misleading if the tumor is unique or voluminous. In such a case a pedicle may develop.

Differential Diagnosis. When the tumors are multiple, exhibit the classical umbilication, and are easily enucleated, differential diagnosis is readily made with respect to milium granules, sebaceous adenomas, and hydradenomas, all of which are embedded in the skin, and with verrucae planes, which rest upon the skin.

In the case of an isolated tumor, differential diagnosis may be difficult with respect to keratoacanthoma, a tumor similarly hemispheric and umbilicated but with a horny, wart-like central crater. When the molluscum tumor is inflamed and crusty, it cannot be distinguished from a botriomycoma or an infected molluscum pendulum except by histological examination.

PATHOLOGY

From a pathological point of view, the picture is absolutely characteristic on microscopic examination, even at low power: the normal epithelium which borders the lesion is lifted up by the small subjacent tumor and folded back deeply at this point so as to form an invaginated tumoral epithelium about a crateriform hollow that corresponds to the clinical picture of umbilication (Fig. 35-10).

This invaginated epidermis pushes back the basement membrane (dermoepidermal junction); its profile is lobulated and festooned. These piriform lobules converge toward the horny center of the tumor, where they taper and merge. This alone is typical and allows differentiation from a wart or keratoacanthoma, especially when the "molluscum corpuscles" are hard to see.

From a more *cytological point of view* the malpighian cells constituting the lobules are very hypertrophied; their cytoplasm is pale, their clear contours are lost. As the cells grow further away from the basement membrane, their cytoplasm becomes more and more acidophilic. In fact they accumulate granules which, under the electron microscope, correspond to viral inclusions. In the stratum granulosum these are extremely abundant: they fill the whole cytoplasm, crowding and pushing back the nucleus; the cell, after becoming globular, forms the typical "molluscum corpuscle," which will later be liberated into the crater (Fig. 35-11).

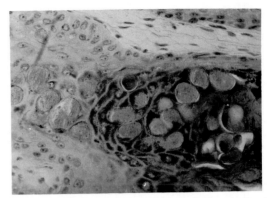

Figure 35-11. Molluscum contagiosum. Detail of the epidermal lesion. × 1150.

ELECTRON MICROSCOPY

Seen under the *electron microscope,* the morphological characteristics of the virus and its cycle of development are spectacular. Indeed the poxviruses lend themselves especially well to ultrastructural studies. They are among the largest viruses (160 to 260 mμ) and, in contrast to most other families of viruses, almost all the stages of viral maturation can be followed morphologically step by step.

Thus the pioneering work of Dourmashkin and Bernhard,[11] confirmed since by Middlekamp and Munger[15] (1964) and Bierwolf et al.,[10] showed that no virus particles are observed in the basal layer and that before the appearance of virus particles proper, plaques of a very finely granular, homogenous substance (the so-called viroplasm) are elaborated at the level of the first cells in the stratum spinosum. This substance is Feulgen positive and corresponds to DNA material of the future virus.

Recently, in studies concerning other poxviruses which follow the same pattern of development, Dales has aptly termed these areas "factory sites" because it is here that viruses will appear and assemble.

It is indeed in the midst of these "factories" that segments of membranes appear and encircle an area of this matrix-like substance. A young slightly ovoid particle, 250 to 300 mμ in size, is thus formed.

As the cells of the pavement epithelium pursue their course toward the upper layers, these particles undergo a series of alterations which terminate in the formation of a complete virus whose central portion (core) is characteristically dumbbell shaped.

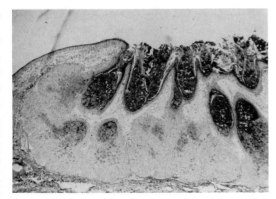

Figure 35-10. Molluscum contagiosum. Histological aspect. × 180.

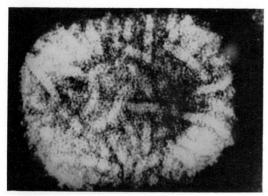

Figure 35-12. Molluscum contagiosum. Causal virus examined under the electron microscope with the negative contrast technique. × 400,000. (Electron micrograph courtesy of Dr. Howatson.)

It is the mass constituted by the accumulation of these viruses in the heart of the viroplasm which makes up the "inclusion bodies" visible in the ordinary microscope which are characteristic of molluscum contagiosum. These inclusion bodies are numerous in each mature tumor.

When the viruses are isolated and examined under the electron microscope, not in thin section within the cell but by the technique of so-called negative staining, the surface structure characteristic of pox-type viruses is seen.

This consists of a criss-crossing of filaments 100 to 120 Å in diameter rolled in counter clockwise spirals which constitute a protein envelope around the central body (DNA) (Fig. 35-12).

From this general description, clinical, histological, and cytological, it appears that diagnosis of mulluscum contagiosum generally poses no problem.

TREATMENT

Treatment consists in scooping out the tumors with a curette and cauterizing the resulting small wound with tincture of iodine, silver nitrate, or 2 per cent zinc chloride.

In the miliary forms, the tumors are too numerous to be removed one by one. Certain systemic treatments can be used, provided they are without danger: sulfonamides, or tetracyclines such as aureomycin at 1 to 1.5 gm. for one or two weeks.

BIBLIOGRAPHY

WARTS

1. Almeida, J. D., Howatson, A. F., and Williams, M. G.: Electron microscope study of human warts; sites of virus production and nature of inclusion bodies. J. Invest. Derm., *38*:337-345, 1962.
2. Ciuffo, G.: Innesto positivo con filtrato di verruca vulgare. G. Ital. Mal. Venereol., *48*:12-17, 1907.
3. Crawford, L. V.: A study of human papilloma virus DNA. J. Molec. Biol., *13*:362-372, 1965.
4. Howatson, A. F.: Viruses connected with tumors and warts. Brit. Med. Bull., *18*:193-198, 1962.
5. Howatson, A. F.: Structure of viruses of the papilloma-polyoma type. J. Molec. Biol., *13*:959-960, 1965.
6. Klug, A., and Finch, J. T.: Structure of viruses of the papilloma-polyoma type. I. Human wart virus. J. Molec. Biol., *11*:403-423, 1965.
7. Rowson, K. E. K., and Mahy, B. W. J.: Human papova (wart) virus. Bact. Rev., *31*:110-131, 1967.
8. Ruiter, M., and Van Mullem, P. J.: Demonstration by electronmicroscopy of an intranuclear virus in epidermodysplasia verruciformis. J. Invest. Derm. *47*:247-252, 1966.
9. Zu Rhein, G. M.: Polyoma-like virions in a human demyelinating disease. Acta Neuropath. (Berlin), *8*:57-68, 1967.

MOLLUSCUM CONTAGIOSUM

10. Bierwolf, D., Randt, A., and Scholz, G.: Vermehrung und Feinstruktur des Molluscum Contagiosum. Arch. Geschwulstforsch., *31*:97-114, 1968.
11. Dourmashkin, R., and Bernhard, W.: A study with the electron microscope of the skin tumor of molluscum contagiosum. J. Ultrastruct. Res., *3*: 11-38, 1959.
12. Grace, J. T., and Mirand, E. A.: Human susceptibility to a simian tumor virus. Ann. N.Y. Acad. Sci., *108*:1123-1128, 1963.
13. Howatson, A. F.: Viruses connected with tumors and warts. Brit. Med. Bull., *18*:193, 1962.
14. Joklik, W. K.: The poxviruses. Bact. Rev., *30*: 33-66, 1966.
15. Middlekamp, J. N., and Munger, B. L.: Ultrastructure and histogenesis of molluscum contagiosum. J. Pediat., *64*:888-905, 1964.
16. Overfield, T. M., and Brody, J. A.: An epidemiological study of molluscum contagiosum in Anchorage, Alaska. J. Pediat. *69*:640, 1966.
17. Wile, U. J., and Kingery, L. B.: The etiology of molluscum contagiosum. Preliminary report of experimental study. J. Cut. Dis., *37*:431, 1919.

PART V

Viral Infections in Which Cardiovascular Manifestations Predominate

36

Viral Infections in Which Cardiovascular Manifestations Predominate

By J. NOUAILLE and M. GAUTIER

Viruses are currently suspected of playing a role in many cardiovascular diseases, including certain chronic diseases without a precise etiology. This paper, however, has intentionally been limited to the clinical description of *acute "primary" myocarditis* and *acute "idiopathic" pericarditis*.

The viral origin of acute "primary" myocarditis has been suspected frequently and has been confirmed in several cases. This section will be followed by a study of endocardial fibroelastosis, which often involves problems of differential diagnosis of myocarditis and difficulties concerning nosological boundaries. Fibroelastosis undoubtedly does not have a single etiology. Recent studies have shown that certain cases may be of viral origin, although this concept is very controversial.

Acute "idiopathic" pericarditis has been demonstrated to have a viral origin in numerous cases.

These sections will be followed, respectively, by studies of myocardial and pericardial involvement during various viral affections. A short supplementary section will deal with cardiac malformations in rubella embryopathies.

ACUTE "PRIMARY" MYOCARDITIS

Acute "primary" myocarditis, is also known as "idiopathic" or "isolated" or Fiedler's myocarditis. These various, partly obsolete, designations are bound to create a confusion in terminology, as they seem to imply an acute inflammation of the myocardium without apparent cause when, in fact, viral origin has been evidenced in various cases. This does not mean that a virus need be the only cause, but it should always be searched for in an acute myocarditis of primary appearance.

The age of onset is variable. Most frequently, it is a disease of newborns and infants, but it can be seen in older children, and some cases in adults have been reported. Sellers and collaborators[43] insist that, beyond the first month of life, when a good many cases can be found as a result of maternal infection at the end of pregnancy, myocarditis occurs irregularly during childhood up to the age of 12 years.

Statistics vary with each author according to whether the data are obtained from departments of obstetrics, pediatrics, or cardiology. Our study in a department of pediatric cardiology covers 55 patients; at discovery of the disease 19 (34 per cent) were less than one year of age, 21 (38 per cent) were one year old, ten (18 per cent) were two years old, two (3 per cent) were three years old, and three (5 per cent) were four years old.

PATHOLOGICAL ANATOMY

Dilation and hypertrophy, particularly of the left ventricle, are seen. Histologically, during the acute phase, impairment is mainly of the myocardium. The impairment is caused by an interstitial infiltration due almost exclusively to mononuclear cells. It is associated with a certain degree of edema, and the myocardial fibers can be necrotic. The endocardium is usually normal, and the pericardium is rarely involved.

Some histological aspects are rarer: we may find disseminated necrotic nodules, not inflammatory or only slightly so, with no infiltration of the neighboring myocardium, which has remained healthy.

The lesions may occasionally predominate in the subendocardial region and, in such cases, be the background for intracavi-

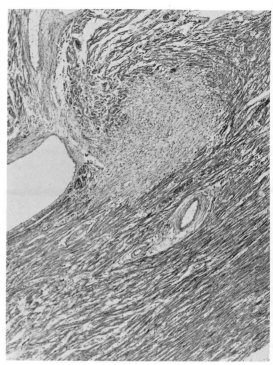

Figure 36-2 Acute myocarditis. Necrotic nodules without inflammatory infiltration. ×70.

tary thromboses (Sanyal), but neither the aortic nor the mitral valve is involved and vascular lesions are lacking.

In a few cases in which Coxsackie infections have been demonstrated, lesions with diffuse cellular necrosis have been found which affected to varying degrees the liver, brain, lungs, kidneys, and other organs.

While the histology of acute myocarditis is well known, there is still some confusion as to the interpretation of the different stages of healing of interstitial myocarditis. It is generally accepted that these inflammatory lesions, together with necrosis of the muscle fibers, may later cause foci of sclerosis. Some aspects of myocardial fibrosis with a minimal inflammatory element have been interpreted as histological stages of healing, although it is not known at what point fibrosis may appear.

Some authors also suggest that fibroelastosis may be a late evolutive aspect of acute myocarditis.

CLINICAL FEATURES

The most typical and often dramatic form is found in the unweaned infant, who,

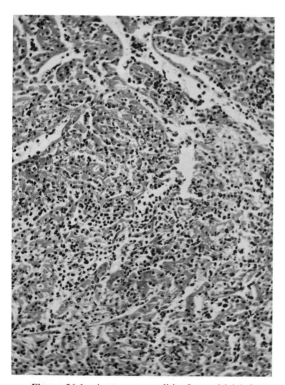

Figure 36-1 Acute myocarditis. Interstitial inflammatory infiltration. ×250.

after being perfectly healthy and eutrophic, abruptly presents the picture of severe cardiac insufficiency.

Although various signs can be misleading diagnostically, three elements point to the heart: dyspnea, tachycardia, and hepatomegaly.

Dyspnea is most often a very marked tachypnea. The respiratory rate may exceed 80 per minute. The infant, obviously very uncomfortable, appears anxious. He is pale, sometimes with a slightly cyanotic or grayish color, covered with sweat, and his appearance can be very alarming. Fairly often, he is in a state of collapse.

Tachycardia is extreme. The pulse, which is weak, is difficult to count, for its speed, confirmed by cardiac auscultation, is 180 to 200 per minute. Cardiac auscultation rarely allows one to perceive anything more than this extremely accelerated and regular rhythm with its dull first sound. A gallop rhythm is frequent but very difficult to perceive and interpret in this accelerated heart. Sometimes a slight systolic murmur can be heard at the apex, but generally auscultation does not give much information.

Hepatomegaly is extremely important, as it reveals the cardiac origin of the tachypnea or tachycardia. The liver is often enlarged. It extends for several fingerbreadths below the costal margin, sometimes below the umbilicus. Palpation is obviously disagreeable and painful, especially when the hepatojugular reflux, often found, is sought.

These signs are often accompanied by edema of the face and the extremities. Oliguria is the rule, and digestive disorders, especially vomiting, are frequent.

Such a picture of serious cardiac insufficiency without fever or often with an inconspicuous elevation in temperature requires, if possible, immediate transfer to the hospital and emergency treatment. Radiological examinations and an electrocardiogram should be executed as soon as possible.

The radiological examination will show that the heart is fully, sometimes enormously, enlarged. The left hand edge may reach the thoracic wall. An important point is that there is no pulmonary hypervascularization, and cardiac insufficiency due to a cardiopathy with a left-to-right shunt can therefore be excluded. Sometimes, however, transparency of the pulmonary fields is diminished by a stasis or edema due to the cardiac insufficiency.

Pleural effusion or even pulmonary localized opacity is fairly frequent.

The electrocardiogram as a rule shows sinus rhythm. This is an important indication which allows the elimination of an acute cardiac failure due to ectopic paroxysmal tachycardia. Descriptions of electrocardiograms vary but they usually agree on two points: the low voltage of the QRS wave in standard and precordial derivations, and modifications of the ST segment and the T wave in the standard and the left precordial leads (flattening or even inversion, albeit slight, of the T wave) accompanied by a positive T wave in the right precordial leads.

Many other anomalies have been described: lengthening of QT; disturbances of auriculoventricular conduction (long PR) or intraventricular conduction giving the appearance of a bundle-branch block. Rhythmic anomalies, occasionally supraventricular tachycardia, or even ventricular tachycardia cause problems of diagnosis. All these signs seem to indicate an infarct or an ischemic lesion in certain precordial derivations. In certain cases the tracings are those of left ventrical overloading with pronounced R waves in V5-V6. The latter appears, as we will see below, much more frequently in fibroelastosis.

To sum up, while the electrocardiogram is often suggestive, it does not necessarily supply the crucial element for diagnosis; it may even confuse the diagnosis. However, it positively localizes the affection in the heart and the myocardium.

EVOLUTION

In a good number of cases the recovery is strikingly rapid after combined treatment by digitalis, diuretics, and corticoadrenal hormones. Within two or three days the condition changes: the heartbeat slows down and the size of the liver becomes normal. Usually, however, it takes weeks and sometimes months for the heart and the electrocardiogram to become normal. One of the first signs of improvement is shown by the electrocardiogram: negativation of T in the right precordial leads while T becomes positive on the left.

During the acute phase there are sometimes complications, in particular embolisms. Even the occurrence of hemiplegia is not exceptional.

Sometimes, treatment cannot prevent

evolution to intractable heart failure and death, which in some forms may occur within a few hours. Even in cases in which the immediate evolution has been favorable, relapses of cardiac failure may occur during the following weeks and months, not necessarily caused by a premature interruption of treatment.

It can even happen that, in spite of an initial improvement, the disease drags on. The heart remains enlarged for months or even for one or two years, and there are successive attacks of cardiac failure. During this period, however, it will be necessary to review the earlier prognosis and the accuracy of the initial diagnosis of acute myocarditis.

Finally, some authors envisage the possibility that an acute myocarditis that was not clinically manifest might be at the origin of so-called chronic cardiomyopathy occurring years later. The viral origin of this still poorly defined entity has not been proved yet but it has not been disproved as a possibility in certain cases.

CLINICAL VARIATIONS

The clinical aspect of onset does not always correspond to the description given above. Very often, onset is less violent. It is known that the infant has not been well for some time and has been coughing for days or even weeks. Since rales have been heard on examination, bronchitis has been assumed. Only when a subsequent clinical examination reveals hepatomegaly is the cardiac disorder recognized.

If this does not occur, the infant who is coughing continually, sometimes even turning slightly cyanotic, will be examined by radiology. The radiological examination shows an enlarged heart, but signs of cardiac insufficiency, in particularly hepatomegaly, are either missing or very discrete.

Sometimes, the enlarged heart is discovered merely by chance during examination for what was believed to be whooping cough or even during examination of an infant who is not well or has digestive disturbances.

Cases have been reported in which the heart had been normal upon first examination and had become enlarged within several days.

Thus the problems of diagnosis arise under very different conditions according to the case.

DIAGNOSIS

When there is acute cardiac failure with an enlarged heart and suggestive electro-cardiographic signs the diagnosis of acute myocarditis must be considered. It will be necessary to eliminate *acute pericarditis* either purulent (pneumococcal, staphylococcal) in the unweaned infant, or viral in the older child. Diagnosis is all the more difficult as the association of pericardial effusion with acute myocarditis is relatively frequent whether the former is part of a generalized edema with pleurisy or a true pericarditis.

Then the other causes of acute cardiac insufficiency must be eliminated:

Noncardiac causes would include acute respiratory syndromes with slowing of the heart, or cardiac insufficiency in acute nephritis, usually accompanied by discrete electrocardiographic signs and very marked edema in the latter, arterial hypertension and more frank urinary signs are present.

An ectopic paroxysmal tachycardic crisis can cause in the infant an abrupt cardiac failure with enlargement of the heart; this stresses the importance of the interpretation of the electrocardiogram.

A congenital cardiac malformation, in particular *coarctation of the aorta,* can bring on abrupt cardiac decompensation. Usually the first manifestations are seen in newborns of about 10 to 15 days old or a little older, and the signs may have various dramatic aspects. The femoral, dorsalis pedis, and posterior tibial pulses are difficult, sometimes even impossible to feel, whereas the radial pulse is normal or even exaggerated. Arterial pressure by the "flush technique" is lower in the legs than in the arms. In the case of cardiac failure, however, all pulses appear weak, especially in the newborn, and the low blood pressure is difficult to take, which often creates a moment of uncertainty.

In some cases, a *cardiopathy with a left-to-right shunt* (ventricular septal defect, patent ductus arteriosus) which can often cause decompensation, in particular during a pulmonary infection, must be eliminated on the basis of auscultation and the radiological aspect of the lungs. Exceptionally a total *aberrant origin of the left coronary artery* may be the cause. This malformation is very rare and as a rule is easy to diagnose by the electrocardiogram, which shows the picture of an anterolateral infarct.

There are some more exceptional diagnoses which are particularly difficult: certain cases of *enlarged "muscular" heart* in which even anatomical verification does not always provide an explanation; cases of *familial cardiomegaly,* the diagnosis of which is based only on the suspicion of earlier cases in the family; cases of *coronary calcification,* in which diagnosis is based on the radiological or histological finding of calcification in other arteries of the body. The rare *glycogen storage disease of the heart* can reveal itself abruptly by a crisis of cardiac insufficiency, but as a rule a certain number of symptoms have already attracted attention: extreme muscular hypotonia, increasing inertia of the newborn leading to quasi-immobility, and macroglossia, which is a frequent and important sign. The electrocardiogram provides a useful element of diagnosis by showing a biventricular hypertrophy predominant on the left side and often a considerable voltage of QRS waves. This diagnosis, often supported by the knowledge of similar cases in the patient's family, is confirmed by muscle biopsy. It can, however, be ruled out after the age of one year, the limit of survival in most cases.

If these different causes have been eliminated, and since rheumatic heart disease is rarely found in very young children (in that case always associated with an endocardial involvement), an isolated enlarged heart probably indicates acute myocarditis, endocardial fibroelastosis, or even myocardial fibrosis, the diagnosis of which is generally made only after histological examination.

Primary Endocardial Fibroelastosis. We have voluntarily expanded this chapter of differential diagnosis of primary acute myocarditis for two reasons: the clinical diagnosis is sometimes difficult, and the importance of viral infections in the still very obscure etiology of endocardial fibroelastosis has been emphasized by several authors. *Pathological anatomy* evidences the complexity of the problem. Basically, there is an *endocardial* lesion composed of fibrosis and elastosis, one often dominant, as their proportions are very variable. These lesions are nearly always localized in the left side of the heart, in the ventricle and the atrium, or in the ventricle alone. The right ventricle is rarely involved.

In their eminent study on 81 cases of chronic fibroelastic myoendocarditis of the newborn and of the infant, Fruhling and collaborators[12] contributed a number of elements on the nature of fibroelastosis, its relation to myocarditis, and its etiology. These authors insist on the practically constant presence of myocardial lesions on histo-

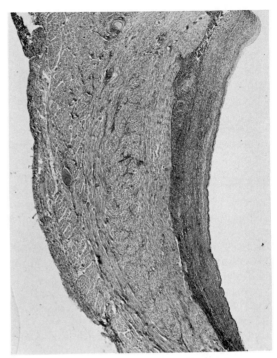

Figure 36-3 Fibroelastosis of the left atrium. ×25.

logical examination. They also assert that the disease, usually called "fibroelastosis of the endocardium," without any degenerative, malformative, or overloading cardiac lesion, might very well be myocarditis, being most frequently interstitial and more rarely degenerative, indicating its inflammatory nature.

In a bacteriological and virological study of 28 cases they found one virus 14 times in at least one organ specimen, 11 times in the heart alone. In 13 cases the virus was a Coxsackie B virus, most often B3 (in three cases the same virus was found in the blood, nose, or feces of the living child).

They emphasize that there are, of course, fibroelastic thickenings of other origin than viral myocarditis. They also consider the possibility that viruses other than those of the Coxsackie group may be found in the myocardium in some cases of fibroelastosis.

Other scientists think that some cases of endocardial fibroelastosis might be the sequelae of myocarditis caused by an enterovirus.[28]

Moreover, Noren and collaborators considered that intrauterine infection with the mumps virus during the first trimester of pregnancy could be an etiological factor in certain cases of fibroelastosis (see Chapter 23).

Undoubtedly, the origin, etiology, and mechanism of formation of fibroelastosis still remain very controversial. There is, however, a striking difference between the histology of acute viral myocarditis, an exclusively inflammatory myocardial lesion, and the histology of fibroelastosis, a predominantly endocardial lesion.

In any case, a viral origin certainly does not account for all cases of fibroelastosis. There is a fibroelastosis "syndrome" in which hemodynamic, anoxic, or other mechanical causes must be taken into consideration. There are, for example, the cases of fibroelastosis which accompany cardiac glycogenesis or an aberrant origin of the left coronary artery. Several cases of cardiac fibroelastosis are known to have occurred in one family.

It is often very difficult to make a differential diagnosis between acute myocarditis and isolated endocardial fibroelastosis. The outcome was used as a basis for diagnosis for a long time: since acute myocarditis can be cured in many cases and since it has been believed that fibroelastosis is nearly without

exception fatal, one was inclined to class as myocarditis all acute primary cardiac insufficiencies in the infant that evolved toward recovery. The problem is certainly more intricate, since some cases of fibroelastosis, histologically confirmed by biopsy in the living patient, have had a clinically favorable evolution.

Moreover, it is necessary to know whether all histological findings of fibroelastosis have the same significance and if the thickness of this alteration does not produce different hemodynamic consequences.

The *clinical picture* often is that of cardiac insufficiency in infants, usually occurring within the first eight months of life. In the study by Fruhling, nearly one-third of the infants were less than three months old and more than half less than six months old, but cases have been known in which the disease has begun in childhood or even later.

The ages of onset in our own series are shown in Table 36-1.

Onset seems to be less sudden than in acute myocarditis. The principal signs are those of all cardiac insufficiencies: dyspnea,

Table 36-1   *Age at Onset in Cases of Proved or Assumed Fibroelastosis*

DECEASED (ANATOMICAL DIAGNOSIS)		
AGE AT ONSET	AGE AT DEATH	AUSCULTATION*
2 days	1 mon.	SS3
1 mo.	8 mo.	0
1 mo.	5 yr.	SS3
2 mo.	4 yr.	SS
3 mo.	4 yr.	SS2
1 yr.	3 yr.	0
4 yr.	7 yr.	SS2
6 yr.	12 yr.	SS3

LIVING (CLINICAL DIAGNOSIS)			
		AUSCULTATION*	
AGE AT ONSET	PRESENT AGE	At Onset	At Present
2 mo.	7 yr.	SS2-3	SS5
2 mo.	2 yr.	0	Clinical cure
2 mo.	18 mo.	0	Clinical cure
2 mo.	7 mo.	0	0
3 mo.	2 yr.	0	0
3 mo.	6 mo.	0	0
4 mo.	2 yr.	0	0
5 mo.	13 mo.	SS2	SS2
5 mo.	9 yr.	SS4	SS1
6 mo.	2 yr.	0	0
6 mo.	1 yr.	0	0
11 mo.	2 yr.	SS2	SS2
12 mo.	30 mo.	0	0

*SS: Systolic murmur (souffle systolique), noted, according to degree of intensity, from 1 to 5.

tachycardia, hepatomegaly, and enlarged heart.

The sounds are often dull, sometimes in gallop rhythm, and a systolic murmur is heard at the apex in many cases, for the mitral valve is often affected. Involvement of the aortic valve is much rarer.

The electrocardiogram often provides the best diagnostic elements (Sellers et al., Kitlak). In the most clear-cut cases, it reveals a ventricular overloading of the left side with an increase in the R wave greater than 20 mm. in the left precordial leads (V5, V6), very often an increase in S in V1, a deep Q wave, greater than 3 mm., in V5 and V6, and a flattening or, even more often, a pronounced inversion of T in V5 and V6. In some cases, the auricular P wave is unusually high. This aspect differs considerably from the usual descriptions of acute myocarditis (low voltage in the standard leads, absence of increased voltage in R_{V6} and S_{V1}, absence of a deep Q wave in V6, and a T wave only flattened or slightly negative in the left precordial leads).

Because tracings may be atypical in either disease, the problem is not simple. Very often, modification in repolarization due to digitalin can make interpretation of tracings difficult. Apparently, not all cases of fibroelastosis yield the same electrocardiographic picture; in our short series of cases these electrocardiographic criteria were rarely found together. Repolarization disturbances in the left precordial leads are not constant, and in the course of the disease signs on the right side can appear, creating an aspect of biventricular overloading.

The clinical and evolutive aspect of fibroelastosis is not uniform. Onset may seem very sudden, creating within a few hours the picture of severe cardiac failure in an infant apparently healthy until then. It may also, as in the case of myocarditis, appear after a period of days, or even weeks, of digestive disorders, failure to grow, or respiratory disturbances. The differential diagnosis may be suggested only upon the discovery of an enlarged heart, without obvious signs of cardiac failure, in an infant or even a small tachypneic child.

The evolution itself can be dramatic, leading to death within a few days, but treatment may also bring about a more or less lasting improvement. Apparently, even in cases showing all the usual diagnostic criteria of fibroelastosis, extended treatment (18 months to two years or more) can bring about cure or at least the disappearance of the functional signs, return to normal size of the heart, and normalization of the electrocardiogram. Manning and Keith believe that 75 per cent of all patients with clinically diagnosed fibroelastosis of the endocardium can survive with extended digitalis treatment. They stop treatment two years after the disappearance of symptoms, maintenance of the cardiothoracic ratio at 55 per cent or less, and the reappearance of positive T waves in the left precordial leads.

Benichoux and collaborators claim similar results with powdering of the pericardium with talc. Diagnosis was then based only on a surgically obtained auricular biopsy.

This demonstrates how difficult it can be to decide whether an infant with cardiac insufficiency and an enlarged heart (even when the heart is back to normal size) has had myocarditis or fibroelastosis. The various arguments that may influence an over-all study are of little help in the single case.

This is why the study of Noren and collaborators, published in 1963, aroused great interest. They describe a positive reaction to mumps antigen in nine children apparently suffering from fibroelastosis. Many studies have since shown highly divergent results. Some authors[44, 47] have found a high percentage of positive reactions, whereas others[15] have not. The reason for this variety of results might be found in the different criteria applied to determine the positive cutaneous reactions. Moreover, no correlation was found with serological tests made simultaneously; these were most often negative. Interrogation has not generally confirmed the supposition that this disease may be due to a mumps infection contracted *in utero*. The interpretation of the cutaneous reaction will undoubtedly be elucidated in the future.

There still are problems of diagnosis in certain cases. Fairly often, primary endocardial fibroelastosis involves the mitral or aortic valve. In this case, diagnosis has to deal with an enlarged heart with a mitral or aortic valve souffle. It is difficult to know whether cardiomegaly and cardiac failure are due to a congenital valvular malformation or, instead, whether a primary endocardial fibroelastosis is involved with extension to a valvular apparatus complex.

There are also rare forms of fibroelastosis of the right ventricle which of course do not manifest the same electrocardiographic signs as the usual fibroelastosis involving the cavities of the left side.

VIRUSES AND MYOCARDITIS

Many viruses have been suspected of being the cause of myocardial involvement, but repeated proof exists only for Coxsackie viruses.

Among them, the most often identified belong to Coxsackie group B. It seems that Coxsackie B viruses, and perhaps types B3 and B4 more often than the others, are responsible for cases in newborns when the mother has been infected by the same virus toward the end of pregnancy. Coxsackie A has rarely been incriminated.

It is known that newborn white mice inoculated with Coxsackie B or type I reovirus contract a systemic disease with myocarditis. The electron microscope shows the virus in the heart.

Possibly, age may have an important influence on infection with Coxsackie B in man as well as in the mouse: the myocardium is most often affected in newborns and infants, whereas generally only the pericardium is affected in older children and adults.

Many viral diseases other than Bornholm's disease may be accompanied by cardiovascular, particularly myocardial, signs. In very rare cases some of these viruses may have been at the origin of apparently isolated myocarditis; in other cases myocardial involvement has occurred in the course of a viral disease. In reference to Pankey's recent general review, we will enumerate the principal viral affections possibly accompanied by myocardial manifestations. Very often, the only manifestation is an electrocardiographic modification which does not necessarily imply an anatomical alteration of the myocardium.

The electrocardiogram during *poliomyelitis* frequently shows irregularities, and some authors have described a good number of cases of myocarditis in the fatal forms of poliomyelitis (Marinesco et al.). However, polioviruses have rarely been isolated from the myocardium. Moreover, most cardiac, and even histological, manifestations are very difficult to interpret because of the general disorders and the repercussions of involvement of the bulbar centers on the myocardium.

During *influenza,* the virus may cause pericarditis but it does not necessarily affect the myocardium. According to Pankey, the higher mortality from influenza among patients with heart disease cannot be explained by myocarditis or pericarditis alone, but toxic effects of the virus may be the cause.

During *infectious hepatitis,* practically the only signs reported have been electrocardiographic abnormalities, most often affecting the T wave.

A recent study by Hoagland reported the possibility of electrocardiographic disturbances during *infectious mononucleosis* (6 per cent of the cases in his study); the majority consisted of modifications of the T wave. One of his patients, however, maintained a nodal rhythm and, ten years later, he had a complete right bundle branch block. Hoagland reported that necropsy studies did not show any significant cardiac involvement during mononucleosis.

Cases of myocarditis during *mumps* have been reported but they seem to be rare. Electrocardiographic abnormalities, however, are rather frequent, particularly in adults.

During *measles,* apart from fairly frequent electrocardiographic abnormalities, real myocardial complications are exceptional, but a few cases have been reported.

One case of myocarditis during *German measles* has been seen in an adult (Bianchi, quoted by Pankey). Recent studies have shown that rubella viruses may play a role in some cases of neonatal myocarditis (see Chapters 27 and 61).

Cases of myocarditis and even pancarditis occurring during *varicella* and also after *smallpox vaccination* have been reported occasionally.

ACUTE "IDIOPATHIC" PERICARDITIS

This disease is also called "acute benign pericarditis." Just as with acute "primary" myocarditis, terminology is not precisely defined and a number of cases with proved viral origin might well be called "viral pericarditis," although this etiology has been proved in only a relatively limited number of cases.

CLINICAL FEATURES

This disease is most frequently seen in young adults. It occurs rarely during adolescence or childhood, and only exceptionally in infancy. It sometimes appears in an "epidemic" environment, e.g., during an epidemic of Bornholm's disease or influenza, but most often cases occur sporadically. It usually occurs a few days or weeks after an infection of the upper respiratory tract, an influenza-like disease, or a pneumopathy.

The onset of pericarditis is marked by fever; respiratory difficulties, occasionally intense; and precordial pain, often fairly violent; this pain can be constrictive and, in the adult, suggests a myocardial infarct. Sometimes, the pain is not purely thoracic but extends to the shoulder or to the abdomen, suggesting a condition requiring surgery.

Very often, a pericardial friction rub can be heard. The heart is enlarged, sometimes barely perceptibly. This is often accompanied either by pleural effusion, the presence of which is rather suggestive, or by parenchymatous condensation.

Electrocardiographic signs correspond to what has been described for all types of acute pericarditis, i.e., anomalies especially of the ST segment.

On the whole, a fairly ordinary picture of acute pericarditis is seen. The usual laboratory examinations are of no major help in the orientation of the etiological investigation: leukocytosis with polymorphonuclear leukocytes is not rare; the sedimentation rate is often accelerated with an increase in fibrinemia; sometimes, these biological reactions are so extremely marked that they misleadingly suggest suppuration. Virological investigations may subsequently provide elements for diagnosis, but not always.

EVOLUTION

Generally, pericarditis evolves spontaneously toward recovery within several weeks, but a few points must be noted.

Evolution is greatly shortened by treatment with corticosteroids, combined with a broad-spectrum antibiotic.

Evolution is often characterized by relapses and recurrences, which vary in number and rhythm. This tendency to recur, common to all pericardial localizations whatever their origin (viral, rheumatic, or other) can be seen over a period of months or even years; the intervals usually get longer and longer as time passes.

Electrocardiographic signs may take a long time to disappear.

Complications may occur; acute compression of the heart ("tamponade") due to an extreme abundance of effusion may necessitate a pericardial tap, but this is very exceptional.

Later on, adhesions may occur and signs of constrictive pericarditis can occur sometimes even fairly rapidly. Therefore, some authors consider the possibility that a viral pericarditis which was not recognized in its acute phase may be the cause of constrictive pericarditis of mysterious etiology which occurs later.

Myocardial involvement thus seems to be fairly frequent during pericarditis. Usually, it is suspected rather than confirmed, as one is limited to electrocardiographic signs which are difficult to interpret. Fatal cases, however, have shown simultaneous lesions of acute myocarditis and of the pericardium. Some authors even use the expressions myopericarditis and perimyocarditis; these terms are rejected by others.

DIAGNOSIS

The diagnosis of pericarditis is most delicate. In the child and infant, the first problem will be to eliminate myocarditis or other causes of an enlarged heart. Once pericarditis is affirmed other possibilities must be eliminated.

In the Infant. Purulent pericarditis, at this age more frequent than idiopathic pericarditis, is a possibility.

In the Child and the Adolescent. Tubercular pericarditis must be eliminated before hormone therapy can be undertaken. The pericarditis of disseminated lupus erythematosus and of Still's disease can be very difficult to diagnose if the pericardial involvement is the first manifestation of the disease, but must also be eliminated. Rheumatic pericarditis is so difficult to diagnose that many cases of viral pericarditis are at first thought to be rheumatic. The absence of arthralgia, of a definite increase in antistreptolysins, and of signs of endocardial involvement provides very valuable arguments, but by no means crucial, as these elements may be absent or appear much later in rheumatic fever. Considering the frequency of severe forms of rheumatic carditis which accompany pericardial involvement, it seems preferable to err by excess in making a diagnosis of rheumatic pericarditis.

In the Adult. In addition to the different kinds of pericarditis, it is possible because of the precordial pain and electrocardiographic alteration relevant to repolarization, to make an erroneous diagnosis of myocardial infarct. An important sign is that in pericarditis the Q wave of necrosis is absent.

VIRUSES AND PERICARDITIS

As with primary myocarditis, several viruses have been suggested as the cause of "idiopathic" pericarditis, in particular *Coxsackie B viruses*, mostly B5 but also the other types B. More rarely, the role of *type A Coxsackie viruses* has been reported.

The *influenza virus* seems to play some role. Hildebrand and collaborators[19] reported a case in which an influenza A2 virus was isolated from the pericardial fluid of a 5-year-old girl who had an acute tamponade syndrome.

Type 3 adenovirus has exceptionally been reported to be the cause of acute pericarditis in the adult.

Among viral infections, it is customary to report pericarditis accompanying Bornholm's disease and pericarditis with influenza. Pericardial signs are still reported during infectious hepatitis, infectious mononucleosis, varicella, and so forth.

Before attributing a viral origin to myocarditis or pericarditis, very strict criteria must be applied, for many viral infections (enteroviruses, respiratory viruses) frequently have no clinical manifestations and the presence of such a virus can be pure coincidence.

CARDIAC MALFORMATIONS IN RUBELLA EMBRYOPATHIES

Congenital cardiopathy is most often part of a picture seen in premature or small full-term newborns. It is certainly the main manifestation of congenital rubella, since it is seen in more than half of the cases, even in two out of three. The given figures vary considerably according to the author. Until recent years the problem was very intricate, on the one hand because of the difficulty in making a definite clinical diagnosis of rubella in the mother, on the other hand because of the existence of unapparent rubella.

The technique of isolating the virus in tissue cultures of monkey kidney cells, where its presence is revealed by its interference with ECHO 11 virus, represents enormous progress. During the 1964-1965 epidemic in the United States this permitted the description of a clinical syndrome, until then unknown, in newborns whose mothers had contracted rubella in the first months of pregnancy. Some of the malformations concern the cardiovascular system: alterations in the renal arteries and lesions of the myocardial fibers.

The more recently acquired possibility of easily titrating hemagglutination-inhibiting antibodies will certainly solve many problems in the coming years.

Before the virus was isolated, the persistence of patent ductus arteriosus was attributed with certainty to rubella if it was associated with cataract or with deaf mutism. This cardiopathy is by far the most frequent. In second place comes pulmonary stenosis, usually valvular. The constriction is slight but can involve the whole pulmonary arterial tree and cause a tiered stenosis of the branches. When the constriction is not great, the association of patent ductus arteriosus and pulmonary stenosis is considered a quasispecific unit of congenital rubella. Other cardiopathies are possible, in particular ventricular septal defect, either isolated or associated with a patent ductus arteriosus, but also any type of cardiopathy.

The reasons why patent ductus arteriosus is seen so often are not evident, as it is not actually a malformation. The rubella virus shows a predilection for vascular endothelium, creating lesions of the intima in the renal and pulmonary arteries. The virus is believed to cause histological impairment of the ductus arteriosus, which is of primary importance to fetal circulation. This impairment hinders normal closing of the ductus in the first weeks of life, as it is well known that viremia exists in the newborn at birth and can last for several months. Inhibition of mitosis at this level, as has been seen with several organs in vitro, is a possibility. This mechanism does not account for more complex congenital cardiopathies such as the tetralogy of Fallot.

The myocardial lesions reported by Korones seem to be much rarer. Histologic examination shows considerable necrosis without inflammation. Infarctus-type electrocardiographic tracings at birth can evolve toward scarring. Neonatal cardiac insufficiency may improve, but the heart remains enlarged. These new facts about rubella are very interesting in themselves, and also because it is likely that other viral infections of the mother can cause similar or identical lesions, particularly cardiac malformations. But all this has not yet been proved.

BIBLIOGRAPHY

1. Aronson, S. R., and Lepow, M. L.: The effect of repeated mumps skin test on skin sensitivity to mumps antigen. Pediatrics, *36*:422, 1965.
2. Bain, H. W., McLean, D. M., and Walker, S. J.: Epidemic pleurodynia (Bornholm disease) due to Coxsackie B-5 virus. The interrelationship of pleurodynia, benign pericarditis, and aseptic meningitis. Pediatrics, *27*:889, 1961.
3. Bell, J. F., and Meis, A.: Pericarditis in infection due to Coxsackie virus group B. type 3. New Eng. J. Med., *261*:126, 1959.
4. Benichoux, R., Lascombes, G., and Gentin, G.: Traitement de la fibro-élastose du nourrisson par le talcage du péricarde. Arch. Franc. Pédiat., *17*:1060, 1960.
5. Burch, G. E., and DePasquale, N. P.: Viral endocarditis. Amer. Heart J., *67*:721, 1964.
6. Cayler, G. G., Taybi, H., Riley, H. D., Jr., and Simon, J. L.: Pericarditis with effusion in infants and children. J. Pediat., *63*:264, 1963.
7. Christian, H. A.: Nearly ten decades of interest in idiopathic pericarditis. Amer. Heart J., *42*:645, 1951.
8. Christiaens, L., Dupuis, C., Nuyts, J. P., Delomez, M., and Itsweire, A.: Le pronostic de la fibro-élastose. (A propos de 12 observations). Arch. Mal. Coeur, *58*:1616, 1965.
9. Fontaine, G.: Les myocardites aigues primitives du nourrisson. Presse Méd., *71*:1477, 1963.
10. Fontan, A., Verger, P., and Battin, J. J.: Péricardite aigue et virus Coxsackie. Intensité des réactions biologiques inflammatoires. Arch. Franc. Pédiat., *21*:561, 1964.
11. Fowler, N. O.: Classification and differential diagnosis of the cardiomyopathies. Progr. Cardiov. Dis., *7*:1-16, 1964.
12. Fruhling, L., Korn, R., Lavillaureix, J. Surjus, A., and Foussereau, S.: La myo-endocardite chronique fibro-élastique du nouveau-né et du nourrisson (fibro-élastose). Données morphologiques, étiologiques et pathogéniques nouvelles. Rapports aves certaines malformations cardiaques. Ann. Anat. Path., (Paris), *7*:227, 1962.
13. Gaillard, L., Cahen, P., Perrin, A., Delphin, D., and Lafond, H.: Myocardite interstitielle primitive d'un type anatomique rare. Pédiatrie, *14*:431, 1959.
14. Gérard, R., Payan, H., and Benyamine, R.: Cardiomégalie primitive et fibro-élastose localisée à l'oreillette gauche chez un adulte jeune. Presse Méd., *69*:1145, 1961.
15. Gersony, W. M., Katz, S. L., and Nadas, A. S.: Endocardial fibro-élastosis and mumps virus. Pediatrics, *37*:430, 1966.
16. Giles, J. P., Cooper, L. Z., and Krugman, S.: The rubella syndrome. J. Pediat., *66*:434, 1965.
17. Grenier, B.: Les myocardites aigues primitives de l'enfant et le virus Coxsackie. Paris, Masson et Cie, 1958.
18. Harvey, W. P., Segal, J. P., and Gurel, T.: The clinical spectrum of primary myocardial disease. Progr. Cardiov. Dis., *7*:17-42, 1964.
19. Hildebrandt, H. M., Maassab, H. F., and Willis, P. W.: Influenza virus pericarditis. Amer. J. Dis. Child., *104*:579, 1962.
20. Hoagland, R. J.: Mononucleosis and heart disease. Amer. J. Med. Sci., *248*:1, 1964.
21. Keith, J. D., Rowe, R. D., and Vlad, P.: Heart Disease in Infancy and Childhood. New York, MacMillan Co., 1958.
22. Kitlak, W.: Zur Diagnostik und Therapie der Myokardose mit Endocardfibroelastose. Arch. Kinderheilk. *171*:276, 1964.
23. Korones, S. B., Ainger, L. E., Monif, G. R. G., Roane, J., Sever, J. L., and Fuste, F.: Congenital rubella syndrome. Study of 22 infants. Amer. J. Dis. of Child., *110*:434, 1965.
24. McCue, C. M.: Three cases of myocarditis in children less than one year of age. Pediatrics, *21*:710, 1958.
25. Manning, J. A., and Keith, J. D.: Fibroelastosis in children. Progr. Cardiov. Dis., *7*:172-178, 1964.
26. Manning, J. A.. Sellers, F. J., Bynum, R. S., and Keith, J. D.: The medical management of clinical endocardial fibro-elastosis. Circulation, *29*:60, 1964.
27. Marinesco, G., Truco, I., Friedman, I., Ciurezo, D., and Draganesco, N.: La myocardite poliomyélitique. Etude anatomo-clinique. Sem. Hop. Paris, *33*:1280 S.P. 212-1289 S.P. 221, 1957.
28. Mehrizi, A., Hutchins, G. M., Mediaris, D. N., Jr., and Rowe, R. D.: Entero virus infection and endocardial fibro-elastosis. Circulation, *32*:Suppl. 2, Abstracts of the 38th Scientific Session, 1965.
29. Nadas, A. S.: Pediatric Cardiology. Philadelphia, W. B. Saunders Co., 1963.
30. Naye, R. L., and Blanc, W.: Pathogenesis of congenital rubella. J.A.M.A., *194*:277, 1965.
31. Noren, G. R., Adams, P., Jr., and Anderson, R. C.: Positive skin reactivity to mumps virus antigen in endocardial fibro-elastosis. J. Pediat., *62*:604, 1963.
32. Pankey, G. A.: Effect of viruses on the cardiovascular system. Amer. J. Med. Sci. *250*:103-114, 1965.
33. Papanicolis, I., Chakacopos, S., Michalopoulos, J., and Gorgoulas, A.: Les myocardites aigues primitives de l'enfance. Arch. Franç. Pédiat., *21*:705, 1964.
34. Pruitt, R. D.: Acute myocarditis in the adult. Progr. Cardiov. Dis., *7*:73-82, 1964.
35. Rabin, E. R., and Melnick, J. L.: Experimental acute myocarditis. Progr. Cardiov. Dis., *7*:65-72, 1964.
36. Rosenbaum, H. D., Nadas, A. S., and Neuhauser, E. B. D.: Primary myocardial disease in infancy and childhood. Amer. J. of Dis. of Child., *86*:44, 1953.
37. Rosenberg, H. S., and McNamara, D. G.: Acute myocarditis in infancy and childhood. Progr. Cardiov. Dis., *7*:179-197, 1964.
38. Sacrez, R., Beauvais, P., and Klein, F.: La fibro-élastose endocardique. Méd. Infant (Paris), *71*:419, 1964.
39. Sanghui, L. M., and Misra, S. N.: ECG abnormalities in epidemic hepatitis. Circulation, *16*:88, 1957.
40. Sanyal, S. K.: Fatal myocarditis in an adolescent caused by Coxsackie virus, group B, type four. Pediatrics, *35*:36, 1965.
41. Saphir, O., Wile, S. A., and Reingold, I. M.: Myocar-

ditis in children. Amer. J. Dis. of Child., *67*:294, 1944.

42. Schneegans, E., Zimmermann, C. H., and Vrousos, E.: Un cas probable de fibro-élastose du nourrisson reconnu du vivant du malade. Evolution. Arch. Franç. Pediat., *2*:987, 1965.

43. Sellers, F. J., Keith, J. D., and Manning, J. A.: The diagnosis of primary endocardial fibro-elastosis. Circulation, *29*:49, 1964.

44. Shone, J. D., Muñoz Armas, S., Manning, J. A., and Keith, J. D.: Mumps antigen skin test in endocardial fibro-elastosis. Pediatrics, *37*:423, 1966.

45. Surjus, A.: Les maladies à virus coxsackie. Etude générale. Path. Biol. Sem. Hop. (Paris), *10*:1587, 1962.

46. Surjus, A., Lausecker, C. H., Reeb, E., and Lavillaureix, J.: Les maladies à virus Coxsackie en Alsace. Epidémiologie et gravité au cours des années 1956 à 1961. Path. Biol. Sem. Hop. (Paris), *11*:149-161, 1963.

47. Vosburgh, J. B., Diehl, A. M., Liu, C., Lawer, R. M., and Fabiyi, A.: Relationship of mumps to endocardial fibro-elastosis. Amer. J. Dis. Child., *109*: 69, 1965.

48. Warembourg, H., Lekiefre, J., and Bertrand, M.: Les myocardo-péricardites grippales. (A propos d'une observation à virus grippal de type A.) Lille Méd., *9*:160, 1964.

49. Wilson, D. R., Lenke, S. C., and Paterson, J. F.: Acute constrictive epicarditis following infectious mononucleosis. Case report. Circulation, *23*:257, 1961.

50. Woodward, T. E., McCrumb, F. R., Carey, T. N., and Togo, Y.: Viral and rickettsial causes of cardiac disease including the Coxsackie virus etiology of pericarditis and myocarditis. Ann. Intern. Med., *53*:1130, 1960.

37

Laboratory Diagnosis During Cardiovascular Manifestations of Viral Infections

By A. BOUE

CRITERIA FOR VIROLOGICAL DIAGNOSIS OF MYOCARDITIS AND PERICARDITIS

The criteria for diagnosis are *virological*—isolation of the virus either from the pericardial fluid or from heart tissues (biopsy, necropsy); *serological*—appearance of antibodies against the virus recognized as being responsible or a significant increase in their titer; and *epidemiological*—several cases of the same syndrome during the same viral epidemic.

Although· numerous viruses have been held responsible for cardiovascular affections, reliable virological proof has been given only as concerns viruses of the Coxsackie B group. Thus, specimen taking for the purpose of establishing a biological diagnosis of Coxsackie B virus infection is what must currently be envisaged. If clinical, or especially epidemiological, consideration can orient the search for other viral infections (influenza, for example), specimens must be taken under conditions described in the chapters concerning those viruses.

Collection of Specimens for Virus Isolation. Since Coxsackie viruses belong to the enterovirus group, specimens taken from the throat and the stools will for the most part be used in a search for the virus.

It is very important to take specimens not only from the patient himself, and this as early as possible, but also from the mother if the patient is a newborn, or from persons in contact with the patient (family, schoolmates).

Elimination of virus in the throat and in the feces may already have ceased by the time a viral origin has been suggested in connection with cardiac manifestations. One can hope to find in the patient's human surroundings subjects infected later or who are still eliminating the virus.

Obviously, it is very important to be able to perform virological examinations on pathological specimens (pericardial effusion fluid) or on cardiac tissue fragments taken at autopsy.

Samples of serum should be taken, the first as early as possible, the second about three weeks later. (See Chapter 3 on enteroviruses for techniques of collection of specimens and conservation).

Interpretation of Results. There is no need to insist on the importance of the isolation of virus either from the pericardial fluid or from heart tissues taken at autopsy. Titration of virus should be done, a high titer of virus confirming the affinity of the virus for these tissues.

Most often, however, the search for a virus can be done only on specimens from the throat or in feces. While a negative result (especially in the case of late specimen taking) does not eliminate the possibility of a viral origin, the isolation of virus poses the problem of the role of the existing viral infection in the cardiac manifestations. In this case, exact typing of the virus is an important element, since observations reported during recent years have shown that Coxsackie B viruses (especially B2 and B5) are most often isolated in the case of cardiac manifestations.

Virus isolation is all the more important in that it permits serological examination which, without virus isolation, would be very difficult to orient. For the study of Coxsackie viruses, serological reactions are specific only for a single type of virus, so that the first necessity is exact identification of the virus.

It is for this reason that a virological study of the surrounding people should be done systematically. Besides the epidemiological interest, it is a means of identifying the virus which has spread throughout the community and can have affected the individual. Knowing the type of the virus makes it possible to titrate the neutralizing antibodies (particularly for the Coxsackie B viruses). The appearance of these antibodies, or a significant increase in their titer, is a sign of viral infection, as is the presence of complement-fixing antibodies.

Besides the data supplied by laboratory examinations, observation of similar cases of cardiac manifestations in the same area during the same viral epidemic is one of the best criteria for affirming the viral origin of such syndromes.

CONGENITAL RUBELLA

We now have at hand laboratory techniques which permit the affirmation of congenital rubella. This diagnosis can be made either by isolating the rubella virus or by serological tests.

Isolating Rubella Virus. It is now known that the virus is present in the throat at birth and during the first months of life. However, it is during the first weeks of life that chances of isolating the virus are greatest. Therefore, a search is to be made only in cases detected very early and after agreement with the laboratory susceptible of isolating this virus (see Rubella: Clinical Features in Chapter 27).

Serological Tests. Normally, antibody transmitted by the mother to the newborn will disappear during the first six months of life. Dudgeon (see Chapter 61) has shown that, in congenital rubella, rubella virus-neutralizing antibodies persist beyond the first six months and into the first years of life, evidence that the child synthesizes antibodies as early as birth and probably during fetal life. The presence of a high titer of these antibodies and their persistence beyond the first six months of life therefore permit retrospective diagnosis of congenital rubella.

With the results of laboratory tests, it is therefore possible to make a differential diagnosis of congenital rubella. This etiological diagnosis can be a great help in comforting parents who are worried about the prognosis for other pregnancies.

PART VI

Viral Infections in Which Respiratory Manifestations Predominate

38

Introduction

By J. COUVREUR

FREQUENCY OF VIRAL RESPIRATORY INFECTIONS

The concept of viral respiratory infection and pneumopathy existed before the actual causal agents were known. Cases of viral pneumopathy were originally diagnosed by excluding bacterial infections, not by isolating pneumotropic viruses. Thus, the picture of primary atypical pneumonia was described and the term came into current usage to refer to a picture that could not be accounted for by any bacterial infection.

The discovery, by Smith, Andrewes, and Laidlaw,[23] of the influenza virus and its culture[4] marked the beginning of a new era in understanding of viral respiratory infections. The observations made by British workers concerning epidemics of "febrile catarrh" among young military recruits and school children drew attention to the clinical syndromes associated with various forms of acute respiratory infection. During World War II, studies carried out by the American Commission on Acute Respiratory Diseases showed that acute respiratory disease (ARD) could be transmitted to volunteers under conditions that suggested viral etiology.[10]

Similar observations were made with regard to virus pneumopathy. Despite the difficulties encountered, it was thought at the time to be possible to distinguish clearly between ARD, the common cold, and virus pneumopathy. The most spectacular progress due to Enders' discovery was probably that made since 1950 in the study of respiratory infections. Since then, it has been recognized that six large groups of viruses are capable of causing infections and almost all of them include a great number of serotypes. Owing to clinical, virological and epidemiological studies carried out in collectivities (military recruits, nurseries, schools, hospitals), and also to inoculation experiments in volunteers, progress has been achieved in the identification of some clinical pictures. However, the manifestations induced by the various agents isolated are often similar. Although the clinician can now recognize some well-defined clinical pictures, such as herpangina, pharyngoconjunctival fever, and fatal adenovirus pneumopathy, he still depends very much on the virologist and the epidemiologist to identify precisely most virus respiratory infections. However, statistical data provided by epidemiologists are of little avail in the study of a particular case. On the whole, the prognosis of respiratory virus infections is excellent, and in current practice study of a given patient generally does not require complex and expensive investigations. Clinical research is pursued less than ecological studies, and the studies undertaken now are mainly aimed at discovering a treatment, and especially at prophylaxis by vaccines able to protect certain groups of exposed subjects.

Viruses are the major cause of respiratory infections. Dingle and Feller[11] estimate that they are the causal agent in 66 per cent of the cases. Because of specific therapies, bacteria now occupy only a modest place, as shown by Beem et al.[3]; in 1960, Evans[12] indicated that bacteria are responsible for only 10 per cent of respiratory infections. In a recent investigation carried out in Great Britain on 1888 children under 16 years of

Table 38-1. *Investigations on the Viral Origin of Respiratory Infections*

Authors	Geographic Location, Period of Study	No. of Cases	Monotypical %	Mixed %	*Myxovirus influenzae*	*Myxovirus parainfluenzae*	*Respiratory Syncytial Virus*	*Adenoviruses*	*Enteroviruses*	*Coxsackie Virus*	*ECHO Viruses*	*Herpes Virus*	*Rhinoviruses*	*Reoviruses*	*Mumps Virus*	*Unidentified*	*Mycoplasma pneumoniae*
Hilleman et al.[17]	Philadelphia, Pa. (U.S.A.) 1959-1960	153 adults / 667 children and infants (10% hospitalized)	19.9 / 30.7	5.1	3.2 / 2.6	1.9 / 5.5	17.2	0.6 / 5.1					14.2 / 4.8	0.1			
Robinson et al.[22]	Atlanta, Ga. (U.S.A.) 1958-1959	125 children and adults	20		4	14.4		0.8		1.6						2.6	
Wenner et al.[27]	Kansas (U.S.A.)	194 hospitalized infants and children	11.9	1.5	1	7.2		2.6								0.6	
Tobin[25]	Manchester (U.K.) 1962-1963	801 hospitalized children	34		2.1	6.4	21	3.6									
Clarke et al.[9]	Bristol (U.K.) 1961-1963	334 (296 children) (general practice and hospital)	38	1.2	7.1	9.5	8.6	5	1.4			3.2				0.2	
Wulf et al.[29]	Kansas (U.S.A.) 1961-1962	114 hospitalized children	51	1.7	13	12	16	4						4	0.8	1.7	
Chanock and Parrott[8]	Washington, D.C. (U.S.A.) 1957-1964	7938 children (in collectivities and hospital patients)	44		<0.5	4	29.6	5.5		0.8			4.4				
Medical Research Council[21]	Great Britain 1961-1964	1888 children and adults (general practice)	24	1.5	1.8	3.2	3	4.5	4.9			1.5	4.1			0.8	
Banatvala et al.[2]	Cambridge (U.K.) 1962-1963	195 children and adults	50.3		28.7	17.9	1.5	2.1									4.6
Gwaltney and Jordan[15]	Virginia (U.S.A.)	286 students above 17 years of age	12.9						0.3	0.6			11.5				0.3

*Diagnosis of viral infection based on isolation of the virus, serology, or both.

age with respiratory infection and living at home, a virus was isolated in 23.6 per cent of the cases and a hemolytic streptococcus, the most common among pathogenic bacteria in children, in 6.7 per cent of the cases. Chanock and Parrott,[8] after seven years of investigations involving 7938 children with respiratory disease reported that a virus was isolated in 44 per cent of the patients but only 8.2 per cent of the control subjects. A significant increase in antibodies was found in 41.7 per cent of the patients and 13.3 per cent of the control subjects.

According to a survey carried out in the United States, between 1957 and 1962, an estimated 227 million respiratory infections per year occurred in the general population. It was estimated that over 90 per cent of the infections were due to nonbacterial agents. In 80 per cent of the cases the patient's activity was decreased, and in 52 per cent of the cases the patient had to remain in bed for at least one day.[28]

Investigations among urban and rural populations have shown that acute respiratory infections are the main cause of morbidity: they represent the motive for 30 to 35 per cent of all visits to or by physicians. An investigation of two private practices repre-

senting fairly well the population of a large British town showed that, during one year, 11.4 per cent of the inhabitants required medical advice concerning an acute respiratory infection. The proportion of patients differed greatly according to age, since it was as high as 51.6 per cent from birth to four years, 24.5 per cent from five to 14, 6.6 per cent from 15 to 39, 6.2 per cent from 40 to 59, and 5.4 per cent for those above 60 years of age. A bacteriological and virological study carried out among these patients provided evidence of a definite viral infection in 54.8 per cent and of a hemolytic streptococcus infection in 7.7 per cent; the etiology remained unknown in 37.5 per cent of the cases. However, a number of the infections of undetermined cause were probably viral, since the authors did not study the rhinovirus group.[2]

ROLES OF THE VARIOUS KNOWN VIRUSES IN RESPIRATORY INFECTIONS

In a given clinical picture, the role attributed to one virus or another depends, as is always the case in virus infections, on the

Table 38-2. *Isolations from Patients Suffering from Various Types of Illness**

Diagnosis	Total	Influenza	Parainfluenza	R.S. Virus	Adenoviruses	Herpes Simplex	Enteroviruses	Rhinoviruses	Unidentified	β-Haemolytic Streptococci	Positive No.	%
Common cold	437	1	15	8	8	6	13	28	4	11	94	21
Feverish cold	341	8	13	6	26	1	14	20	2	7	97	28
Influenza	144	23	2	1	3	1	5	4	2	4	45	31
Sore throat	376	1	4	1	31	7	32	8	2	90	176	47
Croup, A.L.T.B., tracheitis, or laryngitis	127	2	11	3	4	1	3	6	1	6	37	29
Bronchitis	179	0	7	8	8	2	8	4	2	3	42	23
Bronchiolitis	46	0	1	10	1	0	4	3	0	0	19	41
Pneumonia, bronchopneumonia, or primary atypical pneumonia	103	0	4	12	2	5	4	2	0	2	31	30
Otitis media	42	0	1	1	0	1	3	0	1	1	8	19
Other	93	0	3	0	3	5	7	3	1	4	26	28
Total	1,888	35	61	50	86	29	93	78	15	128	575	30

*From Report of the Medical Research Council Working Party on Acute Respiratory Virus Infections.[21]

Table 38-3. *Viruses and Mycoplasmas Which Cause Respiratory Disease in Infants and Children**

	SEROTYPES		RELATIVE IMPORTANCE IN INDICATED SYNDROME†				
Group	*Total No.*	*No. Assoc. with Respir. Illness*	*Bronchiolitis*	*Pneumonia*	*Croup*	*Bronchitis*	*URI*
Myxovirus							
Influenza	3	2 (A & B)	+	+	+	+	++
Parainfluenza	4	4 (1, 2, 3, & 4)	++	++	++++	+++	+++
Resp. syncytial	1	1	++++	++++	++	+++	+++
Adenovirus	31	8 (1, 2, 3, 4, 5, 7, 14, and 21)	++	+++	+	+++	+++
Picornavirus							
Coxsackie A	23	6 (2, 4, 5, 6, 8, 10)					++
Coxsackie B	6	3 (2, 3, 5)					++
Rhinoviruses	60+	60+ (?)	++(?)	++(?)		++	++
Mycoplasmataceae	8	1 (*M. pneumoniae*)	+	++		++	

*From Chanock and Parrott.[8]

†Relative importance graded on a scale of 0 to ++++.

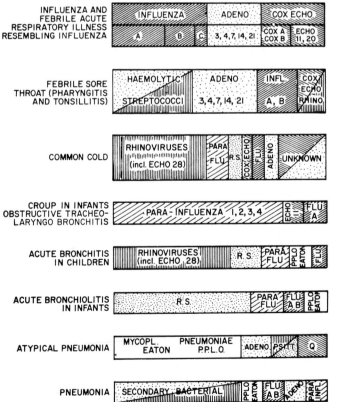

Figure 38-1. Respiratory syndromes and the respiratory viruses. (From Stuart-Harris, C. H.: Respiratory viruses, ciliated epithelium, and bronchitis. Amer. Rev. Resp. Dis., *93*:150, 1966.)

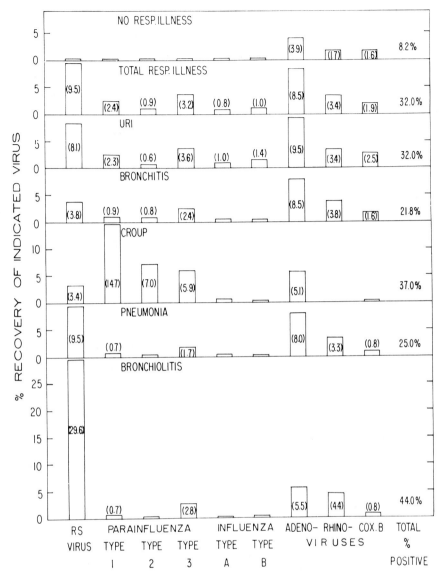

Figure 38-2. Estimate of importance of various viruses in pediatric respiratory disease based upon virus recovery (Children's Hospital of D.C., 1957-1964): 7938 patients with respiratory disease were studied for presence of parainfluenza, influenza, and enteroviruses, 7016 for adenoviruses, 5641 for RS virus, and 1826 for rhinoviruses. (From Chanock, R. M., and Parrott, R. H.: Acute respiratory disease in infancy and childhood: present understanding and prospects for prevention. Pediatrics, *36*:21, 1965.)

virological techniques used, the mode of investigation (prospective or retrospective), and the mode of selection of the subjects (patients in a hospital, patients with a well-defined clinical syndrome). Results vary also according to the geographic location, the year, and the season of the investigation. Finally, age is an essential point, since respiratory infections produce marked clinical signs in the young child. However, despite some divergences, various studies agree in many respects. Table 38-1 sums up several of the most sizable or representative investigations, based on isolation of the virus or identification of the infection involved. By using virus isolation and serological methods conjointly, it is possible to prove the viral etiology in a large number of cases. Thus, taking these two elements as a basis, Chanock and Parrott[8] achieved the most sizable investigation so far (approximately 8000 children for over seven years), and they succeeded in identifying a viral cause for respiratory infections in 44 per cent of the cases.

Influenza myxoviruses play only a small role in general, being responsible for less than 0.5 per cent of respiratory infections, according to Chanock and Parrott, but if an epidemic breaks out during an investigation they may hold the foremost place (Banatvala et al.[2]: 28.7 per cent). According to a generally held opinion, *Myxovirus parainfluenzae* are very important, especially in children: they are the cause of 4 to 18 per cent of the respiratory infections.

The respiratory syncytial virus is now recognized as important in pediatrics, and for Chanock and Parrott it comes first, accounting for 29.6 per cent of the infections.

Adenoviruses are less important: nearly all the investigations have shown them to be the causal agent in fewer than 6 per cent of the cases (2.1 to 5.5 per cent). Enteroviruses seem to play no role or a very small one, although they were found in investigations such as that of the Medical Research Council,[21] aimed at the study of the common cold. In fact, the causal agents of this syndrome include a certain number of enteroviruses.

In investigations concerning lower respiratory tract infections, the herpes virus does not appear as the causal agent, and its role in general is slight: 1.5 per cent in investigations involving infections of the upper respiratory tract. The role of reoviruses has been found to be negligible so far; Wulf et al.,[29] however, found them to be responsible in 4 per cent of the pediatric cases. In fact, the roles of these viruses in respiratory affections has yet to be defined. The number of respiratory viral agents not identified often depends on the battery of technical means applied but hardly exceeds 1 per cent. Banatvala et al. found Eaton's agent responsible for 4.6 per cent of the infections, and Chanock and Parrott for 1 to 10 per cent, according to the year. All the authors cited agree on the existence of combined viral infections, with an incidence of from 1 to 5 per cent.

The difficulty of establishing a clinical diagnosis for a given virus infection is seen with respiratory infections in the absence of an epidemic. In addition, the epidemiological argument is not always sufficient: "What could appear, from the clinical and epidemiologic point of view, as a well defined epidemic of respiratory disease, may in reality be due to several agents, this being revealed by applying suitable laboratory techniques to individual cases."

The great number of agents that may provoke the same clinical picture and their respective importance are indicated, for instance, in the investigation carried out by the Medical Research Council of Great Britain (Table 38-2). Figure 38-1 shows the approximate estimation of Stuart-Harris[24] on the respective roles that the various known

agents play in the clinical pictures usually observed. Figure 38-2 and Table 38-3 show Chanock and Parrott's estimate in this respect.[8]

However, precise diagnosis must not seem a hopeless task to the clinician. For in the study by Banatvala et al.[2] of two general practices, the two physicians established diagnoses that proved to be exact in 89 per cent of the cases of influenza and in 70 per cent of the cases of primary atypical pneumonia.[2]

BIBLIOGRAPHY

1. Adams, J. M.: Acute respiratory disease; etiologic, diagnostic and therapeutic considerations. Pediatrics, *19*:129, 1957.
2. Banatvala, J. E., Anderson, T. B., and Reiss, B. B.: Viruses in acute respiratory infection in a general community. J. Hyg. (Camb.), *63*:155, 1965.
3. Beem, M., Wright, F. H., Fasan, D. M., Egerer, R., and Oehme, M.: Observations on the etiology of acute bronchiolitis in infants. J. Pediat., *61*:864, 1962.
4. Burnet, F. M.: Influenza virus infections of chick embryo by the amniotic route. Aust. J. Exp. Biol. Med. Sci., *18*:353, 1940.
5. Breese, B. B., and Morgan, H. R.: A study of an epidemic of respiratory infection of multiple etiology. New York J. Med., *57*:1918, 1957.
6. Breton, A., Gaudier, B., Ponte, C., and Samaille, J.: Les bronchopneumopathies à virus de l'enfant. Etudes épidémiologique, clinique et paraclinique. Critique des méthodes de diagnostic. 18 Cong. Ass. Pédiatres Langue Fr., Genève, 1961. Basel, Karger, 1961, Vol. 3, pp. 64-119.
7. Chanock, R. M., and Johnson, K. M.: Infectious disease: respiratory viruses. Ann. Rev. Med., *12*:1, 1961.
8. Chanock, R. M., and Parrott, R. H.: Acute respiratory disease in infancy and childhood: present understanding and prospects for prevention. Pediatrics, *36*:21, 1965.
9. Clarke, S. K., Corner, B. D., Gambier, D. M., et al.: Viruses associated with acute respiratory infections. Brit. Med. J., *1*:1536, 1964.
10. Commission on Acute Respiratory Diseases: Clinical patterns of undifferentiated and other acute respiratory diseases in army recruits. Medicine, *26*:441, 1947.
11. Dingle, J. H., and Feller, A. E.: Noninfluenzal viral infections of the respiratory tract. New Eng. J. Med., *254*:465, 1956.
12. Evans, A. S.: Infections with hemadsorption virus in University of Wisconsin students. New Eng. J. Med., *263*:233, 1960.
13. Forsgren, M., Sterner, G., and Wolontis, S.: Antibodies against respiratory viruses among healthy children. Acta Paediat. Scand., *54*:314, 1965.
14. Grieble, H. G., Jackson, G. G., and Dowling, H. G.: Etiology of common respiratory infections in civilian adult population. Amer. J. Med. Sci., *235*:245, 1958.

5. Gwaltney, J. M., and Jordan, W. S.: Rhinoviruses and respiratory illnesses in university students. Amer. Rev. Resp. Dis., *93*:362, 1966.
6. Higgins, P. G., Ellis, E. M., and Boston, D. G.: The isolation of viruses from acute respiratory infections. A study of the isolations made from cases occurring in a general practice in 1962. Monthly Bull. Minis. Health. (London), *22*:71, 1963.
7. Hilleman, M. R., Hamparian, V. V., Ketler, A., Reilly, C. M., McClelland, L., Cornfeld, D., and Stokes, J.: Acute respiratory illness among children and adults. Field study of contemporary importance of several viruses and appraisal of the literature. J.A.M.A., *180*:445, 1962.
8. Huebner, R. J.: New frontiers for virus disease research. J. Hyg. Epidem. (Praha), *6*:34, 1962.
9. Krugman, S., and Ward, R.: Infectious Diseases of Children. St. Louis, C. V. Mosby Co., 1964.
10. Manson, G.: Acute respiratory disease with special reference to pathogenesis, classification and diagnosis. J. Pediat., *43*:599, 1953.
21. Report of the medical research council working party on acute respiratory virus infections. A collaborative study of the aetiology of acute respiratory infection in Britain 1961-4. Brit. Med. J., *2*:319, 1965.
22. Robinson, R. Q., Hoshiwara, I., Schaeffer, M., Gorrie, R. H., and Kaye, H. S.: A survey of respiratory illnesses in a population. I. Viral studies. Amer. J. Hyg., *75*:18, 1962.
23. Smith, W., Andrewes, C. H., and Laidlaw, P. P.: A virus obtained from influenza patients. Lancet, *2*:66, 1933.
24. Sohier, R., Bernheim, M., Chaptal, J., and Jeune, M.: Bronchopneumopathies à virus et à rickettsies chez l'enfant. Monographie Inst. Nat. Hyg., *13*: 175. 1957.
24a. Stuart-Harris, C. H.: Respiratory viruses, ciliated epithelium, and bronchitis. Amer. Rev. Resp. Dis., *93*:150, 1966.
25. Tobin, J. O.: The isolation of respiratory viruses from children in hospital in South East Lancashire. Proc. Roy. Soc. Med., *56*:991, 1963.
26. Ward, T. G.: Viruses of the respiratory tract. Progr. Med. Virol., *2*:203, 1959.
27. Wenner, H. A., Christodoulopoulou, G., Weston, J., Tucker, V., and Liu, C.: The etiology of respiratory illnesses occurring in infancy and childhood. Pediatrics, *31*:4, 1963.
28. Wilder, C. S.: Acute respiratory illnesses reported to the US National Health Survey during 1957 to 1962. Amer. Rev. Resp. Dis., *88*:14, 1963.
29. Wulf, H., Kidd, P., and Wenner, H. A.: Etiology of respiratory infections. Further studies during infancy and childhood. Pediatrics, *33*:30, 1964.

39

Influenza

INFLUENZA: CLINICAL FEATURES

by R. Debré and J. Couvreur

The early history of influenza is lost in the mists of time. Along with the four epidemics of the sixteenth century, related by Hirsch in his "Histoire de la Médecine," there are also those described by Sydenham in the seventeenth century and the five great epidemics of the eighteenth century. The disease was perfectly described during the great epidemics of the nineteenth (1887-1889) and twentieth centuries.

The epidemic of 1888-1889 was a pandemic which may have started in China, then developed in Russia and spread to the whole world. It is thought to have affected 40 per cent of the world's inhabitants. It was during the course of this epidemic, which coincided with the development of bacteriology, that Pfeiffer isolated the bacterium which was to be named after him and which he thought to be the agent of influenza.

In 1918-1919, after several more localized epidemics, a new pandemic took place which affected 80 or 90 per cent of the population and killed 1 per cent, including vigorous young adults. It was recognized during this pandemic that Pfeiffer's coccobacillus was a secondary agent, and the viral nature of the pathogen was finally ascertained by Selter in 1918 and by Nicolle with Lebailly in 1919. The identity of the virus was not established until 1938 by Smith, Andrewes, and Laidlaw, and confirmed by Francis in 1934. Since then, many important studies have enriched our knowledge of *Myxovirus influenzae:* its various types and their variants. Since 1941, in addition to the studies of hemagglutination and Burnet's immunological investigations, many studies carried out in different countries have permitted accurate descriptions of the disease.

Influenza is characterized by (1) dreadful pandemics, often with the country first affected considered as the starting point (Asiatic, Spanish, English influenza, and so forth), resulting in a high fatality rate, involving all mankind, and wreaking more havoc than the bloodiest wars, and (2) less severe and less widespread epidemics affecting population groups, especially in winter in temperate countries. Now, in common language and even in medical terminology, sporadic and so-called seasonal infections are given the name of "influenza"; these infections are usually relatively mild, except for the two extreme ages of life, and are characterized, like pandemic or epidemic influenza, by contagiousness, a short incubation period, an abrupt and violent onset, respiratory tract catarrh, high fever, and severe fatigue. By completely illegitimate extension, sudden episodes of respiratory or digestive disorders are even called "influenza." At present, these traditional habits should be abandoned and the morbid episodes which we have just mentioned should be defined more precisely.

The usual terms "influenza" (created in 1358 by Villani and Segni), recalling the *influence* of the stars (borrowed from astrology by ancient medicine), and "grippe" (an old French word, related to the word "griffe," whose radical is of German origin, designed to suggest the sudden involvement of the patient by the disease), must now be reserved to the morbid phenomena caused by *Myxovirus influenzae* and separated from similar diseases due to other viruses, with special reference to *Myxovirus parainfluenzae,* adenoviruses, respiratory enteroviruses, and common cold viruses. As the pathogens have been identified, we must now call "viroses" the diseases which have been wrongly called "grippe," and follow the term virosis with the name of the responsible agent.

"Grippe," or influenza, owing to the action of its specific viruses, is endowed with a clinical physiognomy and epidemiological characteristics definite enough to permit a rigorously defined nosological frame. This exigence is the more legitimate, as the clinical picture observed in transient and local epidemics of influenza at present is exactly similar to that observed during the pandemics just mentioned.

UNCOMPLICATED INFLUENZA

Incubation is very short: this is a striking feature. It usually ranges from 24 hours to three days and may be even briefer. Abruptly, a previously healthy subject feels acutely ill: he has severe malaise, nausea, headache, and diffuse pains in the limbs; he often has chills, and his temperature quickly increases within a few hours up to 38.5°, 39°, 40° C. or even more. The subject suddenly feels as if he were "seized in the claws" of the disease.

At the height of the disease, headache persists or is more marked, often accompanied by very unpleasant ocular or periorbital pains. A hoarse cough is a manifestation of the tracheobronchial localization. Sometimes the pharynx is tender and the throat red. The tonsils are swollen. Fever remains high, oscillating between 38° C. and 39° to 40° C. from the morning to the evening. Fatigue is intense, and prostration is striking; cough is seldom productive, with at the most a small amount of mucus, often pinkish or blood-striated. The face is often congested and the eyes injected, but there is no nasal catarrh. The physical examination may reveal a few bubbling, often basilar rales; the pulse is moderately accelerated, the urine is scanty and rarely contains albumin. Blood pressure is reduced; the digestive tract is spared, and the appearance of the tongue does not differ from that seen during any pyrexial disorder. The patient is thirsty, but anorexic. Neither the spleen nor the liver is enlarged. The blood count shows few changes: a mild leukopenia seems to be the most common manifestation, and slight hyperleukocytosis suggests a secondary infection of the respiratory tract. The erythrocyte sedimentation rate is not markedly accelerated.

The fever remits after two to four days. It must be emphasized that there is no secondary elevation of temperature and that the so-called influenza V corresponds in reality to a more or less marked superinfection. Usually, the decrease in temperature is progressive; at times there is a true crisis, with a transient secondary rise and then an abrupt fall in temperature accompanied by sweating.

Convalescence is lengthy: the patient remains tired and anorectic. He feels that he has been through a short but severe disease. In general, the prognosis is good, and after two to four weeks the patient recovers completely.

Such is the picture of common, uncomplicated influenza. It is identical in sporadic cases, small epidemics, and great pandemics. However, influenza often results in the development of secondary infections of no gravity, such as labial herpes, transient conjunctivitis, or a laryngotracheobronchitis somewhat more marked than the one mentioned before. Complications may also assume a real importance, as when bronchopneumonia develops.

OTHER LOCALIZATIONS

The question may be asked whether the localization to the upper respiratory tract, the edematous and spastic laryngitides which are accompanied by dysphonia, aphonia, cyanosis, and dyspnea, are due to the influenza virus alone or to associated viruses or to bacterial superinfections. All these possibilities are likely, with a more or less marked predominance according to epidemics or cases.

The same remarks apply to pharyngeal complications (tonsillitis and pharyngitis) and especially to otitides, which seem unquestionably due to secondary bacterial infections and which may be accompanied by all the manifestations and complications (mastoiditis, meningitis) observed in such cases and also by serous or suppurative sinusitis.

The problem of the cardiac complications of influenza has not been settled once and for all. It was mentioned that in common influenza there seems to be no cardiac impairment with the exception of tachycardia, especially during convalescence. Nevertheless, the clinical experience of authors who during influenza epidemics observed electrocardiographic changes and sometimes fatal heart failure, cannot be ignored. Do they represent localizations of the influenza virus or of other associated viruses or indirect complications of viral infections in predisposed subjects whose myocardium was not entirely normal? There is no virological or histological evidence of myocarditis caused by the influenza virus, but the existence of heart failure and its possible severity cannot be denied. This is also true of pericarditis.

Generally speaking, influenza, which favors secondary microbial infections of the respiratory tract, pharynx, and ear, may exert the same deleterious effect on the different tissues of the eye.

BRONCHITIS AND BRONCHO-PNEUMOPATHIES ASSOCIATED WITH MYXOVIRUS INFLUENZAE

Usually, bronchopneumopathies follow the initial catarrh of the upper respiratory tract: dry, hemorrhagic, or congestive rhinopharyngitis or more or less severe laryngotracheitis. They sometimes appear suddenly after one day but often require several days. According to their localization and the intensity of the respiratory involvement, several clinical pictures can be distinguished:

Acute bronchitis is characterized by frequent, obstinate, and productive cough, with foamy expectoration, and persistent irregular fever. On examination, respiratory sounds are normal; persistent ronchi and sibilant rales are heard, and sometimes fixed foci of moist, bubbling rales, especially frequent in the right submamillary area, are noticed. On x-ray examination, bilateral hilar congestion with hilar and diaphragmatic linear opacities can be seen. The disease may last from a few days to several weeks.

Uncomplicated bronchopneumopathy is associated with clinical and radiological signs of parenchymatous involvement. On auscultation, bronchial and subcrepitant rales are heard which are often bilateral and predominantly basilar. Roentgenograms show rounded, parenchymatous, nodular densities, and sometimes systematized subsegmental or segmental opacities that may be associated with a pleural reaction or even a slight serofibrinous effusion. The course is benign but may last from one to several weeks.

A focus of pulmonary condensation may be detected on physical examination: dullness, area of crepitant rales confirmed by x-ray examination. This clinical picture can be related to various aspects usually described under the names of pneumonia,[20] influenzal pulmonary congestion, influenzal splenopneumonia. Until the advent of antibiotics, rapid secondary infection of these foci often made their prognosis very poor; bronchial suppuration with purulent expectoration), lung abscess, and pleural effusion were not uncommon.

Acute dyspneic bronchopneumopathy due to influenza can occur. Its features are variable and some are very dangerous ("malignant influenza"). In spite of dyspnea, there are only discrete auscultatory signs on physical examination. The patient's general condition deteriorates in a few hours, and the facies is livid. Neurological findings are frequently noted: agitation, delirium, carphology, as well as signs of vascular collapse and of anoxia. Occasionally, a hemorrhagic syndrome with renal manifestations (azotemia, proteinuria) is observed. Death may occur within a few days.

In other cases, the disease appears as an *acute pulmonary edema* (edematous pulmonary influenza, Huchard's bronchoplegic edema, "primary influenzal pneumonia" of the English-speaking authors, Graves' asphyxic influenza, or apoplectic pulmonary influenza). The syndrome usually appears during the second or third day of the illness. There is pink expectoration, often blood streaked. an abundant, foamy, occasionally salmon-Examination reveals the presence of many pulmonary endothelial cells. Thoracic resonance is normal, and crepitant rales, heard at first at the bases, spread throughout both lungs within a few hours. Dyspnea is intense. Cyanosis and nervous manifestations appear. Death may occur, sometimes preceded by the formation of pulmonary foci. In bronchoplegic edema, expectoration is scanty. No rales are heard on auscultation and the vesicular breath sounds may disappear. This impressive silence reveals, in some way, a respiratory obstruction due to pulmonary edema.

Pulmonary apoplexia is observed in cases of influenza which are severe from the very onset and whose hemorrhagic tendency has been revealed by epistaxis, purpura, and digestive hemorrhages. Intense dyspnea and cough are accompanied by repeated hemoptyses. Expectoration of foamy red blood, with mucopurulent streaks, reaches 400 to 700 ml. per day. Thoracic resonance is normal, but there are no vesicular breath sounds. The respiratory blockade corresponds to the areas of infarction and emphysema found at autopsy. Death may occur within one to

three days in hyperthermia: it is due to asphyxia and heart failure.

Severe forms of influenza may be accompanied by *pleural manifestations:* dry pleurisy, scanty aseptic effusions. *Extrapulmonary complications* set in and complicate severe forms and sometimes even those that, at the onset, appeared benign.

The course of influenzal pneumopathies varies with the initial symptoms. Uncomplicated bronchopneumopathies are resolved within one or two weeks, but x-ray anomalies may persist longer. Such a mild course was usual during the 1957 epidemic.

The prognosis of acute dyspneic influenzal bronchopneumopathies is much more severe. Statistics of the 1918 epidemic showed a high case fatality rate (25 to 31 per cent in nursling infants).[22] According to some authors, it was as high as 95 per cent, but bacterial superinfection played a role in this high figure. In 1957, no study permitted estimates of the mortality rate, but some observations have shown that the viral infection may induce a fatal respiratory disease independent of any superinfection. When the course is favorable, recovery is protracted, taking from one to several weeks. The possibility of sequelae has hardly been studied. However, it seems that influenza bronchopneumopathy may result in permanent bronchial anomalies, for example, moniliform deformations.

COMPLICATIONS

Complications are essentially due to bacterial infections, the development of which is favored by influenza; Pfeiffer's coccobacillus (*Hemophilus influenzae*) is responsible for severe bronchopleuropulmonary manifestations which may be severe and even fatal. At present, pneumococci, hemolytic streptococci, *Klebsiella pneumoniae*, and above all staphylococci (which are often resistant to many antibiotics) are the predominating pathogens in the complications affecting the respiratory tract and the pleura.

Secondary bacterial infections may have very different manifestations: multiple focal bronchopneumonia, pulmonary abscesses, and pleural empyema. The presently available antibiotic agents shorten and alleviate the various respiratory manifestations, especially in previously healthy and robust subects, although staphylococcic infection is more difficult to control.

The possibility of transient and various rashes associated with influenza cannot be excluded. Attributing digestive, nervous, and urogenital complications to influenza, however, is invalid, as they have not been authenticated during the course of recent epidemics followed by virological examinations.

CLINICAL FORMS

In the healthy adult, the severity of influenza is usually due largely to its complications, especially the respiratory ones. However, there are cases in which the picture of the disease itself seems to be malignant from the onset; in these cases, fever is very high, prostration is extreme, heart failure follows infectious pulmonary edema with a possible hemorrhagic tendency, and death may ensue.

The child, because of the narrowness of the laryngeal tract, may more often present manifestations of acute or hyperacute laryngitis, sometimes with dramatic dyspnea, marked stridor, a painful cough with aphonia, tachycardia, and a rapid deterioration of the general condition. Following this acute stage, during which life is in great peril, a slow improvement may be obtained with eventual recovery.

In the pregnant woman, influenza is poorly tolerated, and acute, dramatic respiratory complications have been frequent in the course of some epidemics. Abortion may be caused by influenza, but its role in the etiology of congenital malformations has not been demonstrated.

Finally, in aged subjects, who are often affected with more or less compensated respiratory and cardiac impairment, the occurrence of influenza may result in rapidly fatal failure, following the aggravation of the physical and functional signs of involvement of the respiratory and circulatory systems.

EPIDEMIC FORMS

The manifestations of influenza vary in incidence or severity according to the patient's previous condition of health, the geographic locale, the mode of selection of the patients considered, and the strain of influenza virus. During a mild epidemic in 1958, Adams recorded a 76 per cent incidence of congestive rhinopharyngitis, a 38 per cent incidence of conjunctivitis, a 20 per cent incidence of bronchial or pulmonary manifestations, and a 7.5 per cent incidence of x-ray anomalies.

According to Stuart-Harris et al.,[30] cough is one of the most frequent symptoms (80 to 93 per cent of the cases), but other thoracic signs are less frequent. The comparative study of four epidemics between 1937 and 1957 showed parenchymatous signs in 0 to 14 per cent of the cases and bronchial signs in 0 to 29 per cent. No objective signs of bronchial or pulmonary impairment were noted in the cases of uncomplicated influenza observed in 1957. This investigation provided two essential elements of information: in the first place, the importance of the role played by bacterial superinfections, in particular those due to staphylococci, in the genesis of fatal pneumonia, and, second, the role of the patient's previous state of health, since most pulmonary complications are observed in debilitated subjects, mainly aged people and persons with cardiopathy or chronic pneumopathy.

LABORATORY AND X-RAY STUDIES

Laboratory and Endoscopic Examinations. These examinations reveal some signs of practical or theoretical interest with regard to the respiratory cytology, the hemogram, and the endoscopic aspect of the respiratory tract.

Since *mononuclear leukocytes* prevail in pharyngeal swabs, the differential diagnosis of influenza from bacterial infections is possible. The presence of inclusions in epithelial cells has been mentioned, but they are not characteristic of influenza. The *blood studies* carried out during the 1957 epidemic have shown that leukopenia is observed in only one-third of the cases, whereas often no appreciable change occurs in the leukocyte count; sometimes, leukocytosis is found without any superinfection.

On *endoscopic examination* the bronchial mucosa is congested and edematous and may bleed on contact with the tube. The openings of the lobar or segmental orifices are reduced. After a few days edema and hypersecretion are exaggerated, which accounts for the obstruction of the small bronchi. Bronchial biopsy has permitted the isolation of the virus and the histological study of the early lesions of the bronchial wall.[3]

X-Ray Study. Since the clinical manifestations of influenza are often scanty, x-ray study is of great interest. A striking fact lies in the consistency of the observations, from the first description by Friedman[12] in 1918 to those of the last epidemic of Asian influenza.[5, 13] They can be classified into five groups: (1) A mere accentuation of bronchovascular markings, localized or diffuse, prevailing in the hilar and basilar areas, discrete in some cases, striking in others, with flocculent opacities of variable size along the bronchovascular axes (hilifuge opacities), (2) Limited, transient, not very dense opacities, with irregular and multiple outlines, often prevailing at the bases. They are 1 to 2 cm. in diameter and may rapidly become confluent. During the 1957 epidemic, these "bronchopneumonic condensation" pictures were unilateral in 41 per cent of the cases and bilateral in 39 per cent with spread to the whole of the two lungs in one-fourth of the latter. In 55 per cent of the cases, lesions were confined to the bases. Usually, they were resolved within an average of three weeks.[13] Occasionally, they may resemble atypical miliaria, with a diffuse micronodular aspect. (3) Lobar or segmental opacities, which are much more rare (5 per cent of the cases). These opacities are often incomplete and nonhomogenous and especially involve the middle lobe, the lingula, or the apical segment of a lower lobe. (4) Lung abscess is due to a superinfection; this has become very rare since the advent of antibiotic therapy. (5) Finally, pleural effusion, which is frequent, occurring in 10 to 20 per cent of the cases; it is most often bilateral and associated with parenchymatous changes. The reaction is then discrete, limited merely to filling of a cul-de-sac, thickening of a scissural line or a triangular opacity of the base of the deep fissure. In other cases, the effusion is considerable but disappears rapidly within seven to 21 days.

Needle aspiration reveals a turbid, albumin-rich fluid; it predominantly contains lymphocytes or eosinophils, but often consists of a mixture of endothelial cells, lymphocytes, and polymorphonuclear leukocytes. Cases of hemorrhagic pleurisy have been reported.

PATHOLOGY OF INFLUENZA BRONCHOPNEUMOPATHY

The direct action of influenza viruses on the respiratory epithelium, independent of any superinfection, has been proved, especially during the 1957 epidemic. The study of the histopathological lesions of influenza should be based only on fatal cases, without any superinfection, from which the influenza virus has been recovered.[2, 10, 16, 24]

It is known that in the experimentally infected ferret, the virus is electively bound to the epithelial cells of the tracheobronchial mucosa. There, it causes extended necrosis with lymphoplasmocytic infiltration of the chorion, followed by regeneration from the basal cells that elaborate, within a few days, a malpighian, then cylindrical epithelium. If the infective dose is high, the initial lesions may spread to the bronchioles and cause death.[29]

In man, degeneration was observed, with necrosis and small hemorrhages of the superficial epithelial layers of the trachea and of the bronchi, which may spread to the bronchioles and the alveolar ducts. These phenomena reach the basal cell layer, which, however, remains intact. Epithelial regeneration from this layer occurs in four to six days and results in an undifferentiated epithelium.

The subepithelial layer is the site of considerable hyperemia. It is infiltrated by inflammatory cells, especially plasma cells. Bronchial glands are more or less degenerated, and many plasma cells are found around them.

According to some authors, influenza may also induce pulmonary lesions, primary edematous or hemorrhagic alveolitis, hyaline membrane, and interstitial pneumonia. However, these aspects of the "influenza" lung are not accepted by other authors, who mention the possible action of nonspecific factors in their genesis, such as bacterial superinfection, agonic phenomena, and hemodynamic or neurovegetative disorders. Thus, necrotizing alveolitis is reported only in some observations, interstitial pneumonia occurs very inconstantly, hemorrhages and alveolar edema are hardly specific, and the significance of the hyaline membrane is questioned.

In some cases of fatal influenza, there exist lesions of the myocardium, whose fibers show nonspecific alterations ranging from partial degeneration to total destruction.[2]

On the whole, the lesions of the tracheal and bronchial epithelium are well individualized. They have been observed in man and experimentally reproduced. On the other hand, the existence of specific pulmonary lesions, both alveolar and interstitial, is not generally accepted as being directly due to the viral involvement, although hyaline membrane, alveolar emphysema, and necrosis of the alveolar walls are often seen.[28]

In any event, pathological observations have led to certain *physiopathological interpretations* of the disease.

They concern, first of all, the local action of the virus: its direct role in the epithelial lesions is accepted. Moreover, it is known that the virus is frequently recovered from tracheal and bronchial specimens taken at autopsy (in 21 per cent of the cases, according to Bowden and French[2]).

It is widely accepted that the influenza virus invades the epithelial cells, multiplies from one cell to another, spreading like a grass fire. Viremia is believed to start from that local lesion. Hers, in his important work, considers hyperemia, hemorrhages, and edema all consequences of the bacterial infection. In fact, they are observed in other infections due to bacteria.[14] In severe, fatal cases, the virus reaches the deep cell layers and develops also in the glandular epithelium.[2] As a matter of fact, not only are swelling, degeneration, and desquamation of the epithelial cells observed, but also infiltration with round cells, including many plasma cells, which invade the subepithelial layer as well. Glandular cells show degenerative changes along with granules stained by hematoxylin and eosin, and plasma cells accumulate in the periglandular areas.

The presence of plasma cells in epithelial glands has led to the elaboration of immunological hypotheses.

Since it is accepted that these cells play an important role in the production of antibodies, the pathological findings seem to support the opinion held by Burnet,[4] who believes that the influenza virus may induce the local formation of antibodies in the invaded tissues. Moreover, it has been proved that the immunity level is related to the antibody titer measured in bronchial and alveolar specimens.[9] It is thus possible that the accumulation of plasma cells in the periglandular areas of the respiratory epithelium is related to the local formation of antibodies.[2]

Finally, the absence of interferon in the pulmonary tissue and the demonstrated presence of viral antigens in alveolar cells[16] suggest not only the direct impairment of the lung by the virus but also, perhaps, a local cause favoring this action.

The mechanism of death is still controversial. Despite the introduction of antibiotics, the role of bacterial superinfection remains important, as shown by bacteriological determinations made at autopsy. Since death is more frequent in subjects suffering from cardiopathy, the role of a vascular disorder is considered. Lastly, anoxia seems to be an important cause of death. It is caused by an alveolocapillary block in which the hyaline membrane plays an important role.[28]

EPIDEMIOLOGY AND DIAGNOSIS

A diagnosis of influenza should not be made in the presence of an isolated case, as the disease is essentially epidemic and assumes the aspect either of a pandemic or of a more or less widespread epidemic. Pandemics take place at distant intervals (1889, 1916, 1957). The following general conclusions can be drawn from their study: the disease appears suddenly and rapidly affects a large number of subjects in a given area of the world; it then spreads out fairly rapidly throughout the world, requiring about six months to spread to the various continents. It affects a large part of the population, ranging in each country from 50 to 80 per cent or more, as many cases remain unrecognized. On the whole, it may present fairly different patterns, according to the specific virus. For instance, as indicated, the pandemic of 1918-1919 was very severe, and resulted in the death of over 20 million people. In contrast, the very diffuse epidemic of 1957 was relatively mild, on the whole. This characteristic is not due exclusively to the advances in treatment and prophylaxis of infection. The pathogenic role of the various responsible virus strains in each pandemic will be discussed in the second part of this chapter. A role must be ascribed to the more or less marked virulence of the bacterial agents responsible for the secondary infections as well.

The occurrence of epidemics limited to

specific geographic areas is more common. They take place at intervals of one to three years. The onset is abrupt, with rapid spread, especially in collectivities (schools, barracks, institutions for aged persons); the epidemic involves a large number of people, then spreads for a few weeks, seldom more than three or four months except in the adjacent region or country. In these cases, influenza is most often benign, much more so than during pandemics. However, it is responsible for a sometimes very striking increase in the fatality rate of aged subjects and young children, although at present microbial superinfection can be largely prevented.

The extreme contagiousness of the disease, which is transmitted from man to man by Flügge droplets, and the widespread susceptibility of man at all ages, accounts for the previously given rule, namely, the physician should consider this diagnosis with skepticism in the presence of an isolated case or of a family outbreak.

The problem of the virus reservoir between the epidemics has not been settled. Is man a healthy virus carrier, or are animals such as pigs, sometimes affected with similar diseases, or other domestic animals, virus reservoirs? No final conclusions with regard to this question have thus far emerged.

There is a good deal of current work on the role of the main types of virus A and B in each epidemic; differences in their pathogenicity are now suspected. For example, myxovirus influenza type A seems to be capable of inducing more widespread and more severe epidemics. Immunity against the influenza and parainfluenza viruses, which plays an important role in the outbreak and development of epidemics, will be studied later. All these considerations are of the greatest importance for the diagnosis as the clinician can seek to establish it.

The widespread practice of diagnosing various gastric, intestinal, cardiac, catarrhal, or respiratory symptoms as variants of influenza should definitely be discarded, and we must again stress that the diagnosis of influenza should be considered by the practitioner only in the presence of multiple cases because of the highly contagious nature of the disease, the great susceptibility of man, and the rapidity of spread.

When the clinician makes a tentative clinical diagnosis of influenza, he may try to ascertain this diagnosis on the basis of labor-atory examination. The essential difficulty lies in the variety of different viruses which may cause acute infections with localization to the respiratory tract: a differential diagnosis can be made only by proper virological investigations. Furthermore, it should be recalled that influenza does not induce the simple nasal catarrh of common cold, and that pharyngitis caused by enteroviruses and adenoviruses is not accompanied by the very marked impairment of the general condition seen with influenza.

Bacterial infections are more easily diagnosed. Guidelines to diagnosis of streptococcal involvement are intense pharyngeal redness, cervical adenopathies, the usual absence of laryngotracheitis, and possibly the polymorphonuclear leukocytosis, to say nothing of a scarlatinous rash. Pneumococcal pneumonia and primary pulmonary staphylococcia are also easy to identify and can be distinguished from influenza with respiratory complications. Diseases due to mycoplasma, ornithosis, and psittacosis have special features which will be described in other chapters.

In spite of all this, a clinical diagnosis of true influenza can only be tentatively considered at the beginning of an outbreak of epidemic virosis in a community.

MANAGEMENT

The prophylaxis of influenza can be considered only on the basis of virology. It is treated in the following pages.

The management of influenza must be reserved and cautious: bed rest, isolation to prevent superinfection, antipyretics such as aspirin, quinine given in small amounts, are generally sufficient. It is not advisable to administer antibiotics or sulfonamides prophylactically. However, if superinfection is suggested by temperature rise, leukocytosis, or manifestations of bronchial or pulmonary impairment, the treatment of infection must be both rapid and energetic, with special regard to the so often resistant staphylococci. The specific pathogen responsible for secondary infection should be sought and identified to permit the use of an effective antibiotic.

In young children, the fear of laryngeal disorders, and, in aged subjects, the possibility of severe pulmonary infection or of congestive heart failure, requires special therapeutic measures. In debilitated patients, diffusible stimulants are indicated; in diabetics and in patients with adrenal insufficiency, the control of the hormonal disorder will require special attention.

BIBLIOGRAPHY

1. Baron, S., and Isaacs, A.: Absence of interferon in lungs from fatal cases of influenza. Brit. Med. J., *1*:18, 1962.
2. Bowden, K. M., and French, E. L.: The pathology of death during influenza epidemics. Med. J. Aust., *45*:553, 1958.
3. Burch, G. E., Walsh, J. J., and Mogabgab, W.: A study of the response of the cardiovascular system to Asian influenza. Amer. Rev. Resp. Dis., *83*: 68, 1961.
4. Burnet, F. M.: Influenza virus infections of the chick embryo by the amniotic route. Aust. J. Exp. Biol. Med. Sci., *18*:353, 1940.
5. Chambatte, C., Laaban, J., Ledédenté, A., and Kermarec, J.: Pneumopathies grippales de l'adulte. Aspects cliniques et diagnostic. Rev. Tuberc. (Paris), *27*:723, 1963.
6. Chanock, R. M., and Parrott, R. H.: Acute respiratory disease in infancy and childhood; present understanding and prospects for prevention. Pediatrics, *36*:21, 1965.
6a. Commission on Acute Respiratory Diseases: Studies on the 1943 epidemic of influenza A. II. Comparison of the clinical and laboratory characteristics of influenza A and undifferentiated acute respiratory disease (ARD). Amer. J. Hyg., *48*: 263, 1948.
6b. Commission on Acute Respiratory Diseases: Studies on the 1943 epidemic of influenza A. VIII. General discussion and summary. Amer. J. Hyg. *48*:332, 1948.
7. Dauer, C. C., and Serfling, R. E.: Mortality from influenza 1957-1958 and 1959-1960. Amer. Rev. Resp. Dis., *83*:15, 1961.
8. Dujarric de la Riviere: Etiologie et prophylaxie de la grippe. Paris, Masson et Cie, 1929.
9. Fazekas de St. Groth, S., and Donneley, M.: Studies in experimental immunology of influenza; production of viral antigens. Aust. J. Exp. Biol. Med. Sci., *28*:31, 1950.
10. Fischer, F., Fjeldborg, N., and Bastrup-Madsen, P.: Fulminating influenzal pneumonia. Nord. Med., *60*:1697, 1958.
11. Forbes, J. A.: Severe effects of influenza virus infection. Med. J. Aust., *2*:75, 1958.
12. Friedman, H. F.: Cited by Galloway and Miller, J.A.M.A., *56*:1847, 1918.
13. Galloway, R. W., and Miller, R. S.: Lung changes in the recent influenza epidemic. Brit. J. Radiol., *32*:28, 1959.
14. Hers, J. F. P.: The histopathology of the respiratory tract in human influenza. Tu Verhandelingen van het instituut voor praeventieve goneeskunde, 26. Leiden, Stenfert-Kroese, 1955.
15. Hers, J. F. P.: Disturbances of the ciliated epithelium due to influenza virus. Amer. Rev. Resp. Dis., *93*:162, 1966.
16. Hers, J. F. P., and Mulder, J.: Rapid tentative postmortem diagnosis of influenza with the aid of cytological smears of tracheal epithelium. J. Path. Bact., *63*:329, 1951.
17. Hers, J. F. P. and Mulder, J.: Broad aspects of the pathology and pathogenesis of human influenza. Amer. Rev. Resp. Dis., *83*:84, 1961.
18. Hilleman, M. R., Werner, J. H., Adair, C. V., and Dreisbach, A. R.: Outbreak of acute respiratory illness caused by RI-67 and influenza A viruses, Fort Leonard Wood, 1952-1953. Amer. J. Hyg., *61*:163, 1955.
19. Liu, C.: Diagnosis of influenzal infection by means of fluorescent antibody staining. Amer. Rev. Resp. Dis., *83*:130, 1961.
20. Menetrier: Cited by Morin.[22]
21. Moreau, R.: Problèmes Actuels de Pathologie Médicale. Paris, Masson et Cie, 1934.
22. Morin, M.: La grippe. In Traité de Médecine. Paris, Masson et Cie, 1948, Vol. 1, pp. 526-561.
23. Neilson, D. B. Sudden death due to fulminating influenza. Brit. Med. J., *1*:420, 1958.
24. Oseasohn, R., Adelson, L., and Kaji, M.: Clinicopathologic study of thirty-three fatal cases of Asian influenza. New Eng. J. Med., *260*:509, 1959.
25. Oswald, N. C., Shooter, R. A., and Curwen, M. P.: Pneumonia complicating Asian influenza. Brit. Med. J., *2*:1305, 1958.
26. Parrott, R. H., Kim, H. W., Vargosko, A. J., and Chanock, R. M.: Serious respiratory tract illness as a result of Asian influenza and influenza B infections in children. J. Pediat., *61*:205, 1962.
27. Robertson, L., Caley, J. P., and Moore, J.: Importance of staphylococcus aureus in pneumonia in the 1957 epidemic of influenza A. Lancet, *2*:233, 1958.
28. Soto, P. J., Broun, G. O., and Wyatt, J. P.: Asian influenzal pneumonitis. A structural and virologic analysis. Amer. J. Med., *27*:18, 1959.
29. Stuart-Harris, C. H.: Twenty years of influenza epidemics. Amer. Rev. Resp. Dis., *83*:54, 1961.
30. Stuart-Harris, C. H., Andrewes, C. H., and Smith, W.: A study of epidemic influenza. With special reference to the 1936-1937 epidemic. Medical Research Council of Great Britain Special Report Series, No. 228. London, 1938.
31. Widal, F.: *In:* Traité de Médecine. Paris, Masson et Cie, 1899, Vol. 2, p. 223.

INFLUENZA: VIROLOGY, EPIDEMIOLOGY, PROPHYLAXIS

by G. CATEIGNE

Influenza is a contagious disease that can develop epidemically at a very rapid rate. It is a specific disease, usually benign, due to a family of viruses whose characteristics are now well known. Clinically, it is chiefly a disease of the upper respiratory tract, but a variety of less common syndromes often occur, including a malignant syndrome.

INTRODUCTION

For many centuries, this disease has been rife in the world. In the 5th century B.C., Hippocrates[40] in the sixth book of "Epidemics" wrote, "a contagious disease raged at Perinthos in Thrace. It began towards the winter solstice. Some cases were of short duration, the others lengthy, there were numerous pneumonias...the throat became inflamed, there was lassitude and were pains in the thighs and in the legs, there was a frequent cough with expectoration; in those whose respiration rate became accelerated, it was very severe, for in this case there was febrile heat...."

Up to the beginning of the sixteenth century, one finds almost no description of epidemic diseases. The first epidemic studied slightly was that of 1557-1558. In 1580 a respiratory infection of pandemic character spread over all Europe. Other epidemics of the same type with abrupt outbreak are described in 1658, 1676, and 1732-1733. It is interesting to note that several times the authors recorded an epizootic infection in certain domestic animals preceding the human epidemic. For example, in 1732: "Before this disease declared itself in man, horses were generally attacked by 'moping,' that is to say, discharge of mucous secretions from the nostrils.... After the epidemic, there reigned pleurisies and pneumonias. The human disease extended to all Europe and to America."

It is difficult to say whether all these epidemics were influenza. However, certain common characteristics can be noted: the rapidity and the intensity of spread of the disease, the successive waves, the severity of the infection.

HISTORICAL ACCOUNT

The nineteenth century witnessed two important epidemics of pandemic proportions: 1837 and 1889-1890. It is almost certain that the 1889-1890 pandemic originated in central Asia. The first cases were described by Heyfelder (May, 1889) in Bokhara and the Russian physicians of the period called the disease "Chinese influenza."

Nearer to our own time, the 1918-1919 pandemic, owing to the fact that it appeared during World War I, was able to spread with extreme rapidity. As in 1889, the scourge came from Asia, from China it seems. From the start of 1918, a generalized epidemic was noted in that country which spread westward in successive, increasingly rapid waves from the borders of Asia across the whole of Europe.

As a result of the movement of troops, the disease spread simultaneously by land and by sea. The first wave, which appeared in Europe in the spring, was relatively mild; the summer was marked by a lull. The second wave, in the autumn, was accompanied by an appalling rate of morbidity and mortality. The 1918-1919 pandemic is estimated to have caused 15 million deaths in the world.

The 1957 pandemic also originated in China at the beginning of the year; it spread rapidly and successively to different regions of Asia. In July, it reached the Middle East, and at the end of the same month the first cases appeared in South America and in Africa. By early August, the disease had spread to all of Latin America; it reached the United States a little later. In Europe, cases were reported in Russia, Scandinavia, Germany, Italy, Rumania, Great Britain, and France. By September, no country seemed to have been untouched. There is no doubt that the summer holidays, with widespread air, sea, and rail travel, permitted rapid diffusion of the infectious agent. The epidemiology of an influenza pandemic differs from seasonal epidemic waves. The epidemic starts in a certain part of the world and extends to all regions of the globe with extreme rapidity, all the greater in our time because of the increase in human travel, without the intervention of climatic and seasonal influences as sixteenth and seventeenth century physicians seemed to believe. The morbidity rate is very high, and the mortality rate is relatively lower during the first wave.

From observations during the last two centuries, influenza pandemics present a certain number of common characteristics which can be summarized as follows: (1) speed and intensity of spread of the disease; and (2) evolution in successive waves giving rise, during the interpandemic periods, to seasonal epidemics with some minor antigenic modifications of the infectious agent.

In our time, spread can occur with extreme rapidity because frontiers have been practically abolished, distances mean little, and contacts between all continents are constant.

BEGINNING OF
VIROLOGICAL RESEARCH

During the major epidemics of influenza that we have just reviewed, the problem of etiology was envisaged in different ways. At the start of the 1918-1919 pandemic, the etiological role of Pfeiffer's bacillus, or *Hemophilus influenzae,* discovered by Pfeiffer in 1892, seemed to be confirmed by the fact that this organism was found, either alone or associated with staphylococci or pneumococci, in specimens from patients with influenza. It was, however, during the 1918 pandemic that the viral origin of the disease was first suspected.

Debré[15a] in 1918, in a study of influenza in the French Armed Forces, demonstrated that patients with influenza were temporarily unable to produce antibodies, most of them being in a state of "anergy."

The author concluded that "these finding as a whole reveal a similarity between influenza and measles; these are the two diseases which produce anergy the most frequently. This biological similarity is perhaps related to an etiological resemblance; it is indeed probable that the unknown agent of influenza is, like the unknown agent of measles, a filterable virus."

We now know that the viruses causing influenza and measles belong to the same group, the myxoviruses.

In August, 1918, Selter[44] in Germany provoked in volunteers a fairly mild form of influenza after inhalation of a filtrate of nasal secretions from a typical case of influenza.

Evidently unaware of the studies being carried out in Germany at this time, Nicolle and LeBailly,[38] in Tunis, and Dujarric de la Riviere,[16] in the French Armed Forces, published simultaneously but independently, in the same issue of the "Comptes rendus de l'Académie des Sciences," their experiments concerning the transmission of influenza to human subjects and to monkeys by means of filtered material (sputum or blood) from patients with clinical influenza. The incubation period, the character of the temperature curve, and the algias observed in the volunteers or the animals indicated the positive value of these research studies. The experiments were reproduced at the Oswaldo Cruz Institute in Rio de Janeiro and also in Japan.

Although none of these investigations had led to isolation of a strain, they opened a new pathway of investigation.

Not until 1933 was the first strain of influenza virus isolated. During this period, Laidlaw, in London, demonstrated that the ferret is sensitive to distemper virus; by analogy, Smith et al.[48] attempted to transmit influenza to this animal by means of material from the pharynx of a patient. This material, filtered and bacteriologically controlled, when inoculated into the ferret provoked a clinical picture corresponding to that of human influenza, and the virus was detected in the turbinate, the trachea, and the lungs of the animal. The strain was maintained by successive passages. The experimenters observed that man and sensitive animals develop specific neutralizing antibodies which persist in the blood. Using the technique perfected by the English authors, numerous other workers succeeded in isolating strains with identical characteristics during human epidemics. From 1933 to 1935, 53 new strains were isolated.

The next step in study of the virus concerned its culture on the chorioallantoic membrane of the embryonated egg, a technique perfected by Burnet in 1935.[5] Since then, this in ovo technique has been used in all countries and the methods have been improved. This subject will be discussed in greater detail later.

Finally, the next stage in study of influenza was initiated with the simultaneous and separate discovery by Hirst in 1941[23] and by McClelland and Hare[31] that the influenza virus agglutinates chicken red cells; since then, we have learned that it agglutinates the red cells of other animal species and of man. These authors observed that the agglutination reflects the virus concentration and that the sera of subjects with influenza inhibit this agglutination; the serum antibodies specifically inhibit the hemagglutination of the homologous virus. On this property is based the hemagglutination-inhibition reaction, one of the methods for the diagnosis of influenza.

BIOLOGICAL AND BIOCHEMICAL CHARACTERISTICS OF INFLUENZA VIRUSES

We shall review briefly some general facts in order to place in the present-day classification the myxoviruses, the group to which the influenza viruses belong.

In virology, the structure and the functional organization of a virus depend on two factors: (1) the infectious element, i.e., the nucleic acid, which is of high molecular weight and which can be either a deoxyribonucleic acid (DNA) or a ribonucleic acid (RNA); and (2) the envelope which surrounds the molecule of DNA or RNA and which permits its conservation intact in a functional state in order to survive extracellularly and to infect a sensitive host.

The essential property of a viral nucleic acid is to deviate the enzyme-synthesizing activity of the cell that it infects and to orient it toward the production of new virus particles. This action on cell metabolism can be exerted at different stages of cellular biosynthesis. The biological and biochemical activity of the viral particle thus depends on the chemical structure of its genetic material, be it a DNA or a RNA, and on the architecture of the envelope. According to the findings of modern biology, DNA is the element of heredity, to which is added exceptionally the RNA of certain viruses. The genetic information is probably coded according to the sequences of nucleotides constituting a given nucleic acid. At present writing, the plant viruses, a large proportion of human and animal viruses, among them the influenza viruses, and certain bacterial viruses are included in this exception (Schaffer[43]). Viral infectious RNA seems thus not to fit into the dogma roughly schematized as follows: DNA→RNA→protein. Such viral RNA can be synthesized independently of a DNA, which implies obligatorily that an RNA controls the synthesis of RNA. The relations between a given virus and the normal constituents of the cell, as well as the number of information elements carried by a viral nucleic acid, are the principal elements in the classification of viruses. But many viruses contain essential nongenetic components. Thus certain myxoviruses, the group to which influenza viruses belong, possess, among others, proteinic constituents that permit them to fix themselves on certain receptors of the membrane of the sensitive cell, and an enzymatic function probably intervening in cell penetration. In influenza viruses, these constituents are closely linked to the normal cellular constituents and are incorporated into the viruses in the final stage of maturation. Despite all the recent work on RNA containing viruses, relatively little is known of the mechanisms by which the information coded by the RNA is transmitted to elaborate the specific viral protein. The literature gives a confused picture as concerns the infectious RNA of the myxoviruses. For the influenza viruses, the results obtained by different investigators are considered to be negative and it must be admitted, up to the present time, that the infectious RNA has not been extracted. Personally, we have attempted for two years, by use of techniques variously modified, to obtain the infectious RNA of influenza viruses (A and A_2 families). The results have always proved negative (unpublished work). The complex structure of these viruses and the high RNA content of the particle are perhaps the reason for this failure.

The basis for the first classification of the myxoviruses was structure, which possesses a biological significance. The criteria initially given by Andrewes et al.[2] in 1935 were as follows: (1) Particle diameter from 800 to 3000 Å; (2) ability to fix on human red cells and those of various lower animal species, the receptor of these red cells being of mucoprotein nature (the suffix "myxo" was given because of the affinity of these viruses for mucins); (3) sensitivity to the action of ether; (4) tropism for the epithelial cells of the respiratory tract.

Since then a provisory revision has been made. The hemadsorption technique, used to demonstrate the viral infection in cells cultured in vitro, has permitted detection and isolation of other viruses which seem to be linked to the myxoviruses, at least by certain criteria. Thus the taxonomists have modified their classification as follows: (1) genetic constituent: RNA with helical symmetry; (2) sensitivity to ether, indicating the lipoid element considered one of the essential constituents of the virus; (3) internal helical nucleoprotein structure; external structure: envelope with protuberances; (4) diameter from 800 to 3000 Å, with considerable variation in the population; (5) maturation of the virus at, or near, the cellular surface, a property common to all members of this group.

This classification includes two main groups: the orthomyxoviruses and the paramyxoviruses. We will consider only the first group, which comprises the human influenza viruses: A, A_1, A_2, B, C, and the animal influenza viruses: avian, porcine, and equine.

Their fundamental structure is helical: a loose envelope surrounds the helically arranged ribonucleoprotein. The diameter of the particles varies between 800 and 1100 Å. Their form is inconstant. There are both spherical and filamentous forms in unequal proportion. The envelope is not rigid; it is composed of a membrane from which project cylindrical protuberances 90 Å long and from 15 to 20 Å in width. These protuberances seem regularly spaced. The particles are stable and do not break spontaneously. The degree of polymorphism varies occasionally from one strain to another for the same virus type. The constituents of these viruses are assembled near, or at, the surface of the host cell immediately before their liberation from the cell. The virion is formed only when the constituents pass through the cell membrane.[36] During this process, a part of the material from the infected cell is incorporated into the virus and serves to constitute its surface components. This phenomenon was demonstrated by different methods by Smith et al. in 1953,[48a] by Hoyle in 1954,[25] by Kates et al. in 1961,[28] and by tagging with radioactive substances by Wecker in 1957.[58] The filamentous particles were especially studied, for, in the opinion of different authors, they were not infectious. In 1957, Valentine and Isaacs[55a] demonstrated the presence of the viral nucleoprotein in the filamentous forms, and in the 1957 pandemic many strains of A_2 Asian type were composed of predominantly filamentous particles. Choppin and Tamm in 1960[13] demonstrated the presence of RNA in these particles as in the spherical forms. By passages in embryonated eggs, the filamentous forms change rapidly and become spherical, without change either in infectiousness or in surface properties. Burnet and Lind in 1957[7] succeeded in maintaining a strain in its fila-

mentous form by egg passages at limit dilutions. These authors think that the change into spherical particles is mutational and could correspond to the variations O→D demonstrated by Burnet, i.e., "original strain" (maintained in the embryonated egg by the amniotic route) transformed into "derived strain" adapted to allantoic cells and no longer pathogenic for man.

If the morphology of the influenza virus is predominantly hereditary, Blough in 1963[4] considered that other factors intervene in regard to this characteristic. Thus the inability of certain cells cultivated in vitro to produce infectious particles (even though the virus constituents are formed in the cell) might be due to the absence of budding at the level of the cell membrane, budding being observed in normal, noninfected allantoic cells. Kilbourne and Murphy in 1960[30] showed that the multiplication rate of the filamentous forms is lower than that of the spherical forms; these authors consider that there may be a relationship between each of these forms and their biological characteristics.

The most precise correlation between the structure of the virus and its power of infection has been demonstrated with the "incomplete" virus, a phenomenon discovered by von Magnus[34] and obtained by inoculation of concentrated virus into the embryonated egg. These particles are irregular in their content and pleomorphic; they appear less dense than those of the normal virus; their surface biological properties are apparently the same, but they are no longer infectious. Despite numerous investigations, the problem remains unsolved.

The internal structure of the virus is constituted by a nucleoprotein which corresponds to the soluble antigen; it determines the type to which the virus belongs: All type A viruses (A_0, A_1, A_2) have an identical nucleoprotein; that of the type B viruses is different, as is that of type C viruses. The nucleoprotein is thus the type-determining factor.

The envelope of the influenza virus is lipoprotein and is responsible for its surface characteristics; the associated protein is the hemagglutinin that is the element determining the strict specificity of a given virus. It is this hemagglutinin that manifests the minor antigenic or mutational variations of influenza strains within a single type.

Numerous studies on the hemagglutina-

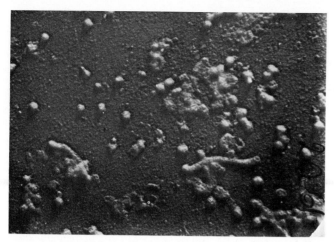

Figure 39-1. Electron microscopic view of influenza virus A_1 (spheres and filaments). × 20,000. (Courtesy of J. Giuntini, Pasteur Institute.)

tion reaction have demonstrated that the phenomenon of virus adsorption on certain red cell receptors also occurs in the sensitive cells; it may be the first mechanism of virus penetration into these cells.

Another phenomenon was demonstrated by Hirst after his discovery of the viral hemagglutination. He showed that the virus, under the influence of an enzyme peculiar to it, can eluate itself from the cell to which it is fixed, provoking the destruction of a constituent of the cellular membrane. The properties of this enzyme are those of a hydrolase which, by acting on the terminal sugar group, liberates a neuraminic acid from the prosthetic group of the red cell mucoprotein or of the sensitive cell on which the virus is fixed. This enzymatic action thus modifies the cell membrane in an important way. More recent work has shown that this enzyme possesses strain specificity.[41]

We shall consider this property again.

LABORATORY DIAGNOSIS OF INFLUENZA

The diagnosis of influenza can be made (1) by isolation of the virus; (2) by serological studies that reveal specific antibodies in the patient's blood; and (3) by "direct" examination with the immunofluorescence technique, the result of this method needing subsequent confirmation either by isolation of the virus or by serological study.

ISOLATION OF THE VIRUS

For isolation of a virus, it is obvious that the specimen plays a major role and that

certain conditions should be met. These conditions concern the date as well as the method of specimen taking and of expedition of the sample. A sufficiently detailed clinical history should always accompany the request for virus isolation.

Specimens. The specimen should be taken at the earliest possible time, i.e., 24 to 48 hours, 72 hours at the latest, after the appearance of clinical manifestations.

The samples that can be taken for a possible isolation are the rhinopharyngeal secretions, the blood, the cerebrospinal fluid, and, in case of death, the liver, the lung, and, accessorily, the other organs.

Two techniques can be employed to sample the *rhinopharyngeal* secretions: throat washing in adults and pharyngeal swabbing in infants and children.

Throat washing in adults consists in having the patient gargle 10 ml. of sterile physiological saline solution to which has been added 1000 I.U. per milliliter of penicillin and 10 mg. per milliliter of streptomycin. The throat-wash liquid is received in a sterile glass which is then placed in a sampling bottle.

For *pharyngeal swabbing in infants and children,* the mucus on the tonsils and the pharynx is removed with a swab, which is plunged in physiological saline (1 ml.) containing the antibiotics already mentioned in the quantities indicated. The swab is squeezed as much as possible into the liquid; the operation finished, the swab is destroyed, and the sample is dispatched.

The *blood* sample should be taken very soon after the appearance of the influenza syndrome. It is taken intravenously (10 ml.) without anticoagulant.

Cerebrospinal fluid samples are obtained

by puncture as soon as nervous system mani-festations appear.

Organs sampled post mortem should be taken three hours, at the latest, after death, under the most sterile conditions possible. The material sampled should be sent frozen.

SENDING OF SAMPLES. The samples should be sent by the most rapid means of transport. They should be packaged with great care. The inner container, whose air-tightness should be verified, must be placed in a resistant container, metallic or wooden, itself put in a resistant small case with cellu-lose or other absorbent wadding. In case of accidental leakage, the virulent material cannot spread to the exterior, and disinfec-tion can be assured easily.

It is preferable, if possible, to use re-frigerated transportation in commercially available isothermic polystyrene boxes. The cold can be obtained by use of ordinary ice or ice plus salt. The whole should be enclosed in a water-tight plastic bag.

Every sample should be accompanied by an information sheet indicating the date and the nature of the sample; the examination requested; the age of the patient, his name, and a reference number; the date of onset of the disease; the clinical diagnosis or the principal clinical signs, the tests already carried out, and the treatments applied. The specimen-containing vial must be labeled in concordance with the information sheet.

Methods of Isolation and Identification. Isolation of the influenza virus is made either in the embryonated egg or in tissue cultures (particularly in cultures of monkey or calf kidney).

CULTIVATION IN OVO. Inoculation of the embryonated egg remains the surest method for isolating influenza viruses, in particular the group A viruses. The adapta-tion is rapid, and identification by serological techniques is rapid.

The identification is made by cross-hemagglutination-inhibition tests between the strain isolated and standard strains of each group and subgroup and homologous sera corresponding to each group. The strain is conserved in lyophilized state.

CULTIVATION IN VITRO. Isolation of the influenza virus by this procedure fails frequently for the group A viruses, but group B viruses are more easily isolated. Group A influenza viruses multiply with difficulty in tissue cultures. As a general rule, the influenza virus conserves its antigenic characteristics (almost without modifications) in the embry-onated egg. In the animal or in tissue culture, important antigenic modifications are ob-served which maintain themselves in repeated passages. These modified strains, inoculated into the embryonated egg, conserve almost entirely the modifications brought about by passage in the animal (mouse, for example) or in cell culture.

Moreover, the influenza virus cultivated in cellular medium in vitro multiplies largely in the form of a nonhemagglutinating, infec-tious particle.

The aptitude for adaptation follows the following order: B virus: easy adaptation; A virus: inconstant adaptation, often of short duration; C virus: no adaptation, has multi-plied so far only in the amniotic cavity of the embryonated egg.

The cytopathogenic effect is also in-constant and cannot serve as a test. The most rapid and the easiest reaction to determine the presence of virus is hemadsorption.

The hemadsorption phenomenon was first observed by Vogel and Shelokov in 1957[56] in an attempt to reveal the influenza virus in monkey kidney cell culture. Hemad-sorption, like hemagglutination, implies a linkage between the viral envelope and red cell mucoprotein receptors.

As concerns myxoviruses, the present concept is that the final constitution of the infectious particle (genetic material and viral envelope) occurs at, or close to, the cell surface and that the liberation of the virus from the cell occurs over a long period. The specific viral material therefore is found at the cell surface for a long time. Because of this fact, the hemadsorption phenomenon can be demonstrated; it has since been shown to be a phenomenon general to cells infected by numerous virus types.

With the influenza viruses, hemadsorp-tion manifests itself very quickly after cellular infection. To reveal the phenomenon, human group O red cells or guinea-pig red cells are generally used.

A positive reaction is characterized by the attachment of the red cells to the cellular layer with rosettes and chains of red cells forming a highly distinctive image easily distinguished from the normal picture given by noninfected cells, which do not fix red cells. The cellular infection can be indicated rapidly by this method. Its specificity is confirmed by inhibition of hemadsorption by a specific immune serum.

VIRAL SEROLOGY

For the viral serology, the blood sample is taken under the same conditions as for general serology. It is necessary to operate *under sterile conditions* and *without use of anticoagulant*. The quantity to be taken is 5 to 10 ml. of blood.

For diagnosis of a present or recent influenza, a single sample is insufficient. Two samples are, in general, necessary; the first should be taken as early as possible in the acute stage of the disease, the second, 15 days after the first. It is thus possible to demonstrate the appearance of, or a significant rise in, the titer of specific antibodies.

Serum specimens must be sent with care and must always be accompanied by the same clinical data as those listed in connection with isolation.

Serological Methods. Use of serological methods is of major importance in diagnosis of influenza. In most cases, they are employed alone to make the diagnosis or to establish the variety of the virus involved.

The most commonly used methods at present are the complement-fixation and the hemagglutination-inhibition reactions, to which we shall add neutralization and immunofluorescence.

At the time of an influenza infection, antibodies of at least two types appear in the patient's blood: (1) antibodies detectable by the complement-fixation reaction, corresponding to a viral nucleoprotein which has no known function in regard to active immunity; and (2) antibodies detectable by hemagglutination inhibition or of neutralization, which correspond to the viral hemagglutinin, which is a surface protein of the virion. These antibodies appear only with the mature viral particle.

The antibodies revealed by the complement-fixation reaction appear early, four to five days after onset of the disease. They disappear rapidly, remaining detectable, on the average, four to five weeks, sometimes less. Subjects vaccinated with an anti-influenza vaccine prepared from the inactivated virus do not elaborate this type of antibody. We will return to this subject in connection with control of vaccination.

COMPLEMENT-FIXATION REACTION. The complement-fixation method was the first to be applied to the serology of influenza. The antigen used consisted of suspensions of virulent organs treated by repeated freezing and thawing. The antigen used is dissociated from the viral particle. It is synthesized in the cell nucleus from the viral ribonucleic acid and appears in the form of spherical particles 10 to 15 mμ in diameter and behaves as a soluble antigen. It is easily obtained from ground-up infected chorioallantoic membranes of embryonated eggs after a short incubation period and treatment by repeated freezing and thawing.

The complement-fixation reaction is practiced on two blood specimens taken under the conditions already specified. The reaction can be considered positive at a level of 1/20 or higher. Comparison of the two serum samples permits affirmation of influenza if there is a marked difference between the levels obtained with the first and the second sample. Nonetheless, if a specimen of the patient's blood was not obtained at the onset of the disease, it is possible to make the serological diagnosis with a serum sample taken toward the twelfth or the fifteenth day. Since this reaction is positive for only a limited time, a negative or decreased antibody level is sought five to six weeks later.

The complement-fixation reaction is an excellent method to establish the diagnosis of influenza, but when the purpose is an epidemiological study, verification in vaccinated subjects, or identification of virus strain, the hemagglutination-inhibition reaction should be used. With the first reaction, it is possible to demonstrate only the family of viruses involved, the antibodies titrated corresponding to the viral nucleoprotein, which is the same for all the type A viruses. It is impossible, by this reaction, to make a precise distinction between the strains A_0, A_1, and A_2, for example, and even less to detect the minor antigenic differences which occur progressively within a member of this family. The same is true for the type B viruses.

HEMAGGLUTINATION-INHIBITION REACTION. We have already discussed the principle of this reaction, which is based on the ability of influenza viruses to agglutinate red cells and on the ability of the sera of patients ill with influenza or of subjects immunized naturally or artificially to inhibit this agglutination. The inhibition is strictly specific; this specificity is due to the hemagglutinin whose plasticity we have seen.

A single reaction cannot give a valid result. During an epidemic period, a large part of the population is concerned, presenting severe, mild, or even inapparent forms. A normal subject may have an antibody titer relatively high as concerns the strain involved. The titer of influenzal antihemagglutinins is therefore relative and never absolute. The titer of the serum sampled at the onset of the disease must be compared with that obtained 15 or 18 days later. The reaction is positive when the second sample shows a titer at least four times higher than the first. Certain subjects, after an influenzal infection, have only a weak concentration of antibodies; thus, it is the difference in titer between the two samples that can shed light on the nature of the infection. However, when a titer of 1/1280 or higher is obtained in a single sample taken late, the reaction can be considered positive.

It can be useful, especially in difficult cases in which the disease evolves with complications, to follow the antibody level by taking more numerous blood specimens. In these cases, we have frequently observed that the antibodies appear relatively late, and the diagnosis of influenza can be affirmed only much after the time limits usually considered sufficient.

The influenza virus makes its mark very early in the life of human beings. During our lifetime we conserve "humoral scars" corresponding to the different influenza infections we have been subjected to; our antibody level is therefore rarely equal to zero. Long-term epidemiological studies have been carried out in subjects of all ages by the hemagglutination-inhibition reaction with the viruses that have emerged at different periods. Such studies have shown that the first "scar" corresponding to the first infection always reflects its presence, occasionally in a very marked way, when a subsequent infection with a different type occurs. The latter provokes in the patient an anamnestic effect, and there is often a high concentration of "old" antibodies due to an infection far in the past, while antibodies corresponding to the new virus may be found at a lower level even after the second week. In this case, a third sample will reveal a lowered level of the old antibodies and an increase in those provoked by the recent infection.

It must be noted that treatment with corticosteroids modifies the immunological response.

NEUTRALIZATION REACTION. Infection by the influenza virus causes the appearance in man of neutralizing antibodies that do not seem to correspond to the antihemagglutinating antibodies.

Neutralizing power is demonstrated above all in the embryonated egg. These tests of virus neutralization, which are highly specific, are lengthy and difficult and little used. They are nonetheless of high value and occasionally necessary.

METHOD USING FLUORESCEIN-MARKED ANTIBODIES. This method consists in revealing an antigen-antibody complex by marking the antibody with a fluorescent stain and examining it under the optic microscope in ultraviolet light. The fluorescence phenomenon is based on the fact that certain substances, excited by a beam of light of short wave length, emit in response a radiation of longer wave length. This procedure can reveal antibodies in patients' serum as well as the virus in the rhinopharyngeal secretions.

DIRECT EXAMINATION OF SAMPLES

Direct examination can be practiced only if the physician has immediate access to the laboratory; it is made on nasal secretions that are placed in contact with fluorescent antisera.

The technique for obtaining the nasal secretions is as follows:

The patient is placed in horizontal position, with the neck bent backward. A 10-ml. pipette is used to introduce into each nostril 5 ml. of physiological saline solution. The patient sits up immediately and lowers his head. The liquid is collected in a Petri dish: it amounts to 4 to 5 ml. Generally, 1 ml. of this sample is put into a sterile ampule that is sealed and stocked in the deep-freezer for virus isolation. The remainder, placed in a tube, is centrifuged at 2000 rpm for five minutes. The supernatant is removed, leaving approximately 0.2 ml. of liquid. The cellular sediment is dispersed in a small volume of saline solution. One drop of the cellular suspension is removed and spread on a microscope object-slide over a surface of 1 cm. diameter. Four to five slides are thus prepared for each washing.

Rhinopharyngeal samples may also be made by swabbing. The smear is then immediately spread on a slide on which have been deposited one to two drops of physiological saline solution.

The positive results present a yellow-green fluorescence. The specificity of this fluorescence is established with the aid of an unmarked control antiserum. The period of the disease during which these results can be observed is limited to two or three days. The fluorescent cells are not observed before the period of pyrexia, since pyrexia usually occurs simultaneously with the desquamation of the ciliated epithelial cells in the rhinopharyngeal passage.

The great simplicity of the method and the rapidity of detection of these cells offers a new diagnostic procedure. This technique cannot permit identification of the strain, and it is also less constant than isolation of the virus and the serological reactions, but it can help the clinician to establish the diagnosis rapidly, subsequent confirmation being obtained either by isolation of the virus or by serological examination.

EPIDEMIOLOGY

From the time when culture of the influenza virus in the embryonated egg became generally used, a relative antigenic uniformity was noted in the different strains isolated from 1933 to 1940 during seasonal epidemics; the antigenic differences observed from one epidemic to another were judged minor.

In 1940, however, Francis[18] isolated a strain which proved to be clearly different from those studied previously. It was then that the strains isolated formerly were designated by the letter "A," whereas the new one was called "B." In 1947, another type made its appearance; this virus, isolated by Taylor,[52] was called influenza "C" virus, while numerous varieties were observed within the types A and B. In 1946, a virus of type A, but distinct from those provoking seasonal epidemics since 1933, was isolated in Australia by Anderson and Burnet[1]; it was designated A_1. In 1947 and 1948, this virus provoked epidemics in America and in Europe, and from this time until 1956 the viruses isolated became, to a greater or lesser degree, different from the initial A_1 1946 strain, and these minor antigenic modifications were observed in almost all countries. The last epidemic of the A_1 substrain was reported in 1957 in Japan. But by February of this

same year, cases of influenza began to appear in South China, where the first Asian strain was isolated; this strain, although still of type A, presented antigenic differences so great in relation to the A and A_1 strains that it provoked a pandemic. It was called Asian A_2 strain. Since 1957, the type A epidemics have been due to the A_2 virus. From 1957 to 1960, the strains isolated presented only slight antigenic differences but since then minor antigenic differences have appeared and increased, so that the slight antigenic differences in regard to the prototype A_2 1957 strain that were scarcely perceptible in 1960 go on accentuating themselves from one epidemic to another.

The seasonal epidemics of type A (A_0, A_1, A_2) have a fairly short cycle, two to three years maximum; they have created more or less extensive centers of morbidity; during the epidemic period, there has always been observed a marked increase in mortality, especially in the aged.

To date, type B influenza has never been associated with a high mortality rate comparable to that observed during a group A epidemic. The centers of morbidity provoked by this virus are, in general, localized; they do not spread to all of a population. The diffusion of type B is therefore much less than that of type A influenza virus, and its cycle is longer (approximately five to six years). Concomitant epidemics of types A and B have been observed.

The strains of type B influenza virus have also shown antigenic differences among themselves, but they do not appear in a regular way as do those observed with type A influenza viruses; these strains overlap, and they have therefore not been classified by family, as have been the A viruses.

The question has been raised whether the C virus provoked major epidemics. Since the first isolation of this virus in 1947 by Taylor,[53] it has been found only in sporadic cases or during type A infections.[19] Searches for antibodies in subjects of very different ages showed that most individuals possessed anti-C antibodies of low level.

ANTIGENIC VARIATIONS

Many hypotheses have been advanced concerning the mechanism of the antigenic variations of influenza viruses.

Several authors, among them Salk in the

United States, without excluding mutations, have thought that influenza is provoked by a family of viruses whose members are more or less linked immunologically; if this is so, it could be that a certain member of this family predominates at a given moment, then declines when the majority of the population has become immune, leaving the place open for another member. As time passes, the population is no longer immune to the old member, and thus becomes vulnerable. According to this hypothesis, there would be only a limited number of antigenic variations; it would thus be necessary to protect the population against the *disease* and not merely against a *variant* responsible for an epidemic.

The results of the investigations of Mulder and Masurel[37] support this hypothesis. Before the epidemic caused by the A_2 1957 strain appeared in Holland, the sera of persons over 75 years of age showed, in a few cases, antibodies specific for the Asian strain, at low levels. In certain of these subjects, vaccination provoked the appearance of an antibody level much higher than the levels obtained in younger individuals or in the aged whose sera did not originally possess antibodies against the A_2 strain. This fact gave the impression of an anamnestic effect, which would signify that the A_2 1957 virus might have an antigenic kinship with that which provoked the 1889 pandemic.

Salk's theory finds here a strong argument, and if the next pandemic involves a virus corresponding to the one which provoked that of 1918-1919, it will be confirmed.

The other theory involves the antigenic modifications of the virus due to external conditions, in particular by passages through partially immunized human beings. The phenomenon of adaptation in influenza viruses, both human and animal, to specific antibodies was revealed in ovo and in vivo in the laboratory animal. Archetti and Horsfall in 1950[3] were the first to adapt different strains of A_0 and A_1 influenza virus to their homologous serum and to heterologous sera. The results observed were surprising enough and indicated the changeability of these viruses. Later, the same adaptation was obtained to the hemagglutination-inhibitors of the virus that are found in the normal serum of different animal species.

The variation in the antigenic constitution of influenza viruses can appear when the host animal species is changed.

In 1958, Choppin and Tamm[12] separated, from a strain of A_2 influenza virus recently isolated from a patient, two types of virus particles, the one sensitive to the corresponding antibodies, the other practically insensitive.

The appearance of a new variant among influenza viruses is thus not necessarily the result of a mutation. It is possible that, from a population of mixed particles, a variant may emerge after successive passages from individual to individual.

In other words, if a subject is infected by a strain which yields only a very small proportion of resistant particles, the particles sensitive to antibodies will be neutralized but those that are resistant will be able to multiply and yield a pure population of resistant particles.

This phenomenon is probably general and permits us to explain partially the changeability of these viruses. But what seems strange is that, on the appearance of a new virus strain that is antigenically different from those preceding, there also appears a variation in sensitivity to qualitatively different serum inhibitors and that these inhibitors are not found in the same animal species. These inhibiting and occasionally neutralizing substances revealed in the normal sera of different animal species cause problems which are still unsolved. It is likely that they play a role in the epidemiology of influenza.

Is the natural immunity to influenza observed in certain species of domestic animals related to the existence of these inhibitors, and, owing to this fact, does an animal species act as virus reservoir?

It is certain that the adaptation of the strain to its inhibitor or to the homologous or heterologous antibodies plays a role in the evolution of influenza viruses, especially as concerns those of the A type, which show a much greater degree of changeability than those of the B group.

It has been generally observed that it is difficult to isolate the influenza virus except during widespread epidemics. It seems that the virus exists in an unstable form.

Is there a relationship between human influenza and the animal influenzas? Those most studied have been influenzas of the pig and the horse.

The important research carried out especially by Shope and co-workers over more than 25 years has contributed substantial facts that permit the supposition that man can transmit the human virus to the pig. Has this animal now become a reservoir? We can state only that the fact has not been demonstrated with certainty.

As regards horse influenza, the recent epidemics both in America and in Europe have been the object of interesting experiments, some of which are under way at present writing, and for which no conclusion can be given. One fact is certain: human influenza is endemic, and the virus therefore persists in man. In the pig "enzooticity" also seems to exist; for the horse, it remains to be demonstrated. It is possible that the pandemics break out after the appearance of a mutant provoked by the transmission of a virus to a different host. The recent investigations by Tumova and Pereira[55] on the genetic interaction of influenza viruses of human and animal origin are of great interest.

Studies still under way suggest that hybridizations between human and animal strains are possible. A strain of avian influenza virus seems to have a neuraminidase with the same specificity as that of the human strain A_2 Hong Kong/68. The hemagglutinin, however, is different.

EPIDEMIOLOGICAL STUDY OF THE IMMUNITY OF A POPULATION

Numerous epidemiological studies have been made with the use of sera from large numbers of persons, grouped according to age, and spread over a great many years. The study has been directed toward individual examinations but also, and above all, has concerned serum pools separated by age groups: infants to preschool children, children from five to 12 years, adolescents to young adults, middle-aged adults, and, finally, the aged.

Thanks to this technique, it has been possible to follow the appearance, evolution, and period of action of a virus of a given type on the population. This study, made in the United States, Australia, and Great Britain at different periods from 1935 to 1964 showed that, for each strain representing an element of a particular family, active at a given period, both the antibody level and the maximal titer observed differ according to the age group, thus showing the specificity of this agent.

It was thus possible to demonstrate an antigenic identity between the virus that provoked the 1918-1919 pandemic and the porcine virus (swine strain) isolated in 1931 by Shope.[46]

The study begun in 1935 by Andrewes, in London, showed that children under 12 years of age did not possess anti-swine virus antibodies, but subjects above 20 years of age presented a very high titer.

Eighteen years later, in 1953, in Sheffield, England, serum pools, grouped by age, were again studied; no anti-swine virus antibodies were found in the groups aged less than 32 years; between ages 32 and 40 years, antibodies were detectible, but the most elevated titers were observed in adults over 40 years of age. Ten years later, in 1963, these antibodies were revealed only in the groups over 40. We have omitted to mention that an epidemic of porcine influenza had occurred in the United States in 1921, but, as in the case of the human epidemic, the virus was not isolated at this period. These serological results led to the hypothesis that the virus agent of the 1918-1919 pandemic was similar to that which provoked the porcine epidemic. Stuart-Harris, in 1935, examined the sera of the adult inhabitants of St. Helena Island, which had been spared in 1918. No anti-swine antibodies were found in these sera, but, after the invasion by the human A_0 influenza virus which raged in 1936, the results were different; the anti-swine antibodies were present in the sera examined.

These studies, over fixed time periods, made it possible to demonstrate that the first infection by an influenza virus in childhood imprints its antigen on the antibody-forming cells and determines the organism's response to the influenza viruses encountered throughout life. This fact has been confirmed by numerous research workers, among them Davenport et al.,[14] Davoli,[15] and Hilleman et al.[22] The experiments of Mulder and Masurel in 1957[37] revealing the presence of anti-A_2 (Asian strain) antibodies in aged persons who could have been in contact with the influenza virus that provoked the 1889-1890 pandemic yielded results favorable to this theory. The specificity of these antibodies could be affirmed by the method of hemagglutinin titration by photometry.

Thus far, the influenza viruses isolated from animals, whether horses, pigs, or birds, have had their particular characteristics, but all belong to the human group A, i.e., the viral nucleoprotein which constitutes the soluble antigen is identical for all these viruses. The viral genome induces specific proteins derived from the host cell.

The experimental investigations carried out in animals have shown that mutations appear with change of host.

We have noted in an earlier section that in 1732, before a human epidemic, an epizootic of an infectious respiratory disease corresponding to that in man occurred in horses. In 1956, an epizootic of equine influenza raged in Czechoslovakia a few months before the human epidemic of A_2 Asian type.

The question therefore arises of a possible virus reservoir, which could be man, or lower animals, or even a parasite; the parasite-carried infection in the pig suggests this possibility.[29, 45, 47] We recently reviewed this question.[9]

The serological studies that we have just summarized thus have contributed extremely valuable information concerning the epidemiology of influenza.

PATHOLOGICAL ROLE OF INFLUENZA VIRUS

The symptomatology is identical whether the influenza infection is of type A, B, or C.

The influenza virus penetrates by the aerial route. The incubation period is generally 48 hours; it may, however, be shorter (24 hours) or longer (72 to 96 hours). It causes a systemic infection that is manifested by the sudden appearance of an infectious syndrome whose principle element is fever. It creates a functional symptomatology, with the appearance of marked nervous system signs, and painful disturbances such as headache, generalized aching, and myalgia. The subject is prostrated with all the manifestations of a toxic state. The temperature often decreases the second day and may return to normal the fourth day. In certain subjects, a second period of pyrexia may be observed on the third or the fourth day, in which case the temperature curve is diphasic, i.e., shows a V curve. During this course the patient is anorexic and a dry cough occurs, with tracheitis, most often accompanied by hoarseness. Certain subjects present vomiting, or the impression of pulsations or lancinating pain in the eyeballs.

A study by Walsh et al. in 1961[57] involving bronchoscopic explorations and biopsies of the tracheobronchial mucosae in 12 patients with uncomplicated influenza showed that the mucosae of the larynx, the trachea, and the bronchi presented an acute inflammatory reaction, with desquamation of the ciliated cells and an exudate of mononuclear subepithelial cells.

Because of this fact, convalescents should wait a few days before resuming normal activities in order to permit reconstitution of the mucosae and thus avert secondary complications. In general, the disease develops to convalescence in four or five days, leaving only asthenia of varying severity and duration.

Apart from the pandemics, the seasonal influenza epidemics always cause a marked increase in the mortality rate, especially in the aged. The complications of influenza are mainly pulmonary; they include all degrees, from bronchitis to bronchiolitis and actual pulmonary involvement with bronchopneumonia, pneumonia with or without pleural reaction, and pulmonary edema. They can be purely viral or postinfluenzal; in the latter case, they are caused by a bacterial superinfection usually due to *Staphylococcus aureus* and *Hemophilus influenzae*. Other complications, especially nervous or cardiac, are not unusual. In patients with low resistance influenza can be rapidly fatal, death probably being due to toxicosis.

Pulmonary Complications. The clinically and radiologically demonstrated pneumopathies that occur during an influenza epidemic are varied and difficult to classify. We shall limit ourselves to purely viral influenzal pneumopathy. It appears very rapidly; the pulmonary signs are diffuse. Occasionally, however, particularly when there is a pleural reaction, extensive foci occur. The signs typical of lobar pneumonia are found only in patients with postinfluenzal pneumonia.[50] Radiological findings may not be what one would expect on the basis of the clinical examination, but the variations observed are numerous. The x-ray abnormalities are slow to disappear, and the patient may remain slightly febrile and greatly asthenic for some time.

This description applies to viral pneumopathy with a normal course. Obviously, it is greatly modified in cases of respiratory insufficiency and cardiac disease.

Cardiac Complications. The action of the influenza virus on the circulatory system was especially studied during the 1957 pandemic. Gibson et al., in 1959,[20] studied 87 students with influenza and concluded that myocarditis specifically linked to the infection provoked by the influenza virus is rare.

Influenza pericarditis represents a form of acute benign pericarditis.

The majority of authors find, in the days preceding the onset of the cardiac involvement, a respiratory system infection often labeled influenza. In France, we have for many years pursued an epidemiological study by means of biological tests and we have been able to demonstrate that in a certain number of cases relatively mild influenza infections can provoke genuine cardiac involvements, including pericarditis.

This work was the subject of a doctoral thesis in medicine at the French National Influenza Center by Letondal[33]; it concerned the analysis of 30 case histories of patients in whom pericarditis appeared in the course of a laboratory-confirmed influenza infection. Repeated radiological and electrocardiographic examinations corroborated this involvement, which can be associated with other localizations (pleuropulmonary, for example) or be masked by a severe influenzal syndrome. The findings of Letondal[33] are paraphrased here:

Pericarditis of influenzal etiology is usually benign. Pain is the most common symptom; the localization may be precordial or retrosternal. It appears abruptly; its intensity is variable; it is increased by deep respiration. At its onset, the pain can misorient the diagnosis toward myocardial infarction.

Biological, radiological, and electrocardiographic examinations confirm the viral diagnosis.

It must be noted that, at the onset of the clinical manifestations, the electrocardiogram may be normal, the electrical signs being delayed in regard to the clinical signs.

The disease evolves toward cure, but fairly often relapses of variable intensity are noted. The relapse can be only painful, or else painful with renewal of the pericardiac rub and increase in cardiac volume.

The differential diagnosis is not always easy. Other than myocardial infarction, there also arise the diagnostic possibilities of acute pericarditis of other etiologies, including rheumatic. Septic pericarditis is suggested in a septicemic picture; lastly, pericarditis due to other viral infections has been demonstrated. The biological tests are of great importance to establish a specific diagnosis.

In consequence of these observations, we can suggest that pericarditis is one of the possible localizations of influenza infection to which there may correspond various pathological processes of variable gravity. However, the mechanism of the numerous electrocardiographic anomalies registered during mild influenza infections requires much more thorough investigation.

Nervous System Complications. The majority of nervous system manifestations of influenzal origin appear during the malignant syndrome, but numerous cases of nervous complications during or after an influenza infection have been described. Certain authors have thought that there was a relationship between the 1918-1919 pandemic and the epidemic of lethargic encephalitis in 1920-1921, but the etiology could not be determined at the time, and it is probable that there was no connection between these two infections.

Cerebral manifestations in the course of a laboratory-confirmed influenza infection give rise to physiopathological problems that are far from being solved.

Between the two pandemics (1918-1919 and 1957), relatively few fatalities followed the nervous complications of influenza.

A study in infants and young children by Marquézy et al. in 1953,[35] in which we participated, showed that, in infants, the clinical picture is usually that of a neurotoxicosis. In certain cases, however, the existence of a perivenous encephalitis was suggested (hemiplegia, lymphocytic meningitis).

The 1957 epidemic presented an unusual number of neurological complications, including encephalitis, meningoencephalitis, meningitis, convulsions, and coma. The A_2 virus was isolated from the cerebrospinal fluid of patients by Flewett and Hoult.[17] These authors observed six cases of convulsions or coma at the acute phase of influenza and two cases of encephalitis. The histopathological study showed lesions resembling those in polioencephalitis and gave reason to believe that the influenza virus was really the agent of these lesions. Hoult and Flewett[24] also observed a case of acute hemorrhagic leukoencephalitis with perivascular demyelinization.

During the same period, in Italy, France, Portugal, and other European countries, as well as in Asia (Japan, India) and in the United States, cases of encephalitis or meningitis presenting the same pictures as those observed in England were described.

During this epidemic, no particular research was undertaken concerning the possible neurotropic properties of these A_2 strains.

Experimentally, Burnet and Lush in 1938[8] succeeded in determining, by repeated passages of a type A strain on the chorioallantoic membrane of chick embryos, a hemorrhagic encephalitis in the embryo. Stuart-Harris in 1939[49] obtained the same results in a shorter lapse of time. Intracerebral inoculation into the newborn mouse of crushed brain matter of the embryo of the twenty-first generation caused a meningoencephalitis. It was possible to conserve this strain with maintenance of its neurotropic properties.

Wilson Smith, during the 1950-1951 influenza epidemic, isolated from a patient a strain of influenza virus that proved, from the start, to be lethal for the chick embryo, causing generalized lesions. On fourth passage, this strain presented a neurotropic affinity, the brains of embryos presenting the picture of a meningoencephalitis.

Cateigne et al. in 1951[10] obtained in the young Cynocephalus baboon, on the sixth day after intracerebral inoculation of an A_1 influenza virus strain recently isolated from a patient, a meningoencephalitic syndrome with characteristic lesions. The histopathological examination, carried out by Bertrand and Mollaret, showed cortical perivascular edema and major alteration of the Purkinje cells. The cerebrospinal fluid of the animal was inoculated into the embryonated egg; the virus was recovered and its specificity demonstrated by the inhibitory power of the patient's serum on the virus.

In a second series of experiments, one of the monkeys inoculated by the nasal route presented a meningeal syndrome at the same time as a pulmonary involvement.

Such experiments show the ability of the influenza virus to develop on contact with nerve tissue and to create cellular lesions of the polioencephalitis type. But the route of intracerebral inoculation is far from being that concerned in human clinical disease. Many clinicians think that the irritation of a nerve cell terminus of the neurovegetative system sets off the clinical picture of an encephalitis without, in fact, the existence of a specific involvement of the central nervous system by the virus. It is true that the overwhelming toxicosis provoked by the influenza virus in certain subjects can set off this picture, but it is not impossible – it is even likely – that certain strains of influenza virus have an action almost "elective" for the nervous system.

Viremia has rarely been demonstrated.

We have set forth briefly the principal complications that may be observed in influenza infections; they occur either as isolated phenomena or in association with each other. During the 1957-1958 pandemic, other less frequent complications were noted, including various forms of hemorrhage such as epistaxis, hematemesis, hemoptysis, hematuria, and purpura, and various syndromes such as splenomegaly, laryngitis, and pancreatitis.[11]

INFLUENZA AND ITS HOST

In general, the course of influenza varies with the subject's age and physiological state.

Table 39-1. *Serological Examination of 4441 Specimens from 2526 Patients from September 1957 through February 1958*

Month	No. of Patients	Positive Reaction to Asiatic Strain %	Positive Reaction to B Strain %	Negative Reaction %	Pulmonary Syndromes %	Nervous Syndromes %	Various Syndromes %
September October 1957	816	43.25	0.36±	56.39	44	19.4	46.4
November December 1957	890	42	0.3 ±	57.7	42.5	30	43.5
January February 1958	820	26.5		73.5	27	27	25.8

Positive results: in no infants aged less than 6 months; 25% of infants aged 6 months to 2 years; 40% of children and adolescents aged 2 years to 19 years; 40% in adults aged 19 to 70 years; 50% in the aged (few in number).

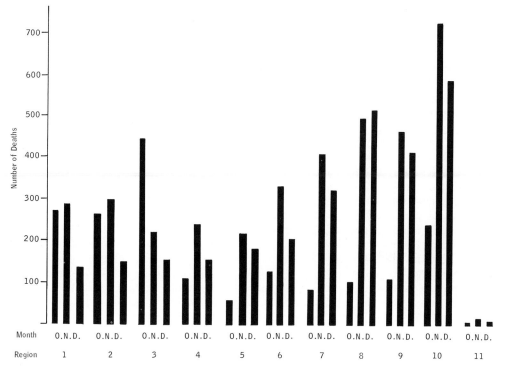

Figure 39-2. Number of deaths in France attributed to influenza during the last three months of 1957. Distribution according to regions. *1*, North Region (4 departments); *2*, Northeast Region (8 departments); *3*, Paris and the Paris region; *4*, East Region (8 departments); *5*, Southeast Region (8 departments); *6*, South Region (9 departments); *7*, Southwest Region (12 departments); *8*, West Region (13 departments); *9*, Northwest Region (8 departments); *10*, Center (17 departments); *11*, Corsica. (The department is the administrative division of French territory; they are of highly variable population density, and they also vary greatly in climate and in extent.) *O.* = October; *N.* = November; *D.* = December. (From Cateigne, G. H., Fauconnier, B., Thibon, M., and Hannoun, C.: La pandemie de grippe A₂ de 1957. Ses caracteristiques et son evolution en France. Ann. Inst. Pasteur, *99*:401-413, 1960.)

Pregnant women, cardiac patients, those with chronic respiratory insufficiencies, and the aged are particulary vulnerable.

Children react differently to the infection according to their age. Children under five years of age, and particularly young infants, are often less severely affected than older children.

The morbidity rate is a little lower in preschool children than in those aged six to eight years. In general, the disease is more severe in adults.[51]

Burnet suggested that the tissues of adults may have been sensitized by antibodies provoked by earlier infections. The intense reactions of adults, with high fever, might indicate either an allergic reaction or an inability of the tissues to tolerate the toxic effects of the influenza virus.[51]

The existence of autoimmunity and its relationship to the disease is a subject of interest to many investigators. Glynn[21] listed the mechanisms that can induce autoimmunity. The most commonly considered are, first, ant genic modifications of the host cell and of the tissue to which the cells belong by physical or chemical factors or by conjugation with haptens or foreign proteins which can form different antigenic determinants and be "considered" foreign by the lymphatic system; and, second, antigenic similarity between the host tissue and the immunizing agent.

Quite recently Isacson[27] turned his attention to the problem of myxoviruses and autoimmunity. Myxoviruses have certain properties that could induce autoimmunity by one of the above-mentioned mechanisms. Experiments have been carried out in animals, but it remains to be shown whether, in human infections, autoimmunization can occur.

One of the unique characteristics of myxoviruses, especially influenza viruses, is that they possess a neuraminidase capable of producing antigenic modifications of the host cells.

Burnet and Anderson[6] observed that the induction of a new cellular antigen by action of a viral or bacterial enzyme on red blood cells might suggest the possibility of a similar action in vivo resulting in the production of autoantibodies corresponding to the "new antigens."

According to Isacson, in the case of mild influenza that produces only cytonecrosis of the ciliated respiratory epithelium, it seems unnecessary to search for an autoimmunologic basis. Viremia is rarely found in the uncomplicated cases, but under certain circumstances the virus has been isolated from the liver, kidney, spleen, and other organs, a fact indicating that this virus has a very extensive distribution potential. Fortunately, in view of the morbidity rate, the simple cases comprise the majority. According to Isacson,[27] certain so-called complications of influenza may result from another simultaneous infection. In the case of influenzal encephalitis, the situation remains obscure owing to the varied nature of the histopathology observed.

However, as concerns the influenza virus, we have seen that the viral particle integrates certain preformed elements of the cell which undergo an antigenic modification through action of the virus that permits the creation of new antigens, perhaps derived from the incorporation of masked antigens (T antigen).[54]

Do these antigens have the property of inducing antibodies to the detriment of the host? Can they induce hypersensitivity reactions? How long do they persist in the organism, and what kind of antibodies do they produce? These questions have only barely been raised.

According to Isacson, in connection with research in patients with myxovirus infections, it can at least be said that the concept of autoimmunity is related to certain pathological manifestations, particularly in cases of postviral encephalomyelitis. The mechanism could be as follows, possibly with a few variations in the case of other complications: After the initial infection and during the incubation period, the virus multiplies in a given point, the nasopharynx; it is then liberated into the blood and circulates widely. The infection may be limited to this stage and manifest itself only by the production of circulating antibodies. Under certain conditions, however, the virus may reach the central nervous system and multiply there. If the multiplication is sufficiently extensive, a "primary" meningoencephalitis may result from the direct action of the virus. In this case, the symptomatology appears early, and histopathological examination does not show disseminated perivenous demyelinization. Isacson states:

An aspect of this type is observed in cases of mumps meningitis. In other cases, the initial multiplication in the CNS may not be sufficiently extensive to be clinically detectable; the virus continues, however, to multiply in the CNS cells, the cellular antigens of which are normally separated from the host's immunological system by physiological barriers and are therefore considered as foreign. Throughout the reconstitution of the viral particle, these antigens are incorporated into the virion and the virus is liberated into the circulation. The virus then reaches the cells producing antibody, not only against the viral antigen but also against the CNS tissue, and there then appear the histopathological pictures typical of demyelinization.

This concept is rather interesting; for this reason we have described it. But autoimmunity in myxovirus infections is far from being an accepted fact. The author believes that strictly controlled experiments could be undertaken, for, according to the theories formulated and the experimental work carried out in animals, it seems possible that the myxoviruses, especially the influenza virus, induce autoimmunity.

PROPHYLAXIS OF INFLUENZA

Disinfection has proved ineffectual against influenza because contagion occurs mainly from sneezing and coughing and it would be impossible to abolish human contacts on the vast scale required.

VACCINATION

The only effective method of prevention is vaccination, the vaccine being prepared from inactivated virus. It has been demonstrated that such vaccine, injected subcutaneously, especially in association with an adjuvant, protects much more effectively than the vaccines at present prepared from live attenuated viruses administered by the nasal route.[39]

All the anti-influenza vaccines in use to

date are prepared from virus inoculated into the allantoic sac of the embryonated egg. The virus multiplies readily in the allantoic cells, and, after its liberation from the cells, it is found in the allantoic fluid. This virulent liquid serves for vaccine preparation, in which the principal stages are concentration and purification of the virus, titration, formaldehyde inactivation, and association with an adjuvant.

The concentration of virus is controlled by quantitative hemagglutination tests. The efficacy of the vaccine is verified by measuring the antibody level in vaccinated mice.

Efforts have been made to adapt the different types of influenza virus to different types of cell cultures in vitro with the purpose of preparing a vaccine in a manner similar to that used, for example, for antipoliomyelitis vaccine. To date, all these attempts have failed to give a sufficient concentration of virus.

When influenza appeared in China early in 1957, the national centers throughout the world were alerted by W.H.O., which advised them as soon as the first strain isolated in China was available. In France, the National Influenza Center at the Pasteur Institute very early initiated its participation in the struggle against this epidemic by preparing a vaccine that was made available to the public in 1957. Since then, vaccination in France continues with use of a quadrivalent vaccine constituted from strains whose characteristics and antigenicity have been particularly studied; the concentration and the purification of each strain are obtained by adsorption on formaldehyde-treated red cells, followed by elution. After titration of the hemagglutinin, adequate dilutions are carried out; the viral particles are inactivated by formaldehyde, then adsorbed on aluminum hydroxide.

Except during pandemics, the best period for vaccination is the autumn. A booster injection at the same period every year yields satisfactory immunity. If, as there is every reason to believe, the minor antigenic variations produced by passage of the virus from partially immunized subjects and which are additive from year to year are, in the main, responsible for seasonal epidemics, especially of type A, a booster injection with a vaccine containing one of the last strains isolated has every chance of protecting sufficiently. The immunity acquired by an acute infection appears to be solid and durable in most individuals, but it is active only in regard to the strain responsible for this disease. Vaccination does not seem to impart as solid an immunity, and this is why booster injections are called for. They have a double purpose: to consolidate the plurivalent immunity acquired, and to provoke specific antibodies for the strain in its current gradual antigenic evolution.

The inoculation of two doses of inactivated vaccine properly spaced (15 to 21 days) is recommended for primary vaccination; a single injection may be given when an epidemic is imminent. When vaccination is carried out at the proper time with respect to appearance of the epidemic and with a vaccine containing the strains required for the immunization, the protection can be of the order of 75 to 80 per cent. These rates have been reported by almost all laboratories, including our own, that have verified the effectiveness of their vaccination within closed communities.

Vaccination against influenza is especially recommended for the aged, persons with respiratory insufficiency, cardiac patients, and pregnant women. In general, it does not produce any systemic reaction. Except in subjects allergic to egg proteins, it has no contraindications other than those, temporary or permanent, common to all vaccinations.

EFFECTIVENESS OF VACCINATION

The value of the vaccine has been determined in several closed communities by two methods. First, serological tests are carried out on four blood specimens, one taken before vaccination and one each taken one month, two months, and three and a half months after the last injection of vaccine. The antibodies are titrated by the hemagglutination-inhibition reaction. Second, the morbidity rate is evaluated.

One study, among others, made by us in a home for the aged in Besançon (France) showed an increase in antibody level for all the strains contained in the vaccine. Three and a half months later, approximately half the subjects had maintained the antibody level acquired one month after vaccination, whereas in the other half this level had diminished to some degree. An influenza epidemic appeared in the winter following the vaccination; the morbidity rate was much lower in the vaccinated subjects than in those not vaccinated. The vaccinated aged persons who had influenza, confirmed by the complement-fixation reaction, were ill only one day with a slight febrile episode; in contrast, in the control group, the mortality rate was 8 per cent.

At present, vaccination against influenza is applied in all countries.

JUSTIFICATION OF VACCINATION

Vaccination against influenza, which should be applied both in adults and in children, is justified because we have no effectual specific therapy against the disease.

Epidemics of pandemic proportions are seen only every 30 or 40 years, but the seasonal epidemics, on a lesser scale, also take a heavy toll of human lives. Influenza is also an economic scourge; it can paralyze the life of a country, and even when it does not attain catastrophic proportions it drains considerable sums from the national economy every year.

Thus effective prophylaxis of influenza remains one of the major goals of the specialists in this field. Substantial improvements will probably be made soon.

CHEMOTHERAPY

It is possible, under certain experimental conditions, to block the synthesis of the virus at one or several stages of the intracellular process, but the substances that interfere with the synthesis of the viral nucleic acid are often so harmful to the cell that harbors the virus that they have no therapeutic value. A great number of substances have been studied, certain of which have shown an antiviral activity in vitro, but in man the results proved to be entirely different. The biguanide derivatives, for example, appeared highly promising but their promise was not fulfilled.

Interferon, a protein synthesized by cells exposed to the action of a foreign nucleic acid, is a natural antiviral substance[26] on which great hope was placed. Extensive investigations have been made, but the successes obtained have not been as great as was hoped. The potency of interferon is weak; it must be administered very early in the infection, or even before; it is difficult to prepare.

The search for a specific antiviral therapy continues.

BIBLIOGRAPHY

1. Anderson, S. G., and Burnet, F. M.: Sporadic and minor epidemic behaviour of Influenza "A" in Victoria 1945-46. Aust. J. Exp. Biol. Med. Sci., *25*:235-243, 1947.
2. Andrewes, C. H., Bang, F. B., and Burnet, F. M.: A short description of the myxovirus group (influenza and related viruses). Virology, *1*:176-184, 1955.
3. Archetti, I., and Horsfall, F. L., Jr.: Persistent antigenic variation of influenza A viruses after incomplete neutralization "in ovo" with heterologous immune serum. J. Exp. Med., *92*:441-462, 1950.
4. Blough, H. A.: The role of the surface state in the morphogenesis of influenza virus filaments. Virology, *19*:112-114, 1963.
5. Burnet, F. M.: Propagation of the virus of epidemic influenza on the developing egg. Med. J. Aust., *2*:687, 1935.
6. Burnet, F. M., and Anderson, S. G.: The "T" antigen of guinea pig and human red cells. Aust. J. Exp. Biol. Med. Sci., *25*:213-217, 1947.
7. Burnet, F. M., and Lind, P. E.: Studies on filamentary forms of influenza virus with special reference to the use of dark-ground microscopy. Arch. Ges. Virusforsch., *7*:413-428, 1957.
8. Burnet, F. M., and Lush, D.: Influenza virus on developing egg. Comparison of 2 antigenically dissimilar strains of human influenza virus after full adaptation to egg membrane. Aust. J. Exp. Biol. Med. Sci., *16*:261-274, 1938.
9. Cateigne, G. H.: Inhibiteurs sériques non spécifiques de l'hémagglutination des virus de la grippe humaine. Relations éventuelles entre les virus grippaux, humains, porcins et équins. Congrès de Pathologie Comparée, Liban, 1966. In: La Grippe. Paris, Editions Médicales et Scientifiques, 1967. Vol. 2, pp. 9-61.
10. Cateigne, G. H., Fauconnier, B., and Brygoo, P.: Etude expérimentale du virus grippal (épidémie de grippe 1950-1951). Sem. Hop. Paris, *1*:90-99, 1953.
11. Cateigne, G. H., Fauconnier, B., Thibon, M., and Hannoun, C.: La pandémie de grippe A₂ de 1957. Ses caractéristiques et son évolution en France. Ann. Inst. Pasteur, *99*:401-413, 1960.
12. Choppin, P. W., and Tamm, I.: Two kinds of particles with contrasting properties in influenza A virus strains from the 1957 pandemic. Virology, *8*:539-542, 1959.
13. Choppin, P. W., and Tamm, I.: Studies of two kinds of virus particles which comprise influenza A₂ virus strains. I. Characterization of stable homogeneous sub-strains in reactions with specific antibody, mucoprotein inhibitors, and erythrocytes. J. Exp. Med., *112*:895-920, 1960.
14. Davenport, F. M., Hennessy, A. V., Stuart-Harris, G. H., and Francis, T., Jr.: Epidemiology of influenza. Comparative serological observations in England and the United States. Lancet, *2*:469-473, 1955.
15. Davoli, R.: Anticorpi verso virus dell' influenza A "Asia" nella popolazione normali. Sperimentale, *107*:358, 1957.
15a. Debré, R.: L'anergie dans la grippe. C. R. Soc. Biol. (Paris), *81*:913-914, 1918.
16. Dujarric de la Riviere, R.: La grippe est-elle une maladie à virus filtrant? C. R. Acad. Sci. (Paris), *167*:606, 1918.

17. Flewett, T. H., and Hoult, J. G.: Influenzal encephalopathy and post-influenzal encephalitis. Lancet, 2:11-15, 1958.

18. Francis, T., Jr.: A new type of virus epidemic influenza. Science, 92:405-408, 1940.

19. Francis, T., Jr., Davenport, F. M., and Hennessy, A. V.: A serological recapitulation of human infection with different strains of influenza virus. Trans. Ass. Amer. Physicians, 66:231, 1953.

20. Gibson, T. C., Arnold, J., Craige, E., and Curnen, E. C.: Electrocardiographic studies in Asian influenza. Amer. Heart J., 57:661, 1959.

21. Glynn, L. E.: In Cruisckshank, R. (ed.): Modern Trends in Immunology. London, Butterworth, 1963, pp. 206-226.

22. Hilleman, M. R., Flatley, F. J., Anderson, S. A., Luecking, M. L., and Levinson, D. J.: Distribution and significance of Asian and other influenza antibodies in the human population. New Eng. J. Med., 258:969-974, 1958.

23. Hirst, G. K.: The agglutination of red cells by allantoic fluid of chick embryos infected with influenza virus. Science, 94:22-23, 1941.

24. Hoult, J. G., and Flewett, T. H.: Influenzal encephalopathy and post-influenzal encephalitis: histological and other observations. Brit. Med. J., 1:1847-1850, 1960.

25. Hoyle, L.: The release of influenza virus from the infected cells. J. Hyg. (Camb.), 52:180-187, 1954.

26. Isaacs, A.: Antiviral action of interferon. Brit. Med. J., 2:353-355, 1962.

27. Isacson, P.: Myxovirus and auto-immunity. Progr. Allerg., 10:256-292, 1967.

28. Kates, M., Allison, A. C., Tyrrell, D. A. J., and James, A. T.: Lipids of influenza virus and their relation to those of the host cell. Biochim. Biophys. Acta, 52:455-466, 1961.

29. Kammer, H., and Hanson, R. P.: Studies in the transmission of swine influenza virus with metastrongylus species in specific pathogen free swine. II. The in vivo association of swine influenza virus with metastrongylus species. J. Infect. Dis., 110: 99-106, 1962.

30. Kilbourne, E. D., and Murphy, J. S.: Genetic studies of influenza viruses. I. Viral morphology and growth capacity as exchangeable genetic traits. Rapid "in ovo" adaptation of early passage Asian strain by combination with PR8. J. Exp. Med., 111: 387-406, 1960.

31. McClelland, L., and Hare, R.: The adsorption of influenza virus. Canad. J. Public Health, 32:530-538, 1941.

32. Lépine, P. R., et al.: Techniques de laboratoire en virologie humaine. Isolements, Identification, Sérologie, Diagnostic. Paris, Masson et Cie, 1964.

33. Letondal, S.: Les péricardites grippales. Thèse Med., Paris, 1964.

34. Von Magnus, P.: Propagation of the PR8 strains of influenza A virus in chick embryos. II. The formation of "incomplete" virus following inoculation of large doses of seed virus. Acta Path. Microbiol. Scand., 28:278-293, 1951.

35. Marquézy, R. A., Bach, C., Debray, P., Hoppeler, A. R., Cateigne, G., and Fauconnier, B.: Les manifestations encéphalo-méningées de la grippe chez l'enfant. Sem. Hop. Paris, 1:119-128, 1953.

36. Morgan, C., Rose, H. M., and Moore, D. H.: Structure and development of viruses observed in the electron microscope. J. Exp. Med., 104:171-182, 1956.

37. Mulder, J., and Masurel, N.: Pre-epidemic antibody against 1957 strains of Asiatic influenza in serum of older people living in the Netherlands. Lancet, 1:810-814, 1958.

38. Nicolle, C., and Lebailly, C.: Quelques notions expérimentales sur le virus de la grippe. C. R. Acad. Sci. (Paris), 167:607-610, 1918.

39. Organisation Mondiale de Santé (World Health Organization): Vaccines against the viruses and Rickettsiae of human illnesses. Geneva, 1966.

40. Oeuvres d'Hippocrate: Epidémies. Livre VI. Javal et Bourdeaux, 1933, Vol. 2, pp. 81-83.

41. Rafelson, M. E., Jr.: The neuraminidases and their action on the glycoproteins and other sialic acid containing compounds. Expos. Ann. Biochim. Med., 24:121-132, 1963.

42. Saillant, M.: Epidémies catharrales. Fac. Med., Paris, 1780.

43. Schaffer, F. L.: Physical and chemical properties and infecting of RNA from animal viruses. Sympos. Quant. Biol., 27:89-99, 1962.

44. Selter, M.: Zur Aetiologie der Influenza. Deutsch. Med. Wschr., 932-933, 1918.

45. Sen, H. G., Kelley, G. W., Uderdahl, N. R., and Young, G. A.: Transmission of swine influenza virus by lungworm migration. J. Exp. Med., 113: 517-520, 1961.

46. Shope, R. E.: Swine influenza I. Experimental transmission and pathology. J. Exp. Med., 54:349-359, 1931.

47. Shope, R. E.: The swine lungworm as a reservoir and intermediate host for swine influenza virus. I. The presence of swine influenza virus in healthy and susceptible pigs. J. Exp. Med., 74:41-47, 1941; II. The transmission of swine influenza virus by the swine lungworm. J. Exp. Med., 74:49-68, 1941; III. Factors influencing transmission of the virus and the provocation of influenza. J. Exp. Med., 77:111-126, 1943; IV. The demonstration of masked swine influenza virus in lungworm larvae and swine under natural conditions. J. Exp. Med., 77:127-138, 1943.

48. Smith, W., Andrewes, C. H., and Laidlaw, P.: A virus obtained from influenza patients. Lancet, 225:66-68, 1933.

48a. Smith, W., Belyavin, G., and Sheffield, F. W.: A host-protein component of influenza viruses. Nature, 172:669-670, 1953.

49. Stuart-Harris, C. H.: A neurotropic strain of human influenza virus. Lancet, 1:497-499, 1939.

50. Stuart-Harris, C. H.: Twenty years of influenza epidemics. Amer. Rev. Resp. Dis., 83:54-61, 1961.

51. Stuart-Harris, C. H.: Influenza and other virus infections of the respiratory tract. London, Edward Arnold, 1965.

52. Taylor, R. M.: Studies on survival of influenza virus between epidemics and antigenic variants of the virus. Amer. J. Public Health, 39:171-178, 1949.

53. Taylor, R. M.: A further note on 1233 (influenza C) virus. Arch. Ges. Virusforsch. 4:485-500, 1951.

54. Thomsen, O.: Ein Vermehrungsfähiges Agens als Veränderer des isoagglutinatorischen Verhaltens der roten Blutkörperchen, eine bisher ungekannte Quelle der Fehlbertimmung. Z. Immunitätsforsch., 32:85-107, 1927.

55. Tumova, B., and Pereira, H. G.: Genetic interaction between influenza A viruses of human and animal origin. Virology, *27*:253-261, 1965.

55a. Valentine, R. L., and Isaacs, A.: The structure of influenza virus filaments and spheres. J. Gen. Microbiol., *16*:195-203, 1957.

56. Vogel, J., and Shelokov, A.: Adsorption-hemagglutination test for influenza virus in monkey kidney tissue culture. Science, *126*:358-359, 1957.

57. Walsh, J. J., Dietlen, L. F., Low, F. N., Burch, G. E., and Mogabgab, W. J.: Broncho-tracheal response in human influenza. Arch. Intern. Med., *108*: 376, 1961.

58. Wecker, E.: Die Verteilung von ^{32}P ein Virus der klassischen Geflügelpest bei verschiedenen Markierungs verfahren. Naturforsch., *12^b*:208-210, 1957.

40

Common Cold

COMMON COLD: CLINICAL FEATURES

by J. Couvreur and J. Celers

For some 20 years, the common cold has given rise to important scientific work. The cold plays an important economic and social role because of the amount of absenteeism it causes. Eighty-five per cent of the population have one to three colds a year.[16]

HISTORY

The cold is part of the clinical picture of many viral respiratory diseases. However, virological studies devoted to the cold confer on it a genuine individuality. Indeed, most often it seems to be associated with a family of viruses which were referred to as coryza viruses, Salisbury strains, enterovirus-like, ERC viruses, or muriviruses and are now called rhinovirus.[1]

As early as 1914, Kruse and Foster suspected that the common cold had a viral origin. Sixteen years later, Dochez and collaborators brought proof of this theory by inducing the disease in chimpanzees and man by inoculating filtrates of nasal origin, obtained from affected subjects with colds. In 1950, culture of a DC virus was obtained in human embryonic tissue. In 1956, two viruses were isolated: the J.H. strain virus of Price and the 2060 virus of Pelon. Their cytopathogenic activity is identical to that of the enteroviruses. Proof of their virological identity was given, and they were called "ECHO 28." This ECHO 28 virus was later related to the rhinovirus group and was the first element of a large family all of whose members are not yet identified.

Other viruses may be responsible for the common cold: adenoviruses, respiratory syncytial virus, parainfluenza myxoviruses, and enteroviruses, among which the Coe virus or Coxsackie A21 plays an important part (see Chapter 44).

The role of the rhinoviruses in the common cold has been established by Andrewes et al.,[1] Hobson and Schild,[15] Hamre et al.,[12] Tyrrell et al.,[35, 36] Johnson and Rosen,[19] Hamparian et al.,[11] and Taylor-Robinson and colleagues.[30, 31, 32]

Clinical study has been renewed by careful and often prospective observation of groups of people[12, 15, 20, 22, 27, 28] and by transmission of the disease to volunteers.[5, 6, 17, 20, 28-31] Some of these experiments followed a precise schema. Volunteers were isolated as much as possible for three or four days before the experiment and for ten days afterward. A virulent filtrate was inoculated intranasally and a close clinical surveillance maintained.

CLINICAL FEATURES

All studies done during epidemics have revealed the multiplicity of different groups and families of viral agents involved. However, no remarkable difference has been seen between the clinical pictures induced in adults by these different viruses that would permit a precise etiologic diagnosis on the basis of signs and symptoms.[13]

Different pictures may be observed, as reported below, according to the host (allergic phenomena) and age. The cold may be much more protean in babies and more severe, with involvement of the lower respiratory tract.[28] This greater severity stems undoubtedly from the fact that children are generally undergoing their first antigenic experience with the virus.[3]

Common Cold due to Rhinoviruses in the Adult. The incubation period is short, 24 hours to three days, and varies according to the virus, being short for enteroviruses and longer for adenoviruses, respiratory syncytial virus, and parainfluenza viruses. Sneezing and rhinorrhea are the first signs. Nasal discharge can increase rapidly: measurements have been made of the number and weight of standard-sized handkerchiefs used by volunteers under study. This number may pass from five to 30 on the second day, and the weight of secretions reaches 85.5 gm. per day.[6] The mucus may become more viscous, then purulent owing to a superinfection. A fairly close parallel is noted between the severity of disease and the abundance of nasal secretion. The nasal mucosa is reddened and edematous, sometimes to the point of more or less completely obstructing the nares. These localized signs are accompanied by general discomfort, as well as by a headache in half of the cases and fever, usually moderate (37.5° to 38.5° C.), in a fifth of them. Myalgia is sometimes present. Other localizations of the cold are often observed: auricular (otalgia, salpingemphraxis, tympanic congestion); ocular (watering eyes, photophobia, injection of the conjunctiva, mucopurulent discharge, swelling of the eyelids); pharyngeal (dysphagia, diffuse erythema, edema of the mucosa). Cough appears early, is very frequent, often paroxysmal, and sometimes incessant. It can suggest a laryngeal involvement which, in children, can go as far as to evoke diphtheritic croup.

Table 40-1 shows the distribution of these different manifestations according to several studies of rhinovirus infection. The evolution of the disease goes toward intensification of all signs, which reach a maximum on the second or third day. Experiments on volunteers have made it possible to distinguish several clinical aspects according to the severity of the disease[6]: One group presents no signs or only a minimal rhinorrhea; in a second group, there are rhinitis with congestion and nasal drip; in a third group, there is general discomfort in addition to the signs present in the second group; finally, in the last group, a definite febrile state occurs.

The disease is short-lived and hardly lasts more than two to five days. Sometimes, however, the nasal drip persists one or two weeks.

Blood studies can show a moderate but significant rise in the number of leukocytes with an increase in the total number of circulating neutrophils during the acute phase. However, this aspect is not very constant. The sedimentation rate remains normal or rises to between 25 and 50 in the first hour.

Bacteria are isolated from the nasal secretions in a very small number of cases, especially if specimens are taken at the beginning of the disease.

Thus the disease is very benign. All severe colds accompanied by marked general signs should make one suspect the presence of an agent other than a rhinovirus.

Common Cold in the Child. Common colds in the child are sometimes more severe. In an appreciable number of cases lower respiratory tract involvement occurs as well as digestive symptoms: loss of appetite, vomiting, diarrhea. It is, however, most likely that the frequency of these comparatively severe forms depends on the etiological agent as well as on the environment, i.e., on the conditions of contamination in which the child is living.

Between 1959 and 1962, Hamparian et al.[11] observed 87 cases of rhinovirus respiratory disease: 59 cases in adults who were university undergraduates or members of the laboratory staff, and 28 cases in children under eight years of age who were outpatients of the neighboring hospital and belonged to a much less favored social group. Whereas only a single adult showed symptoms of bronchitis, approximately 50 per cent of these children had involvement of the lower respiratory tract. The diagnoses were as

Table 40-1. *Respective Frequencies (Percentages) of Various Manifestations during Rhinovirus Infections as Reported in Several Studies on the Common Cold*

Author	Subjects	General Signs				Localized Signs — Eyes				Tympanic Membrane		Nose			Pharynx			Larynx	Respiratory Tract		Digestive Tract	Cervical Adenopathies
		Fever	Headache	Discomfort	Myalgia	Watering Eyes	Photophobia	Conjunctivitis	Ocular Discharge	Reddening	Otorrhea	Mucal Rhinorrhea	Purulent Rhinorrhea	Congestion	Pharyngitis	Edema	Lymphoid Hyperplasia	Involvement	Cough	Stethoscopic Signs	Vomiting-Diarrhea	Presence
Hamre	Young Adults	0–25	37–50									80–88		12–44	57–88				37–57			
Reilly	Adults	20	30	55		5	10	10	5	0	0	90	20	50	50	30	0	20	40	0	5	5
	Children	60	7	20		0	0	47		0	20	67	7	33	33	20	33	7	100	47	33	53
Cate	Adults (inoculated volunteers)	16	66	50	24	18		16		8		100			24				66			26
Forsyth	Adults	22	62	40	25	31						90							86		12–14	

follows: croup (one case), bronchitis (seven cases), bronchiolitis (three cases), broncho-pneumonia (three cases).

On the other hand, in 1961 Bloom et al.,[3] in comparing rhinovirus infections in young Navy recruits and their children living with them under the same conditions, did not notice any difference that might have been caused by age. Symptomatology as well as the frequency rate of virus isolation were fully comparable in the different age groups.

However, if discrepancy in degree of severity according to age may still be contested for rhinoviruses, it has been abundantly proved for other viruses causing infection of the upper respiratory tracts — parainfluenza myxoviruses, respiratory syncytial virus, and adenoviruses (see Chapter 44).

Etiological Forms. As we have mentioned before, it is practically impossible to channel virological research taking clinical symptomatology alone as a starting point; the very same symptoms may be encountered for each type of virus causing infections of the upper respiratory tract. However, thanks to investigations bearing on several dozens of cases, it is possible to find evidence of certain discrepancies in the relative frequency of these different symptoms. Thus, Forsyth et al.[10] have been able to study 121 cases of rhinovirus infections (cf. Table 40-1), 348 cases of adenovirus type 4 infections, and 120 cases of Coxsackie A21 virus infections in the same Army unit of young recruits. They observed in patients with adenovirus type 4 infection a more significantly higher incidence of fever (51 to 81 per cent) and general symptoms, and lower incidence of sneezing and chest pains than usual in rhinovirus infections. This decreased frequency of sneezing and chest pains was also found in subjects infected by Coxsackie A21 virus, who, on the other hand, complained more frequently of conjunctival irritation, but who did not show more marked systemic signs than subjects infected by rhinoviruses.

It should be stressed that virological investigations of the common cold have been unable to identify a virus in more than 20 to 50 per cent of all cases. It is probable that a great number of viruses cannot be identified by present-day techniques. It is equally possible, however, that other factors, particularly factors of allergy, have played a role in the appearance of the syndrome.

Allergic Response. Allergic constitution, the importance of which is also stressed in connection with acute viral laryngitis (cf. Chapter 41), may increase the symptoms of the common cold at the level of both the upper and the lower respiratory tracts (asthmatic bronchitis and attacks of asthma).

Furthermore, the common cold is much more frequent in subjects suffering from a nasal sinus allergy, and it is not always possible to determine with certainty the exact degree of participation of the infectious element. That is to say, the very diagnosis of the "common cold" is sometimes difficult.

DIAGNOSIS

In most cases, however, the diagnosis of the common cold is easy: sneezing, rhinitis, sore throat, and coughing without any significant general symptoms are the first elements of a diagnosis which will be confirmed epidemiologically.

Allergic rhinitis yields the most comparable picture. Theoretically, the circumstances of its appearance, the recurrence and the frequency of attacks, the evidence of persistent symptoms in the intervals between acute attacks, the presence of a family or personal history of allergy, the noncontagious nature of the affection, and its connection with the absorption or inhalation of allergens are among the many elements which should make the diagnosis of characteristic forms easier. However, symptoms are by no means always so clear cut, especially in the child. It may be necessary to look for an itching nose or an itching lip, which may be revealed by facial expressions, or for eosinophils in nasal secretions, and finally, one may have to study the reaction of the patient to antihistamines. As we have seen, an allergic constitution favors the development of the infectious process. Authentic accidents due to allergy complicate the symptomatology of the most clearly demonstrated viral infection, and we are still ignorant of the exact mechanism of these reactions.

Pyogenic rhinitis or rhinopharyngitis is rapidly accompanied by purulent secretions and pulpy exudates at the level of the tonsils, as well as by leukocytosis with polymorphonucleosis, and, finally, by the selective development of a germ which is identifiable by current bacteriological techniques. Streptococcic infections, however, and mainly in the child, are sometimes shown by a reddened throat and a thin mucopurulent discharge. Inversely, congestive otitis is frequent during the course of viral infections of the upper respiratory tract and anterior cervical adenopathy is found so often during the examination of children that it has but little orienting value.

Other virus infections display, at least at their outset, the picture of acute common cold. This is more particularly the case with *measles*, the first symptoms of which should be systematically looked for in the child (cf. Chapter 27). In contrast, influenza does not produce any notable coryza (cf. Chapter 39).

EPIDEMIOLOGY AND PATHOGENESIS

Spontaneous colds usually occur in epidemics. Recrudescence during the winter is obvious. Colds can be observed particularly between November and March, and their frequency sharply diminishes in April. Most authors have noted that, surprisingly enough, an appreciable proportion of the population, 6 to 10 per cent, never have colds.

This notion leads to a discussion of the role of certain factors which favor colds. For centuries, the common cold has been considered to be a complication of chilling. Certain studies seem to have seriously shaken this idea.

By exposing lightly dressed subjects for four hours, some at relatively high temperatures in humid atmospheres and others at cool temperatures in a dry atmosphere, it was established that in noninfected subjects the chill does not activate latent viruses and does not give rise to the clinical syndrome of the common cold. In subjects who are uniformly inoculated and subjected to these environmental variations, chilling does not increase susceptibility, the rate of appearance, or the severity of the clinical syndrome. Fatigue and exercise do not significantly increase susceptibility. Women seem to be resistant during their menstrual periods and more susceptible afterwards. Susceptibility is much more marked in hayfever sufferers. Thus, the variability in the relationships between infection and disease depends not only on the type of virus but also on the host's reactions, previous antigenic stimulations, physiological state at the time of contamination, and, perhaps, hereditary factors such as allergies. The increased number of colds during the winter has causes other than chilling of the subject.[17]

The viruses of the common cold are spread by person-to-person contact, and the Salisbury group has shown that the air in a room in which cold-infected children have played was infectious for volunteers. Quantitative studies have afforded a greater understanding of the mechanism of the spreading of colds.[4] Volunteers were inoculated with Coxsackie A21 virus and their nasal secretions were "marked" with a bacillus (*Bacillus mycoides*). It was thus possible to establish that the material expelled upon sneezing is projected in droplets which fall to the floor, dry up, and are not infectious. Speaking and coughing hardly spread the virus. Much greater quantities of virus are disseminated when patients blow their noses or sneeze, but only 0.1 per cent of these particles survive without being dried out and inactivated. There are enormous differences in the amounts of virus produced by individuals who present identical clinical signs and symptoms. Only a small proportion of them eliminate significant amounts of virus. Then a single droplet emitted during a sneeze is sufficient to infect a volunteer.

Inoculation of the Coxsackie A21 virus via the intestinal tract produces neither a clinical syndrome nor an immunological response. It certainly seems that these latter phenomena are associated with the multiplication of virus in the nasal mucosa. Study of epithelial cells taken from the concha nasalis inferior and studied with the Papanicolaou technique has shown that on the second, fourth, and sixth days after inoculation of volunteers there was a progressive increase in the number of abnormal epithelial cells, analogous to those seen in tissue culture. No lesions seemed to be specific for a given virus. Experiments on volunteers have shown that a certain parallel exists between the local multiplication of virus and the clinical syndrome.[8] Three types of responses can be distinguished. In a large group of subjects, virus multiplication is striking as early as the first or second day after inoculation and the cold is clinically apparent. This evolutionary aspect is called "early high-shedding pattern." In the second, smaller group, the multiplication of virus takes place only after at least three days and remains moderate without being associated with clinical signs. This is the "late low-shedding pattern."

Finally, in a small number of cases, no multiplication of virus is detected and no disease appears. All members of this group have high titers of antibodies at the time of inoculation. However, in the first two groups, no relation was seen between the frequency and extent of the disease and that of the viral elimination. The virus is less often found in pharyngeal than in nasal secretions. It is more frequently found in male subjects.

BIBLIOGRAPHY

1. Andrewes, C. H., Burnet, F. M., Enders, J. F., Gard, S., Hirst, C. K., Kaplan, M. M., and Zhdanov, V. M.: Taxonomy of viruses infecting vertebrates: present knowledge and ignorance. Virology, *15*:52, 1961.
2. Bang, F. B., Bang, B. G., and Foard, M. A.: Responses of upper respiratory mucosa to drugs and viral infections. Amer. Rev. Resp. Dis., *93*:142, 1966.
3. Bloom, H. H., Forsyth, R. R., Johnson, K. M., and Chanock, R. M.: Relationship of rhinovirus infection to mild upper respiratory disease. Result of a survey in young adults and children. J.A.M.A., *186*:38, 1963.
4. Buckland, F. E., Bynoe, M. L., and Tyrrell, D. A. J.: Experiments on the spread of colds. II. Studies in volunteers with Coxsackie virus A21. J. Hyg. (Camb.), *63*:327, 1965.
5. Bynoe, M. L., Horner, J., Schild, G. C., Hobson, D., Kipps, A., and Tyrrell, D. A. J.: Inoculation of human volunteers with a strain isolated from a common cold. Lancet, *1*:1194, 1961.
6. Cate, T. R., Couch, R. B., and Johnson, K. M.: Studies with rhinoviruses in volunteers: production of illness, effect of naturally acquired antibody, and demonstration of a protective effect not associated with serum antibody. J. Clin. Invest., *43*:56, 1964.
7. Dochez, A. R., Shibley, G. S., and Mills, K. C.: Studies on the common cold. IV. Experimental transmission of the common cold to anthropoid apes and human beings by means of a filtrable agent. J. Exp. Med., *52*:701, 1930.
8. Douglas, R. G., Cate, T. R., Gerone, P. J., and Couch, R. B.: Quantitative rhinovirus shedding patterns in volunteers. Amer. Rev. Resp. Dis., *94*:159, 1966.
9. Dowling, H. F., and Lefkowitz, L. B.: Clinical syndromes in adults caused by respiratory viruses. Amer. Rev. Resp. Dis., *88*:61, 1966.
10. Forsyth, B. R., Bloom, H. H., Johnson, K. M., and Chanock, R. M.: Patterns of illness in rhinovirus infections of military personnel. New Eng. J. Med., *269*:602, 1963.
11. Hamparian, V. V., et al.: Epidemiologic investigation of rhinovirus infections. Proc. Soc. Exp. Biol. Med., *117*:469, 1964.
12. Hamre, D., Connelly, A. P., and Procknow, J. J.: Virologic studies of acute respiratory disease in young adults. III. Some biologic and serologic characteristics of seventeen rhinovirus serotypes isolated October, 1960, to June, 1961. J. Lab. Clin. Med., *64*:450, 1964.
13. Hamre, D., and Procknow, J. J.: Virus isolated from natural common colds in the U.S.A. Brit. Med. J. *2*:1382, 1961.
14. Heggie, A. D., Schultz, I., Gutekunst, R. R., Rosenbaum, M., and Miller, L. F.: An outbreak of a summer febrile disease caused by Coxsackie B2 virus. Amer. J. Public Health, *50*:1342, 1960.
15. Hobson, D., and Schild, G. C.: Virological studies on natural common colds in Sheffield in 1960. Brit. Med. J., *2*:1414, 1960.
16. Jackson, G. G., Dowling, H. F., Anderson, T. O., Riff, L., Saporta, J., and Turck, M.: Susceptibility and immunity to common upper respiratory viral infections. The common cold. Ann. Int. Med., *53*: 719, 1960.
17. Jackson, G. G., Muldoon, R. L., Johnson, G. C., and Dowling, H. F.: Contribution of volunteers to studies on the common cold. Amer. Rev. Resp. Dis., *88*:120, 1963.
18. Johnson, K. M., Bloom, H. H., Forsyth, B., Mufson, M. A., Webb, P. A., and Chanock, R. M.: The role of enteroviruses in respiratory disease. Amer. Rev. Resp. Dis., *88*:240, 1963.
19. Johnson, K. M., and Rosen, L.: Characteristics of five newly recognized enteroviruses recovered from human oropharynx. Amer. J. Hyg., *77*:15, 1963.
20. Kendall, E. J. C., Bynoe, M. L., and Tyrrell, D. A. J.: Virus isolation from common cold occurring in a residential school. Brit. Med. J., *2*:82, 1962.
21. Ketler, A., Hamparian, V. V., and Hilleman, M. R.: Characterization and classification of ECHO 28-rhinovirus-coryza-virus agents. Proc. Soc. Exp. Biol. Med., *110*:821, 1962.
22. Kjersgaard, R., Lindbom, G., Dinter, Z., and Philipson, L.: The aetiology of respiratory tract infections in military personnel. 5. The recovery of ECHO 28 from cases with minor respiratory illness. Acta Path. Microbiol. Scand., *59*:537, 1963.
23. McDonald, J. C.: The importance of respiratory viral diseases in western Europe. Amer. Rev. Resp. Dis., *88*:35, 1963.
24. Mogabgab, W. J.: Muriviruses and others associated with mild upper respiratory illnesses in adults. Amer. Rev. Resp. Dis., *88*:246, 1963.
25. Mufson, M. A., et al.: Description of six new rhinoviruses of human origin. Amer. J. Epidem., *81*:32, 1965.
26. Pelon, W.: Classification of the "2060" virus as ECHO 28 and further study of its properties. Amer. J. Hyg., *73*:36, 1961.
27. Pereira, M. S., Hambling, M. H., MacDonald, J. C., and Zuckerman, A. J.: Viruses from the common cold. A survey in Royal Air Force recruits on arrival from civilian life. J. Hyg. (Camb.), *61*:471, 1963.
28. Reilly, C. M., Hoch, S. M., Stokes, J., Jr., McClelland, L., Hamparian, V. V., Ketler, D., and Hilleman, M. R.: Clinical and laboratory findings in cases of respiratory illness caused by coryza viruses. Ann. Int. Med., *57*:515, 1962.
29. Spickard, A., Evans, H., Knight, V., and Johnson, K.: Acute respiratory disease in normal volunteers associated with Coxsackie A-21 viral infection. III. Response to nasopharyngeal and enteric inoculation. J. Clin. Invest., *42*:840, 1963.
30. Taylor-Robinson, D.: Laboratory and volunteer studies on some viruses isolated from common

colds (rhinoviruses). Amer. Rev. Resp. Dis., *88*: 262, 1963.

31. Taylor-Robinson, D., and Bynoe, M. L.: Inoculation of volunteers with H. rhinoviruses. Brit. Med. J., *1*:540, 1964.
32. Taylor-Robinson, D., and Tyrrell, D. A. J.: Serotypes of viruses (rhinoviruses) isolated from common colds. Lancet, *1*:452, 1962.
33. Tyrrell, D. A. J.: Discovering and defining the etiology of acute respiratory viral disease. Amer. Rev. Resp. Dis., *88*:77, 1963.
34. Tyrrell, D. A. J.: Some recent work at the common cold research unit. Proc. Roy. Soc. Med., *59*:637, 1966.
35. Tyrrell, D. A. J., and Bynoe, M. L.: Some further virus isolations from common colds. Brit. Med. J., *1*:393, 1961.
36. Tyrrell, D. A. J., Bynoe, M. L., Hitchcock, G., Pereira, H. G., and Andrewes, C. H.: Some virus isolations from common colds. I. Experiments employing human volunteers. Lancet, *1*:235, 1960.

RHINOVIRUSES: VIROLOGY, EPIDEMIOLOGY, AND PROBLEMS OF PROPHYLAXIS

by D. TAYLOR-ROBINSON

DEFINITIONS

Rhinoviruses are a major cause of upper respiratory disease, and they are considered as a distinct group of viruses, forming a subgroup of the picornaviruses. In 1953, Andrewes and his colleagues[2] induced colds in volunteers with a virus (DC) that had been propagated serially in cultures of human embryo lung; it did not produce a cytopathic effect, but this was demonstrated later.[71] Viruses producing a cytopathic effect were first isolated from persons with colds in monkey kidney cell cultures by Price[53] and by Pelon and colleagues[50]; these viruses were named 2060 and J.H., respectively, and because of their close antigenic relationship they were regarded as one serotype and called ECHO virus 28.[49] Subsequently, it has been shown that this virus has the properties of a rhinovirus and it is now regarded as such. In 1960 Tyrrell and Parsons[74] isolated two rhinoviruses, H.G.P. and F.E.B., in human embryo kidney cell cultures by modifying conventional tissue culture methods. Rhinovirus F.E.B. grew in human embryo kidney cells only and was termed an "H" virus; rhinovirus H.G.P. grew in monkey kidney

cells also and was termed an "M" virus. Subsequently, similar viruses isolated by other workers were termed coryzaviruses by some,[24] and entero-like viruses or muriviruses by others.[35, 43] However, the term rhinovirus is now accepted and widely used and 55 rhinovirus serotypes and one subtype have so far been established.[12]

LABORATORY STUDIES

PHYSICOCHEMICAL PROPERTIES OF RHINOVIRUSES

To appreciate the significance of laboratory tests the properties of rhinoviruses and the ways in which they differ from other picornaviruses are outlined (Table 40-2). The name picornavirus has been given to a family of small, ether-stable, RNA-containing viruses without outer envelopes,[34] and the rhinoviruses are members of the picornavirus family. Estimations of rhinovirus size, based mainly upon ultrafiltration studies,[16, 36, 37] vary from 15 to 31 mμ. The sedimentation coefficients of nine strains were between 125 and 140 S.[17] Electron micrographs indicate that the viruses are spherical,[11, 42] but the substructure has not been defined. Infectious RNA has been extracted from two strains,[15, 37] and many H and M strains have not been inhibited by 5-bromodeoxyuridine, indicating RNA composition.[25] Rhinoviruses are stable at 4° C. for several weeks and survive indefinitely at −70° C.[23] They are ether and chloroform stable[23] and also resistant to fluorocarbon.[24, 74] Therefore, in many respects rhinoviruses resemble enteroviruses, also members of the picornavirus family. However, rhinoviruses differ from enteroviruses in certain other respects. It has been discovered that the buoyant density of some rhinoviruses in cesium chloride is significantly greater than that of other picornaviruses.[11, 14, 42] Whether this is a feature of all rhinoviruses is unknown. In addition, enteroviruses are protected from inactivation at 50° C. by 1 M magnesium chloride, whereas rhinoviruses, although they do not all behave the same, are generally less affected.[17] Enteroviruses can be divided into groups according to their sensitivity to 2-(α-hydroxybenzyl)-benzimidazole (HBB) or to guanidine. In their relative insensitivity to these sub-

Table 40-2. *Properties of Rhinoviruses*

PHYSICOCHEMICAL PROPERTIES
(1) Size: 15-31 mμ.
(2) Shape: Spherical. Fine structure not determined.
(3) Contain RNA because (a) RNA extracted from some.   Similar
                         (b) not inhibited by 5-bromo (or   to
                               5-fluoro) deoxyuridine.   enteroviruses
(4) Resistant to ether, chloroform, and fluorocarbon.
(5) Generally less protected from inactivation at 50° C. by 1 M magnesium chloride than enteroviruses.
(6) Generally insensitive to 2-(α-hydroxybenzyl)-benzimidazole and guanidine hydrochloride.
(7) Buoyant density in cesium chloride 1.4 gm./cc. (enteroviruses 1.34 gm./cc.).
(8) Labile at pH 3.0 - 5.0 (enteroviruses stable).

BIOLOGICAL PROPERTIES
(1) Isolation optimal when tissue cultures are rolled and incubated at 33° C. with medium between pH 6.8 and 7.3. Focal enterovirus-like cytopathic effect.
(2) Isolated in (a) monolayer cultures of human embryo kidney (HEK) cells, human embryo lung (HEL) fibroblasts, and monkey kidney (MK) cells → "M" rhinoviruses.
             (b) monolayer cultures of HEK and HEL cells only → "H" rhinoviruses.
             (c) organ cultures of human nasal and tracheal epithelium and grow subsequently in HEK and HEL cells.
             (d) organ cultures only.
(3) "M" and "H" strains propagated in various malignant cell lines (e.g., HeLa and KB cells).
(4) No growth or detectable damage in suckling or adult mice, guinea pigs, or embryonated chicken eggs.
(5) Hemagglutinins and hemadsorption not demonstrated.
(6) Complement-fixing antigen demonstrated.

stances, rhinoviruses resemble the Coxsackie A viruses rather than the other enteroviruses. However, the results are too variable for these tests to be used in routine rhinovirus diagnosis.[27]

Acid Lability. The test which is most useful for the separation of rhinoviruses from other picornaviruses is based upon the determination of stability at acid pH. Enteroviruses are stable at pH 3 to 5; rhinoviruses are inactivated by incubating for one to three hours at these pH levels.[16, 37] The test is performed in this laboratory in the following manner: virus in tissue-culture fluid is mixed with an equal volume of 0.1 M sodium citrate–citric acid buffer at pH 4.0 and another portion is mixed with the same volume of 0.1 M sodium phosphate buffer at pH 7.0. The mixtures are held at 37° C. for one hour, diluted with an equal volume of 0.5 M phosphate buffer at pH 7.2, and then diluted 1:5 or more in medium and titrated for infectivity.

COLLECTION AND TRANSPORT OF SPECIMENS

Specimens for virus study should be collected as soon as possible after the onset of illness, preferably within four days of the onset; rhinovirus shedding has been shown to persist for at least three to four days,[28, 30, 47]

and virus is rarely found during convalescence.[13, 28] Nasal secretion may be obtained by running a few milliliters of sterile saline (see below) into the nose while the patient mouth-breathes with the head held backward; the head is then tilted forward and the fluid allowed to run into a petri dish held below the nose. This method of collection has been reported to give the highest virus yield.[4, 8] In some individuals, however, particularly children, this is not a practical technique, and nasal and pharyngeal swabbing has been found to be satisfactory,[23, 52] the swabs being broken off into a few milliliters of transport medium contained in a screw-capped bottle. The transport medium may consist of physiological saline to which protein is added to stabilize the virus. Bovine plasma albumin (1 or 2 per cent) may be used for this purpose. Beef heart or veal infusion broths with added albumin are good transport media also. The respiratory infection under investigation may not be due to a rhinovirus but may be caused, for example, by a myxovirus. Myxoviruses are particularly labile and susceptible to freezing and thawing, so that the specimen should not be frozen but should be transported at about 0° C. to the laboratory and, if possible, inoculated within three hours into tissue culture. However, immediate inoculation may not be possible, and the specimen should then be frozen to −70° C. and stored. For rhinoviruses, such a procedure may reduce the isolation rate slightly[4, 52] or, in the experience of others,[23] not at all.

VIRUS CULTIVATION (TABLE 40-2)

Isolation. Rhinoviruses are more difficult to grow in tissue culture than enteroviruses, although they resemble enteroviruses in the cytopathic changes they cause. The isolation of virus strains at the Common Cold Research Unit, Salisbury, was achieved by using rolled monolayer cultures of human embryo kidney (HEK) cells, which were maintained in medium at a pH between 6.8 and 7.3, and incubated at 33° C.[74] The rolling of cultures and the maintenance of low temperature seem to be particularly important conditions for primary isolation. However, those who use human diploid lung fibroblasts do not consider control of the initial pH to be so critical.[23, 36] The production of semicontinuous strains of human diploid lung fibroblasts[29] which are sensitive to some rhinoviruses has provided greater facilities for rhinovirus isolation. In addition, a line of human aorta endothelial cells[51, 52] and a semicontinuous strain of human embryo kidney fibroblasts[60] with rhinovirus sensitivity have been developed recently. Among the diploid cell strains, the WI26 and WI38 cells have been used extensively because they are particularly sensitive to rhinoviruses. Gwaltney and Jordan[23] found that the rhinovirus isolation rate was lower in monkey kidney cells then in HEK cells and, in turn, lower in HEK cells than in WI diploid cells. On the other hand, Taylor-Robinson and Bynoe[63] found that a strain of diploid lung fibroblasts was inferior to HEK cells for the isolation of an H rhinovirus. These findings are compatible with the fact that HEK cell monolayers derived from different embryos vary in their sensitivity,[35] perhaps as much as 100-fold. In addition, a wide variation in the rhinovirus susceptibility of diploid lung fibroblast strains derived from different human embryos has been demonstrated.[6] Therefore, when commencing a rhinovirus isolation program it is important to compare the sensitivity of the cell strain to be used with one of known sensitivity.

Plaques. Porterfield[52a] first reported plaques in cells under overlay, and a plaque assay for all 55 rhinovirus serotypes has been developed[12a] using sensitive HeLa cells.[21a]

Organ Cultures. Even with a variety of tissue cultures the best rhinovirus isolation rate has been about 30 per cent. However, many nasal washings that do not produce cytopathic changes in tissue culture are capable of producing colds in volunteers, indicating that the washings contain viruses. Many of these viruses have now been grown in organ cultures.[70] The organ culture technique allows the relationship of cells one to another to be preserved so that they function in a manner similar to that in the body. By using organ cultures of ciliated human nasal and tracheal epithelium[31] it is often possible to detect rhinoviruses, since the epithelial cells are destroyed so that ciliary movements cease (Fig. 40-1). Some of the rhinoviruses, after a few passages in organ cultures, grow in the more conventional tissue cultures. Others, however, are unable to reproduce in anything but organ cultures of ciliated epithelial cells from the human respiratory tract.[32] Tyrrell and Bynoe[70] reported that it was possible to isolate rhinoviruses from about 75 per cent of persons with colds. The

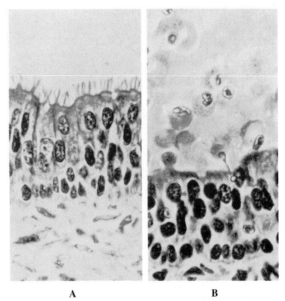

A   B

Figure 40-1. Histopathological changes in organ cultures of human nasal epithelium inoculated with H.S. virus: *A,* uninoculated culture with regular ciliated epithelial-cell surface; *B,* 30 hours after inoculation with rounded and vacuolating ciliated cells with pyknotic nuclei leaving the surface. (Hematoxylin and eosin, ×320.) (From Hoorn, B., and Tyrrell, D. A. J.: Arch. Ges. Virusforsch., *18*:210, 1966; courtesy of the authors.)

most recent observations[68] indicate that, from every nasal washing which is capable of inducing colds in volunteers, a virus may be detected by using the techniques of tissue culture, organ culture, and organ culture combined with electron microscopy.[72] Not every virus detected, however, belongs to the rhinovirus group.[1a]

ANTIBODY MEASUREMENT

Neutralization. Early neutralization tests were difficult to perform, since different batches of monkey kidney and HEK cells varied greatly in virus sensitivity. This problem was overcome by using a microplaque reduction technique.[65] Since the result depends upon the ratio between the number of microplaques produced by rhinoviruses in the presence and in the absence of serum, the result is independent of variations in the sensitivity of the tissue-culture cells. The advent of diploid fibroblast cell strains, which vary much less in their virus sensitivity from one batch to another, has made it possible to perform the usual end-point neutralization test; serial dilutions of serum and 10 to 100 doses of virus are employed.[13, 25, 45, 52, 64] In addition, microneutralization techniques which conserve cells and rhinovirus antisera have been developed,[59a] and would seem to have particular application in laboratories where multiple tests are performed.

Complement Fixation. An ECHO virus 28 (rhinovirus type 1a) complement-fixing antigen has been used by Mogabgab.[44] However, with ECHO virus 28 antiserum, a heterotypically reactive complement-fixing antigen was detected in a suspension of rhinovirus H.G.P. (type 2),[14] suggesting a common complement-fixing antigen within the rhinovirus group. Furthermore, concentrated and purified rhinovirus H.G.P. fixed complement with the sera of most children and adults whether or not the sera contained neutralizing antibody.[11a] In addition, there were no complement-fixing antibody rises in paired sera, although rises were detected by neutralization tests. Therefore, it is not likely that complement-fixing antigen will prove useful in assessing immunity or in diagnosing rhinovirus infections.

Hemaggregation Inhibition. The inhibition of the aggregation of trypsinized red cells by poliovirus, influenza virus, and adenovirus[20] has been successfully performed

with a rhinovirus.[73] The technique may b useful as a means of measuring rhinoviru antibody. Hemagglutination by rhinoviruse has not been demonstrated.[24]

VIRUS DIAGNOSIS AND SEROLOGICAL IDENTIFICATION

The isolation of an ether-stable viru under the conditions previously mentionec from an individual with an upper respirator tract infection, indicates the possibility tha it is a rhinovirus. Confirmation of this ma be made by means of the acid-lability tes described previously. Further identification i dependent upon neutralization tests with type specific antisera. The results of a collaborativ rhinovirus program, which has involved man laboratories and which was set up under th auspices of the W.H.O. and supported by th Vaccine Development Branch of the Unitec States National Institutes of Health, hav shown that there are at least 55 distinct rhino virus serotypes.[12] Each laboratory contribute a new virus and its corresponding antiserun and the neutralization tests performed by eacl laboratory were checked by a Rhinoviru Reference Laboratory at the Children' Hospital, Columbus, Ohio. Future rhinoviru identification will proceed along the sam lines, and each laboratory involved will b required to submit to the collaborative pro gram plaque or limit-dilution purified viru and the corresponding antiserum.[12]

EPIDEMIOLOGY

Since the advent of virological technique for studying respiratory viruses, the combi nation of laboratory methods and epidemi ological observations has added greatly to th knowledge of the role of rhinoviruses an other viruses in respiratory disease. Labora tory studies have comprised both isolatio and serological methods.

TRANSMISSION

The earliest epidemiological studies wer based upon clinical observations only. Vai Loghem[75] recorded that outbreaks of colds occurred simultaneously over a wide geo graphical area and deduced from this tha colds were unlikely to be the result of direc person-to-person transmission. The ability of meteorological changes to induce colds was considered, and support for this idea came subsequently from the studies of other workers.[33, 38] Further, Lidwell and Williams[41] reported that office workers could rarely associate the development of a cold to contact with a fellow worker who had a cold. On the other hand, Paul and Freese[48] studied the inhabitants of Spitzbergen who were totally isolated during the winter months; at this time colds were infrequent. Following the arrival of a ship in the spring the incidence of colds among the population increased dramatically, providing strong evidence that the disease was due to infection transmitted by human contact. Similar observations have been made on the isolated island of Tristan da Cunha.[77] Furthermore, Lidwell and Somerville,[39] who studied the occurrence of colds in several isolated areas of rural England, concluded that the number of colds experienced by a subject increased with exposure to more colds. There seems little doubt, therefore, that person-to-person contact is a factor in the transmission of colds.

INCIDENCE OF INFECTION

Geographic. The world-wide and similar frequency of occurrence of antibodies to two M rhinoviruses has been demonstrated,[62] even in very isolated communities.[5] This indicates a world-wide distribution of rhinoviruses, and there are now reports of isolations from many regions of the world.

Age. In several epidemiological studies[3, 39, 40] it was observed that the frequency of colds decreased with age. These observations are consistent with the findings of various laboratory studies. Neutralizing antibodies to all the rhinoviruses studied, both M and H strains, have been found in the sera of 50 to 70 per cent of adults, the biggest rise in mean antibody titer occurring during adolescence.[36, 58, 65] Children appear to respond to infection with both M and H rhinoviruses by developing antibody titers which equal those observed in adults.[64] This indicates that the lack of antibody in children is a result of fewer infections. The rhinovirus isolation rate in colds of infants and children is apparently lower than in colds of adolescents and adults, although the data are inadequate. Rhinovirus H strains are isolated more frequently than M strains; they comprise 52 to 100 per cent of strains isolated from adults[4, 23, 24, 28] and 63 to 93 per cent of strains isolated from children.[4, 24]

Seasonal. In the clinical epidemiological studies mentioned previously it was shown that colds occurred most frequently in the winter months. The prevalence of different rhinovirus strains and serotypes at different times of the year has also been recorded. Bloom and colleagues,[4] in a Marine camp, isolated predominantly M strains in the winter and spring and predominantly H strains in the autumn. Others observed that early in the winter colds were likely to be due to H rhinoviruses.[28] However, it appears that characteristically the epidemiology of rhinovirus infection may be described as a constantly changing mosaic involving different serotypes. Usually, serotypes prevalent during one period disappear as other serotypes become prevalent.[26, 45, 47]

ASSOCIATION WITH DISEASE

Upper Respiratory Tract. The rhinovirus DC (type 9), propagated by Andrewes and colleagues,[2] was later shown to produce colds in volunteers.[71] Further, Price and colleagues[55] provided epidemiological evidence that ECHO virus 28 (rhinovirus type 1a) was the cause of colds that they observed. Subsequently, other workers[24, 25, 28, 35, 45] have shown that rhinoviruses are recovered significantly more frequently from individuals with common colds than from individuals without colds. These observations in association with several volunteer studies[8, 46, 63, 69] leave no doubt that rhinoviruses are able to cause upper respiratory disease in adults and less frequently in children.

Lower Respiratory Tract. The evidence that rhinoviruses cause more serious illness is scanty. Bloom and colleagues[4] were unsuccessful in their attempts to isolate rhinoviruses from Marine recruits with pneumonia. Some children from whom rhinoviruses were isolated had evidence of lower respiratory tract disease, such as bronchitis and bronchopneumonia,[4, 25, 64] but it was not established that the viruses caused the disease. On the other hand, when a rhinovirus was given to volunteers in aerosol form, those without antibody developed tracheobronchitis with fever and cough, rather than rhinitis.[9] In addition, it seems that some exacerbations of chronic bronchitis are associated with rhinovirus infections.[21, 59] In general, however, it appears that rhinoviruses cause predominantly upper and not lower respiratory disease. Nevertheless, it must be remembered that not all upper respiratory disease is the result of infection by rhinoviruses, especially in children. This must be taken into account in the virological examination of clinical material from individuals with colds.

PROBLEMS OF PROPHYLAXIS

ANTIBODY RESPONSES

Naturally occurring infections and those induced in volunteers by M strain rhinoviruses are almost always associated with a significant antibody response. On the other hand, individuals infected with H rhinoviruses respond less frequently and the antibody titers are lower;[23, 27, 64] furthermore, the level of antibody does not appear to persist as long as in M strain infections.[61] Mogabgab[44] studied complement-fixing and neutralizing antibody responses in persons with naturally acquired disease and concluded that there were many serological cross-reactions between different members of the picornavirus group. He thought it probable that vaccination with a few strains would induce antibody responses to many. This contention now seems unlikely. Although other workers[18, 21b] have observed heterotypic responses with some rhinoviruses, others[7, 37] have not done so and, in general, it seems that heterotypic antibody responses to rhinoviruses occur infrequently.

IMMUNITY

Naturally Acquired Antibody. Considerable data have now accumulated to show that naturally acquired neutralizing antibody is protective in nature. Thus, the intranasal inoculation of volunteers with both M and H rhinoviruses resulted in the development of colds almost entirely in those who did not possess serum antibody or who possessed low levels only.[8, 46, 63] The possession of antibody to other rhinovirus serotypes, apart from the one inoculated, did not prevent illness,[46, 66] indicating the very specific protective nature of naturally acquired antibody.

Vaccines. Apart from naturally acquired antibody, several investigators have shown that formalin-inactivated rhinovirus type 1a

vaccines stimulated neutralizing antibody an that this protected against natural or experi mental illness produced by the same virus.[45, 5] In addition, a live attenuated M rhinoviru given intranasally produced an antibody re sponse and illness, but when given paren terally it stimulated a high titer of antibody without symptoms.[19] Furthermore, the vac cinated volunteers were protected agains illness produced by the same virus giver intranasally.[56] It is clear, therefore, that the antibodies produced by vaccination can pre vent colds induced by the same virus sero type.

Antibody to one rhinovirus does no afford protection against infection produced by another, and multiple colds are apparently the result of multiple infections with viruses of different serotype.[28, 69] Fifty-five rhino virus serotypes have now been numbered. These are the result of relatively short surveys, and it seems likely, therefore, that other serotypes will be found. The steps necessary for the development of a successful vaccine have been outlined,[23, 67] and under certain circumstances this approach may be rewarding eventually. However, since a useful vaccine would need to contain multiple serotypes and be given parenterally because gut infection with antibody production has not been achieved,[10a] the outlook for an effective vaccine is not encouraging.

SPECIFIC ANTIVIRAL AND NONSPECIFIC DRUGS

Cate and colleagues[10] have demonstrated that for a few weeks after infection of volunteers with a rhinovirus, resistance to infection with heterotypic strains occurs. This resistance is possibly mediated by interferon. Lidwell and Williams[41] noted a similar phenomenon in their clinical and epidemiological study. Unfortunately, it has not been possible by prophylactic nasal instillation of interferon to protect volunteers against rhinoviruses or other viruses causing common colds.[67] This is probably due to the inability to maintain a sufficient concentration of interferon within the nose to protect a significant number of cells, since it is washed away by the mucociliary blanket. However, the existence of interferon, which is highly specific in its action, has given hope that it might be possible to find other drugs which have both *in vitro* and *in vivo* antiviral activities. Indeed, a few compounds such as the steroid anti-biotics, Fucidin and cephalosporin P_1, which have shown promise in *in vitro* antiviral tests, have been tested in volunteers, but again, unfortunately, they have not been effective in preventing colds.[1]

The beneficial prophylactic effect of vitamin C on upper respiratory disease has been reported.[57] Recently, a carefully controlled trial in volunteers was undertaken to determine the efficacy of vitamin C in preventing upper respiratory disease caused by several viruses, including rhinoviruses; the number, duration, and severity of colds was the same in those persons who had and who had not taken the drug.[76]

BIBLIOGRAPHY

1. Acornley, J. E., Bessell, C. J., Bynoe, M. L., Godt-fredsen, W. O., and Knoyle, J. M.: Antiviral activity of sodium fusidate and related compounds. Brit. J. Pharmacol. Chemotherap., *31*:210, 1967.

1a. Almeida, J., and Tyrrell, D. A. J.: The morphology of three previously uncharacterized human respiratory viruses that grow in organ culture. J. Gen. Virol., *1*:175, 1967.

2. Andrewes, C. H., Chaproniere, D. M., Gompels, A. E. H., Pereira, H. G., and Roden, A. T.: Propagation of common-cold viruses in tissue cultures. Lancet, *2*:546, 1953.

3. Badger, G. F., Dingle, J. H., Feller, A. E., Hodges, R. G., Jordan, W. S. Jr., and Rammelkamp, C. H., Jr.: A study of illness in a group of Cleveland families. II. Incidence of the common respiratory diseases. Amer. J. Hyg., *58*:31, 1953.

4. Bloom, H. H., Forsyth, B. R., Johnson, K. M., and Chanock, R. M.: Relationship of rhinovirus infection to mild upper respiratory disease. I. Results of a survey in young adults and children. J.A.M.A., *186*:38, 1963.

5. Brown, P. K., and Taylor-Robinson, D.: Respiratory virus antibodies in sera of persons living in isolated communities. Bull. WHO, *34*:895, 1966.

6. Brown, P. K., and Tyrrell, D. A. J.: Experiments on the sensitivity of strains of human fibroblasts to infection with rhinoviruses. Brit. J. Exp. Path., *45*:571, 1964.

7. Buckland, F. E., Doggett, J. E., and Tyrrell, D. A. J.: The specificity of the antibody responses of human volunteers to certain respiratory viruses. J. Hyg. (Camb.), *62*:115, 1964.

8. Bynoe, M. L., Hobson, D., Horner, J., Kipps, A., Schild, G. C., and Tyrrell, D. A. J.: Inoculation of human volunteers with a strain of virus isolated from a common cold. Lancet, *1*:1194, 1961.

9. Cate, T. R., Couch, R. B., Fleet, W. F., Griffith, W. R., Gerone, P. J. and Knight, V.: Production of tracheobronchitis in volunteers with rhinovirus in a small-particle aerosol. Amer. J. Epidem. *81*:95, 1965.

10. Cate, T. R., Couch, R. B., and Johnson, K. M.: Studies with rhinoviruses in volunteers: production

of illness, effect of naturally acquired antibody, and demonstration of a protective effect not associated with serum antibody. J. Clin. Invest., *43*:56, 1964.

10a. Cate, T. R., Douglas, R. G., Jr., Johnson, K. M., Couch, R. B., and Knight, V.: Studies on the inability of rhinovirus to survive and replicate in the intestinal tract of volunteers. Proc. Soc. Exp. Biol. Med., *124*:1290, 1967.

11. Chapple, P. J., and Harris, W. J.: Biophysical studies of a rhinovirus. Ultracentrifugation and electron microscopy. Nature, *209*:790, 1966.

11a. Chapple, P. J., Head, B., and Tyrrell, D. A. J.: A complement fixing antigen from an M rhinovirus. Arch. Ges. Virusforsch., *21*:123, 1967.

12. Collaborative report. Rhinoviruses: A numbering system. Nature, *213*:761, 1967.

12a. Conant, R. M., Somerson, N. L., and Hamparian, V. V.: Plaque formation by rhinoviruses. Proc. Soc. Exp. Biol. Med., *128*:51, 1968.

13. Connelly, A. P., and Hamre, D.: Virologic studies on acute respiratory disease in young adults. II. Characteristics and serologic studies of three new rhinoviruses. J. Lab. Clin. Med., *63*:30, 1964.

14. Dans, P. E., Forsyth, B. R., and Chanock, R. M.: Density of infectious virus and complement-fixing antigens of two rhinovirus strains. J. Bact., *91*:1605, 1966.

15. Dimmock, N. J.: Biophysical studies of a rhinovirus. Extraction and assay of infectious ribonucleic acid. Nature, *209*:79, 1966.

16. Dimmock, N. J., and Tyrrell, D. A. J.: Physicochemical properties of some viruses isolated from common colds (Rhinoviruses). Lancet, *2*:536, 1962.

17. Dimmock, N. J., and Tyrrell, D. A. J.: Some physicochemical properties of rhinoviruses. Brit. J. Exp. Path., *45*:271, 1964.

18. Fawzy, K. Y., Fox, J. P., Ketler, A., Brandt, C. D., Hall, C. E., and Haraway, A. W.: The virus watch program: a continuing surveillance of viral infection in metropolitan New York families. V. Observations in employed adults on etiology of acute upper respiratory disease and heterologous antibody response to rhinoviruses. Amer. J. Epidem., *86*:653, 1967.

19. Doggett, J. E., Bynoe, M. L., and Tyrrell, D. A. J.: Some attempts to produce an experimental vaccine with rhinoviruses. Brit. Med. J., *1*:34, 1963.

20. Drescher, J., and Schrader, K.: Titration of poliovirus and influenza virus by means of the hemagregation test. Amer. J. Hyg., *79*:218, 1964.

21. Eadie, M. B., Stott, E. J., and Grist, N. R.: Virological studies in chronic bronchitis. Brit. Med. J., *2*:671, 1966.

21a. Fiala, M., and Kenny, G. E.: Enhancement of rhinovirus plaque formation in human heteroploid cell cultures by magnesium and calcium. J. Bact., *92*:1710, 1966.

21b. Fleet, W. F., Douglas, R. G., Jr., Cate, T. R., and Couch, R. B.: Antibody to rhinovirus in human sera. II. Heterotypic responses. Proc. Soc. Exp. Biol. Med., *127*:503, 1968.

22. Gwaltney, J. M., Jr.: Micro-neutralization test for identification of rhinovirus serotypes. Proc. Soc. Exp. Biol. Med., *122*:1137, 1966.

23. Gwaltney, J. M., and Jordan, W. S.: Rhinoviruses and respiratory disease. Bact. Rev., *28*:409, 1964.

24. Hamparian, V. V., Ketler, A., and Hilleman, M. R.: Recovery of new viruses (coryzavirus) from cases of common cold in human adults. Proc. Soc. Exp. Biol. Med., *108*:444, 1961.

25. Hamparian, V. V., Leagus, M. B., and Hilleman, M. R.: Additional rhinovirus serotypes. Proc. Soc. Exp. Biol. Med., *116*:976, 1964.

26. Hamparian, V. V., Leagus, M. B., Hilleman, M. R., and Stokes, J., Jr.: Epidemiologic investigations of rhinovirus infections. Proc. Soc. Exp. Biol. Med., *117*:469, 1964.

27. Hamre, D., Connelly, A. P., and Procknow, J. J.: Virologic studies of acute respiratory disease in young adults. III. Some biologic and serologic characteristics of seventeen rhinovirus serotypes isolated October, 1960, to June, 1961. J. Lab. Clin. Med., *64*:450, 1964.

28. Hamre, D., and Procknow, J. J.: Virologic studies on common colds among young adult medical students. Amer. Rev. Resp. Dis., *88*:277, 1963.

29. Hayflick, L., and Moorhead, P. S.: The serial cultivation of human diploid cell strains. Exp. Cell Res., *25*:585, 1961.

30. Higgins, P. G., Ellis, E. M., and Boston, D. G.: The isolation of viruses from acute respiratory infections. A study of the isolations made from cases occurring in a general practice in 1962. Monthly Bull. Minist. Health (London), *22*:71, 1963.

31. Hoorn, B., and Tyrrell, D. A. J.: On the growth of certain "newer" respiratory viruses in organ cultures. Brit. J. Exp. Path., *46*:109, 1965.

32. Hoorn, B., and Tyrrell, D. A. J.: A new virus cultivated only in organ cultures of human ciliated epithelium. Arch. Ges. Virusforsch., *18*:210, 1966.

33. Hope-Simpson, R. E.: Discussion on the common cold. Proc. Roy. Soc. Med., *51*:267, 1958.

34. International Enterovirus Study Group. Picornavirus Group. Virology, *19*:114, 1963.

35. Johnson, K. M., Bloom, H. H., Chanock, R. M., Mufson, M. A., and Knight, V.: Acute respiratory disease of viral etiology. VI. The newer enteroviruses. Amer. J. Public Health, *52*:933, 1962.

36. Johnson, K. M., and Rosen, L.: Characteristics of five newly recognized enteroviruses recovered from the human oropharynx. Amer. J. Hyg., *77*: 15, 1963.

37. Ketler, A., Hamparian, V. V., and Hilleman, M. R.: Characterization and classification of ECHO 28-rhinovirus-coryzavirus agents. Proc. Soc. Exp. Biol. Med., *110*:821, 1962.

38. Lidwell, O. M., Morgan, R. W., and Williams, R. E. O.: The epidemiology of the common cold. IV. The effect of weather. J. Hyg. (Camb.), *63*: 427, 1965.

39. Lidwell, O. M., and Sommerville, T.: Observations on the incidence and distribution of the common cold in a rural community during 1948 and 1949. J. Hyg. (Camb.), *49*:365, 1951.

40. Lidwell, O. M., and Williams, R. E. O.: The epidemiology of the common cold. I. J. Hyg. (Camb.), *59*:309, 1961.

41. Lidwell, O. M., and Williams, R. E. O.: The epidemiology of the common cold. II. Cross-infection and immunity. J. Hyg. (Camb.), *59*:321, 1961.

42. McGregor, S., Phillips, C. A., and Mayor, H. D.: Purification and biophysical properties of rhinoviruses. Proc. Soc. Exp. Biol. Med., *122*:118, 1966.

43. Mogabgab, W. J.: Additional respirovirus type related to GL 2060 (ECHO 28) virus from military personnel. Amer. J. Hyg., *76*:160, 1962.

44. Mogabgab, W. J.: 2060 virus (ECHO 28) in KB ce cultures: Characteristics, complement-fixation an antigenic relationships to some other respirc viruses. Amer. J. Hyg., *76*:15, 1962.

45. Mufson, M. A., Bloom, H. H., Forsyth, B. R., an Chanock, R. M.: Relationship of rhinovirus infec tion to mild upper respiratory disease. III. Furthe epidemiologic observations in military personnel Amer. J. Epidem., *83*:379, 1966.

46. Mufson, M. A., Ludwig, W. M., James, H. D., Jr. Gould, L. W., Rourke, J. A., Holper, J. C., an Chanock, R. M.: Effect of neutralizing antibody or experimental rhinovirus infection. J.A.M.A. *186*:578, 1963.

47. Mufson, M. A., Webb, P. A., Kennedy, H., Gill V., and Chanock, R. M.: Etiology of upper respiratory-tract illnesses among civilian adults J.A.M.A., *195*:91, 1966.

48. Paul, J. H., and Freese, H. L.: An epidemiologica and bacteriological study of the "common cold" ir an isolated arctic community (Spitzbergen). Amer J. Hyg., *17*:517, 1933.

49. Pelon, W.: Classification of the "2060" virus a ECHO 28 and further study of its properties Amer. J. Hyg., *73*:36, 1961.

50. Pelon, W., Mogabgab, W. J., Phillips, I. A., an Pierce, W. E.: A cytopathogenic agent isolate from Naval recruits with mild respiratory illnesses Proc. Soc. Exp. Biol. Med., *94*:262, 1957.

51. Phillips, C. A., Melnick, J. L., and Grim, C. A. Human aorta cells for isolation and propagation o rhinoviruses. Proc. Soc. Exp. Biol. Med., *119*:843 1965.

52. Phillips, C. A., Riggs, S., Melnick, J. L., and Grim C. A.: Rhinoviruses associated with common cold in a student population. J.A.M.A., *192*:277, 1965

52a. Porterfield, J. S.: Titration of some common col viruses (rhinoviruses) and their antisera by a plaqu method. Nature, *194*:1044, 1962.

53. Price, W. H.: The isolation of a new virus associatec with respiratory clinical disease in humans. Proc Nat. Acad. Sci. U.S.A., *42*:892, 1956.

54. Price, W. H.: Vaccine for the prevention in human of cold-like symptoms associated with JH virus Proc. Nat. Acad. Sci., U.S.A., *43*:790, 1957

55. Price, W. H., Emerson, H., Ibler, I., Lachaine, R. and Terrell, A.: Studies of the JH and 2060 viruse and their relationship to mild upper respiratory disease in humans. Amer. J. Hyg., *69*:224, 1959.

56. Report by Scientific Committee on Common Colc Vaccines. Prevention of colds by vaccinatior against a rhinovirus. Brit. Med. J., *1*:1344, 1965

57. Ritzel, G.: Kritische Beurteilung des Vitamins C als Prophylacticum und Therapeuticum der Erkätungskrankheiten. Helv. Med. Acta, *28*:63 1961.

58. Schild, G. C., and Hobson, D.: Neutralizing antibody levels in human sera with the H.G.P. and B632 strains of common cold virus. Brit. J. Exp. Path., *43*:288, 1962.

59. Stenhouse, A. C.: Rhinovirus infection in acute exacerbations of chronic bronchitis: a controllec prospective study. Brit. Med. J., *2*:461, 1967.

59a. Stott, E. J., and Tyrrell, D. A. J.: Some improved techniques for the study of rhinoviruses using HeLa cells. Arch. Ges. Virsuforsch., *23*:236, 1968.

60. Stott, E. J., and Walker, M.: Human embryo kidney fibroblasts for the isolation and growth of rhino-viruses. Brit. J. Exp. Path., *48*:544, 1967.

61. Taylor-Robinson, D.: Laboratory and volunteer

studies on some viruses isolated from common colds (rhinoviruses). Amer. Rev. Resp. Dis., *88:* 262, 1963.

2. Taylor-Robinson, D.: Respiratory virus antibodies in human sera from different regions of the world. Bull. W.H.O., *32:*833, 1965.

3. Taylor-Robinson, D., and Bynoe, M. L.: Inoculation of volunteers with H rhinoviruses. Brit. Med. J., *1:*540, 1964.

4. Taylor-Robinson, D., Johnson, K. M., Bloom, H. H., Parrott, R. H., Mufson, M. A., and Chanock, R. M.: Rhinovirus neutralizing antibody responses and their measurement. Amer. J. Hyg., *78:*285, 1963.

5. Taylor-Robinson, D., and Tyrrell, D. A. J.: Serological studies on some viruses isolated from common colds (rhinoviruses). Brit. J. Exp. Path., *43:*264, 1962.

6. Tyrrell, D. A. J.: Further experiments on viruses isolated from common colds (rhinoviruses). In Pollard, M. (ed.): Perspectives in Virology, Vol. 3. New York, Hoeber, 1963.

7. Tyrrell, D. A. J.: Common Colds and Related Diseases. London, Arnold, 1965.

8. Tyrrell, D. A. J.: Personal communication.

9. Tyrrell, D. A. J., and Bynoe, M. L.: Some further virus isolations from common colds. Brit. Med. J., *1:*393, 1961.

70. Tyrrell, D. A. J., and Bynoe, M. L.: Cultivation of viruses from a high proportion of patients with colds. Lancet, *1:*76, 1966.

71. Tyrrell, D. A. J., Bynoe, M. L., Buckland, F. E., and Hayflick, L.: The cultivation in human embryo cells of a virus (D.C.) causing colds in man. Lancet, *2:*320, 1962.

72. Tyrrell, D. A. J., and Almeida, J. D.: Direct electron-microscopy of organ cultures for the detection and characterization of viruses. Arch. Ges. Virusforsch., *22:*417, 1967.

73. Tyrrell, D. A. J., Head, B., and Dimic, M.: Titration of tuberculin, nucleic acids and viruses by haemaggregation inhibition using a "pattern" test. Brit. J. Exp. Path., *48:*513, 1967.

74. Tyrrell, D. A. J., and Parsons, R.: Some virus isolations from common colds: III. Cytopathic effects in tissue cultures. Lancet, *1:*239, 1960.

75. Van Loghem, J. J.: An epidemiological contribution to the knowledge of respiratory diseases. J. Hyg. (Camb.), *28:*33, 1928.

76. Walker, G. H., Bynoe, M. L., and Tyrrell, D. A. J.: A trial of ascorbic acid in the prevention of colds. Brit. Med. J., *1:*603, 1967.

77. Woolley, E. J. S.: Discussion in Medical problems presented by the Tristan da Cunha community. Trans. Roy. Soc. Trop. Med. Hyg., *57:*24, 1963.

41

Acute Viral Laryngitis

By J. COUVREUR

The term "acute viral laryngitis" may apply in part to a number of different clinical patterns described as acute laryngeal catarrh, acute laryngeal dyspnea, infectious laryngitis, subglottic or supraglottic laryngitis, suffocating laryngotracheobronchitis, croup, nondiphtherial croup, and so forth.

HISTORICAL ACCOUNT

The occurrence of acute laryngitis was noted during the epidemic of influenza in 1918-1919. Beach [4] was the first to observe a laryngeal disease of viral origin in the domestic fowl. On the basis of comparative histo-pathological and pathological information, Burnet and Foley [10] and Arden and Duhing [2] were of the opinion that "nondiphtherial croup" is most often due to a virus. This opinion was shared by Rabe, [32] who, having made a research study of a considerable number of cases, demonstrated that the infection could not be attributed to bacterial contamination except in a small number of cases. Beale et al. [5] and Chanock [11] were the first to isolate a virus from children suffering from acute laryngitis.

Diphtheria was for a long time considered the essential cause of acute laryngeal dyspnea, so much so that the term "croup" remains for French medical practitioners synonymous with laryngeal diphtheria. Later on the intervention of other germs such as streptococcus[21] or *Hemophilus influenzae*[19] was demonstrated. Since the disappearance of diphtheria, it is generally accepted that viruses are now the major causal agents of acute infectious laryngitis.

THE CLINICAL PICTURE OF VIRAL LARYNGITIS

Viral laryngitis occurs most frequently in children between eight months and three years of age and shows a definite predilection for the males (four boys to one girl). There is a clear predominance during the winter season, particularly from November to April, in the Northern Hemisphere.

The onset is generally sudden, the child often waking in the middle of the night. As a rule, however, it is preceded for one or two days by a slight upper respiratory infection. It may be marked for a few hours by hoarseness and coughing. The medical practitioner is generally called in urgently to see the child, whose condition appears to be dramatic: he is seated in bed, agitated, subject to intense dyspnea with extensive substernal, suprasternal, subclavicular, supraclavicular, intercostal, and epigastric traction. Inspiration is noisy and difficult, with stridor. The lips and extremities become cyanosed, and there is a raucous, barking, nonproductive cough. Two symptoms are essential to confirm the laryngeal origin of the dyspnea: the bradypnea on inspiration and the substernal retraction. If the voice remains clear, one can assume that the edema is subglottic even before laryngoscopic examination. Finally, the position of the head, which is held backward, is a symptom in favor of laryngeal dyspnea, although it is not a constant finding. Dyspnea is continuous, with paroxysms of suffocation and anxiety during which coughing and cyanosis become more marked.

The infectious syndrome is constant but of variable intensity. The temperature may reach 39° C. or more, but a viral laryngitis may produce little or no fever.

When the child is treated early, by moist air and antispasmodic drugs, he may respond quickly and favorably. In the absence of any rapid improvement, hospitalization is necessary, particularly in the case of a firs attack.

Direct laryngoscopy should be one of the first examinations to be performed on ad mission. It permits exclusion of anothe cause, such as the presence of foreign bodies and assessment of the lesions; it reveal edema, the localization and general aspec of which should be carefully noted. Depend ing on its localization it is possible to dis tinguish three types of laryngitis: *vestibula laryngitis*, in which the edema infiltrates the lower surface of the epiglottis, the aryteno epiglottic folds, and the top of the arytenoids producing a genuine ring outlining the open ing into the larynx; *subglottic laryngitis*, in which edema forms false cords or less fre quently is horseshoe-shaped with posterior concavity; and *localized or unilateral laryn gitis*, in which the epiglottis, the arytenoids or the false cords are in some cases affected The posterior surface of the epiglottis and the vocal cords are always free of edema, the mucosa adhering directly to the subjacent muscles.

It is important to take account of the general appearance of the edema for the pur pose of diagnosis, prognosis, and treatment It may be white or lilac colored in appear ance. Such edema reacts well to vasocon strictors, and the prognosis is then favorable But when there are signs of bacterial super infection the prognosis is less hopeful: e.g. bright red edema, sometimes ecchymotic fungoid ulcerations on the posterior por tion of the vocal cords and on the interary tenoid commissure, where the lymphoid fol licles are numerous, as well as in the region of the ventricles and false cords, and finally a considerable hypersecretion of laryngea or laryngotracheobronchial origin. The pres ence of crusted lesions requires tracheotomy

THE VIRUSES ASSOCIATED WITH THE CLINICAL PICTURE

The virological surveys of the past few years make it possible to reply — to a certain extent — to three questions. What is the inci dence of viral laryngitis in comparison with that of acute laryngitis as a whole? What are the viruses that cause such laryngitis and for what proportion of cases is each virus re sponsible? Do there exist certain distinctive clinical features peculiar to one or anothe of these viruses that can help to identify it before the laboratory results?

The hypothesis of a viral etiology of "non-diphtherial croup" has received support for years in view of the meager results obtained from extensive systematic bacteriological surveys. In 1948, Rabe[31] reported that, of 347 cases of infectious laryngitis, 86 per cent had nonbacterial etiology. Philipson[26] found that bacteriological examination made on admission permitted isolation of bacterial agents in 36.1 per cent of the 269 cases studied, but the serological examinations (antistreptolysins, antistaphylolysins, complement-fixation reaction of *Hemophilus influenzae*) proved an infection due to the germs isolated in only a few rare cases. Virological investigations, on the other hand, showed the presence of viral infection in 80 per cent of the cases according to Sabin, 64 per cent of the cases according to Vargosko et al.[33]

Since the first isolations carried out in 1956[5, 11] the number of viruses identified which produce an infection associated with laryngitis has increased regularly.

Chanock and Beale were the first to underline the role of a parainfluenza myxovirus "associated with croup" (CA). That of the hemadsorbent viruses HA_1 and HA_2 was demonstrated later.[11] It is known that these hemadsorbent viruses have a particular capacity for adsorbing the red blood cells in cultures of inoculated tissues. These viruses have been regrouped and are now called parainfluenzae myxoviruses types 1 and 3.[1] The CA virus has been classified as parainfluenza 2; HA_1 as type 3; and HA_2 as type 1. The Sendai virus appears to be related to parainfluenza 1. The presence of these parainfluenza myxoviruses has since been regularly confirmed during systematic surveys.[14, 17, 23, 33] They have been incriminated in 36 per cent[11, 33] and even 60 per cent[5] of the cases. In an extensive survey carried out in Melbourne on 299 cases of laryngitis that had required hospitalization and on 615 cases of various respiratory diseases, Lewis et al.[20] isolated a parainfluenza myxovirus in 7.4 per cent of the subjects suffering from laryngitis, in 2.8 per cent of those suffering from respiratory affections, and in 0.3 per cent of the controls. Of the 113 myxoviruses isolated from cases of laryngitis 75 were found to be of type 1, 18 of type 2, and 20 of type 3. A significant increase in the antibody titer was observed in 25 cases out of 29 (i.e., 83

per cent). Infections due to myxoviruses are in fact extremely widespread, and they do not necessarily always cause laryngeal symptoms or even any apparent manifestations. In a survey made in Washington, Chanock observed that 25 per cent of infants and 90 per cent of young adults possessed antibodies that hemagglutinate CA virus. In view of the extent of the infection among the population, the number of cases of laryngitis seems comparatively low.

The virus of influenza (of the Asian strain) was later found in 5 per cent,[22] 19 per cent,[33] and even 65 per cent of the cases.[26] Strain B was also found.[22] An infection due to a virus that has an antigenic relationship with ECHO virus 11 and which so far has been called the "U virus" (Uppsala virus) was demonstrated in 40 per cent of a group of 87 children suffering from subglottic laryngitis.[24, 25, 29] Recognized to be a frequent causal agent of respiratory infection in small children, Morris' CCA virus (i.e., the chimpanzee coryza agent or respiratory syncytial virus) seems to cause laryngitis in only 1 to 2 per cent of the cases.[15] Finally, infections due to adenovirus type 5 and ECHO virus 13 have been reported. Obviously this list is not exhaustive. As is the rule in viral pathology, one can expect variations in the relative importance of the role of these agents from year to year and according to the season and the geographical location.[14]

Long-term surveys may reveal—to a certain extent—decreases in the importance of some of these factors. A survey performed on some 8000 subjects with respiratory infection from 1958 to 1964 in Washington, D.C., now makes possible a better estimate of the frequency of laryngitis due to viruses and of the respective roles played by the different viruses isolated. Viruses isolation was achieved in 37 per cent of the cases of acute laryngitis. The serological examinations made in 340 cases were positive in 53.5 per cent: for respiratory syncytial virus in 5.9 per cent; for *Myxovirus parainfluenzae* of type 1 in 11.5 per cent, of type 2 in 8.2 per cent and of type 3 in 10.6 per cent; for *Myxovirus influenzae* A in 5.3 per cent and for *M. influenzae* B in less than 1 per cent; for adenoviruses in 3.5 per cent; for mixed viral infections in 8.2 per cent. No rhinovirus was isolated, and Coxsackie B viruses were found only episodically (Chanock).

It thus appears all the more difficult to

attempt to foresee what virus is responsible for a given case of acute laryngitis. For this purpose, Parrott[22] carried out a detailed comparison of the clinical manifestations in 47 patients with respiratory infection due to influenza virus type A2 and 32 cases of infection due to influenza B. Of all these subjects, 27 per cent were found to have laryngeal signs. A differential diagnosis with regard to other viral infections seemed impossible except in the case of an epidemic. At the most it was found that the myxoviruses gave rise more readily to associated bronchial signs, producing a symptomatology of acute laryngotracheobronchitis that could prove fatal.[23]

DIFFERENTIAL DIAGNOSIS

It is possible to distinguish three types of laryngeal dyspnea depending on whether the origin is mechanical, allergic, or infectious. Before concluding that the disorder is viral, it is therefore necessary to eliminate any possible mechanical factor—e.g., foreign body, irritation owing to intubation, compression caused by an extrinsic tumor—or allergic cause. The angioneurotic edema of allergic origin is obvious when it succeeds an insect bite or contact with a known respiratory or alimentary allergen, for example, following the administration of iodine in a sensitized subject.

In the presence of an associated infectious syndrome the possibility of a bacterial laryngitis should be eliminated. The latter does not show the same predominance in the nursling infant and is just as frequent in children between three and seven years of age. It does not have the same seasonal occurrence.

The infectious syndrome is more striking. Examination of the pharynx shows it to be encumbered with thick secretions. Laryngoscopy shows that the laryngeal edema is neither white nor lilac colored but bright red, ecchymotic, and very extensive.

Acute epiglottitis, which some do not hesitate to consider a type of laryngitis, has its own particular clinical pattern which facilitates its diagnosis and which it is important to recognize because of its dangerous prognosis. The onset is abrupt, the evolution fulminating within several hours, with rapid respiratory obstruction; the toxic-infectious syndrome appears very serious. Examination shows the epiglottis to be prominent, edematous, and of a cherry red color; difficulties in deglutition are observed as a result of the accumulation of pharyngeal secretions. *Hemophilus influenzae* is frequently the cause and is confirmed by hemoculture. The prognosis is serious, and tracheotomy is often necessary.

Apart from well-defined cases, it is in fact often difficult to assert or to eliminate bacterial infection, especially since the latter is a frequent intercurrent complication of an authentic viral infection.

Finally, before confirming a primary viral laryngitis it is necessary to eliminate the possibility of a secondary viral laryngitis, e.g., accompanying measles, chickenpox, herpes.

The concept of spasmodic laryngitis and the eventual part played by viral infection in such laryingitis can also be discussed. The clinical picture is well known: it is particularly characterized by absence or bare existence of an infectious syndrome and by the repetition of the attacks. The child awakens suddenly in the night, with a noisy laryngeal dyspnea; there are no previous signs. The attacks occur several nights in succession with bouts recurring over several years and ceasing after the child is four to seven years of age. There is no fever, and the attacks are fairly easily subdued by means of simple sedatives or antispasmodics. There is a certain familial tendency toward this syndrome, which is often observed in neurotonic children.

Various hypotheses have been put forward to explain this, such as allergy, predisposition, or "immaturity," but none of these provides a valid explanation. Assuming that certain children are prone to spasmodic laryngitis, it is probable that certain viral infections are capable of triggering these crises. Spasmodic laryngitis is often preceded by a benign respiratory infection. Cramblett[14] reported the case of a child who had attacks successively associated with infections due to CA virus, influenza A, and ECHO 13, and rightly considered that it is not possible to separate "spasmodic croup" from "infectious croup."

To conclude, it should be remembered that acute infectious laryngitis is more frequently associated with a viral infection than with a bacterial infection. However, "the" virus of laryngitis has not yet been isolated.

Laryngitis is associated particularly with infections due to *Myxovirus influenzae,* and much more rarely adenovirus type 5, RS virus, ECHO 11 and 13, and Coxsackie B viruses. However, acute infectious laryngitis due to these viruses is rare in proportion to the number of subjects infected by these same viruses in the general population. No doubt in certain subjects there is a particular predisposition that favors the development of this clinical pattern.

THERAPEUTIC INDICATIONS

The two major objects in treating acute viral laryngitis are to maintain the permeability of the respiratory tract and to avert secondary bacterial infection. The patient must be placed in an atmosphere as humid as possible, cool humidity being preferable to steam. Apprehension should be calmed and good sedation obtained, unnecessary tests being avoided; opiate derivatives and atropine are contraindicated; barbiturates should be used prudently. Perfect hydration must be attained, either by the oral route or, if necessary, intravenously. Antibiotic treatment is obligatory. When the physician is not absolutely certain that he has eliminated *Hemophilus influenzae* infection, it is preferable to employ tetracycline or chloramphenicol.

All cases of acute tracheitis can be life threatening; hence hospitalization should be resorted to quickly if rapid improvement is not notable within a few hours or if a young child is affected by a first crisis of this type. Two therapeutic possibilities can be envisaged in such cases: corticosteroid treatment and tracheotomy. Steroids, by their anti-inflammatory action, can reduce the edema and improve ventilation. Used for only two or three days they have scarcely any secondary effects, but their systematic use is unjustifiable, particularly in benign cases.

Tracheostomy should be applied in certain cases. Its indications are difficult to decide, requiring great experience and the opinion of a laryngologist. It should be considered when, despite a well-conducted medical treatment, traction effect and dyspnea increase and the patient remains agitated. To be kept in mind is the fact that tracheostomy should never be a last-minute measure.

BIBLIOGRAPHY

1. Andrewes, C. H., Bang, F. B., Chanock, R. M., and Zhdanov, V. M.: Para-influenza viruses 1, 2 and 3: suggested names for recently described myxoviruses. Virology, *8*:129-130, 1959.
2. Arden, F., and Duhing, J. V.: Acute laryngotracheobronchitis. Med. J. Aust., *31*:145, 1944.
3. Babb, J. M., Stoneman, M. E. R., and Stern, H.: Myocarditis and croup caused by Coxsackie virus type B5. Arch. of Dis. Child., *36*:551-556, 1961.
4. Beach, R. R.: Bacteriological study of infectious laryngotracheitis in chickens. J. Exp. Med., *54*: 801, 1931.
5. Beale, A. J., et al.: Isolation of cytopathogenic agents from tracheal secretions in cases of acute laryngotracheobronchitis. Amer. Dis. Child, *93*:42-44, 1957.
6. Beale, A. J., McLeod, D. L., Stackiw, W., and Rhodes, A. J.: Isolation of cytopathogenic agents from the respiratory tract in acute laryngo-tracheobronchitis. Brit. Med. J., *1*:302-303, 1958.
7. Berenberg, W., and Kevy, S.: Acute epiglottitis in childhood. A serious emergency, readily recognized at the bedside. New Eng. J. Med., *258*: 870-874, 1958.
8. Blattner, R. J.: Virus group. J. Pediat., *55*:793-796, 1959.
9. Bruckner, S., Ciugarin, M., and Cotarcea, S.: Considérations sur le rôle du virus ECHO type 11 dans les laryngites obstructives aiguës graves de l'enfant (Rapport d'une observation anatomo-clinique avec étude virologique). Ann. Pediat. (Paris), *11*:246, 1964.
10. Burnet, F. M., and Foley, M.: Infection of respiratory tract of chick embryos by viruses of psittacosis and infectious laryngotracheitis. Comparison with influenza virus infections. Aust. J. Exp. Biol. Med. Sci., *19*:235, 1941.
11. Chanock, R. M.: Association of a new type of cytopathogenic myxovirus with infantile croup. J. Exp. Med., *104*:555-576, 1956.
12. Clarke, S. K. R., and Saynor, R.: Hemagglutination-inhibition tests against C.A. virus. Arch. Ges. Virusforsch., *9*:288-294, 1959.
13. Cramblett, H. G.: Isolation of a cytopathogenic agent resembling the CA virus from an infant with croup. Pediatrics, *22*:56-59, 1958.
14. Cramblett, H. G.: Croup. Present day concept. Pediatrics, *25*:1071-1076, 1960.
15. Couvreur, J., Falcoff, E., Chany, C., and Gerbeaux, J.: Une épidémie d'infections respiratoires associées au virus CCA de Morris dans une collectivité d'enfants. Bull. Soc. Med. Hop. Paris, *115*: 1281, 1965.
16. Forbes, J. A.: Croup viruses. Clinical aspects. Med. J. Aust., *2*:769-771, 1960.
17. Kilbrick, S.: Cited by Cramblett.[14]
18. Larson, J. B.: Croup. Pediat. Clin. N. Amer., *8*: 123-126, 1961.
19. Lemierre, A., Meyer, A., and Laplane, R.: Les septicémies à bacille de Pfeiffer. Ann. Med. (Paris), *39*:97, 1936.
20. Lewis, F. A., Lehmann, N. I., and Ferris, A. A.: The haemadsorption viruses in laryngotracheobronchitis. Med. J. Aust., *2*:929-932, 1961.
21. MacNab, J. C. G.: Acute streptococcal infection of trachea in an infant aged 15 months. J. Laryngol. Rhinol. Otol., *30*:336, 1915.

22. Parrott, R. H.: Viral respiratory tract illnesses in children. Bull. N.Y. Acad. Med., *39*:629, 1963.
23. Pereira, M. S., and Fisher, O. D.: An outbreak of acute laryngotracheobronchitis associated with parainfluenza-2-virus. Lancet, *2*:790-791, 1960.
24. Philipson, L.: Recovery of a cytopathogenic agent from patients with non-diphtheritic croup and from day-nursery children. 3. Studies on the haemagglutination and haemagglutination-inhibition of the agent. Arch. Ges. Virusforsch., 8:332-350, 1958.
25. Philipson, L.: Aetiology of non-diphtheritic croup. 2. Virologic investigation. Acta Paediat., *47*: 611-625, 1958.
26. Philipson, L.: The etiology of non-diphtheritic croup: a review. Quart. Rev. Pediat., *14*:13-18, 1959.
27. Philipson, L.: Virologic aspects of the upper respiratory infections in childhood with special reference to non-diphtheritic croup. Acta Paediat., *48*: 89-90, 1959.
28. Philipson, L., and Rosen, L.: Identification of a cytopathogenic agent called U-virus recovered from patients with non-diphtheritic croup and from day-
29. Philipson, L., and Wesslen, T.: Recovery of a cytopathogenic agent from patients with non-diphtheritic croup and from day-nursery children. 1. Properties of the agent. Arch. Ges. Virusforsch., 9:77-94, 1958.
30. Poland, J. D., Welton, E. R., and Chin, T. D. Y.: Influenza virus B as cause of acute croup syndrome. Amer. J. Dis. Child., *107*:54-57, 1964.
31. Rabe, E. F.: Infectious croup: II "Virus" croup. Pediatrics, *2*:415, 1948.
32. Rabe, E. F.: Acute inflammatory disorders of the larynx and laryngotracheal area. Pediat. Clin. N. Amer., pp. 169-182, Feb. 1957.
33. Vargosko, A. J., Chanock, R. M., Huebner, R. J., Luckey, A. H., Kim, H. W., Cumming, C., and Parrott, R. B.: Association of type 2 hemadsorption (Parainfluenza 1) virus and Asian influenza A virus with infectious croup. New Eng. J. Med., *261*:1-9, 1959.
34. Ward, T. G.: Viruses of the respiratory tract. Progr. Med. Virol., *2*:203-234, 1959.

nursery children. Arch. Ges. Virusforsch., 9: 25-30, 1959.

42

Clinical Diagnosis of Bronchopneumopathies Occurring in the Course of Viral Infections

By J. COUVREUR

GENERAL CLINICAL STUDY

ACUTE BRONCHITIS

Most cases of acute bronchitis seem to be of viral origin. The bronchial involvement rarely occurs alone. It is almost always associated with a tracheal mucosal involvement and is often complicated, either at the onset or later, by pulmonary involvement; thus, bronchopneumopathy often succeeds a tracheobronchitis. The bronchitis is often preceded or accompanied by rhinopharyngeal inflammation. Cough is the most important sign. It is a dry, obstinate, often harsh, barking, unremittent cough, worse at night. After one or two days it becomes productive and progressively looser, the expectoration being mucous at first, then purulent in case of superinfection. In children, the cough may be severe enough to cause vomiting. It may be associated with retrosternal or thoracic pain.

Fever is not constant and in any case is moderate, rarely rising above 38.5° C.

The physical examination yields variable results. Although it is often unrevealing at the onset, one to three days later it shows rhonchi, sibilant rales, or severe moist rales throughout the thorax, heard especially in the postero-inferior areas. Palpation reveals fremiti produced by the secretions in the main bronchial trunks. Percussion is negative. There is no parallel between severity of the auscultation signs and the gravity of the disease. In the absence of parenchymatous involvement, acute bronchitis does not last much more than five to six days, but cough and expectoration may persist for one to two weeks, even longer in the presence of such factors as sinusitis, tonsil and adenoid infection, preëxisting bronchial lesions, allergy, general debilitating disease, hypogammaglobulinemia, and so forth.

The bronchial signs are particularly marked and frequent in measles. They may be very serious in adenovirus infections, and the seriousness of the lesions is revealed by histopathological study in fatal cases; even diffuse epithelial necrosis can be found.

In some cases, the bronchial lesions are intense enough to cause partial obstruction, especially in young children whose bronchi are smaller.

Endoscopic study of viral acute bronchitis has never been systematically performed. Occasionally, signs of bronchial inflammation with edema and hyperemia of mucosa have been observed, and sometimes there is an aspect of segmentary edema capable of reducing the caliber of one or several bronchial openings. The presence of purulent secretions suggests bacterial superinfection. The *cytological examination* of bronchial secretions reveals a mixture of mononuclear cells, desquamated bronchial cells, and some polymorphonuclear cells. *Bronchial biopsy* shows edema of the submucosa accompanied by capillary dilations and mononuclear infiltrates. The rarity of polymorphonuclear cells distinguishes the viral infection from a bacterial infection. The action of the virus on the bronchial epithelium has been determined precisely in vitro.[20]

BRONCHIOLITIS

The term "acute bronchiolitis" is often applied to cases of virus pneumopathy in children. It can also include the pictures described as capillary bronchitis, virus pneumonia, and even suffocating cattarh (Laennec, 1832), acute suffocating bronchitis (Rillet and Barthez, 1838), infectious pulmonary edema,[7] or spumous bronchoalveolitis. It must not be regarded as a synonym for acute interstitial pneumonia, which corresponds to a histopathological definition. But a strictly bronchiolar impairment involving neither the bronchial mucosa nor the interstitial tissue of the alveoli[1] is an evident impossibility. It perhaps explains why some French-speaking authors prefer a more clinical terminology when referring to virus bronchopneumopathies and distinguishing those causing dyspnea from those which do not.

Acute bronchiolitis is observed mainly in young children, especially during the first six months of life, whereas primary atypical pneumonia, much less serious in appearance, occurs in older children and in adults. Acute bronchiolitis occurs predominantly in winter or in early spring. Most often it is sporadic, but a higher incidence coincides with epidemics of infection of the upper respiratory tract in older children and adults. Real epidemics may also be observed in collectivities.

The disease is preceded for two or three days by an infection of the upper respiratory tract. Its onset is marked by a rise in temperature that is often abrupt, a dry, persistent cough, and progressive dyspnea. The cough may be pertussis-like. Respiration is difficult, with, at the very beginning, tachypnea, respiratory traction, fluttering of the nasal alae, cyanosis, and, in some cases, a little foam on the lips. The cough may be accompanied by vomiting. Often, the child refuses to drink. The temperature is quite variable, and may be moderate or reach 39° to 40° C. at the onset. Convulsions may occur in the young child. The seriousness of the clinical picture does not parallel the degree of fever. On examination the clearest signs result from extremely severe muscular effort required to breathe. The thorax is distended, and breathing is rapid and superficial. Expiration is often noisy. The intercostal, suprasternal, and substernal inspiratory retraction of the chest walls is evident but less severe than in acute laryngitis because of the pulmonary distention.[17]

Percussion reveals a hyperresonance, auscultation, lowered vesicular murmur and prolonged expiration. Pulmonary or bronchial rhonchi may be absent, but at other times "mucous rhonchi with both big and small bubble-bursting sounds are heard throughout lungs" (Laennec). These subcrepitant disseminated rales are sometimes covered by wheezing or are associated with rhonchi and sibilant rales. When the bronchiolar obstruction is total, an almost absolute respiratory silence may occur that marks some serious forms of influenza.

X-ray examination reveals signs which are usually compatible with an obstructive generalized emphysema: diffuse hyperclarity prevailing at the bases and obvious in the retrosternal areas on profile films, lowering and flattening of the diaphragmatic arches with reduced mobility on fluoroscopy, thoracic enlargement and widening of the intercostal spaces, with horizontal position of the ribs. Occasionally the hilum is accentuated, the bronchovascular shadows are darker, there are local or diffuse macronodular flocculent opacities or a segmentary opacity; pleural reaction is also possible.

The course is most often favorable, even in the cases that appear severe at the onset. The fever decreases quickly within the first 48 hours or more progressively in four or five days, rarely longer. The functional and physical manifestations run parallel. X-ray films may reveal pulmonary densities for a much longer time. However, complications may occur: convulsions in the initial phase of hyperthermia, heart failure, bacterial bronchopneumonia, otitis, pulmonary atelectasis, and dehydration due to hyperventilation, which may be serious.

The mortality due to bronchiolitis is not negligible. The course may be so fulminant that certain forms of respiratory viral disease are regarded as a possible cause of sudden death (see Chapter 59). Moreover, apoplectic forms have been reported accompanied by a hemorrhagic syndrome, nervous manifestations, adrenal insufficiency, and renal involvement with albuminuria and cylindruria.

The mortality is highly variable: 14 per cent and 28 per cent during two epidemics reported by Adams, 14 per cent according to Breton, 1.25 per cent for Jeune. It depends on so great a variety of factors (age, criteria of selection, epidemic in question, virus responsible) that no valid comparison of the groups studied is possible.

PRIMARY ATYPICAL PNEUMONIA (P.A.P.)

The term "atypical" refers to acute pulmonary infections in which clinical, radiological, pathological, or therapeutic characteristics are distinct from those in bacterial pneumonia.

Having been for a long time described and regarded as the prototype of virus pneumonia, "primary atypical pneumonia" has had a surprising destiny, for, after some 18 years of investigation, it proved to be most often related not to a virus but to a mycoplasma—Eaton's agent (see Chapter 45).

Originally, primary atypical pneumonia was differentiated from bacterial pneumonia on clinical and therapeutic grounds. Then it was noted that the picture is often associated with the presence of cold hemagglutinins. Moreover, it was noted that during convalescence 20 to 75 per cent of the patients present agglutinins against the nonhemolytic *Streptococcus salivarus* (streptococcus MG) isolated from lungs of patients having died of pneumopathy and from patients' sputum samples. Later, it was possible to communicate the disease to volunteers (1945). In 1941, Eaton et al. isolated a filterable agent from patients, but it was not until 1959 that, by means of the fluorescent antibody technique, the role of Eaton's agent was demonstrated in primary atypical pneumonia. Finally, it was a surprise to discover that this agent is not a virus: it cultivates on a cell-free agar medium (Chanock, 1962). Eaton's agent is related to the bovine peripneumonia group described by Nocard and Roux in 1898 and belongs to the *Mycoplasma* genus (see Chapter 45).

Although most often associated with Eaton's agent, primary atypical pneumonia has been progressively broken down as other agents were discovered. In some cases the cause has not been found; in others the influenza viruses A, B, and C and parainfluenza 1 and 3, the adenoviruses, the respiratory syncytial virus, and the ornithosis or Q fever agents are capable of producing an absolutely identical picture. Finally, mixed infections can occur.[4]

Endemic primary atypical pneumonia may occur in close groups—families, schools, the army—and also in the general population.

The incubation period lasts seven to 15 days. At the onset, the disease is characterized by malaise and chills, fever of variable degree, and occasionally throat redness or coryza. The most striking element is a dry and stubborn cough which may subsequently turn productive and cause thoracic pain. The fact that physical signs are absent or moderate should be emphasized: there is no dullness, and there may be subcrepitant rales with fine bubble-bursting sounds or moist rales, or occasionally rhonchi and sibilant rales which may not be perceived before the tenth day.

X-ray examination is required for the diagnosis and reveals some anomalies from the onset. It shows a nonhomogeneous, hazy, cloud-like opacity. Nine times out of ten it is located in an inferior lobe, often in the cardiophrenic angle, where hilodiaphragmatic linear opacities can be seen. It may be limited to one segment, rarely to one lobe. It is bilateral in one-fifth of the cases. One of its essential characteristics is its progressive course. The opacities may become more and more apparent over two weeks.

As a rule, the blood count is normal; neither lymphocytosis nor leukopenia is observed. Leukocytosis occurs only in the very febrile cases. The sedimentation rate may range from 20 to over 100 mm. during the first hour.

The course is usually mild but prolonged.

As a rule, the systemic signs disappear within three to ten days, but may persist longer. The physical and the radiological signs persist after the defervescence, lasting for more than one month in one-fifth of the cases.

The clinical picture described at present is often limited to the cases associated with Eaton's agent.

It should be borne in mind that the possible occurrence of hemoptysis, pleural reaction, bronchial ulcerations, hemolytic anemia, and cardiac localization were reported originally, as were severe, sometimes fatal forms involving all the lobes successively.[18]

SEQUELAE

The possible existence of sequelae to virus bronchopneumopathy has often been suggested, but this problem has never been thoroughly studied. The foundation is triple: animal experimentation; clinical observation; and study of patients' respiratory function.

Experimentation in rats has shown that

Table 42-1. *Comparative Frequency of Functional, Clinical, and Radiological Signs in Primary Atypical Pneumopathy Associated with Eaton's Agent, the Adenoviruses, or Undetermined Agents**

	EATON'S AGENT	ADENOVIRUS	UNDETERMINED
Number of Cases Studied	109	23	122
Functional signs			
Headache	84	43	59
Chills	78	65	72
Malaise	74	57	71
Stiffness	45	48	49
Anorexia	36	17	27
Cough	93	91	97
Thoracic pains	42	57	43
Pharyngeal pain	53	65	49
Coryza	49	78	82
Physical signs			
37.8 to 40° C. fever	100	100	100
Rales on auscultation	84	61	73
Cervical adenopathy	18	26	16
Red pharynx	12	43	8
Tonsillar exudate	0.9	17	0.8
Radiological signs			
Pulmonary infiltration right: lower lobe	38	4	24
other	2	3	9
left: lower lobe	43	9	52
other	7	1	4
bilateral:	19	6	9

*After Mufson et al., 1961 (figures given in percentage).

ligature of a bronchus causes progressive development of areas of bronchiectasis. Cultures made from mucopurulent material obtained from the lesions show, fairly regularly, the presence of *Mycoplasma pneumoniae*.[15] If the ligature is brief, bronchial drainage is restored and bronchiectasis does not occur; it becomes irreversible in case of prolonged ligature. It seems that the lesions of the ciliated epithelium and of the elastic and muscular structures are determinants of these irreversible lesions, as well as involvement of nerve endings and of the peribronchiolar ganglionic nerve structures. As will be seen below, such lesions have been observed in severe forms of adenovirus pneumopathies in man. It is imaginable that the systematized, occasionally very persistent opacities observed in certain virus pneumopathies could result in definitive bronchial lesions: the relationship between these two facts is well established.

Clinical observation has shown that originally healthy subjects suffered repeated respiratory manifestations or chronic bronchitis after the viral bronchopneumopathy of influenza, measles, or adenovirus diseases, or after primary atypical pneumonia.

Furthermore, systematic study of the causes of bronchiectasis shows that in a goodly number of cases it seems to have been secondary to an infection other than primary tuberculosis. Thus, of 187 pediatric cases reported by Glauser et al.,[10] 129 were considered secondary to an infection, including three cases which followed measles, four, viral pneumopathy, and 23, a nonspecific infection. However, bronchography during viral pneumopathy or after recovery revealed anomalies, in fact, transitory, in only two of 18 cases.[14]

The respiratory function has been studied in a valid fashion only in varicella pneumopathy, in which persistence of functional consequences during several months has been demonstrated.[3] Such investigations with regard to other viral pneumopathies could be worth while. Lastly, adenoviruses have been found in specimens removed surgically because of bronchial lesions.[16]

In fact, the existence of respiratory sequelae, particularly bronchial lesions, after viral bronchopneumopathies has never been formally demonstrated. This demonstration would require the identification of a definite viral respiratory infection in a subject whose bronchial tree was known to have been normal originally, the exclusion of such factor as bacterial superinfection, and finally th demonstration of bronchial lesions by endos copy, bronchoscopy, functional exploration and even by histopathological study if th occasion presented itself.

Such an investigation requires a consider able material and large means for investiga tion. Perhaps such studies would make i possible to establish the viral origin of som syndromes of pulmonary fibrosis or of chroni bronchopathy the etiology of which is a present unknown.

LABORATORY STUDIES, STUDIES OF RESPIRATORY FUNCTION, RADIOLOGICAL STUDIES

HEMATOLOGICAL ASPECTS

The hematological response has long been regarded as an important element in orienting the diagnosis. A normal or lowered level of leukocytes and the absence of polymorphonuclear cytosis could suggest a viral origin. Experimental studies reveal that the influenza virus induces leukopenia.[27] Among 256 children with virus bronchopneumopathy, Breton noted a leukocyte level below 5000 per cubic millimeter in 10 per cent, between 5000 and 11,000 in 60 per cent, and higher than 11,000 in 30 per cent; in only nine cases did the level exceed 20,000. No correlation was observed between the clinical or radiological types and the blood changes.

A comprehensive controlled study of the blood count was made by Portnoy et al.[19] They compared 246 children with a lower respiratory tract disease with 96 patients without fever or clinical signs of respiratory infection. The existence of a viral respiratory infection was demonstrated in 29 per cent of the former group and 17 per cent of the latter. The respiratory syncytial virus was most frequently isolated in the former group and adenoviruses in the latter. The median white blood cell count for patients with respiratory infections was 14,465 per cubic millimeter (range, 1100 to 60,000); in the control group, it was 9000 (range, 4800 to 23,400). These differences were significant. However, the respective average percentages of polymorphonuclear cells were 44 per cent and

39 per cent and of leukocytes, 40 per cent and 50 per cent (nonsignificant differences). Portnoy et al.[19] endeavoring to establish a relation between the clinical picture and the leukocyte count, obtained, as average figures, 16,725 in pneumopathies, 13,550 in bronchiolitis, and 13,000 in laryngotracheobronchitis, these differences not being significant.

The usual aspects of the white cell count in the child being taken into account, a normal level of leukocytes can be considered the rule in subclinical respiratory virus infections.

In contrast, an appreciable tendency to leukocytosis is observed in some patients with obvious lower respiratory tract infections. The degree of leukocytosis does not seem influenced by the day of the disease, the child's age, or the specific virus involved. Several factors could account for the leukocytosis: hyperthermia, existence of tissue destruction phenomena, or a bacterial superinfection, although the absence of polymorphonuclear cells is an argument against this last diagnosis. The direct action of the virus upon the leukocytes is a possibility; moreover, it is known that the white blood cells play an important part in viral infections[12, 13] (see Introduction). Whatever the hypothesis, leukocytosis can be observed in the respiratory virus diseases and is not characteristic of only the bacterial infections.

The sedimentation rate is often elevated.[24] Thus, among 16 cases of primary atypical pneumonia observed by Berven, this acceleration was marked in 15, with figures ranging between 30 and 125 mm. for the first hour and over 90 in nine cases.

RADIOLOGICAL STUDY

Aside from the investigation carried out by Jeune et al.[14] few comprehensive surveys have been devoted to the radiological aspects of virus bronchopneumopathy. These authors analyzed the data obtained from x-ray films of the thorax of 241 children, newborn to age 16, hospitalized because of their respiratory infection. The serological examination provided arguments in support of adenovirus disease in 36 cases, of influenza in 65, and of ornithosis in 22, and it revealed cold hemagglutinins in 118 cases.

The x-ray pictures were classified into eight categories: normal thoracic picture, hilar intumescence, hilifuge linear opacities, heterogeneous condensations, generalized miliary aspect, dense condensation with a segmentary aspect, segmental opacity suggesting a ventilation disturbance, and aspects of pleural reactions.

The thoracic x-ray picture was normal in 12.8 per cent of cases.

Simple, isolated hilar intumescence was rare: 14 cases (5 per cent), seven during influenza. It was most often associated with other aspects, namely, heterogeneous trails or condensations. When isolated, it may suggest an adenopathy.

The hilifuge linear opacities and the aspects of heterogeneous condensation were most often concomitant but may be successive. They were found in 53 per cent of the abnormal films. In most cases, these pictures extended from hilar and basilar areas. In a tenth of the cases they were confined to the upper half of the pulmonary fields, but were often accompanied by basilar changes. They were bilateral in half of the cases but were generally located on the left side when unilateral. On the right, they often filled in the phrenopericardial angle. Such aspects should be considered suggestive of bronchopneumopathy.

The miliary pictures were rare (3 per cent), and suggested a possible heart failure or an associated asthma. Their viral etiology should not be accepted until the possibility of tuberculosis has been eliminated. They clear up fairly quickly.

The segmental condensations (20 per cent) were rather flocculent. When associated with other pictures, such as hilar tumescence, pleural reaction, or hilifuge linear opacities, they strongly suggest a virus pneumopathy. On the other hand, when isolated and frankly opaque (as occurred in 8 per cent) they are more suggestive of acute bacterial lobar pneumonia.

The pleural pictures (24 per cent of the cases) were most often associated with parenchymatous changes. They were of two kinds: (1) minimal pleural reactions, which were most frequent (21.5 per cent), with a fissural thickening and a picture of edging line, and (2) a filling in of the anterior or posterior cul-de-sac on the lateral views. The latter pictures seemed more frequent in the course of influenza. In no case do they justify punctures.

Pleural effusion was rare. Among the

seven cases studied, three were associated with purulent streptococcic pleurisy, two were aseptic puriform extravasations, and two were serofibrinous pleurisies; only the last can be considered viral pleurisies. On the whole, true nonbacterial pleurisies were exceptional in children with viral pneumopathy (0.8 per cent of the cases) but minor pleural involvement, most often associated with parenchymatous changes, was found in a quarter of the cases.

The association of several types of pictures (35 per cent) was of great value in orienting the diagnosis, especially if the abnormalities were diffuse and bilateral.

One can raise certain questions concerning the radiological aspects of virus bronchopneumopathy. Are these aspects the same in adults and in children? What is their exact incidence? Are certain pictures characteristic of certain viruses? Does the evolution of radiological images run parallel to the clinical syndrome? What elements should be weighed in differential diagnosis?

The pictures of virus pneumopathy seem exactly the same in children and in adults, but the frequency varies with age. This variation in frequency is in accordance with the clinical and epidemiological data showing that bronchopneumopathy due to viral respiratory disease is much more frequent in children.

The incidence of these radiological findings depends not only upon the age but also on the epidemic and the criteria of selection of patients. For instance, it should be mentioned that the children studied by Jeune et al. were all hospitalized, which increases the chances of finding radiological abnormalities.

As for establishing a relation between the type of picture and the responsible virus, it is impossible to suggest an etiological agent without knowing what viruses are prevalent at the time. All authors agree that no radiological aspect is characteristic of any one virus. We saw, when studying the pattern of primary atypical pneumonia, that its radiological aspect, long identified with that of viral pneumopathy, is now regarded as more often associated with involvement by the Eaton agent.

The radiological abnormalities of viral bronchopneumopathy often persist for a long time. Jeune followed up 131 cases. He noted that half of the abnormalities disappeared within less than 11 days and 84 per cent in less than 21 days, whereas 16 per cent persisted beyond that limit. The fact that certain opacities still persisted after one and even two months has been mentioned even in the early descriptions of primary atypical pneumonias, especially in their completely latent form. This persistence suggests the possibility of sequelae, a question we will return to.

In some cases, the differential diagnosis of virus pneumopathy may not be easy. Bacterial pneumonia may be suggested by a dense systematized lobar or segmental picture. Alternating densities and clearer areas may suggest a staphylococcic pulmonary involvement, especially in the presence of pleurisy. The occurrence of a bacterial superinfection does not facilitate the diagnosis, and recourse to hematological, bacteriological, and virological studies, as well as the results of therapy with antibiotics, is often necessary for diagnosis.

Finally, some pictures showing a reticulonodular aspect, segmental opacities associated with an enlarged hilar shadow suggestive of adenopathy, and irregular densities with small clear areas suggest respectively miliary tuberculosis, primary tuberculosis, or ulceronodular tuberculosis. Such cases require checking of tuberculin allergy and radiological, bacteriological, and bronchological studies; occasionally, when a doubt remains, specific antitubercular chemotherapy may be considered.

EFFECTS ON CARDIORESPIRATORY FUNCTION

The few works devoted to the effect of virus pneumopathy on cardiorespiratory function prove that it is appreciable and should not be disregarded. Some examples are given in studies on varicella pneumopathy and on influenza. In varicella pneumopathy, significant modifications of the alveolocapillary exchanges during the acute phase of the disease have been demonstrated. Some anomalies may persist for several months.[3] Soto et al.,[22] from a histological study of nine fatal cases of Asian influenza, concluded that death was due to anoxemia resulting from alveolocapillary blockade. It is obvious that if a virus pneumopathy causes respiratory difficulties which are clinically severe and accompanied by wheezing, an obstructive-type ventilation deficiency will soon become established. In fact, Berven verified, in the late stage of primary atypical pneumonia, a reduction in the capacity of pulmonary gaseous exchanges, anatomic shunts representing 6 to 15 per cent of the cardiac output. Above all, the modifications of respiratory function remain despite normalization of the pulmonary radiographs and may persist for at least six months, although improving progressively.

During the acute phase of the serious cases of bronchopneumopathy, the various lesions, such as bronchial and bronchiolar inflammation, interstitial pneumopathy, even edematous or hemorrhagic alveolitis, are capable of considerably reducing the oxygenation of the blood. Hypoxia is responsible for dyspnea and tachypnea, and later for cyanosis revealing anoxemia.

Two types of responses can be distinguished: respiratory alkalosis and respiratory acidosis. Respiratory alkalosis with reactional hyperventilation can entail a decrease in partial pressure of alveolar CO_2, which may be lower than 30 mm. Hg, and a rise in blood pH, while the alkaline reserve is little altered. The secondary elimination of bases through the kidneys counterbalances this alkalosis and brings the pH back to normal. The hyperventilation may cause a certain degree of dehydration and hemoconcentration.

Respiratory acidosis is seen in severe cases: the respiratory obstruction and the alveolar blockade induce a hypoventilation which cannot be counterbalanced by a superficial tachypnea. The CO_2 pressure rises above 5 mm. Hg and the blood pH may decrease. The alkaline reserve is normal or slightly increased.

These two aspects, respiratory alkalosis and acidosis, may be successive; hypoventilation accompanied by acidosis is a grave sign. Such biological disturbances are found especially in young children, but the extent of the radiological signs and the intensity of the acid-base disturbances do not run parallel.[14] The latter are in no case specific of virus infections. They are due to prolonged perfusion, the nonventilated areas of pulmonary condensation, and disturbances in gaseous exchanges.

PATHOLOGY

The histopathological lesions were described even before the isolation of their causal agents. In 1947, Parker et al. reported that the essential lesions of fatal virus pneumopathy

are bronchitis, bronchiolitis, inflammation of alveolar septa, alternating zones of atelectasis and emphysema, and the presence of plasma, blood corpuscles, and histiocytes within the alveoli. In half the cases there is a hyaline membrane-like aspect within the alveoli. We shall see that such a lesion has been observed in some cases of influenza.[22] Let us recall here that lesions of mainly lymphomonocytic interstitial pneumonia have been reported in 30 to 80 per cent of cases of fatal poliomyelitis. We shall see that the histopathology of adenovirus pneumonia is characteristic and has been intensively studied.

The lesions of primary atypical pneumonia have seldom been studied because of its low mortality. Golden, however, has provided a comprehensive description based on the study of 42 cases. He reported that the pleural surfaces are smooth or bristling with fibrinous exudates. In some cases, an amber-colored effusion is observed. The parenchymal lesions may involve a single lobe or be more diffuse and bilateral. Macroscopically they consist of a miliary-like granuloma. However, whitish nodules are due to a thickening of the alveolar walls full of pus. The nearby pulmonary tissues may be normal or they may be edematous, hemorrhagic, and congestive. The mucosa of the trachea and of the large bronchi is normal or slightly edematous and congestive, only rarely is it greatly inflamed or ulcerated. The principal lesions are located in the bronchioles, the mucosa of which is desquamated in places. Their lumina contain pus, mucus, and desquamated epithelial cells. Bacteria are rare and of different types. The bronchioles are dilated and their walls are mainly infiltrated with mononuclear cells. This infiltration reaches the nearby interstitial tissues, the alveolar walls, and the pulmonary septa. The alveoli still contain some air or are deflated but are free from exudate. Such a description with regard to primary atypical pneumonia clearly shows the predominance of bronchiolar lesions. This predominance has been confirmed by many studies, among which are those of Parker et al.[18]

ROLE OF SOME ETIOLOGICAL FACTORS

AGE

Age is often a decisive factor in the clinical aspects of viral pneumopathy. As a rule, bronchiolitis is observed in the child under two years of age, whereas primary atypical pneumonia is encountered in older children or adults.

In the newborn child, cases of viral or nonviral pneumopathy are very rare. In England, in 1959, the death rate due to pneumopathy among newborn children was 1.03 per 1000, and the total mortality was 15.9 per cent. The problems are not the same during the first and the second weeks of life.

During the first week, viral pneumopathy belongs to a picture of generalized infection of toxic aspect and is rarely recognized because the respiratory troubles—delay in the establishment of vigorous respiratory movements, irregular and noisy respiration with inspiratory retraction of the chest walls, cyanosis, and pallor—tend to be ascribed to various perinatal disorders other than viral infection. However, the pediatrician should bear in mind that herpes, cytomegalic inclusion body disease, varicella, and Coxsackie infections are often attended by respiratory manifestations.

After the first week, the newborn child may have caught a nosocomial infection that, after an asymptomatic interval, is followed by a stage of nasal obstruction and subsequently by severe manifestations. These manifestations result from a diffuse involvement of the respiratory tract.

Involvement of the lower respiratory tract is revealed by a sudden deterioration of the general physical condition, grayish complexion, acceleration and inversion of the respiratory rhythm, and appearance of bilateral and diffuse moist rales. The temperature is either normal or subnormal. Cough is infrequent. The course may be fulminant. However, the mortality is in fact fairly low and, as a rule, progressive improvement is observed; recovery occurs within one or two weeks.

Two facts should be mentioned with regard to neonatal viral pneumopathy.

Adams[1] described several epidemics in nurseries and sporadic cases of pneumopathy characterized by an abrupt onset with cough, rapid spread of the infection to the lower respiratory tract, and abundant pharyngeal exudate. The evolution covered a period of three to ten days, and the mortality reached 20 per cent in premature infants. The diagnosis was based on a pathognomonic element: the presence of many cells containing nuclear inclusions in the pharyngeal specimens from the child and occasionally from surrounding persons. These elements in diagnosis have been criticized; other authors did not find them, and the specificity of the inclusions has been questioned.

Another fact is noteworthy. During an epidemic of eight cases of respiratory infections in premature infants, ECHO virus 9 infection was proved. This virus was isolated from the pulmonary tissue in one fatal case. In four of the eight cases the radiological aspect of cystic emphysema suggested the Wilson-Mikity syndrome. These facts, should they be confirmed, open further perspectives for the study of viral pneumopathy in newborn children.

HOST FACTORS

The importance of the *allergy factor* in the clinical picture of respiratory viral diseases deserves special mention. It has long been known that crises in asthmatic subjects are often due to a respiratory infection. Many studies have been devoted to determining the exact relation between respiratory allergy and infection. It has not been established whether colds, bronchitis, or pneumopathy aggravate allergic reactions already in progress or whether they sensitize respiratory mucosae. In any event, it is certain that, during respiratory viral diseases, allergic subjects are more liable to respiratory obstruction than those who are not allergic. In this respect, the work of Freeman and Todd[9] is important because they took virological data into account to verify a clinical impression. They studied 357 children, most of them under two years of age, with a respiratory infection associated with duly determined adenovirus, parainfluenza, or respiratory syncytial viruses. They observed that 27 per cent of the patients had had an expiratory wheezing during the disease. The incidence of this symptom was 41 per cent between 0 and 12 months, 21 to 26 per cent between 12 and 24 months, 8.4 per cent between two and five years, and 35 per cent after five years of age. Wheezing was observed in 21 per cent of the cases of parainfluenza type 1 and type 3 infection, 52 per cent of the cases of respiratory syncytial virus infection, and 13 per cent of the cases of adenovirus infection. Most important, allergy was much more frequently observed in patients exhibiting wheezing (50 per cent) than in those without this symptom (17 per cent). However, wheezing was less frequently associated with allergy in those under the age of 18 months (39 per cent) than in those above this age (73 per cent). It thus can be assumed that, after 18 months of age, allergy may alter and considerably aggravate the manifestations of respiratory viral diseases.

The *immune state* of the infected subjects is the second important element that can modify the clinical picture. In normal subjects, a previous immunizing experience undoubtedly accounts for the fact that respiratory manifestations due to the respiratory syncytial virus are moderate in adults whereas they are much more apparent in children. These facts account for the frequency of bronchiolitis during the first years of life and their much greater rarity later. The respiratory manifestations, remarkable for their frequency and severity, in patients with agammaglobulinemia or dysgamma-globulinemia are well known. Cytomegalo-virus pneumopathy, which among adults is observed almost solely in subjects with blood disorders or malignant diseases or in those treated with immunodepressant agents, is a clear-cut example of a respiratory disease illustrating perfectly the point in question.

PREËXISTING BRONCHIAL LESIONS

The role played by viruses in the occurrence and persistence of chronic bronchitis has often been discussed. Although some workers were unable to prove that respiratory viruses play any role in acute attacks in chronic bronchitis, others have shown, by means of serological studies, that a relation is probable between these incidents and infections due to syncytial virus,[8] influenza B virus, or parainfluenza viruses.[5, 23] Influenza A virus infection may severely aggravate chronic bronchitis.[25] A longitudinal virological study in subjects with chronic bronchitis and living at home in Glasgow showed not only the role of influenza and parainfluenza viruses but also, and for the first time, that of rhinoviruses. The high titer of these viruses in the expectorate sometimes contrasted with the negative results in nasopharyngeal specimens; this opposition indicates that these viruses may infect the lower respiratory tract in adults. A rhinovirus was associated with 23 per cent of exacerbations of chronic bronchitis and was present in almost 50 per cent of the cases in which symptoms of common cold had preceded or followed such an exacerbation.[8] The respective proportion of viruses infecting patients with chronic bronchitis seems very close to that of the viruses of mild respiratory infections in the normal population. The reasons for peculiar clinical manifestations of viral respiratory infection among subjects with bronchitis are probably related more to factors of allergy and immunity and to the preëxisting bronchial abnormality than to the specific etiological agent. As is known, rhinoviruses may induce colds in volunteers when administered as nasal drops, whereas they may cause bronchitis when experimentally introduced into the lower respiratory tract.[6] It is possible that viruses are introduced directly into the bronchi, avoiding the nasal barrier, in patients with chronic bronchopathy, who often breathe through their mouths. Perhaps, also, viruses causing lesions of the epithelial mucous membranes upset the precarious equilibrium in these subjects by promoting rapid secondary development of infection by pathogenic bacteria.

ASPECTS CHARACTERISTIC OF THE VIRUS TYPE

INFLUENZA PNEUMOPATHY

Influenza is discussed in Chapter 39.

BRONCHOPNEUMOPATHY DUE TO PARAINFLUENZA MYXOVIRUSES

The main characteristics of parainfluenza myxoviruses 1, 2, 3, and 4 are their ability often to provoke respiratory infections, especially in the young child. Types 1 and 3 differ from influenza myxoviruses in that that they are ubiquitous, endemic, and induce infections all the year round.

Three clinical syndromes are associated with them: mild rhinopharyngitis, suffocating laryngotracheitis with or without bronchitis, and acute bronchopneumopathy.[39] According to Chanock, 7 to 16 per cent of respiratory infections in children are associated with this group of viruses. The four types of virus are recovered in pneumopathy. However, the bronchopneumopathy associated with parainfluenza types 1 and 2 is often accompanied by laryngeal manifestations (in 20 per cent of cases), whereas the parainfluenza type 3 infections are more often associated with bronchiolitis or with a bronchopneumopathy than are parainfluenza type 1 infections.[39]

Type 1 Parainfluenza Myxoviruses. Sendai virus is generally considered a member of this subgroup. This virus was isolated from newborn children in 1953 during a nursery epidemic in Japan. The infection manifested itself by severe bronchopneumopathy, with marked functional and physical manifestations, and x-ray pictures showed bilateral pulmonary involvement. The disease was fatal in 12 to 17 cases. Postmortem examination revealed, in all cases, hemorrhagic pneumonia with thickening of the alveolar walls due to hyperplasia of the mononucleated cells contrasting with the discreteness of the bronchial epithelium. This pneumopathy was experimentally reproduced. However, this epidemic has remained unique. Sendai virus has never been isolated in other continents, and the validity of the virological bases of this investigation remains open to discussion.

HA$_2$ virus, antigenically related to Sendai virus, was isolated by Chanock et al.[29, 32] and is associated with a disease fairly similar to that produced by parainfluenza type 3. Studies in volunteers have shown that the incubation period is six to eight days. Bronchopneumopathy due to HA$_2$ virus is comparatively rare and its course is prolonged: eight to ten days. It has no specific clinical features.

Type 2 Parainfluenza Myxovirus (CA). This type is usually associated with acute laryngitis and rarely with pneumopathy. Unlike the other two types, it is encountered sporadically.

Type 3 Parainfluenza Myxovirus. This type causes pneumopathy fairly often, especially in young or even in premature children.[37] A strain isolated in France that seems to have been widespread in 1958[33] caused a hospital epidemic: six children aged from two to 12 months were involved.[36] The manifestations in this epidemic seem representative in regard to those reported by other authors. All the children were febrile: temperatures reached 38.5° to 39°C. in four cases, but the thermic spikes did not last more than one or two days. Cough was constant, and in two cases foam was noted on the lips. Four children showed dyspnea for three to four days; bilateral rhonchi and sibilant rales were heard.

X-ray examination revealed anomalies in four cases: parenchymatous opacities (two cases), unilateral or bilateral decreased transparency and accentuation of hilar shadows (two cases). The clinical picture was complicated by pharyngitis (one case), otitis (three cases), and diarrhea (two cases). Blood count revealed moderate leukocytosis: 8000 to 12,000 cells per cubic millimeter with 64 to 67 per cent lymphocytes, except in one instance of hyperleukocytosis (18,000 cells) with polymorphonuclear cytosis. Illness was mild, and the general physical condition was not altered. A serological study carried out in several hospitals of the Paris area indicated that infection due to EA 102 strain of parainfluenza type 3 myxovirus was associated with 23.8 per cent of respiratory infections in children during the winters of 1956 and 1957. Among these patients, 61.6 per cent manifested clinical and radiological signs of pneumopathy. According to age, the positive results were classified as follows: 26 per cent from 0 to 23 months, 22.2 per cent from 24 months to three years, and 13.6 per cent from three to nine years of age.

After a seven-year investigation, Chanock and Parrott[31] reported that a highly positive serological reaction to parainfluenza type 3 myxovirus had been observed in 10.7 per cent of the cases of bronchitis, 8.1 per cent of the cases of pneumopathy, and 8 per cent of the cases of bronchiolitis, this agent being the parainfluenza virus most often associated with the last-named picture in children.

Moreover, its pathogenicity has been proved in adult volunteers.[40] However, the clinical signs were fairly mild, probably because of previously acquired spontaneous immunity. Under such conditions, the spectrum of clinical effects due to this virus could not be studied with the desired precision.

Type 4 Parainfluenza Myxovirus. This type seems to be less pathogenic for the lower respiratory tract. It has been recovered from only a few patients with such infections.[34] By experimental inoculation of volunteers, only common colds have been obtained, or an upper respiratory tract infection.[40] These common colds could be distinguished from manifestations of rhinovirus infection only by their longer incubation period: four days, on an average. These inoculations into volunteers concerned adults. In children, in contrast, the spontaneous illness more often involves pneumopathy.

BRONCHOPNEUMOPATHY DUE TO RESPIRATORY SYNCYTIAL VIRUS (MORRIS' CCA VIRUS)

In 1956, a virus responsible for coryza epidemics among chimpanzees was recovered from these animals by Morris et al.[68] who named it CCA (Chimpanzee Coryza Agent). Moreover, these authors observed, in one of their laboratory workers, febrile rhinitis and an increase in neutralizing antibodies to this virus. A year later, Chanock and Finberg[49] isolated, in two children with bronchopneumopathy, two strains of syncytial virus with the same characteristics as Morris' virus. They proposed naming it RSV (Respiratory Syncytial Virus). In 1960, Beem et al.[44] provided evidence of the role played by this virus in bronchopneumopathy in children. Since then, epidemiological investigations carried out in Australia, the United States, Canada, Great Britain, and France have shown the importance of this virus in pneumopathy in children. Among all the respiratory viruses, it is the one most often associated with lower respiratory tract infections in children. In a study of nearly 8000 children. Chanock et al.[51] isolated it in 29.6 per cent of cases of bronchiolitis and 9.5 per cent of those of pneumopathy, i.e., in 9.5 per cent of the total number of respiratory diseases. It seems that RS virus is the most important viral respiratory pathogen of infancy. The main clinical studies concerning it are reported in Table 42-2.

The respiratory manifestations of this virus are highly diverse. The average incubation period is four days. It is unanimously agreed that infection may, in a single epidemic, give rise to coryza, bronchiolitis, bronchopneumopathy, or an isolated febrile reaction.[50, 59, 66, 69, 70] However, cases of pneumopathy predominate. Three studies carried out during epidemics in circumscribed collectivities indicated the spectrum of clinical manifestations due to RS virus.[45, 52, 63] The second epidemic, observed during a longitudinal study made in a hospital for children with pulmonary tuberculosis, provided an example approximately typical of all the aspects of RS virus infection[52] reported by clinicians and epidemiologists. Eighty-eight children aged from four months to four years were hospitalized at the time the epidemic occurred. The virus was isolated from 35.7 per cent of 28 subjects. In almost 71 per cent of the 62 children adequately studied by serological methods a significant rise in antibody titer occurred. In order of frequency, the clinical manifestations were fever, 77.2 per cent; bronchial signs, bronchiolitis, or foci of pulmonary condensation, 30.6 per cent; fever without severe clinical manifestations, 23.8 per cent; exudative and erythematous pharyngitis, 19.3 per cent; erythematous pharyngitis, 14.7 per cent; inapparent infection, 10.2 per cent, and croup, 1.1 per cent (Table 42-3).

X-ray examination may reveal a variety of images extending from normal roentgenogram to images of extensive pneumopathy with areas of pulmonary condensation. Rice

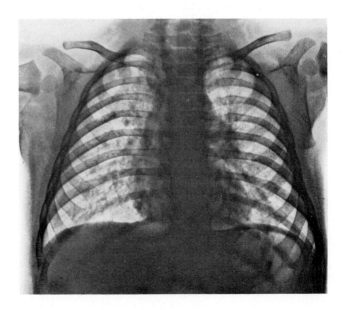

Figure 42-1. RS virus pneumopathy. Male infant aged 6 months. Film made at the thirty-sixth hour of a clinical picture of bronchiolitis of abrupt onset. Bilateral hilar enlargement with dense markings radiating away from the hilus. Emphysema of both bases. The gravity of the clinical picture had suggested pleuropulmonary staphylococcic infection. Titer of neutralizing antibodies, nil on the second day of hospitalization, was higher than $1/160$ on the seventeenth day.

Table 42-2. *Virological and Clinical Data from Main Studies Concerning Respiratory Infections Caused by RS Virus*

Authors	Location and Period of Study	Reason for Investigation	Patients No.	Patients Age	Virus Isolation No. Tested	Virus Isolation No. Positive	Serologic Studies Complement-Fixing Antibodies	Serologic Studies Neutralizing Antibodies	Clinical Manifestations
Morris et al.[68]	Washington, D.C. 1956	Laboratory worker	1	Adult				+	Rhinitis + fever
Chanock and Finberg[49]	1957		2	6 months	2	2		2/2	Bronchopneumopathy, croup
Rowe and and Michaels[74]	U.S.A. 1960		1	6 months	1	1		1/1	Severe bronchopneumopathy with cardiac failure and hepatomegaly
Beem et al.[44]	Chicago October, 1959–June, 1960	Systematic study of respiratory infections in children	291	Infants and children under 12 years	291	41	16/23	14/23	Bronchopneumopathy, bronchitis, pneumopathy
Hamre and Procknow[57]	U.S.A. October, 1960–June, 1961	Study of the "common cold" in students	101	Young adults	101	11		11/11	"Common cold"
Adams et al.[42]	Los Angeles January–March 1961	Epidemic bronchiolitis and pneumonitis	12	Infants, children and adolescents	12	8			Bronchiolitis, pneumopathy
Lewis et al.[66]	Australia 1961	Virological study of respiratory infections in infants	160	Infants	160	45			Croup, pneumopathies, bronchitis, bronchiolitis, rhinitis
Johnson[61]	North Carolina 1961	Virological study of respiratory infections at a military training center	243	Adults	4			15/243 patients 8/247 healthy subjects	Coryza
McClelland et al.[67] Hamparian et al.[56] Reilly et al.[72]	Philadelphia November, 1959–June, 1960	Studies of acute respiratory illness in children	667	Under 8	34	21		115/667	Upper respiratory tract disease; bronchitis, bronchiolitis, bronchopneumopathies
Peacock and Clarke[71]	Bristol 1961	Epidemic bronchiolitis		6 and 7 months	2	2			Bronchiolitis

Author	Location / Date	Study	Number	Age					Clinical diagnosis
Kapikian et al.[63]	U.S.A. 1961	Epidemic pneumopathy	90	5 to 50 months	60	24	73/80	17/41	Fever in 84 children of 90; pneumopathy in 36
Forbes[54]	Australia 1961	Virological study of respiratory infections in children	244	Infants and children under 4 years	237	70			Bronchitis, pneumopathy, bronchopneumopathy
Kravetz et al.[64] Johnson et al.[62]	Bethesda, Md. 1961	Administration of RS virus to 41 volunteers	41	Adults	41	30	22/41		Coryza
Parrott et al.[70]	Bethesda, Md. October, 1957–July, 1960	Serological studies of respiratory infections in children	1038	Infants and children			114/1038		Bronchiolitis, pneumopathy, minor respiratory disease
Chanock et al.[50]	Washington, D.C. March–July, 1960	Systematic study of respiratory infections	346	Infants and children	346	56	16/34	20/34	Bronchiolitis, pneumopathy, minor respiratory disease
Gernez-Rieux et al.[55] Breton et al.[47]	Lille, France February–March, 1960	Epidemic in a premature nursery	12	Premature infants	12	2		5/8	Coryza, cough, x-ray abnormalities
Holzel et al.[59]	Manchester, U.K. January–April, 1962	Study of children with bronchopneumopathies		Infants and children under 4 years		36			Bronchopneumopathy (one fatal case)
Moss et al.[69]	Manchester, U.K. April, 1962	Systematic serological study of children hospitalized with respiratory infections	45	Infants and children	45		15/45	3/3	Bronchitis, bronchopneumopathy
Adams et al.[43]	Manchester, U.K. December, 1961–April, 1962	Study of respiratory infections				38		16	
Couvreur et al.[52]	Paris November–December, 1962	Longitudinal study in a collectivity of children	88	4 months to 4 years	28	10		44/62	Fever, rhinopharyngitis, bronchitis, bronchiolitis
Chanock et al.[51]	Bethesda, Md. 1957–1964	Study of respiratory diseases	5641 2393	Infants Children	9.5% 13.7%				Severe respiratory disease
Sterner	Stockholm 1964	Epidemic in day nursery	15	Infants	13			7/15	Respiratory infection, rhinitis, bronchiolitis
Crone	Sinderland, U.K. 1964	Epidemic of bronchiolitis	170	Infants and children				38/78	Bronchiolitis

Table 42-3. *Clinical, Virological, and Serological data in a Typical RS Epidemic Observed in France*[52]

		Virus Isolation		Serological Study					
Clinical Manifestations	Cases No. (%)	No. Tested	No. Positive	No. Tested	Lack of Antibody	Significant Titer of Antibody	Presence of Antibody in First Specimen	Significant Rise in antibody Titer No. Cases	%
Isolated febrile reaction (with or without cough or coryza)	21 (23.8)	3	1	12		1	2	9	75
Bronchial signs or bronchiolitis or foci of pulmonary condensation	27 (30.6)	7	1	17	2	2	2	11	64
Erythematous pharyngitis without bronchopulmonary signs	13 (14.7)	10	4	12				12	100
Exudative and erythematous pharyngitis	17 (19.3)	3	1	12		3	3	6	50
Croup	1 (1.1)			1				1	
Inapparent infection	9* (10.2)	5	3	8		3		5	62
Total No. (%)	88 (100)	28	10 (35.7)	62	2 (3.2)	9 (14.5)	7 (11.1)	44	70.9

*Three of the nine patients without clinical manifestations were under corticosteroid therapy at the time of the epidemic.

and Loda[73] made a study of 38 infants. They noted anomalies in 34: in 33, interstitial pneumopathy, which, in 21, was generalized to all the lobes; foci of parenchymatous condensation in six, located in the right upper lobe in four; 13 patients showed emphysematous distention; two showed minimal pleural reaction; one showed hilar adenopathy. Thus, the most frequent radiological image is that of interstitial pneumopathy with emphysema, the severity of which parallels that of the clinical signs. However, none of these elements seems specific. Diagnosis may suggest beginnings of staphylococcic pulmonary infection, but pneumatocele, pneumothorax, and pleural involvement are lacking. Signs spontaneously disappeared within less than nine days in all the cases.

Thus, clinical and radiological manifestations of pneumopathy associated with RS virus are not specific. They are noteworthy because of their frequency in young and premature infants, because of the explosive character of the epidemics they cause in collectivities, and because of their gravity.

Several fatal cases have been reported.[43, 54, 59]

By means of an immunofluoresence technique, RS virus was demonstrated in giant cell bronchiolitis.[76]

On the other hand, in older children or adults illness is generally mild, limited to a "common cold" if not totally inapparent. This fact, which has been demonstrated by administering the virus to volunteers,[64] is probably due to prior immunity, since the proportion of subjects with antibodies may attain 93 per cent by age five.

The extensiveness and possible gravity of the infection in young children living in collective conditions would justify a program of specific vaccination in certain groups of exposed subjects. The work done for eight years in Hillman's laboratory produced an apparently utilizable formaldehyde-inactivated vaccine. Given in association with a vaccine against type 1, 2, and 3 myxoviruses, it was well tolerated and gave an excellent level of antibodies in initially seronegative subjects. But this vaccine gives no protection.[11a] It even seems that the presence of serum antibodies aggravates the clinical disease. Kapikian et al. (1969),[22a] for example, found pneumonia in 69 per cent of children vaccinated, against 9 per cent in nonvaccinated children. RS virus hence seems to have a peculiarity: most antibodies that neutralize viruses immunize against reinfection by the same virus, whereas those against RS can aggravate the disease.[11a, 22b] Immunity might depend more heavily on antibodies in respiratory tract secretions than in serum. These facts explain why bronchiolitis due to RS virus is frequent in very young children, despite (or because of) the frequent presence of antibodies transmitted by the mother (cf. Chapter 44).

PNEUMOPATHY DUE TO ADENOVIRUS

After the isolation of the "Adenoid Degenerative Agent" in adenoid tissue by Rowe, Huebner, et al. in 1953[112] and the demonstration of what Enders et al.[97] proposed naming adenoviruses in pharyngoconjunctival fever and follicular and catarrhal conjunctivitis,[80, 112] a series of works made it possible to incriminate them in infections of the lower respiratory pathways.[82, 87, 105, 109, 128, 140, 143, 148]

Table 42-4. *Review of Fatal Cases of Adenovirus Pneumopathy Reported in the Literature*

AUTHOR	COUNTRY	AGE (MONTHS)	CASES, NO.	CLINICAL DIAGNOSIS	VIRUS ISOLATED FROM	ADENOVIRUS TYPE
Kingman (cited by Sterner)	The Netherlands	?	1	Atypical pneumonia	?	?
Chany	France	12-54	4	Acute pneumopathy	Lung, CSF, brain	7a
Matumoto	Japan	3	1	Pneumopathy	Lung	3 and 7 (intermediate)
Henle	U.S.A.	?	1	?	?	1
Pereira	Great Britain	4½	1	Pneumopathy	Trachea, lung	1
Deinhardt	U.S.A.	14	1	Pneumopathy	Lung	1
Huebner	U.S.A.	9½	1	Letterer-Siwe disease	Mesenteric lymph nodes	3
Gerbeaux	France		1	Pneumopathy	Lung	7a
Hsiung	China	4-48	40			3 7
Teng	China	Nursing infants	47	Pneumopathy		3 7
Koch	The Netherlands	?	3	Pneumopathy	Lung	7
Van der Veen	The Netherlands	8	3	Pneumopathy	Lung	7 (2 cases) 3 (1 case)
Kapsenberg	The Netherlands	7-72	5	Bronchopneumopathy, gastroenteritis	?	7
Quenum	Senegal	24	1			
Wright	U.S.A.	9½	1	Pneumopathy, Werdnig-Hoffmann disease	Lung	3
Benyesh-Melnick	U.S.A.	5	1	Pneumopathy, unexplained fever	Lung, spleen, liver, serum	7
Andreoni	Italy	9-11	2	Pneumopathy	Pharynx, trachea, stools	7
Mamykina	U.S.S.R.	?	1	Pneumopathy	?	7a
Collier	U.S.A.	42	1	Whooping cough syndrome	Lung, liver, kidney	5

It was mostly in young military recruits and then in children that adenoviruses were isolated in cases of primary atypical pneumonia and bronchiolitis.

A certain number of fatal cases have been reported. These should be considered first, because they shed light on certain physiopathological and histopathological aspects of the disease.

Fatal Forms. The clinical picture in the fatal forms of adenovirus pneumopathy is that of a generalized infection with predominance of pulmonary localization.[81] Several cases were described in 1957 and 1958; Chany et al.[87] gave the best initial description of four epidemic cases observed in a collectivity in Paris. If only those cases in which the virological diagnosis was established are counted, the total number of fatal cases described is 27 (Table 42-4). This does not include a large series of case reports from China, where lethal epidemics seem to have occurred in 1958-1960. Thanks to the histological criteria of the disease, it has been possible to identify *a posteriori* certain pneumopathies described earlier[106, 116] as probably due to adenoviruses.[87, 127]

The disease in its fatal forms has generally occurred in very young children, aged three to 12 months in most cases; 75 per cent of the children who succumbed in China were less than two years of age. The cases reported have been sporadic, as in the United States, or else they were observed during epidemics of adenovirus pneumopathies, as in the Netherlands, France, and China; some even occurred during familial infections.[104] In certain cases an associated disease may have played a favoring role: Werdnig-Hoffmann disease,[152] Letterer-Siwe disease,[112] immunological anomaly.[81] Malnutrition might be suspected to be at the origin of the Chinese epidemics. However, most often the disease occurred in healthy children.

The *clinical picture* is that of a serious respiratory infection associated with nervous, digestive, and cardiovascular manifestations and occasionally with an exanthem.

The *onset* may be preceded by signs of upper respiratory infection with a febrile state, intense cough, watering eyes, and runny nose, abruptly aggravated after one to three days. More often, the onset is abrupt, with temperature from 39° to 40° C., rapidly progressive dyspnea, resulting occasionally within a few hours in intense respiratory distress with tachypnea, cyanosis, and laryngeal involvement with suprasternal and substernal evidence of intense respiratory traction effect. Paradoxically, the physical signs may remain relatively discrete: on auscultation, only a few rales may be heard at the bases at a time when radiological examination already shows signs of extensive bronchial and parenchymatous involvement. In other cases, the respiratory signs are pronounced. The cough is intense and incessant, there is suprasternal and substernal evidence of intense muscular effort, the beating of the nasal alae is very marked, and moist rales are heard in the entire thorax. Occasionally, a focus of pulmonary condensation is discovered.

Thereafter the temperature remains elevated, oscillating, and uninfluenced by antibiotics. The respiratory distress is intense and can be accompanied by complications: pulmonary, mediastinal, and even subcutaneous emphysema, or discrete pleural effusion.

Nervous system signs[87, 92, 104] are almost a constant finding and should suggest the diagnosis. They appear from the very onset or after two or three days: stupor, irritability, somnolence, convulsions, coma. The electroencephalogram is almost invariably altered.[149] The physiopathology of these signs has been debated. Doubtless they can be attributed in large part to the cerebral anoxia or to electrolytic disturbances. However, the early appearance of these signs, the isolation of the virus from the central nervous system[87, 146] or from the cerebrospinal fluid,[87] and the histopathological lesions of the central nervous system[110, 146] suggest the possibility of involvement of the nervous system by the virus itself.

Digestive signs, including vomiting, diarrhea, intense abdominal pain, and meteorism are very frequent. These phenomena have been related hypothetically to the discovery of the virus in the mesenteric lymph nodes in a fatal case[112] or in cases of mesenteric adenitis.[120]

Cardiovascular signs are usual: tachycardia, deadening of sounds, peripheral collapse, congestive heart failure, edema of the face and of the extremities,[149] and hepatomegaly. The electrocardiogram may show signs of myocarditis[140, 149]; an exudative pericarditis has been reported.

The cardiovascular manifestations are not immediate and often appear only if the disease has been prolonged for a week.[146]

A generalized morbilliform rash is frequent. It may be associated with hemorrhagic manifestations: petechiae and hematomas at injection sites that may be related to hypo-prothrombinemia.[87]

Other elements testify to *diffuse visceral involvement:* albuminuria, cylinduria, azotemia, hepatosplenomegaly, and signs of hepatic insufficiency. Autopsy has confirmed the existence of the lesions that had been suspected clinically: tubular necrosis and interstitial infiltration of the kidney, follicular mucosal and submucosal hypoplasia of the digestive tract, fatty degeneration of the liver and/or interstitial myocarditis. In almost all the viscera, capillary alterations are noted: proliferation of the intima, perivascular infiltration by lymphocytes and monocytes leading to narrowing, and occasionally even to occlusion, of the lumen and occasionally to genuine endarteritis[146] attributed to a viremia the existence of which has been proved.[81]

The blood count does not usually show striking changes: during the Peking epidemic in 1958, the leukocyte count was normal or subnormal in half the cases and moderately increased in a third of cases; the blood picture showed nothing worthy of note.[146] Elsewhere a tendency to monocytosis was noted.[135]

Radiological examination reveals the images associated with serious viral pneumopathy, but lacking specific characteristics. At the onset, it yields pictures of bronchitis or of bronchiolitis with emphysema, or else flocculent parenchymatous opacities that may become confluent. At a late stage, extensive poorly delimited opacities are observed with predominance in the lower lobes. Segmental opacities may also be noted, as may a discrete pleural effusion that had escaped notice on clinical examination. The x-ray film may demonstrate a cardiomegaly.

The *evolution* toward death is generally quick, less than one week, but the disease can be prolonged eight to 15 days. Death can occur owing to the respiratory congestion, either by vascular collapse or heart failure, or with the patient in a coma with convulsive crises. Mortality in the serious cases was 33.60 per cent in Peking in 1958.

The factors possibly responsible for this evolution have been the object of question and controversy. Young age plays an important role, since the majority of fatal cases have been reported in children aged less than one year; no fatal case has been reported in late childhood or in adulthood. The favoring role of an associated disease

mentioned earlier[8, 112, 152] in this chapter is a possibility in certain isolated cases. The role of confinement and/or overcrowding in over-aged and miserable premises has appeared evident in certain epidemics.[87, 135] It could have played a role in the Chinese epidemics. The particular virulence of certain strains of virus may be involved in serious familial epidemics.[104] The problems arising from the association with measles caught the attention of the Chinese authors. In a study elsewhere of 14 cases of fatal measles pneumopathy, type 3 or type 7 adenoviruses were isolated in seven of them.[146] It is to be emphasized, however, that the adenoviruses can simulate the picture produced by measles virus and that diagnostic errors have been made. Lastly, the ill-effects of artificial hibernation have been emphasized, since this treatment had been applied in the four fatal cases initially observed by Chany.

The *pathology* of the pulmonary lesions has been the object of minute descriptions.[81, 87, 103, 107, 110, 123, 133, 146] These lesions present a striking uniformity. Macroscopically, the lungs show an increase in volume. The parenchyma is congestive, and on section it releases a foamy liquid. Pleural petechiae are numerous. Hilar adenopathies are not observed.

On histopathological examination, the essential lesions are of three types: necrotic bronchitis, presence in the bronchial epithelium of cellular inclusions, and interstitial alveolitis.

Necrosis and tissue destruction of the bronchi are present in varying degrees: in certain cases, focal necrosis of the bronchial mucosa is observed, while in others there appears a simple degeneration of the superficial cellular layers with lymphomonocytic infiltration of the bronchial walls. Occasionally, the epithelial necrosis is intense, with parietal and extensive degeneration. The bronchial lumina are filled with large amounts of inflammatory exudates, acidophilic masses, and necrotic debris. The lumina of certain bronchioles may be more or less totally obstructed by large quantities of granulomatous tissue, producing a veritable obstructive bronchiolitis. The parenchyma adjacent to the bronchi is necrotic and destroyed; the alveoli are filled with an inflammatory exudate analogous to that found in the bronchial lumina. Often the bronchiolar and alveolar walls are bordered by a homogeneous acidophilic hyaline membrane. The mucosa of the bronchi and of the neighboring alveoli is the seat of a proliferation and a hypertrophy or of an epithelial metaplasia of variable degree. It is at this mucosal level that the cells with intranuclear inclusions so characteristic of the disease are found.

These *inclusions* appear in the form of irregular masses surrounded by a halo and usually situated in the center of the nucleus. They represent an aggregate of fine granules, in droplets of 1 to 2 μ, stainable with hematoxylin and eosin. Their eosinophilia is slight and yields a steel-blue coloration. Their evolution has been thoroughly studied, particularly through culture on fibroblasts, in which the cytopathogenic effect encountered at autopsy is very exactly reproduced. The cells with inclusions appear 12 hours after inoculation.

At an early stage, the granules are very fine, irregularly disseminated in the nucleus, purple-red on hematoxylin-eosin staining. No anomalies of the chromatin or of the cytoplasm are observed. The disposition of the bronchial epithelial cells is often normal at this stage, and the inclusions can be found in only a few cells.

At a more advanced stage, the inclusion body delimits itself sharply from the nuclear membrane by a slight halo or clear zone. The nucleolus is visible and appears normal. The inclusion becomes more eosinophilic. The nuclear chromatin has almost disappeared or persists only in the form of small granules. It seems that, at this stage, the inclusion body is formed by a conglomerate of the early granules into an irregular mass.[123] It can be sufficiently large to fill the nucleus in its entirety. The cytoplasm is little modified. The cells of the bronchial epithelium containing inclusions are often detached from the basal membrane, but there is still continuity with the adjacent epithelium.

At a final stage, the inclusion body is clearly delimited, rounded, localized in the center of the nucleus, and surrounded by a clear halo separating it from the nuclear membrane. The nucleus shrinks, the inclusion occupies it entirely, and it disintegrates. Having thus reached maturity, the inclusion, on hematoxylin-eosin staining, presents a rather basophilic, homogeneous internal structure. The nucleolus, with rare exceptions, is no longer visible; the cell is deformed. The disintegrated protoplasm remains around the nucleus in the form of a basophilic mass or disappears entirely. The cell is completely detached from a degenerated epithelium.

These cells with inclusions are most often present on the epithelium on the large bronchial trunks. They are not found in the alveolar walls, the interalveolar tissue, or the lymph nodes. They have not been found in the other organs except in one reported case in the liver.[81]

Two types of cells with inclusions have been distinguished.[127] The first, and the rarer, is easy to identify: slightly chromatophilic nucleus, acidophilic inclusion with a clear peripheral zone in which rearrangement of the chromatin produces a rosette form. The second, and the more frequent, is more difficult to identify, for the basophilic inclusion is voluminous, fills the whole area of the nucleus, and is separated from the nuclear membrane by only small clear vacuoles. During the Peking epidemic, typical cells were observed in 27 of the 40 cases examined at autopsy.[110] These cells differ greatly from those observed in herpes, in which the inclusion is more eosinophilic with a clearer, better defined and delimited contour even in the early stages of its development. Benyesh-Melnick and Rosenberg,[81] however, consider that histological differential diagnosis, on the basis of cellular inclusions, between the adenoviruses, varicella and herpes remains difficult.

The lesions of *interalveolitis* comprise a thickening of the alveolar walls that varies from one sector to another and an infiltration with mononuclear cells of average size, with a network rich in reticular fibers without any collagen fiber. The blood capillaries are moderately dilated, occasionally with thrombi. Multinucleated cells may be encountered. Infiltrates with lymphocytes or polymorphonuclear neutrophils are possible, but plasmocytes are not found.

Besides these three orders of lesions, less specific elements may be found: *emphysema, atelectasis, and/or bronchopneumopathy.* In the emphysematous zones, the alveoli and the bronchi are distended without epithelial lesions. In the atelectasic zones, the alveoli are filled with an acidophilic exudate, with occasional presence of lymphocytes, neutrophils, and erythrocytes that have undergone phagocytosis. In the zones of bronchopneumopathy, the bronchial walls are infiltrated by neutrophils, and the epithelial desquamation is extensive, as is peribronchitis. All these lesions can coexist in the same patient in different pulmonary lobules well delimited by interlobular connective tissue. In the

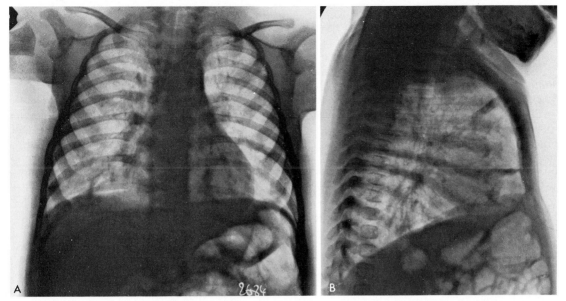

Figure 42-2. Adenovirus pneumopathy. Female infant aged 2½ months. Dyspnea-producing pneumopathy with severe functional signs and diffuse bronchial rales. Stuporous condition. Bilateral conjunctivitis. Paroxysmal cough. Temperature: 38° C. Blood count: 13,000 leukocytes per cubic millimeter with 52 per cent of polymorphonuclear neutrophils. Cerebrospinal fluid: normal. Electroencephalogram: normal. Radiographs made the day of admission (*A* and *B*): signs of diffuse pneumopathy with several opacified foci on the right (ventral segment of the upper lobe, in the middle lobe, basal posterior segment). The child recovered without sequelae.

lobules with isolated involvement, the lesions surrounding the small bronchi are less severe in the peripheral regions. One author considered this observation proof of the bronchial extension of the lesions.[133] In other reported cases, endarteritis-type vascular lesions with true pulmonary emboli[110] call to mind the physiopathological importance of the viremia.

However, Benyesh-Melnick and Rosenberg[81] did not find these lesions in a case studied in finest detail.

Virological study has shown that the fatal forms of adenovirus pneumopathy were most often associated with type 7, more rarely with type 3, and occasionally with type 1. Matumoto et al.[130] reported cases associated

Figure 42-3. Adenovirus pneumopathy. Girl, aged 4½ years. Film made on the fourth day of a febrile state complicated the second day by a renewed elevation of temperature to 39° C., with appearance of signs of condensation at the left base, diarrhea, and conjunctivitis. Hilar distention with nonhomogeneous focus in the left lingula. On the tenth day of illness, persistence of febrile state despite antibiotic treatment; convulsive crisis; then coma, rash, hyperleukocytosis (17,800 white cells per cubic millimeter with 96 per cent of polymorphonuclear leukocytes); negative blood culture. Death occurred, despite assisted respiration, on the eleventh day. Autopsy confirmed adenovirus pneumopathy.

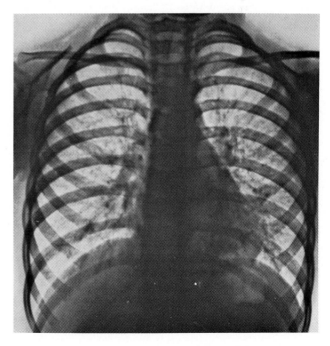

with an intermediate-type virus belonging to both types 3 and 7, with rise of heterotypical antibodies.

The virus can be isolated not only from pharyngeal and rectal samples but also from pulmonary tissue: this was the case in the 44 per cent of cases in the Peking epidemics.[110] The high titer of virus in the viscera was specified by Benyesh-Melnick and Rosenberg,[81] who found it, in order of decreasing concentration, in the liver, the lung and the spleen, the kidney, and the blood serum. The possible diagnostic importance of the in vivo demonstration of cells with inclusions in tracheal washings has been suggested,[152] since the cells have been demonstrated at this level not only at autopsy[87] but also in the sputum.[137]

Usual Forms with Recovery. Although adenovirus infections are widespread throughout the world, they do not always have a clinical expression: far from it, particularly at the level of the lower respiratory tract.

Even when 20 to 70 per cent of the infantile or adult population shows a positive complement-fixation reaction,[125, 140, 142] the infection often remains latent: in 60 per cent of cases according to Loeffler.[128] During epidemics in young recruits in the Netherlands and in the United States, only 10 to 20 per cent of subjects required hospitalization for pneumopathy.[93, 109, 148, 151] In children, epidemics have scarcely been observed except in collectivities.[87, 135] In 125 hospitalized children, Chaney et al.[87] noted 20 cases of pneumopathy of which 12 were due to an adenovirus. On the other hand, investigations in the urban population have shown the rarity of adenovirus pneumopathies. Evans,[99] in a study of 649 subjects with an acute respiratory infection, isolated an adenovirus in only seven of them. The percentage of adenovirus pneumopathies would seem to vary between 1 and 4 per cent in the general population or in university environments and hardly exceeds this proportion even in winter.[99, 115] Certain authors have estimated that 7 per cent of respiratory infections in children are associated with adenovirus infection.[111] The percentage of adenovirus pneumopathies was found to be 5.3 per cent by Sohier et al.,[140] 7 per cent by Chanock et al.,[86] and 9 per cent by Breton et al.[85] Vargosko et al.[150] isolated the virus in 4.3 per cent of children with bronchopneumonia. It is generally agreed that, in adenovirus infections, whereas sore throat is almost always present, tracheobronchitis occurs in only 40 or 50 per cent of such infections in children and pneumopathies in approximately 10 per cent of cases.[120, 144]

The low level of isolations is surprising when one recalls that half of the tonsils sampled in children and young adults have been shown to harbor an adenovirus.[112] It thus seems that exacerbation of these latent infections is rare.[99] The contrast between the frequency of pneumopathies in certain collectivities and their rarity in the general population suggests that interhuman contamination occurs only after prolonged and intense contact, as in barracks or overpopulated premises.

The winter predominance of adenovirus bronchopneumopathies has appeared evident to all authors. Young age is a certain promoting factor: for Chany et al.[87] the frequency of adenovirus pneumopathies was 1.1 per cent between birth and six months, 16.4 per cent between six and 23 months, 10 per cent between two and four years, and 0 per cent after five years.

The role of a preceding irritation of the mucosae is probable and may explain a certain number of cases in which adenovirus pneumopathy complicated authentic influenza, whooping cough, or measles.

Let us recall the fact that, although a certain degree of cross-immunity exists between adenoviruses of different types,[86] protection against heterologous strains is weak and does not apply to all serotypes. A single subject is capable of presenting several successive pneumopathies due to adenoviruses of different types.

Types 3, 4, 7, 8, and 14, especially, are encountered in epidemic pneumopathies both in adults and in children in collectivities.[82, 91, 105, 109, 140, 148] Types 3, 7, and 14 have been isolated from the population outside such collectivities.[80, 83, 101, 102, 119, 147] On the other hand, types 1, 2, and 5 seem to be less pathogenic for the respiratory tract, and their association with pneumopathy seems to be occasional or sporadic.[100, 101, 115, 120, 139, 144, 149] Type 6 adenovirus and the other types not mentioned are rarely found in such cases.

CLINICAL STUDY. The *incubation period* is, on the average, from four to six days and varies between a minimum of two and a maximum of 13 days. Experiments in volunteers showed identical incubation periods for types 1, 3, 4, 5, and 8.[80, 89] The *onset* is, in general, abrupt, sometimes occurring in a patient in apparently complete good health, occasionally after a few days' infection of the upper respiratory tract.

The clinical picture is wanting in specificity, and it must be emphasized from the outset that, very often, if does not suggest the diagnosis. In a systematic investigation, the diagnosis was made in only a single case.[99] Van der Veen observed no difference between pneumopathies associated with an adenovirus and those in which this association was not demonstrated. For Ginsberg, the clinical picture is confounded with that of primary atypical pneumonia. Sohier considers that the picture is that of an "infectious state with influenza-like symptomatology" without specific characteristics.

It appears that the three essential clinical elements are the syndrome of infection, the cough, and the bronchopulmonary signs.

The infectious syndrome is a constant and comprises hyperthermia above 39° C. with intense malaise, headaches, shivering, generalized painful stiffness, myalgias, rachialgias, thoracic or abdominal pains, anorexia, and intense asthenia confining the patient to bed or requiring hospitalization.

The cough is intense, distressing, at first dry then productive, often associated with a hoarseness that indicates laryngeal involvement. Cough may occur in paroxysms and suggest whooping cough.[87, 88, 134]

The bronchopulmonary signs are observed in the severe forms: dyspnea, disseminated rales of bronchitis or of bronchoalveolitis, and, more rarely, focal signs.

The pneumopathies due to adenoviruses seem more often to create dyspnea than the other viral pneumopathies in children. Jeune et al.[114] noted dyspnea in 14 of 36 adenovirus infections, as against 13 in 65 due to influenza and 32 in 118 due to parainfluenza viruses.

Certain of the associated manifestations can be useful for orientation of the diagnosis, but they are inconstant. Unilateral or bilateral conjunctivitis is occasionally accompanied by a periorbital edema. The oculonasal catarrh and the congestive, occasionally exudative, pharyngitis, which may be accompanied by cervical adenopathies, are often the first signs of the disease. A rash has often been noted that may be morbilliform.[84, 87, 132, 140] Before attributing such a rash to the adenovirus, it is, however, obligatory to eliminate a reaction to a medicinal agent or an associated disease: roseola infantum, rubella, measles, or ECHO virus infection.

The gastrointestinal disturbances (abdominal pains, vomiting, and diarrhea) should recall the fact that adenoviruses have been isolated from the mesenteric lymph nodes.[120] Splenomegaly may be found in an appreciable number of cases.[140] Also noteworthy is the possibility of epistaxis, microscopic hematuria, or albuminuria, occasionally in considerable amount (up to 4 gm. per liter).[140] Exceptionally, signs of pericarditis or of myocarditis have been reported.[87] A relatively benign adenovirus infection, if it occurs in certain particular physiopathological contexts, can produce sudden heart failure when cardiopathy is present, or suggest a relapse of rheumatic fever.[90] Lastly, the sudden appearance of meningoencephalitic symptoms mentioned in connection with the fatal forms, either at the onset or after several days' evolution, should be considered both as a serious argument in favor of the diagnosis and as an index of gravity. The electroencephalogram is almost always disturbed in such cases.

Results of hematological examination are of no great help in diagnosis. Smears can reveal either a relative leukopenia or a leukocytosis of 10,000 to 15,000 cells per cubic milliliter, with polymorphonuclear predominance. A blood count showing more than 50 per cent of mononuclear cells has been reported.[87, 140] On the other hand, the association of paroxysms of coughing with a very elevated leukocytosis (close to 120,000 cells per cubic millimeter with 69 per cent lymphocytes) has led to the misdiagnosis of whooping cough.[88] The sedimentation rate may be notably accelerated in the first hour.[145]

The frequency of radiological modifications has given rise to variable estimates according to the mode of selection of the groups of patients examined. Jeune and his co-workers,[114] who attached particular interest to study of this problem, studied 44 cases of virologically confirmed adenovirus bronchopneumopathies and found a normal x-ray picture in only five of them. Opacities radiating out from the hilus (ten cases) constituted the most frequent aspect. The study also revealed pictures of nonhomogeneous infiltration (seven cases), hilar adenopathies (6 cases), signs of pleural reaction (seven cases), miliary aspect (three cases), and dense condensation (six cases). No case of ventilation disturbance was observed.

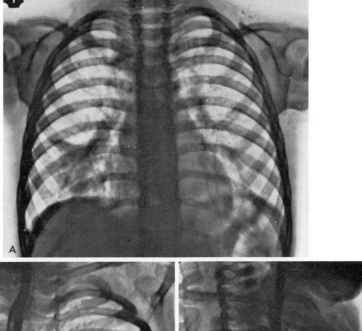

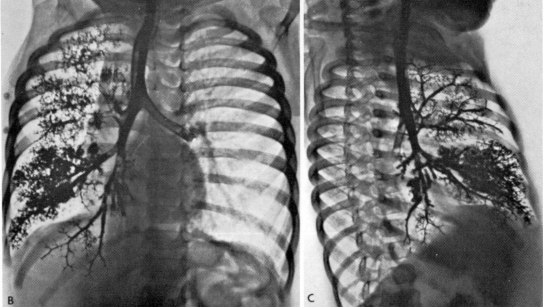

Figure 42-4.   Adenovirus pneumopathy with bronchial sequelae. Infant aged 17 months admitted for bronchopathy. Fever from 38.5° C. to 40.6° C. three days' duration. Productive cough. Focus of congestion at the right base. Diarrhea. Abdominal meteorism. Marked somnolence. Leukocytosis of 10,000 cells per cubic millimeter with 50 per cent of polymorphonuclear neutrophils.

A, Standard radiograph; right basal posterior and right apicodorsal foci. Bilateral hilar distention. The pneumopathy persisted more than a month despite administration of corticosteroid and antibiotic therapy. Bronchoscopy made the thirtieth day of illness showed diffuse, not very intense bronchitis especially marked on the right, where there was some fluid, purulent secretion.

B and *C*, Bronchographies made 2½ months after onset of the disease: global involvement of the right inferior lobar bronchus, showing rigidity, amputation effect, and partial defect in opacification. Dilation in the area tributary to the basal posterior bronchus. Since the illness, during a 2 year follow-up, the child has had repeated right-sided bronchitis, necessitating sessions of kinesiotherapy. The electroencephalograms have, moreover, shown the presence and the persistence of anomalies; numerous paroxysmal posterior slow waves of wide amplitude, predominant on the left with presence of temporoparietal spikes on the right. Thrusts of spike waves on hyperpnea.

The evolution is often characterized by the tenacity of the disease. The temperature may remain at 39° to 40° C. for one to six days, then cede abruptly, or by lysis in a few days.[84] In certain epidemics the febrile state lasted two to 12 days,[144] and its persistence for 69 days has been reported.[129]

The physical signs are at their maximum during the period of defervescence and often take more than a week to disappear. The lengthy persistence of the radiological signs must be especially emphasized; these persist several weeks after disappearance of the physical signs. In 17 cases in children, normalization of the thoracic image was observed in less than ten days in nine, in 11 to 20 days in six, and in 21 to 30 days in two.[114]

The possibility of bronchial or pulmonary *sequelae* must be considered. Van der Veen[149] noted that, among 16 subjects, seven who had had no pathological incident before the disease were subsequently victims of repeated respiratory infections with productive cough. McFarlane and Sommerville[131] isolated a type 2 adenovirus from the bronchial lesions in a patient who had undergone exeresis for bronchiectasis. Breton et al.[84] suggested the possibility of segmentary relapsing bronchitis consequent to an adenovirus infection.

Bronchography has permitted discovery of important bronchial alterations: stenosis or dilatation. In certain fatal cases, the pathological study revealed dilated bronchi filled with a purulent material in association with multiple abscesses and with aspects of atelectasis.[110] The role attributable to the adenovirus infection in certain bronchial sequelae thus deserves consideration, but intervention of bacterial superinfection cannot be eliminated. Controlled studies should be directed toward an understanding of the sequelae of adenovirus pneumopathies.

Pathogenesis. The clinical aspects of the pathogenesis of adenovirus disease are illustrated especially by experiments with virus inoculation into volunteers. Trials of inoculation into the nose, the pharynx, or the conjunctival sac have produced only infection of the upper respiratory tract or the conjunctiva.[80, 111] Administration of the virus by aerosols makes it possible to obtain pneumopathies and a disease identical with that provoked by spontaneous infections. Couch et al.,[89] by administering in aerosols a type 4 adenovirus to 15 volunteers, obtained a disease in nine of them: isolated

pharyngitis in one, and infectious syndrome with general malaise in eight, accompanied by tracheobronchitis in four, with radiological manifestations of pneumopathy in two subjects. The clinical manifestations in the last-mentioned disease were those of primary atypical pneumonia.

In contrast, the intramuscular injection of a mixture of adenoviruses of types 3, 4, and 7, in another study, provoked an acute respiratory disease that manifested itself two to three days after the inoculation and lasted four to five days. The disease involved the upper respiratory tract, producing inflammation of the pharynx, the nose, and the ears, with hyperplasia of submucosal lymphatic tissue, of the conjunctiva and of the pharynx, and cervical adenopathies associated with a febrile state. Pneumopathy, however, was not observed, the disease resembling spontaneous pharyngoconjunctival fever.[109]

Prophylaxis. In the absence of specific treatment, vaccines have been prepared with adenoviruses of types 4 and 7 or of types 3, 4, and 7.[98] Their use in military camps significantly reduced the frequency of infections. Use of a vaccine prepared with types 4 and 7 enabled Hilleman et al.[109] to reduce by 98 per cent the frequency of respiratory adenovirus diseases. Kozinn et al.,[122] administering a polyvalent vaccine comprising types 1, 2, 3, 4, 5, and 7 to children with repeated respiratory infections, obtained an inconstant immunological response and no clinical result whatever.

Varicella Pneumopathy

The proved existence of pulmonary complications, occasionally fatal, of varicella suffices to revise the concept held by Trousseau (1869) that "no physician has seen a patient die of varicella." Before the introduction of antibacterial chemotherapy, Bullowa and Wishik[156] had already reported 21 cases of "pneumonia" in a series of 2534 cases of varicella (0.8 per cent), but most of them seemed to result from bacterial superinfection. Waring et al.[192] were the first to provide a clinical and pathological description of the varicella-involved lung. Since then, the number of reported cases has increased steadily. These reports have made it possible to establish a precise picture of the different aspects of the disease and particularly of its histopathological aspects.[159, 162, 167, 175, 176, 186, 187]

The frequency of this complication varies greatly. Whereas in 1955 Endress and Schnell[163] collected 18 published cases of which seven were fatal (31.6 per cent mortality), Weinstein and Meade[193] reported an average frequency of 5.1 per cent which rose to 16.5 per cent in the adult, and Krugman et al.[175] reported 33 per cent in the adult and 0 per cent in the child. In fact, when radiological signs of pulmonary involvement are systematically sought during varicella, much higher frequencies are discovered: 27.3 per cent in cases in children, according to Binder.[154] These divergencies arise from the rather frequent latency of lung involvement by varicella, especially in the child,[168, 169] in whom it can nonetheless be fatal.[183, 163] Pneumopathy is also part of the picture of malignant varicella observed during corticosteroid therapy and of the varicella due to fetal contamination[178] or congenital varicella.[184]

Clinically, the onset is marked by a cough that appears one to five days after the rash. The cough is dry and tiring. Toward the third day, it becomes tenacious, occasionally with bloody sputum. Hemoptysis, occurring in certain reported cases, can be moderately abundant. Thoracic pain and dyspnea occur in half the cases. Cyanosis may appear. The temperature may attain 38° to 40° C. It has generally been emphasized that the gravity of the disease parallels the intensity of the exanthem: the exanthem, very extensive, occasionally confluent, hemorrhagic in serious cases, is almost always accompanied by oropharyngeal lesions. The disease may worsen toward the fourth day, be complicated by signs of rightsided heart failure[186] and of prostration. However, in general, the meagerness of results of physical examination contrasts with the intensity of the functional signs. Physical examination may be entirely negative or may reveal more or less diffuse bronchial, but rarely parenchymatous, signs. The blood count shows a discrete leukocytosis in more than half the cases, but the differential is normal. The sedimentation rate may be greatly accelerated (82 mm. in the first hour has been reported[177]) or it may be normal.[158]

Radiological examination is a major factor in the diagnosis. In a number of cases, it shows only an accentuation of the hilar shadows and bronchovascular images. For Binder et al.,[154] who observed these modifications in 27.3 per cent of cases of varicella, there is nothing specific about them; they are identical with those of the lung in measles, often without showing any clinical manifestation. In contrast, the micronodular or occasionally macronodular images are highly uniform and constitute the essential element in pulmonary varicella.[174, 176, 187, 189, 192] They are superimposed on increased bronchovascular markings. Their size is variable, from 2 to 15 mm. in diameter. Occasionally well delimited, in other cases the nodules seem to melt into the surrounding parenchyma. These modifications are often highly transitory, and, in certain cases, some infiltration zones undergo attenuation at the same time that others appear during the evolution. Occasionally, the nodules show a tendency to coalescence, particularly at the bases, where aspects of poorly delimited zones of condensation may be noted. The lesions extend to the whole lung but predominate in the hilar regions and diminish in number and intensity toward the periphery. Emphysema, segmentary opacities, and mediastinal anomalies are absent. Pleural effusion is possible; as a rule, it is discrete and without clinical expression, but is occasionally considerable.[175] The nodules persist for three to 18 days and are seen, on an average, for nine days. It seems[174] that nodular images may appear very early, at the moment of the exanthem, but they are detectable in general only after three to six days. They may persist for a long time. In a case reported by Levin[177] the nodules that had a diameter of 6 to 15 mm. were sufficiently dense to have suggested metastatic carcinoma. They continued to evolve for 13 days after onset of the varicella; toward the thirtieth day, half of them appeared on the x-ray films to be excavated. They began to diminish toward the fortieth day, and the radiological picture appeared normal only toward the third month. As a rule, the evolution is toward complete clearing. Nonetheless, the possibility of *multiple nodular calcifications* has been raised,[172, 173] and it would certainly seem that the disease can be responsible for aspects of calcified miliaria. The histological proof has been furnished, and long-term radiological follow-up of adults with varicella has contributed a supplementary argument. Knyvett[173] observed 88 such cases. The calcifications appeared late, at least two years after the disease, after three to four years in 10 cases, five to eight years in 24, and after nine years or more in the other cases.

Knyvett also reported five cases of calcifications in children. These calcifications, in general, measure 1 to 2 mm. in diameter and are disseminated throughout the whole parenchyma. They become denser with the years. They may be counted by tens or even hundreds. Certain calcifications may, in time, attain 5 mm. in diameter. A search for histoplasmosis or tuberculosis always yields a negative result.

These findings have given a new dimension to the importance of varicella involvement of the lung. The same is true concerning the *effects on respiratory function.* Thus Bocles et al.[155] found disturbances in the alveolocapillary gaseous exchanges in all of the seven cases they studied. Ventilatory insufficiency might well play an important part in the irreversible respiratory distress in the fatal cases. It is tenacious, certainly. In only three of the seven cases described by Bocles et al. did ventilatory function return to normal in the months following the disease, and these authors estimated that the disturbances might last eight years. The same disturbances are seen in patients having a history compatible with pulmonary varicella, but not in patients with uncomplicated varicella.

In terms of *evolution,* the lung disease has been tentatively classified into three categories: serious disease with a radiological picture of extensive severe lesions; serious disease with radiologically discrete lesions; mild, even subclinical, disease detectable only radiologically. Usually, the functional and systemic signs disappear in four to six days despite the persistence of the radiological images. In a few cases, especially in the adult, death may occur as a result of respiratory insufficiency, shock, or heart failure. Abundant hemoptysis, pulmonary edema, and subcutaneous emphysema signify a poor prognosis. Death may be sudden; it was so in 15 cases in a series of 22.[157]

The *pathological lesions* of the lung are constant in fatal cases of varicella. They present great uniformity.[158, 159, 162, 167, 171, 173, 175, 183, 187, 192]

To the naked eye, the pleural surfaces are strewn with small, round, purple nodules 2 to 4 mm. in diameter. A few purpural stains may be disseminated on the pleural surfaces, and a unilateral or bilateral serofibrinous effusion may be noted. The lung is strewn with small nodules analogous to those on the pleura, entirely distinct one from the other. The mucosae of the trachea and the main bronchial trunks are strewed with lesions that are often hemorrhagic, the centers of which are ulcerated and filled with bloody mucus.

The histopathological lesions are constant at a time when the macroscopic lesions may be absent. Three essential elements can be distinguished: foci of necrosis, exudates, and intranuclear inclusions. The foci of necrosis comprise, at the center, an eosinophilic, amorphous granular material surrounded by an inflammatory reaction with mononuclear elements. Occasionally, the pathologist may note calcareous deposits in the caseous material. These disseminated foci are considered pathognomonic by some workers.[173] They may be found in the bronchial walls and, more rarely, in the tracheobronchial lymph nodes. A fibrinous exudate with leukocytes and numerous macrophages fills the alveoli. The alveolar walls are bordered by round or cuboid, occasionally multinucleated, cells. At the periphery, the alveoli are often bordered by an eosinophilic hyaline membrane. The acidophilic intranuclear inclusions are found at the periphery of the necrotic foci in the parenchymatous cells still preserved, in the bronchial or tracheal epithelium, and in the endothelium of the vessels. They are intranuclear, frankly acidophilic, and surrounded by a clear halo that separates them from the nuclear membrane, itself thickened by margination of the chromatin. The inclusion is single; it is identical with that observed in the cutaneous lesions. The lesions of arteriolitis are frequent. The rest of the histological study shows cells with inclusions in the spleen, the liver, the adrenal glands, and the mediastinal lymph nodes, vesicles on the surface of the liver and spleen, and, occasionally, encephalitic lesions.

However particular the radiological aspect of the varicella-involved lung may be, certain authors consider that these nodular lesions are not specific,[164] and, to establish the diagnosis, require that autopsy reveal cells with inclusions. Another study[194] demonstrated the possibility of making the diagnosis during life; cells with intranuclear inclusions were found in the sputum from the sixth to the eighth day of hospitalization for respiratory distress of an asthmatic with mild varicella rash that reached its acme on the sixth day, at which time radiological signs of pulmonary condensation appeared. The expectorations were collected in 70 per cent alcohol. The sediment was studied both in smears and after embedding in paraffin blocks.

With regard to *conditions of appearance,* some investigators consider varicella to be a disease inoculated into the lungs. The virus is thought to be transmitted by the air route.[191] After local multiplication in the respiratory tract, it is disseminated by the blood. Having reached the level of the epithelial cell, it may provoke characteristic lesions not only at the level of the skin but also in the lungs and other viscera. The respiratory signs appear at a period when the virus is multiplying actively in the organism. Perivascular and peribronchial edema explains the nonspecific radiological images. However, Nelson and St. Geme[182] called attention to the surprising absence of the virus from the respiratory tract before and during the exanthem.

Certain factors that may promote the pulmonary complications of varicella have been emphasized. These complications seem to occur more frequently in the course of malignant blood diseases treated by antimetabolites or cortisone.[176] The role of corticosteroid therapy has been much discussed.[170] Whereas certain authors see it as an aggravating factor, others have emphasized its clearly beneficial action. The third opinion is that it has not modified the evolution of varicella.[168] Certain case reports have suggested a favoring role of preëxisting pulmonary lesions, especially tuberculosis,[153] but the closer supervision to which tubercular patients are submitted perhaps merely facilitates the discovery of the disease. In pulmonary varicella there is no sexual predominance, and, despite the existence of fatal cases in pregnant women, pregnancy does not seem to play an unfavorable role.[165]

In the absence of specific *treatment* and even of prophylaxis of pulmonary varicella, it is opportune to prevent bacterial superinfection by antibiotics, to humidify the atmosphere, and to improve pulmonary ventilation. Artificial ventilation by respirator associated with oxygen therapy can save certain patients.[161]

PNEUMOPATHY DUE TO HERPES ZOSTER

The term zosterian pneumopathy was introduced by Herbeuval et al. in connection with three cases of intercostal herpes zoster associated with a unilateral pulmonary focus. However, as early as 1902, Curtin[196] had reported four cases of zoster associated with pleurisy, and innumerable case reports have called attention to a pleural rub concurrent with zoster and having the same localization. The visceral localizations of herpes zoster, and especially the pulmonary ones, have been the object of only scattered reports. This fact may arise either from their rarity or from their benignancy and their predominately subclinical character. According to certain investigations,[199, 206] they may be more frequent than they are thought to be. In any event, the real frequency of herpes zoster pneumopathies can not be defined precisely at present. It can only be stated that a generalized eruption has been reported in only 3 per cent of cases of zoster.[197, 202]

In a complete review of the literature in relation to a personal case, Pek and Gikas[201] collected 22 cases. A pleural rub was noted in seven cases, a pleural effusion in one case. Five patients had bronchial or pulmonary signs on auscultation. X-ray of the thorax revealed pulmonary anomalies in eight of 12 cases. It can be considered that nine of 22 subjects had a pneumopathy. The case observed by Pek and Gikas[201] is very clear: their patient, whose chest x-ray picture was normal before the onset of zoster, showed respiratory signs nine days after onset of the rash. On the eleventh day, the x-ray film showed disseminated nodular opacities that became confluent on the fifteenth day in a voluminous focus. The disease was fatal. Of the 22 patients, three died. In the two cases in which complete histopathological study was made, intranuclear inclusions characteristic of zoster or of varicella were seen in the pulmonary tissue and lesions of pneumopathy. One case was of generalized zoster with necrotic and hemorrhagic pulmonary lesions.

The clinical differential diagnosis between foci of pulmonary condensation, most often observed on the same side as the zoster, arises in regard to the deglutition bronchopneumopathy that can always be suspected in a subject in whom the thoracic excursion is weaker on the affected side owing to the pain syndrome.

To be emphasized is the frequency of malignant disease in patients who present herpes zoster pneumopathy: of 22 cases of such pneumopathy, nine were in patients with diseases of this type (Hodgkin's disease, leukosis, etc.). On bronchoscopy, Andrews[195] observed bronchial vesicles concurrent with the exanthem; this fact is useful in understanding the syndrome. The fact that certain analogies exist between lung involvement by varicella and that by herpes zoster is not surprising. The appearance, within a few days, of zoster, varicella, and massive atelectasis has been noted in one case.[203]

PNEUMOPATHY DUE TO MEASLES

It has long been known that catarrh of the upper respiratory tract is part of the clinical picture of measles in its preeruptive phase. The notion of pneumopathy in measles is old enough for it to be the earliest known of viral pneumopathies.[207, 208, 211, 213–215, 219–222, 224, 225]

It would be useless to linger on the frequency of the cough, rhonchi, and sibilant rales and occasionally of moist rales detected especially at the bases. The clinical data have been completed by the radiological description of the measles-involved lung. It is characterized by two elements: (1) accentuation of the hilar shadows in connection with discrete hypertrophy of the interbronchial lymph nodes, and (2) opacities radiating out from the hilus which indicate a peribronchial inflammatory reaction.

These aspects may occasionally be associated with a reaction in the interlobar spaces or micronodular perihilar opacities. Large opaque areas that may be seen correspond to massive foci or to atelectasis that may involve all the lobes, with a predilection for the inferior ones.[210]

These radiological changes occur early, at the initial febrile phase, as soon as the oculonasal catarrh appears. The mediastinal adenopathies reach their maximum at the time of the rash. In 80 per cent of patients with pulmonary foci, these foci develop before or during the exanthem.[213] They may become accentuated subsequently.

The radiological changes are often slow to disappear, lasting one to three weeks and occasionally more, long after the apparent clinical cure. Their intensity contrasts with the usual discreteness of the functional and physical manifestations of the pneumopathies.

In the adult, the lung involvement by measles yields appreciably the same images as in the child.

The reported frequency of these radiological manifestations varies according to the author. The opacity of the hilar and mediasti-

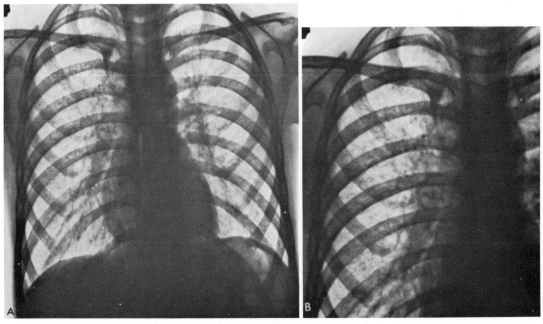

Figure 42-5.   Miliary aspect during measles. Five year old boy. Typical measles. Persistence of 40° C. fever four days later. Subcrepitant rales at the right lung base. Leukocytosis of 14,600 cells per cubic millimeter with 50 per cent of polymorphonuclear leukocytes. *A*, Standard radiograph made five days after onset of the exanthem. Bilateral hilar distention with miliary-appearing dissemination. Rapid recovery: the miliaria disappeared within 5 days. *B*, Enlargement of the upper right quarter of the film.

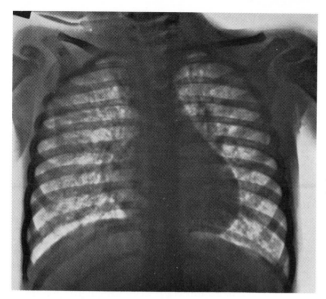

Figure 42-6. Measles bronchopneumopathy Girl, aged 21 months. Typical measles. Severe functional respiratory signs with tachypnea of 90 per minute, diffuse bronchial signs, and cyanosis. Film made the day after appearance of the exanthem. Aspect of diffuse pneumopathy with reticulonodular seeding extending to both pulmonary fields.

nal lymph nodes varies from 64 per cent[210] to close to 100 per cent.[214] The frequency of dense pulmonary foci runs from 25 per cent[225] to 77 per cent.[224]

Serotherapy seems to be susceptible of modifying and attenuating the pulmonary complications of measles but seems to have no action on the hilar adenopathies. The pneumopathies are rare in adults, in whom their occurrence is associated with a malignant or debilitating disease. The difficulties in the formation of immunity in such cases have been demonstrated.[218]

The physiopathology of the lung in measles has been elucidated not only by the attentive and prolonged radiological study of the patients but also by pathological studies made in the exceptional cases in which death occurred in the early stage of measles, fortuitously[207] or under particular circumstances.[223]

The thoracic anomalies in measles involve two elements, the lung and the reticuloendothelial system, the lesions in these two systems being completely distinct. The involvement of the reticuloendothelial system is responsible for adenopathies, sometimes moderate, sometimes massive. These adenopathies often disappear rather quickly while the pulmonary x-ray images persist.

The bronchial lesions, which predominate, are characterized by thickening of the submucosal layer infiltrated by mononuclear cells and by an intense peribronchial lymphoid reaction. These lesions may go as far as necrosis.

In the parenchyma, nodular congestive formations, clear-cut particularly at the bases,

are manifest. The foci, with rounded form and clean edges, are characterized by a coagulation necrosis in which are seen, without inflammatory reaction, cells more or less destroyed and lacking a nucleus, appearing as more or less acidophilic cytoplasmic masses with the alveolar septa infiltrated by mononuclear cells, and the alveoli gorged with serous fluid in which float macrophages and lymphocytes.

At the level of the bronchial epithelium, of the septal cells, and of the macrophages, intranuclear and intracytoplasmic inclusions attract attention. The existence of giant cells with inclusions is, as a matter of fact, considered by many as characteristic of the measles-involved lung. Interstitial pneumonia with giant cells was described by Hecht[211] in 1910 in children. Subsequently, this pneumonia was noted in subjects who had died of measles, and histological similarities were noted between the pneumonia described by Hecht in man and the pneumonia in distemper in the dogs. The existence of serological cross-reactions between measles virus and distemper virus gave rise to the idea that an analogous virus was responsible for giant cell pneumonia in the human species. MacCarthy et al.[217] established the proof of the intervention of the measles virus by isolating it from children with this syndrome. These observations were subsequently confirmed, particularly by localization of the viral antigen in the cells by the fluorescent antibody technique.[212]

Thus the presence of epithelial giant cells with intranuclear and intracytoplasmic inclusions in an interstitial pneumonia is considered characteristic of infection by measles virus. However, nonbacterial pneumopathies without these characteristic pictures may be observed after measles. Moreover, these interstitial pneumonias may occur without an exanthem or a febrile state.[209] It is in these cases that the demonstration of measles virus takes on all its value.

Pneumopathy due to Mumps

The association of a pneumopathy with mumps has been demonstrated, but it is rare.[226, 228, 230] Meyer et al.[230] encountered it in only five of approximately 3500 cases of mumps. They reported, in another study, seven cases of pleuropneumopathies associated with biological signs of mumps with or without parotitis. The patients were aged 11 to 65 years. Two were children aged 11 and 13 years. The systemic signs were sometimes severe; the fever was sometimes high. Cough was a constant finding. The onset, on occasion, was marked by violent thoracic pain. One case of hemoptysis was noted.

In almost every case, radiological examination showed a dense opacity, lobar or segmentary, with various localizations. In a few cases, the films showed images with a fuzzy contour, rounded or more or less oval, disseminated in one lung, or, in one case, in both lungs. A more or less discrete pleural participation was constant.

The evolution was slow. Recovery was complete, but the clinical and radiological signs disappeared progressively, in 10 days to two months.

The physiopathology of these manifestations remains imprecise. The direct involvement by the virus of the parenchyma that has been demonstrated in the mouse[231] is a possibility. However, the duly proved existence of pulmonary infarcts during mumps[227, 233] should not be forgotten. It may be related to a thrombophlebitis of the lower limbs or to a thrombophlebitis of the spermatic veins in the case of orchitis.

Whatever the truth may be, owing to the rarity of cases and in the absence of well-documented virological observations, the reality of mumps pneumopathy remains entirely a matter of conjecture at present.

Pneumopathy due to Enteroviruses

The cases in which the association of an enterovirus with a pneumopathy has been demonstrated are rare. Certain cases, however, are demonstrative enough.

Coxsackie Virus and Pneumopathy. During an epidemic of 15 cases of *Coxsackie A9* virus infection observed in Boston in 1959, Lerner et al.[244] noted the association of vesicular exanthem with pneumopathy in three cases or with a laryngotracheobronchitis in one case. One of these cases was fatal in a 16-month-old child with cough, dyspnea, and a focus of condensation in the right upper lobe. Autopsy revealed peritracheobronchial adenopathies, hemorrhagic zones in the pleura, inflammation of the alveolar septa, desquamation with necrosis of the bronchial epithelium, and alternation of zones of emphysema with those of atelectasis compatible with the diagnosis of virus pneumopathy. Above all, the virological study of the pulmonary tissue revealed a very high titer of virus, leaving practically no doubt as to the reality of local multiplication of virus.

Two further cases of fatal interstitial pneumonia, characterized by a mononuclear infiltration of the alveolar walls and an alveolar exudate with formation of hyaline membrane, were reported in children aged four and 17 months. A *Coxsackie B5* virus was isolated from the pulmonary tissues in both of these cases.[239]

During a limited systematic investigation made in Washington, D.C., the proof of the association with a *Coxsackie B5* infection was made in 3 per cent of cases of bronchiolitis and in 3 per cent of cases of pneumonia.[246]

Four cases of pneumopathy with recovery in children aged three to nine years were attributed to a *Coxsackie B2* virus on the basis of serological evidence.[236] The role of *Coxsackie B1* viruses in the school environment has been considered.[245] However, though the importance of the Coxsackie B viruses is thought to be real by some investigators,[228, 240] it is contested by others.[242]

ECHO Viruses and Pneumopathy. In an epidemic of pneumopathy in which the radiological pictures recalled those of the Wilson-Mikity syndrome in four of the eight cases, one patient died after an 88-day evolution and an *ECHO 19* virus was isolated from the pulmonary tissue.[234]

Also in a collectivity, an epidemic of *ECHO 13* virus infection was observed that involved signs of acute bronchitis or of bronchiolitis in four of the 13 cases at a time when no other viral or bacterial cause could be demonstrated,[241] while radiological anomalies of the lung were observed in six of 20 children with gastroenteritis associated with an *ECHO 20* virus. In yet another study, seven cases of acute bronchitis, of bronchopneumopathy or of pneumopathy were linked to infections by *ECHO virus 4, 7, 9, or 11 or to an unidentified enterovirus.*[237]

Thus observations of bronchopneumopathies associated with enteroviruses are scarce. It is to be remarked that those reported have concerned children almost exclusively. The relationships between these viruses and the respiratory disease need to be clarified. It has been emphasized that numerous enteroviruses multiply poorly at best in respiratory epithelium.[242] But no large-scale controlled study has been devoted to this problem; the few examples mentioned here show sufficiently that it merits attention.

PNEUMOPATHY DUE TO CYTOMEGALOVIRUS

Among the viscera involved, it was especially in the lung of a stillborn premature infant that Jesionek and Kiolemenoglou[256] described for the first time the cytomegalic inclusion cell.

The studies have multipled in number since discovery of the cytomegalovirus by Smith, Rowe, and Weller, and they have confirmed the importance of the role played by the pulmonary localization both in children and in adults.

The *pathological* elements of cytomegalic pneumopathies are now well defined. Three aspects, variable according to age, have been described: an accompanying pneumopathy in the generalized forms in the newborn; primary cytomegalic pneumopathy in the infant, and the miliary form often encountered in the adult.

In the *generalized forms* in the newborn and the infant, the cytomegalic pneumopathy is an "accompanying pneumopathy."[264] The macroscopic aspect is not characteristic. Pleura, larynx, trachea, and bronchi are normal. There are no thoracic adenopathies. The lung is well ventilated and not infiltrated. Violaceous plaques of infarction produce a spotted aspect, and, on section, pressure yields only a serosanguineous fluid. Histological examination shows little alteration of the bronchi: their epithelial covering is not ulcerated and there is no necrobiosis. The bronchial walls show congested vessels. The parenchyma is the seat of an intense vascular congestion with slight thickening of the interalveolar walls due to the vascular congestion and the edema. Foci of hemorrhagic, edematous, macrophagic alveolitis are common, with cytomegalic cells here and there in the alveolar or the bronchial lumina. Certain cytomegalic cells border the alveolar wall. They are also encountered at the level of the bronchial epithelial covering and in the mucus glands. This description was applicable in its entirety to 14 cases in a series of 32 generalized forms of the disease.[264]

In *primary cytomegalic pneumopathy,* the pulmonary lesion is isolated or predominant. This form is not observed in the newborn. It is encountered in the infant with a manifest respiratory syndrome and was found in six of 32 cases of the generalized disease.[264] The macroscopic lesions are not striking. The lung may be congested and poorly ventilated. On section, the surface is granular, yellowish gray; on pressure, it yields only a serosanguineous fluid.

Histological examination shows the bronchial alterations: the bronchial lumen is encumbered with cellular debris in which figure a great number of polymorphonuclear and mononuclear inflammatory cells. The bronchial wall is thickened, congestive, and infiltrated by numerous cells, many of which are eosinophilic. These cells occasionally form lymphoid masses. The bronchial epithelial covering is neither ulcerated nor necrotic. The peribronchial mucus glands are normal or infiltrated by mononuclear cells. The pulmonary parenchyma is the seat of an interstitial pneumonia, frequently pure, without alveolar exudate. The interalveolar walls are considerably thickened by a vascular congestion, a proliferation of fixed histioconjunctive elements, and an inflammatory infiltration with mononuclear cells. Alveolitis is absent, and the interstitial pneumonia appears pure. Occasionally, the inflammatory reaction presents in the form of voluminous lymphoid nodules with a clear center. In the plaques of pure interstitial pneumonia, a few cells with cytomegalic inclusions border the interalveolar walls. The areas of pure interstitial pneumonia are separated from each other by near-normal pulmonary tissue.

As the disease evolves, the size of the alveolar cavities may be reduced by the interstitial inflammatory reactions. The alveolar covering epithelium becomes cuboid. A lymphoid infiltration develops that progressively surrounds and compresses the small bronchioles and favors atelectasis. At this stage, the cells with inclusions are rarer and more difficult to reveal. Some are discovered either in the alveolar cavities or in the bronchial mucous glands.

However, this picture characteristic of purely interstitial pneumopathy, without alveolitis is rare. The pathologist may see a macrophagic, fibrinohemorrhagic, or fibrinoleukocytic alveolitis and find cells with inclusions in the alveolar exudate.

In the adult especially, the infection may present an appearance of fibrinous pneumopathy characterized by a *miliary necrosis*.[271] The lungs appear to be riddled with nodules 3 to 10 mm. in diameter; these are firm, with an elastic consistency, well delimited, disseminated or confluent, often peripheral or subpleural. They are associated with various lesions of bronchopneumopathy, with congestive hyperemia, and with nonspecific lesions. In section, their surface everts; they appear dark red with a necrotic, grayish or yellow exudate and present an umbilicated aspect. The histological features depend on the age of the lesions.[271] At the beginning, discrete foci of hemorrhagic necrosis are noted in which the alveolar spaces are filled with a network of fibrin, red cells, mature granulocytes, histiocytes, and cellular debris. These foci are limited by hyperplastic alveolar cells, many of which bear the characteristic inclusion. The alveolar cells appear turgescent in the cellular layer or free in the blood or the fibrinous intra-alveolar exudates. A hyaline membrane is often found. The associated presence of *Pneumocystis carinii* is frequent.[253, 260, 263, 264, 266] At a late stage, a tendency toward organization of the cellular exudate, development of an interstitial fibrosis, and cellular reactions of chronic inflammation appear. It has thus been said that the pneumopathy due to cytomegalovirus resembles the interstitial fibrosis of the hyaline membrane and that it has features in common with Hamman-Rich fibrosis.[249]

Clinical Aspects. Long considered to be a "disease of pathologists," cytomegalic pneumopathy can now be diagnosed in an increasing number of patients during their lifetime.

In the newborn and the infant, Turgeon[273] noted the great frequency of this interstitial pneumonia in the generalized forms of the disease and did not hesitate to consider it the essential manifestation at this age. Of 132 cases collected from the literature and compared by Medearis,[267] 84 presented the clinical or pathological signs of respiratory involvement, this involvement having appeared essential in 13, among which were eight instances of interstitial pneumonia, two of bronchopneumopathy, one of tracheobronchitis, and two of chronic pneumopathy. In a series personally observed by Le Tan Vinh comprising 34 cases, 20 were of pneumopathy, six of which were of primary predominant pneumopathy. The proportion of interstitial pneumonia reached 80 per cent in Seifert's experience. Thus it can be expected that these pulmonary lesions will sometimes be manifested by clinical signs. Study of the different case histories published[247, 250, 258, 262, 263, 264, 266, 267, 275] shows that the forms with respiratory predominance begin between seven weeks and three months of age with a stubborn, occasionally paroxysmal cough. Next appears dyspnea of progressive severity, with tachypnea and epigastric traction. Apyrexia is a constant finding except in the presence of bacterial superinfection. The course, usually brief, has occasionally lasted several weeks or even several months. The symptomatology reaches completion more or less rapidly, and death occurs with a picture of more or less acute asphyxia with cyanosis. This picture is not as characteristic as that of *Pneumocystis carinii* pneumopathy. The physician must habitually think of the diagnostic possibility of cytomegalic inclusion disease in all cases of subacute pneumopathy in infants, the cause of which has not been elucidated. Other signs of the disease, such as hepatosplenomegaly and/or icterus, can orient the diagnosis.

The pulmonary x-ray picture can be normal.[247] In other cases, radiography reveals reticulonodular images or diffuse reticular images often predominating at the summits. Emphysema is severe, particularly in the retrosternal region. All considered, although the reticular aspect may be suggestive, it is neither specific nor constant.

In adults, the pulmonary localization appears as the most frequent and the most serious localization in acquired cytomegalovirus infection.[254, 259, 265] In the young infant the cytomegalic inclusions are found in the viscera in the following order of decreasing frequency: salivary glands, kidney, liver, lung, pancreas, thyroid, adrenal glands, and brain. In the adult, however, this order is modified as follows: lung, adrenal glands, liver, and digestive tract.[274] The frequency of the disease remains low. Wong, in 1872 serial autopsies and more than 17,000 surgical biopsies, found 14 cases, nine of them on autopsy and five on biopsy. He gathered 41 cases from the literature. In the total of 55 histologically verified cases, he noted pulmonary involvement in 34, adrenal involvement in 19, and hepatic involvement in 14.

Cytomegalic inclusion pneumopathy in the adult is as a rule observed in connection with a debilitating disease: hypogammaglobulinemia,[260] Hodgkin's disease,[270] leukosis,[248, 252] lymphosarcoma, anemia refractory to treatment, ulcerative colitis, chronic pneumopathy, cancer of the lung, bedridden state, serious bacterial infection. Most patients have in common a weakening of natural defense mechanisms due to some condition which results in medullary insufficiency with or without reticuloendothelial involvement, immunosuppressive therapy, or radiotherapy.

The particular frequency of the disease in subjects who die some time after renal transplant throws a new light on certain aspects of the disease. Hill found pneumopathy at autopsy in 26 of 32 such subjects; 15 of the 26 had pulmonary inclusions, cytomegaly being found in the other organs in only three.

Kanich found a generalized inclusion disease in eight of 25 cases in recipients of renal homografts. The disease occurred in the patients in whom immunosuppressive drugs had been used. The lung was the elective site of the lesions, and in three cases death was due to an interstitial pneumonia related to the disease.

Often the virus is found only in the lung and cannot be isolated from other organs. The quantity of virus isolated in the pulmonary tissue has no direct correlation either with the number of cytomegalic cells or with the extent of the pulmonary lesions.

It can be estimated that, so far, the diagnosis of cytomegalovirus pneumopathy has been made in vivo only in cases in which cytomegaly was demonstrated in biopsy fragments, i.e., the five cases of Wong; survival occurred in four of them. In the light of the observations made in the subjects having undergone kidney transplant, a picture of progressive dyspnea with secondary exudative manifestations, followed by increasing respiratory insufficiency over several weeks,

can suggest the diagnosis. The original disease may mask the cytomegalovirus pneumopathy. In a case history reported by Capers, the respiratory phenomena were the most prominent: first to be observed were radiological signs of upper lobe involvement, with dyspnea, thoracic pains without physical signs, then appearance of a condensation focus in the lower left lobe and disseminated bronchial rales, followed by pleural rub associated with a prolonged subfebrile state. Pleurisy was demonstrated by thoracentesis.

To confirm the diagnosis, it is possible to search for cells with inclusions in gastric washings and sputum samples, rarely studied so far for want of clinical arguments. Study of the urine has lesser chances of being useful, owing to the relative rarity of renal involvement. The existence of radiological signs of interstitial pneumopathy or of miliary images might constitute an argument for the diagnosis. Results of serological examination are of slight value owing to the great frequency of latent infections in the general population. Rowe indeed pointed out that 80 per cent of the population shows positive serological results after the age of 35 years. The presence of the virus in the expectoration, the saliva, the urine, or gastric washings would, on the other hand, have real value, as would the discovery of cells with inclusions in a biopsy specimen. Certain clinical data show that transfusion of fresh blood,[257] existence of mononucleosis with negative Paul-Bunnel-Davidsohn reaction, and liver involvement[257, 261] may constitute arguments in favor of cytomegalovirus infection.

Many *physiopathological aspects* of the disease are not yet clearly elucidated. It appears that the respiratory manifestations observed in infants can probably be attributed to the disease. The intratracheal inoculation of cytomegalovirus has produced an interstitial pneumonia in the pig and in the rat. In man, the histopathological and clinical differences between the expression of the disease in the infant and in the adult might well result not only from differences in the terrain but also, in the adult, from an antecedent infection by the virus. Indeed, in the child, the inclusions predominate in the epithelial cells whereas in the adult they are found above all in the mesenchyma, endothelium of vessels, and macrophages.[274] Association of cytomegalovirus disease with a *Pneumocystis carinii* infection, aspergillosis, nocardiosis, or a bacterial infection is frequent and may cause the presence of inclusions to be overlooked. The association with whooping cough has been known for years. McCordock and Smith[269] noted as early as 1934 the presence of inclusions in 45 per cent of fatal cases of whooping cough in 40 consecutive autopsies. Hamperl[253] found the visceral lesions of the disease in 31 cases; in 30 of these there were inclusions in the lung. Feyrter,[251] however, found them only once in more than 100 cases. Thus the relationship between inclusions and whooping cough remains obscure and necessitates further research work.

It should be recalled as well that, in the subjects having undergone kidney transplant, the virus may be isolated from the pulmonary tissue without pneumopathic lesions being observed. These lesions might thus occur only when the virus titer is high or owing to particular circumstances that remain to be elucidated.

PNEUMOPATHY AND INFECTIOUS MONONUCLEOSIS

Like all the other viscera, the lungs can be involved in the course of infectious mononucleosis. In fact, a low percentage of patients present a cough that may be paroxysmal with clinical and radiological signs impossible to distinguish from those of "primary atypical pneumonia." It is, however, important to eliminate a concomitant viral infection before attributing the pulmonary involvement to the mononucleosis.

Systematic radiological examination of patients with infectious mononucleosis revealed anomalies in 2.7 per cent or 16 per cent of cases according to the series of cases studied.[282, 284, 286] The picture is of diffuse pulmonary infiltration, of hilar lymph nodes of increased volume with bilateral opacities radiating away from the hili. In certain cases, the clinical signs are discrete despite extensive radiological signs.[286] Two cases of pleurisy with effusion of considerable degree have been reported,[280, 285] one being unilateral, the other, bilateral. Briggs, Bellomo, and Zauner[278] reported a hemorrhagic effusion and Hansen[281] an x-ray picture of miliary type.

One reported case of pneumopathy characterized by diffuse foci of intracellular infiltration was verified at autopsy.[277]

PRINCIPLES OF TREATMENT

Given the absence of specific antiviral agents, the symptomatic treatment of respiratory viral disease remains one of the primary considerations. Its directive principles are to relieve the patient, to maintain good hydration, to reduce the bronchial or bronchiolar obstruction, to correct the anoxemia and prevent acidosis, to prevent secondary infections, and to control the pulmonary complications and their sequelae.

The great majority of viral bronchopneumopathies are not an indication for hospitalization, but isolation of the patient and bedrest are desirable.

The cough, when it is severe, must be calmed with codeine derivatives. Use of antitussive derivatives of phenothiazine, which is rather widespread at the moment, should be prudent, as they may contribute to thickening the secretions. It is necessary to ease the thoracic pain and the insomia. The fever, which is a normal response to the infection, should not be combated except when it is very high. Use of aspirin in *high* dosage may favor acidosis; the corticosteroids should not be used solely for their action on the fever (see below). Care should be taken to ensure a correct carbohydrate intake to avert ketosis. It is not essential to assure a sufficient caloric intake in the acute phase except in the infant.

Hydration should be sufficient to maintain proper diuresis. In the adult, intake of 2500 to 3000 ml. of liquid per day is required. Intravenous perfusion under control of ionograms is occasionally required in children.

Humidification of the ambient air and vapor therapy are widely utilized. Water vapor reduces the density and the viscosity of the secretions. It is particularly useful in cases of laryngeal involvement and indispensable after tracheotomy. It should be remembered that the particles, to reach the alveoli, should be on the order of 1 μ. Also, most of the numerous nebulizers utilized have no efficacy whatever. The addition of hydroscopic substances such as 10 per cent propylene glycol is questionable; it might stabilize the water particles and retard evaporation.

The main indication for *oxygen therapy* is cyanosis. Oxygen in 40 per cent to 60 per cent concentration can be administered intermittently.

Digitalization is rarely indicated except

when the fragility of the terrain renders it obligatory; indications are: increase in volume of the liver, the appearance of triple-time rhythm, heart rate above 200 beats per minute, or pulmonary edema.

Bronchial or bronchiolar obstruction can be decreased by humidification, mucolytic drugs, relief of the bronchial spasm by small doses of barbiturates, theophylline, isoproterenol, or ephedrine. One purpose is to avert or to overcome the localized bronchial obstructions formed by mucous agglomerates. An obstruction lasting over a month can indeed induce a dilatation of the bronchi. In order to favor expectoration and removal of bronchial obstruction, kinesitherapy may be indicated.

Antibiotics are widely utilized in viral bronchopneumopathies. While the physician is of course aware that they are ineffective against the disease, he believes that they prevent superinfection. The physician who prescribes a course of tetracycline for a patient with measles believes that he is protecting his patient against secondary bacterial complications. Antibiotic therapy should not, however, be systematic. It has been proved that the suppression of the normal flora of the respiratory pathways favors superinfection. Controlled experiments with continuous or intermittent antibiotic therapy in the common cold and influenza in the healthy subject have proved their prophylactic uselessness. It has never been formally proved that this method could prevent bacterial superinfections in measles in the normal child, and for certain authors[290] antibiotics have no place in the initial treatment of respiratory diseases of viral origin. Hence antibiotics should be utilized only when indicated: when there exist a pulmonary focus and a hyperleukocytosis or when the patient's state justifies special precautions: for example, in chronic pneumopathy, cardiopathy, or pregnancy.

On the other hand, in severe cases of influenza, the frequency and the gravity of staphylococcic superinfection should cause the physician to consider using the therapeutic agents most active against staphylococci.

Use of *corticosteroids* in viral bronchopneumopathies remains highly controversial. Their anti-inflammatory action seems to justify their use in the obstructive forms and most especially in cases of bronchiolitis in the young child and in pulmonary edema. The advantages should be weighed against certain disadvantages: they hinder establishment of immunity, favor sodium retention, and can aggravate heart failure. Certain authors, after prospective or retrospective investigations, have emphasized the favorable action of steroids and have considered that they relieved the patient and shortened the course. Others have considered that they did not modify the course in the least. The authors of a minutely controlled study established that the divergencies of opinion resulted from the variability of the parameters utilized to determine the efficacy of this therapy.[288] They themselves considered that in children the intramuscular administration of methyl prednisolone in a dose of 5 mg per kilogram the first day and of 2.5 mg per kilogram the second did not modify the course in any way. In fact, all writers agree that corticosteroid therapy is not harmful. It is better never to utilize it as a routine treatment, but it seems that in certain toxic and exudative forms, when bronchiolitis worsens despite the usual treatment, it can help to change the course of the disease. It can be useful in treating a persistent bronchial obstruction. Thus reserved for particular cases, corticosteroid therapy retains its indications.

Use of *gamma globulins* in sufficient dosage may be justified, especially in the young child.

Treatment of the *bronchiolitis of the infant* merits special mention. In the great majority of cases it has an excellent prognosis that should not be altered by unwise therapeutic measures.[295] The baby should be fed often and in small quantities without trying to impose a precise time schedule for feedings; perfusion may be necessary for rehydration. Oxygen in high concentration can dry the respiratory mucosa. It should never be administered systematically but as required to reduce the cyanosis. Humidification is of major importance to relieve cough and dyspnea. The bronchodilators (sympathomimetic drugs and aminophylline) are generally ineffective and perhaps dangerous. If the dosage is increased because of their inaction, toxic phenomena (tachycardia, excitation, vomiting, cardiovascular collapse) may result. The "asthmatiform" aspect of the clinical picture often leads to use of antihistaminics or cough sedatives that may lead to unfortunate secondary effects. The corticosteroids have no major ill effects if they are used for a brief period, but their efficacy has not been demonstrated. An antibiotic cover is desirable, particularly to prevent staphylococcus superinfection.

The benign character of bronchiolitis in the infant is not absolute. According to some authors[291] mortality attains 5.5 per cent. The gravity of the disease is mainly the result of abrupt episodes of apnea that may mark the disease from its onset and that necessitate emergency resuscitation.[292] These forms require artificial ventilation with tracheal intubation, which should be preferred to tracheostomy. The last-mentioned indeed represents operative shock and risk of pneumothorax. Simple aspiration under bronchoscopy cannot suffice, for it cannot be repeated and the bronchial obstruction is too distal to be accessible to this maneuver. Artificial ventilation is impossible to envisage except in a specialized service. It should be accompanied by supervision of the ionogram and the blood gases and by correction of possible anemia by blood transfusion. An intubation for 48 hours generally suffices to pass the most dangerous period.[292]

Present research work on the therapy of respiratory viral diseases is oriented in two directions: protection of the patient by interferon or the direct action of certain chemical agents on the virus. The action of products such as para-α-ethiony-paraphenyl phenacylamine benzoic acid on the influenza virus inoculated into the mouse permits some hope in this respect.

BIBLIOGRAPHY

General Clinical Study:
Laboratory Studies; Etiological Factors

1. Adams, J. M.: Congenital pneumonitis in newborn infants. Amer. J. Dis. Child., 75:544, 1948.
2. Berven, H.: Studies on the cardiopulmonary function in the post-infectious phase of "atypical" pneumonia. Acta Med. Scand. 171:1, 1962.
3. Bocles, J. S., Ehrenkranz, N. J., and Marks, A.: Abnormalities of respiratory function in varicella pneumonia. Ann. Int. Med., 60:183, 1964.
4. Breese, B. B., and Morgan, H. R.: A study of an epidemic of respiratory infection of multiple etiology. New York J. Med., 57:1918, 1957.
5. Carilli, A. D., Gohd, R. S., and Gordon, W.: A virologic study of chronic bronchitis. New Eng. J. Med., 270:123, 1964.
6. Cate, T. R., Couch, R. B., and Johnson, K. M.: Studies with rhinovirus in volunteers. Production of illness, effect of naturally acquired antibody

and demonstration of protective effect not associated with serum antibody. J. Clin. Invest., 43:56, 1964.
7. Debré, R., Semelaigne, G., and Cournand, R.: Oedème du poumon infectieux subaigu et curable chez le nourrisson. Bull. Soc. Pédiat., 1926, p. 72.
8. Eadie, M. B., Stott, E. J., and Grist, N. R.: Virological studies in chronic bronchitis. Brit. Med. J., 2:671, 1966.
9. Freeman, G. L., and Todd, R. H.: The role of allergy in viral respiratory tract infections. Amer. J. Dis. Chil., 104:330, 1962.
10. Glauser, E. M., Cook, C. D., and Harris, G. B. C.: Bronchiectasis: a review of 187 cases in children with follow-up pulmonary function studies in 58. Acta Paediat. Scand., Suppl. 165, 1966.
11. Golden, A.: Pathologic anatomy of "atypical pneumonia etiology undetermined." Arch. Path., 38:187, 1944.
12. Gresser, I., and Chany, C.: Isolation of measles virus from the washed leucocytic fraction of blood. Proc. Soc. Exper. Biol. Med., 113:695, 1963.
13. Gresser, I., and Chany, C.: Multiplication of poliovirus type I in preparation of human leukocytes and its inhibition by interferon. J. Immunol., 92:889, 1964.
14. Jeune, M., Sohier, R., Beraud, C., Bethenod, M., and Nivelon, J. L.: Les aspects radiologiques des broncho-pneumopathies virales chez l'enfant. 18 Cong. Ass. Pédiatres Langue Française, Genève, 1961. Basel, Karger, 1961, Vol. 3, pp. 170-197.
15. Klineberger-Nobel, E.: Pleuropneumonia-like Organisms (P.P.L.O.). The Mycoplasmataceae. New York, Academic Press, 1962.
16. McFarlane, P. S., and Sommerville, R. G.: Nontuberculous juvenile bronchiectasis: a virus disease? Lancet, 11:770, 1957.
17. Nelson, W. E.: Viral or probable viral infection. In: Nelson, W. E. (ed.): Textbook of Pediatrics. 8th ed. Philadelphia, W. B. Saunders Co., 1964.
18. Parker, F., Joliffe, L. S., and Finland, M.: Primary atypical pneumonia; report of 8 cases with autopsies. Arch. Path., 44:581, 1947.
19. Portnoy, B., Hanes, B., Salvatore, M. A., Eckert, H. L.: The peripheral white blood count in respivirus infection. J. Pediat., 68:181, 1966.
20. Reimann, H. A.: The viral pneumonias and pneumonias of probable viral origin. Medicine, 26:167, 1947.
21. Sommerville, R. G.: Epidemic kerato-conjunctivitis. An adenovirus infection. J. Hyg. (Camb.), 56:101, 1958.
22. Soto, P. J., Brown, G. O., Wyatt, J. P.: Asian influenzal pneumonitis. A structural and virologic analysis. Amer. J. Med., 27:18, 1959.
23. Stark, J. E., Heath, R. B., and Curwen, M. P.: Infection with influenza and parainfluenza viruses in chronic bronchitis. Thorax, 20:124, 1965.
24. Sterner, G.: Adenovirus infection in childhood. An epidemiological and clinical survey among Swedish children. Acta Paediat. Scand., Suppl. 142, 1962.
25. Stuart-Harris, C. H.: Field studies in relation to chronic bronchitis. Proc. Roy. Soc. Med., 49:776, 1957.
26. Stuart-Harris, C. H.: Respiratory viruses, ciliated epithelium and bronchitis. Amer. Rev. Resp. Dis., 93:150, 1966.

27. Voisin, C., Martin, G., and Aerts, C.: Effets toxiques des virus de la grippe sur les leucocytes du cobaye. Etude micro-cinématographique au contraste de phase. Path. Biol. (Paris), *8*:1453, 1960.

PARAINFLUENZA

28. Andrewes, C. H., Bang, F. B., Chanock, R. M., and Zhdanov, V.: Parainfluenza viruses 1, 2 and 3; suggested names for recently described myxoviruses. Virology, *8*:129, 1959.
29. Chanock, R. M., et al.: Newly recognized myxoviruses from children with respiratory disease. New Eng. J. Med., *258*:207, 1958.
30. Chanock, R. M., Bell, J. A., Parrott, R. H.: Natural history of parainfluenza infection. The Gustav-Stern symposium. In: Pollard, M. (ed.): Perspectives in Virology. Minneapolis, Burgess Publishing Co., 1961, pp. 126-139.
31. Chanock, R. M., and Parrott, R. H.: Acute respiratory disease in infancy and childhood: present understanding and prospects for prevention. Pediatrics, *36*:21, 1965.
32. Chanock, R. M., Parrott, R. H., Cook, M. K., Andrews, B. E., Bell, J. A., Reichelderfer, T., Kapikian, A. Z., Mastrota, F. M., and Huebner, R. J.: Newly recognized myxoviruses from children with respiratory disease. New Eng. J. Med., *258*:207, 1958.
33. Chany, C., Robbe-Fossat, F., and Couvreur, J.: Enquête sérologique sur le rôle épidémiologique d'un virus respiratoire nouvellement reconnu: souche E.A. 102 des myxovirus parainfluenzae type 3. Bull. Acad. Nat. Med. (Paris), *143*:110, 1959.
34. Kapikian, A. Z., Chanock, R. M., Reichelderfer, T. E., Ward, T. G., Huebner, R. J., and Bell, J. A.: Inoculation of human volunteers with parainfluenza virus type 3. J.A.M.A., *178*:537, 1961.
35. Lefkowitz, L. B., and Jackson, G. G.: Dual respiratory infection with parainfluenza and rhinovirus. The pathogenesis of transmitted infection in volunteers. Amer. Rev. Resp. Dis., *93*:519, 1966.
36. Lelong, M., Vialatte, J., Cotlenko, M., Chany, C., and Nodot, A.: Isolement d'un virus produisant des syncytiums en culture cellulaire (myxovirus parainfluenzae type 3) à l'occasion d'une petite épidémie de crèche à manifestations respiratoires aiguës bénignes. Arch. Franc. Pediat., *15*:145, 1959.
37. Moscovici, C., Laplaca, M., and Amer, J.: Respiratory illness in prematures and children. Illness caused by parainfluenza type 3 virus. Amer. J. Dis. Child., *102*:91, 1961.
38. Parrott, R. H., Vargosko, A. J., Kim, H. W., Bell, J. A., and Chanock, R. M.: Myxoviruses: parainfluenza. Amer. J. Public Health, *52*:907, 1962.
39. Parrott, R. H., Vargosko, A., Luckey, A., Kim, H. W., Cumming, C., and Chanock, R. M.: Clinical features of infection with hemadsorption viruses. New Eng. J. Med., *260*:731, 1959.
40. Tyrrell, D. A. J., Bynoe, M. L., Petersen, K. B., Sutton, R. N. P., and Pereira, M. S.: Inoculation of human volunteers with para-influenza virus type 1 and 3 (HA 2 and HA 1). Brit. Med. J., *2*:909, 1959.
41. Van der Veen, J., and Smeur, F. A. A. M.: Infections with parainfluenza viruses in children with respiratory illnesses in Holland. Amer. J. Hyg., *74*:326, 1961.

RESPIRATORY SYNCYTIAL VIRUS

42. Adams, J. N., Imagawa, D. T., and Zike, K.: Epidemic bronchiolitis and pneumonitis related to respiratory syncytial virus. J.A.M.A., *176*:1037, 1961.
43. Adams, M. O., Thompson, K. M., Tobin, J. O.: Respiratory syncytial virus infection in the North-West of England. Arch. Ges. Virusforsch., *13*: 268, 1963.
44. Beem, M., Wright, F. H., Hamre, D., Egerer, R., and Oehme, M.: Association of the chimpanzee coryza agent with acute respiratory disease in children. New. Eng. J. Med., *263*:523, 1960.
45. Berglund, B.: Studies on respiratory syncytial virus infection. Acta Paediat. Scand., Suppl. 176, 1967.
46. Berkovich, S., and Taranko, L.: Acute respiratory illness in the premature nursery associated with respiratory syncytial virus infections. Pediatrics, *34*:753, 1964.
47. Breton, A., Samaille, J., Gaudier, B., Gérard-Lefebvre, and Ponte, C.: Isolement du virus syncytial (virus C.C.A. de Morris) au cours de manifestations respiratoires bénignes épidémiques chez des prématurés. Arch. Franc. Pediat., *18*:459, 1961.
48. Chanock, R. M.: Association of a new type of cytopathogenic myxovirus with infantile croup. J. Exper. Med., *104*:555, 1956.
49. Chanock, R. M., and Finberg, L.: Recovery from infants with respiratory illness of a virus related to champanzee coryza agent (C.C.A.). II. Epidemiologic aspects of infection in infants and small children. Amer. J. Hyg., *66*:291, 1957.
50. Chanock, R. M., Kim, H. W., Vargosko, A. J., Deleva, A., Johnson, K. M., Cummings, C., and Parrott, R. H.: Respiratory syncytial virus. I. Virus recovery and other observations during 1960 outbreak of bronchiolitis, pneumonia and minor respiratory diseases in children. J.A.M.A., *176*:647, 1961.
51. Chanock, R. M., Parrott, R. H., Vargosko, A. J., Kapikian, A. Z., Knight, V., and Johnson, K. M.: Respiratory diseases of vital etiology. IV. Respiratory syncytial virus. Amer. J. Public Health *52*:918, 1962.
51a. Chanock, R. M., Roizman, B., and Myers, R.: Recovery from infants with respiratory illness of a virus related to chimpanzee coryza agent (CCA). I. Isolation, properties and characterization. Amer. J. Hyg., *66*:281, 1957.
52. Couvreur, J., Chany, C. H., Falcoff, E., and Gerbeaux, J.: Une épidémie d'infections respiratoires associée au virus C.C.A. de Morris dans une collectivité d'enfants. Bull. Mem. Soc. Med. Hop. Paris, *115*:1299, 1964.
53. Doggett, J. E., and Taylor-Robinson, D.: Serological studies with respiratory syncytial virus. Arch. Ges. Virusforsch., *15*:601, 1965.
54. Forbes, J. A., et al.: Epidemic bronchiolitis caused by a respiratory syncytial virus: clinical aspects. Med. J. Aust., *48*:933, 1961.
55. Gernez-Rieux, C., Breton, H., Samaille, J., Gaudier, B., Lefebvre, and Lelong, M.: Isolement

du virus respiratoire syncytial (C.C.A. de Morris) au cours d'une épidémie de manifestations respiratoires bénignes chez des prématurés. Arch. Ges. Virusforsch., *13*:265, 1963.

56. Hamparian, V. V., Ketler, A., Hilleman, M. R., Reilly, C. M., McClelland, D. I., Cornfeld, D., and Stokes, J.: Studies of acute respiratory illnesses caused by respiratory syncytial virus. I. Laboratory findings in 109 cases. Proc. Soc. Exp. Biol. Med., *106*:717, 1961.

57. Hamre, D., and Procknow, J. J.: Viruses isolated from natural common colds in the U.S.A. Brit. Med. J., *2*:1382-1385, 1961.

58. Hilleman, M. R., Hamparian, V. V., Ketler, A., Reilly, C. M., Clelland, L., Cornfeld, D., and Stokes, J.: Acute respiratory illness among children and adults. Child study of contemporary incidence of several viruses and appraisal of the literature. J.A.M.A. *180*:445, 1962.

59. Holzel, A., Parker, L., Paterson, W. H., White, L. I. R., Thompson, K. M., and Tobin, J. O.: Isolation of respiratory syncytial virus from children with acute respiratory disease. Lancet, *1*:295, 1963.

60. Jamieson, S. R., Alexander, J. G., and Teal, J.: Respiratory syncytial virus epidemic. Public Health, *80*:194, 1966.

61. Johnson, K. M.: Natural reinfection of adults by RSV. Possible relation to mild upper respiratory disease. New Eng. J. Med., *267*:68, 1962.

62. Johnson, K. M., Chanock, R. M., Rifkind, D., Kravetz, H. M., and Knight, V.: Respiratory syncytial virus. IV. Correlation of virus shedding serologic response and illness in adult volunteers. J.A.M.A., *176*:663, 1961.

63. Kapikian, A. Z., Bell, J. A., Mastrota, F. M., Johnson, K. M., Huebner, R. J., and Chanock, R. M.: An outbreak of febrile illness and pneumonia associated with respiratory syncytial virus infection. Amer. J. Hyg., *74*:234, 1961.

64. Kravetz, H. M., Knight, V., Chanock, R. M., Morris, J. A., Johnson, K. M., Rifkind, N. D., and Utz, J. P.: Respiratory syncytial virus. III. Production of illness and clinical observations in adult volunteers. J.A.M.A., *176*:657, 1961.

65. Lafleur, L., Poirier, R., and Martineau, B.: Étude du virus respiratoire syncytial et autres virus dans les infections des voies respiratoires à l' Hôpital Sainte-Justine. Un. Med. Canada, *93*:521, 1964.

66. Lewis, F. A., Rae, M. L., Lehmann, N. I., and Ferris, A. A.: A syncytial virus associated with epidemic disease of the lower respiratory tract in infants and young children. Med. J. Aust., *48*:932, 1961.

67. McClelland, L., Hilleman, M. R., Hamparian, V. V., Ketler, A., Reilly, C. M., Cornfeld, D., and Stokes, J.: Studies of acute respiratory illness caused by respiratory syncytial virus. I. Epidemiology and assessment of importance. New Eng. J. Med., *264*:1169, 1961.

68. Morris, J. A., Blount, R. E., and Savage, R. E.: Recovery of cytopathogenic agent from chimpanzees with coryza. Proc. Soc. Exp. Biol. Med., *92*:544, 1956.

69. Moss, P. D., Adams, M. O., and Tobin, J. O.: Serological studies with respiratory syncytial virus. Lancet, *1*:298, 1963.

70. Parrott, R. H., Vargosko, A. J., Kim, H. W., Cum-

ming, C., Turner, H., Huebner, R. J., and Chanock, R. M.: Respiratory syncytial virus. II. Serologic studies over a 34 month period of children with bronchiolitis, pneumonia and minor respiratory diseases. J.A.M.A., *176*:653, 1961.

71. Peacock, D. M., and Clarke, S. K. R.: Respiratory syncytial virus in Britain. Lancet, *2*:466, 1961.

72. Reilly, C. M., Stokes, J., McClelland, L., Cornfeld, D., Hamparian, V. V., Ketler, A., and Hilleman, M. R.: Studies of acute respiratory illness caused by respiratory syncytial virus. III. Clinical and laboratory findings. New Eng. J. Med., *264*: 1176, 1961.

73. Rice, R. P., and Loda, F.: A roentgenographic analysis of respiratory syncytial virus pneumonia in infants. Radiology, *87*:1025, 1966.

74. Rowe, D. S., and Michaels, R. H.: Isolation of the respiratory syncytial virus from a patient with pneumonia. Pediatrics, *26*:623, 1960.

75. Sandiford, B. R., and Spencer, B.: Respiratory syncytial virus in epidemic bronchiolitis of infants. Brit. Med. J., *2*:881, 1962.

76. Shedden, W. I., and Emery, J. L.: Immunofluorescent evidence of respiratory syncytial virus infection in cases of giant cell bronchiolitis in children. J. Path. Bact., *89*:343, 1965.

77. Tobin, J. O.: The isolation of respiratory viruses from children in Hospital in South East Lancashire. Proc. Roy. Soc. Med., *56*:991, 1963.

ADENOVIRUS

77. Andreoni, O., and Rossi, G.: Su due casi mortali di pneumopatia correlati all'adenovirus tipo 7. Minerva Pediat., *17*:1504, 1965.

79. Barr, J., Kjellen, L., and Svedmyr, A.: Hospital outbreak of adenovirus type 3 infections. Acta Paediat. (Stockholm), *47*:366, 1958.

80. Bell, T. M., Turner, G., MacDonald, A., and Hamilton, D. A.: Type 3 adenovirus infection. Lancet, *3*:1327, 1960.

81. Benyesh-Melnick, M., and Rosenberg, H. S.: The isolation of adenovirus type 7 from a fatal case of pneumonia and disseminated disease. J. Pediat., *64*:83, 1964.

82. Berge, T. O., England, B., Mauris, C., Shuey, H. E., and Lennette, E. H.: Etiology of acute respiratory disease among service personnel at Fort Ord, California. Amer. J. Hyg., *62*:283, 1955.

83. Breckoff, E.: Bericht über eine durch das APC-virus hervorgerufene Epidemie. Deutsch. Med. Wschr., *81*:1149, 1956.

84. Breton, A., Gaudier, B., Ponte, C., and Martin, G.: Bronchite segmentaire à rechutes chez deux soeurs. Rôle étiologique possible d'une infection chronique à virus APC. Arch. Franc. Pediat., *14*:1075, 1957.

85. Breton, A., Gaudier, B., Ponte, C., and Samaille, J. Les bronchopneumopathies à virus de l'enfant. Étude épidémiologique, clinique et paraclinique. Critiques des méthodes de diagnostic. 18 Congrés de l'Association des Pédiatres de Langue Française, Genève, 1961. Basel, Karger, Vol. 64, p. 223.

86. Chanock, R. M., Vargosko, A., Luckey, A., Cook, M. K., Kapikian, A. Z., Reichelderfer, T., and Parrott, R. H.: Association of hemadsorption

viruses with respiratory illness in childhood. J.A.M.A., *169*:548, 1959.

87. Chany, C., Lepine, P., Lelong, M., Le Tan Vinh, Satge, P., and Virat, J.: Severe and fatal pneumonia in infants and young children associated with adenovirus infections. Amer. J. Hyg., *67*: 367, 1958.

88. Collier, A. M., Connor, J. D., and Irving, W. R.: Generalized type 5 adenovirus infection associated with the pertussis syndrome. J. Pediat., *69*:1073, 1966.

89. Couch, R. B., Cate, T. R., Fleet, W. F., Gerone, P. J., and Knight, V.: Aerosol-induced adenoviral illness resembling the naturally occurring illness in military recruits. Amer. Rev. Resp. Dis., *93*: 529, 1966.

90. Cramblett, H., Kasel, J., Langmark, M., and Wilken, F.: Illness in children infected with an adenovirus antigenically related to types 9 and 15. Pediatrics, *25*:822, 1960.

91. Dascomb, H. E., and Hilleman, M. R.: Clinical and laboratory studies in patients with respiratory disease caused by adenoviruses (RI - APC - ARD agents). Amer. J. Med., *21*:161, 1956.

92. Deinhardt, F., May, R. D., Calhoun, H. H., and Sullivan, H. E.: The isolation of adenovirus type 1 from a fatal case of viral "pneumonitis." A.M.A. Arch. Int. Med., *102*:816, 1958.

93. Dingle, J. H., and Feller, A. E.: Noninfluenzal viral infection of the respiratory tract. New Eng. J. Med., *254*:465, 1956.

94. Dinter, Z., Ekelund, H., Laurell, G., Lindrom, G., Löfström, G., Philipson, L., and Wesslen, T.: Aetiology of respiratory tract infection in military personnel. I. Virological findings. Acta Path. Microbiol. Scand., *53*:375, 1961.

95. Dreizin, R. S., Boldyreva, A. S., Isachenko, V. A., and Kniazeva, L. D.: Outbreaks of adenovirus infections in Gorki. Probl. Virology, *5*:196, 1960.

96. Drouhet, V.: Étude d'un virus APC (adenovirus) isolé d'un cas de pneumopathie mortelle. Ann. Inst. Pasteur, *93*:138, 1957.

97. Enders, J. F., Bell, J. A., Dingle, J. H., Francis, T.: Hilleman, M. R., Huebner, R. J., and Payne, A. N. M.: Proposal of the term "adenoviruses" as the group name for the newly recognized respiratory tract viruses (AD - RI - APC - ARD agents). Science, *124*:119, 1956.

98. Evans, A. S.: Adenovirus vaccine. J.A.M.A., *162*: 1178, 1956.

99. Evans, A. S.: Latent adenovirus infections of the human respiratory tract. Amer. J. Hyg., *67*:256, 1958.

100. Felici, A., Ginevri, A., and Franco, F.: Etude étiologique des inflammations aiguës des voies aériennes supérieures chez les nourrissons. Ann. Inst. Pasteur, *98*:229, 1960.

101. Forssell, P., Halonen, H., Stenström, R., Jansson, E., and Wager, O.: An adenovirus epidemic due to types 1 and 2. Ann. Paediat. Fenn., *8*:35, 1962.

102. Fukumi, H., Nishikawa, F., Mizutani, H., Yamaguchi, Y., and Nanba, J.: An epidemic of adenovirus type 3 infections among school children in an elementary school in Tokyo. Jap. J. Med. Sci. Biol., *11*:129, 1958.

103. Gerbeaux, J., and Habib, R.: Pneumopathies à adénovirus. Rev. Tuberc., *27*:736, 1963.

104. Gerbeaux, J., Hebert-Jouas, J., Masse, N., and

Beauchef, A.: Epidémie familiale de maladie à virus du groupe APC chez trois enfants (un cas mortel). Etude clinique, anatomique et virologique. Bull. Soc. Med. Hop. Paris, *73*:519, 1957.

105. Ginsberg, H. S.: Newer aspects of adenovirus infection. Amer. J. Public Health, *49*:1480, 1959.

106. Goodpasture, E., Auerbach, S., Swanson, H., and Cotter, E.: Virus pneumonia of infants secondary to epidemic infections. Amer. J. Dis. Child., *57*:997, 1939.

107. Habib, R.: Pneumonie ä virus A.P.C. In: Journées Pédiatriques. Paris, Lanord, 1957, pp. 13-16.

108. Henle, W., Henle, G., Hummeler, K., and Lief, F. S.: The changing aspects of the serodiagnosis of viral infections. J. Pediatrics, *59*:827, 1961.

109. Hilleman, M. R., Flatley, F. J., Anderson, S. A., Lueking, M. L., and Levinson, D. J.: Antibody response in volunteers to adenovirus vaccine and correlation of antibody with immunity. J. Immun., *80*:299, 1958.

110. Hsiung, C. C.: Adenovirus pneumonia in infants and children. Pathologic studies of 40 cases. Chin. Med. J., *82*:390, 1963.

111. Huebner, R. J., Rowe, W. P., and Chanock, R. M.: Newly recognized respiratory tract viruses. Ann. Rev. Microbiol., *12*:49, 1958.

112. Huebner, R. J., Rowe, W. P., Ward, T. G., Parrott, R. H., and Bell, J. A.: Adenoidal-pharyngeal-conjunctival agents. New Eng. J. Med., *251*: 1077, 1954.

113. Jen, K. F., Tai, Y., Lin, Y. C., and Wang, H. Y.: The role of adenovirus in the etiology of infantile pneumonia and pneumonia complicating measles. Chin. Med. J., *81*:141, 1962.

114. Jeune, M., Sohier, R., Beraud, C., Bethenod, M., and Nivelon, J. L.: Les aspects radiologiques des bronchopneumopathies virales chez l'enfant. 18 Congrès de l'Association des Pédiatres de Langue Française, Genève, 1961. Basel, Karger, 1961, pp. 170-195.

115. Jordan, W. S.: Occurrence of adenovirus infections in civilian populations. Arch. Intern. Med., *101*: 54, 1958.

116. Kaplan, M., Grumbach, R., Strauss, P., and Guillard, J.: Coqueluche maligne chez un enfant de 11 mois avec nécrose diffuse de la muqueuse bronchique sans atteinte notable du parenchyme pulmonaire. Arch. Franc. Pediat., *13*:880, 1956.

117. Kapsenberg, J. G.: Een epidemic big Kinderen, veroorzaakt door Adenovirus type 7. I. Verschignselen big Patienten, big voie Vitscheiding van dit virus is Vastgesteld. Nederl. T. Geneesk., *105*:65, 1962.

118. Kawai, K.: Pathology and pathologic anatomy of adenovirus infection (based on three autopsy cases of infantile pneumonia). Jap. J. Exp. Med., *29*:359, 1959.

119. Kendall, E. J. C., Cook, G. T., and Stone, D. M.: Acute respiratory infections in children. Isolation of Coxsackie B virus and adenovirus during a survey in general practice. Brit. Med. J., *2*:1180, 1960.

120. Kjellen, L., Sterner, G., and Svedmyr, A.: On the occurrence of adenoviruses in Sweden. Acta Paediat. (Stockholm), *46*:164, 1957.

121. Koch, L. M., and Van Gelderen, H. H.: Een epidemie van Adenovirus pneumonie. Maandschr. Kindergeneesk., *27*:402, 1959.

122. Kozinn, P. J., Wiener, H., and Burchall, J. J.: Ef-

fectiveness of adenovirus vaccine in children with repeated acute respiratory illnesses. J. Pediat., *59*:669, 1961.

123. Kusano, N., Kawai, K., and Aoyama, Y.: Intranuclear inclusion body in fatal infantile pneumonia due to adenovirus. Jap. J. Exp. Med., *28*:301, 1958.

124. Lamy, M., Frezal, J., and Cohen-Solal, J.: Pneumopathie chronique associée à une infection par adénovirus. Arch. Franc. Pediat., *20*:612, 1963.

125. Laplaca, M.: Osservazioni sulle variazioni degli anticorpi f.c. per gli adenovirus nei bambini ospiti di una collettivita a contatto continuo, a distanza di otto mesi. Riv. Ital. Ig., *18*:118, 1958.

126. Lelong, M., et al.: La pneumonie à virus du groupe. A.P.C. chez le nourrisson. Isolement du virus. Les lésions anatomo-histologiques. Arch. Franc. Pediat., *13*:1092, 1956.

127. Le Tan Vinh: Quelques aspects anatomo-pathologiques des bronchopneumopathies à virus. 18 Congrès Association Pédiatres Langue Française, Genéve, 1961. Basel, Karger, 1961, Vol. 3, pp. 198-226.

128. Loeffler, H.: Epidemiologie der viruskrankheiten. Praxis, *48*:585, 1959.

129. Mamykina, L. G.: Particularities of the clinical picture and the course of adenoviral pneumonia in children. Vop. Okhr. Materin. Dets., *7*:10, 1962.

130. Matumoto, M., et al.: Isolation of an intermediate type of adenovirus from a fatal case of infantile pneumonia. Jap. J. Exp. Med., *28*:305, 1958.

131. McFarlane, P. S., and Sommerville, R. G.: Nontuberculosis juvenile bronchiectasies: a virus disease? Lancet, *1*:770, 1957.

132. Neva, F. A., and Enders, J. F.: Isolation of a cytopathic agent from an infant with a disease in certain aspects resembling roseola infantum. J. Immun., *72*:315, 1954.

133. Ninomiya, S.: A fatal case of infantile pneumonia due to adenovirus pathological findings. Jap. J. Exp. Med., *28*:297, 1958.

134. Olson, L., Miller, G., and Hanshaw, J. B.: Acute infectious lymphocytosis presenting as a pertussis like illness: its association with adenovirus type 12. Lancet, *1*:200, 1964.

135. Osada, R., and Hanayama, R.: A fatal case of infantile pneumonia due to adenovirus; clinical findings. Jap. J. Exp. Med., *28*:293, 1958.

136. Pereira, H. G., and Kelly, B.: Studies on natural and experimental infection by adenoviruses. Proc. Roy. Soc. Med., *50*:755, 1957.

137. Pierce, C. H., and Knox, A. W.: Ciliocytophthoria in sputum from patients with adenovirus infection. Proc. Soc. Exp. Biol. Med., *104*:492, 1960.

138. Quénum, C., Aubry, L., and Richir, C.: Sur un cas mortel de bronchopneumopathie dûe à des virus APC avec inclusions cytomégaliques. Ann. Anat. Path. (Paris), *8*:417, 1963.

139. Rowe, W. P., Huebner, R. J., and Bell, J. A.: Definition and outline of contemporary information on the adenovirus group. Ann. N.Y. Acad. Sci., *67*:255, 1957.

140. Sohier, R. P., Bensimon, P., Chardonnet, Y., et al.: Une épidémie d'infections à adénovirus. Rev. Hyg. Med. Soc., *5*:423, 1957.

141. Sommerville, R. G.: Epidemic kerato-conjunctivitis. An adenovirus infection. J. Hyg. (Camb.), *56*:101, 1958.

142. Squeri, L., Pernice, A., and Ioli, A.: L'indagine sierologica ai fini epidemiologici nelle infezioni da adenovirus. Riv. Ist. Sieroter. Ital., *34*:427, 1959.

143. Sterner, G.: Infections with adenovirus type 7 in children and their relationship to acute respiratory disease. Acta Paediat. (Stockholm), *48*:287, 1959.

144. Sterner, G.: Adenovirus infection in childhood. An epidemiological and clinical survey among Swedish children. Acta Paediat. (Stockholm), Suppl. 142, 1962.

145. Suzuki, S., et al.: The role of adenoviruses as the etiological agent of sporadic acute respiratory infections especially that of "virus pneumonia" in a civilian population. Jap. J. Exp. Med., *29*: 601, 1959.

146. Teng, C. H.: Adenovirus pneumonia epidemic among Peking infants and preschool children in 1958. Chin. Med. J., *80*:331, 1960.

147. Tyrrell, D. A. J., Balducci, D., and Zaiman, T. E.: Acute infections of the respiratory tract and the adenoviruses. Lancet, *2*:1326, 1956.

148. Van der Veen, J.: Infections with adenovirus in Europe. Ann. Soc. Belg. Med. Trop., *38*:891, 1958.

149. Van der Veen, J.: Adenovirus and viral pneumonia in children. J. Hyg. Epidem. (Praha), *6*:85, 1962.

150. Vargosko, A. J., Chanock, R. M., Kim, H. W., and Parrott, R.: Contribution of adenovirus infection to childhood respiratory tract illness. Amer. J. Dis. Child., *102*:501, 1961.

151. Ward, T. G., Huebner, R. J., Rowe, W. P., Ryan, R. W., and Bell, J. A.: Production of pharyngoconjunctival fever in human volunteers inoculated with A.P.C. viruses. Science, *122*:1086, 1955.

152. Wright, H. T., Jr., Beckwith, J. B., and Gwinn, J. L.: A fatal case of inclusion body pneumonia in an infant infected with adenovirus type 3. J. Pediat., *64*:528, 1964.

VARICELLA

153. Bastin, R., Binard, C., and Phav-Sany: Les manifestations pulmonaires au cours de la varicelle. Presse Med., *71*:1873, 1963.

154. Binder, L., Fekete, F., and Schläffler, E.: Pulmonary radiological changes in varicella. Acta Paediat. Acad. Sci., Hung., *2*:149, 1961.

155. Bocles, J. S., Ehrenkranz, N. J., and Marks, A.: Abnormalities of respiratory function in varicella pneumonia. Ann. Intern. Med., *60*:183, 1964.

156. Bullowa, J. G. M., and Wishik, S. M.: Complications of varicella. I. Their occurrence among 2534 patients. Amer. J. Dis. Child., *49*:923, 1935.

157. Burton, G. G., Sayer, W. J., and Lillington, G. A.: Varicella pneumonitis in adults: frequency of sudden death. Dis. Chest, *50*:179, 1966.

158. Carstairs, L. S., and Emond, R. T. D.: Chickenpox virus pneumonia. Proc. Roy. Soc. Med., *56*:267, 1963.

159. Claudy, W. D.: Pneumonia associated with varicella: review of the literature and report of a fatal case with autopsy. Arch. Intern. Med., *80*: 185, 1947.

160. Combe, P., Boineau, N., and Zannettacci, M.: Manifestations pulmonaires de la varicelle au cours de la primo-infection tuberculeuse du nourrisson. Considérations générales sur le poumon varicelleux. Arch. Franc. Pediat., *16*: 855, 1959.

161. DiMasse, J. D., Groover, R., and Allen, J. E.: Artificial respiration in the therapy of primary varicella pneumonia. New Eng. J. Med., *261*:553, 1959.

162. Eisenbud, M.: Chickenpox with visceral involvement. Amer. J. Med., *12*:740, 1952.

163. Endress, Z. T., and Schnell, F. R.: Varicella pneumonitis. Radiology, *66*:723, 1956.

164. Felson, B.: Acute miliary diseases of the lungs. Radiology, *59*:32, 1952.

165. Fish, S. A.: Maternal death due to disseminated varicella. J.A.M.A., *173*:978, 1960.

166. Fitz, H., and Meiklejohn, G.: Varicella pneumonia in adults. Amer. J. Med. Sci., *232*:489, 1956.

167. Frank, L.: Varicella pneumonitis: report of a case with autopsy observations. Arch. Path. (Chicago), *50*:450, 1950.

168. Gerbeaux, J., Couvreur, J., Crémer, V., M'Bargha, P.: Le poumon dans la varicelle chez l'enfant. Rev. Med. (Paris), *10*:557, 1964.

169. Gerbeaux, J., and Crémer, V.: Aspects radiologiques des localisations pulmonaires au cours de la varicelle. J. Radiol. Electr., *45*:398, 1964.

170. Hildreth, E. A.: Corticosteroids and varicella pneumonia, or skepticism. The chastity of intellect. Ann. Intern. Med., *55*:531, 1961.

171. Johnson, H. N.: Visceral lesions associated with varicella. Arch. Path. (Chicago), *30*:292, 1940.

172. Knyvett, A. F.: Complicated chickenpox. Med. J. Aust., *44*:91, 1957.

173. Knyvett, A. F.: The pulmonary lesions of chickenpox. Quart. J. Med., *35*:313, 1966.

174. Kriss, N.: Chickenpox pneumonia. Radiology, *66*: 727, 1956.

175. Krugman, S., Goodrich, C. H., and Ward, R.: Primary varicella pneumonia. New Eng. J. Med., *257*:843, 1957.

176. Le Tan Vinh, Canlorbe, P., Gentil, C., and Lelong, M.: La varicelle maligne pluriviscérale. Un cas avec mise en évidence des foyers de nécrose et des inclusions acidophiles intranucléaires. Sem. Hop. Paris, *33*:3989, 1957.

177. Levin, H. G.: A case of chicken-pox pneumonia with x-ray findings suggesting metastatic carcinoma. New Eng. J. Med., *257*:461, 1957.

178. Lucchesi, P. F., La Boccetta, A. C., and Peale, A. R.: Varicella neonatorum. Amer. J. Dis. Child., *73*:44, 1947.

179. McCarthy, O.: Primary varicella pneumonia. Brit. Med. J., *2*:1155, 1959.

180. Mermelstein, R. H., and Freireich, A. W.: Varicella pneumonia. Ann. Intern. Med., *55*:456, 1961.

181. Nakao, T.: Primary varicella pneumonia. Tohoku J. Exp. Med., *72*:249, 1960.

182. Nelson, A. M., and St. Geme, J. W., Jr.: On the respiratory spread of varicella-zoster virus. Pediatrics, *37*:1007, 1966.

183. Nicolaïdes, N. J.: Fatal systemic varicella: a report of three cases. Med. J. Aust., *44*:88, 1957.

184. Oppenheimer, E. H.: Congenital chickenpox with disseminated visceral lesions. Bull. Johns Hopkins Hosp., *74*:240, 1940.

185. Raush, L. E., Grable, T. J., and Musser, J. H.: Atypical pneumonia complicating severe varicella in an adult. New Orleans Med. Surg., G. *96*: 271, 1943.

186. Rosecan, M., Baumgarten, W., and Charles, B. H.: Varicella pneumonia with shock and heart failure. Ann. Intern. Med., *38*:830, 1953.

187. Sargent, E. N., Carson, M. J., and Reilly, E. D.: Roentgenographic manifestations of varicella pneumonia with post-mortem correlation. Amer. J. Roentgen., *98*:305, 1966.

188. Saslaw, S., Prior, J. A., and Wiseman, B. K.: Varicella pneumonia. Arch. Intern. Med., *91*: 35, 1953.

189. Southard, M. E.: Roentgen findings in chickenpox pneumonia. Amer. J. Roentgen., *76*:533, 1956.

190. Tan, D. Y. M., Kaufman, S. A., and Levene, G.: Primary chickenpox pneumonia. Amer. J. Roentgen., *76*:527, 1956.

191. Thomson, F. H.: The aerial conveyance of infection with a note on the contact infection of chickenpox. Lancet, *190*:341, 1916.

192. Waring, J. J., Neubuerger, K., and Geever, E. F.: Severe forms of chickenpox in adults, with autopsy observations in a case with associated pneumonia and encephalitis. Arch. Intern. Med., *69*:384, 1942.

193. Weinstein, L., and Meade, R. H.: Respiratory manifestations of chickenpox. Special consideration of the features of primary varicella pneumonia. Arch. Intern. Med., *98*:91, 1956.

194. Williams, B., and Capers, T. H.: The demonstration of intranuclear inclusion bodies in sputum from a patient with varicella pneumonia. Amer. J. Med., *27*:836, 1959.

HERPES ZOSTER

195. Andrews, R. H.: Pneumonia and bronchial vesiculation associated with herpes zoster; with reference to other visceral associations of zoster. Brit. Med. J., *2*:384, 1957.

196. Curtin, R. G.: Herpes zoster and its relation to internal inflammations and diseases, especially the serous membranes. Amer. J. Med. Sci., 1902, pp. 123-264.

197. Downie, A. W.: Chickenpox and zoster. Brit. Med. Bull., *15*:197, 1959.

198. Gais, E. S., and Abrahamson, R. H.: Herpes zoster and its visceral manifestations. Amer. J. Med. Sci., *197*:817, 1939.

199. Head, H., and Campbell, A. W.: Pathology of herpes zoster. Brain, *23*:353, 1900.

200. Herbeuval, R., Remy, M., and Pierson, M.: Les pneumopathies zostériennes. J. Franc. Med. Chir. Thorac., *4*:466, 1950.

201. Pek, S., and Gikas, P. W.: Pneumonia due to herpes zoster; Report of a case and review of the literature. Ann. Intern. Med., *62*:350, 1962.

202. Taylor-Robinson, D.: Herpes-zoster occurring in a patient with chickenpox. Brit. Med. J., *1*:1713, 1960.

203. Thiodet, J., Fourrier, A., et al.: Varicelle, zona et troubles de la ventilation pulmonaire. Algérie Med., *60*:718, 1956.

204. von Bärensprung, F. G. H.: "Die Gurtelkrank." Ann. Char. Kranken Berl., *9*:40, 1961.

205. Wilson, F. W., and Matlock, T. B.: Herpes zoster

pneumonitis: case report. Dis. Chest, *40*:74, 1961.

206. Wyburn-Mason, R.: Visceral lesions in herpes zoster. Brit. Med. J., *1*:678, 1957.

MEASLES

207. Bastin, R., Morin, H., and Lubetzki, J.: Les comlications respiratoires de la rougeole. Rev. Prat., 1955. *5*:657, 1955.
208. De Mattia, R., Maestri, O., Di Nola, F., Rapellini, M., and Angela, G. C.: Il pomone nel morbillo. Minerva Med., *2*:1089, 1952.
209. Enders, J. F., et al.: Isolation of measles virus at autopsy in cases of giant-cell pneumonia without rash. New Eng. J. Med., *261*:875, 1959.
210. Fawcitt, J., and Parry, H. E.: Lung changes in pertussis and measles in childhood: review of 1894 cases with follow up study of pulmonary complications. Brit. J. Radiol., *30*:76, 1957.
211. Hecht, V.: Die Riessenzellen Pneumonia im Kindesalter eine Historis experimentelle Studie. Beitr. Path. Anat., *48*:263, 1910.
212. Koffler, D.: Giant cell pneumonia, Fluorescent antibody and histochemical studies on alveolar giant cells. Arch. Path. (Chicago), *78*:267, 1964.
213. Kohn, J. L., and Koiransky, H.: Successive roentgenogram of chest of children during measles. Amer. J. Dis. Child., *38*:258, 1929.
214. Kohn, J. L., and Koiransky, H.: Roentgenographic reexamination of chests of children from six to ten months after measles. Amer. J. Dis. Child., *41*:500, 1931.
215. Kohn, J. L., and Koiransky, H.: Further roentgenographic studies of the chests of children during measles. Amer. J. Dis. Child., *46*:50, 1933.
216. Le Tan Vinh: Quelques aspects anatomopathologiques des bronchopneumopathies à virus. 18 Congrès. Association Pédiatres Langue Française, Genéve, 1961. Basel, Karger, 1961, Vol. 3, pp. 198-226.
217. MacCarthy, K., Mitus, A., Cheatham, W., and Peebles, T.: Isolation of virus of measles from three fatal cases of giant cell pneumonia. Amer. J. Dis. Child., *96*:500, 1958.
218. Mitus, A., et al.: Persistence of measles virus and depression of antibody formation in patients with giant-cell pneumonia after measles. New Eng. J. Med., *261*:882, 1959.
219. Naussac, H., Fath, A., and Verneyre, H.: Les images radiologiques diffuses des pneumopathies infectieuses de l'enfant: miliaires et réticulomiliaires non tuberculeuses de la rougeole et de la coqueluche. J. Med. Lyon, *42*:765, 1961.
220. Pegni, U.: Observazioni clinice in 64 casi de morbillo nell' adulto. Rass. Clinico. Sci. Ist. Biochim. Ital., *31*:19, 1955.
221. Quinn, J. L.: Measles pneumonia in an adult. Amer. J. Roentgen., *91*:560, 1964.
222. Sedallian, P., Maral, P., L'Hermuzière, J. de, and Traeger, J.: Le poumon dans la rougeole. Pédiatrie, *1*:112, 1950.
223. Simpson, C. L., and Pinkel, D.: Pathology in leukemia complicated by fatal measles. Pediatrics, *21*:436, 1958.
224. Toscano, F., and Pisani, G.: Considérations radiocliniques sur le poumon rougeoleux. Pédiatrie, *8*:563, 1953.
225. Weinstein, L., and Franklin, W.: Pneumonia of measles. Amer. J. Med. Sci., *217*:314, 1949.

MUMPS

226. Binechvar, A., et al.: A case of pleurisy after mumps. Acta Med. Iran, *3*:45, 1960.
227. Cottel, C. E., and Hanser, M. H.: Pulmonary infarction complicating mumps. Northwest Med., *51*:40, 1952.
228. Huseyin, K.: Pleurisy due to mumps. Acta Med. Turc., *1*:45, 1948.
229. Ledoux, G.: Contribution à l'étude des pleurésies ourliennes. Thèse No. 23, Paris, 1952.
230. Meyer, A., Bastin, R., Lajouanine, P., Brunel, M., and Magloire, C.: Pleuropneumopathies associées aux oreillons. Rôle éventuel du virus ourlien. Bull. Soc. Med. Hop. Paris, *114*:1075, 1963.
231. Ogawa, K.: Pulmonary condensation caused by myxovirus of mumps in mice. Virology, *9*:714, 1959.
232. Turiaf, J., and Marland, P.: Pneumopathie à virus ourlien. Bull. Soc. Med. Hop. Paris, *114*:1095, 1963.
233. Young, L. J., and Cowley, R. G.: Pulmonary infarction complicating mumps. A.M.A. Arch. Intern. Med., *97*:249, 1956.

ENTEROVIRUSES

234. Butterfield, J., Moscovici, C., Berry, C., and Kempe, C. H.: Cystic emphysema in premature infants. A report of an outbreak with the isolation of type 19 ECHO virus in one case. New Eng. J. Med., *268*:18, 1963.
235. Cramblett, H. G., et al.: Respiratory illness in six infants infected with newly recognized ECHO virus. Pediatrics, *21*:168, 1958.
236. De Ritis, L.: Broncopneumopatia da probabile infezione da virus Coxsackie. Riv. Clin. Pediat., *71*:228, 1963.
237. De Sanctis-Monaldi, T., Benedetto, A., Frugoni, G., Lotti, A., and Jacoangeli, C.: Maladies respiratoires aiguës à virus ECHO. Observation clinique et étude virologique. Sem. Hop. (Paris), *43*:577, 1967.
238. Eckert, H. L., Portnoy, B., and Salvatore, M.: Summer pneumonia in infants associated with group B Coxsackie virus infection. Clin. Res., *13*:101, 1965.
239. Flewett, T. H.: Histological study of two cases of Coxsackie B virus pneumonia in children. J. Clin. Path., *18*:743, 1965.
240. Holzel, A., Parker, L., Patterson, W. H., Cartmel, D., White, L. L. R., Purdy, R., Thompson, K. M., and Tobin, J. O.: Virus isolations from throats of children admitted to hospital with respiratory and other diseases, Manchester, 1962-4. Brit. Med. J., *1*:614, 1965.
241. Hooft, C., et al.: Clinical findings during an ECHO virus type 13 endemic infection. Helv. Paediat. Acta, *18*:230, 1963.
242. Johnson, K. M., Bloom. H. H., Forsyth, B., Mufson, M. A., Webb, P. A., and Chanock, R. M.: The role of enteroviruses in respiratory disease. Amer. Rev. Resp. Dis., *88*:240, 1963.
243. Kendall, E. J. C., Cook, G. T., and Stone, D. M.:

Acute respiratory infections in children. Isolation of Coxsackie B virus and adenovirus during a survey in a general practice. Brit. Med. J., *2*: 1180, 1960.

244. Lerner, A. M., Klein, J. O., Levin, H. S., and Finland, M.: Infections due to Coxsackie virus group A, type 9 in Boston, 1959, with special reference to exanthems and pneumonia. New Eng. J. Med., *263*:1265, 1960.

245. Niitu, Y.: Coxsackie B1 virus associated with atypical pneumonia found in a mass chest x-ray survey among school children in Sendai in 1960. Sci. Rep. Res. Inst. Tohoku Univ. (Tuberculosis, Leprosy, Cancer), *12*:75, 1965.

246. Vargosko, A., Kim, H., Parrott, R. H., and Chanock, R. M.: Association of Coxsackie B5 with minor respiratory tract illness in children. Amer. J. Dis. Child., *104*:539, 1962.

CYTOMEGALOVIRUS

247. Bacala, J. C., and Burke, R. J.: Generalized cytomegalic inclusion disease. Report of a case and review of literature. J. Pediat., *43*:712, 1953.

248. Bodey, G. I., Wertlake, I. T., Douglas, G., and Levin, R. H.: Cytomegalic inclusion disease in patients with acute leukemia. Ann. Intern. Med., *62*:899, 1965.

249. Capers, T. H., and Lee, D.: Pulmonary cytomegalic inclusion disease in an adult. Amer. J. Clin. Path., *33*:238, 1960.

250. Emanuel, I., and Kenny, G. E.: Cytomegalic inclusion disease of infancy. Pediatrics, *38*:957, 1966.

251. Feyrter, F.: Ueber die pathologische Anatomie der Lungenver anderungen beim Keuckhusten. Frankfurt Z. Path., *35*:213, 1927.

252. Gottman, A. W., and Beatty, E. C.: Cytomegalic inclusion disease in children with leukemia or lymphosarcoma. Amer. J. Dis. Child., *104*:180, 1962.

253. Hamperl, H.: Pneumocystis infection and cytomegaly of the lungs in the newborn and adult. Amer. J. Path., *32*:1, 1956.

254. Hanshaw, J. B., and Weller, T. H.: Urinary excretion of cytomegaloviruses by children with generalized neoplastic disease. Correlation with clinical and histopathologic observations. J. Pediat., *58*:305, 1961.

255. Hill, R. B., Rowlands, D. T., and Rifkind, D.: Infectious pulmonary disease in patients receiving immunosuppressive therapy for organ transplantation. New Eng. J. Med., *271*:1021, 1964.

256. Jesionek and Kiolemenoglou: Ueber einen Befund von protozoenartigen Gebilden in den Organen eines hereditärluetischen Fötus. Munchen. Med. Wschr., *51*:1905, 1904.

257. Kaariainen, L., et al.: Cytomegalovirus. Mononucleosis. Isolation of the virus and demonstration of subclinical infections after fresh blood transfusion in connection with open heart surgery. Ann. Med. Exp. Fenn., *44*:297, 1966.

258. Kalfayan, B.: Inclusion disease in infancy. A.M.A. Arch. Path., *44*:467, 1947.

259. Kanich, R. E., and Craighead, J. E.: Cytomegalovirus infection and cytomegalic inclusion disease on renal homotransplant recipients. Amer. J. Med., *40*:874, 1966.

260. Kramer, R. I., Cirone, V. C., and Moore, H.: Interstitial pneumonia due to pneumocystis cari-

nii, cytomegalic inclusion disease and hypogammaglobulinemia occurring simultaneously in an infant. A case report with necropsy findings. Pediatrics, *29*:816, 1962.

261. Lamb, S. G., and Stern, H.: Cytomegalovirus mononucleosis with jaundice as presenting sign. Lancet, *2*:1003, 1966.

262. Lamy, M., Aussanaire, M., Jammet, M. L., and Nezelof, C.: La maladie des inclusions cytomégaliques. Bull. Mem. Soc. Med. Hop. Paris, *68*:960, 1952.

263. Le Tan Vinh: La maladie des inclusions cytomégaliques. A propos de six observations personnelles. Ann. Pediat. (Paris), *33*:514, 1957.

264. Le Tan Vinh: Quelques aspects anatomo-pathologiques des broncho-pneumopathies à virus. 18 Congrès de l'Association des Pédiatres de Langue Française, Genève, 1961. Basel, Karger, 1961, Vol. 3, p. 198.

265. McMillan, G. C.: Fatal inclusion disease pneumonitis in an adult. Amer. J. Path., *23*:995, 1947.

266. Margileth, A. M.: The diagnosis and treatment of generalized cytomegalic inclusion disease of the newborn. Pediatrics, *15*:270, 1955.

267. Medearis, D. N.: Cytomegalic inclusion disease. An analysis of the clinical features based on the literature and six additional cases. Pediatrics, *19*:467, 1957.

268. Medearis, D. N.: Observations concerning human cytomegalovirus infection and disease. Bull. Johns Hopkins Hosp., *114*:181, 1964.

269. McCordock, H. A., and Smith, M. C.: Intranuclear inclusions; incidence and possible significance in whooping cough and in a variety of other conditions. Amer. J. Dis. Child., *47*:774, 1934.

270. Nezelof, C., Gaquiere, A., and Brousse, A.: Les inclusions cytomégaliques chez l'adulte. Première observation française et revue de la littérature. Presse Med., *69*:1845, 1961.

271. Peace, R. J.: Cytomegalic inclusion disease in adults. A complication of neoplastic disease of hemopoietic and reticulohistiocytic systems. Amer. J. Med., *24*:48, 1958.

272. Seifert, G.: Zur Pathologie der Cytomegalie. (Einschlusskörperchenkrankheit, Speicheldrüsenviruskrankung. Arch. Path. Anat., *325*:596, 1954.

273. Turgeon, C.: La maladie des inclusions cytomégaliques. Ann. Anat. Path., *2*:563, 1957.

274. Wong, T., and Warner, N. E.: Cytomegalic inclusion disease in adults. Report of 14 cases with review of literature. Arch. Path. (Chicago), *74*:403, 1962.

275. Wyatt, J. P., Saxton, J., Lee, R. S., and Pinkerton, H.: Generalized cytomegalic inclusion disease. J. Pediat., *36*:271, 1950.

276. Wyatt, J. P., Simon, T., Trumbull, M. L., and Evans, M.: Cytomegalic inclusion pneumonitis in an adult. Amer. J. Clin. Path., *33*:353, 1953.

INFECTIOUS MONONUCLEOSIS

277. Allen, F. H., and Kellner, A.: Infectious mononucleosis: an autopsy report. Amer. J. Path., *23*: 463, 1947.

278. Briggs, J. F., Bellomo, J., and Zauner, R. J.: Hemorrhagic pleural effusion complicating infectious mononucleosis. Dis. Chest, *30*:557, 1956.

279. Brusa, P. and Carletti, B.: Pneumopatia in corso di

mononucleosi infettiva. Minerva Pediat., *10*: 1211, 1958.

280. Eaton, O. M., Little, P. F., and Silver, H. M.: Infectious mononucleosis with pleural effusion. Arch. Intern Med., *115*:87, 1965.

281. Hansen, F. F.: Miliare pneumonie bei infektiösen Mononukleose. Arch. Kinderheilk., *153*:262, 1956.

282. McCort, J. J.: Infectious mononucleosis with special reference to roentgenologic manifestations. Amer. J. Roentgen, *62*:645, 1949.

283. Perugini, S., and Fontanini, F.: Su di un epidemia di mononucleosi infettiva a localizzazione prevalentemente do polmonare. G. Mal. Infett., *9*: 525, 1957.

284. Smith, J. D.: Complications of infectious mononucleosis. Ann. Intern. Med. *44*:861, 1956.

285. Vander, J. B.: Pleural effusion in infectious mononucleosis. Ann. Intern. Med., *41*:146, 1954.

286. Wechsler, H. F., Rosenblum, A. H., and Sills, C. T.: Infectious mononucleosis. Report of an epidemic in an army post. Ann. Intern. Med., *25*:113, 1946.

TREATMENT

287. Austrian, R.: Current status of therapy in the pneumonias. J.A.M.A., *163*:1040, 1957.

288. Avery, M. E., Galina, M., and Nachman, R.: Mist therapy. Pediatrics, *39*:160, 1967.

289. Dabbous, I. A., Tkachyk, J. S., and Stamm, S. J.: A double blind study on the effects of corticosteroids in the treatment of bronchiolitis. Pediatrics, *37*:477, 1966.

290. Davis, S. D.: Antibiotic prophylaxis in acute viral respiratory diseases. Amer. J. Dis. Child., *109*: 544, 1965.

291. Heycock, J., and Noble, T.: 1230 cases of acute bronchiolitis in infancy. Brit. Med. J., *2*:879, 1962.

292. Joly, J. B., Huault, G., Amsili, J., Lemerle, J., and Thieffry, S.: Place de l'intubation et de la ventilation artificielle dans le traitement des bronchoalvéolites graves du nourrisson. A propos de 7 observations. Arch. Franc. Pediat.,*24*:303, 1967.

293. Palmer, K. N. V.: Sputum liquefiers. Brit. J. Dis. Chest, *60*:177, 1966.

294. Sussman, S., Grossman, M., Magoffin, R., and Schieble, J.: Dexamethasone (16-alpha-methyl, 9-alpha-fluoroprednisolone) in obstructive respiratory tract infections in children. A controlled study. Pediatrics, *34*:851, 1964.

295. Wright, F. H., and Beem, M. O.: Diagnosis and treatment. Management of acute viral bronchiolitis in infancy. Pediatrics, *35*:334, 1965.

43

The Clinical Diagnosis of Viral Pleurisies

By J. COUVREUR

The existence of viral pleurisies has been suspected ever since aseptic pleural effusions were noticed during the 1918 influenza epidemic[12] and in the epidemic of primary atypical pneumonia in 1942-1943.[16]

The frequency of pleurisies in viral respiratory tract infections has been variously assessed. Some authors have estimated the frequency to be less than 5 per cent, others have found it to be 25 per cent. These considerable discrepancies are connected with the criteria for the diagnosis of pleurisy. Virus pleurisies are rarely sufficiently severe to produce obvious clinical signs. On the other hand, systematic radiological examinations with lateral views make it possible to detect a greater number of pleural reactions. Thus, a serofibrinous pleurisy was found in five cases and a localized pleural reaction in two cases in a series of 48 virus pneumopathies in adult patients[14, 15] and in six of 480 cases of virus pneumopathies observed in another series.[7]

CLINICAL ASPECTS

Viral pleurisies may have four clinical aspects: serofibrinous effusions in the chest cavity; encysted-appearing local effusions; accompanying pleural reactions; effusions associated with viral pericarditis.

Effusions in the Pleural Space. Effusions in the pleural space are rarely sufficiently severe to yield an obvious clinical syndrome. The latter is usually discrete: dry and painful cough, localized chest wall pain, decrease in the percussion note ranging from dull to flat at the base of a hemithorax, disappearance of the palpable fremitus and the breath sounds, and, occasionally, pleural rub.

Radiographs show a more or less extended dimness of the diaphragmatic cul-de-sac. They make it possible to assess the spread of the effusion and to look for associated pulmonary lesions. Bilateral pleurisies have also been noted.

Thoracentesis confirms diagnosis by yielding fluid of greatly varying aspects: serofibrinous and transparent, blood-tinged, or cloudy. Albumin content may reach 30 gm. per liter. The sediment shows, in variable proportions, polymorphonuclear cells, neutrophils, lymphocytes, and endothelial cells, none of the cellular groups exceeding 60 to 70 per cent of the total.[14] The polymorphonuclear cells are not altered even when the liquid is puriform. A high proportion of eosinophilic polymorphonuclear cells (30 to 84 per cent) has been noted, and it is not impossible that certain eosinophilic pleurisies could have a viral origin. It would seen that no search for viruses has been yet undertaken in this type of effusion.

Blood count does not show anything noteworthy, although moderate leukocytosis (around 12,000 per cubic millimeter), accompanied by average polymorphonucleosis (75 per cent) has been noted.[10]

The effusion usually regresses within one to two weeks, but the evolution may last five to six weeks. It does not leave any radiological signs.

The differential diagnosis is established essentially in connection with tuberculous pleurisy and bacterial pleural superinfections possibly masked by antibiotic therapy. It should be borne in mind that, in comparison with tuberculous pleurisy, nonlocalized viral pleurisies are infrequent in the adult and exceptional in the child. It should be the main concern of the clinician to attempt to establish the existence of tuberculous pleurisy, because it may be triggered in a tuberculous patient by an intercurrent viral respiratory infection.

Isolated Local Effusions. Isolated local effusions are even more infrequent. A few cases have been reported, all connected with an influenza infection.[15] Their clinical features — violent outbreak with a febrile state and localized chest pain — were nonspecific. Radiographs and, more particularly, lateral views may give a lead to the diagnosis: as a rule, it is a right-sided interlobar effusion and appears to be isolated without any signs of parenchymatous involvement. The fluid may abound in eosinophils. A case of profuse extravasation amounting to 500 ml. has been reported. The evolution is favorable; spontaneous resorption occurs within 10 to 30 days without after-effects.

Accompanying Pleural Reactions. Accompanying pleural reactions are comparatively frequent. They give few clinical signs. X-rays of the thorax show the filling out of a costodiaphragmatic sinus and the evident thickening of an interlobar fissure associated with pictures of the causal pneumopathy. These reactions are frequently bilateral, but do not justify a puncture. They are very often accompanied by a clear-cut rise in blood sedimentation rate.

Pleural Effusions with Pericarditis. Finally, certain pleural effusions may be associated with pericarditis. The viral origin of these exceptional pleuropericarditis syndromes, in which the pleural effusion is usually bilateral, has been suspected for a long time. It has been possible to provide in several cases the evidence of the viral origin, particularly in influenza A myxovirus infections.[15] The pericarditis either is dry or causes a moderate effusion. It is often masked by pleurisy. The clinical picture may be alarming, with dyspnea, cyanosis, and high and protracted fever. Cure occurs progressively, without after-effects, within four to six weeks.

ETIOLOGICAL ASPECTS

Influenza. Noted as early as 1918, influenza pleurisies were thoroughly studied during the 1957 epidemic. The pleural reaction frequently occurs during an influenza pneumopathy—in 10 to 20 per cent of the cases. In several cases the influenzal origin of pleurisies of the pleural cavity, interlobar pleurisies, hemorrhagic effusions, or eosinophilic pleurisies has been demonstrated.[2, 10, 14, 15]

Adenovirus Infections. Adenovirus and influenza infections are most often responsible for viral pleurisies. The radiological examination of 44 patients with adenovirus bronchopneumopathies revealed a pleural reaction in seven.[7] Occasionally, the effusion was demonstrable by puncture. In the severe and fatal cases of bronchopneumopathy pleural reaction may be extensive. Chany noted pleurisy in three of 27 such cases. During the epidemic reported in China, autopsies revealed an effusion in a third of the 50 cases examined. In another case, reported by Benyesh-Melnick, there was a thickening of the pleura with diffuse infiltrates of mononuclear cells and hemorrhagic zones. In still another fatal case, viral inclusions were revealed by the Hotchkiss-MacManus technique in the pleural fluid aspirated before death (cf. Chapter 42).

Varicella. Pleurisy is not unusual in varicella-infected lungs. Anatomical examinations have shown blisters on the pleura histologically similar to the cutaneous lesions. Several cases associated with an effusion have been reported (cf. Chapter 42). Finally,

of 22 cases of herpes zoster with pulmonary complications, collected by Pek, seven were associated with pleural rub or with effusion.

Mumps. Pleurisy is the respiratory manifestation most often associated with mumps. However, it is comparatively infrequent. Huseyin[6] observed 25 cases of pleural involvement in 1359 cases of mumps. Other authors[9] have reported seven cases of pleural pneumopathy. Pleural involvement was constant, and in four cases the effusion was fairly abundant. A few other cases have also been reported.[1, 8] Turiaf[13] observed one case of pleurisy associated with a significant increase in mumps complement-fixing antibodies in 174 cases of viral pleurisy. The existence of antigenic relations between the mumps virus and certain myxoviruses should be remembered.

Pleurisy associated with the clinical or biological symptoms of mumps infection may be accompanied by well-marked systemic signs and high fever. It is sometimes discovered on the occasion of violent chest pain followed by rebellious dry cough. The effusion may be sufficiently voluminous to be easily recognizable. The pleural fluid contains 28 to 53 gm.[8, 9] of albumin and shows a mixed cellular content: 53 to 75 per cent of polymorphonuclear cells and 24 to 35 per cent of endothelial cells. The fluid is sterile and its formula evolves toward lymphocytosis. The pleurisy disappears within one to three weeks; it may leave after-effects. However, the

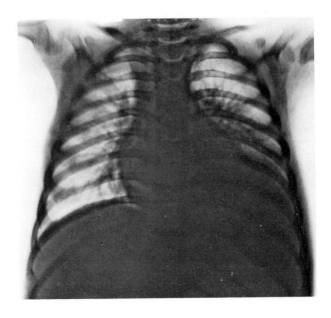

Figure 43-1. Adenovirus pleurisy. Boy, aged 6 years. Left pulmonary focus complicated by pleural reaction. Complete clearing on the eighth day without bacterial superinfection. This child (brother of the patient in Figure 42-3) had a significant rise in titer of complement-fixing antibodies.

pleural participation is more often discrete and is accompanied by parenchymatous localizations.

The physiopathology of these pleural involvements is still a matter of debate. The direct viral involvement of the pleura has been suggested, but so far proof of it is lacking. The possibility of a pulmonary infarctus should not be forgotten, especially because of the painful and abrupt onset. The occurrence of pulmonary infarction in mumps has been demonstrated,[3, 17] and thrombophlebitis is a known complication of mumps.[4] Also, the possibility of an effusion following a latent involvement of the pancreas should not be discarded.

Coxsackie Virus Infections. The clinical picture of pleurodynia caused by Coxsackie viruses (most often group B, occasionally group A) has been known for a long time. It has a characteristically abrupt onset accompanied by paroxysmal chest pains. In a quarter of the cases there is a prodromal period of one to ten days with headaches, loss of appetite, a general feeling of discomfort, and muscular pains. Chest pains occur in attacks and are accentuated by the respiratory movements. Coughing can be violent and the pain sometimes excruciating. As a rule, there is no chest pain between attacks. In half of the cases the disease is accompanied by abdominal pains and vomiting, which may suggest a surgical emergency; the retrosternal localization of the pain can also suggest inflammation of the coronary arteries. Fever may rise as high as 40° C. Examination reveals a pleural friction rub in a quarter of the cases. Palpation of the upper abdomen is painful, but this superficial pain suggests a muscular cause. The radiographs of the thorax are normal. The febrile state and the painful syndrome improve within one day to two weeks, the average period being three and a half days. There are no after-effects.

Cytomegalovirus Infection. A clear-cut case of pleurisy was reported during a cytomegalovirus infection (cf. Chapter 42).

Primary Atypical Pneumonia. Pleurisy may be part of the picture of primary atypical pneumonia. Van Ravensway et al.,[16] who were the first to report this finding, encountered it in 9.7 per cent of their cases. Other authors have not observed it in laboratory-confirmed cases of infection by the Eaton agent (cf. Chapter 42).

BIBLIOGRAPHY

1. Binechvar, A., et al.: A case of pleurisy after mumps. Acta Med. Iran, *3*:45, 1960.
2. Boucher, H., et al.: Pleurésies virales et pleurésies au cours des viroses pulmonaires. Rev. Lyon Med., *8*:969-977, 1959.
3. Cottel, C. E., and Hanser, M. H.: Pulmonary infarction complicating mumps. Northwest Med., *51* 40, 1952.
4. Crosnier, R., Darbon, A., et al.: Phlébite ourlienne Bull. Soc. Med. Hop. Paris, *68*:669, 1952.
5. Dupré, N., et al.: Aspects cliniques des adénoviroses dans l' Est de la France. Presse Med., *71*:2439-2441, 1963.
6. Huseyin, K.: Pleurisy due to mumps. Acta Med Turc., *1*:45, 1948.
7. Jeune, M.: Cited in Chapter 42.
8. Ledoux, G.: Contribution à l'étude des pleurésies ourliennes. Thèse No. 23, Paris, 1952.
9. Meyer, A., Bastin, R., Lajouanine, P., Brunel, M. and Magloire, C.: Pleuropneumopathies associées aux oreillons. Rôle éventuel du virus ourlien. Bull. Soc. Med. Hop. Paris, *114*:1075, 1963.
10. Michon, P.: Les épanchements pleuraux d'origine virale. A propos de 45 observations. Bull. Soc. Med. Hop. Paris, *75*:33-42, 1959.
11. Ogawa, K.: Pulmonary condensation caused by myxovirus of mumps in mice. Virology, *9*:714, 1959.
12. Richet, M., and Barbier: Epanchements aseptiques de la plèvre au cours des infections pulmonaires grippales. Bull. Soc. Med. Hop. Paris, *42*:1016, 1918.
13. Turiaf, J., and Marland, P.: Pneumopathie à virus ourlien. Bull. Soc. Med. Hop. Paris, *114*:1095, 1963.
14. Turiaf, J., et al.: Les pleurésies et les péricardites virales. Poumon Coeur *15*:449-470, 1959.
15. Turiaf, J., Blanchon, P., and Gallaudac, C.: Deux cas de pleurésie interlobaire sérofibrineuse autonome à virus grippal. Bull. Soc. Med. Hop. Paris, *73*: 241, 1957.
16. Van Ravensway, A. C., et al.: Primary atypical pneumonia: clinical aspects: study based on 1862 cases seen at Station Hospital, Jefferson Barracks, Missouri, from June 1, 1942, to August 10, 1943. J.A.M.A., *124*:1, 1944.
17. Young, L. J., and Cowley, R. G.: Pulmonary infarction complicating mumps. A.M.A. Arch. Intern. Med. *97*:249, 1956.

44

Virological Studies, Epidemiology, and Prophylaxis of Virus Infections in Which Respiratory Manifestations Predominate

PARAMYXOVIRUSES: PARAINFLUENZA AND RESPIRATORY SYNCYTIAL VIRUSES

by R. M. CHANOCK

PARAINFLUENZA VIRUSES

DEFINITION

The parainfluenza virus group contains four distinct serotypes. These viruses are RNA-containing, medium-sized (150 to 250 mμ), ether-sensitive viruses which replicate in the cytoplasm. They exhibit helical symmetry and possess a lipoprotein outer envelope studded with projections. Parainfluenza viruses share many biophysical and biological properties with the influenza viruses, but they differ from them in several important respects. They are larger than influenza viruses, have a wider nucleoprotein inner helix, and unlike the influenza viruses are capable of hemolyzing certain types of erythrocytes. Also in distinction to the influenza viruses, certain of the parainfluenza viruses can cause cell fusion under appropriate conditions. In addition, the parainfluenza viruses have common antigens which are not shared by the influenza viruses. The viruses of Newcastle disease and mumps share the foregoing properties, including antigenic relationships, with the parainfluenza viruses.

The first human parainfluenza virus to be recognized was the CA (croup-associated) virus, which was isolated in 1955 from infants with croup (acute laryngotracheobronchitis). This syndrome had previously been called "viral croup" because of failure to recover pathogenic bacteria from most patients. CA virus was recognized by the characteristic syncytial cytopathic effect it produced in monkey kidney or human amnion tissue culture. Subsequently three additional antigenically distinct parainfluenza viruses were recovered in tissue culture from infants and children with respiratory disease. These viruses produced minimal if any cytopathic effect during initial passage in tissue culture, but they could be recognized by the occurrence of hemadsorption when guinea pig erythrocytes were added to infected tissue culture. For this reason these viruses were initially called "hemadsorption" viruses. Subsequently these viruses were brought together and classified as parainfluenza viruses. Type 2 hemadsorption virus was designated type 1 parainfluenza virus, CA virus was classified as type 2 parainfluenza virus, and type 1 hemadsorption virus was designated type 3 parainfluenza virus. Type 4 parainfluenza virus was originally thought to be antigenically homogeneous; however, subsequent studies indicated the existence of two separate subtypes within the type 4 serotype—subtypes A and B.

Viruses sharing the biological and biophysical properties of the parainfluenza viruses have been recovered from a number of animal species. Sendai virus was recovered from mice and also later from pigs. In addition simian virus 5 (SV-5) and simian virus 41 (SV-41) were isolated from monkeys and shipping fever virus (SF-4) from cows. Each of the viruses recovered from these animal species is antigenically related to one of the human parainfluenza virus types. Sendai virus is antigenically related to type 1 parainfluenza virus, SV-5 and SV-41 viruses to type 2 parainfluenza virus, and SF-4 to type 3 parainfluenza virus. It has been suggested that Sendai virus be classified as a murine subtype of type 1 parainfluenza, SV-5 and SV-41 viruses as simian subtypes of type 2 parainfluenza, and SF-4 virus as a bovine subtype of type 3 parainfluenza virus.

PROPERTIES

The parainfluenza viruses (types 1, 2, and 3) are pleomorphic and vary in size from 120 to 800 mμ when examined by the phosphotungstic acid negative staining technique. Thus, they are larger than the influenza viruses, which measure 80 to 120 mμ when examined by the same method. The parainfluenza virion contains a coiled inner helical component which is surrounded by an envelope studded with numerous spike-like projections. The inner helix is single stranded and has a diameter of 15 to 18 mμ and a hollow core of 5 mμ. The inner helix of the influenza viruses is considerably narrower— 9 mμ. The chemical nature of the parainfluenza inner helix has not been determined by direct analysis; however, studies with nucleic acid inhibitors suggest that it consists of ribonucleoprotein.

Parainfluenza viruses are relatively unstable at temperatures of 37° C. and above. Each of the four virus types can be stored without loss of infectivity for several years at −60° C. if protein, such as 5 per cent chicken serum or 0.5 per cent bovine albumin, is incorporated in the suspending medium. The parainfluenza viruses are rapidly inactivated at pH 3.0. Infectivity is also completely destroyed by exposure to 20 per cent ether for 18 hours at 4° C., indicating that lipid is essential for the integrity of the virion.

Parainfluenza viruses agglutinate certain fowl and mammalian red cells. Except for type 4 virus, moderate to high levels of hemagglutinins are produced in infected tissue cultures. Hemagglutinating subunits consisting of envelope material and its spike-like projections are released from parainfluenza type 1 virus when it is treated with ether. Such subunits are unstable in ether, but they can be stabilized by Tween 20 or 80. Irreversible binding of virus antigen to erythrocytes occurs when type 2 *(simiae)* virus is incubated at 37° C. with chicken red cells. Erythrocytes which this virus had adsorbed to and then eluted from (a) agglutinate fresh red cells and (b) are agglutinated when exposed to high dilutions of serum containing antibody for type 2 *(simiae)* virus. At present it is not clear whether the virion or only its hemagglutinating subunit is irreversibly bound to the erythrocyte.

Type 1 *(muris)* virus exhibits neuraminidase activity. Following disruption of the virion by ether the neuraminidase activity is associated with the hemagglutinating subunits. Types 1, 2, and 3 *(hominis)* viruses each exhibit enzymatic activity, presumably neuraminidase.

An hemolysin has been demonstrated for type 1 *(hominis* and *muris)*, 2 *(hominis)*, and 3 *(hominis)* viruses. Type 1 *(muris)* hemolysin has been characterized most completely. This hemolysin is associated with the virion and its activity is mediated through the same red cell receptors as are concerned with hemagglutination. Red cells are rendered insusceptible to hemolysis when receptors are removed by receptor-destroying enzyme (RDE) or the action of nonhemolytic myxoviruses. Hemolysin may be lipid in nature, since treatment of the virion with ether releases hemagglutinating subunits which lack hemolytic activity. Hemolysin has been extracted from type 1 *(muris)* virus by a number of lipid solvents, and the active material is thought to be a lysophosphatide. There is also some evidence that the hemolysin might be a phosphoesterase.

Final assembly of parainfluenza viruses occurs at or near the cell membrane. The helical nucleocapsid is formed in the cytoplasm and becomes aligned under those regions of the host cell's unit membrane which acquire virus surface projections. The virus is then released by a budding process from the cell surface.

The latent period between parainfluenza type 1, 2, or 3 virus infection and the appearance of newly formed infectious virus is approximately six to nine hours. Parainfluenza viruses do not exhibit autointerference following high multiplicity infection. In simian renal cells infection does not generally lead to cell death. Rather, infected cells survive and produce virus over a prolonged interval. The best studied parainfluenza virus–host cell interaction is that involving type 2 *(simiae)* virus and simian renal cells. In this moderate type of virus-cell interaction, infection does not lead to depression of cellular DNA, RNA, or protein synthesis. The synthesis of type 1 *(muris)* virus RNA differs from that of the host cell in that it is not inhibited by actinomycin D.

Tissue culture cells infected with any of the parainfluenza viruses can absorb certain types of erythrocytes when they are added to such cultures. This phenomenon is known as hemadsorption and is attributable to the presence at the cell surface of virus-specific projections (hemagglutinin) which react with receptors on the red cell. Maturation and release of virus at the membrane of simian renal cells occurs over a long interval, and hemadsorption can often be demonstrated in the same tissue culture for one to two weeks.

Virus specific antigens detectable by immunofluorescence are produced in infected cells. In most cell systems parainfluenza antigens are limited to the cytoplasm; however, type 1 *(muris)* and type 3 *(hominis)* viruses can also produce antigens in the nucleus. Eosinophilic cytoplasmic inclusions develop in simian renal cells infected with type 1, 2, 3, or 4 virus. Type 3 virus can also produce eosinophilic nuclear inclusions. Both nuclear and cytoplasmic inclusions are rich in RNA.

EPIDEMIOLOGY

Type 1, 2, and 3 parainfluenza viruses have a wide geographical distribution. The three types have been identified in most areas where appropriate tissue culture and hemadsorption techniques have been applied to the study of childhood respiratory tract disease. Thus far type 4 viruses have been recovered only in the United States and Great Britain.

Primary parainfluenza type 3 infection generally occurs early in life and usually precedes that of the other types. Most infants acquire type 3 neutralizing antibody by two years of age. Acquisition of type 1 and type 2 neutralizing antibodies occurs at a slower rate, but a majority of children possess such antibodies by the sixth to tenth year.

Each of the four parainfluenza virus types can cause acute respiratory tract disease in man. This etiological relationship is indicated by two observations. First, each of the virus types has been recovered significantly more often from patients with respiratory disease than from comparable individuals free of such illness. Second, type 1, type 2, and type 3 virus have each produced upper respiratory tract infection and illness when administered to adult volunteers.

The parainfluenza viruses are most important as respiratory tract pathogens during infancy and childhood. Each of the viruses causes a spectrum of effects in this age group which range from inapparent infection to life-threatening lower respiratory tract involvement. Studies in different parts of the world indicate that type 1, 2, and 3 viruses are associated with approximately one-third of cases of croup or, as it is sometimes called, acute laryngotracheobronchitis. Type 1 is the most important of the parainfluenza viruses in the croup syndrome. In addition to croup, type 1, 2, and 3 viruses are also responsible for smaller but appreciable segments of the other acute respiratory disease syndromes of infancy and childhood. Illness produced by type 4 virus is usually mild and limited to the upper respiratory tract. Parainfluenza viruses have been recovered from many adults with upper respiratory tract disease.

In large urban communities, type 1 and type 3 viruses often exhibit an endemic pattern, i.e., these viruses can be recovered from children with respiratory tract disease during most months of the year. When this occurs seasonal peaks may be observed in the fall, winter, or spring. Type 1 or type 3 virus infection may also assume an epidemic pattern. Such epidemics usually last two to three months and are preceded and followed by periods of markedly decreased prevalence. Type 1 virus can, on occasion, assume an epidemic pattern over a large geographic area. Type 2 infections have a predilection for fall and winter and occur more sporadically than type 1 and type 3 infections. On occasion type 2 may exhibit epidemic behavior. Type 2 and type 3 viruses appear to spread more rapidly from person to person than type 1 virus. Type 3 virus outbreaks in semiclosed nursery populations are often explosive and resemble those produced by influenza A or B virus. Type 3 virus spreads more effectively from person to person than type 1 or type 2 virus. In semiclosed populations the former virus characteristically infects all children initially free of neutralizing antibody, whereas the latter viruses infect only 40 to 60 per cent of seronegative individuals at risk.

PHYSIOPATHOLOGY

The effect of parainfluenza virus upon the host ranges from silent infection to serious respiratory tract disease such as pneumonia or croup. Response to infection is influenced to a considerable degree by age and immunological status. Lower respiratory tract involvement occurs most often during primary infection and is less likely to occur during subsequent reinfection when antibody is present.

Parainfluenza viruses are capable of causing respiratory disease without the cooperative action of pathogenic bacteria. However, bacterial superinfection may occur, resulting in an altered disease picture in which suppuration complicates the changes produced by the virus itself.

Initially in parainfluenza virus infection the mucous membranes of the nose and throat are involved. Paranasal and eustachian tube obstruction may also occur. In many patients the inflammatory process descends into the lower respiratory tract and produces limited changes in the bronchi. If more extensive changes occur in the lower tract there is a tendency for type 1 and type 2 infections to involve the larynx and produce the croup syndrome; there may also be extensive involvement of the trachea and bronchi with accumulation of inspissated mucus resulting in additional obstruction of the airway. When type 3 virus produces severe disease there is a tendency for extension to occur into the lungs and small bronchi with the development of bronchopneumonia.

The risk of febrile disease during primary type 3 infection has been estimated to be 78 per cent and that of pneumonitis or

bronchitis 33 per cent. Febrile illness occurs during approximately one half of primary type 1 virus infections and during two thirds of primary type 2 virus infections. Croup however, develops during only a small proportion of such infections; during a series of prospective longitudinal studies in children only one of 45 type 1 virus infections and one of 31 type 2 virus infections were associated with croup.

IMMUNITY

Severe respiratory tract disease caused by type 1, 2, or 3 parainfluenza virus generally occurs in the first three to five years of life. This finding suggests that primary infection confers upon the host a relative resistance to subsequent severe parainfluenza virus illness.

Reinfection of adults as well as children with parainfluenza viruses has been recognized on a number of occasions, particularly with type 3 virus. Although the frequency of reinfection is not known, it is probable that many individuals have repeated experience with type 3 virus. In a series of sequential outbreaks of type 3 infection in a nursery population, it was observed that 17 per cent of children infected during one outbreak were reinfected during subsequent outbreaks, although the interval between outbreaks was not longer than nine months. Illness usually occurs less often and is less severe during reinfection than during primary infection.

In one study of type 3 virus infection in infants and young children serum neutralizing antibody was found to correlate with resistance to infection and illness. However, resistance associated with serum neutralizing antibody was not complete but only partial. One third of infants and children with high serum antibody levels became reinfected. Although reinfection occurred an effect of antibody was observed, since the period of virus shedding was shorter than during primary infection. Moderate levels of serum antibody did not provide complete protection against febrile illness, since such illness occurred approximately 40 per cent as often as during first infection.

Recent studies in adult volunteers indicate that neutralizing antibody in respiratory tract secretions plays a greater role in resistance to parinfluenza virus infection than does antibody in serum. In experimental type 1 virus infection neutralizing antibody in nasal secretions was almost completely protective whereas serum neutralizing antibody provided very little resistance to reinfection. Neutralizing antibody in nasal secretions is predominantly IgA, whereas neutralizing antibody in serum is predominantly IgG.

LABORATORY STUDIES

Naturally occurring strains of type 2 virus usually produce focal syncytial changes in primary simian tissue cultures, whereas strains of type 1, 3, or 4 virus usually do not produce a cytopathic effect. Strains of the latter viruses are easily recognized when infected cultures are tested for hemadsorption. During subsequent passages in primary simian tissue culture type 3 virus strains induce the formation of elongated stellate cells and occasional syncytial changes, whereas type 1 and type 4 strains produce, at most, minimal rounding and degeneration of cells. When parainfluenza viruses are serially propagated in heteroploid human cell lines (HeLa, HEp-2 etc.), type 2 and type 3 viruses produce marked syncytial changes, whereas type 1 virus fails to produce a cytopathic effect.

Naturally occurring strains of parainfluenza viruses grow poorly or not at all in the embryonated hen's egg. Egg-adapted variants of type 1, 2, or 3 parainfluenza virus grow at a slower rate than the influenza viruses; parainfluenza virus–infected eggs generally require four to six days of incubation for development of maximal titer. When administered by the intranasal route parainfluenza viruses infect guinea pigs without producing overt disease. Hamsters are also sensitive to intranasal infection with type 1, 2, or 3 virus. One TCD_{50} of each of these viruses is sufficient to infect the hamster. This animal undergoes a silent infection without obvious signs of disease, although virus replication occurs in the lung to a level of 10^5 to 10^7 TCD_{50} per gram of tissue.

Specific antigens are present on the envelope of the parainfluenza viruses. Thus, parainfluenza type 1, 2, 3, and 4 viruses react in a specific manner when tested with the appropriate antisera by tissue culture neutralization, hemadsorption-inhibition, or hemagglutination-inhibition. In addition specific antigenic activity has been demonstrated for the hemagglutinating subunits of type 1 *(muris)* parainfluenza virus which are released from the surface of the virion by ether disruption. Soluble, nonhemagglutinating, specific complement-fixing antigens have been prepared from type 1, 2, and 3 viruses by ether treatment and subsequent red cell adsorption of hemagglutinins. The soluble nonhemagglutinating antigen of type 1 *(muris)* virus is associated with the inner helical component of the virion, and it is probable that similar antigens of the other parainfluenza viruses are of the same nature. Unlike the influenza A and B viruses, the parinfluenza viruses do not share a common soluble complement-fixing antigen.

Type 1, 2, and 3 *(hominis)* viruses appear to be antigenically homogeneous, i.e., only one serotype has been recognized for each of the three types. In addition, these viruses appear to be antigenically stable. Thus far major periodic alterations in antigenic structure, characteristic of the influenza A and B viruses, have not been detected.

The parainfluenza viruses share related antigens. Despite antigenic relatedness these viruses can be easily differentiated by complement fixation, hemagglutination inhibition, or tissue culture neutralization using sera from previously infected guinea pigs. The two subtypes of type 4 parainfluenza virus can not be distinguished by complement fixation; however, they can be differentiated by tissue culture neutralization or hemadsorption inhibition.

LABORATORY DIAGNOSIS

The clinical features of parainfluenza illness are not sufficiently distinctive to permit differentiation from disease caused by other respiratory tract pathogens. For this reason the diagnosis of parainfluenza illness can be established only by the appropriate laboratory tests. Simian renal tissue culture is the most sensitive system for recovery of parainfluenza viruses. Human embryonic kidney cultures are also satisfactory, while human diploid fibroblast cell strains and human heteroploid cell lines are considerably less sensitive than simian renal cultures. Naturally occurring type 1, 3, and 4 strains usually do not produce appreciable cytopathic effect in monkey tissue culture, but they can be recognized by the occurrence of hemadsorption when guinea

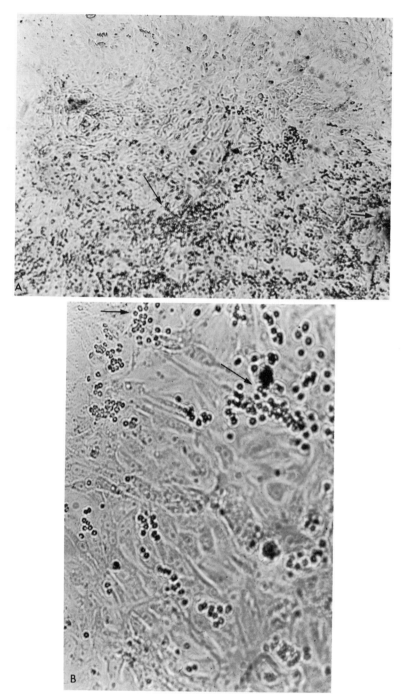

Figure 44-1. *A* and *B*, Parainfluenza virus type 3 revealed on the fifth day of incubation in monkey kidney cell culture by the hemadsorption phenomenon (arrows) utilizing guinea pig erythrocytes. (Courtesy of V. Drouhet.)

pig erythrocytes are added to the cultures. Most type 2 isolates can be recognized by a characteristic syncytial cytopathic effect, but detection is generally more rapid by hemadsorption. The majority of type 1 and type 3 isolates from children can be detected by hemadsorption by the fifth day after inoculation of tissue culture. Strains of types 2 and 4 usually require a longer incubation interval before hemadsorption is detectable, generally ten days or more. Isolates from adults commonly require a longer incubation interval than do strains from children. This probably reflects the small quantity of virus shed by adults, most of whom undergo reinfection rather than primary infection.

The serological response of man to parainfluenza infection is commonly less specific than that of infected animals. In part this results from man's prior experience with other members of the parainfluenza group and mumps virus, whereas experimental infection of laboratory animals generally represents first exposure to antigens of the group. Heterotypic antibody (complement fixing, hemagglutination inhibiting, and/or neutralizing) responses are not unusual following childhood infection and are most often observed to type 3 virus. Adults infected with one of the parainfluenza viruses commonly develop heterotypic antibody responses, which is not surprising in view of their extensive prior experience with antigens of the group. Infected individuals may also develop an antibody response to the related animal parainfluenza viruses as well as mumps virus. Such human heterotypic antibody responses occur in an unpredictable fashion. In addition, patients with mumps infection often develop a rise in antibody for one or more of the parainfluenza viruses.

The majority of children infected with type 1, 2, or 3 virus develop homologous neutralizing and hemagglutination-inhibiting antibodies. The complement fixation technique is efficient for recognition of type 2 and 3 virus infections, whereas many mild type 1 virus infections are not detected by this test. Because of the frequent occurrence of heterotypic antibody responses following parainfluenza virus infection, sometimes in the absence of a homotypic response, it is not possible to identify the infecting virus type with certainty by serological methods. This can be accomplished only by virus isolation.

PROBLEMS OF PROPHYLAXIS

At present specific control measures are not available; however, experimental vaccines for types 1, 2, and 3 virus have been prepared which stimulate the development of serum neutralizing antibody in young infants who lack such antibody. Whether such vaccines will protect against naturally acquired disease remains to be determined. Since antibody in respiratory tract secretions appears to offer greater protection than serum antibody against experimental parainfluenza virus infection, and since infection is more effective than inactivated vaccine in stimulating the former type of antibody, consideration should be given to the development of attenuated vaccines which could be administered intranasally.

Immunization is most urgently needed for the young infant and young child who develop the most severe type of illness during primary infection. Older children and adults, when they undergo reinfection, constitute the major source of infection for infants and young children. For this reason it would be desirable to develop immunoprophylactic procedures for the prevention of such reinfection and thus decrease the level of virus in the community.

RESPIRATORY SYNCYTIAL VIRUS

DEFINITION

Respiratory syncytial virus is a medium-sized (120 to 300 mμ) ether-sensitive virus which has helical symmetry and contains RNA as its genetic material. Its fine structure resembles that of the parainfluenza, mumps, and measles viruses. Although RS virus has not been shown to hemagglutinate nor grow in the embryonated hen's egg, its biophysical properties indicate that it should be grouped together with the paramyxoviruses.

The virus was first recovered in 1955 from a chimpanzee with "common cold"–like illness during an outbreak of such disease in a group of laboratory chimpanzees. Shortly thereafter it was recovered from a child with pneumonia and a child with croup. At this time its characteristic syncytial cytopathic effect in tissue culture was first noted. Initially the virus was named the chimpanzee coryza agent (CCA). Subsequently, the name respiratory syncytial virus, descriptive of its association with respiratory disease and of its cytopathic effect in tissue culture, was proposed and generally accepted. During the past 12 years this virus was shown to play an important role in severe lower respiratory tract illness of infancy and childhood in many parts of the world. In fact, it now appears to be the single most important viral respiratory pathogen of infancy.

PROPERTIES

Virus particles negatively stained with phosphotungstic acid have a diameter of 120 to 300 mμ. The general organization of the negatively stained virus is similar to that of the parainfluenza and Newcastle disease viruses, i.e., a coiled inner component surrounded by a spike-armed envelope. The inner helical component is approximately the same width as the inner helix of the parainfluenza viruses. Both viral filaments and spheres develop at the surface of the infected cell, but are not demonstrable within the cell itself.

The density of the virus in sucrose is 1.18 to 1.19 and in cesium chloride 1.23. The chemical nature of the inner component has not been determined by direct analysis; however, failure of FUDR and IUDR to inhibit virus replication suggests that it is ribonucleic acid.

RS virus is very unstable at temperatures of 37° C. and above. In addition, approximately 90 per cent of infectivity is lost following slow freezing. The virus is stable, however, when it is rapidly frozen and then stored at −70° C. RS virus is rapidly inactivated at pH 3.0. Infectivity is also completely destroyed by exposure to 20 per cent ether for 18 hours at 4° C.

Unlike the parainfluenza viruses, RS virus has not been grown in the embryonated hen's egg nor has hemagglutination or hemadsorption been demonstrated.

Using the immunofluorescence technique, virus-specific antigen(s) can be visualized in the cytoplasm but not the nucleus of infected cells. Such antigen is first detectable ten hours following infection, the time when newly formed virus is first demonstrable. Electron microscopic studies indicate that final assembly of the virus occurs at the host cell membrane. Consistent with this view is the finding that large amounts of virus-specific antigen can be visualized at the cell membrane of unfixed infected cells studied by immunofluorescence.

Prominent introcytoplasmic eosinophilic inclusions are usually found in infected human heteroploid tissue culture cells. These inclusions are characteristically surrounded by a clear zone and are more numerous in syncytia than in single cells.

EPIDEMIOLOGY

Two findings indicate that RS virus causes respiratory tract disease in man. First, in epidemiological studies the virus has been recovered significantly more often from infants, children, or adults with respiratory disease than comparable individuals free of such illness. Second, the virus has produced upper respiratory tract disease when administered to adult volunteers. RS virus can cause respiratory disease without the cooperative action of pathogenic bacteria; the frequency of pathogenic bacteria in the nasopharynx of patients with RS virus lower respiratory tract illness does not differ significantly from that of comparable healthy individuals.

RS virus is most important as a respiratory tract pathogen during the first half year of life. In addition, the most serious RS illnesses occur in early infancy. In a number of large urban populations the virus has been associated with 32 to 75 per cent of bronchiolitis illnesses and 9 to 39 per cent of pneumonia illnesses of infancy and childhood. These types of illness are often life threatening. RS virus also has been associated with other types of acute febrile respiratory disease, i.e., bronchitis and pharyngitis, during infancy and childhood. RS virus illness in adults is usually mild, afebrile, and limited to the upper respiratory tract.

RS virus has a wide geographic distribution. It has been recovered in most countries where the appropriate tissue culture techniques have been used to study respiratory disease in infants and young children.

Primary infection occurs early in life, usually before two to four years of age. Characteristically, in large urban populations RS virus produces yearly epidemics of infection among infants and small children. In this behavior it differs from the other respiratory tract myxovirus pathogens which become epidemic every two to four years (influenza A and influenza B viruses) or exhibit a mixed endemic-epidemic pattern (paranfluenza viruses). RS virus epidemics are sharply circumscribed, generally last three to five months, and are quite extensive. The epidemics may occur in the fall, winter, or spring but never in the summer.

Coincident with each of the yearly RS virus epidemics there is a marked increase in lower respiratory tract disease in infants and young children. This temporal association is most striking for bronchiolitis and bronchopneumonia in infants six months of age or less. During months of RS virus prevalence mean monthly admissions of young infants to the hospital for these conditions are often six times or more greater than during periods when the virus is quiescent in the community.

RS virus spreads rapidly and effectively from person to person. This is particularly evident during outbreaks of infection in semiclosed populations of infants and young children. During such outbreaks essentially all infants and children who lack serum neutralizing antibody become infected within a two- to three-week period. The incubation period from exposure to onset of illness is approximately four to five days.

PHYSIOPATHOLOGY

The effect of RS virus upon the host ranges from inapparent infection to severe respiratory tract disease such as bronchiolitis or pneumonia. Response to infection is influenced by age and immunological status. Bronchiolitis or pneumonia caused by RS virus occurs in most instances during the first year of life.

Several findings suggest that an immunological reaction may play an important role in the pathogenesis of RS virus lower respiratory tract disease. First, serum neutralizing antibody is quantitatively transferred from the mother to the infant. Such transplacentally transmitted antibody is present at a detectable level in the infant's serum until six to eight months of age. Second, neutralizing antibody is present in serum at the onset of most RS virus lower respiratory tract illness which occurs during the first six months of life. Third, RS virus bronchiolitis or pneumonia occurs most commonly during the first four months of life and thereafter decreases in incidence in an inverse fashion with increasing age. Based upon these considerations it has been suggested that passively acquired serum neutralizing antibody may be an important ingredient in the genesis of RS virus bronchiolitis of infancy.

Initially in RS virus infection there is involvement and inflammation of the mucous membranes of the nose and throat. Paranasal and eustachian tube obstruction may also occur. In a significant proportion of infections in early infancy and in a minority of instances in later life there is extension of the inflammatory process into the trachea, bronchi, bronchioles, and the parenchyma of the lung. In young infants there is a tendency for necrotizing bronchiolitis and pneumonitis to occur. Bronchiolar obstruction results in focal areas of atelectasis or emphysema. The clinical picture may be dominated by obstructive bronchiolitis, pneumonitis, or a combination of the two patterns. Inflammation and edema of the larynx may occur, but this condition is less frequently observed than bronchiolitis or pneumonia.

In fatal illnesses caused by RS virus the most prominent changes are necrotizing or interstitial pneumonitis, peribronchiolar lymphocytic infiltration, necrosis of tracheobronchiolar epithelium, atelectasis, and emphysema. Cytoplasmic inclusions may be present in affected areas of the lung.

IMMUNITY

Severe respiratory tract disease caused by RS virus generally occurs during infancy or early childhood. This pattern suggests that infection confers upon the host a relative resistance to subsequent severe RS virus illness. Although the basis for such resistance is not completely understood, it is probable that serum neutralizing antibody does not play a major role. In young infants it is possible to assess the protective effect of serum neutralizing antibody free of an effect of locally induced antibody in the respiratory tract. Maternal antibody is quantitatively transferred to the infant and persists at detectable levels until six to eight months of age. Since RS virus lower respiratory tract disease occurs most commonly during the first four months of life and then decreases in incidence with increasing age, it is clear that serum neutralizing antibody per se does not provide effective protection. If such antibody were protective one would observe a relative deficit of RS virus–induced illness during the first few months of life when maternally transmitted antibody is at its highest level.

First infection with RS virus does not

appear to provide complete protection against the effects of a second infection occurring within one to three years. Young children with low to moderate levels of serum neutralizing antibody frequently develop lower respiratory tract involvement during re-infection.

RS virus infection and associated upper respiratory tract disease occur under natural conditions in adults despite the presence of moderate to high levels of serum neutralizing antibody. Similarly, adult volunteers given RS virus become infected and develop mild illness although antibody is present in serum.

One can only speculate about the capacity of RS virus to successfully evade the host's resistance mechanisms and to produce significant illness during reinfection. RS virus characteristically induces formation of syncytia in tissue culture. This property, plus the fact that the virus enters the body, infects, and produces its pathogenic effect in the same tissue, i.e., the respiratory tract epithelium, suggests a basis for its successful evasion of host defense mechanisms. Direct attack upon respiratory tract epithelium minimizes the protective role of serum neutralizing antibody, while syncytium formation permits incorporation of uninfected cells into the disease process under conditions which minimize the effectiveness of serum or locally produced antibody in halting extension of infection and tissue damage.

LABORATORY STUDIES

RS virus grows in a variety of primary, diploid, and heteroploid human cell cultures. Considerable differences in sensitivity to RS virus exist among various sublines of heteroploid cells. The virus also grows in primary simian and bovine kidney cultures. Characteristically, syncytial areas develop in infected cell culture; however, the extent of this type of change is influenced by the virus strain, the tissue culture medium, and the host cell. In addition to syncytium formation a variable proportion of affected cells round up and degenerate singly without fusing with other cells in the monolayer.

Generally titration end-points for tissue culture–adapted strains of RS virus in human heteroploid cell cultures are reached within five to 12 days. Infectivity can be measured in Petri dish cultures of human heteroploid or diploid fibroblast cells by plaque assay or in roller tube cultures using cytopathic effect as the criterion of infection. With tissue culture–adapted RS strains new infectious virus is first detected ten to 12 hours following infection of human heteroploid (HEp-2) cells, whereas syncytia do not develop until ten to 24 hours later.

A number of species of animals can be experimentally infected with RS virus. These include chimpanzees, baboons, monkeys, ferrets, mink, chinchillas, guinea pigs, hamsters, and mice. Only the chimpanzee exhibits signs of illness. In chimpanzees, RS virus–induced disease is mild, unassociated with fever, and limited to the upper respiratory tract.

During asymptomatic infection of the hamster RS virus grows to high titer in the lung. In the ferret virus grows poorly in the lungs but multiplies to a high titer in the nasal turbinates. In addition, multinucleated cells containing eosinophilic cytoplasmic inclusion bodies form in the respiratory epithelium of infected ferrets.

RS virus is unrelated antigenically to other myxoviruses. Specific antigen(s) is present on the envelope of the RS virion, since the virus reacts in a specific manner when tested by the neutralization technique. Gel diffusion studies indicate that at least three diffusible antigens are formed in RS-infected cells. The relationship of these antigens to the subunits which make up the virus is not known.

Two serologically distinct complement-fixing antigens have been identified in infected tissue culture suspensions: antigen A and antigen B. These antigens are associated with the virion and are also found in a soluble form, i.e., not sedimentable at $78,000 \times g$. Antigen A and antigen B possess different biophysical properties and can be separated by chromatography or isopycnic centrifugation. Both antigens elicit the development of complement-fixing antibodies in inoculated animals; however, only antigen A stimulates the development of neutralizing antibody. The latter finding suggests that antigen A occupies a surface position on the virion.

At least four RS virus serotypes can be distinguished by tissue culture neutralization; however, the total extent of antigenic variation is not known since only a limited number of strains have been studied. The four serotypes share a common soluble complement-fixing antigen, but they differ from each other in a reciprocal fashion in neutralization tests with post-infection ferret sera. Differences among serotypes are minimal, however, when such strains are compared using paired sera from infants with primary RS infection. It is not known why infants develop a broader antibody response than ferrets. It has been suggested that this difference reflects the extent of infection in the two hosts—extensive in the infant and limited to the upper respiratory passages in the ferret.

LABORATORY DIAGNOSIS

Diagnosis of RS infection can be made by virus isolation and/or demonstration of a rise in antibody during convalescence. Virus is present in the nasal and pharyngeal secretions of infected individuals and can be isolated with greatest efficiency when specimens are inoculated directly into cell cultures without prior freezing. It is possible, however, to isolate a large proportion of strains from frozen specimens when veal infusion broth with 0.5 per cent bovine albumin is used as the collecting medium.

Human heteroploid cell cultures (HeLa, HEp-2, etc.) represent the most sensitive host systems for recovery of natural virus. Characteristic syncytial cytopathic changes develop three to 14 days after inoculation of clinical specimens containing RS virus. Since sublines of HeLa and HEp-2 differ considerably in sensitivity to RS virus, it is essential that cultures of a sensitive subline be used in virus isolation attempts. Primary human embryonic kidney and human diploid fibroblast cultures can also be used for virus isolation.

Isolates are most easily identified by complement fixation using serum obtained following infection of ferrets or guinea pigs. Subsequently, strains can be separated into distinct serotypes by tissue culture neutralization using highly specific animal sera.

Except in early infancy complement fixation and tissue culture neutralization are relatively efficient (80 to 90 per cent) serological procedures for diagnosis of RS infection. Infants less than seven months of age develop neutralizing and complement-fixing antibodies less often following RS infection than do older individuals. In addition, a greater concentration of antigen is required for detection of complement-fixing antibodies during early life. In young infants infection is most accurately determined by virus isolation.

PROBLEMS OF PROPHYLAXIS

At present specific control measures are not available; however, experimental inactivated vaccines have been prepared which stimulate the development of serum neutralizing antibody in young infants. Since serum antibody may play a role in the pathogenesis of RS virus bronchiolitis in early infancy, consideration should be given to the development of a method of immunization which would stimulate the development of neutralizing antibodies in the respiratory tract secretions. Possibly, this could be achieved either by an attenuated strain of virus or a large quantity of highly purified inactivated viral antigen given intranasally.

BIBLIOGRAPHY

PARAINFLUENZA VIRUSES

1. Abinanti, F. R., Chanock, R. M., Cook, M. K., Wong, D., and Warfield, M.: Relationship of human and bovine strains of myxovirus parainfluenza 3 (26371). Proc. Soc. Exp. Biol. Med., *106*:466-469, 1961.
2. Banatvala, J. E., Anderson, T. B., and Reiss, B. V.: Parainfluenza infections in the community. Brit. Med. J., *1*:537-540, 1964.
3. Beale, A. J., McLeod, D. L., Stackiw, W., and Rhodes, A. J.: Isolation of cytopathogenic agents from the respiratory tract in acute laryngotracheobronchitis. Brit. Med. J., *1*:302-303, 1958.
4. Bloom, H. H., Johnson, K. M., Jacobsen, R., and Chanock, R. M.: Recovery of parainfluenza viruses from adults with upper respiratory illness. Amer. J. Hyg., *74*:50-59, 1961.
5. Brandt, C. D.: Cytopathic action of myxoviruses on cultivated mammalian cells. Virology, *14*:1-10, 1961.
6. Bukrinskaya, A. G., and Blyumental, K. V.: The role of parainfluenza viruses in etiology of false croup. Vop. Virus, 7:567-572, 1962.
7. Bukrinskaya, A. G., and Zhdanov, V. M.: Shortening by actinomycin D of latent period of multiplication of Sendai virus. Nature, *200*:920-921, 1963.
8. Canchola, J., Vargosko, A. J., Kim, H. W., Parrott, R. H., Christmas, E., Jeffries, B., and Chanock, R. M.: Antigenic variation among newly isolated strains of parainfluenza type 4 virus. Amer. J. Hyg., *79*:357-364, 1964.
9. Chanock, R. M.: Association of a new type of cytopathogenic myxovirus with infantile croup. J. Exp. Med., *104*:555-576, 1956.
10. Chanock, R. M., Bell, J. A., and Parrott, R. H.: Natural history of parainfluenza infection. In: Pollard, M. (ed.): Perspectives in Virology. Minneapolis, Burgess Publishing Co., 1961, Vol. 2, pp. 126-138.
11. Chanock. R. M., Johnson, K. M., Cook, M. K.,

Wong, D. C., and Vargosko, A.: The hemadsorption technique, with special reference to the problem of naturally occurring simian parainfluenza virus. Amer. Rev. Resp. Dis., *83*:125-129, 1961.

12. Chanock, R. M., Parrott, R. H., Cook, M. K., Andrews, B. E., Bell, J. A., Reichelderfer, T., Kapikian, A. Z., Mastrota, F. M., and Huebner, R. J.: Newly recognized myxoviruses from children with respiratory disease. New Eng. J. Med., *258*:207-213, 1958.

13. Chanock, R. M., Parrott, R. H., Johnson, K. M., Kapikian, A. Z., and Bell, J. A.: Myxoviruses: Parainfluenza. Amer. Rev. Resp. Dis., *88*:152-166, 1963.

14. Chanock, R. M., Smith, C. B., Friedewald, W. T., Parrott, R. H., Forsyth, B. R., Coates, H. V., Kapikian, A. Z., and Gharpure, M. A.: Resistance to parainfluenza and respiratory syncytial virus infection – implications for effective immunization and preliminary study of an attenuated strain of respiratory syncytial virus. Pan American Health Organization, International Conference on Vaccines. *In*: First International Conference on Vaccines against Viral and Rickettsial Diseases of Man. Washington, D.C., Pan American Health Organization, 1967, sci. pub. 147, pp. 53-61.

15. Chanock, R. M., Wong, D. C., Huebner, R. J., and Bell, J. A.: Serologic response of individuals infected with parainfluenza viruses. Amer. J. Public Health, *50*:1858-1865, 1960.

16. Chany, C., and Cook, M. K.: Sur un facteur induit par le virus entrainant la formation de syncytium en culture cellulaire. Ann. Inst. Pasteur, *98*:920-924, 1960.

17. Chany, C., Robbe-Fossat, F., and Couvreur, J.: Enquête sérologique sur le rôle épidémiologique d'un virus respiratoire nouvellement reconnu: souche EA 102 des myxovirus parinfluenzae type 3. Bull. Acad. Nat. Med. (Paris), *143*:106-110, 1959.

18. Choppin, P. W., and Stoeckenius, W.: The morphology of SV virus. Virology, *23*:195-202, 1964.

19. Compans, R. W., Holmes, K. V., Dales, S., and Choppin, P. W.: An electron microscopic study of moderate and virulent virus-cell interactions of the parainfluenza virus SV5, Virology, *30*:411-426, 1966.

20. Cook, M. K., Andrews, B. E., Fox, H. H., Turner, H. C., James, W. D., and Chanock, R. M.: Antigenic relationships among the "newer" myxoviruses (parainfluenza). Amer. J. Hyg., *69*:250-264, 1959.

21. Cook, M. K., and Chanock, R. M.: In vivo antigenic studies of parainfluenza viruses. Amer. J. Hyg., *77*:150-159, 1963.

22. Craighead, J. E., Cook, M. K., and Chanock, R. M.: Infection of hamsters with parainfluenza 3 virus. Proc. Soc. Exp. Biol. Med., *104*:301-304, 1960.

23. DeMeio, J. L.: Adaptation of parainfluenza 2 (croup-associated) virus to the embryonated hen's egg. J. Bact., *85*:943-944, 1963.

24. DeMeio, J. L., and Walker, D. L.: Demonstration of antigenic relationship between mumps virus and hemagglutinating virus of Japan. J. Immunol., *78*:465-471, 1957.

25. Demont, G., Berkaloff, A., and Colobert, L.: Cytological manifestations of the infection of KB cells with parainfluenza 1 myxovirus (Sendai virus). Ann. Inst. Pasteur, *104*:26-42, 1963.

26. Fukumi, H., Nishikawa, F., and Kitayama, T.: A pneumotropic virus from mice causing hemagglutination. Jap. J. Med. Sci. Biol., *7*:345-363, 1954.

27. Fukumi, H., Nishikawa, F., and Sugiyama, T.: An epidemic due to HA2 virus in an elementary school in Tokyo. Jap. J. Med. Sci. Biol., *12*:307-317, 1959.

28. Hamparian, V. V., Hilleman, M. R., and Ketler, A.: Contributions to characterization and classification of animal viruses. Proc. Soc. Exp. Biol. Med., *112*:1040-1050, 1963.

29. Hermodsson, S.: Effect of ultrasonic vibration on the haemagglutinating activity of some parainfluenza viruses. Nature, *188*:1214, 1960.

30. Holmes, K. V., and Choppin, P. W.: On the role of the response of the cell membrane in determining virus virulence. J. Exp. Med., *124*:501-520, 1966.

31. Horne, R. W., and Waterson, A. P.: A helical structure in mumps, Newcastle disease and Sendai viruses. J. Molec. Biol., *2*:75-77, 1960.

32. Hosaka, T., Hosokawa, Y., and Fukai, K.: A new device for preparing subunits of myxovirus. Biken J., *2*:367-370, 1959.

33. Hsiung, G. D., Isacson, P., and McCollum, R. W.: Studies of a myxovirus isolated from human blood. J. Immunol., *88*:284-290, 1962.

34. Hull, R. N., Minner, J. R., and Smith, J. W.: New viral agents recovered from tissue cultures of monkey kidney cells. Amer. J. Hyg., *63*:204-215, 1956.

35. Jensen, K. E., Peller, B. E., and Dulworth, W. G.: Immunization against parainfluenza infections. Antigenicity of egg adapted types 1 and 3. J. Immunol., *89*:216-226, 1962.

36. Johnson, K. M., Chanock, R. M., Cook, M. K., and Huebner, R. J.: Studies of a new human hemadsorption virus. I. Isolation, properties and characterization. Amer. J. Hyg., *71*:81-92, 1960.

37. Kapikian, A. Z., Bell, J. A., Mastrota, F. M., Huebner, R. J., Wong, D. C., and Chanock, R. M.: An outbreak of parainfluenza 2 (croup-associated) virus infection. Association with acute undifferentiated febrile illness in children. J.A.M.A., *183*:324-330, 1963.

38. Kim, H. W., Canchola, J. G., Vargosko, A. J., Arrobio, J. O., DeMeio, J. L., and Parrott, R. H.: Immunogenicity of inactivated parainfluenza Type 1, Type 2, and Type 3 vaccines in infants. J.A.M.A., *196*:819-824, 1966.

39. Kim, H. W., Vargosko, A. J., Chanock, R. M., and Parrott, R. H.: Para-influenza 2 (CA) virus: etiologic association with croup. Pediatrics, *28*:614-621, 1961.

40. Kuroya, M., Ishida, N., and Shiratori, T.: Newborn virus pneumonitis (type Sendai). II. The isolation of a new virus possessing hemagglutinin activity. Yokohama M. Bull., *4*:217-233, 1953.

41. Lepine, P., Chany, C., Droz, B., and Robbe-Fossat, F.: Cytopathogenic effect of two newly recognized myxovirus strains: mechanism of syncytial formation. Ann. N.Y. Acad. Sci., *81*:62-72, 1959.

42. Lewis, F. A., Lehmann, N. I., and Ferris, A. A.: The haemadsorption viruses in laryngotracheobronchitis. Med. J. Aust., *48*:929-932, 1961.

43. Maassab, H. F., and Loh, P. C.: Fluorescent antibody studies in tissue culture of parainfluenza 3 infection (27371). Proc. Soc. Exp. Biol. Med., *109*:897-900, 1962.

44. McClelland, L., Hampil, B., Hamparian, V. V., Potash, L., Ketler, A., and Hilleman, M. R.: Laboratory and field investigations of bovine myxovirus parainfluenza 3 virus and vaccine. II. Development and appraisal of potency of SF-4 (shipping fever) virus vaccine. J. Immunol., *87*:134-138, 1961.

45. McLean, D. M., Bach, R. D., Larke, R. P. B., and McNaughton, G. A.: Myxoviruses associated with acute laryngotracheobronchitis in Toronto, 1962-63. Canad. Med. Ass. J., *80*:1257-1259, 1963.

46. Marston, R. Q., and Vaughan, E. R.: Parainfluenza 3 – assay and growth in tissue culture. Proc. Soc. Exp. Biol. Med., *104*:56-60, 1960.

47. Mogabgab, W. J., Dick, E. C., and Holmes, B.: Parainfluenza 2 (CA) virus in young adults. Amer. J. Hyg., *74*:304-310, 1961.

48. Neurath, A. R.: A component splitting diisopropyl fluorophosphate in Sendai and Newcastle disease virus preparations; its possible identity with haemolysin. Acta Virol. (Praha), *9*:25-33, 1965.

49. Parrott, R. H., Vargosko, A. J., Kim, H. W., Bell, J. A., and Chanock, R. M.: Acute respiratory diseases of viral etiology. III. Myxoviruses: parainfluenza. Amer. J. Public Health, *52*:907-917, 1962.

50. Parrott, R. H., Vargosko, A., Luckey, A., Kim, H. W., Cumming, C., and Chanock, R. M.: Clinical features of infection with hemadsorption viruses. New Eng. J. Med., *260*:731-738, 1959.

51. Potash, L., Tytell, A. A., Sweet, B. H., Machlowitz, R. A., Stokes, J., Jr., Weibel, R. E., Woodhour, A. F., and Hilleman, M. R.: Respiratory virus vaccines. I. Respiratory syncytial and parainfluenza virus vaccines. Amer. Rev. Resp. Dis., *93*:536-548, 1966.

52. Rabe, E. F.: Infectious croup: I. Etiology. Pediatrics, *2*:255-265, 1948.

53. Rebel, G., Fontanges, R., and Colobert, L.: Nature lipidique des substances responsables de l'activité hèmòlytique de myxovirus parainfluenzae 1 (virus Sendai), Ann. Inst. Pasteur, *102*:137-152, 1962.

54. Reichelderfer, T. E., Chanock, R. M., Craighead, J. E., Huebner, R. J., Turner, H. C., James, W., and Ward, T. G.: Infection of human volunteers with type 2 hemadsorption virus. Science, *128*:779-780, 1958.

55. Reisinger, R. C., Heddleston, K. L., and Manthei, C. A.: A myxovirus (SF-4) associated with shipping fever of cattle. J. Amer. Vet. Med. Ass., *135*:147-152, 1959.

56. Rott, R., Waterson, A. P., and Reda, I. M.: Characterization of "soluble" antigens derived from cells infected with Sendai and Newcastle disease viruses. Virology, *21*:663-665, 1963.

57. Sokol, F., Blaskovic, D., and Krizanova, O.: Subunits of myxoviruses. II. Properties of haemagglutinins of Newcastle disease, para-influenza 1 and mumps viruses. Acta Virol. (Praha), *5*:153-159, 1961.

58. Taylor-Robinson, D., and Bynoe, M. L.: Parainfluenza 2 virus infections in adult volunteers. J. Hyg. (Camb.), *61*:407-417, 1963.

59. Traver, M. I., Northrop, R. L., and Walker, D. L.: Site of intracellular antigen production by myxo-viruses. Proc. Soc. Exp. Biol. Med., *104*:268-273, 1960.

60. Tyrrell, D. A. J., Bynoe, M. L., Petersen, K. B., Sutton, R. N. P., and Pereira, M.: Inoculation of human volunteers with parainfluenza viruses types 1 and 3 (HA 2 and HA 1). Brit. Med. J., *2*:909-911, 1959.

61. Tytell, A. A., Torop, H. A., and McCarthy, F. J.: Plaque formation by myxovirus parainfluenza type 2 in grivet monkey kidney cells. Proc. Soc. Exp. Biol. Med., *108*:723-725, 1961.

62. Van der Veen, J., and Smeur, F. A. A. M.: Infections with parainfluenza viruses in children with respiratory illnesses in Holland. Amer. J. Hyg., *74*:326-331, 1961.

63. Waterson, A. P., and Hurrell, J. M. S.: The fine structure of the parainfluenza viruses. Arch. Ges. Virusforsch., *12*:138-142, 1962.

64. Waterson, A. P., Jensen, K. E., Tyrrell, D. A. J., and Horne, R. W.: The structure of parainfluenza 3 virus. Virology, *14*:374-378, 1961.

RESPIRATORY SYNCYTIAL VIRUS

65. Adams, J. M., Imagawa, D. T., and Zike, K.: Epidemic bronchiolitis and pneumonitis related to respiratory syncytial virus. J.A.M.A., *176*:1037-1039, 1961.

66. Armstrong, J. A., Pereira, H. G., and Valentine, R. C.: Morphology and development of respiratory syncytial virus in cell cultures. Nature, *196*:1179-1181, 1962.

67. Beem, M., Egerer, R., and Anderson, J.: Respiratory syncytial virus neutralizing antibodies in persons residing in Chicago, Illinois. Pediatrics, *34*:761-770, 1964.

68. Beem, M., Wright, F. H., Hamre, D., Egerer, R., and Oehme, M.: Association of the chimpanzee coryza agent with acute respiratory disease in children. New Eng. J. Med., *263*:523-530, 1960.

69. Beem, M., Wright, F. H., Fasan, D. M., Egerer, R., and Oehme, M.: Observations on the etiology of acute bronchiolotis in infants. J. Pediat., *61*:864-869, 1962.

70. Bennett, C. R., Jr., and Hamre, D.: Growth and serological characteristics of respiratory syncytial virus. J. Infect. Dis., *110*:8-16, 1962.

71. Berglund, B., Forssell, P., and Harvo-Noponen, M.: An outbreak among children of respiratory illness caused by respiratory syncytial virus. A serological and clinical study. Acta Paediat. Scand., *54*:519-525, 1965.

72. Chanock, R. M., and Finberg, L.: Recovery from infants with respiratory illness of a virus related to chimpanzee coryza agent (CCA). II. Epidemiologic aspects of infection in infants and young children. Amer. J. Hyg., *66*:291-300, 1957.

73. Chanock, R. M., Kim, H. W., Vargosko, A. J., Deleva, A., Johnson, K. M., Cumming, C., and Parrott, R. H.: Respiratory syncytial virus. I. Virus recovery and other observations during 1960 outbreak of bronchiolitis, pneumonia, and minor respiratory diseases in children. J.A.M.A., *176*:647-653, 1961.

74. Chanock, R. M., Parrott, R. H., Johnson, K. M., Mufson, M. A., and Knight, V.: Biology and ecology of two major lower respiratory tract pathogens – RS virus and Eaton PPLO. In:

Pollard, M. (ed.): Virology. Vol. 3. New York, Hoeber Division of Harper & Row, 1963.

75. Chanock, R. M., Parrott, R. H., Vargosko, A. J., Kapikian, A. Z., Knight, V., and Johnson, K. M.: Respiratory syncytial virus. Amer. J. Public Health, *52*:918-925, 1962.

76. Chanock, R. M., Roizman, B., and Myers, R.: Recovery from infants with respiratory illness of a virus related to chimpanzee coryza agent (CCA). I. Isolation, properties and characterization. Amer. J. Hyg., *66*:281-290, 1957.

77. Chanock, R. M., Smith, C. B., Friedewald, W. T., Parrott, R. H., Forsyth, B. R., Coates, H. V., Kapikian, A. Z., and Gharpure, M. A.: Resistance to parainfluenza and respiratory syncytial virus infection—implications for effective immunization and preliminary study of an attenuated strain of respiratory syncytial virus. Pan American Health Organization, International Conference on Vaccines. In press.

78. Coates, H. V., and Chanock, R. M.: Experimental infection with respiratory syncytial virus in several species of animals. Amer. J. Hyg., *76*: 302-312, 1962.

79. Coates, H. V., Forsyth, B. R., and Chanock, R. M.: Biophysical studies of respiratory syncytial virus. I. Density of respiratory syncytial virus and associated complement-fixing antigens in a cesium chloride density gradient. J. Bact., *91*: 1263-1269, 1966.

80. Coates, H. V., Kendrick, L., and Chanock, R. M.: Antigenic differences between two strains of respiratory syncytial virus (28221). Proc. Soc. Exp. Biol. Med., *112*:958-964, 1963.

81. Disney, M. E., Sandiford, B. R., Cragg, J., and Wolff, J.: Epidemic bronchiolitis in infants. Brit. Med. J., *1*:1407-1411, 1960.

82. Forbes, J. A., Bennett, N. McK., and Gray, N. J.: Epidemic bronchiolitis caused by a respiratory syncytial virus: clinical aspects. Med. J. Aust., *48*:933-935, 1961.

83. Forsyth, B. R., Coates, H. V., and Chanock, R. M.: Biophysical studies of respiratory syncytial virus. II. Identification of two soluble complement-fixing antigens of respiratory syncytial virus. J. Bact., *91*:1270-1276, 1966.

84. Freeman, G. L., and Todd, R. H.: The role of allergy in viral respiratory tract infections. Amer. J. Dis. Child., *104*:330-334, 1962.

85. Hamparian, V. V., Hilleman, M. R., and Ketler, A.: Contributions to characterization and classification of animal viruses. Proc. Soc. Exp. Biol. Med., *112*:1040-1050, 1963.

86. Hamre, D., and Procknow, J. J.: Viruses isolated from natural common colds in the United States. Brit. Med. J., *2*:1382-1385, 1961.

87. Holzel, A., Parker, L., Patterson, W. H., White, L. L. R., Thompson, K. M., and Tobin, J. O.: The isolation of respiratory syncytial virus from children with acute respiratory disease. Lancet, *1*:295-298, 1963.

88. Johnson, K. M., Bloom, H. H., Mufson, M. A., and Chanock, R. M.: Natural reinfection of adults by respiratory syncytial virus. Possible relation to mild upper respiratory disease. New Eng. J. Med., *267*:68-72, 1962.

89. Johnson, K. M., Chanock, R. M., Rifkind, D., Kravetz, H. M., and Knight, V.: Respiratory syncytial virus. IV. Correlation of virus shedding, serologic response, and illness in adult volunteers. J.A.M.A., *176*:663-667, 1961.

90. Jordan, W. S., Jr.: Growth characteristics of respiratory syncytial virus. J. Immunol., *88*:581-589, 1962.

91. Kapikian, A. Z., Bell, J. A., Mastrota, F. M., Johnson, K. M., Huebner, R. J., and Chanock, R. M.: An outbreak of febrile illness and pneumonia associated with respiratory syncytial virus infection. Amer. J. Hyg., *74*:234-248, 1961.

92. Kisch, A. L., and Johnson, K. M.: A plaque assay for respiratory syncytial virus (28111). Proc. Soc. Exp. Biol. Med., *112*:583-589, 1963.

93. Kisch, A. L., Johnson, K. M., and Chanock, R. M.: Immunofluorescence with respiratory syncytial virus. Virology, *16*:177-189, 1962.

94. Kravetz, H. M., Knight, V., Chanock, R. M., Morris, J. A., Johnson, K. M., Rifkind, D., and Utz, J. P.: Respiratory syncytial virus. III. Production of illness and clinical observations in adult volunteers. J.A.M.A., *176*:657-663, 1961.

95. Lewis, F. A., Rae, M. L., Lehmann, N. I., and Ferris, A. A.: A syncytial virus associated with epidemic disease of the lower respiratory tract in infants and young children. Med. J. Aust., *48*: 932-933, 1961.

96. McClelland, L., Hilleman, M. R., Hamparian, V. V., Ketler, A., Reilly, C. M., Cornfeld, D., and Stokes, J., Jr.: Studies of acute respiratory illnesses caused by respiratory syncytial virus. 2. Epidemiology and assessment of importance. New Eng. J. Med., *264*:1169-1175, 1961.

97. Morris, J. A., Blount, R. E., Jr., and Savage, R. E.: Recovery of cytopathogenic agent from chimpanzees with coryza (22538). Proc. Soc. Exp. Biol. Med., *92*:544-549, 1956.

98. Moss, P. D., Adams, M. O., and Tobin, J. O.: Serological studies with respiratory syncytial virus. Lancet, *1*:298-300, 1963.

99. Parrott, R. H., Vargosko, A. J., Kim, H. W., Cumming, C., Turner, H., Huebner, R. J., and Chanock, R. M.: Respiratory syncytial virus. II. Serologic studies over a 34-month period of children with bronchiolitis, pneumonia, and minor respiratory diseases. J.A.M.A., *176*:653-657, 1961.

100. Sandiford, B. R., and Spencer, B.: Respiratory syncytial virus in epidemic bronchiolitis of infants. Brit. Med. J., *2*:881-882, 1962.

101. Tyrrell, D. A. J.: Discovering and defining the etiology of acute respiratory viral disease. Amer. Rev. Resp. Dis., *88*:77-84, 1963.

102. Waterson, A. P., and Hobson, D.: Relationship between respiratory syncytial virus and Newcastle disease—parainfluenza group. Brit. Med. J., *2*:1166-1167, 1962.

ADENOVIRUSES

by B. FERIGNAC AND C. CHANY

INTRODUCTION

Adenoviruses were discovered as a result of the application of tissue culture techniques to virology. In 1953, Rowe et al.[58] observed that explants of adenoid tissues maintained in vitro degenerated "spontaneously." They showed that this degeneration was due to the presence in their explant cultures of a latent virus.

Similar viruses were subsequently isolated from pharyngeal secretions and from fecal material in the course of epidemics of acute respiratory tract infections.[26] These viruses were called adenoviruses[15] mainly on the basis of historical considerations. The ease with which these viruses were isolated and the use of serological methods permitted their subsequent grouping and identification. Epidemiological studies based on serological techniques established the causal relationship between infections with these viruses and the various clinical manifestations observed in patients.

The difficulty of interpreting only epidemiological data remains linked to the absence of clinical manifestations specific for adenovirus infection and to the large number of inapparent infections.

In 1953 Hilleman and Werner isolated adenoviruses from young recruits in military camps during epidemics of respiratory disease.

Neva and Enders[47] recovered similar viruses from children with mild febrile diseases associated with conjunctivitis and a morbilliform eruption. Lastly, in 1957, Lelong et al.[39] described a pneumoencephalitis due to adenovirus infection and identified the pathological lesions. A parallel study was undertaken of various physiochemical and biological properties of adenoviruses. The specific cytological lesions induced by these viruses in vitro were described by Barski and Cornefert[4] and by Lépine et al.[41] Our knowledge of the structure of the virion has benefited from advances in the techniques of electron microscopy.[27, 46] The different antigenic components of the virion have been investigated by Ginsberg,[18] Pereira,[50] and Pereira and Valentine.[53] Hemagglutination by adenoviruses was described by Rosen.[55] More recently, Trentin has demonstrated the oncogenicity of adenovirus type 12 for the hamster. This observation was promptly confirmed and extended to other adenovirus types by several other investigators.[64, 71, 72] So far the oncogenic nature of adenoviruses has been demonstrated only in the animal. The virus-induced tumors do not contain virions or structural viral antigens.[42] These tumor cells do, however, contain a complement-fixing antigen. This antigen was named T (for tumor) antigen by Huebner et al.[31] The T antigen, which was discovered in connection with adenoviruses, has also been found in cells infected with other oncogenic viruses. It is therefore of considerable importance, since it permits the identification of the transformation-inducing agent in non-virus-producing cells.

STRUCTURE OF THE VIRION

Electron microscopic examination of ultrathin sections reveals the presence within

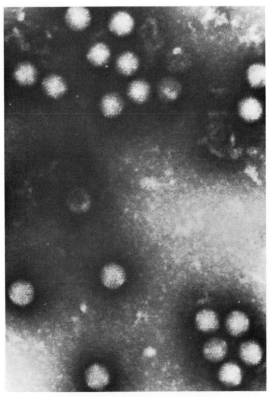

Figure 44-2. Adenovirus 7 with negative staining. Cubic symmetry and icosahedral structure of the capsid with capsomeres. (× 200,000.) (Courtesy of Dr. N. Granboulan.)

the cell of spherical virions with a diameter of 60 to 80 mμ. By x-ray diffraction techniques, chemical analysis, and electron microscopy (negative staining) the virion is shown to have an icosahedral structure.[27, 46] An icosahedron is a polyhedron with 20 equilateral triangular faces, 30 edges, and 12 apices. When the axis of symmetry passes through the apices five successive similar images are observed, and when the axis of symmetry passes through the centers of the faces there are three similar images. When the virion is rotated on an axis of symmetry which passes through the edges, two similar images are observed. Thus the polyhedron has a five, three, two cubic symmetry.

The capsid of the virion is antigenic and comprised of proteins. It is divided into 252 capsomeres. Pereira and Valentine[53] showed the presence on the 12 apical capsomeres of a filament with a terminal enlargement. This filament represents the hemagglutinin. The virion is not enclosed in an envelope. The genetic material of adenoviruses is deoxyribonucleic acid (DNA). The DNA molecule can be visualized under the electron microscope after rupture of the virion by osmotic shock by the Kleinschmidt technique.

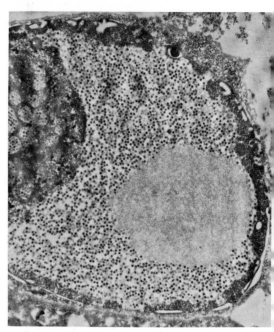

Figure 44-4. Adenovirus 5 in the nucleus of a KB cell. Protein crystal. ($\times$ 18,000.) (Courtesy of Dr. N. Granboulan.)

Studies using light microscopy and electron microscopy clearly demonstrate that synthesis of virions occurs exclusively in the nucleus. The viral particles are aligned therein in crystalline array.[35] The nuclei of infected cells also contain clearly visible proteins, especially in the case of adenovirus 5, which form eosinophilic crystals under the light microscope.[44]

ANTIGENIC CONSTITUTION

By chromatography on DEAE-cellulose, three distinct soluble antigens, A, B, and C, were isolated from adenovirus-infected cells.[37]

A antigen is group specific, whereas C antigen is type specific.

B antigen contains the "cell-detaching factor" responsible for the early detachment of infected cells from the cultures flasks. The fractions corresponding to the B and C antigens possess hemagglutinating activity. Examination of the different fractions by electron microscopy has revealed that the A antigen contains the basic capsid structure: the capsomeres of the faces, numbering 240. They are called hexons because they are surrounded by six others. As previously mentioned, the 12 apical capsomeres are prolonged by a fiber which constitutes the hemag-

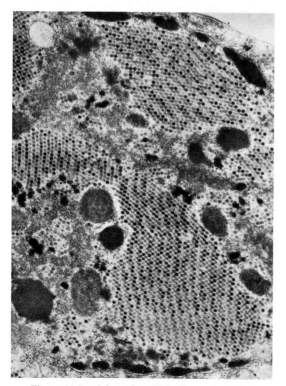

Figure 44-3. Adenovirus 12 in the nucleus of a KB cell. Pseudo-crystalline arrangements. ($\times$ 40,000.) (Courtesy of Dr. N. Granboulan.)

glutinin. Each of the capsomeres is surrounded by five others and is therefore called a penton. These pentons contain the B antigen. C antigen represents the filament originating at the pentons and as stated above possesses the hemagglutinating properties.[20]

PHYSIOCHEMICAL PROPERTIES

For practical reasons it is important to determine the sensitivity of adenoviruses to inactivation by various chemical means (antiseptics, pH) and physical agents. Adenoviruses have no lipid envelope and are therefore resistant to ether.[32] They are also resistant to chloroform and to deoxycholate. Virus type 3 is inactivated by hypochlorite.[12] Type 1 is rapidly inactivated by 1 M nitrous acid at pH 4.4 to 4.8. Types 4 to 20 are resistant to inactivation under the same conditions. The infectivity of the virus is destroyed by ultraviolet irradiation. However, marked differences in the sensitivity to ultraviolet irradiation have been noted among the various types of adenoviruses.[69] By placing the virus suspension in a thin layer in a Petri dish 68 cm. from a lamp of 11 ergs per square millimeter per second, Wassermann obtained complete inactivation in 30 minutes. In spite of initial variations in the inactivation curves it was found that the inactivation slope of all these curves was essentially the same.

Adenoviruses are resistant to fairly large variations of pH and temperature. While infectivity is destroyed by heating from five minutes to two and a half hours at 56° C., a temperature of 36° C. for seven days or of 22° C. for 14 days does not cause any significant loss of infectivity for adenovirus types 1 to 4.

Adenoviruses types 1 to 4 retain their maximal infectivity at pH 6 to 9.5 at room temperature. All these viruses are less stable, however, at an alkaline pH than at an acid pH. Thus, viral suspensions kept for 30 minutes at room temperature at a pH of 1.5 to 2.5 still retain some infectivity. At the same temperature, complete inactivation occurs in 30 minutes at a pH of 10.[19]

VIRAL MULTIPLICATION

Adenoviruses multiply in vitro in cells of human origin, which may be primary explants (amnion, thyroid, kidney) or continuous cell lines of cancerous origin (HeLa or KB cells). The cells of choice for culturing these viruses are human embryo kidney cells.

CYTOPATHIC EFFECT

Fresh Preparations. Early lesions can be observed two to three hours after inoculation of the cultures. These are characterized by retraction of the cell sheet and its separation from the glass surface. The extent of this effect varies according to the type of adenovirus and the size of the inoculum. As previously mentioned, this effect is due to a viral protein (cell-detaching factor), which forms part of the B antigen.

The characteristic intranuclear lesion, which is related to multiplication of the virus, is clearly visible only at the end of the infectious cycle. Under low magnification, small foci of cell destruction are observed, which soon spread throughout the whole cell sheet. This is accompanied by the cell retraction phenomena described above.

Preparations Fixed and Stained with Hemalum-Eosin. Characteristic lesions are observed in the cell nuclei.[4, 41] The differences in the appearance of the lesions can to some extent distinguish the type of adenovirus involved.

First, small crystals of eosinophilic protein appear. The nucleus then becomes progressively filled with Feulgen-positive basophilic material which seems to leave the nucleolus intact. When the lesions have reached an advanced stage, the nucleus is globular, deformed, and contains a central basophilic inclusion surrounded by a clear vesicular zone. Actually, these vesicular lesions are fixation artefacts, but their characteristic appearance is useful for establishing the diagnosis.

With types 1, 2, 5, and 6, retraction is considerable and the vesicles are distributed irregularly over the surface of the nucleus. The protein crystals are particularly clear in the case of adenovirus 5.[45]

In types 3, 4, and 7 retraction is slight and the vesicles are distributed regularly around the periphery of the inclusion.

MULTIPLICATION CYCLE

The length of the multiplication cycle averages 30 hours. At the end of four to six hours maximal absorption has taken place. The virus penetrates into the host cell by

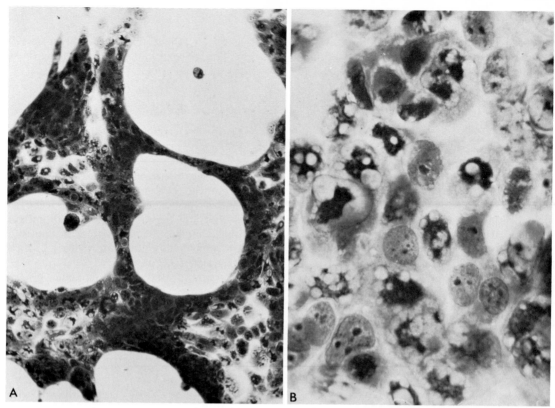

Figure 44-5. Adenovirus type 2 in HeLa cells: *A*, considerable retraction of the culture (× 18); *B*, intranuclear basophilic mass and vesicles irregularly distributed at the surface of the nucleus (× 600).

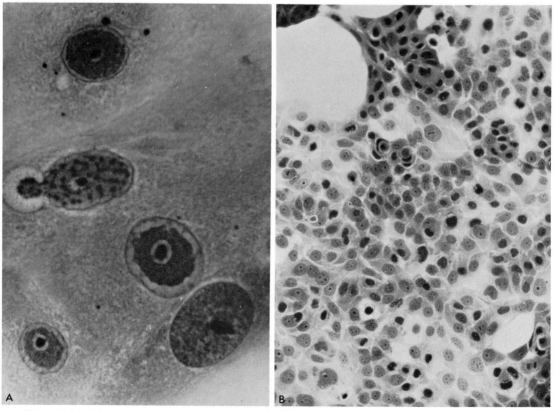

Figure 44-6. Adenovirus type 7: *A*, slight retraction (× 18); *B*, intranuclear basophilic mass which apparently does not affect the nucleolus — vesicles distributed regularly around the inclusion (× 600).

pinocytosis.[13] After penetration, the virus accumulates in vesicles enclosed in a membrane of cellular origin. After penetration into the cell, the viral particle loses its capsid. The nucleic acid released from the virus induces the synthesis of all the viral components. The synthesis of a precursor of viral DNA begins ten hours after infection.[10] Intimately related to this synthesis is the synthesis of specific viral antigens two to three hours later.

Lastly, infectious viral particles appear four to six hours after the onset of DNA synthesis and two to three hours after synthesis of viral antigen.[16] The virions synthesized within the nucleus are released with difficulty, which explains the long delay (minimum of 14 days) before plaques begin to appear on monkey kidney cells. Kjellén obtained a mutant of adenovirus 5 which produces plaques in five to six days on HeLa cells.

DIAGNOSIS

The number and variety of respiratory viruses preclude the possibility of a clinical diagnosis without the aid of the laboratory, since various clinical manifestations may be associated with several viruses, and a wide variety of clinical signs may be associated with a given virus. Samples are obtained from the rhinopharynx, the conjunctiva, and the anus by means of a swab. The swab is immediately immersed in a nutrient medium, squeezed, and discarded. The virus can also be detected in the urine, in the blood,[25] and in lymph nodes by tissue culture. It has been isolated from fragments of various organs, particularly lung tissue. Postmortem specimens should be procured as early as possible to avoid bacterial contamination and destruction of the virus due to liberation of proteolytic enzymes from the tissues.

Early sampling is an important diagnostic element. It has been shown that throat samples obtained during the first day of illness gave 86 to 100 per cent positive results, whereas when the samples were obtained on the sixth to tenth day of illness the proportion dropped to only 15 per cent.[36] The virus is frequently isolated from the stools during the first two weeks and can be found until the third or fourth week. The samples can be stored in the transport medium at $-20°$ C. or lower.

Human epithelial cells are the most sensitive to cytopathogenic effect of the virus. In some instances this effect is slow to appear and cultures should therefore be kept for at least 30 days. It may at times be useful to perform "blind" transfers toward the tenth to twentieth day.[24] In some instances adenoviruses may be associated with other viruses, and the simultaneous multiplication of adenoviruses and myxovirus parainfluenzae[68] and of adenoviruses and poliovirus[9] has been reported. Identification after isolation consists in three successive steps: study of the cytopathogenic effect, diagnosis of the adenovirus group, identification of the serotype.

The presence of characteristic cellular lesions suggests the diagnosis of adenoviruses, and this diagnosis can be subsequently confirmed by serological tests. The next step is to look for the soluble group antigen. This antigen is obtained from cells infected by one of the adenoviruses, the virions being eliminated by ultracentrifugation. A standard immune serum of human or animal origin is used as reference. The serotype remains to be identified. As 30 human serotypes have been described,[51, 57] it is usually too long and costly to attempt to identify the virus by the neutralization reaction for all the known types. The differences observed in nuclear lesions produced by types 1, 2, and 5 and by types 3, 4, and 7 can be used as guides. It is preferable to determine in the first place the hemagglutinating properties of the virus[55] and to determine the type by inhibition of hemagglutination.

Adenoviruses have been divided into four subgroups: (1) those which agglutinate monkey erythrocytes (3, 7, 11, 14, 16, 20, 21, 25, 28); (2) those which agglutinate rat erythrocytes (8, 9, 10, 13, 15, 17, 19, 22, 23, 24); (3) those which agglutinate rat erythrocytes in presence of heterotypic human serum (1, 2, 4, 5, 6); and (4) serotypes 12, 18, and 31, which do not seem to cause hemagglutination. It has now been shown that these serotypes behave like those of the third group but that hemagglutination is always weak.

When the subgroup has been determined, identification is continued by the hemagglutination-inhibition test. This test is carried out with the erythrocytes utilized in the determination of the subgroup. The reference immune serum is prepared in the rabbit or the horse. It must be preabsorbed before use by kaolin and the red cells utilized. The hemagglutination inhibition test is carried out at room temperature. Cross reactions between the various serotypes have been observed.

SEROLOGICAL DIAGNOSIS

Serological tests have a twofold interest. They permit establishment of a diagnosis by demonstrating a rise in the antibody titer of the serum. There are three principal tests: the complement-fixation reaction, hemagglutination, and the neutralization test.

Fixation of Complement. Diagnosis is based on the presence of the group antigen.

PREPARATION OF THE ANTIGEN. The antigen may be prepared by three methods. A first method consists in maintaining the infected cells at 37° C. and harvesting two or three days after complete cellular degeneration has occurred.[2] It is also possible to use a high dose of virus to obtain complete degeneration in 24 to 48 hours[10, 23] or to allow degeneration to proceed slowly in four to five days.[59, 70] The cells are ruptured by successive cycles of freezing and thawing. This theoretically should release the intracellular antigen. However, electron microscopic control has revealed that this treatment is inadequate to disrupt the nucleus and release the virion. Cell fragments are then eliminated by low-speed centrifugation.[2]

PERFORMANCE AND INTERPRETATION OF THE TEST. Two samples of blood are collected, the first during the acute phase of the disease and the second seven to ten days later. The reaction is considered positive when the second serum contains four times more complement-fixing antibody than the first, provided that the antibody titer of the two sera are determined in the same test. Higher titers are obtained when the antigen employed is the type antigen or related to it.

Complement-fixing antibodies appear to rise in the blood between the fourth and fifth day following the onset of the disease. Maximal titers are obtained between the seventh and sixteenth day in adults, and usually later in children. It should be borne in mind, however, that the onset of an infection due to a different adenovirus can produce an anamnestic reaction because of the presence of a common group antigen.

In some cases adenoviruses have been isolated but antibodies have not been detected in the serum. Thus, adenoviruses types 1, 2, 3, 5, and 6 have been recovered from the mesenteric lymph nodes of apparently healthy subjects, but neither neutralizing nor complement-fixing antibodies were detected in their serum.[7] Similarly, such antibodies were not detected in children who succumbed to a type 3 adenovirus infection.[49]

In addition to its diagnostic interest, the test is of epidemiological interest, since it permits an investigation of the incidence of adenovirus infections among different populations.

T ANTIGEN. The T antigen represents a special type of complement-fixing antigen. It is a nonstructural antigen that is synthesized in the early stage of the infectious cycle. By fluorescent microscopy it has been localized in the nucleus and the cytoplasm as fluorescent filaments.[42] As we shall see later, this antigen can persist in cells that have been modified by the oncogenic adenoviruses, thus permitting the retrospective determination of the virus that induced the modification, even though the complete virion is not synthesized.

Hemagglutination Test. This previously described test is used chiefly for typing adenoviruses.

As for the hemagglutination-inhibition test, it is not usually employed for serological diagnosis.

Neutralization Reaction. The neutralization reaction consists in testing the neutralizing effect of a serum on the cytopathogenicity of a known adenovirus.[18, 23, 59] A metabolic or colorimetric test has been developed for the detection of neutralizing antibodies.[34, 40] This method, which is used for the typing and identification of adenoviruses, is applicable to serological diagnosis. Neutralizing antibodies usually appear six to seven days after the onset of the infection.

PATHOLOGY

Pulmonary lesions have been the most striking.[11, 14, 17, 63] At times only a few lesions are present; at other times, numerous lesions are observed, predominantly at the level of the bronchial and tracheal epithelium. These lesions are characterized by massive necrosis of the epithelium. Necrotic debris may obstruct the bronchial lumen and cause respiratory difficulties. Occasionally necrotic cells are observed among the alveolar endothelial cells. As in vitro, it is the nucleus of these cells which shows characteristic adenoviral lesions. Owing to the relative specificity of these lesions, the anatomical

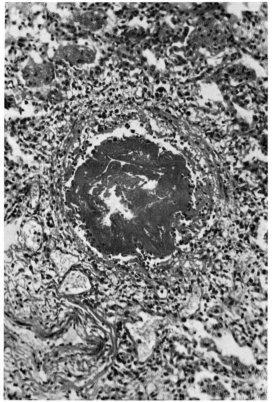

Figure 44-7. Bronchiole. The epithelial lining is completely necrotic and the lumen is obstructed by a hyaline mass. (Hematoxylin and eosin, × 250.) (Courtesy of Dr. Le Tan Vinh.)

site suggests a diagnosis of adenovirus pneumopathy. These lesions recall those of infantile pneumonia described by Goodpasture et al.[22] In some cases perivascular lymphocytic infiltrations have been observed in the brain.[11]

Examination of lymph nodes during certain forms of mesenteric adenitis has revealed the presence of follicular hyperplasia, proliferation of mononuclear cells, and an increase in the number of reticular cells.

Epidemic keratoconjunctivitis is characterized by marked conjunctival edema, followed by exudation of mononuclear cells, mainly lymphocytes. Later, a pseudomembrane containing degenerated epithelial and mononuclear cells may cover the conjunctiva.[60]

EXPERIMENTAL PATHOGENICITY

Adenoviruses do not seem to be pathogenic for most laboratory animals.[26, 59] How-

ever, specific antibodies appear in the serum of guinea pigs, rats, and hamsters after a single inoculation of adenovirus.[59] By injection of large quantities of type 5 virus, Pereira et al.[50a] produced fatal infections in newborn hamsters and observed under the electron microscope the presence of viral particles in hepatic cells.

Oncogenic Potency of Adenoviruses. In 1962 Trentin et al.[64] demonstrated the formation of malignant tumors in animals inoculated with adenovirus 12, the first virus of human origin known to be oncogenic in animals. Subcutaneous injection of large doses of virus in hamsters less than 24 hours old caused the appearance of sarcomatous tumors at the site of injection.[71, 72] The specificity of the oncogenicity of adenovirus 12 (or other oncogenic adenoviruses) is demonstrable by the inhibition of induction of tumors by a specific antiviral serum. These tumors can be transplanted and cultivated in vitro. All attempts to isolate virus from the tumors or from cultures of

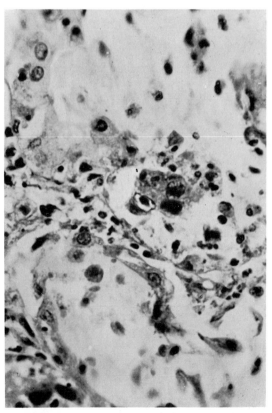

Figure 44-8. Trachea. Group of mucous glands in the trachea, with inflammatory infiltration and necrosis. In the center is a group of three cells; the lowermost has a well characterized acidophilic intranuclear inclusion. (Hematoxylin and eosin, × 450.) (Courtesy of Dr. Le Tan Vinh.)

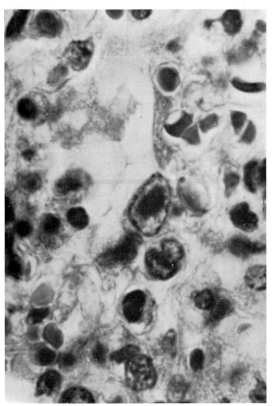

Figure 44-9. Lung. Note, in the center, an acidophilic intranuclear inclusion in a cell lining an alveolus. (Hematoxylin and eosin, × 750.) (Courtesy of Dr. Le Tan Vinh.)

tumor cells have failed.[62] These cells contain the T antigen. The serum of tumor-bearing hamsters contains antibodies which fix complement in the presence of this antigen. No antibodies against structural antigens are detected; hence, the virion is probably not synthesized in the tissues of this animal. It is assumed that the cells of tumors cultivated in vitro or in vivo contain a fragment of the genome of the virus which controls the synthesis of certain nonstructural viral antigens. However, the modified cell does not produce complete virions[29, 31] or any structural antigens.[42] The current but unverified hypothesis is that the viral DNA incorporated into the cellular genome is defective or incompletely expressed.[38] Adenoviruses 18 and 31 are also oncogenic for hamsters.[30] Adenovirus type 7 was recently found to be oncogenic for newborn hamsters,[21] but with a lower incidence than serotypes 12 and 18. Moreover, tumors induced by type 12 develop in 26 to 216 days and those induced by type 18 in 70 to 280 days, whereas the time is 231 to 405 days for type 7.

Interaction Between Infections Due to

Adenoviruses and Those Due to Other Viruses. It has long been known that adenovirus infections can be associated with those by other viruses or bacteria. A recrudescence of adenovirus epidemics has frequently been noted during influenza epidemics. Association with measles or with pertussis has also been reported.[22, 63]

In vitro, adenoviruses interfere but little, if at all, with other viruses. Adenoviruses multiply in cells infected by other viruses, such as Myxovirus parainfluenzae 3. Similarly, the simultaneous infection of the same cell by adenovirus 12 and SV 40 results in the multiplication of both viruses within the same nucleus. The presence of both types of virions has been demonstrated by electron microscopy.[28, 43, 54]

In some cases a stimulating interaction has been observed between an adenovirus and other antigenically different viruses. For instance, adenovirus 12 stimulates multiplication of the K virus of the rat, in rat embryo cells. The latter is a small DNA virus (diameter 20 mμ).[8]

Some as yet unidentified viruses, which

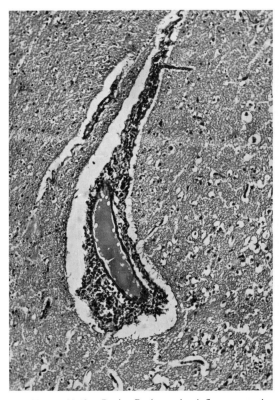

Figure 44-10. Brain. Perivascular inflammatory infiltration. (Hematoxylin and eosin, × 250.) (Courtesy of Dr. Le Tan Vinh.)

morphologically resemble K virus, have been found in a few stocks of adenovirus. These viruses apparently cannot multiply unless they are accompanied by adenoviruses. They have provisionally been called AAV (adeno-associated-viruses). The stimulation of rat K virus by adenovirus 12 is probably related to the anti-interferon action of adenovirus 12. This anti-interferon action is attributed to a viral antigen called "stimulon," which blocks the inhibiting action of interferon.

SV 40 facilitates the multiplication of adenovirus 12 in monkey kidney cells, provided the cells are infected simultaneously by the two viruses. Part of the virus population contains, in an adenovirus capsid, the SV 40 genome, and the adenovirus genome. The cells transformed by these hybrids contain the T antigen of both adenovirus 12 and SV 40 virus. This mixed virus population, containing at the same time SV 40 virus, adenovirus 12, and the SV 40—adenovirus 12 hybrid, induces tumors in animals more rapidly than the two virus populations separately.[28, 43, 54]

EPIDEMIOLOGY

Adenoviruses have been isolated throughout the world. A few important factors in the occurrence of respiratory tract diseases may be listed as follows.

Age and Sex. Age seems to have some influence on the severity of adenovirus diseases. For instance, respiratory tract infections, particularly those due to types 7 and 3, are less severe in adults than in young children. Some serotypes (4, 7, 14, 21) are found more commonly in adolescents and young adults.

Sex does not seem to have any influence on the incidence of adenovirus infections, at least among children.[7]

Seasonal Variations. Seasonal variations in the occurrence of adenovirus infections are a well-known phenomenon. The fever-pharyngitis-conjunctivitis syndrome is seen most frequently during the summer months, which suggests that swimming may be a factor. On the whole, the number of adenovirus infections increases during the winter and spring, as compared with a low incidence in summer. This seasonal variation is particularly noticeable in temperate climates and is less marked in tropical regions.

Predominance of Certain Serotypes. Serotypes 3, 4, 7, 14, and 21 are responsible for epidemics of respiratory tract diseases, whereas the other types are met with only sporadically or occasionally and in small foci. Types 14 and 21 have been found only in limited geographical regions: serotype 14 in Holland and in Great Britain,[1, 67] serotype 21 in Russia,[73] Holland,[66] India,[65] and Great Britain. Keratoconjunctivitis due to type 8 is endemoepidemic in Japan and many Oriental countries.

Studies on the presence of antibodies among the population of the United States, Holland, Hungary, the Congo, and Japan indicated that adenovirus infections occur early in life. Of the first 7 serotypes, types 1 and 2 seem to be the most frequently responsible for these infections in early life, types 3 and 5 being somewhat less frequent. By age five, all children seem to have been infected with at least one type of adenovirus and at least 50 per cent with four types.

Studies have shown that adenoviruses are responsible for 2 to 25 per cent of respiratory tract diseases in children, but that they have a much less important role among adults.

Miscellaneous Factors. The living conditions of a population can favor the outbreak of adenovirus epidemics. Such epidemics are frequently observed in collectivities such as military camps or barracks and among children in hospital wards, day nurseries, and schools.[3, 5, 11] Certain factors, such as malnutrition, unsanitary conditions, or the coexistence of other virus infections such as influenza or measles, would seem to be responsible for an increased susceptibility to adenoviruses.

In the case of keratoconjunctivitis, irritation of the eye by dust or fragments of metal seems to be a promoting factor.[33] Similarly, it has been suggested that swimming, particularly in pools, might be a source of adenovirus conjunctivitis.[48] In the majority of cases no abnormal physiological conditions have been found to be associated with the outbreak of these diseases.

BIBLIOGRAPHY

1. Andrews, B. E., and McDonald, J. C.: Epidemiological studies of adenovirus infection. Proc. Roy. Soc. Med., *50*:753-755, 1957.
2. Balducci, D., Zaiman, E., and Tyrell, D. A. J.: Laboratory studies of APC and influenza C viruses. Brit. J. Exp. Path. *37*:205-218, 1956.

3. Barr, J., Kjellen, L., and Svedmyr, A.: Hospital outbreak of adenovirus type 3 infections. A clinical and virologic study on 38 patients partly involved in a nosocomial outbreak. Acta Pediat. (Stockholm), *47*:365-382, 1958.

4. Barski, G., and Cornefert, F.: Aspects distinctifs des lésions cellulaires causées in vitro par différents types d'adénovirus. Etude de 20 souches appartenant à 6 types d'adénovirus. Ann. Inst. Pasteur, *94*:724-731, 1958.

5. Bell, J. A.: Epidemiology of pharyngo-conjunctival fever. Amer. J. Ophthal., *43*:36-40, 1957.

6. Bell, T. M., and Steyn, J. H.: Viruses in lymp nodes of children with mesenteric adenitis and intussusception. Brit. Med. J., *2*:700-702, 1962.

7. Bell, J. A., Ward, T. G., Huebner, R. J., Rowe, W. P., Suskind, R. G., and Paffenberger, R. S., Jr.: Studies of adenoviruses (APC) in volunteers. Amer. J. Public Health, *46*:1130-1146, 1956.

8. Bernhard, W., Kasten, F. H., and Chany, C.: Etude cytochimique et ultrastracturale de cellules infectées par le virus K du rat et le virus H. C. R. Acad. Sci. (Paris), *257*:1566-1569, 1963.

9. Binn, L. N., and Hilleman, M. R.: Detection of poliovirus 1 in monkey kidney cultures inoculated with overwhelming dose of adenovirus 4. J. Infect. Dis. *103*:127-128, 1958.

10. Binn, L. N., Hilleman, M. R., Rodriguez, J. E., and Glabere, R. R.: Antigenic relationships among adenoviruses with appraisal of reliability of complement fixation test for typing isolates. J. Immun., *80*:501-508, 1958.

11. Chany, C., Lépine, P., Lelong, M., Le Tan Vinh, Satgé, P., and Virat, J.: Severe and fatal pneumonia in infants and young children associated with adenovirus infections. Amer. J. Hyg., *67*:367-378, 1958.

12. Clarke, N. A., Stevenson, R. E., and Kabler, P. W.: The inactivation of purified type 3 adenovirus in water by chlorine. Amer. J. Hyg., *64*:314-319, 1956.

13. Dales, S.: An electron microscope study of the early association between two mammalian viruses and their hosts. J. Cell. Biol., *13*:303-322, 1962.

14. Deinhardt, F., May, R. D., Calhoun, H. H., and Sullivan, H. E.: The isolation of adenovirus type 1 from a fatal case of viral pneumonitis. Arch. Intern. Med., *102*:816-819, 1958.

15. Enders, J. F., Bell, J. A., Dingle, J. H., Francis, T., Jr., Hilleman, M. R., Huebner, R. J., and Payne, A. M. M.: Adenoviruses; group name proposed for new respiratory-tract viruses. Science, *124*:119-120, 1956.

16. Flanagan, J. F., and Ginsberg, H. S.: Synthesis of virus specific polymers in adenovirus infected cells: effects of 5-fluordeoxyuridine J. Exp. Med., *116*:141-157, 1962.

17. Gerbeaux, J., Heber-Jouas, J., Masse, N., and Beauchef, A.: Epidémie familiale de maladie à virus du groupe APC chez 3 enfants (un cas mortel). Etude clinique, anatomique et virologique. Bull. Soc. Med. Hôp. Paris, *73*:519-529, 1957.

18. Ginsberg, H. S.: Characteristics of the new respiratory viruses (adenoviruses). I. Qualitative and quantitative aspects of the neutralization reaction. J. Immun., *77*:271-278, 1956.

19. Ginsberg, H. S.: Characteristics of the new respiratory viruses (adenoviruses). III. Stability to temperature and pH alterations. Proc. Soc. Exp. Biol. Med., *93*:48-52, 1956.

20. Ginsberg, H. S., Pereira, H. G., Valentine, R. C., and Wilcox, W. C.: A proposed terminology for the adenovirus antigens and virion morphological subunits. Virology, *28*:782-783, 1966.

21. Girardi, A. J., Hilleman, M. R., and Zwickey, R. E.: Tests in hamsters for oncogenic quality of ordinary viruses including adenovirus type 7. Proc. Soc. Exp. Biol. Med., *115*:1141-1150, 1964.

22. Goodpasture, E. W., Auerbach, S. H., Swanson, H. S., and Cotter, E. F.: Virus pneumonia of infants secondary to epidemic infections. Amer. J. Dis. Child., *57*:997-1011, 1939.

23. Grayston, J. T., Johnston, P. B., Smith, M. E., and Loosli, C. G.: An improved technique for the neutralization test with adenovirus in Hela cells cultures. J. Infect. Dis., *99*:188-198, 1956.

24. Grayston, J. T., Loosli, C. G., Smith, M., McCarthy, M. A., and Johnston, P. B.: Adenoviruses. I. The effect of total incubation time in Hela cells cultures on the isolation rate. J. Infect. Dis., *103*:75-85, 1958.

25. Gutekunst, R. R., and Heggie, A. D.: Viremia and viruria in adenovirus infections. Detection in patients with rubella or rubelliform illness. New Eng. J. Med., *264*:374-378, 1961.

26. Hilleman, M. R., and Werner, J. R.: Recovery of new agent from patients with acute respiratory illness. Proc. Soc. Exp. Biol. Med., *85*:183-188, 1954.

27. Horne, R. W., Brenner, S., Waterson, A. P., and Wildy, P.: The icosahedral form of an adenovirus. J. Molec. Biol. *1*:84-86, 1959.

28. Huebner, R. J., Chanock, R. M., Rubin, B. A., and Casey, M. J.: Induction by adenovirus type 7 of tumors in hamsters having the antigenic characteristics of SV 40 virus. Proc. Nat. Acad. Sci. U.S.A., *52*:1333-1340, 1964.

29. Huebner, R. J., Pereira, H. G., Allison, A. C., Hollinshead, A. C., and Turner, H. C.: Production of type-specific C antigen in virus-free hamsters tumor cells induced by adenovirus type 12. Proc. Nat. Acad. Sci. U.S.A., *51*:432-439, 1964.

30. Huebner, R. J., Rowe, W. P., and Lane, W. T.: Oncogenic effects in hamsters of human adenovirus types 12 and 18. Proc. Nat. Acad. Sci. U.S.A., *48*:2051-2058, 1962.

31. Huebner, R. J., Rowe, W. P., Turner, H. C., and Lane, W. T.: Specific adenovirus complement fixing antigens in virus-free hamster and rat tumors. Proc. Nat. Acad. Sci. U.S.A., *50*:379-389, 1963.

32. Huebner, R. J., Rowe, W. P., Ward, T. G., Parrott, R. H., and Bell, J. A.: Adenoidal-pharyngeal conjunctival agents. A newly recognized group of common viruses of the respiratory system. New Eng. J. Med., *251*:1077-1086, 1954.

33. Jawetz, E., Thygeson, P., Hanna, L., Nicholas, A., and Kimura, S. J.: The etiology of epidemic keratoconjunctivitis. Amer. J. Ophthal., *43*:79-83, 1957.

34. Johnston, P. B., Grayston, J. T., and Loosli, C. G.: Adenovirus neutralizing antibody determination by colorimetric assay. Proc. Soc. Exp. Biol. Med., *94*:338-343, 1957.

35. Kjellén, L., Lagermalm, G., Svedmyr, A., and Thorsson, K. G.: Crystalline-like patterns in the nuclei of cells infected with an animal virus. Nature, *175*:505-507, 1955.

36. Kjellén, L., Zetterberg, B., and Svedmyr, A.: An epidemic among Swedish children caused by adenovirus type 3. Acta Paediat. (Uppsala), *46*: 561-568, 1957.

37. Klemperer, H. G., and Pereira, H. G.: Study of adenovirus antigens fractionated by chromatography on DEAE cellulose. Virology, 9:536-545, 1959.

38. Latner, A. L., Gardner, P. S., Turner, D. M., and Brown, J. O.: Effect of possible oncogenic virus (adenovirus type 12) on lactate dehydrogenase in tissue culture. Lancet, *1*:197-201, 1964.

39. Lelong, M., Lépine, P., Alison, F., Le Tan Vinh, Satgé, P., and Chany, C.: La pneumonie à virus APC chez le nourrisson. Isolement du virus. Les lésions anatomo-histologiques. Arch. Franc. Pediat., *13*:1092-1096, 1956.

40. Lennette, E. H., Neff, B. J., and Fox, V. L.: A colorimetric method for the typing of adenovirus. Amer. J. Hyg., 65:94-109, 1957.

41. Lépine, P., Chany, C., Maurin, J., and Carré, M. C.: Etude des virus APC (adénovirus). II. Evolution des lésions cellulaires provoquées par les virus APC in vitro. Ann. Inst. Pasteur, 92:728-734, 1957.

42. Levinthal, J. D., Ahmad-Zadeh, C., Van Hoosier, G., Jr., and Trentin, J. J.: Immunofluorescence of human adenovirus type 12 in various cell types (30 791). Proc. Soc. Exp. Biol. Med., *121*:405-414, 1966.

43. Lewis, A. M., Jr., Prigge, K. O., and Rowe, W. P.: Studies of Adenovirus SV 40 hybrid viruses. IV. An adenovirus type 2 strain carrying the infection SV 40 genome. Proc. Nat. Acad. Sci. U.S.A., 55:526-531, 1966.

44. Morgan, C., Godman, G. C., Breitenfeld, P. M., and Rose, H. M.: A correlative study by electron and light microscopy of the development of type 5 adenovirus. I. Electron microscopy. J. Exp. Med., *112*:373-382, 1960.

45. Morgan, C., Godman, G. C., Rose, H. M., Howe, C., and Huang, J. S.: Electron microscopic and histochemical studies of an unusual crystalline protein occurring in cells infected by type 5 adenovirus. Preliminary observations. J. Biophys. Biochem. Cytol., 3:505-508, 1957.

46. Morgan, C., Howe, C., Rose, H. M., and Moore, D. H.: Structure and development of viruses observed in the electron microscope. IV. Viruses of the RI-APC group. J. Biophys. Biochem. Cytol., 2:351-360, 1956.

47. Neva, F. A., and Enders, J. F.: Isolation of a cytopathogenic agent from an infant with a disease in certain respects resembling roseola infantum. J. Immun., 72:315-321, 1954.

48. Ormsby, H. L., and Aitchison, W. S.: The role of the swimming pool in the transmission of pharyngeal-conjunctival fever. Canad. Med. Ass. J., 73:864-866, 1955.

49. Parker, W. L., Wilt, J. C., and Stackiw, W.: Adenovirus infections. Canad. J. Public Health, *52*: 246-251, 1961.

50. Pereira, H. G.: Typing of adenoidal pharyngeal conjunctival (APC) viruses by complement fixation. J. Path. Bact., 72:105-109, 1956.

50a. Pereira, H. G., Allison, A. C., and Niven, J. S. F.: Fatal infection of new-born hamsters by an adenovirus of human origin. Nature, *196*:244-245, 1962.

51. Pereira, H. G., Huebner, R. J., Ginsberg, H. S. and Van der Veen, J.: A short description of the adenovirus group. Virology, *20*:613-620, 1963.

52. Pereira, H. G., and Kelly, B.: Latent infection of rabbits by adenovirus type 5. Nature, *180*:615-617, 1957.

53. Pereira, H. G., and Valentine, R. C.: Antigens and structure of the adenoviruses. J. Molec. Biol., *13*:13-20, 1965.

54. Rabson, A. S., O'Conor, G. T., Berezesky, I. K., and Paul, F. J.: Enhancement of adenovirus growth in African green monkey kidney cell cultures by SV 40. Proc. Soc. Exp. Biol. Med., *116*:187-190, 1964.

55. Rosen, L.: Hemagglutination by adenoviruses. Virology, 5:574-577, 1958.

56. Rosen, L.: A hemagglutination-inhibition technique for typing adenoviruses. Amer. J. Hyg., 71:120-128, 1960.

57. Rosen, L., Hovis, J. F., and Bell, J. A.: Further observation on typing adenovirus and a description of two possible additional serotypes. Proc. Soc. Exp. Biol. Med., 110:710-713, 1962.

58. Rowe, W. P., Huebner, R. J., Gilmore, L. K., Parrott, R. H., and Ward, T. G.: Isolation of a cytopathogenic agent from human adenoids undergoing spontaneous degeneration in tissue culture. Proc. Soc. Exp. Biol. Med., 84:570-573, 1953.

59. Rowe, W. P., Huebner, R. J., Hartley, J. W., Ward, T. G., and Parrott, R. H.: Studies on the adenoidal-pharyngeal-conjunctival (APC) group of viruses. Amer. J. Hyg., 61:197-218, 1955.

60. Sohier, R., Chardonnet, Y., and Prunieras, M.: Adenovirus — status of current knowledge. Progr. Med. Virol., 7:253-325, 1965.

61. Sohier, R., Prunieras, M., and Chardonnet, Y.: Recherches cytochimiques préliminaires sur le cycle intracellulaire des adénovirus. Path. Biol. (Paris), 8:885-893, 1960.

62. Strohl, W. A., Rouse, H. C., and Schlesinger, R. W.: In vitro cultivation of malignant cells derived from adenovirus-induced hamster tumors. Virology, *21*:513-516, 1963.

63. Teng, C. H.: Adenovirus pneumonia epidemic among Peking infants and preschool children in 1958. Chin. Med. J., 80:331-339, 1960.

64. Trentin, J. J., Yabe, Y., and Taylor, G.: The quest for human cancer viruses. Science, *137*:835-841, 1962.

65. Van der Veen, J.: The role of adenoviruses in respiratory disease. Amer. Rev. Resp. Dis., 88:167-180, 1963.

66. Van der Veen, J., and Dijkman, J. H.: Association of type 21 adenovirus with acute respiratory illness in military recruits. Amer. J. Hyg., 76:149-154, 1962.

67. Van der Veen, J., and Kok, G.: Isolation and typing of adenoviruses recovered from military recruits with acute respiratory disease in the Netherlands. Amer. J. Hyg., 65:119-129, 1957.

68. Verville, E., Connor, J. D., and Sigel, M. M.: Double infection of tissue culture cells with CA virus and adenovirus. Virology, *13*:261-262, 1961.

69. Wassermann, F. E.: The inactivation of adenoviruses by ultraviolet irradiation and nitrous acid. Virology, *17*:335-341, 1962.

70. Werner, G. H.: Complement fixing antibodies in guinea pigs immunized with type 3 adeno-pharyn-

go-conjunctival virus. J. Bact., *72*:568-569, 1956.

71. Yabe, Y., Samper, L., Taylor, G., and Trentin, J. J.: Cancer induction in hamsters by human type 12 adenovirus. Effect of route of injection. Proc. Soc. Exp. Biol. Med., *113*:221-224, 1963.

72. Yabe, Y., Trentin, J. J., and Taylor, G.: Cancer induction in hamsters by human type 12 adenovirus. Effect of age and of virus dose. Proc. Soc. Exp. Biol. Med., *111*:343-344, 1962.

73. Zhdanov, V. M., and Dreizin, R. S.: A group of strains of a new serological type of adenoviruses (adenovirus 19). Vop. Virus. *1*:88-95, 1961.

RESPIRATORY ENTEROVIRUSES AND REOVIRUSES

by F. BRICOUT

REOVIRUSES

PROPERTIES

Following the research work by Sabin, the reoviruses were excluded from the group of ECHO viruses to form a well-defined group of their own, being particularly characterized by their size (75 mμ); they produce a cytopathogenic effect in a great number of cell cultures.

These viruses are called reoviruses as a reminder of their dual respiratory and enteric tropism. Three serotypes, which are antigenically differentiated by tests of seroneutralization and inhibition of hemagglutination, are included within one group by their complement-fixation reaction.

They resemble the enteroviruses in their physicochemical properties; they are resistant to ether and are destroyed by heating to 56° C. for 45 minutes, and their half-life, at least in the case of reovirus type 1, is two days at 24° C. and 19 hours at 37° C., reoviruses types 2 and 3 being considerably more thermolabile.

EPIDEMIOLOGY

Frequency of Isolation of the Viruses. The frequency with which the reoviruses have been isolated seems fairly low, and if this were the basis used to estimate the extent of reoviral infections, they would appear to be relatively rare. At least certain surveys tend to suggest this.

Only a few cases of infections due to reoviruses have been published so far, and at present the pathogenic role of these viruses is not well known.

Gelfand et al.[2] carried out 12,041 virological examinations over a period of two years in healthy children in six different American towns and isolated reoviruses in 17 cases; these were equally distributed between the three different serotypes: five instances of reovirus type 1, six of reovirus type 2, and six of reovirus type 3.

In 5000 examinations for viruses in the throat and feces of children hospitalized in a Parisian hospital for a supposedly viral syndrome,[1] only four reoviral infections were noted, two due to type 1, and two to type 3.

In both cases the frequency of isolation of reoviruses was approximately one in 1000.

As in the case of the enteroviruses, there seems to be a seasonal influence, the high point also being the summer-autumn period; the cases noted by Gelfand et al. were in fact distributed in the following manner: 8 per cent from January to March, 6 per cent from April to June, 24 per cent from July to September, and 62 per cent from October to December.

The infections reported essentially affected children, but there did not appear to be any predominance with regard to sex.

There are only a few descriptions of sporadic cases of reoviral infection, and not many research studies have been devoted to epidemics due to these agents. Nevertheless, epidemics of reovirus type 1 and of reovirus type 3 occurring in a community of children studied by Rosen et al.[11, 12] and an epidemic of reovirus type 2 described by Lerner et al.[4] have made it possible to establish certain conclusions:

The reoviruses can be isolated from the throat and feces of infected patients. It is preferable to look for the viruses in the stools. The duration of excretion of the virus in the stools appears to be somewhat variable. Sometimes it is very short, three to five days, but it can also extend over two weeks or even five weeks. The duration of this viral excretion or the quantity of viruses eliminated, or both, are generally less in infected subjects whose serum already contains homologous antibodies, signifying a previous infection.

These conclusions were confirmed by nasal inoculation of adult volunteers with strains of reoviruses of human or bovine origin.[3, 10] In all the cases the clinical symptomatology was poor and nonsystematized, so that a clear-cut clinical picture of these infections could not be established any more than had been possible in epidemics in children. The virus was always found in the stools of the volunteers and occasionally in the throat swabs of the subjects who had received type 1 reovirus; virus was never found in the urine samples. Excretion of the virus extended from the first or second day to the thirteenth day following inoculation.

Serological Studies. In contrast with the relatively low frequency with which reoviruses are isolated, the frequency with which the antireovirus antibodies are found in human sera proves irrefutably the worldwide distribution of these viruses.

The reoviruses, like the other viruses, possess antigenic properties that induce the formation of specific antibodies in the infected organism.

These antibodies appear after a more or less constant period whatever the type of reovirus used. By means of inoculations of volunteers and successive systematic titrations of the antibodies, the time of their appearance has been found to be about the tenth day following inoculation.

The increase in antibodies continues during the second week, and this high con-centration is maintained for 24 weeks in the case of experimental infections. The concentration of antibodies then remains level over a fairly long period before decreasing slowly.

Lerner et al.[4] studied the frequency of occurrence of antibodies for reovirus type 2 in 235 sera from subjects of various ages selected at random; they were able to observe a progressive increase with age in the percentages of sera containing the antibody: 20 per cent at one year of age, 50 per cent at 10 years of age, and 90 per cent in subjects over 40 years of age.

A comparable study of 163 sera sampled in the Paris region and in Brittany provided the same indirect proof of the wide distribution of the three serotypes of reoviruses. Figure 44-11 shows a progressive increase in the percentage of positive sera, particularly with regard to reovirus type 3, up to 20 years of age; the subsequent decrease can probably be explained by the small number of samples studied in this very large age group.

The distribution of reoviruses estimated on the basis of serological tests seems just as extensive as that of the enteroviruses. However, during purely serological surveys of this type one should take into account the possibility that heterotypic reactions take

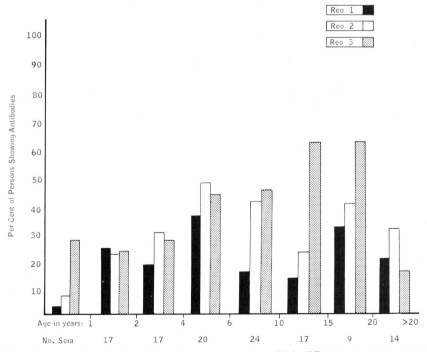

Figure 44-11. Presence of antibodies for reoviruses types 1, 2, and 3 in different age groups among 163 subjects in the Paris region and in Brittany.

place, a fact which has been widely demonstrated. Following primary infection in volunteers by the type 1 reovirus,[3, 10] there is not
only an increase in the antibodies inhibiting
hemagglutination of the homotypic virus but
in addition there is very often a slight increase
in the antibodies for the two other serotypes.
Similarly, an infection due to reovirus type
2[3, 10] is often followed by an increase in the
antibodies for type 3 and sometimes for type
1. Moreover, infection by reovirus type 3[3, 10]
occasionally gives rise to antibodies against
reovirus type 2.

Antibodies for the three different serotypes of reovirus are often found in the same
subject. These may reflect, particularly in the
adult or older child, a prior triple infection;
but although a low percentage of one of these
serotypes may be due to a previous infection,
it may also be the result of a heterotypic
reaction. Preëxisting heterotypic antibodies
favor the occurrence of a heterotypic response, which probably consists of an anamnestic reaction. The heterotypic antibodies
may even appear in some instances before
the homologous antibodies, as has been
demonstrated by experimental inoculation of
animals. The subject's age also plays a part,
and heterotypic responses occur more readily
in adults than in children[6]; here again it is
probably a case of anamnestic reactions.
Finally, the degree of the homotypical reaction also plays a role; when it is very high
the heterotypic responses are more frequent
and more pronounced.

It is also important in the case of infants
to take into account passive transfer of antireovirus antibodies. It has in fact been proved[4]
that these antibodies can pass through the
placenta and may remain in the child's blood
for three to four months. This fact has been
confirmed in cattle, where antibodies may persist up to the fifth month.[9]

It remains true, nevertheless, that although few epidemics of infections due to
reoviruses have been demonstrated, these
viruses are very widely distributed. It is
therefore highly probable that the reoviruses
give rise to benign epidemics during which the
infections remain mostly inapparent or
so benign that they do not justify hospitalization or tests for isolating the virus.

Reservoirs of Viruses. In a great many
viral diseases, the reservoir of viruses is
exclusively human. The reoviruses present a
particular problem because of their wide
distribution throughout the animal kingdom.

These viruses have been isolated from
various animal species, both wild and domestic, e.g., the African and Asian monkeys,
mice, dogs, cats, and cattle.[7]

Serological studies confirm the susceptibility of these animals to infection, and the
presence of antibodies against the three different serotypes has been demonstrated in the
serum of numerous animals. The reoviruses
responsible for animal infections are identical
in every respect to the human reoviruses,
particularly with regard to their physicochemical and antigenic properties; this identity is
confirmed by the successful inoculation of
calves with reoviruses of human origin[8, 9]
and, conversely, of adult volunteers with
reoviruses derived from cattle.[3]

It has not been proved that animals play
a part in human infections. The contrary has
not been definitely proved either, although the
reoviruses have been isolated and serological
proof of viral infection has been observed
mostly in animals that are in contact with
man. The research studies of Stanley and
Leak[13] on the reoviral infection of the quokka,
an Australian marsupial (Setonyx), suggested
that the animal infections originate from
man. These animals live in a region that is
barely inhabited; whereas the quokkas in
captivity show the presence of antibodies in
the proportion of 70 to 100 per cent depending on the serotype, this proportion is lower
in those animals that are only occasionally in
contact with man, and drops to 17 to 34
per cent, depending on the serotype, in the
case of free-living animals that are never in
contact with man.

However, the size of the animal reservoir
of reovirus is such that one cannot disregard
this as a possible factor in the propagation
of the infection. Recently, reoviruses have
even been observed in the mosquito.[5] A
multiplication cycle has not been observed
in these insects, and it is probable that their
role is that of passive vector, a role that may
not be negligible but concerning which precise data are lacking so far.

LABORATORY STUDY

Sampling. Whenever a reoviral infection is suspected, it is important to take a
sample from the throat and stools as early as
possible after the onset of the disease.

The samples can be taken by means of
sterile cotton swabs slightly moistened preferably with transport solution or else with

isotonic sodium chloride solution; swabs of the throat and of the pharynx or the rectum are carefully taken.

The swabs are then squeezed into 2 ml. of transport solution and dispatched as quickly as possible to the laboratory. They should be kept away from heat, i.e., maintained in carbon dioxide snow, if the transport time is likely to exceed several hours.

A stool sample can be substituted for the rectal swab; it should be sent to the laboratory under the same conditions described above.

If the samples cannot be dispatched to the laboratory immediately, they should be kept in a deep freezer at $-20°$ C. or in the freezer compartment of a refrigerator, so as to keep them as cold as possible.

After the tenth day of infection one can no longer count on isolating the virus responsible for the disease; if a reovirus is then isolated it is more than likely that this is a sign either of a superinfection or of the temporary presence of a virus in the alimentary canal.

At the same time as the samples taken for the purpose of isolating the virus, it is essential to take a blood sample of 3 to 5 ml. which should be sent to the laboratory together with the swabs; care should be taken to send only serum if the transit time is likely to be long, so as to avoid hemolysis in the specimen sent to the laboratory.

Finally, a second blood sample should be taken about two weeks after the first and dispatched in the same way.

Results. Failure to isolate the virus does not definitely eliminate the viral origin of the infection under consideration: the sample may have been taken with faulty technique or too late or transported under unfavorable conditions.

Isolation of a reovirus is not sufficient in itself to confirm the origin of the infection; it is quite possible to isolate this virus from a normal subject in good health, or else its presence might represent superinfection.

Therefore, to confirm the etiology of the infection it is necessary to ascertain an increase in the level of homologous antibodies. These can be titrated by means of complement fixation, a reaction that is easy to carry out but which is only group specific for the three different reoviruses. Titration of the neutralizing antibodies takes longer but is sensitive and specific for the type. Finally, following viral infection there is an increase in the antibodies inhibiting hemagglutination of the homotypic virus, a reaction that is easy to perform and specific for the type but which frequently shows a simultaneous increase in the heterotypic antibodies.

Whatever the reaction used, infection is indicated only if the level of antibodies is at least four times higher in the second serum sample than in the first. It should be remembered that the frequency with which antibodies are found in the human population is very high and hence it is absolutely necessary to have two sera as a means of comparison.

Isolated serological tests, without isolation of the virus itself, are of no value in confirming a recent infection. The result can only be of interest from the epidemiological point of view, and by itself cannot confirm the part played by the virus in a supposedly viral infection.

There is a further possible limitation in the interpretation of the results of investigations on viruses, particularly reoviruses: namely, the isolation of a reovirus associated with an increase in the homotypic antibodies simply signifies that the virus has multiplied within the organism. The virus is not necessarily responsible for the clinical syndrome and may only constitute an additional factor. That is to say, one should be extremely prudent with regard to any clinical syndrome during which a reoviral infection has been demonstrated. It is still difficult to specify the exact part played by reoviruses in human pathology, and, except in the presence of a coherent epidemic, the results should be interpreted with the utmost caution.

IMMUNITY

Epidemiological studies, as well as inoculations into volunteers, have demonstrated the part played by antibodies in the phenomena of immunity. It appears that these serum antibodies are the basis of immunity and their presence protects the subject against reinfections. Their passage through the placenta provides protection for the newborn infant for three to five months.

It is probable that the levels of antibodies in the serum of adults are maintained at more or less high levels as a result of the reinfections that are more often than not inapparent because of the very presence of these antibodies.

TREATMENT AND PROPHYLAXIS

There is no specific treatment of reoviral infections; therapy is reduced to symptomatic treatment.

Taking into account the probable benignity of reoviral infections, their brevity, and the length of time required by the laboratory to confirm their diagnosis, it does not seem likely that an etiological treatment will be forthcoming in the more or less near future.

RESPIRATORY ENTEROVIRUSES

PROPERTIES

The properties of the enteroviruses have been thoroughly discussed in other chapters and will not be discussed again here.

EPIDEMIOLOGY

A certain number of enteroviruses seem to possess a respiratory tropism. They most often cause upper respiratory tract infection, but the possibility of an enteroviral origin of a pleuropulmonary infection should also be born in mind.

In a recent general review of the part played by enteroviruses in human pathology, Kibrick[18] noted the following etiological patterns: *upper respiratory infections*: Coxsackie viruses A21, A24, and the strains responsible for herpangina; Coxsackie B2, B3, B5; and ECHO 1, 3, 6, 19, 20, and probably ECHO 25; *croup*: Coxsackie A9, Coxsackie B5, ECHO 11; *pleuropulmonary infections*: Coxsackie A9, Coxsackie B4 and others, ECHO 9, 19, 20.

Certainly the myxoviruses and the adenoviruses play a preponderant part in respiratory viral infections, but the proportion of respiratory infections due to enteroviruses is by no means negligible. Wenner et al.[26] observing 25 young children during upper respiratory infections, noted the following percentages of increase in antibodies: anti-ECHO 11 in 36 per cent of the children, anti-ECHO 20 in 8 per cent, anti-ECHO 25 in 4 per cent, and anti-Coxsackie A21 in 8 per cent.

Generally speaking, the respiratory symptoms of enteroviral infections occur mainly in the summer-autumn period, as do the other symptoms due to these viruses.

However, various epidemics in nurseries that have been studied by Rosen et al.[24] showed that the enteroviruses could be introduced into a collectivity of this type at any time of the year and that propagation of the infection was always just as rapid. In fact, contagion from one child to another in this type of closed institution takes place extremely rapidly, and within four weeks after introduction of the virus practically all the children are contaminated. The persistence of the virus in the nursery can be explained by the successive infections of new arrivals.

This communal infection is due to the long period of elimination of the enteroviruses: 80 per cent of the children excreted the enterovirus in their stools for at least one week, 50 per cent for at least two weeks, 33 per cent for three weeks or more. The virus is also frequently found in the throat, but less regularly than in the stools. Furthermore, it does not seem possible to isolate these enteroviruses from the throat before they are found in the stools, nor do they seem to persist in the pharynx for less time than in the stools.

Again, in a general way, and according to the studies carried out on infections in nurseries, the virus is usually found in the stools 24 to 48 hours after the clinical onset of the disease.

The considerable variety of viruses responsible for infections of this type does not enable one to study the general epidemiological problems involved in greater detail. (The epidemiology of the ECHO and Coxsackie viruses has been dealt with in other chapters.) Indeed, the epidemiology of these respiratory enteroviruses is identical, on the whole, with that of the neuromeningeal, digestive, or cutaneous diseases caused by enteroviruses. However, of these viruses, two deserve to be studied in greater detail, as they differ considerably from the others; these are Coxsackie virus A21 (Coe virus) and ECHO virus 28.

Epidemiology of Coxsackie Virus A21. This virus, which is identical to Lennette's Coe virus, has been identified during the course of various epidemics of upper respiratory infections, accompanied or unaccompanied by pyrexia; these epidemics essentially affected military groups.[14, 17, 19]

One fact is worth stressing: Although Coxsackie A21 is an enterovirus that is altogether comparable in its characteristics with other type A Coxsackie viruses, it is isolated much more easily from the pharynx than from the stools.

From the end of August to November, 1960, a widespread epidemic due to Coxsackie A21 affected an American military training camp consisting of troops in training and military personnel permanently stationed at the camp.[14] A certain number of facts were comparable as far as these two military groups were concerned: the virus was isolated far more frequently from the throat than from the stools, the rectal samples being positive in only 15 per cent of the subjects whose throat samples were positive; and elimination of the virus was fairly prolonged, with it sometimes being excreted more than two weeks.

On the other hand, the epidemic itself assumed different aspects depending on whether it affected the young military trainees or the remainder of the camp population. Among the young recruits, the virus was isolated in 50 per cent of the patients and in 38 per cent of healthy subjects. During the first three weeks of the epidemic, the proportion of viral isolation was particularly high in the group of ill subjects, and then gradually decreased until at the end of the epidemic the number of viral isolations in the control group and in the patients was comparable.

In the group of military personnel permanently stationed in the camp, there were only 26 per cent of viral isolations among the patients and the virus was isolated in only 6 per cent of the control subjects in this group. Unlike the first group, this group did not show more frequent viral isolations among the patients than among the controls at the onset of the epidemic, the percentage of viral isolations being more or less parallel.

Another important difference is worth mentioning: when the epidemic had ceased there were 85 per cent seroconversions among the young military recruits, whereas over 50 per cent of the other military personnel lacked anti-Coxsackie A21 antibody.

This serological study showed that the majority of the population lacked these antibodies at the onset of the epidemic. As the epidemic gradually spread, the proportion of sera containing these antibodies increased, and there were fewer patients among the subjects who already possessed these antibodies than among the others, thus confirming the association of Coxsackie virus A21 infections with the respiratory disease.

In the group of recruits, the epidemic probably was terminated by the arrival of new immune subjects who had apparently been infected during their period of training in another camp. But in the other group at the end of the epidemic more than half of the subjects did not show the presence of antibodies. Hence it seems that contagion of Coxsackie virus A21, which occurs via the air, is probably slight and that the factors of immunity other than antiviral antibodies must interfere in the determination of natural infection in different social groups.

Analysis of a certain number of other epidemics due to Coxsackie A21 did not provide any further conclusions concerning this immunity. According to McDonald et al.[19] who examined over 1000 throat samples from November, 1958, to March, 1964, during respiratory infections, and approximately 1200 paired samples of serum, 8 per cent of the infections were considered to be due to Coxsackie viruses A21; 34 per cent of them thought to be associated with another viral infection, on the basis of results of serological tests. On the other hand, on the basis of viral isolations alone, there appeared to be only 3 per cent of Coxsackie A21 infections.

By comparing the serum antibodies for the Coe virus with homologous viral isolations, McDonald et al.[19] reached the same conclusions as Chanock: subjects showing antibodies in the early serum sample are less frequently affected clinically than subjects who do not possess these antibodies, a fact which confirms the protective role of the antibodies. However, the presence of antibodies neutralizing the virus has not always prevented infection.

Several tests involving nasal administration of the virus to volunteers[25] provided the following data:

In most of the subjects in the group without measurable homologous antibodies, an influenza-like disease appeared 24 to 48 hours after inoculation and lasted two to four days; the virus could be isolated from the patients' throats for three to six weeks, thus confirming the long period of elimination of this virus, whereas in the stools it was isolated only occasionally but for the same length of time.

Most of the inoculated subjects in the group with an intermediate titer of serum antibodies showed a syndrome of common cold with profuse rhinorrhea and few systemic manifestations.

Volunteers in the group with a high titer

of serum antibodies at the time of inoculation showed no increase in nasal secretion.

A fourfold rise in hemagglutination-inhibiting and neutralizing antibody occurred in a majority of volunteers with no measurable, or intermediate titers of antibody 12 to 15 days after challenge. The rise was considerably greater in subjects who had some antibody when challenged.

Both oral administration by means of capsules and direct inoculation of the intestinal tract in subjects with no homologous antibody produced no illness, no antibody production, no positive throat cultures, and only transient intestinal infection as judged by stool culture (rectal swabs were less often positive).

Although in many studies it is apparent that in general the enteroviruses more often affect children than adults, and that adults are contaminated by children, it seems clear that this is not the case for the Coxsackie virus A21. The majority of epidemics due to this virus have been described in adults and especially in soldiers. Furthermore, it was clearly evident from the epidemic studied by Chanock and co-workers[14, 17] that infection due to Coxsackie virus A21 is infrequent in children.

Epidemiology of ECHO Virus 28. Infections due to ECHO 28 have given rise to considerable interest with regard to the characteristics in tissue culture of this virus, which differ considerably from those of the other ECHO viruses, as do its pathogenicity and epidemiology. Indeed, in the opinion of a certain number of authors, this virus is a member of the rhinovirus group. Nevertheless, it does seem that in a chapter concerning the epidemiology of the respiratory enteroviruses it is necessary to say a few words about this virus.

A more complete study of it is to be found in the chapter concerning rhinoviruses (40).

Studies of epidemics, especially in military groups, and of inoculations of adult volunteers have contributed to a better understanding of the pathogenicity and of the epidemic pattern peculiar to this virus.

On the basis of serological surveys the ECHO virus 28 seems fairly widely distributed. Homologous antibodies are found in 6 per cent of children less than five years of age,[22] and according to statistics this percentage reaches 23 per cent in young children,

51 per cent in adolescents, and 65 per cent[22] to 68 per cent[23] in adults.

Infections due to ECHO virus 28 seem to be rare during the summer months but are encountered fairly regularly during the other seasons.

Epidemics due to this virus hence show a rather unusual character: their manifestations are usually minimal and affect only a fraction of a given population.

During an epidemic, 30 per cent of the subjects under observation by Holper et al.[15] and 36 per cent by Mogabgab[20] during the winter of 1958-1959 and in November and December 1959 showed an increase in anti-ECHO 28 antibodies.

It would seem that infections due to ECHO virus 28 are air borne, as is the case for Coxsackie A21 infections, since the virus is practically never isolated from the stools but solely from the nasopharynx.

On the other hand, although these infections may involve all the strata of a given population, it seems that adolescents and adults are more frequently infected than young children. Moreover, and this seems somewhat unusual, the spread of this virus within the family circle seems rather limited,[22, 23] as witnessed by the rarity of secondary cases in a family and the prevalence of the serum antibodies according to age.

Finally, the percentage of asymptomatic infections seems remarkably high, which may explain the paradoxically rather limited nature of these epidemics of ECHO virus 28.

The research studies of Price et al.[22] on natural infections as well as those of Jackson et al.[16] on the inoculation of volunteers permitted a better understanding of the epidemiology of this virus.

The incubation period is extremely short, and the symptomatology is generally evident after 24 hours and continues for two to five days. The virus is isolated solely from the pharynx and only during the first two to four days of infection.

As in the case of natural infection, inoculation by nasal administration to volunteers reproduced the disease in only 30 per cent of the subjects. However, there was infection even in the subjects who did not show any symptoms, as proved by virus isolations and the increase in homologous antibodies. The presence of these antibodies confers a certain immunity, but the latter is not complete, since natural infections may occur in subjects possessing these antibodies. Similarly, 5 per cent of the volunteers who received a second instillation of virus between four weeks and eight months after the first infection again showed clinical symptoms of this infection. But during this second experiment with ECHO 28, the subjects who had shown a clinical symptomatology the first time did not eliminate the virus, as opposed to those who had no visible symptoms the first time.

The antibodies seem to persist for six to nine months, sometimes even much longer, before decreasing.[22]

The epidemiological studies of Price again showed that, in contrast to the other enteroviruses, there was no difference in the extent of infections, as shown by the percentage of subjects possessing antibodies, whether they came from well-to-do populations or those in poor economic conditions; indeed the percentage of subjects possessing these antibodies increased with age in the same proportions in both groups.

To conclude, as concerns Coxsackie virus A21 or ECHO virus 28, both these viruses play an incontestable part in the origin of respiratory infections. However, they differ from the other enteroviruses by their almost exclusively pharyngeal elimination, their unusual distribution pattern, the fact that there are other factors involved than the neutralizing antibodies that can explain the immunity of certain subjects, and finally the fact that children seem less subject to infection by these viruses than they are to the other enteroviruses, the myxoviruses and the adenoviruses.

It is not feasible, with regard to the respiratory enteroviruses, to review the epidemiological characteristics of the other enteroviruses. The epidemiology of the ECHO viruses and Coxsackie virus A and B has been dealt with elsewhere (Chapters 15 and 22).

In all events, the epidemiological problems involved with regard to enteroviruses showing respiratory manifestations, other than the Coxsackie virus 21 and the ECHO virus 28, are common to all the other enteroviruses in every respect. In their case there reappears the pathogenic role essentially apparent in childhood (e.g., epidemics of croup due to ECHO virus 11[21]), adults becoming reinfected through contact with the children, but generally showing a minor

disease. These viruses are to be found just as frequently in the stools as in the throat rather than almost exclusively in the throat. They do not remain as long in the throat as the Coxsackie virus A21 does; the increase in the antibodies is more rapid and detectable from the tenth or fifteenth day of infection. Finally, these infections have a definite predilection for the summer-autumn period.

LABORATORY STUDIES

Sampling. The samples taken with a view to isolating respiratory enteroviruses should be taken as early as possible. Throat swabs and rectal swabs are taken, the swabs being subsequently squeezed into transport medium, i.e., Hank's-type medium, and dispatched to the laboratory as quickly as possible, maintained away from heat (cf. Chapter 3).

As always in diagnostic virology, it is always necessary, in addition, to take two serum samples, one at the onset of infection and the other after two weeks. It is sometimes advisable to take a third sample of serum, as the antibodies, particularly in the case of Coxsackie virus A21, have a tendency to appear rather later, often only in the third week of infection.

The virological techniques used to detect respiratory enteroviruses are very different according to the type of virus concerned. In fact, the enteroviruses do not all multiply in cell cultures, nor under the same conditions of culture. For this reason it is important to send, in addition to the request for viral isolation, any data that can orient the search. Thus if a clinical symptom associated with the respiratory infection suggested a Coxsackie infection, then newborn mice would be immediately inoculated.

That is to say, the clinician is well advised to include his clinical observations with his request in as great detail as possible.

Results. As is the case for the reoviruses, the simple isolation of a virus is of no value in itself. Even during an epidemic of respiratory infections during which, for example, a Coxsackie A21 is repeatedly isolated, other viruses may be concerned and frequently there are multiple infections,[19] so that isolation of a virus should not by itself be considered sufficient. It is always necessary in addition to perform serological tests and to observe a significant increase in the amounts of homologous antibodies to the virus isolated. It should be remembered that the increase in antibodies may be slow and appear only three weeks after the onset of infection.

To ask a virology laboratory to perform a serological test without search to detect the virus is useless if the enteroviral origin of a respiratory syndrome is suspected. In fact, there is no group-specific serological reaction for the enteroviruses. The seroneutralization tests or titration of antibodies by a complement-fixation reaction are only specific for the type. That is to say, it is not possible by any of the methods available to titrate the antibodies against all the enteroviruses that might be the cause of the respiratory syndrome. Also, there is an important obstacle to these investigations should they be attempted. On the one hand, a certain number of antigenic relationships between certain enteroviruses, detectable especially by the complement-fixation reaction, may make it difficult to interpret the serological reactions. On the other, the presence of viral strains that are slightly different antigenically from the prototype strains makes it clearly impossible, during the course of infection by any one given enterovirus, to detect an increase in the antibodies in the serum of the infected subjects if these antibodies are titrated against the prototype strain and not against the so-called prime strain responsible for the infection. Finally, anamnestic reactions, particularly in adults, are always possible, and an increase in the antibodies of an enterovirus does not necessarily signify a concomitant viral infection by this virus.

Thus, as far as the enteroviruses are concerned, one should be particularly careful and always remember that a considerable number of these viruses are likely to give rise to a respiratory symptomatology; that these infections are frequently quiescent; that their role in respiratory pathology is far less frequent than that of myxoviruses or adenoviruses; that during epidemics they are frequently associated with other viruses, in particular the adenoviruses, respiratory syncytial viruses, and parainfluenza viruses; and, finally, that there is no serological reaction specific to the group and that isolation of the virus together with a comparative homologous serological study in two serum samples provides a proof of multiplication of the viral agent within the organism.

Suffice it to say that, except during a definite epidemic, when a single serotype of enterovirus is consistently isolated more often in the affected population than in control subjects, one should remain extremely cautious before concluding that an enterovirus isolated in a single case of respiratory disease has played a pathogenic role.

IMMUNITY

As is the case for the majority of viral affections, the serum antibodies are the basis of immunity. Primary infections that are more or less spectacular contrast considerably with inapparent reinfections in subjects who already possess homologous antibodies. Inoculations to volunteers possessing antibodies frequently fail, thus confirming the protective role of the antibodies. However, the epidemiology of the Coxsackie virus A21 shows that there are other factors involved in the resistance to infection. These factors are at present unknown but may be related to age, the fact of living in a community, or even climate.

TREATMENT AND PROPHYLAXIS

At present there is no specific treatment against respiratory enteroviruses. There are a number of chemical substances that inhibit the multiplication of these viruses in vitro, but their use in human pathology is not current practice.

Interferon may prove to be an efficient weapon in combating viral infection, particularly respiratory virosis, but at present it is impossible to obtain it in sufficiently large quantities and the attempts at treatment that have already been carried out are insufficient to judge its efficacy. Hence, one is obliged to resort to symptomatic treatment, which should always be as limited as possible.

The use of current antibiotics is without effect, but it might be advisable, especially in young children, to prescribe them in addition to the symptomatic treatment, not for their specificity but to fight possible superinfection.

There remains the problem of prophylaxis; this has been attempted by vaccination, particularly in the case of ECHO virus 28, but this method does not seem to have wide possibilities. Indeed, the number of viruses that cause respiratory infections is far too great for vaccination to be possible against all these pathogenic agents. Furthermore, the enteroviruses play a relatively minor part, and this part is shared by a large number of serotypes.

Consequently, all the problems would need to be resolved as concerns the large-scale production of these vaccines; their efficacy would have to be proved, but also their innocuousness and the absence of contamination by a latent virus. Moreover, at least for the present, it is quite illusory to think of attempting to control the spread of the enteroviruses in general, and of the respiratory enteroviruses in particular. The latter, as we have already seen, are mainly transmitted by the air route; among town dwellers, it would seem impossible to prevent their pullulation. Hence it is natural to return to the thought of chemotherapy. Antiviral chemotherapy is still in its infancy, and nothing proves unjustified the hope that in the years to come interferon or antimetabolites may be used in human pathology and thus reduce the considerable number of working days lost because of respiratory enteroviruses.

BIBLIOGRAPHY

REOVIRUSES

1. Bricout, F., Regnard, J., and Duval, J.: Pouvoir pathogéne et diffusion des réovirus. Ann. Pediat. (Paris), *12*:43-48, 1965.
2. Gelfand, H. M., Holguin, A. H., Marchetti, G. E., and Feorino, P. M.: Enterovirus infections in healthy children. Amer. J. Hyg., *78*:358-375, 1963.
3. Kasel, J. A., Rosen, L., and Evans, H.: Infection of human volunteers with a reovirus of bovine origin. Proc. Soc. Exp. Biol. Med., *112*:978-981, 1963.
4. Lerner, A., Cherry, J., Klein, J., and Finland, M.: Infections with reoviruses. New Eng. J. Med., *267*:947-953, 1962.
5. Parker, L., Baker, E., and Stanley, N. F.: The isolation of reovirus type 3 from mosquitoes and a sentinel infant mouse. Aust. J. Exp. Med. Sci., *43*:167-170, 1965.
6. Rosen, L.: Serologic grouping of reovirus by hemagglutination inhibition. Amer. J. Hyg., *71*:242-265, 1962.
7. Rosen, L.: Reoviruses in animals other than man. Ann. N.Y. Acad. Sci., *101*:461-465, 1962.
8. Rosen, L., and Abinanti, F.: Natural and experimental infection of cattle with human types of reovirus. Amer. J. Hyg., *71*:250-257, 1960.
9. Rosen, L., Abinanti, F., and Hovis, J.: Further observations on the natural and experimental infection of cattle with reovirus. Amer. J. Hyg., *77*:38-48, 1963.

10. Rosen, L., Evans, M. E., and Spickard, A.: Reovirus infections in human volunteers. Amer. J. Hyg., *77*:29-37, 1963.
11. Rosen, L., Hovis, J., Mastrota, F., Bell, J., and Huebner, R.: An outbreak of infection with a type 1 reovirus among children in an institution. Amer. J. Hyg., *71*:266-274, 1960.
12. Rosen, L., Hovis, J., Mastrota, F., Bell, J., and Huebner, R.: Observation of a newly recognized virus (Abney) of the reovirus family. Amer. J. Hyg., *71*:258-265, 1960.
13. Stanley, N. F., and Leak, P. J.: The serologic epidemiology of reovirus infection, with special reference to the Rottnest Island quokka. Amer. J. Hyg., *78*:82-88, 1963.

RESPIRATORY ENTEROVIRUSES

14. Bloom, H. H., Johnson, K. M., Mufson, M. A., and Chanock, R. M.: Acute respiratory disease associated with Coxsackie A21 virus infection. II. Incidence in military personnel: observations in a nonrecruit population. J.A.M.A., *179*:120-125, 1962.
15. Holper, J. C., Miller, L. F., Crawford, Y., Sylvester, J. C., and Marquis, G. S., Jr.: Further studies on multiplication, serology and antigenicity of 2060 and JH viruses. J. Infect. Dis., *107*:395-401, 1960.
16. Jackson, G. G., Dowling, M. F., and Mogabgab, W. J.: Infectivity and interrelationships of 2060 and JM viruses in volunteers. J. Lab. Clin. Med., *55*:331-341, 1960.
17. Johnson, K. M., Bloom, H. H., Mufson, M. A., and Chanock, R. M.: Acute respiratory disease associated with Coxsackie A21 virus infection. I. Incidence in military personnel: observations in a recruit population. J.A.M.A., *179*:112-119, 1962.
18. Kibrick, S.: Current status of Coxsackie and Echo viruses in human disease. Progr. Med. Virol., *6*:27-70, 1964.
19. McDonald, J. C., Miller, D. L., Zuckerman, A. J., and Pereira, M. S.: Coe (Coxsackie A21) virus, parainfluenzae virus and other respiratory virus infection in the RAF, 1958-1960. J. Hyg. (Camb.), *60*:235-248, 1962.
20. Mogabgab, W. J.: Additional respirovirus type related to GL 2060 (Echo 28) virus, from military personnel, 1959. Amer. J. Hyg., *76*:160-172, 1962.
21. Philipson, L.: Association between a recently isolated virus and an epidemic of other respiratory disease in a day nursery. Arch. Ges. Virusforsch., *9*:25-30, 1954.
22. Price, W. H., Emerson, H., Ibler, I., Lachaine, R., and Terrell, A.: Studies of the JH and 2060 viruses, and their relationship to mild upper respiratory disease in humans. Amer. J. Hyg., *69*:224-249, 1959.
23. Rake, G. W., Sharma, R., and Werner, G. H.: Studies on the 2060 JH viruses. II. Seroepidemiological survey of infections with the 2060 agent in a group of families. Arch. Ges. Virusforsch., *12*:58-68, 1962.
24. Rosen, L., Bell, J. A., and Huebner, R. J.: Enterovirus infection of children and a Washington, D.C., welfare institution. In: Rose, H. M. (ed.): Viral

Infections of Infancy and Childhood. New York, Hoeber Division of Harper & Row, 1960, pp. 114-127.

25. Spickard, A., Evans, H., Knight, V., and Johnson, K. H.: Acute respiratory disease in normal volunteers associated with Coxsackie A21 viral infection. III. Response to nasopharyngeal and enteric

inoculation. J. Clin. Invest., *42*:840-852, 1963.

26. Wenner, H. A., Christodoulopoulou, G., Weston, J., Marsh, A., and Liu, C.: The epidemiology of acute respiratory diseases. II. Risk of infection among infants and family associates from viruses accompanying respiratory illnesses. Pediatrics, *28*: 886-907, 1961.

45

Nonviral Infections with Predominant Respiratory Manifestations

PSITTACOSIS AND ORNITHOSIS

by F. Dekking

The almost identical infectious agents causing psittacosis and ornithosis are not viruses, since they contain both RNA and DNA, whereas, by definition, in viruses the genetic material of the infectious particle consists of either one or the other, never both. They are probably related to the Rickettsiae. They are nevertheless included in this book, because the methods used to study them are those of virology, and because the infection in man produces a so-called "atypical" pneumopathy closely resembling viral pneumopathy.

CLINICAL ASPECTS

In man these agents cause an acute infectious disease of the respiratory tract, mostly characterized by a dry, nonproductive cough. The patient may be very ill, with high fever, sweating, severe, sometimes nearly intolerable headache, and a drowsiness which at times develops into coma or mental confusion. This is the classic picture of pneumotyphus of Ritter (1880).

Examination of the chest by auscultation and percussion usually reveals no signs of pneumonia, but x-ray examination shows a triangular shadow, which may migrate on subsequent days and may be large without producing any physical sign.

Because of the dull mental condition and the lack of physical signs of pneumonia, most patients are brought to the hospital with the diagnosis of typhoid fever.

The patient may present a picture of a severe toxic state and may die of myocarditis within a few days. Encephalitis has been described as a complication but is exceptional. On the other hand, in some patients bronchitis may be the only manifestation of the disease, which then resembles a mild influenza-like disorder.

As a rule the clinical picture at present is much less severe than that to be expected from the classic descriptions, perhaps because the mild forms are more frequently recognized, or, more specifically, owing to a change, more apparent than real, due to "dilution" of serious forms in a much higher number of attenuated or even subclinical forms now detected by the laboratory. The change may, however, be real: the present extensive dissemination among wild and domesticated birds may have created strains attenuated by rapid and repeated passages in this large population. Such endemicity tends to select the least virulent strains, as was seen in Australia when myxomatosis was introduced into a virgin rabbit population: in a few years mortality fell from some 95 per cent to about 50 per cent.

Without specific treatment the disease lasts several weeks, and convalescence lasts several months, but even in adequately treated patients convalescence may be long.

CAUSATIVE AGENT

Like viruses, the causative agent, a round particle 450 mμ in diameter, is an obligate intracellular parasite; it does not grow on artificial media, and it can infect most laboratory animals (especially mice), embryonated eggs, and, less efficiently, various tissue culture systems. The agent belongs to a very large group of related microbes, infectious for birds, mammals, and man. The agents of lymphogranuloma venereum, trachoma, and inclusion conjunctivitis (TRIC) belong to this group, as well as the agents of numerous diseases in domestic animals (cats, sheep, horses, and cattle, in particular).

The particles are surrounded by a weak, thermolabile, strain-specific antigen which covers a strong, thermostabile carbohydrate antigen. For serological tests a boiled suspension of infected tissue is used as antigen; it gives strong, but only group-specific, complement-fixation reactions. All members of the group produce a strain-specific toxin. By use of antitoxic sera, it is possible to distinguish these agents by a method that is exact but subtle and laborious to execute. Especially in psittacosis, the toxin is responsible for a large part of the clinical picture.

Although under natural conditions the agent coated by excreta survives at room temperature for about a week, under laboratory conditions infectious material is labile and should be kept frozen at $-20°$ C., or preferably at $-70°$ C. The boiled antigen is stable for several years. The particles stain well with all rickettsial stains (Giemsa, Castaneda, Macchiavello) and can be studied with the ordinary microscope. Typically, the particles are found in large intracellular colonies.

LABORATORY DIAGNOSIS

From human material the agent can be isolated in mice, eggs, and tissue culture, in that order of preference. The agent is found in sputum and blood and in the viscera at autopsy, but sputum and blood, especially, usually contain few infective particles. Isolation is much easier from the spleen, liver, and kidney of birds and from their droppings. The isolation procedures are time consuming and not very rewarding in human material.

Smears are of little practical value, except in heavily infected material.

The complement-fixation test is the method of choice. As antibody titers may remain high for ten years or longer, serological examination of a single specimen has a very limited diagnostic value and a rising titer should always be demonstrated. The fact that infection by other members of the group—lymphogranuloma venereum, enzootic abortion of ewes, bovine encephalomyelitis, and so forth—can give similar serological reactions should always be kept in mind. In TRIC infections the titers are low.

Neutralization tests are not practicable.

EPIDEMIOLOGY

The agent of psittacosis is found in psittacine birds (budgerigars, and others) and in canaries, among other pet birds; the agent of ornithosis is found in pigeons, chickens, ducks, and so forth. The agents differ in their virulence for man and the mouse, the psittacosis agent being the more virulent of the two. Distribution of both is worldwide. The agents are widespread in nature and especially abundant in aviaries and bird farms. They tend to cause lifelong latent infection, and even perfectly healthy birds may excrete the microbe continuously or intermittently, excretion being triggered by adverse conditions or the breeding season. The young birds are infected in the nest. It can be stated that nearly all cage birds have been infected once; most of them will carry the agent, and a sizable proportion will excrete it at one time or another. The droppings carry the agent, and infection takes place by inhalation of infective dust from the cage floor. The infectivity for man is low: multiple cases within the same household are rare, except when the source of the infection is a recently imported parrot.

Although man can carry the microbe for many years in his throat, man-to-man infections are an extreme rarity.

DIFFERENTIAL DIAGNOSIS

Clinical differentiation from other respiratory infections caused by viruses, *Rickettsia burneti,* or *Mycoplasma pneumoniae* is almost impossible, but the severe headache and the typhoid-like mental condition are rarely seen in the other infections, nor is the usually very high sedimentation rate.

Adequate therapy with tetracyclines causes the temperature to return to normal within 24 hours: this prompt reaction is seen only in psittacosis and ornithosis, and in infections with the Eaton agent; it distinguishes these from viral pneumopathies.

Previous contact with birds is another helpful criterion, but often the patients are not aware of such contact.

An absolutely certain diagnosis can be based only on the complement-fixation test, performed on two serum samples: one from the first week of the disease, and the second taken two or three weeks later. Such a test should form part of a complete battery of antigenic tests, including tests for the maximum number of respiratory viruses, psittacosis, Q fever, and the Eaton agent.

PREVENTION AND TREATMENT

The only sensible and effective prevention is to discourage the keeping of birds in the home. An attempt can be made to put an end to the carrier state of the birds by adding tetracyclines to their drinking water, but although successes have been described, it seems that failures are common.

Vaccination in birds or in man is not a practical possibility, because immunity is poor, and second infections in man are not rare: some subjects may have psittacosis twice or even three times at a few years' interval.

The specific treatment consists of 500 mg. of tetracycline four times a day, for four days.

BIBLIOGRAPHY

1. Beaudette, F. R. (ed.): Psittacosis: Diagnosis, Epidemiology, and Control. New Brunswick, N.J., Rutgers University Press, 1955.
2. Horsfall, F. L., and Tamm, I. (eds.): Viral and Rickettsial Infections of Man. Philadelphia, J. B. Lippincott Co., 1965.
3. Van der Hoeden, J.: Zoönoses. New York, American Elsevier Publishing Company, 1964.

Q FEVER

by P. Giroud and M. Capponi

Q fever, described for the first time in 1937 by Derrick[3] with the name of Query fever, is a rickettsial disease* provoked by *Rickettsia burnetii (Coxiella burnetii).*

Rickettsiae are microorganisms having both two types of nucleic acid and enzymes that permit a metabolic activity. They cannot, therefore, be confounded with viruses despite their inability to develop in artificial media. Q fever is discussed here because, in one of its best-known forms, it presents a radiological and clinical picture much like that of viral respiratory diseases and in this respect often poses difficult problems of differential diagnosis.

CLINICAL FEATURES

Form with Pulmonary Signs. The *incubation* period of the disease ranges from 11 to 26 days (average, 18 days). Short incubation periods have been described when contamination was massive and longer ones when the contamination was minimal. If the possible moment of contagion is known, it is easy to specify the length of incubation, as the onset of illness is usually sharply marked.

The disease *begins abruptly;* in some cases the patient can specify not merely the day, but even the hour of onset. Fever rises rapidly to 40° C. (104° F.) and sometimes higher. Profuse sweating, cephalalgia, arthralgia, and diffuse myalgia accompany it.

---

*Q fever should not be confused with Queensland fever, which belongs to the spotted-fever group and is caused by *R. australis.*

n the moderate form of the disease, fever asts about a week with daily remissions. The temperature curve takes on a serrated aspect. In the relapsing type, which is very common, after several days of hyperthermia, a remission may suggest that the disease is at an end. But a few days later the temperature rises again to about 39° C. (102.2° F.), describes a few oscillations, and then becomes lastingly normal.

Cephalalgia, either frontal or occipital and sometimes retro-orbital, may be accompanied by slight stiff neck but without true Kernig's sign. A lymphocytic reaction has sometimes been noted in the spinal fluid.

Anorexia is usual; it is often accompanied by nausea and vomiting, and sometimes by intestinal disorders.

Hepatomegaly and *splenomegaly* are detected irregularly.

A *thoracic rash* is fairly frequent. It can be localized on the shoulders. Often it is barely apparent and fleeting; sometimes it is scarlatiniform.

Usually toward the fifth or sixth day the cough appears with a sensation of thoracic constriction and occasionally even moderate dyspnea, that suggest a search for a genuine *respiratory localization.* The extent of this localization is extremely variable. In the series of cases reported by Derrick in 1937, no signs of pneumopathy were seen. In other reported cases the clinical signs were those of acute pneumococcal lobar pneumonia; in others foci of fine crepitant rales were heard, particularly at the end of inspiration. However, pulmonary involvement is often a discovery made in systematic radiological examination. The most diverse aspects have been described: hilifuge linear opacities, subclavian infiltration, infiltration of the lung bases, heterogeneous condensations, and/or a more or less opaque segmental or lobar picture. These aspects are very suggestive of viral pneumopathy. However, during Q fever, highly localized, homogeneous condensations, suggestive of pneumococcal pneumonia, are said to be much more frequent. The pleural images are sometimes associated with parenchymatous modifications, creating fissural thickening, a picture of bordering line, and sometimes even a discrete filling-in of the anterior or posterior cul-de-sac.

The usual *laboratory examinations* provide few characteristic elements. The leukocyte and erythrocyte counts are not notably altered. Usually leukopenia occurs at the onset and moderate leukocytosis at the end of the disease. In children an earlier and more marked leukocytosis may be found. In general only relative lymphocytosis with slight anemia is observed.

Sedimentation rate is moderately increased, in relation to the fever, and returns to normal with defervescence.

In rare cases, slight albuminuria has been reported.

The course is essentially benign. The duration of the disease is from one to two weeks. The fever falls abruptly or in swift lysis. Radiological signs persist for 10 to 15 days on the average. Recovery is total, without sequelae. However, asthenia often continues several weeks, with weight loss.

Relapses, essentially febrile, but on occasion with a labile pulmonary infiltration, can be expected.

Fatal cases are exceptional. A 1 per cent mortality rate has been reported in some regions in which epidemics of Q fever occurred. However, this is a relatively high rate, rarely observed.

Complications. Complications are exceptional. Other than the usual asthenia and weight loss of 7 to 10 kg., complications may, however, occur: they are vascular, endocarditic, or ocular.

The affinity of *R. burnetii* for *blood vessels* has been described by all authors, especially by us in France. Even arteriolar thrombosis with gangrene has been reported. Numerous cases of endocarditis due to Q fever have been described in Scotland, autopsy confirming this etiology, which had already been indicated by the serological results. In these cases, isolation of the pathogenic agent in the guinea pig left no room for doubt. However, the Scottish authors emphasized that earlier lesions due to rheumatic fever might have acted as a predisposing factor as concerns this localization of the rickettsial disease, a factor not always present.

Ocular complications are not exceptional. Uveitis is the most common. Of 2000 sera from a lesser number of patients who presented ocular diseases in Paris, 127 were positive for *R. burnetii.* It is possible that in these cases the initial disease was unrecognized, that either diagnosis of Q fever was not considered or that this disease was subclinical.

Mild or wholly subclinical Q fever can leave sequelae in all the blood vessels and provoke certain *disorders during gestation.* In a study of women who aborted for other than hormonal or mechanical reasons, 33 of 658 sera gave a reaction positive for *R. burnetii.* Among women who had malformed children, 5 of 47 sera were positive for *R. burnetii.*

Pleural and especially *hepatic* localizations must be mentioned among the complications. There can be signs of hepatic congestion and even jaundice. True necrosis with no apparent etiology other than *R. burnetii* infection has also been described. In Italy, fairly frequent hepatic complications have been reported; the supposition is that a precirrhotic state preceded the infection. It is interesting to note that the guinea pig inoculated with *R. burnetii* often shows hepatic modifications.

Clinical Forms. Although the disease is fairly monomorphous, different clinical forms can be distinguished.

The pure *febrile form* is the most typical form of Q fever, as Derrick described it. Attention should be called to the prolonged febrile forms, in which the persistent hyperthermia suggests brucellosis in certain cases.

Minor forms, and even subclinical forms, probably exist, especially in endemic zones.

In relation to host factors, the child presents a particular form, in which, especially in very young children, signs of encephalitis may be seen; the mother may be ill but not the infant, or vice versa. A form occurs in the aged in which cardiac complications are unusually frequent.

The possibility of meningeal forms should be mentioned.

THE PATHOGENIC AGENT

R. burnetii is the smallest member of the rickettsia group, usually measuring 0.25 by 1 μ, but it is very polymorphous. Spearshaped, bipolar, and diplobacillar aspects have been described; its size can then reach 1.5 to 2 μ.

It is gram negative and selectively stained by Giemsa's method. Its life is strict-

ly intracellular. It has a double or triple envelope and contains both types of nucleic acid, RNA and DNA.

It possesses a certain number of characteristics that distinguish it so clearly from other Rickettsiae that it has been proposed that the genus *Coxiella* be created for it; hence its second name, *Coxiella burnetii.* It is filterable with Berkefeld N filters and is particularly resistant to physical and chemical agents. It does not induce the formation of agglutinins against the Proteus strains, so that the Weil-Felix reaction cannot be used for the diagnosis of Q fever. It can survive and propagate independently of arthropods with no intermediate vector.

The peculiar resistance of *R. burnetii* to physical and chemical agents should be emphasized; it is greater than that of the other rickettsiae, but also greater than that of most non-spore-forming microorganisms. *R. burnetii* can subsist in ordinary drinking water for 30 to 36 months, in skimmed milk for 42 months, and in butter and in frozen or salted meat for more than a month. It resists pasteurization at 61.7° C. for 30 minutes. It is destroyed in 24 hours in yogurt and in a few minutes by boiling. It is preserved indefinitely by lyophilization or congelation at −70° C.

R. burnetii multiplies well in the yolk sac of the embryonated egg, in cultures of chick embryo tissue, and in a great variety of mammalian tissue cultures. Most small laboratory animals (rats, mice, hamsters, rabbits, guinea pigs) are easily infected by various routes: nasal, ocular, or peritoneal inoculation, for example.

Q fever confers a long-lasting immunity. Complement-fixing and agglutinating antibodies develop during convalescence.

EPIDEMIOLOGY

Q fever is a *zoonosis* widespread among wild animals, especially rodents: rabbits, rats, mice, and voles, but also among bats, hedgehogs, bandicoots, and so forth. In Czechoslovakia and in Russia, the role of birds as a virus reservoir has also been discussed. However, for man, domestic animals are the main source of contamination: in decreasing order of frequency, sheep, goats, cattle, horses, and swine. The disease rages in certain herds in an endemic form, and apparently healthy animals can eliminate considerable quantities of this rickettsia in their milk, urine, feces, and, particularly, the placenta.

Q fever is only rarely transmitted to man by bites of acarids, although Derrick incriminated ticks in his initial case reports. Contamination often occurs at the time of professional contact with infected animal products. Thus Q fever is most frequent among breeders, veterinarians, butchers, slaughter-house workers, laboratory personnel, and so forth.

The routes of inoculation are various: subcutaneous introduction through minute skin erosions, conjunctival inoculation, ingestion of raw milk, and, in most cases, inhalation of contaminated dust (e.g., infection of postal workers who have manipulated sacks inadvertently transported in railway wagons used for cattle). Cases of interhuman contamination have been reported but remain rare.

Distribution of the disease is therefore closely linked to the animal reservoirs of *R. burnetii*. It is endemic in certain regions where infection of wild animals maintains the source of contamination of domestic herds (Australia, the United States, Africa, Great Britain, France, the countries bordering the Mediterranean, Central Europe, and Russia). Epidemic outbreaks appear either when nonimmunized populations enter endemic zones ("Balkan influenza" during World War II and among Europeans arriving in Africa), or when contaminated animals are transferred into disease-free areas.

CLINICAL DIAGNOSIS

Diagnosis of the disease is based on clinical and radiological signs and, especially, on epidemiological facts and the results of laboratory investigations.

During the first few days of illness, the pure febrile form and the pulmonary form pose problems of diagnosis common to all acute febrile disorders. In particular, influenza, typhoid fever, meningitis, infectious hepatitis, and even brucellosis may come to mind. The long train of associated signs, the course, and, lastly, the results of laboratory tests make elimination of bacterial infections fairly easy. Consideration of the anicteric forms of infectious hepatitis may lead to performing different tests for hepatic involvement. But influenza is the disease that poses the most difficult problems of differential diagnosis. Isolated cases of influenza are rare, however, and the existence of an epidemic, the extent of the systemic signs, the rapidity of evolution, and the appearance of specific hemagglutination-inhibiting antibodies enable diagnosis.

Appearance of the pulmonary signs suggests diagnoses as varied as acute lobar pneumococcic pneumonia, ornithosis, psittacosis, "atypical pneumonia," and viral pneumopathy.

The presence of polymorphonuclear leukocytosis and the isolation of the pathogenic agents from the blood or sputum permit recognition of bacterial pneumonia. The elements in favor of diagnosis of other diseases appear in other chapters of this book. We shall only mention that the radiological pictures in Q fever are more often suggestive of acute lobar pneumococcic pneumonia than of viral pneumopathy or "atypical pneumonia."

Aside from these negative arguments, certain signs orient the clinician more or less directly toward a diagnosis of Q fever: the polymorphous character of the clinical picture, and, especially, the *epidemiological contact* (profession, travel in an endemic area, evidence of a circumscribed group of cases centered around presumably contaminated material). Such findings render laboratory investigation obligatory, as it alone can affirm the etiological role of *R. burnetii*.

LABORATORY DIAGNOSIS

Direct demonstration of Rickettsiae is not to be hoped for, although sputum and blood may contain them and although inoculation of laboratory animals, preferably guinea pigs, may be revealing. But even if *R. burnetii* has already been isolated in several cases, especially from the blood (where, in a manner more theoretical than practical, *R. burnetii* may be detectable by Coons' technique, for example) reliance should be placed on the serological results, which are indispensable for the diagnosis. In Q fever antibodies are detectable fairly early, in contrast to their much later appearance in diseases of the spotted-fever group. From the tenth day after onset of the disease, agglutinating antibodies appear, and their level rises rapidly.

As the Weil-Felix test is always negative, a search for agglutinating antibodies should be made with the technique described in 1942 by Giroud and Giroud and applied to Q fever since 1950. A positive reaction with low titers and without a rising curve suggests an earlier infection.

R. burnetii agglutinating antibodies are sensitive and highly specific. If the antibody titer rises rapidly and if strong doses of antibiotics do not hinder antibody formation, Q fever is suggested. Even a low antibody titer (1/20) followed by increasing titers is incontestable evidence. Very high titers, in the order of 1/1280, can be observed, but usually the response is in the range of 1/80 to 1/160.

Used in parallel with the microagglutination technique, two methods are of interest: Coons' technique of indirect immunofluorescence, and the complement-fixation reaction.

Coons' technique can be applied by any laboratory with the formalin-treated antigen used for the microagglutination test. It often yields responses closely parallel to those of microagglutination; thus, by its high specificity, it confirms the results given by the agglutinins.

The complement-fixation test has its usefulness: it affords confirmation, by results of a third test, of results of the two previous reactions and permits better precision in situating the onset of the disease, for appearance of complement-fixing antibodies follows, with a slight delay, that of the agglutinating and of the fluorescent antibodies.

Can diagnosis by a test of allergy also be considered? Q fever is an allergy-producing disease. With a highly attenuated antigen, preferably phenol-treated, it is entirely feasible to determine the intradermal reaction. But a test of allergy made with too high doses presents the danger of a focal and a systemic reaction; moreover the test is of only epidemiological value and is not diagnostic.

Other tests described, such as the radioisotope test, are seldom used. The radioisotope test confirms results obtained by the allergic reactions.

Thus, when the laboratory finds a low titer of *R. burnetii* antibodies in an early serum sample and a titer significantly higher in the later sample, the increase is proof of the etiology of the disease. On the other hand, a reaction that is positive in the early sample but subsequently disappears should simply be considered to represent a booster reaction involving earlier antibodies.

As concerns anatomic pathology, it is diagnostically useless except in connection with autopsy because few biopsies are practicable during Q fever. *R. burnetii* strains have often been isolated from the guinea pig in cases of fatal Q fever endocarditis. In such cases hyaline thrombus of the valves with microcolonies of rickettsia, vegetations, and a slight inflammatory reaction have been described, as in the lungs. In other cases, edema, a hyperergic reaction, granulation tissue, and so forth have been seen.

TREATMENT

Once the diagnosis has been established, treatment of the disease is simple. *R. burnetii* is sensitive to broad-spectrum antibiotics, especially chlortetracycline and oxytetracycline. Chloramphenicol, Rovamycin, and the cyclines are usually active. However, because *R burnetii*, unlike other Rickettsiae, is highly resistant, very strong doses of these antibiotics given over a long period are required to eliminate the microbe. One schedule of treatment for adults is 2 gm. per day by mouth for some 12 days, then a pause, and continuation of treatment at the same dose for another 10 days or so.

Low doses of corticosteriods, in combination with the antibiotics, can be useful.

PROPHYLAXIS

In endemic zones it is indispensable to take all the precautions capable of reducing the risk of food contamination: *boiling of milk or pasteurizing it* either at 62.8° C. for 30 minutes or at 71.7° C. for 15 seconds.

In areas where the disease is not established, control of the transport of domestic animals is desirable.

Isolation of patients does not seem indispensable, but careful *disinfection* of their excreta is recommended.

Various types of vaccines (attenuated or inactivated) are being studied. When they have proved their efficacy and innocuousness they could present some interest in man, especially for subjects who run a high professional risk of contamination. But, in general, Q fever is a disease that responds well to antibiotic therapy and in which the dangers of immunization at present seem greater than those of nonimmunization.

In view of the serious effect of Q fever on cattle, in which the most frequent complications of this type of disease are abortion and infertility, in France the only form of vaccination that it has seemed possible to consider has been immunization of the animals themselves. Vaccination of animals with a strain of *R. burnetii* and a strain of neorickettsia (group Bedsonia) has been proposed. This is the vaccine formula adopted by the Pasteur Institute.

BIBLIOGRAPHY

1. Capponi, M.: Valeur de l'immunofluorescence indirecte pour le diagnostic sérologique des rickettsioses. Ann. Inst. Pasteur, *111*:458-469, 1966.
2. Combiesco, D.: Fièvre Q (typhus pulmonaire, rickettsioses pulmonaires). Arch. Roum. Path. Exp. Microbiol., *16*:37-55, 1957.
3. Derrick, E. H.: "Q" fever, a new fever entity. Med. J. Aust., *2*:281-299, 1937.
4. Giroud, P.: Ce que l'on sait et ce que l'on voudrait savoir de la fièvre Q ou maladie de Derrick et Burnet. Bull. Soc. Vét. Pratique de France, Vol. 35, Juillet-Octobre, 1951, seance du 10 octobre, 1951.
5. Giroud, P., and Capponi, M. G.: La fièvre Q ou maladie de Derrick et Burnet. Collection de l'Institut Pasteur, Paris, Flammarion, 1966.
6. Giroud, P., and Giroud, M. L.: Agglutination des rickettsies, test de séro-protection et réaction d'hypersensibilité. Bull. Soc. Path. Exot., *37*:84, 1944.
7. Giroud, P., and Jadin, J.: Comparaison entre différents tests pour le diagnostic de la fièvre Q. Réactions allergiques, fixation du complément et agglutination des rickettsies. C. R. Acad. Sci., *230*:2347-2348, 1950.
8. Ormsbee, R. A.: "Q" fever rickettsia. In: Horsfall, F. L., and Tamm, I.: Viral and Rickettsial Infections of Man. Ed. 4. Philadelphia, J. B. Lippincott Co., 1965, pp. 1144-1160.
9. Porte, L., and Capponi, M.: Syndrome encéphalitique chez un enfant présentant au décours de sa maladie une réaction positive vis-à-vis de R. burneti. Bull. Soc. Path. Exot., *47*:480-481, 1954.

MYCOPLASMA PNEUMONIAE PNEUMOPATHIES

by R. Caravano

Some 30 years ago, an entity with a characteristic anatomicoclinical appearance and usually associated with a biological syndrome[5, 13, 14, 22, 27] was identified within the large group of infectious nonspecific pulmonary condensation syndromes. This syndrome, which could not be linked to a known germ, has been described under various names, the most common being primary atypical pneumonia, virus pneumonia, or cold agglutinin pneumonia.

The more thorough study of epidemics in the Armed Forces during World War II made it possible to specify their clinical and biological characteristics and also showed that the disease is transmissible by a filtrate of bronchial secretions or throat washings. The ineffectiveness of treatment with sulfonamide drugs and penicillin was also established.[11, 12] These features seemed to suggest a viral etiology. The isolation of the causal agent by Eaton in 1944 appeared definitively to confirm this view.[15] This filterable microorganism, which multiplied only in tissue culture and was penicillin- and streptomycin-resistant, was indeed considered a virus for years. However, the favorable results of treatment with antibiotics other than penicillin and streptomycin aroused doubt as to the viral etiology of the disease. The problem was elucidated in 1962 by Chanock et al.,[6] who first succeeded in cultivating Eaton's agent in an artificial medium and in identifying it as a Mycoplasma.

Hence the pneumopathies due to *Mycoplasma pneumoniae* described here are treated essentially from the viewpoint of their clinical and radiological similarities to the bronchopulmonary diseases of viral origin.

MYCOPLASMA

The identification of a Mycoplasma as the true agent of "atypical pneumonia" was the first reliable evidence of the part played in human pathology by a member of this microbiological group, which had been discovered some 70 years earlier. The role in veterinary pathology of other members of the group had been fully established since 1910, the year when Bordet[2] and Borrel[3] confirmed the earliest description by Nocard,[25] of the first known of these agents, the cause of bovine peripneumonia, a disease well known to stock breeders and justly feared. Later, Bridré and Donatien[4] isolated a similar organism from animals with contagious agalactia. All these organisms were first assembled in a fairly homogeneous bacteriological group then called pleuropneumonia organisms (PPO). Subsequently, these and a large number of similar organisms, isolated from many animal species, in which they may act either as pathogens or as apparently harmless saprophytes, were grouped under the name of pleuropneumonia-like organisms (PPLO). All of the PPO-PPLO are now considered to form a microbiological "group," the taxonomy of which has not yet been firmly established, but which has received officially the name Mycoplasma.

With suitable research techniques, mycoplasma can be isolated fairly frequently from man, particularly from the upper respiratory tract[24] and the genital tract.[23] Many of these organisms are undoubtedly saprophytes. But their pathogenic role seems likely in certain cases, particularly in some cases of nonspecific urethritis in man. However, for the time being, primary atypical pneumonia is the only disease in man to be linked with certainty to a mycoplasma.

Mycoplasma are very difficult to culture in artificial media. In low-concentration agar media, they grow in small colonies, usually visible under low-power microscopic magnification, that present a highly distinctive appearance: the center, deeply embedded in the gel, is dense and opaque; it is surrounded by a clearer areola, with a dentate aspect, formed by large globules.

Mycoplasma are poorly stained by the usual aniline dyes, and more complex methods must be used, such as the hot Giemsa or the Dienes technique. As mycoplasma grow poorly in liquid media, and as they also are extremely sensitive to conditions in the medium, their elementary forms are not well known. The smallest element capable of reproduction, called elementary body, passes through bacterial filters. The electron microscope reveals a limiting membrane, formed by two or three layers, with the characteristics of a cytoplasmic membrane,[28] but no formation similar to the cell wall of bacteria.

This group comprises serologically different species. Several methods have been used to find antigenic differences: direct agglutination, agglutination of sensitized latex particles, and the complement-fixation test. A very interesting property of mycoplasma is that the growth of a given species is inhibited by the homologous immune serum.

Mycoplasma pneumoniae has the general characteristics of the members of the group and several individual ones. Its colonies are more homogeneous and rarely show the typical "fried egg" appearance; it is the only human mycoplasma causing slight hemolysis in blood media.[9] Its culture is difficult and requires addition to the media of horse serum and yeast extract. The specific antigens of *Mycoplasma pneumoniae* that are not found in other species of human origin (there is no group antigen) are revealed by the complement-fixation test,[7] which has superseded the immunofluorescence test.[10] The homologous immune serum inhibits growth of *Mycoplasma pneumoniae* both in experimental animals and in agar or cell cultures.[19]

PNEUMOPATHY CAUSED BY MYCOPLASMA PNEUMONIAE

CLINICAL FEATURES

The disease affects all age groups but seems more frequent among children and young adults and is infrequent among children under age five.

The incubation period, established by inoculation into volunteers, lasts from one to three weeks. It seems to be better defined (one to two weeks) in patients who react with a pneumopathy of the pneumonic type than in those in whom the respiratory disease takes on a different character.[11, 12, 14, 27]

The onset is not as abrupt as in pneumococcal lobar pneumonia. It may be marked either by systemic symptoms—general discomfort, headache, fever, prostration, and anorexia—or by symptoms affecting the upper respiratory tract—sore throat and rhinitis. Thoracic respiratory symptoms appear a few days later. The cough, which is dry and often paroxysmal at the beginning, aggravates the headache that is one of the most constant symptoms. After three to five days expectoration appears. The sputum is first mucous, then mucopurulent; rarely it is streaked with blood. At this stage, the patient frequently complains of dull chest pain, often retrosternal.

Fever varies in intensity. The patient appears not to be seriously ill. The pulse rate is moderately accelerated, but respiratory frequency is normal.

Generally speaking, physical findings are few. At the outset an ordinary pharyngeal erythema may sometimes be noticed. Respiratory signs may be limited to a decrease in the vesicular breath sounds. When the disease has developed fully, the most characteristic sign is the presence of foci of subcrepitant rales, but without other signs of hepatization (neither souffle nor dullness). When expectoration becomes more abundant, coarse moist bronchial rales are heard.

The length of the course varies widely. Fever disappears progressively, most often after one or two weeks but occasionally it may last as long as six weeks. The disease is rarely fatal: 2 per 1000 is the maximum mortality in the most disfavored groups of patients; death most often results from cardiovascular complication. Convalescence is slow and is frequently accompanied by pronounced asthenia.

RADIOLOGICAL SIGNS

The extraordinary contrast between the paucity of clinical symptoms and signs and the extent of the radiological lesions is one of the striking characteristics of pneumopathy caused by *Mycoplasma pneumoniae*. The first radiological signs appear on the second to the fifth day after onset. They consist in condensation images which are frequently much more extensive than the physical examination indicated; they do not have the regularity, the segmentary limitation, or the density of pneumonic hepatization. The opacities are irregular, cloudy, and ill defined. They involve more than one lobe in half of the cases. They often radiate away from the hilus in trails along the bronchovascular axes. The picture is extremely variable; new centers appear with the development of the disease, while earlier ones are modified. Another characteristic peculiarity is the slow resorption of these centers: residual opacities may persist several weeks after clinical cure.

PATHOLOGICAL ANATOMY

Because the disease is rarely fatal, there have been no anatomical observations since the disease was specifically linked with *Mycoplasma pneumoniae*. Earlier examinations in fatal cases in which the clinical picture resembles that produced by *Mycoplasma pneumoniae*[26] suggested that the condensation seen by x-ray had resulted not from exudative alveolitis, as in pneumococcal lobar pneumonia, but from cellular infiltration and peribronchial edema.

Superimposed atelectatic foci have been found. This anatomical image fits the aspect and the evolution of the radiological pictures.

EPIDEMIOLOGY

Pneumopathy caused by *Mycoplasma pneumoniae* appears to be endemic throughout the world. Epidemics have been noted in hospitals[13, 18, 20, 22, 27] and in the Armed Forces.[5, 13, 21] The study of these grouped outbreaks was what led to precise knowledge of this disease. However, epidemics seem to have become rare in the last 20 years. The exact incidence is unknown. During World War II it approached 10 per 1000 annually in the United States Army. Chanock et al.[8] proved serologically that in the Armed Forces *Mycoplasma pneumoniae* was at the origin of 28 per cent of febrile disorders of the upper respiratory tract and of 56 per cent of cases of "atypical pneumonia," but this percentage varied widely in function of epidemiological conditions.

In current civilian practice, the cases most often observed are individual and caused by direct contact. Limited epidemics are obviously possible in certain collectivities.

Transmission is probably direct, and the portal of entry appears to be the upper respiratory tract. The length of the infectious period is unknown; possibly there exist chronic carriers able to infect receptive subjects.

The incidence of the disease is higher in winter. Although it is higher in children and young adults, no age group is entirely spared. Immunity, if it exists, is not absolute, since repeated infections have been observed.

DIAGNOSIS

The "diphasic" onset (involvement first of the upper respiratory tract and then of the lower respiratory pathways) suggestive of "viral" pneumopathies, the nondeterioration of general physical condition, the paucity of physical signs (particularly the lack of signs of condensation) contrasting with the extent of radiological signs, and the aspect of the radiological pictures themselves make it easy to eliminate diseases such as pneumococcal pneumonia and bacterial bronchopneumonias.

On the other hand, nothing in the clinical picture or its course enables the practitioner to connect with certainty an "atypical pneumonia" with *Mycoplasma pneumoniae.* Pulmonary diseases such as coccidioidomycosis and histoplasmosis may cause difficulties in diagnosis if there are no associated cutaneous signs. The same applies to rickettsial disease not accompanied by a mark of insect bite, as is precisely the case for Q fever, the pneumopathy of which closely resembles that due to *Mycoplasma pneumoniae.*

Other pneumopathies to be eliminated are mainly those due to agents of the psittacosis group, to influenza and parainfluenza viruses, to the respiratory syncytial virus, and to adenoviruses. Epidemiological evidence is not constant and is merely a guideline. The only possibility of a firm etiological diagnosis lies in biological examinations.

Direct Isolation It is possible to isolate *Mycoplasma pneumoniae* directly from throat swabs or washings or from sputum as long as there has been no treatment. The microorganism remains in the respiratory tract for a long time (up to 45 days after the clinical onset). The method of inoculating embryonated eggs or tissue cultures has yielded good results, but its practice is limited because of the spontaneous dissemination of *saprophytic mycoplasma* in almost all eggs and almost every current cell strain.[1] Inoculation into the animal (cotton rat) is difficult. The current method therefore remains isolation in a special medium containing a high proportion of horse serum and fresh yeast extract, slightly solidified by an atoxic jellifying substance and with addition of crystal violet or antibiotics (penicillin-streptomycin) to reduce the development of associated flora.

Unfortunately, the isolation and handling of mycoplasma and their identification require considerable experience. Moreover, the method is slow; it may take from two to three weeks. Diagnosis of the species is serological; since it is based on growth inhibition by the homologous protective serum, such serum must obviously be available.

Nonspecific Serological Tests. Non-specific serological tests, which are easily carried out but necessarily of limited value, have been known for a long time and are an integral part of the conventional description of "primary atypical pneumonia."

COLD AGGLUTININS. Cold agglutinins for group O erythrocytes appear in approximately half of the subjects affected; the percentage varies considerably from one group of patients to another. The level begins to rise from the seventh to the tenth day and attains its maximum between the third and the fourth weeks. A fourfold increase in the initial level during convalescence is considered significant. If only an isolated titration is available, a level of at least 1/32 is required. Cold agglutinins may appear during hepatic diseases, blood dyscrasias, protozoan infections (malaria, trypanosomiasis), and also, unfortunately, in adenovirus pneumopathies, in which this biological sign is, however, less frequent (maximum 17 per cent).

AGGLUTINATION OF MG STREPTOCOCCUS. Streptococcus MG is a serological variety of *Streptococcus viridans,* found by Horsfall. There is no conclusive evidence of any link between this organism and *Mycoplasma pneumoniae* pneumopathy, and its agglutination by the serum of patients with this disease is possibly a phenomenon of coantigenicity, similar to that of the agglutination of certain Proteus organisms in rickettsial diseases. The agglutination of streptococcus MG at a significant level is rare in other diseases; this fact would make it a more reliable test if it were not extremely irregular: agglutinins for streptococcus MG are found in from 25 to 75 per cent of authentic cases of infection due to *Mycoplasma pneumoniae.*

Specific Serological Tests. Specific serological tests have the obvious advantage of greater accuracy but are not practicable by most laboratories, the antigen (*Mycoplasma pneumoniae* itself) being difficult to prepare. There are two serological methods.

THE IMMUNOFLUORESCENCE TECHNIQUE. This is the most sensitive but technically the most difficult. It consists in checking with an ultraviolet microscope the agglutination of *Mycoplasma pneumoniae,* sensitized by an antiglobulin serum marked with fluorescein, by the serum examined at increasing dilutions. The levels thus defined re high enough but because of the equipment required this technique is beyond the means of most laboratories.

THE COMPLEMENT-FIXATION TEST. This test is based on the conventional system of complement serology and uses *Mycoplasma pneumoniae* as antigen. It does not require the expensive equipment of the previous technique but may present technical difficulties. Only levels higher than 1/16, indicating strong fixation of complement should be retained. Results of the complement-fixation test are slightly less regular than those of the preceding one (positive in only 80 per cent of cases).

It is preferable in both instances to note a distinct rise between the phase of the clinical outset and convalescence, because some previous disease may have left a detectable residual level.

TREATMENT

Since neither the degree of immunity against *Mycoplasma pneumoniae* nor its basis is known, no active immunization measure is available. Contamination being essentially (if not exclusively) direct and interhuman, quarantine in dubious cases may prove helpful if the outset of an epidemic is suspected.

Since in "atypical pneumonia" due to *Mycoplasma pneumoniae* penicillin and streptomycin are ineffective, an effective antibiotic should be chosen from the tetracycline group. Although the disease is usually not dangerous and regresses spontaneously, suitable antibiotic therapy reduces its intensity and significantly shortens the duration of systemic and local signs and symptoms. In the more severe cases that seem to justify specific treatment, the physician may administer 2 gm. of tetracycline daily in four doses for five to six days. Dimethlychlorotetracycline may be used with the same results at a dose of 300 mg. three times a day for six days.

When the titer of cold agglutinins is very high, physical methods of cooling the patient to reduce the fever should be avoided because of the risk of acute hemolysis.

BIBLIOGRAPHY

1. Barile, M. F., Malizia, W. F., and Riggs, D. B.: Incidence and detection of PPLO in cell cultures by fluorescent antibody and cultural procedures. J. Bact., *84*:134, 1962.
2. Bordet, J.: La morphologie du microbe de la péripneumonie des bovidés. Ann. Inst. Pasteur, *24*: 161, 1910.
3. Borrel, P.: Le microbe de la péripneumonie. Ann. Inst. Pasteur, *24*:168, 1910.
4. Bridré, J., and Donatien, A.: Le microbe de l'agalaxie contagieuse du mouton et de la chèvre. Ann. Inst. Pasteur, *39*:925, 1925.
5. Campbell, T. A., Strong, P. S., Grier, G. S., and Lutz, R. J.: Primary atypical pneumonia; a report of 200 cases. J.A.M.A., *122*:929, 1943.
6. Chanock, R. M., Hayflick, L., and Barile, M. F.: Growth on artificial medium of an agent associated with atypical pneumonia and its identification as a PPLO. Proc. Nat. Acad. Sci., *48*:41, 1962.
7. Chanock, R. M., James, W. D., Fox, H. H., Turner, H. C., Mufson, M. A., and Hayflick, L.: Growth of Eaton PPLO in broth and preparation of complement-fixing antigen. Proc. Soc. Exp. Biol. Med., *110*:884, 1962.
8. Chanock, R. M., Mufson, M. A., Bloom, H. H., James, W. D., Fox, H. M., and Kingston, J. R.: Eaton agent pneumonia. J.A.M.A., *175*:213, 1961.
9. Clyde, W. A., Jr.: Hemolysis in identifying Eaton's PPLO. Science, *139*:55, 1963.
10. Clyde, W. A., Jr., Denny, F. W., and Dingle, J. H.: Fluorescent-stainable antibodies to the Eaton agent in human primary atypical pneumonia transmission studies. J. Clin. Invest., *40*:1638, 1961.
11. Commission on Acute Respiratory Diseases: The transmission of primary atypical pneumonia to human volunteers. Bull. Johns Hopkins Hosp., *79*:97, 1946.
12. Commission on Acute Respiratory Diseases: Experimental transmission of minor respiratory illness to human volunteers by filter-passing agents. J. Clin. Invest., *26*:957, 974, 1947.
13. Dingle, J. H., Abernethy, T. J., Badger, G. F., Buddingh, G. J., Feller, A. E., Langmuir, A. D., Ruegsegger, J. M., and Wood, W. B.: Primary atypical pneumonia, etiology unknown. Amer. J. Hyg., *39*:67, 1944.
14. Dingle, J. H., and Finland, M.: Virus pneumonias. II. Primary atypical pneumonias of unknown etiology. New Eng. J. Med., *277*:378, 1942.
15. Eaton, M.D., Meiklejohn, G., and van Herick, W.: Studies on the etiology of primary atypical pneumonia. I. A filterable agent transmissible to cotton rats, hamsters and chick embryos. J. Exp. Med., *79*:649, 1944.
16. Eaton, M. D., Meiklejohn, G., van Herick, W., and Corey, M.: Studies on the etiology of primary atypical pneumonia. II. Properties of the virus isolated and propagated in chick embryos. J. Exp. Med., *82*:317, 1945.
17. Favour, C. B.: Infections associated with an epidemic of primary interstitial pneumonia. New Eng. J. Med., *230*:537, 1944.
18. Gallagher, J. R.: Bronchopneumonia in adolescents. Yale J. Biol. Med., *7*:23, 1934.
19. Jensen, K. E., Neal, E. J., and May, P. A.: Suppression of growth of Eaton mycoplasma by immune sera. Fed. Proc., *22*:325, 1963.
20. Johnson, R. T., Cook, M. K., Chanock, R. M., and Buescher, E. L.: Family outbreak of primary atypical pneumonia associated with the Eaton agent. New Eng. J. Med., *262*:817, 1960.

21. Kingston, J. R., Chanock, R. M., Mufson, M. A., Helmann, L. P., James, W. D., Fox, H. H., Manko, M. A., and Boyers, J.: Eaton agent pneumonia. J.A.M.A., *176*:118, 1961.

22. Kneeland, Y., Jr., and Smetana, H. F.: Current bronchopneumonia of unusual character and undetermined etiology. Bull. Johns Hopkins Hosp., *67*:229, 1940.

23. Morton, H. E., Smith, P. F., and Leberman, P. R.: The cultivation of PPLO from the human genitourinary tract with reference to their possible venereal transmission. Amer. J. Syph., *35*:14, 1951.

24. Morton, H. E., Smith, P. F., Williams, N. B., and Eickeberg, C. F.: Isolation of PPLO from human saliva; a newly detected member of the oral flora. J. Dent. Res., *30*:415, 1951.

25. Nocard, M. L.: Le microbe de la péripneumonie des bovidés. Ann. Inst. Pasteur, *12*:240, 1898.

26. Parker, F., Jr., Jolliffe, L. S., and Finland, M.: Primary atypical pneumonia. Report of 8 cases with autopsies. Arch. Path., *44*:581, 1947.

27. Reimann, H. A.: An acute infection of the respiratory tract with atypical pneumonia. A disease entity probably caused by a filterable virus. J.A.M.A., *111*:2377, 1938.

28. Van Iterson, W., and Ruys, A. C.: The fine structure of mycoplasmataceae. J. Ultrastruct. Res., *3*:282, 1960.

PART VII

Viral Infections with
Involvement of the
Hematopoietic and
Lymphatic System

46

Viruses and Leukemias

By J. BERNARD

This study is purposely confined to a critical examination of the methods used and the data obtained from them. These methods can be grouped under three main headings: (1) study of animal leukemias; (2) epidemiological study of human leukemias; and (3) observations and research made on human leukemias.

STUDY OF ANIMAL LEUKEMIAS

Spontaneous Leukemias in Animals

Leukemias may occur spontaneously in numerous animal species. The better known are those occurring in fowl, mice, and cattle.

Leukemias in Fowl. First mentioned in 1896 by Caparini, fowl leukemia was transmitted experimentally in 1908 by Ellerman and Bang, who at this early date proved its viral nature.

Clinicopathological Aspects. Three forms of leukemia are found in fowl:

Erythroblastosis, which occurs in nature as a sporadic, noncontagious disease, is fairly infrequent. It is accompanied by anemia and severe erythroblastemia and results in death within two or three weeks.

Myeloblastosis, which is rarer, was recognized more recently. The invasion of the blood and tissues is by myeloblasts and undifferentiated hemoblasts.

Lymphomatosis, or lymphoid leukemia, generally aleukemic, is frequent, so frequent

in fact that, by devastating stock farms, it occasionally presents economic problems. It occurs in four different forms, occasionally associated: (1) visceral lymphomatosis, (2) neurolymphomatosis with paralysis (3) ocular lymphomatosis, and (4) osteopetrosis.

Natural Transmission. Essentially *vertical transmission via the egg* is involved. The disease is passed from one generation to another but may remain quiescent during several successive generations and then appear misleadingly as a sporadic disease. This form of transmission has been proved by germ-free raising of fowl from a highly contaminated breed hatched from eggs the shells of which had been carefully sterilized and the chicks isolated from birth. Viral particles were found in eggs from the breed contaminated by erythroblastosis.

Another form of transmission, *horizontal transmission by contact,* has been proved only in lymphomatosis. Birds from a healthy breed, when placed in contact with those of a lymphomatous breed, become infected via their digestive and respiratory systems from the droppings of the virus carriers. Isolation of the animals during the first month of life (age of maximum sensitivity to the virus) is thus one of the best methods of prophylaxis.

Spontaneous Leukemias in Rodents. These leukemias, which are rare in the rabbit and the hamster and are sometimes found in the rat (in which they are mainly myeloid), are best known in the mouse. The frequency of the disease in nature is unknown but is probably low. However, none of the numerous pure breeds of mice used in laboratory work is completely free of leukemia. It appears as a rule after age seven months.

CLINICOPATHOLOGICAL ASPECTS. As concerns leukemia in mice and in man, the following similarities and differences deserve mention:

Leukemias of mice closely resemble the leukemias of man.

The distinction between leukemias and sarcomas in mice is nevertheless illusory, and a whole range of forms exists between these two diseases.

Acute leukemias analogous to acute human leukemias are rare.

Lymphoid leukemias represent the great majority of the leukemias of the mouse. They are leukemic or very often aleukemic. At autopsy the lymphoid infiltration found is generalized or limited to certain organs (thymus, lymph nodes, spleen).

The other forms are either rare (myeloid leukemia, occasionally chloroleukemia) or exceptional (monocytic and plasma-cell leukemia).

NATURAL TRANSMISSION. This never seems to occur by horizontal contagion. Healthy animals raised in the same cage as leukemic animals are not infected. Vertical transmission is manifest. It has long been known that animals of leukemic parentage are more often affected than others, and pure breeds have been isolated that are characterized by the high frequency of leukemia.

Spontaneous Leukemias in Cattle. The increasing frequency of leukemia in cattle in certain stock-breeding countries (e.g., Germany and the Scandinavian countries) is an object of attention at present. France is less affected, but nonetheless 1000 deaths per year among cattle are due to leukemia.

CLINICOPATHOLOGICAL ASPECT. The bovine type of leukemia is almost invariably a lymphoid leukemia with a chronic course. Aleukemic forms are frequent as well as lymphosarcomas. Myeloid leukemias are exceptional.

NATURAL TRANSMISSION. The existence of a *vertical* form of transmission is generally rejected but cannot be entirely dismissed.

Contagiousness (*horizontal* transmission), which was long rejected, seems possible in view of recent epizootiological investigations (limited epizootic diseases following introduction of an animal in the incubation phase into a herd). Geographical study shows an uneven distribution of cases with a predominance in certain regions. The infectious nature of bovine leukemia, at present regarded as probable, has not, however, been proved.

Spontaneous Leukemias in Other Species. Leukemias may also be observed in wild animals (leukemias in deer in the regions where bovine leukemias occur), in livestock, (horses and pigs), and in other domestic animals (especially dogs and cats). The mechanism of natural transmission is unknown.

EXPERIMENTAL TRANSMISSION OF SPONTANEOUS LEUKEMIAS IN ANIMALS; TRANSMISSION BY ACELLULAR MATERIAL; LEUKEMOGENIC VIRUSES

Transmission of leukemia by inoculation of an acellular filtrate obtained from crushed leukemic tissues has succeeded in four species, chicken, mouse, rat, and cat. The leukemias induced in this way develop from the cells of the infected animal itself. Thanks to these experiments it was possible to attribute the spontaneous leukemias of these species to a subcellular agent, subsequently identified as a virus.

Acellular Transmission of Leukemias in Fowl. The acellular transmission of erythroblastosis is relatively easy (1908), as is that of myeloblastosis. Such transmission of lymphomatosis is more difficult. Recent experiments have attempted to isolate the various agents of the different forms often associated in nature.

Acellular Transmission of Murine Leukemias; Gross's Leukemia. The transmission of a leukemia to newborn C3H mice by inoculation of the filtrate from leukemic tissue of AK2 mice was successfully performed by Gross in 1951. He thus demonstrated for the first time the viral etiology of a murine leukemia.

Gross virus is now well known, and its virulence has been enhanced.

Other Murine Viral Leukemias. Other murine leukemogenic viruses have been described in recent years, such as Graffi virus (chloroleukemia), Moloney virus (lymphoid leukemia), Schwartz virus (spontaneous leukemia of Swiss mice), Friend virus (malignant reticulopathy), and Rauscher virus (lymphoid leukemias preceded by an erythroblastic phase).

These murine leukemic viruses can be classified under two headings, depending on the circumstances of their initial isolation: (1) viruses derived from a murine leukemia (Gross, Schwartz), (2) viruses isolated from different nonleukemic tumors (sarcoma 37, Erlich's carcinoma, and so forth—Graffi, Friend, Moloney).

DOUBTS AND CERTAINTIES CONCERNING THE VIRAL ETIOLOGY

After being long confined solely to erythroblastosis in fowl, the etiological role of viruses appears highly important since the work done by Gross. A viral etiology has been proved in the following cases: fowl erythroblastosis, myeloblastosis, and lymphomatosis; spontaneous leukemias in AKR and C58 mice; the experimental murine leukemias of Gross, Schwartz, Graffi, Friend, Moloney, and Rauscher; spontaneous leukemia of the rat; and spontaneous leukemia of the cat.

However, no virus has yet been demonstrated in the spontaneous leukemias of guinea pigs, dogs, cattle, or pigs.

Viral etiology is by no means incompatible with the effect of other factors such as irradiation. Irradiation probably intervenes by activating a virus already present in the mouse, although in a latent nonpathogenic state. An acellular filtrate prepared from the tissues of a mouse that has been rendered leukemic by irradiation is capable of inducing a leukemia in nonirradiated receivers of the same strain. Two agents, i.e., two viruses that can be activated by irradiation in this way, are known today (Kaplan virus, Gross X passage). Their existence shows that a leukemia can both be viral and be induced by irradiation. However, no virus has yet been isolated in chemically induced leukemias.

STUDY OF LEUKEMIC VIRUSES

One remarkable fact is that the viruses isolated from animal leukemias belong to the same group and have numerous characteristics in common.

1. They are all RNA viruses (cf. Chapter 62).

2. Their size varies between 80 and 120 $m\mu$, and their structure (central "nucleoide" surrounded by two "membranes") is the same for all of them. The murine and fowl leukemia viruses are rapidly inactivated by heat but can survive at $-70°$ C. for several months.

3. In all, the mode of formation (on contact with the cell membrane) is the same, and none is free within the cell; all are contained in a vacuole. Viral particles, relatively rare in leukemic cells, are present in considerable number in other apparently nonmalignant cells and in the plasma.

4. Today we know how to culture all the leukemic viruses on embryonic or homologous hematopoietic cells, but study is impeded by the fact that none of them induces optically detectable lesions in the cells on which it grows.

5. The viruses seem to be weakly antigenic. No passive immunity has yet been obtained. On the other hand, active immunity certainly exists; it has led to study of vaccination against certain fowl leukemias and Friend's leukemia of the mouse.

6. *Vertical* transmission predominates. *Horizontal* transmission from one individual to another plays a lesser role.

7. In their natural state leukemia viruses have strict specificity for the target animal. The species barrier (e.g., from the mouse to the rat) has been overcome in the case of strains hyperactivated by repeated experimental passages.

Numerous unknowns subsist in the etiology of animal leukemias, but from study of the more favorable cases, i.e., those in which a virus has been isolated, it would appear that the phenomena involved are highly complex and require the association of at least three different factors: (1) a virus present from the first few days of life, and which may be activated by an extrinsic aggression such as irradiation; (2) genetic sensitivity of the host; (3) favorable physiological conditions, among which the state of the thymus and/or of the endocrine glands, are thought probably to be the most important. Thus the part played by the humoral medium and environment is emphasized.

EPIDEMIOLOGICAL STUDY OF HUMAN LEUKEMIAS

Epidemiology (taken in the broadest sense of the word, as indicated by its etymology and Anglo-American usage) takes into account the uneven frequency and distribution of human leukemias.

Sometimes this uneven frequency is explained and the reasons for it are used in discussion of the etiology, and sometimes it is merely recorded. Here, we shall limit ourselves to a study of the uneven geographical distribution of leukemias.

UNEVEN GEOGRAPHICAL DISTRIBUTION OF LEUKEMIAS; LEUKEMIA "EPIDEMICS"; THE SURPRISING CONCENTRATIONS OF LEUKEMIAS NOTED IN CERTAIN AREAS AT CERTAIN PERIODS

The history of leukemia gives a few examples of remarkable concentrations of leukemias in certain areas that are also limited to certain periods. For instance, the abrupt appearance of leukemia in eight children (seven of them girls) within four years in an extremely limited population, in Niles, Illinois, far exceeds the probabilities of chance and seems to be linked to the intervention of special factors that could not be determined.

African Sarcomas. In numerous animal species, especially mice and cattle, leukemias and sarcomas of hematopoietic tissues are closely related to each other. It seems legitimate to utilize here, at least as a subject of reflection, the data provided by recent research on African sarcomas, especially since Burkitt's disease, like other hematopoietic sarcomas, may pass through two stages, one apparently nonleukemic and the other leukemic, and since, in the regions where Burkitt's disease is prevalent, the leukemias of young children are extremely rare. The hypothesis has been proposed that Burkitt's disease in these regions is the homologue of acute leukemia.

The remarkable research work by Burkitt has established:

1. The anatomoclinical originality of sarcomas, which electively involve the maxillary bones, then the kidneys, ovaries, thyroid, and parotid glands.

2. The extremely limited age group of the victims; almost always children aged seven to eight years, no case having been reported before age one year, and practically no cases after age 16 years.

3. The geographical distribution of the sarcomas. Preliminary study showed that the tumors depend on altitude, latitude, and humidity; a more attentive analysis revealed two essential factors: the temperature and the vegetation. Tumors occur only when the temperature is higher than 17° C. and in a zone of dense vegetation. These data suggest the participation of an arthropod vector and of a virus. The role of a herpes-like virus (EB) is strongly suspected.

PERMANENT GEOGRAPHY OF LEUKEMIAS

Geographical Distribution of Leukemias; Unevenness of the Over-All Incidence. Two general facts seem to be certain:

1. The over-all incidence of leukemias varies considerably according to countries. Unquestionably, there exists a clear-cut inequality in the frequency of leukemias in different parts of the world. Even when only countries with a health organization that makes it possible to compile comparable statistical data are taken into account, three classes can be distinguished: (a) countries having a high incidence of leukemia — the United States, Denmark, Israel (Jewish population); (b) countries of medium incidence — Great Britain, Italy; (c) countries of low incidence — Japan.

Clemmesen noted that the variations are particularly noticeable among older persons, especially those aged over 50 years.

2. The frequency of leukemias seems to be related in part to urban living. This observation has been made particularly in the United States and in Denmark.

Furthermore, within any one given country, the frequency of leukemia varies from one region to another. In the United States, the leukemia rate is far higher in Minnesota than in the other states, and among the Eastern states, Vermont, or, to be more precise, its northern half, has an abnormally high rate.

Unequal Distribution of the Clinical Forms. The most remarkable fact is the extreme rarity of chronic lymphoid leukemias in the Far East. The documents published by Japanese authors are significative. This rarity of chronic lymphoid leukemias is not due to the shorter life expectancy of the populations concerned.

Geographical Inequality of Distribution According to Age. The high incidence of acute leukemias in children between three and six years of age which has been particularly emphasized by Occidental hematologists is neither a universal phenomenon nor a consistent one. It has been recognized in Great Britain since 1920 and became clear cut after 1940. It is evident in the white population of the United States only since 1940. This high frequency of acute leukemia in young children has not been found in the Far East, in Africa, or in the Negro population of the United States.

OBSERVATIONS ON HUMAN LEUKEMIAS

THE SEARCH FOR THE VIRUS OF HUMAN LEUKEMIAS

A reasonable hypothesis, difficulties of experimental procedure, insufficiency of controls, and sufficiency of the claims—these proposals describe fairly well an uncertain situation; the observer is torn between two opposite fears: the fear, too often justified, of being misled by peremptorily announced false results, and the fear of not recognizing the new study that provides the proof so long awaited.

Electron Microscopy. This state of mind applies to the observation under the electron microscope of apparently viral images. Long limited to relation of a few observations made by this method in ganglia or medullary cells, the study has recently been encouraged by the discovery of plasmatic viremia in murine leukemias. Formations resembling viruses have been observed in the plasma of leukemic patients. On the one hand the experienced observer hesitates to assert that these are in fact viruses, since he must regretfully recognize the imperfect methods, and the frequent errors (cellular debris, platelets, granules, PPLO); if, indeed there is a virus he hesitates still more to allot to it a leukemogenic role (certain viruses first taken to be leukemogenic have subsequently been identified as the virus of cytomegalic inclusions, encephalitic viruses, and so forth). On the other hand, he grasps at the hope that such observations, once confirmed, might have the value of an orienting factor and thus permit the selection of cases worth a more complete study. The rarity of positive observations is remarkable, and it is difficult to tell whether it is evidence of artifact, whether it is genuine, or

whether it must simply be explained by our incompetence, the virus not having been sought where it is when it is there and as it presents itself.

Inoculation of Animals. It is perhaps with regard to the inoculation of animals that the contrast between certain optimistic experimental results and present reality is the most striking.

When we consider the diversity of possible errors, we may be justifiably surprised by the lack of caution and by the speed shown in making certain affirmations. A certain bone lesion in a young monkey is proposed as a tumor and appears to affirm the transmissibility of Burkitt's disease, when in reality the lesion was only dysplastic. A leukemia in a mouse, attributed to an inoculated human virus, is in fact due to a murine virus; in the most lenient hypothesis, this virus may have been enhanced by the human material inoculated, but it is more likely that the murine leukemia is intercurrent and has no connection with the inoculation attempt.

Erroneous claims are unfortunate; unsuccessful results are far from discouraging. The second simply constitute an invitation to modify unsatisfactory methods in one of two ways: from the viewpoint of precision, by using germ-free animals, and from the viewpoint of efficiency, by using the animals most closely related to man. It was in this line of thought that we suggested recourse to anthropoids, in particular newborn chimpanzees.

Tissue Cultures. Tissue cultures (i.e., direct culture of leukemic cells or inoculation of varied cell cultures with leukemic extracts) have been widely used for three purposes, namely, to observe the cytopathogenic effect, to observe cellular transformation in vitro, and to obtain an increase in the pathogenicity of a possible virus. Here again, failures have been numerous. Some short-lived hopes have not been confirmed. For instance, the causal agent cultured by Negroni in bone marrow in a case of acute leukemia was in fact a mycoplasma, and the interpretation of agents bearing a resemblance to viruses, discovered by Epstein and by Grace in certain cultures of leukemic cells, remains highly doubtful.

It is worth noting the relative frequency with which mycoplasma or PPLO's are discovered by the different methods in use. These organisms, which are much closer to bacteria than to viruses, are probably not etiological agents. Their possible role as adjuvants has been suggested, but their incidence varies from laboratory to laboratory, and the PPLO's reported in the United States do not so far seem to have been observed in French research centers.

Nucleic Acids. Research directed toward the nucleic acids has yielded little fruit. The only positive datum, that of Harel et al., who succeeded in inducing a mesothelioma by inoculation of RNA from leukemic lymph nodes, could not be repeated by these workers themselves.

Immunology. Modest results and high hopes could sum up the situation of immunology as applied to the study of possible viruses of human leukemias. In practice immunology without a known antigen must be applied, a fact that poses two difficulties: either the experiments cannot even be undertaken, or else they can be criticized. A good example is provided by the recent work by Finck. Leukemic human plasma rich in apparently viral particles was used as antigen. A rabbit antiserum was obtained. After adsorption by normal human antigens and tagging with fluorescein, this serum reacted specifically with the blood cells and marrow cells of leukemic patients. A cross reaction may be observed between these human cells and an analogous antiserum prepared against the virus of Rauscher's leukemia.

These very interesting observations do not make it possible to dismiss the presence in leukemic tissues of a contaminant such as a PPLO whose frequent association with the virus of Rauscher's leukemia we have also noted.

Two explanations could account for these failures. Either the leukemias of primates are not due to a virus (or to several viruses), or else the methods used that are suitable for other vertebrates are not applicable to man.

Changes or improvements in the methods will perhaps be inspired by examination of the possible forms of these possible viruses.

THE POSSIBLE VIRUSES OF HUMAN LEUKEMIAS

First hypothesis: This virus, or these viruses, may be solely leukemogenic and strictly human.

Most (or all) viruses responsible for animal leukemias are indeed specific for one species and do not induce disorders other than the leukemias. These different viruses, as we have seen, belong to the same class and possess the same general characteristics, characteristics that might also be those of a possible human virus.

Second hypothesis: The virus of an animal leukemia may be transmitted to man. Studies of the epizootics of bovine leukemias and of the comparative geography of human and bovine leukemias have not contributed a decisive element.

Theoretically, the virus of an animal leukemia passes the species barrier only with great difficulty. However, it was seen earlier that the virus of certain leukemias of the mouse can be leukemogenic in the rat, and that the virus of Rous sarcoma can cause tumors in mammals (including monkeys) and is able to transform human cells in culture.

Third hypothesis: A known and a latent virus in man could under certain circumstances cause a leukemia.

The virus of herpes simplex, as we ourselves have shown, causes numerous chromosomal modifications, but its incidence in leukemic patients, just as that of other common viruses (e.g., the herpes zoster virus, the agent of cytomegalic inclusion disease, and adenoviruses), is generally attributed to a weakening of the immunological defense mechanisms.

The supposed relations between outbreaks of measles and the seasonal incidence of leukemias have not been confirmed, and the similarities postulated between the possible causal agent of human leukemia and the possible causal agent of infectious mononucleosis remain uncertain. New data, however, have recently shown the role of EB virus in the etiology of infectious mononucleosis. EB virus is found especially often in Burkitt's tumor. (Cf. Chapters 50 and 62.)

Systematic research undertaken by Chany, Cook, and ourselves, in 1961, on latent viruses in leukemic children revealed—in comparison with a control group—the rarity of enteroviruses in the leukemic children but no other differences. However, one cannot overlook the "orphan" viruses of the arbogroup. Instead of a leukemia in search of a virus, perhaps in this instance a virus is in search of a leukemia.

Fourth hypothesis: A virus that is nononcogenic with regard to its species may be leukemogenic in man. A nononcogenic virus, when placed in an unusual medium where it develops with difficulty, may subsequently become oncogenic. However, the only known examples (SV 40, and adenoviruses 12 and 18) concern the DNA viruses responsible for solid experimental tumors, and not the RNA viruses, the only ones known to be responsible for spontaneous tumors and leukemias.

A few more hypotheses can be mentioned with regard to the form of the virus:

Is there *a complete virus* in its vegetative form or one in masked form as suggested by the rarity of the viral images obtainable with the electron microscope?

Is there *an active virus or, instead, a defective virus* that requires the assistance of a helper virus? This defective form, described in the case of Rous virus, has not as yet been reported for the leukemogenic viruses.

Hence the failures are not surprising. What a list of difficulties! Difficulties arise from the different properties of the possible viruses of humam leukemias, which are probably rare, fragile, perhaps masked, and certainly only slightly antigenic. Difficulties result from the presence in the leukemogenic tissues of more conspicuous agents, e.g., other viruses or mycoplasma, which may be blameless or accomplices. Finally, difficulties result from the obvious impossibility of carrying out experimental investigations in the human being comparable to those that enabled Gross's discovery in the mouse. The example of Gross shows precisely that a change in method may suddenly provide the proof long awaited in vain.

What changes, what new orientations could be envisaged in the case of man? Further exploration is probably worthwhile in two directions: research for sensitive cells of sensitive animals, and immunological investigations.

The discovery of *sensitive cells* would enable us to make proper use of tissue culture methods. This is not a vain hope; Rauscher's virus, for example, which develops rather miserably on most cell media, multiplies vigorously, we demonstrated, in a mixed tissue culture of mouse spleen cells and thymus cells.

The only *animals* used as receivers have so far been rodents and, in a few experiments, the lower monkeys. It would be useful to extend this list to include various other animal species, e.g., cattle because of a possible similarity of their leukemias to those of man, pigs, and the higher anthropoids, especially chimpanzees, since in rodent leukemias the species barrier was overcome only in closely related species.

Since the known leukemia viruses are produced on the membrane of the cells in which they multiply, by means of fairly strong antiviral antibodies, it should be possible to recognize the viral antigen by *immunofluorescence or by cytotoxicity.*

Since, as Klein demonstrated, the leukemic cells of the mouse transformed by a virus possess one or several additional antigens, linked to the presence of the virus but different from the viral antigen, it should be possible to identify these new antigens despite the weakness of their reactions. This demonstration has been undertaken by Huebner using a complement deviation between tumor extract and serum from animals with tumors, in the case of certain oncogenic DNA viruses, and even more recently, in the case of Rous virus and certain fowl leukemia viruses.

Perhaps these direct and indirect research investigations ought to be aimed more specifically in terms of the data obtained from the study of human leukemias: rational data, e.g., the various cell forms have not been the object of systematic exploration, and some one of them may prove to be more accessible; naïve data: e.g., the high temperature is perhaps occasionally directly related to a specific virus; more accurate data: e.g., certain leukemias, such as leukemias with thymic tumor and congenital leukemias, are perhaps of particular importance. It is probably useful to take into account the various stages in the course of the disease, the so-called preleukemic conditions, and the beginning and end of the remission period, and also useful to direct the investigations not only to the patients with leukemia but also to their parents and persons around them, particularly when several leukemias are observed in the same family or the same human group.

BIBLIOGRAPHY

1. Ageenko, A. I.: Leukemias induced in rat with extracts from human leukemic tissue. Acta Un. Int. Cancr., *18*:140, 1962.

2. Almeida, J. D., Hasselback, R. C., and Ham, A. W.: Virus-like particles in blood of two acute leukemia patients. Science, *142*:1487, 1963.

3. Benyesh-Melnick, M., Dessy, S. I., and Fernbach, D. J.: Cytomegaloviruria in children with acute leukemia and in other children. Proc. Soc. Exp. Biol. Med., *117*:624, 1964.

4. Benyesh-Melnick, M., Smith, K. O., and Fernbach, D. J.: Studies on human leukemia. III. Electron microscopic findings in children with acute leukemia and in children with infectious mononucleosis. J. Nat. Cancer Inst., *33*:571, 1964.

5. Bergolz, V. M.: Transmission of human leukemia to mice. Progr. Exp. Tumor Res., *1*:86, 1960.

6. Bernhard, W.: The detection and study of tumor viruses with the electron microscope. Cancer Res., *18*:491, 1958.

7. Bessis, M., and Thiery, J. P.: Etude au microscope électronique des hématosarcomes humains. Nouv. Rev. Franç. Hémat., *1*:703, 1961; *2*:387, 577, 1962.

8. Bostick, W. L., and Hanna, L.: Characteristics of virus isolated from Hodgkin's disease lymph nodes. Cancer Res., *15*:650, 1955.

9. Braunsteiner, H., Fellinger, K., and Pakesch, F.: On the occurrence of virus-like bodies in human leukemia. Blood, *15*:475, 1960.

10. Burger, C. L., Harris, W. W., Anderson, N. G., Bartlett, T. W., and Kniseley, R. M.: Virus-like particles in human leukemic plasma. Proc. Soc. Exp. Biol. Med., *115*:151, 1964.

11. Dalldorf, G., and Bergamini, F.: Unidentified filtrable agents isolated from African children with malignant lymphoma. Proc. Nat. Acad. Sci., *51*:263, 1964.

12. Dalton, A. J., Moloney, J. B., Porter, G. E., and Freie-Mitchel, E. Z.: Studies on murine and human leukemia. Trans. Ass. Amer. Physicians, *77*:52, 1964.

13. De Carvalho, S.: Cytopathogenicity of RNA-rich particles from human leukemic and tumor cells for human amniotic cells. Proc. 3rd Canadian Cancer Conf., 1959, p. 329.

14. De Long, R.: Production of leukemia in mice with cell-free filtrates from human leukemias. J. Lab. Clin. Med., *56*:891, 1960.

15. Dmochowski, L., Grey, C. E., Sykes, J. A., Schullenberger, C. C., and Howe, C. D.: Studies on human leukemia. Proc. Soc. Exp. Biol. Med., *101*:585, 1959.

16. Dmochowski, L., Sinkovics, J. G., Sykes, J. A., and Schullenberger, C. C.: Biological studies on human leukemia. Ann. Rep. Univ. Texas, 1960, p. 57.

17. Dmochowski, L., Taylor, H. G., Grey, C. E., Designer, E., Dreyer, D. A., Sykes, J. A., Langford, P. L., Rogers, T., Schullenberger, C. C., and Howe, C. D.: Viruses and mycoplasma (PPLO) in human leukemia. Cancer, *18*:1345, 1965.

18. Epstein, M. A., Achong, B. G., and Barr, Y. M.: Virus particles in cultured lymphoblasts from Burkitt's lymphoma. Lancet, *1*:702, 1964.

19. Epstein, M. A., Heule, G., Achong, B. G., and Barr, Y. M.: Morphological and biological studies on a virus in cultured lymphoblasts from Burkitt's lymphoma. J. Exp. Med., *121*:761, 1965.

20. Fink, M. A., Malmgren, R. A., Rauscher, F. J., Orr, H. C., and Karon, M.: Application of immunofluorescence to the study of human leukemia. J. Nat. Cancer Inst., *33*:581, 1964.

21. Fink, M. A., Karon, M., Rauscher, F. S., Malmgren, R. A., and Orr, H. C.: Further observations on the immunofluorescence of cells in human leukemia. Cancer, *18*:1317, 1965.

22. Friend, C., Darchun, V., De Harven, E., and Haddad, J.: The incidence and classification of spontaneous malignant diseases of the hematopoietic system in Swiss mice. Ciba Foundation Symposium on Tumour Viruses of Murine Origin. London, Churchill, 1962, p. 193.

23. Girardi, A. J., Hayflick, L., Lewis, A. M., and Somerson, N. L.: Recovery of mycoplasmas in the study of human leukemia and other malignancies. Nature, *205*:188, 1965.

24. Girardi, A. J., Hilleman, M. R., and Zwickey, A. E.: Search for virus in human malignancies. 2. In vivo studies. Proc. Soc. Exp. Biol. Med., *111*:84, 1962.

25. Girardi, A. J., Slotnick, V. B., and Hilleman, M. R.: Search for virus in human malignancies. I. In vitro studies. Proc. Soc. Exp. Biol. Med., *110*:776, 1962.

26. Grace, J. T., Horoszewicz, J. S., Stim, T. B., Mirand, E. A., and James, C.: Mycoplasmas (PPLO) and human leukemia and lymphoma. Cancer, *18*:1369, 1965.

27. Grace, J. T., Mirand, E. A., Millian, S. J., and Metzgar, R. S.: Experimental studies of human tumors. Fed. Proc., *21*:32, 1962.

28. Grist, N. R., and Fallon, R. J.: Isolation of viruses from leukemic patients. Brit. Med. J., *2*:1263, 1964.

29. Hayflick, L., and Koprowski, H.: Direct agar isolation of mycoplasmas from human leukemic bone-marrow. Nature, *205*:713, 1965.

30. Huth, E., and Bruester, H.: Virusartige bei der akuten Leukämie der Kinder (vorrangige Mitteilung). Folia Haemat., *5*:162, 1961.

31. Inman, D. R., Woods, D. A., and Negroni, G.: Electron microscopy of virus particles in cell cultures inoculated with passage fluid from human leukemic bone marrow. Brit. Med. J., *1*:929, 1964.

32. Katzman, R. A.: Studies on the induction of leukemia in Swiss mice by cell-free filtrates from human tissues. J. Lab. Clin. Med., *60*:579, 1962.

33. Lacour, F., Lacour, J., Harel, J., and Huppert, J.: Transplantable malignant tumors in mice induced by preparations containing ribonucleic acid extracted from human and mouse tumors. J. Nat. Cancer Inst., *24*:301, 1960.

34. Leplus, R., Debray, J., Pinet, J., and Bernhard, W.: Lésions nucléaires décelées au microscope électronique dans une cellule de lymphomes malins chez l'homme. C. R. Acad. Sci., *253*:2788, 1961.

35. Magrassi, F., Corraggio, F., Turisi, E., Coto, V., Cocco, F., Catalono, G., and Fantoni, V.: Isolation and biological characterisation of viruses derived from human leukemia. In I. Virus nelle leucemie dei mammiferi. Symp. Rome, 16-17 Juin 1963. Acad. Nat. dei Lincei Ann., *361*:241-260, 1964.

36. Mettenleiter, M. W., Manheim, J. H., and Borchardt, P. R.: Isolation of viral agents from human blood and their relationship to lymphatic leukemia. Oncologia, *16*:307, 1963.

37. Moore, A. E.: In Cancer. Gordon Research Conferences. New Hampshire, 1961.

38. Murphy, W. H., Ertel, I. J., Zarafonetis, C. J. D.:

Virus studies of human leukemia. Cancer, *18*: 1329, 1965.

39. Murphy, W. H., and Furtado, D.: Isolation of viruses from children with acute leukemia. Univ. Mich. Med. Bull., *29*:201, 1963.

40. Negroni, G.: Isolation of viruses from leukaemic patients. Brit. Med. J., *1*:927, 1964.

41. Nicolau, C. T., and Goresco, I. D.: Induction de la leucose chez des souris H par injection d'extraits acellulaires de moelle osseuse de leucose aiguë humaine. Bull. Assoc. Franç. Canc., *48*:539, 1961.

42. Parnes, V. A., and Suntzova, V. V.: Induction of leukemia in mice by administration of material from leukemic subjects. Pat. Fiziol. Eksp. Ter., *3*:14, 1959.

43. Porter, G. H., Dalton, A. J., Moloney, J. B., and Mitchel, E. Z.: Association of electron dense particles with human acute leukemia. J. Nat. Cancer Inst., *33*:547, 1964.

44. Postnikova-Medvedev, cited in Zilber, L. A.: The role of viruses in the origin of leukemia in animals and man. Bull. WHO, *26*:597, 1962.

45. Prince, A. M., and Adams, M. R.: Virus-like particles in human plasma and serum from leukemic, hepatic and controls patients. Fed. Proc., *49*:175, 1965.

46. Riman, J., and Veselv, I.: Experiments on the heterotransmission of hemoblastosis. Neoplasma, *4*:91, 1957.

47. Schmidt, F.: Zur heterologen Ubertragung von Krebs und Leukämiemateriel des Menschen auf Laboratoriumstiere. Z. Krebsforsch., *63*:532, 1960.

48. Schmidt, P. J., Basile, M., and MacGinniss, M. H.: Mycoplasma (pleuropneumonia-like organisms) and blood group I. Associations with neoplastic disease. Nature, *205*:371, 1965.

49. Schwartz, S. O., Spurrier, W., Yates, L., and Maduros, B. P.: Studies in leukemia. XV. The induction of leukemias in Swiss mice with human leukemic brain extracts. Blood, *15*:758, 1960.

50. Smith, K. O., Benyesh-Melnick, M., and Fernbach, D. J.: Studies on human leukemia. II. Structure and quantitation of myxovirus-like particles associated with human leukemia. J. Nat. Cancer Inst., *33*:557, 1964.

51. Stewart, S. E., and Irwin, M. L.: Cellular proliferation in primary tissue cultures induced with substance derived from cell-free concentrates from human neoplastic material. Cancer Res., *20*:766, 1960.

52. Stewart, S. E., Lovelace, E., Whang, J. J., and Ngu, V. A.: Burkitt tumor: tissue culture, cytogenetic and virus studies. J. Nat. Cancer Inst., *34*:319, 1965.

53. Sykes, J. A., Dmochowski, C., Schullenberger, C. C., and Howe, C. D.: Tissue culture studies on human leukemia and malignant lymphoma. Cancer Res., *22*:21, 1962.

54. Timofeevskii, A. D.: Globular virus-like bodies in human tumors. Acta Un. Int. Cancr., *15*:748, 1959.

55. Whitaker, J. A., Bovis, R., Andrews, S. L., and Sulkin, S. E.: Focal cellular alteration in stable amnion cells produced by inoculation with human leukemia brain extracts. Cancer Res., *23*:519, 1963.

47

Thrombocytopenic Purpuras

By J. BERNARD

This chapter comprises four parts: (1) a description of Thai hemorrhagic fever, a model of viral thrombocytopenia; (2) a description of rubella thrombocytopenia; (3) a review of thrombocytopenias occurring during various recognized viral infections; and (4) a discussion of arguments in favor of the viral origin of so-called idiopathic thrombocytopenic purpura.

THAI HEMORRHAGIC FEVER

Thai hemorrhagic fever has a double value as an example: it is certainly a clear-cut example of a viral thrombocytopenia, and it is probably the first example, in man, of bone marrow changes due to a virus.

EPIDEMIOLOGY

History and Geography. First observed in 1954 almost simultaneously in Thailand and the Philippines, Thai hemorrhagic fever was defined during the great 1958 epidemic in Bangkok. Since then, it has been the object of much study, which the epidemic paroxysms of 1960 and 1962 renewed. Despite these studies, the history and the geography of the disease are not yet completely known. It is known to be both endemic (a certain number of cases are seen each year) and epidemic, especially, occurring more frequently during some years and during certain months of these years (especially between June and October).

For instance, of 2418 patients hospitalized in Bangkok in 1958, 2200 were affected during the months of July, August, and September. Since 1961, not one month has passed in Bangkok in which at least one case has not been seen. Between 1961 and 1965, 16,000 Thai and Chinese children were involved in Bangkok; 1000 of them died. The geographic distribution covers a large portion of Southeast Asia.

The greatest number of cases has been seen in Thailand, particularly in Bangkok, Dhonburi, and the neighboring provinces. Cases are much less frequent in the other provinces.

In the Philippines, hemorrhagic fever is known mainly on the island of Luzon.

The disease was also observed in Malaysia, in Singapore in 1960 and in Penang in 1962, and in Saigon and Calcutta in 1963.

Age and Sex. The sexes are affected equally. The disease affects children particularly, especially small children, as is evidenced by these statistics from Thailand in 1958: The number of cases in children less than one year old was 199; in those one year old, 165; two years old, 239; three years old, 310; four years old, 279; five years old, 292; six years old, 226; seven years old, 170; eight years old, 145; nine years old, 99; ten years old, 90; 11 years old, 65; 12 years old, 60; and 13 years old and over, 32.

Vector. The vector responsible is *Aedes aegypti*. All studies carried out in Thailand, as well as in the Philippines, found a close correlation between the distribution of *Aedes aegypti* and that of the hemorrhagic fever. The viruses responsible for the disease have been isolated over and over from *Aedes aegypti*.

VIROLOGY

The responsible viruses belong to the group of dengue viruses, described in Chapter 58. Here we shall mention only certain features peculiar to the hemorrhagic fever.

Several varieties of dengue viruses have been isolated. Type 2 seems most often associated with hemorrhagic fever. The appearance of antibodies is early, massive and perhaps explains the difficulty of finding the virus at autopsy. The fact that these antibodies react with all viruses of the same group might explain the frequent difficulties in identification of the causative type.

The Chikungunya virus, responsible in Africa for epidemics closely resembling dengue (see Chapter 58), is found fairly frequently in Thai hemorrhagic fever.

Serological studies performed in Bangkok after the 1958 epidemic showed that 50 to 60 per cent of the children under four years of age had been infected either by a dengue virus or by the Chikungunya virus. These facts explain, at least in part, the distribution of the disease over the years, according to age.

CLINICAL PICTURE

General Description. A very high fever, as high as 40° C. (104° F.), and an intense malaise prostrating the infant are the initial manifestations of the disease. Vomiting, diarrhea, cough, and dyspnea are frequent. The conjunctivae are red; rashes are not infrequent. The signs of collapse (algidity, hypotension) are often alarming.

Hemorrhages and Thrombocytopenia. Hemorrhages are not constant but very frequent. Petechiae, ecchymoses, and epistaxis are the most common manifestations. Hematemesis and intestinal hemorrhage are seen in the most serious cases. Hemorrhage of the meninges and the central nervous system is not common.

The frequent polyadenopathy, moderate hepatomegaly, and, more rarely, splenomegaly can complete the resemblance between this disease and a primary blood disease.

The erythrocyte count and the hemoglobin level are at times increased by hemo-concentration or, at others, diminished after hemorrhages.

Leukopenia (3000 to 4000 cells per cubic millimeter) is usual. Moderate leukocytosis (10,000 to 12,000 cells per cubic millimeter) is occasionally observed.

The thrombocytopenia is defined by the following characteristics: It is very frequent, if not constant. It occurs early but not immediately, appearing on the second or third day of disease. It is moderate (60,000 to 70,000 cells) or severe. A thrombocyte level below 40,000 carries an unfavorable prognosis. It is ephemeral, lasting only a few days. It is accompanied by the usual biological disorders (prolonged bleeding time, Rumpel-Leede phenomenon, lack of clot retraction). It is associated with hemorrhages in some cases and latent in others.

The descriptions of the *myelogram* are not all concordant. During the thrombocytopenic period, the bone marrow is active, and the megakaryocytes are abundant and present in all their forms and in all the stages of their maturation.

During the short prethrombocytopenic period, a clear-cut decrease in the number of megakaryocytes is sometimes reported. At other times the changes are moderate, but in all cases, the bone marrow is hypoplastic. Arrested erythroblast maturation, occasionally with a megaloblastic aspect of some erythrocytes, has been described.

The rapid evolution of the disease and the brief prethrombocytopenic and thrombocytopenic periods explain these difficulties in part, but it certainly seems that the bone marrow is impaired early and for a very short time. The appearance of the bone marrow during the thrombocytopenic stage is probably already that of repair.

The bone marrow is one of the target organs in Thai hemorrhagic fever. It is not known whether bone marrow lesions are due to direct impairment of the medullary cells by the virus or whether the virus acts indirectly by way of immunological disorders; antiplatelet antibodies have been discovered in certain cases.

General Course. The rapidity and the gravity of the disease are striking. The mortality rate ranges, according to the epidemic, from 5 to 10 per cent. Collapse and hemorrhages (associated or separately) are the usual causes of death. Mild forms of the disease are not rare. Only so-called symptomatic therapy (treatment of collapse, transfusions) is effective.

RUBELLA THROMBOCYTOPENIA

NEONATAL RUBELLA THROMBOCYTOPENIA

Like the thrombocytopenia in Thai hemorrhagic fever, neonatal rubella thrombocytopenia is highly important. It constitutes the second known example of a human thrombocytopenia assuredly (or at least very probably) due to a definite virus.

Thrombocytopenia of newborn infants from mothers with rubella was long the subject of only sporadic reports. Its real frequency was recognized during the rubella epidemic in the United States in 1964. This frequency, which may vary according to the epidemic and according to the virus, was very high during the American epidemic. Thrombocytopenic purpura held a place—close after cardiac lesions and ahead of cataracts—second on the list of disorders in infants infected by maternal rubella. Thrombocytopenic purpura was seen in 13 of the 20 newborn infants in a series reported by Banatvala et al. The purpura occurred either alone or with other disturbances.

It is seen at birth and can take one of several forms: petechiae, ecchymoses, or hematomas. Purpura can spread all over the body or be localized on the shoulders, the face, or the trunk. The hemorrhagic elements can be at different stages, some reddish-blue, others with yellow and green shades.

The liver and the spleen are normal or are hypertrophied in a fair number of cases.

Thrombocytopenia is found at birth in all cases of purpura. It may be severe (3300 thrombocytes per cubic millimeter in one case) but most often is moderate (50,000 to 100,000 cells per cubic millimeter).

The bone marrow has not always been examined rigorously enough. In the cases studied, megakaryocytes were scarce in some cases, and numerous and mainly immature in others; in still others they appeared to be normal. It is hard to know whether these differences are real or chronological.

The duration of purpura is short (a few days), whereas the duration of thrombocytopenia is more variable (a few days to a few weeks).

The heart lesions that were not recognized at birth can become manifest during recovery from thrombocytopenia.

In the vast majority of cases, the rubella virus could be isolated from the throat of newborn infants with rubella. It has been found in various viscera, including the spleen, the lymph nodes, and the bone marrow.

The physiopathology of neonatal thrombocytopenia remains obscure. The role of rubella virus seems unquestionable, but the mechanism of its action remains unknown, and one can only cite the hypotheses proposed: (1) direct action of the virus on the megakaryocytes or on the platelets; (2) thrombocytolysis in the spleen; or (3) conflict between an antiplatelet antibody in the maternal serum and a virus-platelet complex in the infant.

THROMBOCYTOPENIA IN OLDER CHILDREN AND ADULTS WITH RUBELLA

This kind of thrombocytopenia presents problems comparable to those associated with thrombocytopenia occurring during other virus diseases, discussed in the following section.

THROMBOCYTOPENIA OCCURRING DURING OTHER KNOWN OR PROBABLE VIRUS DISEASES

It is generally agreed that there is a cause-and-effect relationship between certain diseases of viral origin and the thrombocytopenic purpura that eventually accompanies them.

Virus diseases of this group, other than rubella, which we have just discussed, are: measles, chickenpox, cytomegalic inclusion disease, mumps, infectious mononucleosis, and epidemic hepatitis.

The data on which the above-mentioned relationship is based and which are the center of discussion are the following:

Thrombocytopenia occurs most frequently in the course of these viral infections. This peculiar frequency is probably authentic even though extensive comparative statistics are lacking. But it should be noted that this frequency is low. Thrombocytopenia is, for example, one of the rarest complications of mumps or of chickenpox.

The chronological development of thrombocytopenia must be taken into consideration. Thrombocytopenia develops early and is recognized either at the onset or during the first week of the viral disease. This chronology does not rule out the possibility of a coincidence.

The course of thrombocytopenia is acute and rapidly regressive, recovery occurring without recurrence. This evolution is not constantly observed in thrombocytopenia associated with virus diseases, and it is not peculiar to them.

Thus it is reasonable to admit the existence of thrombocytopenias due to mumps, chickenpox, infectious mononucleosis, and so forth, but it is difficult to provide conclusive evidence. Coincidences should always be considered (more in very common diseases such as measles than in less common ones such as infectious mononucleosis), and the possibility that one of the drugs (quinine, sulfonamides, and others) given to treat the infection may be responsible for the thrombocytopenia should be kept in mind.

The particular problem of neonatal purpura associated with cytomegalic inclusion disease is considered in Chapter 60.

ARGUMENTS IN FAVOR OF THE VIRAL ETIOLOGY OF SO-CALLED IDIOPATHIC THROMBOCYTOPENIC PURPURA

The viral origin of so-called idiopathic thrombocytopenic purpura is often assumed. The arguments put forward are diverse and of unequal value.

Etiological Data. Acute thrombocytopenia is most often observed in children and is particularly frequent during the spring and fall.

Clinical Data. The thrombocytopenia is preceded by sore throat, coryza, and adenoiditis with a frequency considered high by some authors. It begins abruptly, this suddenness being opposed to the progressiveness of the onset of the chronic forms.

Serological Data. Certain authors have from time to time reported positive reactions to certain viruses (adenovirus 12 and others).

Experimental Data. (1) Certain myxoviruses (influenza and Newcastle disease virus) impair platelets in vitro and disturb their functions (clot retraction, thromboplastin). (2) Some viruses responsible for murine leukemia are found with a particular frequency in megakaryocytes even when the number of platelets is normal.

These data are vague and insubstantial, and it is at present impossible to answer the important questions posed.

Is the hypothesis of a viral origin of these thrombocytopenias founded? If so, should this viral origin be considered valid for all acute thrombocytopenias, or, more restrictively, for only some of them, or, more generally, for certain chronic thrombocytopenias as well? Should one or several viruses be incriminated? Are they rare or common viruses? What is the viral mechanism (megakaryocytic, directly thrombocytolytic, immunological)?

Direct and systematic virological investigations have been started only recently. They may provide elements that will permit at least partial answers to these questions.

BIBLIOGRAPHY

THAI HEMORRHAGIC FEVER

1. Bierman, H. R.: Thai hemorrhagic fever. Med. Arts. Sci., *17*:98-100, 1963.
2. Bierman, H. R., and Nelson, E. R.: Hematodepressive virus diseases of Thailand. Ann. Intern. Med., *62*:867-884, 1965.
3. Chaudhuri, R. N., et al.: Clinical hematological observations on a recent outbreak of dengue-like fever in Calcutta with or without hemorrhagic manifestations. J. Indian. Med. Assoc., *43*:579-584, 1964.
4. Chew, A., Leng, G., Yuen, H., Teik, K., Kiat, L., Hong, L., and Wells, R.: A hemorrhagic fever in Singapore. Lancet, *1*:307-310, 1961.
5. Dasaneyavaja, A., and Pongsupat, S.: Observations on Thai hemorrhagic fever: J. Trop. Med. Hyg., *64*:310-314, 1961; *66*:35-41, 1963.
6. Goldsmith, R. S., Wong, H. B., Paul, F. M., Chan, K. Y., Loh, T. E., and Chan, K. C.: Haemorrhagic fever in Singapore. A changing syndrome. Lancet, *1*:333-336, 1965.
7. Hammon, W., Rudnick, A., Sather, G., et al.: New hemorrhagic fevers of children in the Philippines and Thailand. Trans. Assoc. Amer. Physicians, *73*:140-155, 1960; Science, *131*:1102-1103, 1960.
8. Hanam, E.: "Singapore hemorrhagic fever"—a clinical review. Singapore Med. J., *5*:73-76, 1965.
9. Kundu, S., Mukherjee, P., and Bakshi, K.: Calcutta haemorrhagic fever. Observations on 15 cases. J. Indian Med. Assoc., *43*:464-469, 1964.
10. Lim, K. A., et al.: Recent studies of haemorrhagic fevers in Singapore. Singapore Med. J., *2*:158-161, 1961.
11. Lim, K. A., et al.: Dengue-type viruses isolated in Singapore. Bull. WHO, *30*:227-240, 1964.
12. Lim, L. E., and Tan, E. C.: A guide to the diagnosis and treatment of Philippine hemorrhagic fever J. J. Philipp. Med. Assoc., 40:787-793, 1964.
13. Na-Nakorn, S., Suingdumrong, A., Pootrakul, S., and Bhamarapravati, N.: Bone marrow studies in Thai hemorrhagic fever. WHO Seminar on Mosquito-Borne Haemorrhagic fevers in Southeast Asia and Western Pacific Regions. 19-26 Oct., 1964.
14. Nelson, E. R., and Bierman, H.: Dengue fever: a thrombocytopenic disease? J.A.M.A., *190*:99-103, 1964.
15. Nelson, E. R., Bierman, H. R., and Chulajata, R.: Hematologic findings in the 1960 hemorrhagic fever epidemic in Thailand. Amer. J. Trop. Med., *13*:642, 1964.
16. Nelson, E. R., and Chulajata, R.: Danger signs in Thai hemorrhagic fever (dengue). J. Pediat., 67:463-470, 1965.
17. Piyaratn, P.: Pathology of Thailand epidemic hemorrhagic fever. Amer. J. Trop. Med., *10*:767-772, 1961.
18. Rudnick, A., Tan, E., Lucas, J. K., and Omar, M. B.: Mosquito-borne haemorrhagic fever in Malaya. Brit. Med. J., *1*:1269-1272, 1965.
19. Sarkar, J., Chatterjee, S., and Chakravarty, S. K.: Further progress in the study of haemorrhagic fever in Calcutta. Bull. Calcutta Sch. Trop. Med., *12*:102-103, 1964.
20. Sarkar, J., Chatterjee, S., and Chakravarty, S. K.: Reappearance of hemorrhagic fever in Calcutta in 1964. Preliminary report of virological investigations. Bull. Calcutta Sch. Trop. Med., *12*:151-152, 1964.
21. Smadel, J. E.: Hemorrhagic fever. In: Rivers, T., and Horsfall, F.: Viral and Rickettsial Infections of Man. 3rd ed. Philadelphia, J. B. Lippincott Co., 1959, pp. 400-404.
22. Symposium on Hemorrhagic Fever, Bangkok, Thailand. Seato Medical Research Monograph No. 2.
23. Symposium on Haemorrhagic Fever. Indian J. Med. Res., Vol. 52, 1964.
24. Weiss, H., and Halstead, S. B.: Studies of hemostasis in Thai hemorrhagic fever. J. Pediat., 66:918-926, 1965.

RUBELLA THROMBOCYTOPENIA

25. Adkins, A. T., and Fernbach, D. J.: Thrombocytopenic purpura following rubella. J.A.M.A., *193*:243-245, 1965.
26. Banatvala, J., Horstmann, D., Payne, M., and Gluck, L.: Rubella syndrome and thrombocytopenic purpura in newborn infants: clinical and virologic observations. New. Eng. J. Med., *273*:474-478, 1965.
27. Berge, T., Brunnhage, F., and Nilsson, L.: Congenital hypoplastic thrombocytopenia in rubella embryopathy. Acta Paediat., *52*:349-352, 1963.
28. Cochran, W., Cornfield, M., and Friedberg, D.: Congenital rubella and thrombocytopenia: report of two cases with initial and follow-up viral cultures. Pediatrics, *36*:268-270, 1965.
29. Cooper, L. Z., Green, R. H., Krugman, S., Giles, J. P., and Mirick, G. S.: Neonatal thrombocy-

topenic purpura and other manifestations of rubella contracted in utero. Amer. J. Dis. Child., *110*:416-427, 1965.

30. Cooper, L. Z., Green, R. H., Krugman, S., Giles, J. P., and Mirick, G. S.: Thrombocytopenic purpura and other manifestations of rubella contracted in utero. J. Pediat., *67*:983, 1965.

31. Ferguson, A. W., and Cantab: Rubella as a cause of thrombocytopenic purpura. Pediatrics, *25*:400-408, 1960.

32. Lokietz, H., and Reynolds, F.: Postrubella thrombocytopenic purpura: report of nine new cases and review of published cases. Lancet, *1*:226-230, 1965.

33. Rausen, A., London, R., Mizrahi, A., and Cooper, L.: Generalized bone changes and thrombocytopenic purpura in association with intra-uterine rubella. Pediatrics, *36*:264-268, 1965.

34. Rudolph, A., Yow, M., Philips, C., Desmond, M., Blattner, R., and Melnick, J.: Transplacental rubella infection in newly born infants. J.A.M.A., *191*:843-845, 1965.

35. Sjögren, I., Bonnevier, J., and Killander, A.: Purpura, thrombocytopenia, hyperlipemia and hepatosplenomegaly in rubella embryopathy. Acta Paediat., *54*:616, 1965.

36. Steen, E., and Torp, K.: Encephalitis and thrombocytopenic purpura after rubella. Arch. Dis. Child., *31*:470, 1956.

37. Svenningsen, N. W.: Thrombocytopenia after rubella (report of two cases). Acta Paediat. Scand., *54*:97-100, 1965.

38. Wallace, D. C.: A case of thrombocytopenic purpura due to rubella. Med. J. Aust., *2*:97-98, 1964.

39. Wallace, S.: Thrombocytopenic purpura after rubella. Lancet, *1*:139-141, 1963.

THROMBOCYTOPENIA OCCURRING DURING OTHER KNOWN OR PROBABLE VIRUS DISEASES

40. Alagille, D.: Les thrombopénies apparaissant au cours des infections virales. Entr. Bichat Méd. Paris, Expansion Scient. Franç. (Publisher) 1961, pp. 575-578.

41. Auban, H., and Combes, B.: Purpura thrombopénique au cours des maladies infectieuses de l'enfant. Toulouse Méd., *59*:483, 1958.

42. Bloom, G. E., Canales, L., and Fairchild, J.: Thrombocytopenic purpura with infectious mononucleosis: two cases in children with review of the literature. Amer. J. Dis. Child., *106*:415-418, 1963.

43. Carter, R. L.: Platelet levels in infectious mononucleosis. Blood, *25*:817-821, 1965.

44. Chamberlin, R. T.: Secondary thrombocytopenic purpura: infectious mononucleosis or nitrofurantoin therapy. J. Maine Med. Assoc., *54*:54-56, 1963.

45. Charkes, N.: Purpuric chickenpox: report of a case, review of the literature and classification by clinical features. Ann. Intern. Med., *54*:745-759, 1961.

46. Clarke, B. F., and Davies, S. H.: Severe thrombocytopenia in infectious mononucleosis. Amer. J. Med. Sci., *248*:703-708, 1964.

47. Cohen, H., Weiss, G., and Appelbaum, E.: Thrombocytopenic purpura secondary to German measles: varicella encephalitis (2 cases). Arch. Pediat., *77*:138-150, 1960.

48. Darbon, A., Portal, A., and Ratignier, A.: Un cas de purpura thrombocytopénique au cours d'une hépatite virale. Bull. Soc. Méd. Milit. Franç., *54*:33-35, 1960.

49. Douglas, W. A.: Infectious mononucleosis with thrombocytopenic purpura in a child. Med. J. Aust., *46*:564-566, 1959.

50. Durand, C., Gavezotti, B., and Pigney, J.: Purpura thrombopénique aigu après une varicelle commune. A propos d'une observation avec anticorps anti-plaquettes dans le sang circulant. Sem. Hôp. Paris, *40*:1227-1229, 1964.

51. Famma, P., Paton, W., Bostock, M.: Thrombocytopenic purpura complicating mumps. Brit. Med. J., *2*:1244, 1964.

52. Giraud, P., Orsini, A., Pinsard, N., et al.: Purpura thrombopénique postvaricelleux. Pédiatrie, *19*:861-864, 1964.

53. Grossman, L. A., and Wolff, S. M.: Acute thrombocytopenic purpura in infectious mononucleosis. J.A.M.A., *171*:2208-2210, 1959.

54. Hyatt, H. W.: Thrombocytopenic purpura complicating epidemic parotitis in a child. Arch. Pediat., *78*:143-150, 1961.

55. Lee, R. C.: Thrombocytopenic purpura in infectious mononucleosis. A case report. Med. Bull. U.S. Army Europe, *21*:13-14, 1964.

56. Lymburner, R. M., and Malcolmson, C. H.: Thrombocytopenic purpura complicating infectious mononucleosis. Canad. Med. Assoc. J., *83*:652, 1960.

57. Maupin, B., and Monteil, R.: Les plaquettes dans la mononucléose infectieuse. Nouv. Rev. Franç. Hémat., *1*:333-335, 1961.

58. Meyer, T. L., Jr.: Case analysis clinic: postinfectious thrombocytopenic purpura and its management. Amer. J. Surg., *99*:118-119, 1960.

59. Ottaviani, P., Mandelli, F., and Deriu, L.: Porpora trombocitopenica acuta da autoanticorpi in corso di rosolia. Policlinico (Prat.), *71*:1250-1252, 1964.

60. Ougier, J., Cahen-Castel, A., and Schlienger, F.: Purpura thrombopénique sévère après mononucléose infectieuse: échec de la corticothérapie nécessitant une splénectomie. Sem. Hôp. Paris. *35*:3115-3117, 1959.

61. Radel, E., and Schorr, J. B.: Thrombocytopenic purpura with infectious mononucleosis: report of 2 cases and a review of the literature. J. Pediat., *63*:46-60, 1963.

62. Radojcic, B., and Kramer, M.: Thrombocytopenische Purpura bei infektiöser Mononukleose. Proc. 8th Congress of the Europ. Soc. Hemat. Wien, 1961. Basel, Karger, 1961.

63. Santella, S. M.: Gastro-intestinal hemorrhage secondary to thrombocytopenia as a complication of mumps. St. Vincent Hosp. Med. Bull., *5*:22-24, 1963.

64. Schumacher, R. H.: Infectious mononucleosis complicated by chronic thrombocytopenia. J.A.M.A., *177*:515-516, 1961.

65. Seringe, P., and Arnal, M.: Purpura thrombopénique aigu morbilleux. Echec de la corticothérapie et des transfusions. Guérison par exsanguino-transfusion. Sem. Hôp. Paris, *36*:3347-3352, 1960.

66. Smith, D. S., Abell, J., and Cast, I.: Auto immune haemolytic anemia and thrombocytopenia complicating infectious mononucleosis. Brit. Med. J., *1*:1210-1211, 1963.

67. Zimprich, H.: Beitrag zu dem postinfektiösen Thrombopenien im Kindesalter. Neue Osterr. Z. Kinderheilk. 6:379-384, 1961.

VIRAL ETIOLOGY OF THROMBOCYTOPENIC PURPURA

68. Delon, J., Rollier, M., et al.: Sur trois cas de purpura infectieux thrombocytopénique avec réaction fortement positive à l'adénovirus. Maroc. Méd., 40:709-710, 1961.
69. Hirsch, E. O., and Dameshek, W., "Idiopathic" thrombocytopenia: review of 89 cases with particular reference to the differentiation and treatment of acute (self-limited) and chronic types. Arch. Intern. Med., 88:701, 1951.
70. Meindersma, T., and De Vries, S.: Thrombocytopenic purpura after smallpox vaccination. Brit. Med. J., 1:226-228, 1962.
71. Pratesi, G., Bolognesi, G., and Fremiotti, A.: Dimostrazione di anticorpi antipiastrine in un caso de porpora trombocitopenica secondaria a rosolia. Recent. Progr. Med., 37:21, 1964.
72. Bentégeat, J., Verger, P., Marc, Y., and Nouaille-Degorge, P.: De l'étiologie virale des purpuras thrombopéniques aigus de l'enfant. Ann. Pédiat., 12:373-382, 1965.

48

Hemolytic Anemias

By J. BERNARD AND J. COLOMBANI

CLASSIFICATION

Viruses, unlike certain bacterial agents, do not seem capable of directly inducing hemolysis. The hemolytic anemias observed during viral infection depend on an immunological mechanism: antierythrocytic autoantibodies can be demonstrated in most cases observed.

The most common clinical picture is that of an acute hemolytic anemia with cold antibodies. Hemolysis is found in association with "viral" pneumopathy. Although the "viral" origin of the infection has been demonstrated in the epidemic cases, this is not so in the sporadic ones. In a few rare cases, a definite viral etiology (influenza A) could be demonstrated serologically.

Much rarer still is an attack of paroxysmal cold hemoglobinuria with hemolysis due to a biphasic hemolysin: the viruses of measles, chickenpox, and mumps, and the possible virus of infectious mononucleosis, have been considered responsible for the hemolytic crisis.

In other cases hemolytic anemia occurs, and immunohematological examinations show either cold agglutinins of low titer or an isolated positive Coombs test. Hemolytic crises of this type occasionally complicate infectious mononucleosis, influenza, infection due to Coxsackie viruses, or ornithosis.

These cases in which immunological hemolytic anemia is related to a precise viral etiology perhaps constitute privileged examples, i.e., the other cases of "idiopathic" immunological hemolytic anemias perhaps only await proof of their viral origin. The part played by the "virus modifier" either of the erythrocyte or of immunologically competent cells in the theories of autoimmunization is known.

These different aspects are considered successively.

ACUTE HEMOLYTIC ANEMIA WITH COLD AUTOANTIBODIES (TYPE: SECONDARY TO "VIRAL" PNEUMOPATHY)

FREQUENCY

The frequent production of high-titer anti-erythrocyte cold antibodies during "atypical primary pneumonia" (i.e., the so-called viral pneumopathy) was clearly recognized for the first time in 1943.[38] The occasional association of an erythrocytic autoagglutination had been previously recognized during respiratory infections, but no connection between these two facts had been established.

The first cases reported[13, 38] of acute hemolytic anemia associated with viral pneumopathy were not at first considered a consequence of the viral infection. Further cases rapidly revealed that the viral pneumopathy could be complicated (although rarely) by an acute brief hemolytic anemia.

It is now evident that the hemolytic anemia is the result of the formation of high-titer cold autoagglutinins with a wide thermal amplitude that are highly hemolytic. These antibodies are of the same nature as those frequently observed in a transitory form during the viral infection.

It is not possible to decide whether the appearance of cold agglutinins is related to a particular type of viral pneumopathy. It does seem, however, that the frequency of cases is highly variable: of the cases observed during World War II, a high titer of cold agglutinins was found in 50 per cent,[21, 22, 54] whereas in the cases observed from 1950 to 1956 the frequency was only 22 per cent.[19] At present the rarity of cases of hemolytic anemia appears to be related to the rarity of epidemics of "viral" pneumopathy. Dacie[12] observed ten cases of hemolytic anemia from 1948 to 1960. It is impossible to estimate the over-all frequency of hemolytic manifestations in cases of viral pneumopathy.

An important reservation should be expressed here. A chronological disagreement exists between, on the one hand, the immunological and hematological descriptions of hemolytic anemia and, on the other, the progress in etiological research. A "pleuropneumonia-like organism," *Mycoplasma pneumoniae,* appears to be responsible for most cases of atypical pneumonia previously attributed to a virus (cf. Chapter 45).

Recent studies of Schmid and Barile showed that most of the strains of mycoplasma isolated from tumors and leukemias and *Mycoplasma pneumoniae,* directly alter the I antigen of red blood cells and render them I negative. It is tempting to establish a link between this fact and the anti-I cold agglutinins of atypical pneumonia.

CLINICAL SYMPTOMS

The disease occurs in both sexes and most often in adults.

The onset of hemolysis is situated 15 to 20 days after the beginning of the infection. It installs itself abruptly. The patient, whose respiratory infection was progressing toward recovery, again shows great lassitude, with icterus and pallor in relation with the hemolysis and subsequent anemia.

Hemoglobinuria may be observed.[13, 29, 36, 45] The spleen is palpable in most cases.

A rare but typical complication of the disease is gangrene of the extremities.[8, 44] One explanation may be the occurrence of thrombosis secondary to an intravascular autoagglutination. Raynaud's syndrome, classic during these hemolytic anemias, seems to result from the same mechanism, as does the acrocyanosis occasionally observed.[28]

HEMATOLOGY

Autoagglutination in vitro, during blood sampling, is constant, and hematological examinations are exact only if the material (pipette, counting chamber, slides) is heated to between 37 and 40° C.

Anemia is often intense and progressive. Counts of approximately one million cells per cubic millimeter may be observed. There is a certain degree of polychromatophilia and spherocytosis. Erythrophagocytosis may be seen. Osmotic resistance is slightly reduced.

An increase of *leukocytosis* is noted that is sometimes considerable, of the order of 40,000 cells per cubic millimeter.[13, 23, 36] The number of neutrophilic granulocytes increases, with presence of a few myelocytes occasionally.

In a case reported by Moeschlin et al.,[35] a severe granulocytopenia and moderate thrombocytopenia followed the hemolytic period. The leukopenia, which persisted a year, was attributed to an antileukocytic autoimmunization.

The percentage of bilirubin is generally increased during the acute phase of hemolysis, as well as plasma hemoglobin and methemalbumin. The haptoglobin level is reduced to zero.

Search for an anomaly of the serum globulins[9] that could be related to the cold antibody was unsuccessful. Only a moderate over-all increase in the alpha and gamma globulins was found.

SEROLOGY

The serological picture in hemolytic anemia secondary to a viral pneumopathy closely resembles that in cold agglutinin disease idiopathic or secondary to a malignant disease (e.g., chronic lymphoid leukosis, Hodgkin's disease). It is distinguished essentially by the transitory nature of the anomalies.

The tests should be carried out on the serum and blood cells of the patient sampled and separated at a warm temperature (37 to 40° C.). A sample taken at laboratory temperature would enable the reaction between antigen (red blood cells) and antibody (serum) to take place. If, on the other hand, the serum is separated from the blood cells without the blood being allowed to cool, the antibody in the serum then is absolutely comparable to that circulating in the patient's blood. The results of in vitro studies thus reflect exactly the properties of the antibody and its activity in vivo.

1. *Increase in the titer of the complete cold agglutinins* (agglutinant in a saline medium) is found. Cold antibodies of low titer, i.e., less than 1/16, are observed in the normal state. In the cases of hemolytic anemia reported the titer has been between 1/512 and 1/32,000 at 4° C.[12, 14, 15] It is to be noted that the highest titer was observed in a case complicated by gangrene of the extremities. The evolution of the titer of cold agglutinins consisted in an extremely rapid increase to a maximum level at the time of the acute hemolytic crisis; then the titer decreased over several weeks, and at the same time hemolysis ceased. Several months were required for a complete return to normal.

2. *The increase in thermal amplitude* of these antibodies is regular. Thermal amplitude is defined as the temperature extremes between which the antibody remains active. The physiological cold antibody is always inactive between 10 and 15° C. The pathological antibody may be active at temperatures of the order of 30° C. or more.

It is conceivable that it is the increase in thermal amplitude that confers to the antibody its pathogenicity, thus making possible intravascular agglutination in the superficial blood vessels of the uncovered parts of the body exposed to cold. The triggering of hemolytic crises by cold is commonly observed in these patients.

The pathogenic significance of the temperature range of the antibody, rather than the titer of agglutination at 4° C., was emphasized by Dacie[12] in a case in which clinical cure coincided with a reduction in thermal amplitude while the agglutination titer had barely decreased.

3. *Existence of a hemolysin* can be shown. In the presence of complement (C') the patient's serum has the power to lyse normal red blood cells or the patient's own red blood cells in vitro. This hemolysin has an optimum activity at pH 6.5 and 20° C. This optimum temperature is a compromise between the optimum temperature of action of the antibody (4° C.) and that of C' (25 to 37° C.), both of which are necessary for hemolysis. Hemolysis does not occur at 37° C. In certain cases the hemolysin is easily demonstratable only with regard to the red blood cells of patients with paroxysmal nocturnal hemoglobinuria.

It is this hemolysin that, under a cooling effect, provokes an intravascular hemolysis responsible for hemoglobinuria. A fall in the level of C' is observed simultaneously, in relation with its consumption in vivo by the immunological reaction.

4. *Existence of a direct Coombs test of the non-gamma globulin type:* this denomination signifies that the reaction is obtained by means of a Coombs serum (i.e., an animal anti-human-globulin serum) previously neutralized by human gamma globulins. Hence it can be concluded that the globulin substance covering the red blood cells is not a gamma globulin. Later studies showed that the globulins fixed to the red blood cells are fractions of C' (C'4, which is a beta$_{1E}$ globulin, and/or C'3a, which is a beta$_{1C}$ globulin). The Coombs test result is therefore due to the fixation in vivo not of the antibody itself but of fractions of C'. This fixation is nevertheless probably related to a previous sensitization by the cold antibody. It has been demonstrated[27] that fixation of the antibody to the red blood cell is less marked than that of C' and that the latter remains fixed even when the antibody level is high.

5. *Blood group specificity.* Various blood group specificities have been demonstrated with regard to the antibodies of acquired hemolytic anemias.[41] The antibodies of cold agglutinin disease generally possess an anti-I specificity.[53] The Ii blood group system is defined by the presence of two antibodies, anti-I and anti-i. The I antigen is

extremely widespread (only one subject was I negative among 4600 individuals). The antigen is not present on the red blood cells of the newborn and develops during the first few months of life.

The four cases of cold antibodies secondary to viral pneumopathy that were studied for their anti-I specificity revealed the following results:[12] an anti-I specificity was observed in two cases; the I-positive and I-negative adult red blood cells were agglutinated in two cases with the same intensity, but the red blood cells of the newborn were agglutinated to a lesser extent. These cases suggest a particular specificity, possibly related to I.

PROGNOSIS AND COURSE

The prognosis of hemolytic anemias secondary to viral pneumopathy is generally good, in view of the extremely transitory character of the hemolysis. Although a few rare fatal cases have been reported,[20, 29] complete recovery is the usual outcome after a period of several weeks.

The patient should be kept in bed and kept constantly warm. Transfusions are sometimes necessary in the case of intense anemia. The blood transfused should be warmed immediately before its perfusion. Corticosteroid hormones are useless in general; splenectomy is never indicated.

ETIOLOGY AND PATHOGENESIS

In most cases the diagnosis of viral pneumopathy (primary atypical pneumonia) is established in terms of the clinical and radiological picture, the epidemiology, and the negative results of bacteriological tests.

In certain cases a definite virus has been rendered responsible for the hemolytic anemia: e.g., various viruses of epidemic influenza[32, 51] and the possible virus of infectious mononucleosis.[34]

TRANSITORY PAROXYSMAL COLD HEMOGLOBINURIA SECONDARY TO A VIRAL DISEASE

This syndrome is clinically defined by a hemoglobinuric crisis set off by cold and, serologically, by a biphasic antibody (cold-warm) that hemolyzes the red blood cells in presence of C'.[12]

THE HEMOLYTIC CRISIS

After exposure to cold, the patient has pain in the lumbar region, cramps in the limbs, and chills. Body temperature rises at the same time that urticaria, cyanosis, and Raynaud's syndrome occur. Hemoglobinuria appears. The crisis lasts several hours; then everything returns to normal. Apart from this typical form, incomplete crises may be observed with, at the minimum, an isolated hemoglobinuria.

HEMATOLOGY

There is noticeable anemia only in the case of prolonged or repeated crises. At the time of the crisis a transitory leukopenia is observed. Pictures of erythrophagocytosis may be seen.

SEROLOGY

The Donath-Landsteiner test consists in incubating together the patient's serum with red blood cells (either normal or from the patient) and C' (either human or from the guinea pig) successively at 4° C. and 37° C. Hemolysis is observed at the end of the warm phase in the positive cases.

During the cold phase the antibody sensitizes the red blood cells and the C' begins to be fixed. During the warm phase C' continues to be fixed while at the same time the antibody increases. The sequence of fixation of the various factors of C' in the presence of Donath-Landsteiner antibody is identical with that found in the classic system Forssman antigen-anti-Forssman antibody: successively C'1-C'4-C'2-C'3. The optimum pH of the reaction is between 7.0 and 7.5. In the absence of C' the Donath-Landsteiner antibody is weakly agglutinating.

ETIOLOGY

The following viral or presumed viral diseases are known to be responsible:

Chickenpox:[31] a hemolytic crisis appeared during the incubation period of the disease.

Infectious mononucleosis:[17] severe hemolytic crisis with hemoglobinuria occurred two weeks after a respiratory infection. At the same time that the Donath-Landsteiner test became positive a titer of cold agglutinins of 1/256 was observed. The patient recovered completely after an extremely severe illness of about two months.

Measles:[12] a case that was thoroughly studied by Dacie evolved in one month toward recovery and complete disappearance of all the serological signs. A phenomenon recognized in the case secondary to chickenpox,[31] a transitorily positive Wassermann reaction, was observed in the acute phase of the disease.

Mumps:[10] paroxsysmal hemoglobinuria followed the infection.

ACUTE HEMOLYTIC ANEMIAS WITH ATYPICAL SEROLOGY

These cases, most often observed as a complication of infectious mononucleosis, maintain a certain clinical homogeneity, but the serological picture is more varied than in the previous cases.

The clinical picture is that of acute hemolytic anemia of extremely abrupt onset with hemoglobinuria on occasion. Hemolysis usually occurs ten to 15 days after onset of the infectious episode. At other times the two diseases seem to be simultaneous. Pallor, icterus, and splenomegaly constitute the clinical signs.

Apart from moderate anemia, hematological examination in most instances reveals the leukocytic disorders of infectious mononucleosis. The reaction of Paul, Bunnell, and Davidson is positive. The immunohematological examination makes it possible to distinguish the cases in which the titer of complete cold agglutinins is abnormal

Table 48-1. *Relationship Between the Serological Type of Hemolytic Anemia and the Causal Virus**

	Cold Agglutinins ≥ 1/512	Paroxysmal Cold Hemoglobinuria, Donath-Landsteiner Hemoglobinuria	Cold Agglutinins ≥ 1/32 ≤ 1/256	Cold Agglutinins < 1/32, Positive Direct Coombs Tests	Doubtful or Positive Serological Tests	Insufficient Serological Tests
'Viral" pneumopathy	20, 21, 22, 54(a) 19, 12(b)					
Infectious mononucleosis	34	17	11, 13, 16 25, 39, 33, 43	26, 30, 42	2, 18(g), 40, 47(g)	1, 4
Influenza	32(c) 51(d)			37(c) 3(d)		
Coxsackie A				5, 52		
Measles		12 12(e)		12(e)		
Chickenpox		31				
Mumps		10				
Ornithosis				24		
Herpes				48(f)		

*The numbers refer to the bibliography.
(a) Numerous epidemic cases (World War II).
(b) Rare sporadic cases.
(c) Influenza A.
(d) "Asiatic" influenza.
(e) Successively Donath-Landsteiner hemolysin then hemolytic anemia with positive direct Coombs test.
(f) Anti-e specificity.
(g) Two cases.

(1/32 to 1/256) but, however, never attains the figures observed in cases secondary to viral pneumopathy. The cases reported concern only infectious mononucleosis.[11, 13, 16, 25, 33, 39, 43]

In other instances the antierythrocyte autoimmunization is detected only by the presence of a positive Coombs reaction. Several cases have been reported during infectious mononucleosis,[26, 30, 42] influenza,[3, 37] Coxsackie A virus infection,[5, 52] measles,[12] ornithosis,[24] and herpes.[48]

In still other instances the immunohematological examination produces doubtful results[1, 4, 18, 40] or negative results[2, 47] during infectious mononucleosis, without these cases being distinguishable from the previous ones.

The prognosis and evolution in these cases are analogous to those with cold autoantibodies.

For a recapitulation of all these data see Table 48-1.

ROLE OF THE VIRUS IN DETERMINING AUTOIMMUNIZATION

Three hypotheses can be envisaged to explain the hemolysis during viral infection.

1. The virus fixes itself on the surface of the red blood cell. The antiviral antibody, by combining with its antigen on the erythrocytes, destroys them. This hypothesis seems to have been verified experimentally in the dog.[46] In man, on the other hand, observation does not confirm this supposition since in most cases the antiviral antibodies appear after the hemolytic crisis.[5]

2. The virus modifies the red blood cells either by direct action or by enzymatic action. These modified erythrocytes become antigenic for the patient's organism, which consequently produces antibodies. No experiment has yet demonstrated this theory. Furthermore, it does not explain why the antibodies produced have the ability to react with normal (nonmodified) erythrocytes and occasionally have a blood group specificity.[48]

3. The virus modifies the antibody-producing cells, which then become capable of producing antierythrocyte autoantibodies. This purely theoretical concept fits into the clonal theory of immunity of Burnet.[6, 7, 50]

So far there has been no experimental confirmation of this hypothesis.

BIBLIOGRAPHY

1. Appelman, D. H., and Morrison, M. M.: Concomitant infectious mononucleosis and hemolytic anemia. Blood, 4:186, 1949.
2. Bean, R. H. D.: Haemolytic anaemia complicating infectious mononucleosis with report of a case. Med. J. Aust., 1:386, 1957.
3. Beickert, A., and Sprossig, M.: Immunhämatologische und virologischserologische Beobachtungen bei erworbener hämolytischer Anämie im Verlaufe einer "asiatischen" Grippe. Klin. Wschr., 37:146, 1959.
4. Berte, S. J.: Acute hemolytic anemia in infectious mononucleosis. New York J. Med., 51:781, 1951.
5. Betke, K., Richarz, H., Schubothe, H., and Vivell, O.: Beobachtungen zu Krankheitsbild, Pathogenese und Atiologie der akuten erworbenen hämolytischen Anämie (Lederer-Anämie). Klin. Wschr., 31:373, 1953.
6. Burnet, M.: Auto-immune disease. I. Modern immunological concepts. Brit. Med. J., 2:645, 1959.
7. Burnet, M.: Auto-immune disease. II. Pathology of the immune response. Brit. Med. J., 2:720, 1959.
8. Carey, R. M., Wilson, J. L., and Tamerin, J. A.: Gangrene of feet and hemolytic anemia associated with cold hemagglutinins in atypical pneumonia. Harlem Hosp. Bull., 1:25, 1948.
9. Christenson, W. N., and Dacie, J. V.: Serum proteins in acquired haemolytic anaemia (auto-antibody type). Brit. J. Haemat., 3:153, 1957.
10. Colley, E. W.: Paroxysmal cold haemoglobinuria after mumps. Brit. Med. J., 1:1552, 1964.
11. Crosby, W. H., and Rappaport, H.: Reticulocytopenia in autoimmune hemolytic anemia. Blood, 11:929, 1956.
12. Dacie, J. V.: The Haemolytic Anaemias. Part 2: The Auto-Immune Haemolytic Anaemias. 2nd ed. New York, Grune & Stratton, 1962.
13. Dameshek, W.: Cold hemagglutinins in acute hemolytic reactions in association with sulfonamide medication and infection. J.A.M.A., 123:77, 1943.
14. Dausset, J.: Immuno-hématologie biologique et clinique. Paris, Flammarion, 1956.
15. Dausset, J., and Colombani, J.: The serology and the prognosis of 128 cases of autoimmune hemolytic anemia. Blood, 14:1280, 1959.
16. Di Piero, G., and Arcangeli, A.: Anemia emolitica acquisata con auto-anticorpi incompleti a freddo in corso di mononucleosi infettiva. Haematologica, 43:91, 1958.
17. Ellis, L. B., Wollenman, O. J., and Stetson, R. M.: Auto-hemagglutinins and hemolysins with hemoglobinuria and acute hemolytic anemia, in an illness resembling infectious mononucleosis. Blood, 3:419, 1948.
18. Evans, R. S., and Weiser, R. S.: The serology of auto-immune hemolytic disease: observations on forty-one patients. Arch. Intern. Med., 100:371, 1957.

19. Finland, M., and Barnes, M. W.: Cold agglutinins. VIII. Occurrence of cold isohemagglutinins in patients with primary atypical pneumonia or influenza viral infection, Boston City Hospital, June 1950 to July 1956. Arch. Intern. Med., *101*: 462, 1958.

20. Finland, M., Peterson, O. L., Allen, H. E., Samper, B. A., and Barnes, M. W.: Cold agglutinins. II. Cold isohemagglutinins in primary atypical pneumonia of unknown etiology with a note on the occurrence of hemolytic anemia in these cases. J. Clin. Invest., *24*:458, 1945a.

21. Finland, M., Peterson, O. L., Allen, H. E., Samper, B. A., Barnes, M. W., and Stone, M. B.: Cold agglutinins. I. Occurrence of cold isohemagglutinins in various conditions. J. Clin. Invest., *24*:451, 1945b.

22. Florman, A. L., and Weiss, A. B.: Serologic reactions in primary atypical pneumonia. J. Lab. Clin. Med., *30*:942, 1945.

23. Ginsberg, H. S.: Acute hemolytic anemia in primary atypical pneumonia associated with high titer of cold agglutinins. New Eng. J. Med., *234*:826, 1946.

24. Goudemand, M., Voisin, C., and Marchandise, C.: Anémie hémolytique aiguë au cours d'une ornithose. Sem. Hôp. Paris, *38*:2235, 1962.

25. Green, N., and Goldenberg, H.: Acute hemolytic anemia and hemoglobinuria complicating infectious mononucleosis. Arch. Intern. Med., *105*:108, 1960.

26. Hall, B. D., and Archer, F. C.: Acute hemolytic anemia associated with infectious mononucleosis. New Eng. J. Med., *249*:973, 1953.

27. Harboe, M.: Interaction between ^{131}I trace-labelled cold agglutinin, complement and red cells. Brit. J. Haemat., *10*:339, 1964.

28. Helwig, F. C., and Freis, E. D.: Cold autohemagglutinins following atypical pneumonia producing clinical picture of acrocyanosis. J.A.M.A., *123*:626, 1943.

29. Horstmann, D. M., and Tatlock, H.: Cold agglutinins: diagnostic aid in certain types of primary atypical pneumonia. J.A.M.A., *122*:369, 1943.

30. Huntington, P. W., Jr.: Hemolytic anemia in infectious mononucleosis; case report. Delaware Med. J., *23*:165, 1951.

31. Kaiser, A. D., and Bradford, W. L.: Severe haemoglobinuria in a child, occurring in the prodromal stage of chickenpox. Arch. Pediat., *46*:571, 1929.

32. Laroche, C., Milliez, P., Dreyfus, B., Dausset, J., and Leprat, J.: Ictère hémolytique aigu postgrippal. Bull. Soc. Med. Hôp. Paris, *67*:779, 1951.

33. Mengel, C. E., Wallace, A. G., and Mc Daniel, H. G.: Infectious mononucleosis, hemolysis and megaloblastic arrest. Arch. Intern. Med., *114*:333, 1964.

34. Mermann, A. C.: Acute hemolytic anemia with infectious mononucleosis. U.S. Armed Forces Med. J., *3*:1551, 1952.

35. Moeschlin, S., Siegenthaler, W., Gasser, C., and Hassig, A.: Immunopancytopenia associated with incomplete cold hemagglutinins in a case of primary atypical pneumonia. Blood, *9*:214, 1954.

36. Neely, F. L., Baria, W. H., Smith, C., and Stone, C. F., Jr.: Primary atypical pneumonia with high titer of cold hemagglutinins, hemolytic anemia and false positive Donath-Landsteiner test. J. Lab. Clin. Med., *37*:382, 1951.

37. d'Oelsnitz, M., Vincent, L., and Lippmann, C.: Ictère hémolytique et hémoglobinurie d'origine grippale. Arch. Franç. Pédiat., *16*:391, 1959.

38. Peterson, O. L., Ham, T. H., and Finland, M.: Cold agglutinins (autohemagglutinins) in primary atypical pneumonias. Science, *97*:167, 1943.

39. Punt, K., and Verloop, M. C.: Even geval van acute haemolytische Anaemie bij mononucleosis infectiosa. Nederl. T. Geneesk., *99*:3128, 1955.

40. Rossi, V.: Anemia emolitica in corso di mononucleosi infettiva: osservazioni sieroimmunologiche. Boll. Soc. Ital. Emat., *6*:12, 1958.

41. Salmon, C.: La spécificité des auto-anticorps d'anémie hémolytique acquise. Rev. Franç. Etud. Clin. Biol., *9*:532, 1964.

42. Sawitsky, A., Papps, J. P., and Wiener, L. M.: The demonstration of antibody in acute hemolytic anemia complicating infectious mononucleosis. Amer. J. Med., *8*:260, 1950.

43. Smith, D. S., Abell, J. D., and Cast, I. P.: Auto-immune haemolytic anaemia and thrombocytopenia complicating infectious mononucleosis. Brit. Med. J., *1*:1210, 1963.

44. Stats, D., Wasserman, L. R., and Rosenthal, N.: Hemolytic anemia with hemoglobinuria. Amer. J. Clin. Path., *18*:757, 1948.

45. Stewart, J. W., and Friedlander, P. H.: Haemoglobinuria and acute haemolytic anaemia associated with primary atypical pneumonia. Lancet, *11*:774, 1957.

46. Stewart, W. B., Petenyi, C. W., and Rose, H. M.: Survival time of canine erythrocytes modified by influenza virus. Blood, *10*:228, 1955.

47. Thurm, R. H., and Bassen, F.: Infectious mononucleosis and acute hemolytic anemia: report of two cases and review of the literature. Blood, *10*:841, 1955.

48. Todd, R. M., and O'Donohue, N. V.: Acute acquired haemolytic anaemia associated with herpes simplex infection. Arch. Dis. Child., *33*:524, 1958.

49. Unger, L. J., Wiener, A. S., and Dolan, D.: Anémie auto-hémolytique chez un nouveau-né. Rev. Hémat., *7*:495, 1952.

50. Van Loghem, J. J.: Concepts on the origin of autoimmune diseases. The possible role of viral infection in the aetiology of idiopathic auto-immune diseases. Series Haemat., *9*:1, 1965.

51. Ventura, S., and Aresu, G.: Grave anemia immuno-emolitica in decorso di influenza cosidetta "Asiatica". Rass. Med. Sarda, *59*:1, 1957.

52. Vivell, O.: Ergebnisse virologischer Studien bei Fällen von akuter hämolytischer Anämie (Lederer-Brill). Mschr. Kinderheilk., *102*:113, 1954.

53. Wiener, A. S., Unger, L. J., Cohen, L., and Feldman, J.: Type-specific cold auto-antibodies, as cause of acquired hemolytic anemia and hemolytic transfusion reactions: biologic test with bovine red cells. Ann. Intern. Med., *44*:221, 1956.

54. Young, L. E.: Clinical significance of cold hemagglutinins. Amer. J. Med. Sci., *211*:23, 1946.

49

Acute Infectious Lymphocytosis
(Carl Smith's Disease)

By J. C. JOB

In 1941 Carl Smith described, under the name of infectious lymphocytosis, an acute epidemic blood disease characterized by a large number of normal circulating lymphocytes, and by the discretion of the clinical manifestations (especially absence of splenomegaly and lymph node enlargement), and an extremely benign course. Similar reports published about the same time[19, 22] seem to indicate that the disease had, until then, been confounded with infectious mononucleosis.

Even today the definition of Carl Smith's disease remains cytological and clinical. The viral nature of this disease is only probable and has not been demonstrated.

CLINICAL DESCRIPTION

Incubation Period. The duration of the incubation period is ill delimited but is probably between 12 and 21 days.[21] In a few cases it seems to last longer.[16a]

Symptoms. Acute lymphocytosis is *most often latent*, being discovered fortuitously by examination of the blood of apparently normal subjects or on routine hematological screening of the family or the schoolmates of patients.

The main clinical fact is of negative order: *absence of splenomegaly, adenopathies, purpura, and hemorrhage*. It distinguishes Carl Smith's disease from infectious mononucleosis and malignant hemopathy. There are, however, a few exceptions to this rule. But small or average-sized cervical adenopa-

thies are common enough in children for a coincidence to be possible.

When symptoms occur, they are most often those of *catarrhal rhinopharyngitis:* coryza, pharyngitis, cough, and congestive otitis, occasionally conjunctivitis as well, with high or low fever.

Abdominal signs and symptoms are a little less frequent. These include abdominal pains, tenderness of the abdominal wall, diarrhea, and fever, variably associated, which may simulate enteritis, colitis, typhoid fever, or occasionally appendicitis. Hepatomegaly is found in a few cases, and needle biopsy of the liver has shown histiocytic nodules.[5]

Meningeal symptoms are still rarer. They comprise a more or less clear-cut meningeal syndrome with headache, vomiting, neck and back pain, spinal rigidity, Kernig's sign, and even muscular hypertonicity. In three cases[16a, 22] convulsive seizures have been reported. The cerebrospinal fluid is clear, with high albumin content and moderate pleocytosis, and a mixed cellular reaction with polymorphonuclear and lymphocytic cells.[7] Clinical symptoms of meningitis have been observed in the absence of biological signs, and, conversely, routine lumbar punctures performed during epidemics of infectious lymphocytosis have occasionally revealed latent meningitis.

In a few cases a *rash* can occur: of macular,[10, 23] herpetic,[21] or erythema multiforme type.[13]

In some other cases *pulmonary involve-*

672

ment occurs with varied clinical signs: cough, dyspnea, sibilant rales, or rhonchi. On x-ray examination various changes have been reported: atelectasis,[15] emphysema,[14] hilar adenopathies,[6, 12] multiple pulmonary opacities,[17] and thickening of the perihilar bronchial shadows,[14, 16a] as in atypical pneumonia.

Fever may be the only symptom without any associated manifestations, and it has been reported that asthenia can also be the only symptom of the disease.[3]

Course. Carl Smith's disease is always benign and generally shortlived. The symptoms, whatever they may be, disappear within a few days. Relapses seem to be highly exceptional.

HEMATOLOGICAL DISTURBANCES

Since the clinical symptoms are never characteristic and can even be nonexistent, blood examination alone leads to diagnosis of the disease. The considerable abnormalities revealed are occasionally a striking surprise in subjects apparently well or barely ill.

Blood. The regularly occurring and characteristic element is marked lymphocytic hyperleukocytosis. The leukocyte count is over 20,000 cells per cubic millimeter; it usually attains 50,000 and occasionally more than 100,000 cells per cubic millimeter, the highest leukocyte counts being found in the youngest subjects.[21]

This hyperleukocytosis represents increase in the number of lymphocytes, the proportion of which exceeds 80 per cent and can reach 97 per cent.[8, 21] The number of polynuclear neutrophils and monocytes remains normal in absolute value or is hardly modified. The level of eosinophils in absolute value or even in percentage can increase at the same time as that of the lymphocytes or, more often, later. The essential fact is that the lymphocytes in Carl Smith's disease are always normal mature lymphocytes, most of them small with dense chromatin and with scanty, bluish cytoplasm. Some abnormalities in the form of the lymphocytes can occur, and, in a few cases, the presence of young forms has been reported, but truly pathological cells are never seen.

Bone Marrow. The myelogram is usually normal. An excess of medullar lymphocytes, all normal and mature, has been reported in several cases,[21] but the question can be raised as to what extent this medullary lymphocytosis may have resulted from dilution of the bone marrow by the blood.[3] In any case, the bone marrow picture has no similarity to that in acute leukemia.

Lymph Nodes. Several case reports have included lymph node biopsies. This procedure revealed sinusal reticuloendothelial hyperplasia with hyaline degeneration of lymphoid follicles[21] or, on the contrary, follicular hyperplasia at the periphery of the node.[1] But neither aspect is in any way characteristic.

Course. The duration of lymphocytosis is variable, usually being from two to five weeks,[21] sometimes as long as seven weeks,[9, 10] and even ten weeks.[4] In any event, it disappears little by little spontaneously; after recovery, blood count is normal.

DIAGNOSIS

The diagnosis of acute infectious lymphocytosis requires consideration of acute leukemia, infectious mononucleosis, and various forms of lymphocytosis. In fact, all three can be eliminated easily enough.

Acute Leukemia. No type of acute leukemia really resembles Carl Smith's disease, in which the circulating leukocytes are normal lymphocytes, the red cells and platelets are present in normal quantities, and the bone marrow remains normal. Chronic lymphoid leukemia, in so far as it occurs mainly in elderly people and is associated with spleen and lymph node hyperplasia, can also be easily distinguished from acute infectious lymphocytosis.

Infectious Mononucleosis. Adenopathies and splenomegaly are the rule. The blood count usually shows moderate leukocytosis (10,000 to 20,000 white cells) comprising, in part, large mononuclear cells with a clear cytoplasm and an atypical appearance, and others with a highly basophilic cytoplasm; these cells differ greatly from the small lymphocytes of Carl Smith's disease. In addition, a positive result of the Paul-Bunnell test is a major argument in favor of the diagnosis of infectious mononucleosis.

Diverse Forms of Lymphocytosis. In the course of *whooping cough*, the level of circulating lymphocytes sometimes reaches values comparable to those observed during Carl Smith's disease. Usually, clinical signs permit the diagnosis, although the physician must take into account the possibility that pulmonary or bronchial involvement in infectious lymphocytosis can simulate whooping cough.[16a] If doubt subsists, bacteriological evidence of *Bordetella pertussis* in the rhinopharyngeal mucus provides a certain diagnosis.

Rhinopharyngeal infections that hang on in infants or young children are sometimes associated with lymphocytosis. Prolonged slight fever and discrete signs of pharyngeal inflammation can orient diagnosis. But mainly the relatively slight hyperleukocytosis and the less acute course make it possible not to confound this syndrome with Carl Smith's disease.

EPIDEMIOLOGY

Acute infectious lymphocytosis *occurs mainly in children* under ten years of age. Cases in adolescents and adults are infrequent.[16a]

The *epidemic character* of the disease is undeniable. The epidemics are limited, involving a school, a family, or a collectivity of children. Sporadic cases seem rarer than epidemics. Routine blood testing of persons surrounding the patient reveals other cases, latent ones in particular, and often provides the essential evidence for diagnosis of acute infectious lymphocytosis.

The *contagiousness*, however, seems to be fairly low.[11, 19] Contamination seems to occur by direct contact.[20a] The latent period between the different cases in an epidemic is no more than several weeks.[12]

The disease has been observed everywhere in the world. It does not seem to be seasonal.

ETIOLOGY AND PHYSIOPATHOLOGY

Because of its acute and self-limited character, the infectious aspect of its clinical manifestations, and particularly its epidemicity, acute lymphocytosis has been considered, ever since its description by Carl Smith in 1941, to be an *infectious disease.*

However, no proof of the infection has ever been given, and its *viral origin* is a hypothesis based solely on the negative results of bacteriological investigations.

Seeding of blood and pharyngeal mucus on the most varied bacteriological media has never brought to light any particular pathogenic agent; blood cultures are always negative and the pharyngeal flora common.

The possibility that *B. pertussis* or *B. parapertussis* has a role in the origin of acute infectious lymphocytosis was initially considered but soon rejected because of the clinical and epidemiological differences between whooping cough and Carl Smith's disease and especially because of the negative results of bacteriological investigations.

Serological reactions for salmonellosis, brucellosis, rickettsial infections, influenza, ornithosis, lymphocytic choriomeningitis, and toxoplasmosis, the Paul-Bunnell test, the search for cold agglutinins—all have been negative. A serological reaction of hemagglutination inhibition was positive with an antigen of fecal origin,[16a] but only three patients and two controls were studied.

Inoculation of different laboratory animals[16a] and cultures attempted on the yolk sac of the chick embryo[16, 16a] have all failed. Nevertheless, Marinesco[16a] inoculated hens and believed that he had so induced a disease with leukocytosis and signs of neural involvement.

The presence of a *poliomyelitis virus* in the pharynx of patients with infectious lymphocytosis and the coincidence with poliomyelitis have been reported.[2] In all likelihood the association was fortuitous.

It does not seem that acute infectious lymphocytosis has been investigated further since the introduction of tissue culture techniques for virus cultivation in vitro. Nevertheless, three cases have been reported[18] of a disease clinically resembling whooping cough with a very high lymphocyte count and a slight rise in the eosinophil count, in absence of *B. pertussis* in the pharyngeal mucus and of antibodies against whooping cough. Adenovirus 12 was isolated from the pharyngeal mucus, and there was a rise in the level of the corresponding serum antibodies. The question arises as to whether the disease was really Carl Smith's disease or a similar infection.

The *mechanism of the blood lymphocytosis* also remains unknown. The bone marrow is normal, which excludes the possibility of a medullary origin. The spleen is not enlarged, which makes a splenic origin unlikely; moreover, the disease has been observed in a splenectomized patient.[8] The superficial lymph nodes are not hyperplastic, and their histological appearance is normal, which makes an enhancement of lymphopoiesis at this site unlikely. Surgical exploration performed in a few cases did not show abdominal adenopathies. The rarity of thoracic localizations makes the hypothesis of a mediastinal or peribronchial origin of the lymphocytes improbable.

PROPHYLAXIS AND TREATMENT

The extreme benignity of the disease and its clinical manifestations makes any attempt at prophylaxis or treatment almost useless. The antibiotics used in a few cases (penicillin, tetracycline) did not have any evident effect on the clinical or hematological course of the disease.

BIBLIOGRAPHY

1. Barnes, G. R., Yannet, H., and Lieberman, R.: A clinical study of an institutional outbreak of infectious lymphocytosis. Amer. J. Med. Sci., *218*:646-654, 1949.
2. Beloff, J. S., and Gang, K. M.: Acute poliomyelitis and infectious lymphocytosis: simultaneous appearance in a summer camp. J. Pediat., *26*:586-592, 1945.
3. Bernard, J.: La lymphocytose infectieuse aiguë (maladie de Carl Smith). Pédiatrie, *4*:583-591, 1949.
4. Birge, R. F., and Hill, L. F.: Acute infectious lymphocytosis. Amer. J. Clin. Path., *45*:508-512, 1945.
5. Chaptal, J., Brunel, D., Salvaing, J., and Jean, R.: Sur un cas de lymphocytose infectieuse aiguë avec réaction méningée biologique. Montpellier Méd., *37*:501-502, 1950.
6. Crisalli, M., and Terragna, A.: La malattia di Smith (linfocitosi infettiva acuta). Revisione della letteratura e presentazione di tre casi. Minerva Pediat., *10*:849-863, 1958.
7. Debre, R., Grenet, P., and Mathe, G.: Lymphocytose infectieuse. In: Encyclopédie Médico-Chirurgicale, Maladies Infectieuses. 1956, p. 8057.
8. Debré, R., Mande, R., Lévy, F. M., and Boissière, H.: La lymphocytose infectieuse aiguë. Arch. Franç. Pédiat., *5*:155-160, 1948.
9. Descovich, C., and Santarsiero, M.: La malattia di Smith (linfocitosi infettiva acuta). Clin. Pediat., *45*:233-259, 1963.
10. Duncan, P. A.: Acute infectious lymphocytosis. New Eng. J. Med., *233*:177-179, 1945.
11. Dunn, H. G.: Acute infectious lymphocytosis. Report of a group of cases in a day nursery. Brit. Med. J., *1*:78-83, 1952.
12. Finucane, D. L., and Philips, R. S.: Infectious lymphocytosis. Amer. J. Dis. Child., *68*:301-307, 1944.
13. Howard, J. E.: Acute infectious lymphocytosis. Rev. Chile Pediat., *22*:566, 1951.
14. Keizer, D. P. R.: Note sur la lymphocytose infectieuse aiguë. Arch. Franc. Pédiat., *6*:595-598, 1949.
15. Lemon, B. K., and Kaump, D. H.: Infectious lymphocytosis: epidemic report. J. Pediat., *36*:61-68, 1950.
16. Marie, J., See, G., and Job, J. C.: Forme pulmonaire de la lymphocytose infectieuse aiguë ou syndrome pneumo-lymphocytaire primitif d'étiologie inconnue. Bull. Mém. Soc. Méd. Hôp. Paris, *67*:761-768, 1951.
16a. Marinesco, G.: La lymphocytose infectieuse aiguë. Masson et Cie, Paris, 1965.
17. Moyer, J. B., and Fisher, G. S.: Acute infectious lymphocytosis. Blood, *5*:668-677, 1950.
18. Olson, L. C., Miller, G., and Hanshaw, J. B.: Acute infectious lymphocytosis presenting as a pertussis-like illness. Its association with adenovirus type 12. Lancet, *1*:200-201, 1964.
19. Reyersbach, G., and Lenert, T. F.: Infectious mononucleosis without clinical signs or symptoms. Amer. J. Dis. Child., *61*:237, 1941.
20. Ryder, R. J. W.: Acute infectious lymphocytosis. Amer. J. Dis. Child., *110*:299-301, 1965.
20a. Scalettar, H. E., Maisel, J. E., and Bramson, M.: Acute infectious lymphocytosis. Amer. J. Dis. Child., *88*:15, 1954.
21. Smith, C.: Acute infectious lymphocytosis. Advances Pediat., *2*:64-91, 1947.
22. Thelander, H. E., and Shaw, E. B.: Infectious mononucleosis. Amer. J. Dis. Child., *61*:1131, 1941.
23. Yuskis, A. S.: Acute infectious lymphocytosis in an adult. Review of the literature and report of case. J.A.M.A., *132*:638-640, 1946.

50

Infectious Mononucleosis

By G. DUHAMEL

Infectious mononucleosis is a disease in which the epidemiology and the hematological, serological, and clinical manifestations strongly suggest a viral origin. Yet, despite strong presumptions, this origin has not been formally proved.

Hence, for want of a specific etiology, the definition of the disease remains purely descriptive: it is an acute febrile infectious disease, occurring in minor epidemics, involving the lymph nodes predominantly, accompanied by blood lymphomonocytosis, and often but not always producing characteristic serological modifications.

Clinical knowledge of the disease dates back to Pfeiffer, who in 1889 described "glandular fever." In 1907 Türk noted the hematological abnormalities. In 1920 Sprunt and Evans suggested the name "infectious mononucleosis," thus stressing the importance of the hematological changes. In 1928 Chevallier grouped its various aspects under the name "benign acute lymphadenitis."

The serological stage opened in 1932 with Paul and Bunnell, who showed that the patients' blood contained heterophilic antibodies. The specific characteristics of these antibodies were defined by Davidsohn in 1937.

Concurrently, the etiology of the disease was sought, and in 1929 Nyfeldt incriminated *Listeria Monocytogenes*. But a viral etiology was suspected early and led to numerous attempts to transmit the disease to monkeys and even to man (Van den Berghe and Liessens, Sohier and Lépine, Wising, and others). The Japanese authors Misao and Kobayashi incriminated a Rickettsia

(1953). More recently, Henle et al.[21a] attributed an essential role to a virus of the herpes group: *the EB virus*.

EPIDEMIOLOGY

Mononucleosis occurs preferentially in young persons between the ages of 15 and 25 years (in 80 per cent of the cases reported by Rugg-Gunn). It is rare past age 40. Moreover, we shall see that the specificity of the forms in young children is fairly often dubious.

The disease is equally frequent in both sexes and is found in all races. The disease is not rare but its epidemicity confers on it a rather peculiar distribution. It most often occurs in sporadic cases or is occasionally endemic, with a recrudescence in the spring and fall stressed in classic descriptions.

The contagiousness of infectious mononucleosis is apparently erratic. Many reports on mononucleosis in closed communities of young people (students or soldiers) indicate a low degree of contagiousness, even when the young people shared the same room, but other publications report small epidemics in these same communities.

An analysis of the probable circumstances of contamination partially explains these discrepancies. The principal condition required for transmission of the disease seems to be *direct contact,* especially by saliva. Several well documented and often picturesque cases furnish examples of this mode of contamination, stressing the importance of kissing on the mouth in the transmission of the disease, for which reason it has occasionally been called "kissing disease."

However, other familial or regional epidemics suggest that other methods of contamination are possible: by projection of drops of saliva; indirect contamination by dishes and perhaps food; venereal contamination, explaining the rare forms at the inguinal level; and inapparent forms explaining the sporadic cases.

Ignorance of the causative agent of the disease means that these epidemiological notions remain fragmentary; but the data can be summarized in the following propositions: (1) The causative organism is probably fragile, since its transmission chiefly requires direct contact. (2) Incubation of the disease seems to be six weeks on the average. (3) Apart from the apparent forms, there are inapparent ones in healthy carriers capable of transmitting the disease.

CLINICAL DATA

Typical Form

In its usual form infectious mononucleosis combines an infectious syndrome, a buccopharygeal syndrome, and hypertrophy of the lymphatic organs.

The infectious syndrome usually marks the onset of the disease, either abruptly with a high fever or with a progressively febrile general malaise. *Fever* is the central element. At times it remains steady at 40° C. (104° F.), with prostration, or it oscillates irregularly, but usually it is moderate, not exceeding 38° C. (100.4° F.). It is diversely accompanied by muscular aches and pains and cephalalgia.

Asthenia is always marked. In the moderately febrile forms it is surprisingly severe. It persists throughout the course of the disease and convalescence.

The buccopharyngeal syndrome of mononucleosis includes sore throat with highly diversified and often misleading aspects. Usually the sore throat is simply erythematous or erythematopultaceous with diffuse redness of the soft palate, tumefaction of the tonsils, and dysphagia, but it sometimes appears as pseudomembranous angina with extensive and adherent pseudodiphtheric false membranes. More rarely, the sore throat is ulcerous or even necrotic. Rhinitis with a seropurulent nasal discharge often accompanies sore throat.

The adenopathies offer the best criterion for the clinical diagnosis, for they nearly always are out of proportion with the sore throat, either by their volume or by their extensiveness. Severe adenopathies during sore throat should always suggest mononucleosis.

In the cervical region, the lymph nodes are firm and slightly tender, without periadenitis. They are bilateral, most often involving the jugular and submaxillary chains and fairly often the spinal nodes. The adenopathies always involve several contiguous lymph nodes. They never become purulent. In some cases they precede and in others succeed the sore throat.

Axillary adenopathies more rarely accompany those in the cervical region. Inguinal adenopathies and deep-seated adenopathies are exceptional.

Splenomegaly is seen in about two-thirds of cases. The spleen is moderately increased in volume, with a palpable lower margin. It is slightly tender. Forms of the disease with voluminous splenomegaly are exceptional. In mononucleosis the spleen is fragile, and its rupture is a classic but rare complication of the disease (Janbon). Splenomegaly is often accompanied by mild hepatomegaly.

Associated with these major signs are less constant minor ones: *conjunctivitis,* indicating extension of the nasopharyngeal inflammation: morbilliform or rubelliform *exanthema* (Lemierre); *purpuric syndrome* with thrombocytopenia (Maupin).

In a young patient febrile sore throat associated with marked adenopathies should suggest mononucleosis and indicate making the hematological and serological tests that, if they yield positive results, confirm the diagnosis and eliminate a possible malignant hemopathy.

Atypical Forms

Although mononucleosis in its usual form seems to have a special affinity for the lymphatic system, visceral localizations are by no means rare. When such localizations predominate, they modify the clinical picture and render diagnosis difficult. Moreover, they emphasize the relationship between mononucleosis and other virus diseases with a predilection for the same viscera. Among such localizations, the first in importance are the hepatic and the neuromeningeal forms.

Hepatic Localizations. Hepatic localizations were suspected early, as Pfeiffer had already noted the increase in liver volume and Chevallier the frequency of icterus. They have since then given rise to fairly numerous statistical and physiopathological studies (Nyfeldt, Cohn, and Lidman, Cachin, and Cattan).

Forms with jaundice are seen in about 5 to 6 per cent of cases (Cachin), icterus appearing during or after the sore throat. But jaundice may sometimes be the only symptom of the disease and may simulate epidemic hepatitis. Search for a few adenopathies, the blood picture typical of mononucleosis (even though it sometimes occurs in infectious hepatitis), and especially the Paul-Bunnell heterophil reaction should lead to diagnosis of the disease.

Forms without jaundice, which are much more frequent, have been demonstrated by routine liver function tests during mononucleosis.

The flocculation reactions are often perturbed, and this disturbance accompanies an increase in serum gamma globulins. The results of the Bromsulphalein test and of the galactose tolerance test are also abnormal.

Interference with prothrombin synthesis has been evidenced by prolonged prothrombin time in Quick's test. Tests specific for cell impairment, such as transaminase determinations, often show striking but transient abnormalities.

But systematic punch biopsies, mainly, have revealed alterations, often clinically silent, in the hepatic cells: uneven vacuolation of the nucleus or of the cytoplasm; swelling of Kupffer's cells; presence of monocytoid cells in the sinusoids (Cattan). However, hepatic sequelae of these lesions appear to be rare.

Neuromeningeal Localizations. Meningeal manifestations of mononucleosis are fairly frequent. Sprunt and Evans drew attention to them. They accompany the infectious syndrome and give rise to a few minor signs of meningeal irritation that, because of their brief course, cause no worry.

But *meningeal signs* can occupy the forefront of the clinical picture and thus justify examination of the cerebrospinal fluid. The fluid is always clear and bacteriologically sterile. Albumin level is moderate-ly elevated. Sugar and chloride levels are normal. The cell count is variable, in some cases barely increased and in others greatly increased. The cytological characterization of the mononucleosis syndrome by means of these cells is impossible. The cerebrospinal fluid gives a negative result in the Paul-Bunnell test.

It should be noted that changes in the cerebrospinal fluid have been observed on systematic examination in absence of any clinical sign (Smidt and Nyfeldt).

Encephalitis, whether or not it is associated with meningeal signs, represents a rarer manifestation that does not always carry a benign prognosis. It usually causes torpor, which may progress to coma; more rarely it causes convulsive seizures. The various cases reported show a wide distribution of localizations: cortical, cerebellar, in the nuclei of the cranial nerves, and in the medulla oblongata. Death by suffocation was reported in one case by Lemierre, Morin, and Alison.

Among these highly polymorphic neurological localizations may also be mentioned ocular or facial paralysis and a Guillain-Barré syndrome (Samuels).

In every case the hematological examination and the serological tests are the means of relating these manifestations to mononucleosis.

Other Visceral Localizations. Among the less frequent localizations are *pulmonary localizations,* consisting of labile infiltrations suggesting a possible diagnosis of atypical pneumonia (MacCort) with increase in either case of the cold agglutinin titer; *cardiac localizations,* which are exceptional, with tachycardia, myocarditis, or pericarditis (Gardner); and *pancreatic, testicular,* or *gastrointestinal* localizations.

COURSE OF THE DISEASE

In its usual form, mononucleosis is a benign disease with spontaneous recovery in 10 to 20 days. However, emphasis should be laid on the severity of asthenia, which may last for several weeks and justifies a long convalescence. *Relapses* are possible. The *complications* are the result of visceral localizations. Rupture of the spleen is an exceptional accident.

The neuromeningeal forms are the only ones that can cause immediate accidents either as the result of the somatic impact of disturbances in consciousness or as the result of a bulbar accident.

THE HEMATOLOGICAL SYNDROME

The hematological syndrome of mononucleosis has successively been understood in various ways. First considered as a proliferation of abnormal monocytes by some (Sprunt and Evans) and of lymphoid cells by others (Türk), this hematological syndrome is now defined by the presence of *large hyperbasophilic cells* evidencing a particular antigenic stimulation.

These hyperbasophilic cells are not absolutely pathognomonic of infectious mononucleosis. They are also found in other types of infections, particularly virus diseases, so that the present tendency is to recognize a *mononucleosis syndrome* (Jean Bernard and Mathé), of which infectious mononucleosis is considered to be the best-characterized manifestation.

This mononucleosis syndrome includes an increase in the count both of normal monocytes and of large and small lymphocytes, and the presence of hyperbasophilic mononuclear cells. This increase in the mononuclear count results in *hyperleukocytosis,* the white blood cell level varying from 15,000 to 30,000 cells per cubic millimeter, rarely more. The other blood cell series are normal, a fact constituting a valuable diagnostic indication.

Hyperbasophilic Mononuclear Cells. Despite their polymorphism, the cells fit into the following general description.

They are fairly large, 15 to 20 μ in diameter. The nucleus is oval or kidney shaped and often adheres to the border of the cytoplasm. The aspect of the chromatin varies. In some cells it is fine and regular or even "combed," the nuclear structure hence being similar to that of a monocyte; in others it is more condensed with an incipient block formation, the nuclear structure resembling that of a lymphocyte or a plasmocyte. A few nuclear atypias with voluminous nucleoli and mitoses are occasionally noted. In practice, an experienced eye rarely mistakes such cells for leukoblasts.

The most characteristic feature of these cells, however, is their highly basophilic cytoplasm, this basophilia being evidence of their high ribonucleic acid content. Treated with Giemsa's stain, the cytoplasm is dark blue, with a lighter colored centrosomic zone. This shade is much more intense than the pale blue of the cytoplasm of large lymphocytes. It does not have the violet tinge of plasmocyte cytoplasm. The strong pyroninophilia of this cytoplasm is evidence of its high RNA content. The cytoplasm appears homogeneous or slightly irregular. It never contains granulations. It extends more or less widely around the nucleus in the larger cells or forms a ring around it in the smaller ones.

According to their morphological type, these cells have been considered differently by cytologists. In their condensed form, they correspond to Türk's irritation cells. In their more extended form some authors have called them monocytoid cells or have considered them to be plasmocytes or proplasmocytes (Misao). Others, considering that they are usually present in virus diseases, called them "virocytes" (Litwins and Leibowitz), but in view of the numerous nonvirus diseases in which they are found, this term is not now considered applicable (Jean Bernard and Mathé).

In the light of present data on the physiology of the lymphatic system, these hyperbasophilic cells appear similar to lymphoid cells that have been altered by an antigenic stimulus. These same cells appear in cultures of lymphocytes stimulated by phytohemagglutinin or by an antigen, a fact which emphasizes their probable lymphoid origin. They might also represent a plasmocyte precursor, the role of which in the genesis of serum antibodies is known, but on a morphological basis this possibility does not apply to mononucleosis cells either in the blood or in the hematopoietic system.

The proportion of these cells in the blood varies from 5 to 30 per cent.

Monocytes and Lymphocytes. The blood level of normal monocytes is above normal (10 to 20 per cent), with slightly atypical forms with a contorted or notched nucleus.

The percentage of large and small lymphocytes is also above normal.

The total of mononuclear cells in the blood represents 60 to 80 per cent of the leukocytes. This mononucleosis appears from the onset of sore throat and can persist several weeks or even two to three months after recovery. It subsequently disappears progressively.

Granulocytes. Although the percentage of polynuclear cells may seem to be subnormal, their absolute number usually remains normal.

Erythrocytes and Platelets. The count is normal in the great majority of cases. However, *hemolytic anemias* have been reported during mononucleosis (Limarzi, Berte). The reports have concerned hemolytic anemia with autoantibodies, often of the cold type (Perrier and Rousso).

Also, a few cases reported were associated with thrombocytopenic purpura (Maupin).

Myelogram. The myelogram is always normal in mononucleosis. Although a slightly elevated proportion of histiocytes or of mononuclear cells is sometimes found, the very small number of such cells and the absence of nuclear abnormalities in any event permits rejection of a diagnosis of malignant hemopathy.

Lymph Node Punch Biopsy. Smears from lymph nodes show an increase in the proportion of histiocytes and of young reticular cells and also a moderately large number of hyperbasophilic cells with the same characteristics as those of the blood. Mitoses seem to be fairly numerous; but, here as well, there is no sign of cellular anarchy.

SEROLOGY

The reaction described by Paul and Bunnell in 1932, which was soon afterward rendered more precise by Davidsohn's test, seemed destined to satisfy clinicians as to the specificity of mononucleosis. A serological proof had apparently been added to results of clinical and hematological examination and thus seemed to complete the proof of a long-suspected entity.

In fact, the want of serological proof in clinically and hematologically evident mononucleosis and the fact that the serological tests are not absolutely specific caused debate to shift to the *serologically negative forms,* in which, although they are now more clearly defined, some uncertainty remains, particularly in the forms occurring in children.

Principle of the Reaction

The *Paul-Bunnell test* reveals in the patient's serum heteroantibodies that agglutinate sheep erythrocytes at a high titer. In normal serum the titer of this antibody does not exceed 1/20; in mononucleosis it is active up to a titer of 1/600 and sometimes 1/2000 or more.

This property is not specific, however, as it is also present in Forssman's heteroantibody, a common antibody that can develop during any kind of infection or after an injection of serum.

Davidsohn's reaction defines more closely the particular nature of the heteroantibody of mononucleosis. This antibody is not absorbed by guinea pig kidney antigen as is Forssman's antibody, but is absorbed by beef erythrocyte antigen.

The Paul-Bunnell-Davidsohn reaction therefore consists in determining the rate of agglutination of sheep erythrocytes by the patient's serum at increasing dilutions, before and after incubation successively with guinea pig kidney and beef red-cell antigens.

This test, the technique of which is fairly simple, becomes positive toward the eighth to tenth day after the onset of the disease, but the increase in antibody titer is occasionally delayed; if the result is doubtful, the test should be repeated 10 to 15 days later.

The high antibody titer persists for several months after the disease and then diminishes progressively.

Value of the Paul-Bunnell-Davidsohn Test

False-positive reactions are exceptional (Demanche.) The problem of *negative reactions,* on the other hand, deserves some comment from the serological standpoint. The percentage of negative reactions in clinically and hematologically evident mononucleosis is variable, but always considerable: 17 per cent was found by Thomsen, 20 per cent by Hobson, and 30 per cent by Gardner and Paul. Comparison of the various reports brings out the following facts:

First, the Paul-Bunnell-Davidsohn test is frequently negative in blood group A patients with evident mononucleosis, so that in practice the blood group should always be specified along with the result of the Paul-Bunnell-Davidsohn test.

Second, all reports agree that the test is usually negative in children under age five years (e.g., reports of Hobson and of Vahlquist), which raises the question whether the disease in children and in adults is identical.

Third, the value of the test varies in different countries. In Japan, Misao showed that the Paul-Bunnell-Davidsohn test is positive during a rickettsial infection the causative agent of which he considers to be responsible for mononucleosis. In Europe, on the other hand, the serum of patients with mononucleosis does not contain antibodies against rickettsia (Giroud). Here again it would seem that one serological reaction brings to light the differences in etiology behind the same signs and symptoms.

MISCELLANEOUS REACTIONS

Other serum phenomena have been observed during mononucleosis. Their practical interest has not been confirmed. Antibovine hemolysins have been found (Mikkelson), as have positive Weil-Felix reactions (Misao); the titers of agglutinins against papain-treated sheep erythrocytes are inversed in regard to those observed in the Paul-Bunnell-Davidsohn test (Eyquem).

The papain-treated erythrocyte reaction has been suggested for rapid slide diagnosis of mononucleosis. Papain selectively destroys the erythrocytic receptors of sheep red cells for the antibodies of mononucleosis. Agglutination of papain-treated erythrocytes is slower than that of normal sheep erythrocytes during mononucleosis. It therefore suffices to compare on a microscope slide the agglutination of the normal and the treated erythrocytes by a drop of the patient's blood to obtain an immediate answer (Schneider).

It should be remembered that in mononucleosis certain serological reactions for syphilis may be transiently positive.

DIAGNOSIS

The problem of diagnosis of mononucleosis presents itself differently when the symptoms have motivated a hematological study or have not.

CLINICAL DIAGNOSIS

In a patient with a *febrile sore throat,* clinical judgment alone might go astray in the direction of a diagnosis of essential sore throat, seasonal infectious sore throat, Vin-

cent's angina, or even angina diphtheritica if there are adherent or extensive false membranes.

In practice, such diagnoses do not bear the scrutiny of a well thought out examination, which cannot miss the severity and the extent of the adenopathies; this element leads to hematological examination.

Infectious mononucleosis must be considered in the presence of an *acute hepatitis* appearing in a young person. The role of mononucleosis is also to be suspected during *"atypical pneumonia"* with cold agglutinins.

The possibility of the diagnosis may not come to mind at first in the presence of a *meningeal* or *encephalomeningeal syndrome,* as mononucleosis is not a frequent cause of meningitis with clear cerebrospinal fluid or of a neurological syndrome. In such cases, an initial rhinopharyngitis, adenopathies, and splenomegaly should attract attention and point to the necessity of a hematological study and then of serological tests.

HEMATOLOGICAL DIAGNOSIS

Usually, the symptoms observed lead initially to making a hematological study, and the diagnostic problem is centered on the *mononucleosis syndrome.*

The problem of a *malignant hemopathy* is appropriately recalled by the incorrect diagnosis of "acute leukemia followed by recovery" published by Türk in 1907. It is rare, however, that the circulating hyperbasophilic cells suggest, by their abundance and their dysmorphosis, a *leukoblastosis.* This diagnostic error is conceivable only in the rare forms complicated by anemia or an immunological thrombocytopenia. In case of doubt, a myelogram, which shows a normal bone marrow, ends any possible confusion. Mononucleosis is a benign disease, and the Paul-Bunnell-Davidsohn test confirms the diagnosis.

DIAGNOSIS OF SEROLOGICALLY NEGATIVE FORMS

A positive Paul-Bunnell-Davidsohn reaction leaves no doubt as to the diagnosis. Repeatedly negative reactions settle nothing, as several diseases can manifest themselves by a mononucleosis syndrome.

Acquired Toxoplasmosis. This frequent protozoan disease closely simulates infectious mononucleosis; only the serological reactions that characterize toxoplasmosis have made it possible to attribute to it numerous syndromes that were originally considered to be forms of Paul-Bunnell-negative mononucleosis (Siim, and Couvreur and Desmonts).

Acquired toxoplasmosis manifests itself by adenopathies that are predominantly cervical and spinal initially but may subsequently spread to the axillary, epitrochlear, and inguinal regions.

The infectious syndrome that may mark their appearance is usually very moderate, consisting merely of febricula and muscle pain; often it is absent. The usual absence of sore throat is a valuable sign in the differential diagnosis. Lymph node enlargement remains moderate in volume. In some cases an exanthem with pinkish maculae accompanies the syndrome of adenopathy. There is no splenomegaly.

Hematological changes are strikingly similar to those in mononucleosis, with an increase in circulating mononuclear cells and the presence of hyperbasophilic cells. However, it should be noted that leukocytosis is not as great; frequently the white blood cell count is normal. Moreover, eosinophilia of 6 to 10 per cent is usual and is of some value in orienting the diagnosis. But, as in infectious mononucleosis, histiocytes and hyperbasophilic cells are found in smears from biopsied lymph nodes and the myelogram is normal.

Diagnosis rests primarily on the determination of serum antibodies by the Sabin-Feldman toxoplasma dye test and secondarily on complement fixation. The dye test is significant only at titers of 1/1000 or more. Lower titers have been found in 85 per cent of subjects and corresponded to toxoplasma infection that had remained inapparent. In the case of doubtful results, repetition of the test with a serum sample taken two weeks after the first one confirms, by increase in the antibody titer, the diagnosis of an active present infection.

Rubella. Rubella can give rise to confusion by the sore throat, the polyadenopathies, and the blood changes that may accompany it. However, the cutaneous manifestations are usually more conspicuous than in mononucleosis, and the hematological changes consist mostly of a fairly characteristic plasmocytosis. The epidemiological context should be considered. In case of serious doubt, virological and serological investigations permit a firm diagnosis.

Rickettsioses. Differential diagnosis with rickettsial diseases rarely needs to be considered in the Occident. In Japan, however, Misao and Kobayashi described a disease which has all the characteristics of mononucleosis, including a positive Paul-Bunnell-Davidsohn test; the etiological agent is a rickettsia which they called *R. sennetsui.* This organism is pathogenic for the mouse. Retransmission from the mouse to volunteers causes a typical mononucleosis with a positive result of the Paul-Bunnell-Davidsohn test. Investigations carried out in Europe on this rickettsia failed to show any protective action for the mouse by the serum of patients with mononucleosis (Babudieri, Giroud). The European disease and the Japanese disease are therefore not identical.

Epidemic Hepatitis. The frequency of clinically evident or purely biological liver impairment in mononucleosis sometimes renders difficult the differential diagnosis of virus hepatitis when the result of the Paul-Bunnell-Davidsohn test is negative. In epidemic hepatitis a mononucleosis reaction in the blood can occur that is in all respects similar to that of mononucleosis (Havens and Marck). Adenopathies, however, are exceptional and gastrointestinal disturbances much more frequent in hepatitis.

The patient's serum often has a high sheep cell-agglutinating power; these agglutinins, however, are absorbed by human liver but not by beef red cell extract (Eaton, Murphy, and Hanford). The antibodies formed in epidemic hepatitis would therefore appear to be of a different type from those of mononucleosis. The clinical and biological convergences of the two diseases nevertheless suggest a possible relationship between the viruses that produce them.

Unresolved Problems in Paul-Bunnell-Davidsohn-Negative Mononucleosis. Whereas certain mononucleosis syndromes can thus be differentiated, mononucleoses are frequently observed that are fully characterized both clinically and hematologically and yet remain *Paul-Bunnell-Davidsohn-negative* during their whole course.

In a study carried out by Hobson, Lawson, and Wigfield on two homogeneous groups of patients (242 serologically positive and 100 serologically negative), the authors conclude that, despite the great clinical and hematological similarity between the two groups, the differences are sufficient to suggest that the etiology is different. The serologically negative forms appear to have a less seasonal epidemicity, a less severe clinical course, and less pronounced hematological signs than the serologically positive forms.

A majority of the serologically negative forms are seen in children under five years of age. These forms, which frequently are atypical as regards the degree of their nasopharyngeal signs, correspond to the "glandular fever" described by Pfeiffer. They probably include, along with true mononucleoses, closely related virus diseases that have not yet been characterized.

In adults, the problem of serologically negative forms will remain unsolved as long as the infectious agent has not been identified. Though serologically positive mononucleosis can be regarded as an autonomous disease (even though serological variations from one country to another seem to suggest the existence of particular varieties of virus), a certain number of mononucleosis syndromes probably represent only convergence of phenomena leading to a common hematological reaction.

An example is furnished by the mononucleosis syndromes observed after thoracic surgery (Bastin) that suggest, without means of differentiation or certitude, transmission of a virus by transfusion or an immunological type of mononucleosis reaction resulting from the graft of the blood donor's lymphoid cells (Scherz).

PATHOLOGY

The histological lesions produced by infectious mononucleosis in the lymph nodes, which are often biopsied, are fairly well known, as are those in the spleen, which is examined in the rare cases complicated by rupture. Punch biopsies have also helped to define more clearly the hepatic lesions. The lesions are less well known in the case of other viscera, as a fatal outcome is exceptional (Custer and Smith).

LYMPH NODES

The lesions cause a nonspecific lymphoreticular hyperplasia. Usually the appearance is that of a node under antigenic stimulation. The marginal follicles are increased in volume and have a large round clear center (secondary follicles). Newly formed follicles develop more deeply in the pulp. The clear centers are composed of large reticular cells, with a clear nucleolated nucleus. Mitoses are numerous but not anarchic. In the central pulp of the node, the number of reticular cells disseminated among the lymphocytes is increased; histiocytes are found, as are plasmocytes in fairly large number. The endothelium of the sinuses is severely tumefied.

More rarely, reticular hyperplasia is more disorderly and forms streaks which partly conceal the normal structure of the lymph node; however, visualization of the reticulin network by use of the silver technique reveals no major changes in the framework of the node, and the capsule always remains intact.

In all cases staining with methylpyronine green shows numerous cells with highly pyroninophilic cytoplasm, i.e., rich in RNA, corresponding to the hyperbasophilic cells shown by other staining techniques.

The adenopathy never progresses toward suppuration.

SPLEEN

The lymphoid follicles are moderately hyperplastic; on the other hand, proliferation in the pulp is striking. Billroth's cords are widened and contain not only lymphocytes but also reticular cells and histiocytes, many of which turn out to be hyperbasophilic mononuclear cells. The endothelial cells lining the sinuses are voluminous. The structure of the reticular network remains normal.

Several authors have described subadventitious impairment of splenic arterioles and venules with edema and infiltration by hyperbasophilic mononuclear cells causing separation of the vessels from their connective axis, which may perhaps explain their fragility and the sudden complications by hemorrhage and rupture of the spleen (Smith and Custer; Janbon, Bertrand, and Dorst).

LIVER

We have mentioned the frequency of hepatic lesions revealed by punch biopsy even in the absence of any clinical manifestation. These lesions combine an infiltration of the portal spaces and the sinuses by mononuclear cells, and more variable hepatocytic lesions: clarification, vacuolation, and mitoses. These lesions usually heal without sequela (Bennike).

OTHER VISCERA

In the forms with neurological complications infiltration by mononuclear cells of the meninges, nerve roots, and vessels has been observed, as well as diffuse hemorrhagic suffusions (Allen and Kellner). Similar lesions have been observed in the myocardium (Brien) and in the lungs (Ziegler).

ETIOLOGY: EXPERIMENTATION

Although clinical and epidemiological data and disease relationships strongly favor a viral etiology for mononucleosis, it must be admitted that no definite laboratory or experimental proof has as yet been furnished.

Among the microorganisms that were once thought to be responsible for the disease, we shall merely mention *Listeria monocytogenes*, which Nyfeldt (1929) demonstrated in the throat and blood of patients with mononucleosis and which, when inoculated into rabbits, causes leukocytosis with a relative neutropenia. But mononucleosis serums do not agglutinate listeria, and injection of listeria into man does not cause production of heterophilic antibodies (Sohier).

Attempts to inoculate the disease in monkeys and in man, though not entirely conclusive, have supplied the most instructive information regarding the etiology of the disease.

In 1939 van de Berghe and Liessens inoculated a *Macaca rhesus* monkey with blood taken from a patient on the fifth day of a typical mononucleosis. Three weeks later the animal presented monocytosis with production of heterophilic antibodies. After filtration through a Seitz filter, the animal's serum produced the same monocytic reaction when inoculated into another animal. The virus, when maintained on tissue culture and inoculated into the monkey, reproduces a monocytic leukocytosis; but the serological reactions are not constant. Attempts at inoculation of mice have remained unsuccessful.

In 1940, by inoculation of the rhesus monkey with the blood of a serologically positive patient, Sohier, Lépine, and Sautter also produced monocytosis with minimal fever but without production of heterophilic antibodies. Blood obtained from the monkeys ten days later was injected into a young demented patient who showed no evident clinical signs but in whom the Paul-Bunnell-Davidsohn reaction became positive 16 days later.

In 1939 Wising inoculated two rhesus monkeys intraperitoneally and subcutaneously with a suspension of fresh glandular extract from a patient. On the fifteenth day the animals presented adenopathies, mononucleosis, and fever. Five successive passages were successfully accomplished by means of lymph nodes from the animals. In 1942 Wising injected into six volunteers a suspension of glandular extract from six patients with mononucleosis. No clinical or hematological changes were produced in any of the receivers. On the other hand, when he transfused the blood of patients to five other volunteers, after an incubation period of 20 days he obtained in one of them a clinical and hematological picture typical of mononucleosis, but the Paul-Bunnell-Davidsohn test result remained doubtful.

If these experiments as a whole furnished a few positive facts, others, in contrast, had negative results. Thus, in 1942 Bang inoculated monkeys with blood, lymph node homogenates, or throat washings from patients with mononucleosis without obtaining any result. Similarly, Evans inoculated 17 volunteers with blood or lymph node extracts without producing any clinical, hematological, or serological manifestation.

Among these attempts, mention should be made of a curious observation by Taylor, who noted an intercurrent infectious mononucleosis in a patient with acute leukemia. Injection of the patient's blood into five other leukemic patients resulted each time in remission of the leukemia and appearance of heterophilic antibodies. However, the monocytic type of the acute leukoses concerned lessens the value of this observation.

After these experiments and their fragmentary results, the announcement by the Japanese authors Misao and Kobayashi in 1953 of the discovery of a rickettsia that might be responsible for mononucleosis inspired fresh investigations. In a very thorough experimental study these authors isolated from the blood, bone marrow, and lymph nodes of patients with mononucleosis a large virus which they considered to be related to the genus Rickettsia and which they called *R. sennetsui*. The organism is pathogenic for the mouse, in which it causes adenopathies and splenomegaly. The animals die within 10 to 20 days after inoculation. The organism can be grown in tissue culture and in the embryonic sac of the chick embryo. Under the microscope it appears as intracellular and extracellular round or oval granulations 200 to 400 mμ in diameter. The nuclei and cytoplasm of the carrier cells are often vacuolated. Inoculation of this material into 11 volunteers produced a typical mononucleosis, but it does not seem that the serological change was observed in all cases.

These experiments were repeated in Europe by Babudieri, who obtained, by inoculating monkeys with *R. sennetsui*, a fairly characteristic mononucleosis with a weakly positive Paul-Bunnell-Davidsohn reaction. The serological reactions produced by *R. sennetsui*, however, appear to be different from those in European mononucleosis. In the latter the patients' serum does not neutralize a suspension of these rickettsia, and serological cross reactions with Proteus OX-K or with psittacosis virus have shown affinities different from those observed by the Japanese authors.

All these data seem to prove that if, in Japan, *R. sennetsui* is in fact responsible for a certain type of infectious mononucleosis, this agent is not responsible in Europe.

The difficulties, the failures and also the mistakes we have mentioned explain that the conclusions drawn by Henle and his associates from their remarkable research work are greeted with a certain reserve.

This research team,[16a, 21a] by use of immunofluorescence tests and the electron microscope, revealed a virus in the leukocytes of patients with biologically and clinically characteristic infectious mononucleosis. This virus is an EB virus, i.e., a herpes-type virus named for the cell line in which it was first detected: this cell line was established by Epstein and Barr from a Burkitt lymphosarcoma and bears their initials.

Henle and his associates reexamined the serums systematically collected from 1958 to 1962 from college freshmen by Niederman et al.[34a] in view of an epidemiological study of infectious mononucleosis.

In each of the 29 patients who had the disease during the investigation, the development of antibodies against EB virus was demonstrated. These antibodies, absent from pre-illness serum specimens, usually appeared early in the disease, rose to peak levels within a few weeks, and remained at relatively high levels during convalescence. They appeared to be clearly distinct from heterophilic antibodies and, unlike them, were reported to persist for years, probably for life. Tests on serums from 50 randomly selected college freshmen revealed EB virus antibodies in 12, two of whom had a history of clinical infectious mononucleosis. Of 38 without demonstrable antibodies, none had had infectious mononucleosis, but the illness developed in three of these subjects within the next two years.

These two series of facts represent strong arguments in favor of the role of the EB virus (or of a virus antigenically closely related to it) in the etiology of infectious mononucleosis as it appears typically in adolescents and young adults. However, the role of a single virus in both mononucleosis and Burkitt's sarcoma casts a doubt on the specific pathogenicity of the virus.

TREATMENT

The course of mononucleosis is generally benign, and recovery occurs spontaneously in 8 to 15 days in most cases. Hence many authors advise refraining from therapeutic attempt and merely applying simple measures of nasopharyngeal hygiene. Frequent gargling, or irrigation of the throat if sore throat is extensive, suffices to prevent local superinfections and to relieve respiratory discomfort and dysphagia.

Nevertheless, even in the mild forms convalescence is long, and it is nearly always necessary to prescribe four to six weeks' convalescence after the acute stage of the disease. The hematological changes persist several weeks, and at times several months, after clinical recovery, and normal equilibrium in the differential leukocyte count returns very slowly.

In the more severe forms *corticosteroid therapy,* recommended by Janbon and Bertrand in 1953, produces striking results.

Such therapy should be reserved for forms presenting impairment of general physical condition, high fever, and stuporous prostration; for forms with large and extensive adenopathies; and for forms with hepatic and meningeal complications. It is also indicated in relapses, which are not rare.

Deltacortisone (prednisone) is prescribed at an oral dosage of 15 to 20 mg. daily for a fairly short course of 8 to 12 days. Action on fever is extremely rapid, and temperature returns to normal within 48 hours. The stuporous prostration of severe forms disappears. Sore throat diminishes in two or three days, and adenopathies in three to five days. Convalescence is clearly shortened, and the usual asthenia is absent. The effect on the differential blood count is more difficult to evaluate. Leukocytosis, when present, seems to diminish under the effect of the treatment; monocytosis, on the other hand, persists. The result of the Paul-Bunnell-Davidsohn test is not influenced.

Association of corticosteroids with antibiotics is indicated if the sore throat is severe or if there is superinfection, but corticosteroid therapy alone is usually adequate to cause regression of these symptoms and, according to certain authors, its indications are therefore fairly broad, provided the treatment is not prolonged.

BIBLIOGRAPHY

1. Allen, F. H., Jr., and Kellner, A.: Infectious mononucleosis; autopsy report. Amer. J. Path., 23:463, 1947.
2. Babudieri, B.: Rapports sérologiques entre Rickettsia sennetsui de Misao et l'agent étiologique de la mononucléose infectieuse européenne. Nouv. Rev. Franç. Hémat., 1:337, 1961.
3. Bang, J.: Experiments with the transfer of infectious mononucleosis to monkeys with negative results. Acta Med. Scand., 111:291, 1942.
4. Bastin, R., Lapresle, C., and Dufrène, F.: Syndrome fébrile avec réaction sanguine mononucléosique après chirurgie thoracique. Presse Méd., 73:63, 1965.
5. Bennike: Les atteintes hépatiques dans la mononucléose. Thesis. Copenhagen, 1959.
6. Bernard, J., and Mathé, G.: Un usurpateur, le virocyte. Rev. Franç. Etud. Clin. Biol., 2:115, 1957.
7. Berte, S. J.: Acute hemolytic anemia in infectious mononucleosis. New York J. Med., 51:781, 1951.
8. Cachin, M.: Les manifestations hépatiques de la mononucléose infectieuse. Sem. Hôp. Paris, 25:861, 1949.
9. Cattan, R., Rey, M., and Maghsondnia, H.: Mononucléose infectieuse ictérigène. Renseignements fournis par la biologie et la ponction-biopsie. Nouv. Rev. Franç. Hémat., 1:329, 1961.
10. Chany, C.: Revue critique de l'étude expérimentale de la mononucléose infectieuse. Nouv. Rev. Franç. Hémat., 1:309, 1961.
11. Chevallier, P.: L'adéno-lymphoïdite aiguë bénigne avec hyperleucocytose modérée et forte mononucléose. Rev. Path. Comp., 28:835, 1928.
12. Cohn, C., and Lidman, B.: Hepatitis without jaundice in infectious mononucleosis. J. Clin. Invest., 25:145, 1946.
13. Couvreur, J., and Desmonts, G.: Toxoplasmose acquise et mononucléose infectieuse. Diagnostic différentiel et fréquence respective. Nouv. Rev. Franç. Hémat., 1:345, 1961.
14. Custer, R., and Smith, E.: Pathology of infectious mononucleosis. Blood, 3:830, 1948.
15. Davidsohn, I.: Serologic diagnosis of infectious mononucleosis. J.A.M.A., 108:289, 1937.
16. Demanche, R.: Le diagnostic de la mononucléose infectieuse. Valeur des réactions sérologiques. Presse Méd., 57:1614, 1939.
16a. Diehl, V., Henle, G., Henle, W., and Kohn, G.: Demonstration of a herpes group virus in cultures of peripheral leukocytes from patients with infectious mononucleosis. J. Virol., 2:663-669, 1968.
17. Eaton, M. D., Murphy, W. D., and Hanford, V. L.: Heterogenetic antibodies in acute hepatitis. J. Exp. Med., 79:539, 1944.
18. Eyquem, A.: Sérologie de la mononucléose infectieuse. Nouv. Rev. Franç. Hémat., 1:312, 1961.
19. Gardner, H. T., and Paul, J. R.: Infectious mononucleosis at New Haven Hospital, 1921-1946. Yale J. Biol. Med., 19:839, 1947.
20. Giroud, P., Capponi, M., and Dumas, N.: Rapports de la mononucléose infectieuse et des rickettsioses. Nouv. Rev. Franç. Hémat., 1:340, 1961.
21. Havens, W. P., Jr., and Marck, R. E.: Leukocytic response of patients with experimentally induced infectious hepatitis. Amer. J. Med. Sci., 212:129, 1946.
21a. Henle, G., Henle, W., and Diehl, V.: Relation of Burkitt tumor associated herpes-type virus to infectious mononucleosis. Proc. Nat. Acad. Sci. U.S.A., 59:94-101, 1968.
22. Hobson, F. G., Lawson, B., and Wigfield, M.: Glandular fever: a field study. Brit. Med. J., 1:845, 1958.
23. Janbon, M., and Bertrand, L.: Mononucléose infectieuse et cortisone. Sang, 24:378, 1953.
24. Janbon, M., Bertrand, L., and Dorst, V.: Un accident trop peu connu de la mononucléose infectieuse: la rupture de rate. Presse Méd., 68:1003, 1960.
25. Kissel, P., Arnould, G., and Leval, P.: Les formes nerveuses de la mononucléose infectieuse. Sem. Hôp. Paris, 28:387, 1952.
26. Lemierre, A., Morin, M., and Alison, M.: Graves accidents de suffocation dans deux cas de mononucléose. Bull. Mém. Soc. Méd. Hôp. Paris, 64:61, 1948.
27. Lépine, P.: Epidémiologie de la mononucléose infectieuse. Nouv. Rev. Franç., Hémat., 1:305, 1961.
28. Limarzi, L. R., Paul, J. T., and Poncher, H. G.: Blood and bone marrow in infectious mononucleosis. J. Lab. Clin. Med., 31:1079, 1946.

29. Litwins, J., and Leibowitz, S.: Abnormal lymphocytes ("virocytes") in virus diseases other than infectious mononucleosis. Acta Haemat., *5*:223, 1951.

30. MacCort, J. J.: Infectious mononucleosis with special reference to roentgenologic manifestations. Amer. J. Roentgen., *62*:645, 1949.

31. Mathé, G.: Le syndrome mononucléosique. Vie Méd., *38*:35, 1957.

32. Maupin, B., and Monteil, R.: Les plaquettes dans la mononucléose infectieuse. Nouv. Rev. Franç., Hémat., *1*:333, 1961.

33. Mikkelsen, W., Tupper, C., and Murray, J.: The ox cell hemolysin test as a diagnostic procedure in infectious mononucleosis. J. Lab. Clin. Med., *52*:648, 1958.

34. Misao, T., Kobayashi, Y., and Shirakawa, M.: La mononucléose infectieuse (fièvre ganglionnaire). Sang, *28*:785, 1957.

34a. Niederman, J. C., McCollum, R. W., Henle, G., and Henle, W.: Infectious mononucleosis. Clinical manifestations in relation to EB virus antibodies. J.A.M.A., *203*:205-209, 1968.

35. Nyfeldt, A.: Recherches expérimentales et cliniques sur la mononucléose infectieuse. Folia Haemat., *47*:144, 1932.

36. Paul, J., and Bunnell, W.: The presence of heterophil antibodies in infectious mononucleosis. Amer. J. Med. Sci., *183*:90, 1932.

37. Perrier, C. V., and Rousso, C.: Un cas de mononucléose avec anémie hémolytique et test de Coombs positif. Schweiz. Med. Wschr., *89*:766. 1959.

38. Pfeiffer, E.: Fièvre ganglionnaire. Jahrb. Kinderh., *29*:257, 1889.

39. Rugg-Gunn, M.: Infectious mononucleosis. A review of the condition as seen in the Royal Navy. Proc. Roy. Soc. Med., *47*:759, 1954.

40. Samuels, M.: Infectious mononucleosis complicated by Landry's paralysis, necessitating recourse to the artificial lung. Calif. Med., *86*:271, 1957.

41. Scherz, R., and Montgomery, R.: Survival of transfused donor mononuclear leukocytes during open heart surgery. New Eng. J. Med., *269*:1236, 1963.

42. Schmidt, V., and Nyfeldt, A.: Ueber Mononucleosis infectiosa und Meningoencephalitis. Acta Oto-laryng. 26:680, 1938.

43. Schneider, M.: Diagnostic sérologique sur lame de la mononucléose infectieuse. Rev. Franç. Etud. Clin. Biol., *10*:759, 1965.

44. Siim, J.: Clinical and diagnostic aspects of human acquired toxoplasmosis. In: Human Toxoplasmosis. Copenhagen, Munksgaard, 1960.

45. Smith, E., and Custer, R.: Rupture of spleen in infectious mononucleosis; clinico-pathological report of 7 cases. Blood, *1*:317, 1946.

46. Sohier, R., Lépine, P., and Sautter, V.: Recherches sur la transmission expérimentale de la mononucléose infectieuse au singe et à l'homme. Ann. Inst. Pasteur, *65*:50, 1940.

47. Sprunt, T., and Evans, R.: Reactionary mononuclear leukocytosis in acute infections (infectious mononucleosis). Bull. Johns Hopkins Hosp., *31*:410, 1920.

48. Taylor, A.: Effects of glandular fever infection in acute leukemia. Brit. Med. J., *1*:63, 1953.

49. Thomsen, S.: Etude sur la mononucléose infectieuse basée sur 549 cas. Copenhagen, Munksgaard, 1942.

50. Türk: Septische Erkrankungen bei Verkummerung des granulozyten System. Wien. Klin. Wschr. *20*:6, 1907.

51. Vahlquist, B., Ekelund, H., and Iveteras, E.: Mononucléose infectieuse et pseudomononucléose infectieuse chez l'enfant. Méd. Hyg., p. 499, 1958.

52. Van den Berghe, L., and Liessens, P.: Transmission de la mononucléose humaine au Macacus rhesus. Résistance du virus aux basses températures. C. R. Soc. Biol., *132*:90, 1939.

53. Wising, P.: Some experiments with lymph gland material from cases of infectious mononucleosis. Acta Med. Scand., *98*:328, 1939.

54. Ziegler, E.: Infectious mononucleosis: report of a fatal case with autopsy. Arch. Path., *37*:196, 1944.

51

Cat-Scratch Disease

By J. C. JOB

In 1950, under the name of "maladie des griffes de chat," Robert Debré and his associates described an infectious adenitis of a particular type; over a period of more than 20 years they had observed some ten cases.[11] They had succeeded in differentiating this disease entity on the basis of clinical data, from tuberculous adenitis, sodoku adenitis, tularemia, and lymphogranuloma venereum and from various other disorders with lymph node localizations. In 1947 they had occasion to compare their observations with those of Lee Foshay, who gave them the antigen with which he was obtaining a specific intradermal reaction in patients with a comparable disorder. The same results were obtained in France with Foshay's antigen and with an antigen prepared in Paris, a fact that made it possible to confer on the disease its biological individuality. The disease is the same as that called "benign inoculation lymphoreticulosis" by Mollaret et al.[28]

Since these initial descriptions, the disease has proved to be fairly frequent, and the occurrence of various visceral manifestations has been described. Although the infectious nature of this type of adenitis appears to be certain and its viral origin highly probable, the agent has not been isolated.

CLINICAL FEATURES

COMMON FORM[12]

The common form of the disease associates the local adenitis that is the principal manifestation of the disease with a discrete and inconstant *lesion of cutaneous inoculation* and an infectious syndrome on occasion.

The incubation period is not always easy to determine precisely. It is clear when, at a known date, the subject was, for example, clawed by a cat, if the interval between the initial lesion and the appearance of adenitis can be determined. Daniels believes that the initial lesion can appear three to 14 days after the contamination. The adenitis appears two to six weeks after this lesion. In certain cases adenitis appears more rapidly (in a week) or more slowly (in one or even two months). As a general rule, the incubation period before appearance of the adenitis averages three weeks.

The primary lesion, or cutaneous inoculation lesion, is visible in a little less than half of the cases and may easily pass unrecognized: it is a tiny inconspicuous macula or pink papule, from 2 to 10 mm. in diameter, occasionally situated on the line made by the claw stroke. A vesicle, an ulceration, or a tiny crust may form at its center. This lesion is ordinarily unique; exceptionally several such lesions have been found. The site is usually the hand, the forearm, the face, the neck, or, in short, the uncovered areas that can be clawed. In connection with the clinical forms, we shall call attention to the cases in which the site of the primary lesion was an exceptional cutaneous area or the mucosa. The primary lesion usually persists until the adenitis is constituted and then disappears. The intradermal injection of the specific antigen occasionally provokes a focal reaction at the site of the initial inoculation lesion, which then reappears when it was on the way toward disappearance.

The adenitis, on the other hand, is constant and may comprise the whole disease. It is regional and occasionally involves a main lymph node with two or three smaller ones. Its localization is axillary in nearly half of the cases, the hand being by far the most frequent site of inoculation. A little less often it is cervical and more rarely inguinal, epitrochlear, pretragal, or occipital. A level-to-level type of adenitis is not rare: epitrochlear and axillary, or submaxillary and carotid, or inguinal and retrocrural, for example. The lymph nodes in the area close to the primary lesion are sometimes less inflamed than those more distant (subclavicular, for example). Apart from this possibility, the adenitis rarely concerns several lymphatic areas. It is never bilateral.

In general, the adenitis is discreetly inflammatory: it is usually indolent or nearly painless. The volume of the inflamed lymph nodes varies from that of a cherry to that of an orange, small lymph nodes surrounding the most voluminous one. The lymph nodes involved are firm, the adenitis evolves slowly toward resorption in a few weeks or, in about half of the cases, becomes surrounded by periadenitis and finally suppurates. In exceptional cases, the adenitis drags on[12] or else recurs.[40]

Signs of infection vary greatly. In nearly a third of cases they are absent. Usually development of the adenitis is accompanied by moderate pyrexia, asthenia, and weight loss for one or two weeks. High or prolonged fever, even chills, and a significant deterioration of general physical condition are less frequent. There is no parallel between the volume of the adenitis and the degree of deterioration of general physical condition. Occasionally, intradermal injection of the specific antigen provokes a febrile general reaction.

The *course* of this common form of the disease is benign. The cutaneous inoculation lesion fades away, leaving a cicatricial macula for a few days. In half the cases the adenitis regresses spontaneously without suppuration. In the other half, the involved lymph nodes suppurate and fistulas form through the thinned-away violaceous skin; thick, viscous, yellowish pus issues from the aperture. With its thin edges and irregular opening, the fistula resembles that in tuberculous adenitis, but it heals rapidly and completely in a few weeks and leaves no durable scar. The lymph node suppuration may occasionally become encysted and the enlargement of the node may persist for months without evolving further, until puncture or incision liberates the pus and permits healing. The fever and other systemic signs ordinarily persist one to three weeks. More prolonged forms are exceptional.

OTHER CLINICAL ASPECTS

Highly diverse clinical manifestations have been proved to be connected with cat-scratch disease insofar as they appear at the same time as a typical adenitis or during its abatement in patients with a clearly positive intradermal reaction to the specific antigen and in the absence of any detectable coincidental cause. The knowledge of inoculation by a cat scratch or a history of contact with a cat is, moreover, an important aid in diagnosis.

Rash. *Maculopapular and maculovesicular eruptions* are the least infrequent: generalized or localized, they appear at the initial stage of adenitis and disappear within a few hours or days, but they can recur. *Erythema nodosum* is still less frequent but is typical because of its site and the bruise-like appearance of the nodular elements.[12, 21, 25] It may be accompanied by fever and arthralgia and even by splenomegaly.

Pharyngeal Forms. In a few rare cases the disease initially appears under the guise of an acute febrile sore throat, which is secondarily complicated by foci of suppurating cervical adenitis or by a lateral pharyngeal abscess. Only a positive specific intradermal reaction and negative results of bacteriological investigation permit the diagnosis of cat-scratch disease in such cases. The same reservations apply to the buccal form, in which the clinician detects an initial lesion in the form of a small indurated ulceration in the mouth.

Ocular Forms. Inoculation of the disease at the eyelid level causes a localized blepharitis and may be accompanied by a pretragal adenitis. Conjunctival inoculation, doubtless more frequent, produces a unilateral follicular or phyctenular conjunctivitis accompanied by pretragal adenitis or adenitis at the submaxillary angle. Cat-scratch disease can thus give rise to Parinaud's syndrome.

Thoracic Forms. Mediastinal adenopathies, isolated or associated with axillary adenitis, and "atypical pneumonia" with a subacute course have been justifiably attributed to cat-scratch disease[12, 25, 26, 35, 39] because of tests clearly positive for this disease and the negative results of all the other investigations.

Abdominal Forms. An attack of pain with defensive contraction or tumefaction of the iliac fossa suggesting appendicitis has led to the operative discovery of inflammatory mesenteric adenopathies. The involved lymph nodes had the histological structure seen in cat-scratch disease, and the diagnosis was later confirmed by the results of the usual biological tests. As a general rule, mesenteric adenitis results from a pasteurella infection, and the physician must be very circumspect before he asserts a diagnosis of cat-scratch disease under such circumstances.

Neuromeningeal Forms. The neuromeningeal manifestations of cat-scratch disease are the only serious accidents observed in the course of this disease. Their frequency is not negligible; at least 20 cases are known.[5, 9, 12, 22, 33, 37, 38, 43] In some cases they are contemporaneous with the adenitis; in others they commence several days or weeks after the lymph node involvement. The initial picture is that of ordinary, more or less febrile cat-scratch disease. No promoting factor and no prodrome has been detected.

Most frequent is encephalitis, with somnolence or coma; focal or generalized convulsions may occur and sometimes assume the aspect of status epilepticus. Signs of focal involvement, such as hemiplegia, localized paresis, deviation of the head and of the eyes, and athetoid movements, are usually noted. The electroencephalogram shows severe changes: ample, generalized slow waves. The cerebrospinal fluid may be normal or shows a cellular reaction with predominance of lymphocytes and moderate increase in albumin level. Despite the gravity of this picture, the course is usually benign, with disappearance of most signs and symptoms in a few days or weeks and return to normal of the electroencephalogram in a few months.

We reported the case of a small boy with suspected cat-scratch disease who died in coma. We were unable to prove the etiology, nor was it proved in the few other reported cases with a fatal outcome. Hence the prognosis can be considered to be favorable.

In general the disease lasts three to six weeks; occasionally it drags out for several months or even a year or two, and this exceptionally prolonged course constitutes an evident difficulty in diagnosis.

Other accidents have been observed: encephalomyelitis, neuritis, and perhaps meningitis with clear cerebrospinal fluid.[12]

The association of peripheral adenitis with neuromeningeal accidents constitutes an indispensable diagnostic criterion; the positivity of the specific intradermal reaction and the negativity of the results of other biological investigations are necessary criteria but not at all sufficient in themselves.

Other Associated Disorders. Thrombocytopenic purpura[2, 3, 19] thyroiditis[14, 36] and alterations of bone suggesting osteitis[1, 8] have been reported in subjects with cat-scratch disease. Although these phenomena appeared with the adenitis and disappeared with it, that they were due to cat-scratch disease is uncertain.

Inapparent Forms. The existence of such forms is highly probable, for certain subjects in frequent contact with cats have a positive intradermal reaction without ever having presented adenitis.[12, 16, 24] Before asserting the diagnosis of cat-scratch disease in a case of adenitis, the physician should remember this possibility and the fact that the patient might have had an antecedent positive reaction.

THE PATHOGENIC AGENT

The *infectious character* of cat-scratch disease seems certain in view of its clinical and histological features and of its mode of transmission. The absence of visible microorganisms in the pus, the sterility of cultures in a great variety of bacteriological media, the negative results of inoculations into the usual species of laboratory animals are all demonstrated.[12] It is hence likely that the pathogenic agent is a virus or a mycoplasma.

The pathogenic agent of cat-scratch disease has not been isolated. In collaboration with Costil and Gerbeaux, then with Boué, we made numerous unsuccessful attempts to inoculate the disease into animals by the subcutaneous, intradermal, corneal, or intracerebral route. We have used the adult, and the newborn mouse, the cortisone-treated mouse, the rabbit, guinea pig and hamster, the monkey (*Aethiops sabaeus*), the ferret, the cat, and the dog. We have attempted dozens of times to inoculate the agent into the yolk sac of the embryonated egg, and as many times to grow it in cell cultures (fibroblasts, HeLa cells, human cancerous cells). These trials utilized material from lymph node samples (pus or ground lymph nodes sampled at different stages of the disease) but also samples from the claws of cats in which the disease had been inoculated and their saliva. All these attempts were fruitless or provoked nonspecific lesions that were not serially transmissible.

Mollaret, Reilly, Bastin, and Tournier[29, 30] published in 1950 and 1951 three observations that led them to relate the pathogenic agent of cat-scratch disease to the Miyagawanella group. They found, first, a common serological reaction between cat-scratch disease and lymphogranuloma venereum; second, in the reticular cells of the involved lymph nodes, basophilic granulations stainable by Giemsa's technique; and, third, in two *Aethiops sabaeus* monkeys a disease comparable to that in man and, in another *Aethiops sabaeus,* a positive specific intradermal reaction.

We have not been able to reproduce the transmission by inoculation that these authors achieved, and the corpuscles they saw have not been found either by other investigators[10, 17, 44] or by ourselves.[12] In a later work Mollaret et al.[31] reported that inoculation of the disease into the monkey had succeeded in seven of 22 animals and that passage from monkey to monkey had proved possible in two animals. The more thorough present knowledge of mycoplasma should lead to new research.

Dodd et al.[15, 41] reported a hemagglutination reaction of rabbit red cells, by pus diluted to 1/256, in cat-scratch disease. This reaction is inhibited by the serum of certain patients up to a dilution of 1/64 and seems to be specific. The hemagglutinating agent appeared to be a virus, antigenically related to the herpes virus but not transmissible to tissue cultures, the rabbit cornea, or the embryonated egg.*

LABORATORY DIAGNOSIS

However typical an adenitis due to cat-scratch disease may be as regards its clinical characteristics and the conditions in which it appeared, the etiology can be identified with certitude only by the result of the specific intradermal reaction and should also be confirmed by histological examination in every case possible. The results of other tests authorize only presumptions.

INTRADERMAL REACTION WITH THE SPECIFIC ANTIGEN[11, 12, 24, 42]

This reaction was worked out by Lee Foshay and further perfected by Robert Debré and his associates. The antigen is a 1/10 dilution of aspirated lymph node pus that has been tyndallized, to which penicillin has been added, and which has been kept under refrigeration; its sterility must have been verified. The technique of the reaction comprises the strictly intradermal injection of 0.10 ml. of antigen into the arm or forearm. The reaction is read four days later.

The reaction is positive when the injection produces a rose-colored, well delimited, raised and indurated papule, with a minimum diameter of 6 mm. but a maximum diameter that may exceed 10 mm.; this papule is occasionally surrounded by a pink areola or may show a small blister at its center. Ordinarily the papule persists three or four days, but if the reaction is strong it may persist as long as two weeks.

A transitory focal reaction may occur, i.e., reactivation of the cutaneous inoculation lesion and increase in volume of the adenitis. A systemic febrile reaction occasionally accompanies the intradermal reaction.

The reaction seems to be highly specific. It is generally negative in control subjects. Positive reactions have been noted with a certain frequency in healthy subjects only when they have been in habitual contact with cats.

The specificity of the intradermal reaction seems to be further confirmed not only by our experience and that of numerous other authors, but by a statistical study by Kalter. Among 250 intradermal tests made in cases of suspected cat-scratch disease, Kalter obtained 210 positive reactions, 15 doubtful ones, and 25 negative reactions. Among the 25 negative reactions, 18 in fact corresponded to bacterial adenitis and seven to cancer. Among the 210 subjects with a positive reaction, 205 had been scratched by cats or were in intimate contact with cats; only five had had no contact with cats.

The cutaneous allergy to the specific antigen usually appears from the onset of the adenitis but may appear two or three weeks later. It may not be demonstrated by one antigen and be positive with a preparation from a different lot; this discordance perhaps results from antigenic plurality.

Specific cutaneous allergy may last more than five years[12] and even last as long as 28 years.[34] Hence arises the need for prudence in the interpretation of the association of atypical pathological manifestations with a positive intradermal reaction that may simply evidence a former cat-scratch disease. Inversely, the intradermal reaction can rectify retrospectively the diagnosis of a healed adenitis.

The diversity of patients' responses to the different samples of pus utilized by Mollaret et al.[32] in the intradermal reaction led these authors to distinguish different antigenic types and hence to subdivide the disease; they further isolated an autonomous entity called regional subacute lymphoplasmodial adenopathy (previously called Type B in their classification).

---

*Other pathogenic agents have been isolated from lymph node material in adenitis similar to that in cat-scratch disease, but the diagnosis had not been firmly established. An agent belonging to the Chlamydiaceae[7] was thus isolated. A photochromogenic mycobacterium has been incriminated[4] on highly criticizable bases.[6, 13] These data should not be taken into account.

COMPLEMENT-FIXATION REACTION

This test was performed by Mollaret et al.[29] with the antigen obtained from the lymphogranuloma venereum agent cultured on the yolk membrane of the incubated embryonated egg; they used the technique ordinarily applied in diagnosis of lymphogranuloma venereum. The reaction is positive in less than half of cases of cat-scratch disease.[20] Its level exceeds 1/10 only when the adenitis has suppurated. The reaction is late appearing (six weeks after onset of the adenitis) and it occurs during a rather short period.

BLOOD TESTS

The changes in white cell count are slight. Initial leukopenia, followed by a lymphocytic reaction and then by polynuclear leukocytosis contemporaneous with the suppuration has been reported. Sedimentation rate may be slightly accelerated, with an hourly index below 50. In other cases the blood count and the differential white cell count are normal.

LYMPH NODE PUNCTURE

Lymph node puncture is worthwhile whatever may be the clinical characteristics of the adenitis. When pus is obtained, it is greenish yellow, of even density, and highly viscous; it contains moderately altered polymorphonuclear leukocytes. The absence of visible microorganisms after use of various staining techniques, the sterility of cultures on the different media utilized in bacteriology and mycology, the failure of attempts to inoculate guinea pigs and mice all represent important elements confirming the diagnosis.

When puncture does not show pus, a smear made with a droplet of lymph node fluid occasionally presents an aspect of simple lymphatic hyperplasia. More often, however, the picture is polymorphous with predominance of lymphocytes, large clear mononuclear cells, and even giant multinuclear cells similar to the Langhans cell. The cell picture yielded by lymph node puncture is hence that of a nonspecific subacute or granulomatous inflammation.

LYMPH NODE BIOPSY[12, 17]

Biopsy is justified when the diagnosis is uncertain. It shows that several lymph nodes are involved, with periadenitis; they contain more or less extensive areas of suppuration.

The histological structure of the involved lymph nodes is always fundamentally modified. Lesions of several types usually coexist in the same lymph node and represent several successive stages of the same disease process.

At the *initial stage* biopsy may show hyperplasia of the reticulum in the form of plaques of large, rounded or polygonal cells, with clear protoplasm and large, pale, irregular nuclei. Around these cells are lymphocytes and plasmocytes, and rare polymorphonuclear leukocytes. The capillary endothelium is tumefied.

At the *next stage* granulomatous foci appear. They are arranged in concentric zones: a lymphocytic crown, then a band of epithelioid cells with a few giant cells, and, in the center, a zone of acidophilic necrosis. This aspect is the most characteristic.

The *final stage* is represented by confluence of the foci of necrosis, which become purulent. Their suppuration tends to overflow the lymph node capsule and to invade the surrounding tissue. The absence of fibrin has been demonstrated.

EPIDEMIOLOGY

The *frequency* of cat-scratch disease is not negligible, although it is difficult to ascertain and doubtless varies at different periods. Since the first descriptions in France in 1945, the use of the specific intradermal reaction has made it possible to detect numerous cases. The disease has been found the world over, always with identical characteristics.

The *age* of patients is highly variable. Receptivity to the disease probably does not vary either with age or with sex. The fact that children seem to be more often concerned than adults, and women more than men, probably stems simply from the fact that they play with cats more often.

The disease is perhaps more frequent during certain *seasons:* autumn and winter.[42]

The existence of familial *epidemics* is well known. At the origin of most of these epidemics is the family cat, coddled and petted by every one.[12, 42] It is striking that the pet cat contaminates all the members of the family almost simultaneously, as though it could transmit the agent during only a limited time.

The possibility of an *endemic focus* has been reported,[12] with multiple cases separated in time and lacking any direct connection between them but grouped in a limited urban area.

The *vector and inoculator role of the cat* is certain.[10, 12, 20] A study of 390 cases[12] revealed, in 83 per cent, recent and usually repeated contacts with one or several cats. The fact was known with certainty, or the trace of an inoculation by cat scratch existed in 54 per cent of cases, and a cat bite was ascertained in 6 per cent. Even higher proportions were found in other series of cases.[10, 20]

There are, however, authentic cases in which no contact with a cat could be discovered. It does not seem that contact with other animals can be incriminated. However, the inoculation lesion can result from cutaneous erosions by the thorns of plants (6 per cent of cases), by fragments of wood, metal, or bone (5 per cent of cases), or from insect bite (2 per cent of cases). In 27 per cent of cases the mode of inoculation has been impossible to ascertain.

These facts suggest that the pathogenic agent of the disease, even though it is usually transported by cats, exists elsewhere in nature. The cat can be supposed to be its principal vector but not the true reservoir. This hypothesis has not, however, been demonstrated. Examination of cats recognized as the inoculators of the disease has never revealed significant pathological data. Nor has research in birds and Muridae, the main prey of cats, been more rewarding.

Search for a virus on the claws or hair of inoculator cats or in their saliva, by means of inoculation into the monkey *Aethiops sabaeus* has yielded negative results.[12] The healthy cat is hence the usual transmitter of the disease. The pathogenic agent usually penetrates by effraction (a scratch or bite), or occasionally perhaps by contamination by infectious hair (in the thoracic and pharyngeal forms). In a case of inguinal adenitis (pseudovenereal form) reported in a couple, venereal contamination of one member was incriminated but was not demonstrated.

DIFFERENTIAL DIAGNOSIS

COMMON FORMS

The diagnosis of cat-scratch disease should be considered in the presence of a subacute regional adenopathy. Two characteristics are of real value in orienting the diagnosis: the relation with a cat scratch, or the mark left on the skin, or habitual and intimate contact with a cat, and the sterility of the pus collected by puncture. The negative result of culture should call to mind the possible diagnosis of cat-scratch disease. Only the result of the specific intradermal reaction, however, can confirm the diagnosis.

Adenitis due to common pyogenic bacteria is the most usual cause of error, especially when it has been "cooled off" by antibiotic treatment. The adenitis can then be subacute and be accompanied by a minimal cutaneous lesion, a normal blood count and sterile pus.

Tuberculous adenitis can be considered when the tuberculin reactions are positive. Proof of the absence of *Mycobacterium tuberculosis* from the pus and a fairly rapid evolution toward healing without scar then constitute the strongest arguments in favor of cat-scratch disease and against tuberculosis. To tuberculous adenitis due to *M. tuberculosis* must be added—to avert erroneous diagnosis—adenitis due to other mycobacteria. In all these instances the favorable course without lasting fistula and the result of the specific intradermal reaction guide the clinician.

Hodgkin's disease can be considered when the adenopathy is not clearly inflammatory. The presence of fever and moderate polynucleosis may lead to a wrong diagnosis. Moreover, biopsy in adenitis due to cat-scratch disease can show reticular hyperplasia and a mixed infiltration as in Hodgkin's disease. Here again the specific intradermal reaction is necessary to avert misdiagnosis.

The *other malignant adenopathies* (metastatic tumors, sarcomas, Brill-Symmers disease) present no real danger of confusion: the result of biopsy and the evolution leave no doubt.

Lymphogranuloma venereum comes to mind only in the adult in case of an inguinal localization. The histological similarity and the existence of a common serological reaction constitute a resemblance, but in each disease the intradermal reaction is specific.

Tularemia, usually inoculated by the hare and the rabbit but occasionally by the cat, has a more acute course and, especially, can be distinguished by serodiagnosis.

The other human diseases due to *other Pasteurella organisms* that can be transmitted by the cat cause a frankly inflammatory inoculation lesion, regional lymphangitis, and subacute adenitis. The intradermal reaction with a culture filtrate of these bacteria is positive, and the intradermal reaction for cat-scratch disease is negative.

Sodoku, usually inoculated by rat bite but occasionally by cat bite, produces an acute cutaneous-lymphatic syndrome with lymphangitis, repeated attacks of fever, and intense anemia with splenomegaly. The revelation of the spirochete by inoculation into the guinea pig fixes the diagnosis.

Pluriregional adenopathies such as those in infectious mononucleosis, toxoplasmosis,[18] sarcoidosis, syphilis, brucellosis, and mycoses are rarely a cause of difficulty in differential diagnosis of cat-scratch disease.

UNUSUAL FORMS

Each one of the clinical signs and symptoms that may accompany cat-scratch disease (eruptions, pharyngeal, and ocular localizations, thoracic and abdominal manifestations) gives rise to particular problems. Only the association with adenitis and the connection with inoculation by a cat or contact with a cat suggest the exact cause. In atypical cases even more than in the common forms, the specific intradermal reaction is indispensable to the diagnosis.

It must, however, be reemphasized that a positive intradermal reaction in a subject who presents one or another of these atypical manifestations does not constitute, in itself and in isolation, a sufficient proof if a characteristic adenopathy is not also present. The persistence of positive cutaneous reactions in subjects who had adenitis due to cat-scratch disease (recognized or misdiagnosed) some years earlier presents the risk of erroneous attribution to this disease of other diseases occurring subsequently.

PROPHYLAXIS AND TREATMENT

No *prophylaxis* can be envisaged in this benign, relatively infrequent disease of which the pathogenic agent is unknown. Isolating the patient is useless, for interhuman contamination does not occur. Moreover, the cat responsible for the contamination doubtless remains contagious during only a brief period. It hence suffices to isolate the cat for a few weeks.

Lymph node puncture is not only a means of diagnosis but also a means of treatment that often suffices in the common form. It should be made with a large-caliber needle, introduced into the healthy skin and directed toward the center of the adenopathy. When the pus is thick and difficult to aspirate, the physician can resort to washing with sterile isotonic saline solution. Two or three successive punctures may be necessary until the suppuration ceases.

Different *antibiotics* have been employed. It seems that tetracycline or its derivatives should receive preference: the dosage is from 40 mg. to 50 mg. per kilogram of body weight per 24 hours for eight to ten days. This treatment usually eliminates fever and the signs of infection but has little effect on the suppuration. Chloramphenicol is as effective, but its use carries too great risks for it to be recommended in such a benign disease. Penicillin and streptomycin seem to be less effective.

Surgical exeresis of the involved lymph nodes may be indicated when antibiotic treatment has failed; or syringe aspiration has been incomplete and the adenitis evolves toward fistulization; or the disease is prolonged beyond three weeks. The surgeon can completely remove the involved lymph nodes or perform a simple curettage of the foci of suppuration. Postoperative recovery is usually rapid.

Use of *corticosteroids* is rarely necessary and their effect on cat-scratch disease has not been exactly determined. Injection in situ, by lymph node puncture, of 1 ml. to 2 ml. of a solution of corticosteroids for local use (hydrocortisone, prednisone, methylated or fluorated derivatives) seems to accelerate healing. Use of corticosteroids by the systemic route (prednisone: 1 mg. to 2 mg. per kilogram of body weight per 24 hours) is reserved for the complicated forms.

THERAPEUTIC INDICATIONS

In the common form, lymph node puncture is often sufficient. Persistence of the suppuration necessitates repetition of punctures and perhaps the injection of corticosteroids in situ as well. Severe or prolonged signs of infection are the principal indication for antibiotic treatment.

Manifestations, besides adenitis, involving other systems, and particularly neuromeningeal accidents, are indications for immediate treatment by tetracycline, associated with symptomatic therapy and perhaps with corticosteroids by the systemic route.

BIBLIOGRAPHY

1. Adams, W. C., and Hindman, S. M.: Cat-scratch disease associated with an osteolytic lesion. J. Pediat., *44*:665, 1954.
2. Belber, J. P., Davis A. E., and Epstein, E. H.: Thrombocytopenic purpura associated with cat-scratch disease; response of cat-scratch disease to steroid hormones. Arch. Intern. Med., *94*:321, 1954.
3. Billo, O. E., and Wolff, J. A.: Thrombocytopenic purpura due to cat-scratch disease. Case reports of three brothers who were continuously exposed to eleven farm cats. J.A.M.A., *174*:1824, 1960.
4. Boyd, G. L., and Craig, G.: Etiology of cat-scratch fever. J. Pediat., *59*:313, 1961.
5. Brooksaler, F.: Cat scratch disease with encephalopathy. Amer. J. Dis. Child., *107*:185, 1964.
6. Carithers, H. A.: Unclassified mycobacteria in the etiology of cat-scratch fever: A skin test evaluation. Pediatrics, *31*:1039, 1963.
7. Cervonskij, V. I., Terskih, I. I., and Beklesova, A. J.: Isolation and study of agent of benign lymphoreticulosis of man (cat-scratch disease). Vop. Virus., *8*:264, 1963.
8. Collipp, P. J., and Koch, R.: Cat-scratch fever associated with an osteolytic lesion. New Eng. J. Med., *260*:278, 1959.
9. Coutel, Y., Thomet, G., and Morel, H.: Manifestations encéphalitiques au cours d'une maladie des griffes du chat. Arch. Franç. Pédiat., *21*:747. 1964.
10. Daniels, W. B., and MacMurray, F.: Cat scratch disease. Report of one hundred sixty cases. J.A.M.A., *154*:1247, 1954.
11. Debré, R., Lamy, M., Jammet, M. L., Costil, L., and Mozziconacci, P.: La maladie des griffes du chat. Sem. Hôp. Paris, *26*:1895, 1950.
12. Debré, R., and Job, J. C.: La maladie des griffes du chat. Acta Paediat., *43*(suppl. 96):1-86, 1954.
13. Debré, R., and Job, J. C.: Etiology of cat-scratch fever. J. Pediat., *60*:472, 1962.
14. Decourt, J., and Gennes, J. L. de: Thyroïdite subaiguë, avec suppuration aseptique, au cours d'une lymphoréticulose bénigne d'inoculation. Bull. Soc. Méd. Hôp. Paris, *77*:305, 1961.
15. Dodd, M. C., Graber, C. D., and Anderson, G.: Hemagglutination of rabbit erythrocytes by pus from cases of cat-scratch fever. Proc. Soc. Exp. Biol. Med., *102*:556, 1959.
16. Gifford, H.: Skin test reactions to cat-scratch disease among veterinarians. Arch. Intern. Med., *95*:828, 1955.
17. Hedinger, C.: Zur Histopathologie der sog. Katzenkratskrankheit, einer benignen Viruslymphadenitis (Maladie des griffes du chat, lymphoréticulose bénigne d'inoculation). Schweiz. Z. Allg. Path. Bakt., *15*:622, 1952.
18. Jeune, M., Euzeby, J., Vialtel, M., Carron, R., and Fournier, P.: Toxoplasmose acquise à forme ganglionnaire survenue chez trois frères et simulant une maladie des griffes de chat. Lyon Mèd., *201*:699, 1959.
19. Jim, R. T. S.: Thrombocytopenic purpura in cat-scratch disease. J.A.M.A., *176*:1036, 1961.
20. Kalter, S., Prier, J., and Prior, J. T.: Recent studies on the diagnosis of cat-scratch fever. Ann. Intern. Med., *42*:562, 1955.
21. Kaplan, M., Salet, J., Grumbach, R., et al.: Deux cas familiaux et simultanés d'érythème noueux par lympho-réticulose bénigne d'inoculation (maladie des griffes du chat). Bull. Soc. Méd. Hôp. Paris, *77*:171, 1961.
22. Kaplan, M., Straus, P., and Devaux, J. P.: Accidents encéphalitiques au cours de la maladie des griffes de chat. A propos d'une observation. Arch. Franç. Péd., *18*:1044, 1961.
23. Lambert, H., and Hausser, E.: Une hépatite anictérique, nouvelle complication possible de la maladie des griffes de chat. Rev. Méd. Suisse Rom., *85*:689, 1965.
24. McGovern, J., Kunz, L., and Blodgett, M.: Nonbacterial regional lymphadenitis ("cat-scratch fever"). An evaluation of the diagnostic intradermal test. New. Eng. J. Med., *252*:166, 1955.
25. Marini, C., and Tonelato, V.: Su di un caso di linforeticolosi benigna d'inoculazione con manifestazioni pleuropolmonari ed eritema nodoso (forma atipica della cosiddetta malattie da graffio di gatto). Acta Paediat. Lat., *12*:161, 1959.
26. Meyer, A., and Fréour, P.: Adénopathies médiastinales transitoires coexistant avec une réaction positive à l'antigène de la lymphoréticulose bénigne d'inoculation (maladie des griffures de chat). J. Franç. Méd. Chir. Thorac., *8*:163, 1954.
27. Meyer, P., and Moeschlin, S.: Das Lymphdrüsenpunktat der Katzenkratzkrankheit. Schweiz. Med. Wschr., *88*:1070, 1958.
28. Mollaret, P., Reilly, J., Bastin, R., and Tournier, P.: Une maladie ganglionnaire nouvelle: adénopathie régionale spontanément curable avec intradermoréaction et lésions histologiques particulières. Presse Méd., *58*:282, 1950.
29. Mollaret, P., Reilly, J., Bastin, R., and Tournier, P.: Réaction de fixation du complement dans la lymphoréticulose bénigne d'inoculation. C. R. Soc. Biol., *144*:1493, 1950.
30. Mollaret, P., Reilly, J., Bastin, R., and Tournier, P.: La découverte du virus de la lymphoréticulose bénigne d'inoculation. Presse Méd., *59*:681, 701, 1951.
31. Mollaret, P., Reilly, J., Bastin, R., and Tournier, P.: Le virus de la lymphoréticulose bénigne d'inoculation. Bilan personnel actuel. Presse Méd., *64*:1177, 1956.
32. Mollaret, P., Reilly, J., Bastin, R., and Tournier, P.: L'adénopathie régionale subaiguë lymphoplasmodiale (ex-type B de la lymphorétic-

ulose bénigne d'inoculation): les sept observations actuellement connues. Presse Méd.,
64:2149, 1956.

33. Paxson, E. M., and McKay, R. J.: Neurologic
symptoms associated with cat-scratch disease.
Pediatrics, *20*:13, 1957.

34. Peterman, M. G.: Cat-scratch disease: report of a
case in 1925. J. Pediat., *44*:563, 1954.

35. Sheldon, G. C., and Smellie, H.: Cat-scratch
disease with pneumonia. Brit. Med. J., *2*:446,
1957.

36. Shumway, M., and Davis, P. L.: Cat-scratch thyroiditis treated with thyrotropic hormone. J.
Clin. Endocr., *14*:742, 1954.

37. Smith, R. E., and Darling, R. M.: Encephalopathy
of cat-scratch disease. Amer. J. Dis. Child.,
99:107, 1960.

38. Steiner, M. M., Vuckovitch, D., and Hadawi, S.
A.: Cat-scratch disease with encephalopathy.
Case report and review of the literature. J. Pe-
diat., *62*:514, 1963.

39. Tessier, R., Berge, C., Servantie, X., and Chas-

saigne, R.: Lymphoréticulose bénigne d'inoculation (adénite suppurée axillaire et image hilo-
pulmonaire). J. Méd. Bordeaux, *136*:824, 1959.

40. Townsend, E. H., and Cravitz, L.: Cat-scratch
disease. Recurrence after three years. Amer. J.
Dis. Child., *110*:213, 1965.

41. Turner, W., Bigley, N. J., Dodd, M. C., and Anderson, G.: Hemagglutinating virus isolated
from cat scratch disease. J. Bact., *80*:430, 1960.

42. Warwick, W. J., and Good, R. A.: Cat-scratch
disease in Minnesota. 1. Evidence for its
epidemic occurrence. 2. The family epidemics. 3.
Evaluation of the intradermal skin test to cat-
scratch disease antigen. Amer. J. Dis. Child.,
100:228, 1960.

43. Weinstein, L., and Meade, R. H.: The neurological
manifestations of cat-scratch disease. Amer. J.
Med. Sci. *229*:500, 1955.

44. Winship, T.: Pathologic changes in so-called cat-
scratch fever. Review of findings in lymph
nodes of 29 patients and cutaneous lesions of 2
patients. Amer. J. Clin. Path., *23*:1012, 1953.

52

Diseases Caused by Chlamydiaceae; Lymphogranuloma Venereum

By J. C. LEVADITI

OVER-ALL CHARACTERISTICS OF CHLAMYDIACEAE*

Very different contagious diseases (trachoma, lymphogranuloma venereum, or-nithosis, psittacosis, and other disorders) are caused by agents with characteristics suf-ficiently distinctive for them to be grouped in the nomenclature in the family now known as Chlamydiaceae (Rake, 1955), placed between Rickettsiae, to which they are allied, and viruses from which they are definitively separated.[9]

---

*Synonyms for Chlamydiaceae include agents of the psittacosis-lymphogranuloma-tracheoma group, and Bedsoniae.

Three types of penetration can be distin-guished from a biological viewpoint within the group, on the basis of the degree of dis-semination in the host.

The first type is strictly epithelial. The best example is the trachoma agent, which invades essentially the ocular or genital mucosa without really penetrating the body more deeply. Related to this type are sap-rophytic and pathogenic microorganisms of man and animals that have not yet been transmitted experimentally or have been iso-lated recently.

The second type is exemplified by the lymphogranuloma venereum agent. It is characterized by invasion of reticulohistiocy-tic tissues and cells, with propagation and

Table 52-1. *Proposed Classification System for Chlamydiaceae (Rake, 1955) Order Rickettsiales**

FAMILY	GENUS	SPECIES	
I. Rickettsiaceae			
	Colesiota	*Conjunctivae*	
	Ricolesia	*Conjunctivae*	
	Colettsia	*Pecoris*	
	Epi- or endocellular		
	Have not been cultivated		
	Too little known to be classified		
	The first two only are pathogenic		
II. Chlamydiaceae		*Trachomatis*	
Visible under the optic		Rigid intracytoplasmic inclusions	*C. trachomatis*
microscope (450 ± 100 mμ in diameter)		Presence of glycogen	*C. oculogenitalis*
RNA + DNA + glu-	*Chlamydia†*	Sensitivity to sodium sulfadiazine	*M. lymphogranulomatosis‡*
cides + lipids + protides	Intracellular		*M. bronchopneumoniae*
Enzymatic system	May be propagated in	*Psittaci*	*M. psittaci*
Common thermostable	the yolk sac of	Nonrigid, irregularly	*M. ornithosis*
group antigen	chick embryos	shaped intracyto-	*M. felis*
Present division	Pathogenic	plasmic inclusions	*M. louisianae*
Susceptibility to anti-		No detectable glycogen	*M. illinii*
bacteria drugs		Resistant to sodium	*M. opossumi*
Not known to be trans-		sulfadiazine	*M. ovis*
missible by arthropods			*M. bovis*
			M. pecoris
III. Bartonellaceae			

*Data from Bergey's Manual of Determinative Bacteriology. 7th ed. Baltimore, Williams & Wilkins, 1957; reviewed by Page.[9]

†Usual abbreviation, P.L.T.

‡Before the trachoma agent was cultivated the species preceded by M were grouped in the genus *Miyagawanella.* They have sometimes been misnamed *Bedsonia,* a genus not recognized by the International Committee for Nomenclature.

localization in the regional lymph nodes of the site of the primary lesion. The inoculation chancre is transitory and regresses spontaneously.

The best-known agents of the third group are those of ornithosis and psittacosis. They are disseminated by the blood and cause an initial respiratory, digestive, or genital disease without evident lymphatic localization.

The agents of ornithosis and psittacosis are maintained in nature by an animal reservoir constituted by numerous species of wild and domestic birds. The strains are much less strictly specialized, and their ability to infect man varies in function of the host bird and the strain, as well as chance local conditions of contact between man and bird.

Chlamydiaceae form a distinct biological group with common characteristics:

They are obligate intracellular parasites in the tissues of vertebrates: man, mammals, and birds. They have not so far been found in invertebrates and do not seem to be transmitted by arthropods.

They multiply in no known culture medium in the absence of living cells. They are visible under the optic microscope (average diameter: approximately 450 mμ). They have a spherical form and show the various aspects of binary fission.

Their chemical composition is complex: it comprises glycolipoprotein, enzymes, and the two nucleic acids, DNA and RNA.

They have a limiting membrane with a chemical composition similar to that of the cell well of gram-negative bacteria.

They always have a common, heat-resistant antigenic fraction that is rapidly detected by allergic or serological reactions.

They are sensitive in general to antibiotics, especially to tetracyclines, to certain sulfonamides, and to penicillin, thus revealing a physiology analogous to that of bacteria.

This group of common characteristics, principally the simultaneous presence of both nucleic acids, has given rise to the suggestion that these pathogenic agents be classified under the name Chlamydiaceae in the class Schizomycetes—that is to say, as bacteria. However, the techniques used to study them are those of virology, a fact justifying their place in this book.

LYMPHOGRANULOMA VENEREUM (Nicolas-Favre Disease)

Sometimes called subacute inguinal lymphogranulomatis or "the fourth venereal disease," lymphogranuloma venereum is often referred to by French-speaking authors as Nicolas-Favre disease.

It is caused by a member of the present Chlamydiaceae family called *Miyagawanella lymphogranulomatosis* by Brumpt in 1938. Its most frequent localization is in the inguinal lymph nodes, but it can adopt other sites as in esthiomene and ulcerovegetative anorectitis.[5]

In 1913, Durand, Nicolas, and Favre[2] reported that various previously observed symptoms constituted a distinct disease entity. In fact, the disease was not new. Navy physicians were already familiar with climatic bubo; Trousseau had given a precise description of the symptoms, and its venereal origin had been suspected by Rost, a German Navy doctor, in 1912. The identity of the diseases described earlier was demonstrated by Phylactos in 1922 in a doctoral thesis inspired by Favre.

This first period of clinical observation and study of the pathology of the disease was succeeded by the experimental phase that proved its specific character.

In 1925 Frei[3] provided the immunological proof of the entity of the disease by the test for cutaneous hypersensitivity that bears his name. In collaboration with Koppel, he used this test to identify certain noninguinal forms of the disease: the reaction is positive in anorectitis as well as in esthiomene (described by Jersild in 1920).

Hellerström and Wassén[4] reported in 1930 the experimental reproduction of the disease by intracerebral inoculation into monkeys of the fluid from lymph nodes excised in cases of lymphogranuloma venereum. This procedure resulted in a fatal specific meningitis reproduced by serial passage in the monkey.

In 1935, Miyagawa et al.[7] reported the first studies of the pathogenic agent under the microscope; the forms described, later called elementary bodies, characterize this agent during one phase of its developmental cycle. The name Miyagawanella was given to the agent by Brumpt in 1938 in honor of Miyagawa who first saw it.

CLINICAL DATA

The onset of the disease is hardly noticeable. From ten to 20 days before adenitis appears, and shortly after venereal contamination, a *fugitive initial chancre* usually marks the onset. This adenogenic venereal ulcer, studied especially by Sézary and by Bory, resembles in form a minimal lesion of genital herpes. It is often solitary, is small and nonpruriginous, painless as a rule, and short lasting. It may not occur. Rarely, it takes a papular form and is then more lasting. Cases of extragenital chancre are known, some of them due to an accidental prick by a contaminated instrument. The chancre of lymphogranuloma venereum may simulate chancre-like ulceration or syphilitic chancre and be accompanied by lymphangitis of the penis and nodules at intervals along the lymphatic channels, or by amicrobial urethritis. In practice, this genital lesion is almost never recognized before inguinal adenopathy leads to attempt to detect it in the case history. Moreover, sometimes no chancre occurs.

Inguinal bubo, which is more frequent in men than in women, appears two to three months after the infecting contact. It is manifested by discomfort and tenderness followed by regional tumefaction. A single lymph node and then several nodes increase in volume and harden; at the same time periadenitis unites them in a tender nodular mass, which remains mobile, however, and does not adhere to the underlying tissues at this stage. The skin becomes violaceous, and this plurinodular mass softens at separate points, forming abscesses and multiple fistulas from which flows filaceous, viscous pus.

This adenopathy is unilateral but may

become bilateral. It often corresponds to iliac adenitis palpable behind the crural arch, which never suppurates. Without treatment the evolution of these fistulas once dragged out for several months or several years, leaving sclerous, adherent scars. At present, treatment can arrest the course of the adenopathy before any suppuration.

Use of biological methods has permitted the detection of a whole series of *unrecognized localizations*. The early forms may be venous (if the inflammation starting from the inguinal lymph nodes reaches the femoral vein), articular (simple relapsing arthrosis more frequently than true arthritis), or cutaneous (of the erythema nodosum or the polymorphous erythema type) occasionally accompanied by high fever and splenomegaly.

Protracted forms are known. The lymphogranulomatous epididymitis seen by Sicard and Léger remains exceptional. Genitoanorectal forms are, however, less unusual; most of them result from sodomitical contamination. The disease can take the form of simple inflammatory stricture of the rectum, of an anogenitorectal syndrome, of vulvar esthiomene, or even of purely vulvular lesions, all of a chronic character.

It is uncertain whether the infection is transmissible by the placentary route.

THE MICROBE: MIYAGAWANELLA LYMPHOGRANULOMATOSIS[8]

In 1936, Miyagawa and his associates discovered fine, rounded "granulocorpuscles" that were either free or embedded in the cytoplasm of certain cellular elements in Giemsa-stained smears of pus; they represented the agent of the disease.

Currently, with use of the Macchiavello staining technique, these elements are seen in the initial lesions or in recent buboes. They appear as ruby-red granules against the blue background of the smears stained by this method. As the lesions enter the chronic phase, the corpuscular elements (elementary bodies) become less numerous and finer, and their staining affinities diminish. In later stages, the corpuscles are no longer detected, although the pus continues to be infectious.

The results obtained by ultrafiltration, ultracentrifugation, and radon irradiation indicate that the diameter of the elementary body is approximately 450 mμ, which is in agreement with the results of light and electron microscopy.

The microbe is extremely sensitive to physical and chemical agents. Ultraviolet radiation rapidly destroys it. The agent survives ten days at + 4° C. and for months at −20° C. or −70° C.; it can be preserved for years after lyophilization. Immersion in dilute buffered glycerin solution is known to keep most viruses alive at low temperature, whereas the lymphogranuloma venereum agent loses its pathogenicity within a few days under these conditions. This difference constitutes another fact distinguishing the agent from viruses.

Culture. In 1940, Rake et al.[10] inoculated the virulent material into the yolk sac of the embryonated hen's egg according to the technique utilized by Cox for culture of rickettsia. Miyagawanella pullulates under these conditions, and serial passages are possible. Elementary bodies abound, and by use of differential ultracentrifugation Smadel prepared suspensions of these bodies in a concentration sufficient for the complement-fixation reaction to enter into current diagnostic practice.

Orfila[8] observed a weak cytotoxic effect in tissue culture and reconstituted the microbe's cycle of intracellular development. After the appearance of an initial body, then of an inclusion body, the elementary bodies become visible first within an iodophilic hydrocarbon matrix and then in an immense vacuole from which they are liberated into the culture medium. The structure and the chemical composition of the elementary bodies are typical of Chlamydiaceae.

Experimental Pathogenicity. When the agent is inoculated intracerebrally, the monkey reacts with acute meningitis, stiff neck, and tremor, but without actual paralysis. Death, preceded by a comatous state and often by attacks of convulsions, occurs within a few days. Subacute, chronic, or inapparent forms are rare. Although the strains isolated have shown difference in virulence in the laboratory, it is nonetheless certain that their pathogenicity for man remains identical and that neither "neurovirulence" nor a "fixation phenomenon" appears as it sometimes does in the case of certain viruses.

Species other than the monkey are also receptive. The rabbit, which is relatively resistant, has been utilized to test the pathogenicity of a strain. The guinea pig is sensitive to subcutaneous inoculations made in the inguinal and the intratesticular region and to intradermal inoculation. It reacts with a transient regional adenitis.

In 1932 Constantin Levaditi and his associates transmitted the disease to the mouse by intracerebral inoculation. Some mice die rapidly. Others survive a long time, and the brain remains virulent until death, a characteristic that can be utilized to preserve strains of the agent.

LABORATORY DIAGNOSIS

Allergic Skin Reaction. In the *Frei test for cutaneous hypersensitivity,* the antigens used in practice are human, simian, and vitelline. Although the last-mentioned has the advantage that it can be prepared in large quantities in hens' eggs, it has the disadvantage of eliciting nonspecific reactions in subjects sensitized to egg constituents, from which fact arises the requirement to utilize control antigens prepared from normal yolk sacs.

TECHNIQUE OF THE TEST. Whatever the antigen used, an injection of 0.1 to 0.3 ml. is made intradermally on the anterior surface of the forearm. The reaction should be read between 48 hours and four days later.

NEGATIVE REACTION. The day after the injection and the days following, the skin shows only a diffuse pinkish tinge. On the fourth day there is no papule and no feeling of nodular texture to the touch. The only trace is the punctiform mark left by the intradermal injection on a perfectly supple skin area.

POSITIVE REACTION. After 48 hours, occasionally even from the twenty-fourth hour on, a papule 7 to 20 mm. in diameter forms. It is dark red, indurated, and raised, and is often surrounded by a paler erythematous ring. The reaction attains its maximum intensity the fourth day. It disappears in seven to ten days as a rule, but may last as long as three weeks. During this period, the reaction takes the aspect of an indurated red papule, giving the tactile sensation of infiltrated skin. When the reaction is intense, after the fourth day a central pruriginous pustule appears; it bursts and becomes covered with squama, but heals without scarring.

DOUBTFUL REACTION. In the rare doubtful reactions a pinkish macula, which is occasionally urticarial, appears after 48 hours or, exceptionally, on the fourth day. It disappears rapidly and never yields on palpation the peculiar sensation of deeply infiltrated skin.

Cutaneous allergy occurs, at the earliest, 30 to 40 days after onset of the infection. As the allergic state sets in, the Frei test reaction, which was negative earlier, becomes doubtful and then positive. The allergy persists many years after recovery and can hence be used in retrospective diagnosis.

Lymph Node Puncture. The pus obtained by puncture of a suppurated nonfistulated lymph node should be sent to the laboratory under refrigeration. The results of cytological study and the presence of elementary bodies are a confirmation of the clinical diagnosis that is established with certainty by experimental inoculation, especially of embryonated eggs. Furthermore, the pus constitutes a valuable antigenic material.

Histological Diagnosis. Study of a lymph node is considered only when diagnosis is particularly difficult. The node is removed under sterile conditions and is sectioned. Part of it is fixed with formalin or Bouin's fluid in view of histological examination. The remainder, which is placed in a tube plunged in an ice bath, is used in an attempt to isolate the strain and should be sent as quickly as possible to the laboratory.

Serological Diagnosis. The *complement-fixation test* should be made at the same time as the Frei intradermal test.

The antigen is prepared from yolk sacs collected six days after inoculation. These sacs are first washed, crushed, treated with phenol, and boiled. Then differential centrifugation yields suspension of elementary bodies in which the specific antigens persist. For serological tests it is indispensable to utilize control antigens prepared in an identical manner but from normal yolk sacs.

The reaction is positive when the titer is at least 1/40, although three sources of error arise.

First, the sera of subjects sensitive to certain components of normal egg yolk yield positive reactions with both the specific antigens and the control antigens.

Second, certain sera from syphilitics in the first serological phase of the disease yield a transiently positive reaction.

Third, all the members of the group (i.e., the agents of psittacosis, ornithosis, and lymphogranuloma venereum) have thermostable antigens in common. This fact is important from a theoretical viewpoint. Hence a positive reaction cannot be fully interpreted except in the light of the clinical information. These cross-reactions do not limit the value of the test. On the contrary, they permitted the establishment of relationship between diseases once considered to be entirely different and even integration of the agents of new diseases into the Chylamydiaceae family.

EPIDEMIOLOGY

Lymphogranuloma venereum exists in all climates but is more frequent in hot regions.

In Europe it is highly infrequent, and in France it has become a great rarity. Nonetheless the disease persists in the tropical and subtropical coastal regions of both the Old World and the New. It seems to be imported into ports by sailors arriving from contaminated areas.

Normal and abnormal sexual relations are the principal source of contamination in this disease. In general venereal transmission occurs by the intermediary of symptom-free subjects, especially women. The source of contamination has been proved experimentally either by demonstration of the agent in the secretions of asymptomatic subjects or by determination of the antigenic properties of the secretions. Lymphogranuloma venereum is subject to obligatory declaration in France.

DIFFERENTIAL DIAGNOSIS

The differential diagnosis is posed in different terms in function of the localization.

That of inguinal bubo presents the most difficult problem. The adenogenic ulcer can simulate chancroid or a lesion of primary syphilis, which resembles it in some forms of syphilis.

Diagnosis of tubercular bubo is a problem belonging more to the past than to the present. Differentiation from chancroid bubo or from cat-scratch disease may be more demanding. The second of these diseases has certain characteristics in common with lymphogranuloma venereum (see Chapter 51), and the agent is possibly related to the Chlamydiaceae group, as may also be the agent of inclusion-body urethrocervicitis (see Chapter 53).

The adenitis in tularemia due to *Francisella tularensis* (formerly *Pasteurella tularensis*) may require differentiation. Usually contamination of animal origin (by a wild rabbit, especially) can be discovered by careful history taking. Moreover, the site of the adenitis is nearly always cervical or subaxillary. Culture of the bacterial agent and the result of the agglutination test or of the intradermal reaction to tularine establish the diagnosis.

PATHOLOGY

Variants of the primary lesion are related to the localization and to the structure of the organs involved, but they always have a similar histological type: that of the specific nodular inflammation. At the moment of their full development before onset of any complication, the lymph nodes are first cribbled with nodules and then by microabscesses with irregular contours that give them a porous look. The center of the nodules shows a suppurated necrosis with pus rich in degenerated polymorphonuclear cells. It is surrounded by a crown of epithelial cells juxtaposed in palisades, near which a few giant cells may be seen. Among the lymphoid cells at the periphery are plasma cells and polymorphonuclear leukocytes (eosinophils, especially). Periadenitis is indicated by sclerotic inflammatory plaques extending beyond the lymph node capsule, linking the involved nodes and reaching far into the cells of the adipose tissue.

These lesions differ entirely from those of inguinal granuloma, a disease unknown in Europe that occurs especially in the Negro populations of the southern United States; it is related to Hodgkin's disease and is characterized by Donovan bodies.

PHYSIOPATHOLOGY

The agent of lymphogranuloma venereum multiplies in mesenchymal cells and provokes lesions at the inoculation site and in the regional lymphatic organs. It is transported by the lymph, which is virulent, as well as by blood cells, and thus reaches the organs rich in reticulohistiocytic cells, without, however, crossing the blood-brain barrier. This mechanism of diffusion and the lack of neurotropism confirm the agent's tissular affinity for the reticulohistiocytic system, and, more generally, for the mesenchyma, a fact that relates the agent to rickettsia and bacteria.[7]

TREATMENT

Since the discovery of sulfonamides and, especially, antibiotics, treatment has become really effective[1] Although penicillin and chloramphenicol have some action, the current preference is for Aureomycin in 2 gm. daily dosage for at least two to three weeks, a therapy that yields the most improvement and averts suppuration. Certain cases of lymphogranuloma venereum still defy all available treatment.

BIBLIOGRAPHY

1. Degos, R.: Dermatologie. Paris, Editions Médicales Flammarion, 1953, pp. 1024-1025b.
2. Durand, M., Nicolas, J., and Favre, M.: Lymphogranulomatose inguinale subaiguë d'origine génitale probable, peut-être vénérienne. Bull. Soc. Méd. Hôp. Paris, 35:274, 1913.
3. Frei, W.: Eine neue Hautreaktion bei "Lymphogranuloma inguinale." Klin. Wschr., 4:2148-2149, 1925.
4. Hellerström, S., and Wassén, E.: Meningo-enzephalitishe Veräderungen bei Affen nach intracerebraler Impfung mit Lymphogranuloma inguinale. 7ème Congrès Inter. Derm. et Syph., Copenhagen, 1930, pp. 1147-1150.
5. Levaditi, C., and Lepine, P.: Maladie de Nicolas-Favre. In: Les ultra-virus des maladies humaines. 2nd ed. Paris, Librairie Maloine, 1948, vol. 2, pp. 1027-1149.
6. Levaditi, J.: La maladie de Nicolas-Favre expérimentale. Thèse. Paris, Maloine & Cie, 1936.
7. Miyagawa, Y., et al.: Studies on virus of lymphogranuloma inguinale Nicolas, Favre and Durand. Jap. J. Exp. Med., 13:1, 1935. On virus of lymphogranuloma inguinale. Jap. J. Derm. Urol., 39:105, 1936.
8. Orfila, J.: Chapter XXXII. In: Techniques de laboratoire en virologie humaine. Paris, Masson et Cie, 1964, pp. 748-765.
9. Page, L. A.: Revision of the family Chlamydiaceae Rake (Rickettsiales); unification of the psittacosis-lymphogranuloma venereum-trachoma group of organisms in the genus Chlamydia Jones, Rake and Stearns, 1945. Intern. J. System. Bact., 16:223-252, 1966.
10. Rake, G., McKee, C. M., and Shaffer, M. F.: Agent of lymphogranuloma venereum in yolk-sac of developing chick embryo. Proc. Soc. Exp. Biol. Med., 43:332, 1940.

PART VIII

Viral Infections with Urogenital Manifestations

53

Viral Infections with Urogenital Manifestations

By P. RENARD AND J. CELERS

The genital disorders that are today ascribed to viral infections have long been known; Hippocrates described such disorders in association with inflammation of the parotid glands. Since the successive discovery of numerous viruses, various etiologies have been described. Mumps virus, however, remains the essential agent of genital involvement of viral origin. Urinary manifestations, on the other hand, are highly exceptional in viral infections, whereas they are a frequent—even an essential—feature of infections due to agents of the psittacosis-lymphogranuloma-trachoma group.

MUMPS[7]

ORCHITIS

Orchitis is secondary to the viremia in mumps; the virus has been found in the infected testis. Local traumatism seems to favor this complication, but what actually determines this localization is unknown. The usual incidence of orchitis in epidemics is estimated to be between 18 and 25 per cent. It varies from one epidemic to another. In the armies stationed in Europe in 1918, Wesselhoeft[54] found an incidence of 27 per cent during April, but it was only 5 per cent during the following months for a nearly identical number of cases. The extremes of 1 per cent and of 75 per cent have been reported.

Orchitis appears in mumps especially in adolescents and young adults. Search of the literature has revealed rare cases in children: aged ten years (Werner), nine years (Fabre-Philip), eight years (Werner), and five years (Rodriguez Castro), and even in infants, aged six and seven months (Connelly).[11]

Usually, the testicular localization is unilateral. The percentages of bilateral forms also vary with the epidemics, representing 5.4, 14.8, 16.7, 17, and 33 per cent of cases of orchitis in different reports.

As a rule, orchitis succeeds parotitis, from the fourth to the eighth day after onset of mumps. In the 2500 cases studied by Eagle over a four-year period, onset of orchitis was most often noted four or five days after the onset of parotitis. Orchitis may also precede parotitis by one to nine days, or follow its onset by 12 or even 21 days; Stengel reported a case of orchitis that appeared on the forty-fourth day. The fact that orchitis may be the only localization of mumps should be borne in mind. Wesselhoeft collected 64 such cases.

Onset. Pain in the testis may be the first sign of orchitis, but more usually a recurrence of fever is the sign of this impending localization. Chills, general discomfort, headache, and severe asthenia mark this phase. Occasionally, the picture may be alarming. "In some cases it is that of extreme agitation with delirium, intense fever (41° C.), carphology, vomiting, incontinence of serous feces as in typhoid fever at its worst moments or in malignant scarlet fever toward its onset; in others a picture of collapse predominates, with anxious, pallid, strained facies, a rapid pulse of low and irregular pressure, and coldness and cyanosis of the extremities" (Trousseau). Although these phenomena appear serious, they recede as soon as painful tumefaction of the testis sets in.

Fully Developed Orchitis. The degree of pain varies from simple discomfort with a sensation of heaviness to excruciating pain radiating toward the thigh, the inguinal region, and the perineum, and even involving the lower abdomen.

This pain is the more severe the more quickly it sets in. It can then become intolerable, forcing groans from the most stalwart patient and making rest of any sort impossible. It is set off by examination of the genital apparatus, by the slightest movement, and even by contact with the bed sheet.

The tumefaction of the testis doubles or triples the volume of the organ without changing its form. The tunica vaginalis testis contains fluid. The scrotum is distended, edematous, and red.

Epididymitis is frequent. It may accompany the orchitis or sometimes may precede it; occasionally, it is an isolated phenomenon. Ramond and Goubert found epididymitis in 20 of 115 cases in an epidemic. Candel noted involvement of the testis and of the epididymis in at least 85 per cent of the 78 cases that he studied. Mumps epididymitis, as a rule, is painful, is moderately firm, and sometimes yields a distinct sensation of induration.

In 1965 Coran and Perlmutter[12] reported the following case of epididymitis without orchitis. A Negro, aged 17, was hospitalized after four days of intense left-sided pain in the scrotum, with fever. Ten days before hospital admission, he had had an infection of the upper respiratory tract. A week later, micturition became frequent and imperious. He denied any recent sexual relationship. His mother had had mumps a month earlier. The testes were of normal volume and not distended. The epididymis, however, was four times more voluminous than normal, and congested, with exaggerated local tenderness. The prostate was normal. Two days later, the epididymis was still swollen and tender, although the testis remained normal. Fever fell progressively three days later. Within two weeks, the epididymis was normal. This case of epididymitis without orchitis was accompanied by an eight-fold increase in antibodies against mumps.

Funiculitis may accompany orchitis and epididymitis, but as a rule it is isolated. Mumps orchitis is usually unilateral, but most exceptionally both testes are involved simultaneously, with consequent marked accentuation of the local and systemic signs. When the orchitis is bilateral, involvement of one gland is usually followed by a two-day interval before signs of contralateral involvement appear. Occasionally one side appears even to have healed completely when the other testis becomes involved. If this last-mentioned involvement occurs late, it may be accompanied by a recrudescence of fever.

The Course. Fever persists in the neighborhood of 38° C. (100.4° F.) for two to ten days. In close to half the cases, it falls progressively by lysis, or in the others disappears rapidly, with an exceptional attack of polyuria.

The local signs begin to regress from the fourth or the fifth day.

The late consequences of this localization of mumps give rise to widely divergent evaluations.

Testicular atrophy, greatly feared by military physicians, has been considered throughout history to be the scourge of mumps. It begins inconspicuously and progresses slowly. A reduction in testicular volume appears clearly only four to six months after the acute episode. Bellow and Masters indicated that this atrophy may progress still further during many months and even years, so that a follow-up of ten years is indispensable to evaluate the definitive consequences of mumps orchitis. At the end of its evolution, the volume of the testis may be half or a third of normal. In a reported case, the testis was reduced to the size of a kidney bean, hard and insensitive on palpation.

The frequency of such sequelae defies accurate assessment. Authors with considerable experience have never encountered even a single case.

The frequency of sterility secondary to mumps-induced testicular atrophy is, if possible, even more difficult to estimate. Among 700 sterile men, Young found only ten with a history of mumps orchitis. A study by Bellow and Masters of 79 sterile couples disclosed a history of unilateral or bilateral orchitis in 15; it proved azoospermia in nine and oligospermia in six. Mumps as a cause of sterility in men hence remains uncommon.

Treatment. *Prophylactic suspension of the scrotum* by means of a special apparatus is applied as soon as mumps appears in adolescents or young adults, whatever its localization.

From the onset of orchitis, the scrotum is *rigorously immobilized* by means of a small thin board. The patient should be kept absolutely at rest. Local application of ice relieves pain. Analgesics such as aspirin and quinine hydrobromide are prescribed in function of the degree of pain and the patient's age. The intensity of the pain has been considered to justify use of morphine in certain cases.

Mumps orchi-epididymitis may be reduced or prevented by the prophylactic action of *gamma globulins prepared from convalescent serum*, when they are injected during the first 48 hours of mumps.

As early as 1925 de Lavergne and Florentin[33] reported the results of prophylactic use of convalescent serum in mumps. The injections were made subcutaneously, as early as possible, in a dose that was successively: 10 ml. (fractionated in two doses of 5 ml.), 15 ml. (10 ml. plus 5 ml.), and then 20 ml. (15 ml. plus 5 ml.).

Globally, in the 107 cases of untreated mumps there were 25 of orchitis and nine of meningeal reaction; in the 103 cases of treated mumps, there were five of orchitis and two of meningeal reaction. These results as a whole indicated the value of the method. The earliest results were bettered, for the five cases of orchitis occurred in the first 85 patients, who received 10 or 15 ml. of serum, whereas in the 28 later cases in which a dose of 20 ml. of serum was injected, no sign of orchitis appeared.

In 1945 Gellis et al.[26] confirmed these results and contrasted the entire ineffectiveness of standard gamma globulins to the high rate of protection obtained with gamma globulins derived from convalescent serum and injected during the first 24 hours of parotitis.

The role of *diethylstilbestrol* is debatable. In 1946 Savran[45] treated preventively 77 patients with 4 mg. of diethylstilbestrol per day for five days: testicular complications occurred in 3.9 per cent, whereas they occurred in 16.8 per cent in 168 controls with mumps. From 1946 to 1948 Norton treated 45 patients preventively with 15 mg. of diethylstilbestrol daily for five to seven days:

orchitis occurred in 15.6 per cent of this group and in 16.7 per cent of the control group.

Analysis of the results of diethylstilbestrol used with a curative purpose by Norton in 47 patients, as compared with 42 non-treated controls, showed a reduction of the febrile period and in the intensity of pain. The doses utilized during five to seven days were 3 mg. per day for seven patients and 15 mg. per day in the other 40.

Corticosteroids and ACTH were later proposed for treatment of mumps orchitis. Smith and Bisher[48] studied the results in three groups of patients: 34 given symptomatic treatment alone; 20 given this treatment in association with ACTH; and 31 given symptomatic treatment associated with cortisone. Cortisone in a dose of 300 mg. per day for three or four days had a definite analgesic effect. It did not, however, reduce the fever, diminish the testicular intumescence, or prevent the orchitis from becoming bilateral. Identical results were reported by Kocen and Critchley.[32] Moreover, the action of cortisone on spermatogenesis does not seem to be entirely elucidated, and the fact that it could favor secondary atrophy is conceivable. Hence the wise course is to wait until late follow-up of the patients so treated gives more precise information.

Surgical treatment (albugineotomy under anesthesia) has been proposed, for it permits reducing the pain.

OTHER UROGENITAL LOCALIZATIONS

Mumps Prostatitis. Prostatitis may or may not accompany testicular involvement. It is manifested by a feeling of heaviness at the base of the bladder, the urethral elimination of a more or less opaque yellowish discharge during a few days, and, on rectal touch, perception of an enlarged, distended, painful prostate. Rarely, this prostatitis may lead to urinary retention. More often it remains discreet and is detected only by systematic examination.

The prostatitis begins toward the sixth day and lasts eight to ten days. More rarely, it appears at the onset of mumps.

Wesselhoeft,[54] who made a special effort to demonstrate it, found it in 5 per cent of men with mumps. He even believed that it could be one of the causes of sterility following mumps.

Gerner,[27] who examined 126 patients with epidemic mumps, noted in 21 (16.7 per cent) an increase in volume and sensitivity of the prostate with difficulty in voiding urine, pain in the lumbar region, and fever.

Mumps Ovaritis. The possibility of ovaritis in the adult woman with mumps is estimated to be approximately 5 per cent, but it may be more frequent as it is difficult to diagnose, especially in mild forms. Ovaritis has also been reported in girls before puberty.

The ovaritis may be unilateral or bilateral. It produces pain of variable intensity (dull in some cases but, in others, acute), disturbances of the menses, and metrorrhagia. Palpation reveals a rounded, painful, tumor-like mass in the iliac fossa. The ovaritis may be followed by menstrual irregularity for several months; the condition ends by spontaneous recovery. No case of sterility consequent to mumps ovaritis has been proved.

Mumps Urethritis. Urethritis was reported by Barthez and Saune in five adolescents with mumps orchitis and by Spence in a boy aged 11 years the day before onset of orchitis.

UROGENITAL DISTURBANCES DURING OTHER VIRAL INFECTIONS

Genital involvement of proved viral origin must be clearly distinguished from that in which the etiology is doubtful, either because the circumstances of clinical observation did not permit confirmation or denial of the laboratory diagnosis or because the agent responsible for the disease could not be isolated.[42] The first group is represented by the genital disorders in infections due to Coxsackie viruses, varicella, variola, and herpes,* as well as the exceptional cases reported in infection by bat salivary-gland virus and Armstrong's lymphocytic choriomeningitis. The second group is represented by the urogenital disturbances reported in

---

*Aside from the cutaneomucosal manifestations of genital herpes already described and that we shall not detail further, we remind the reader of the particular association between a high frequency of antibodies against type 2 herpes virus and carcinoma of the cervix uteri (cf. Chapter 34).

epidemics of "dengue" and of "influenza" and those in infectious mononucleosis.

COXSACKIE VIRUS INFECTIONS

Genital involvement of two sorts may occur during Coxsackie virus infections. The first, orchitis, is associated with Coxsackie B viruses; the types B_2, and, especially, B_4 and B_5 are incriminated. The second is vaginal ulceration associated with the pharyngeal lesions of herpangina, which is usually due to Coxsackie A viruses.

Orchitis. Orchitis is an infrequent but well known complication of Bornholm's disease. In 1896 Bacher[4] described it in epidemic myalgia. During the 1931 Swedish epidemic, which involved more than 800 patients, Huss[30] reported 50 cases of orchitis.

Orchitis in Bornholm's disease, as in mumps, usually occurs after puberty. Its frequency, a subject of widely divergent estimates, seems to vary from one epidemic to another even if only the statistics for adult men are taken into account. In 1947 Jamieson and Prinsley[31] described orchitis as an uncommon complication in an epidemic in Aden: it occurred in 12 of 30 male patients. In 1951, Warin et. al.[52] established a 10 per cent frequency of orchitis (three in 30 cases) in adult men in an epidemic in Oxford, England, which comprised a total of 277 cases.

The testicular involvement is probably linked to the spread and the multiplication in situ of Coxsackie B viruses. Craighead,[14] who made a testicular biopsy in a 25-year-old patient in whom orchitis developed on the fourteenth day of pleurodynia, found not only histological lesions comparable to those in mumps orchitis but also Coxsackie B_5 virus in relatively large quantity.

Orchitis is not associated solely with the myalgic forms of Coxsackie virus disease. Artenstein et al.[2] found four cases of orchitis in 180 patients with Coxsackie B virus infection examined from 1955 through 1960: two cases occurred during regression of pleurodynia; the third appeared in a young boy with Coxsackie B virus meningitis; the fourth was not accompanied by any systemic sign, but a simultaneous and parallel rise occurred in antibodies against the Coxsackie types B_2, B_3, B_4, and B_5.

Usually, however, the testicular involvement appears during the regression of pleurodynia. It begins most often between the eighth and the fourteenth day. Occasionally its onset is later: cases have been reported in which orchitis set in up to 36 days after onset of the Coxsackie virus disease.

In some cases the course of the Coxsackie infection is interrupted; in others the disease evolves in two phases, the onset of orchitis being preceded by a remission of several days.

Pain is the first and occasionally the only sign of the testicular involvement. Sometimes a recrudescence of the systemic signs and of painful thoracic signs precedes it. Usually the orchitis remains unilateral; when it is bilateral, a few days separate the involvement of one testis from that of the other. An increase in volume of the testis and the epididymis is detected within a short time, but its occurrence is irregular, and its degree is always moderate. Orchitis regresses in three to 20 days, usually without sequelae.

Treatment should be confined to local measures, associated with analgesics if necessary. The danger of treatment by cortisone or its derivatives of orchitis due to Coxsackie viruses should encourage reticence in view of the aggravation of Coxsackie B infections by corticosteroid hormones in laboratory animals.

Genital Ulcerations. Genital ulcerations were first observed by Mitchell and Dempster[37] during herpangina due to Coxsackie A_{10} in a girl aged seven years. The ulcerations, surrounded by a red border, were small, circular, and grayish white, situated on the cutaneomucosal surface of the labia majora pudendi. The lesions were painless and discovered only by systematic examination. They disappeared in four days. The Coxsackie A_{10} virus was isolated from these lesions, whereas search for herpes virus did not reveal it.

VARICELLA

Aside from genital localizations of the cutaneomucous eruption in chickenpox, the possibility of *orchitis* should be borne in mind.

The first case cited by Wesselhoeft and Pearson had been described by Sabrazès[44] in 1927. A man, aged 20 years, vaccinated against smallpox some months earlier, presented an eruption of chickenpox primarily on the arms and legs, on December 24, 1917. Almost from the onset of the disease, the patient had pain in the right testis. The testis increased in volume to the size of a hen's egg; the left testis and epididymis also became involved. Then remissions and exacerbations of the pain and swelling accompanied by fever succeeded one another for 18 days. Fluid appeared in the scrotum on the right on December 29. On January 11, 1918, the fever finally fell, and the testes rapidly decreased in volume and in sensitivity.

The patient in the second case of Wesselhoeft and Pearson[55] was a man, aged 46 years, exposed to chickenpox 17 days before onset of a typical eruption and pulmonary involvement. He was treated with penicillin and streptomycin. Nine days after the onset he had pain in the right testis, which swelled and became painful to touch, with increase in volume of the epididymis and temperature of 38.9° C. The degree of orchitis remained moderate, for the testis never became hard, was never severely painful, and only doubled in volume. Within a week it became normal. But six and one half months after the onset of the orchitis, the testis appeared diminished in volume by a third, and softer and less sensitive than the noninvolved left testis. The authors described this case as the first example of partial testicular atrophy as a sequel to a complication of varicella.

The third case report[41] concerned a seven-year-old boy. On June 23 an eruption was noted with slight systemic signs. June 25 serious disturbances appeared. The patient vomited continuously for three hours, and severe abdominal pain affected the umbilical area and both iliac fossae with a maximum in the left iliac fossa. He appeared intoxicated; temperature was 39.8° C. June 28 the child seemed severely ill, but the abdominal pain was less severe. Constipation was absolute. The left testis and epididymis were very painful and their volume was four times greater than normal. On June 30 the patient remained ill and nervous but, despite somnolence and a toxic state, consciousness was clear. Temperature and pulse became normal, and the orchitis began to be resolved. Slight pain and muscular resistance remained only in the umbilical region. On January 1 (some five months later) the left testis was completely atrophied.

These three cases must be related to the

results of autopsy of a four-and-a-half-year old boy who died of chickenpox.[9] Gross examination revealed a few petechiae in the testes; the microscope exposed intranuclear inclusions in the endothelium of the capillaries and small arteries of the testes and in the seminal canal.

SMALLPOX

Testicular lesions in smallpox were described in 1859 and have often been confirmed since then. Chiari[10] found testicular lesions post mortem in 45 of 63 smallpox victims most of whom were adults.

Councilman and his co-workers observed, on occasion, a diffuse testicular involvement and the absence of spermatogenesis of the tubular cells. Symptomatic orchitis was recognized in only four of the 432 patients with smallpox examined by Curshman.[16]

No case of orchitis was found by Teissier during 20 years at the Claude Bernard Hospital in Paris, a large center of care of infectious diseases.

Dixon,[19] moreover, observed no correlation between the microscopic lesions found at autopsy in the testes in smallpox and the clinical descriptions of orchitis, the etiology of which, in his opinion, is hence not established.

INFREQUENT VIRUS INFECTIONS WITH LABORATORY CONFIRMATION

Lymphocytic Choriomeningitis. In 1961, Lewis and Utz described the first case, and apparently the only one, of Armstrong's disease that associated meningoencephalitis, parotitis, and orchitis. These localizations appeared successively, the parotitis on the fourth day of the meningitis and the orchitis on the seventeenth day. The testicular involvement remained unilateral, doubling the volume of the gland. It regressed in a few days, along with the other symptoms, but left severe atrophy. The origin of the disease was exactly determined by means of laboratory examination that excluded a herpes infection and proved Armstrong's disease by isolation of the virus from the patient's blood and cerebrospinal fluid as well as by a rise in serum complement-fixing antibodies from 1/8 to 1/64.

Infection by Bat Salivary Gland Virus.[49] The reported cases concerned laboratory infections that simultaneously affected five subjects during research on the bat salivary gland virus (an arbovirus isolated in the United States and linked to group B because of its immunological relationships with the other members of this group). The five patients, who represent the only cases known so far, showed fairly severe general systemic signs. Three had signs of an associated localization: abacterial meningitis in one, orchitis in two, and ovaritis and pneumopathy in one. The etiological diagnosis was established by serological tests: appearance during the course of the disease of complement-fixing, hemagglutination-inhibiting and neutralizing antibodies.

EPIDEMICS WITH REPORTED UROGENITAL INVOLVEMENT

"Influenza" Epidemics. The epidemics of "influenza" to which cases of orchi-epididymitis were attributed antedate 1932, and the elements required to attribute the facts observed to the influenza virus are wanting. The etiological diagnosis is supported solely by negative data: sterile cultures in bacteriological media and failure to induce tuberculosis in the guinea pig by the fluid obtained by puncture.[1, 3, 5, 6, 17, 21, 24]

"Dengue" Epidemics. During epidemics of "dengue," pain in the groin and the testes has been reported among the multiple painful phenomena[43] in the dengue syndrome. Dooley[20] found these algesic manifestations in one of a series of 11 cases of attenuated forms.

Weyrauch and Gass observed more severe signs in United States military personnel stationed in the South Pacific islands in 1943. Of 141 subjects, eight (5.7 per cent) showed urogenital disorders in the absence of any clinical or epidemiological evidence of mumps or filariasis. Five of these eight patients had orchitis. The symptoms appeared in four during the febrile period and, in the fifth, two months later, but in most a recrudescence of the local signs occurred during convalescence. Although the clinical signs and symptoms—increase in volume and pain—remained moderate, the involvement evolved toward bilateral testicular atrophy in one case and unilateral atrophy in two. In three other patients, hemospermia was noted during convalescence; its exact origin could not be determined.

INFECTIOUS MONONUCLEOSIS

In 1944,[35] two patients were reported with the diagnosis of orchitis in the course of infectious mononucleosis. In one of them, a characteristic febrile episode was followed by atrophy of one testis. A month later the other testis showed progressive increase in volume that persisted until hospital admission six months after the original illness. The length of the course is long for infectious mononucleosis. The other patient with unilateral orchitis had no increase in volume of the spleen or of the lymph nodes but a positive reaction (1/512) to the Paul-Bunnell test.

In 1963, Grégoire et al.[28] cited the case of a patient who first presented balanitis characterized by burning sensation on urination, a purulent exudate, and edema of the prepuce such that it was impossible to uncover the glans and to examine the underlying lesions. Smears of the pus revealed severely altered polymorphonuclear leukocytes. Microbiological examination showed an abundant microbial flora comprised of spirilla, numerous fusiform bacilli, and *Trichomonas vaginalis*. Darkfield microscope examination showed no treponema.

Fever appeared 17 days later, without chills and without signs other than extreme asthenia and attacks of abundant sweating. In particular the patient had no digestive or articular sign, no eruption, and no sore throat. Blood culture revealed hemolytic streptococci that were probably contaminants.

The patient presented an appearance of great weariness, with a temperature of 39° C. and an erythematous rash on the face, neck, and upper thorax. The conjuctivae were slightly subicteric. Ptosis of the liver was detected, but liver volume was normal. The examiner noted superficial and diffuse inguinal, axillary, and subclavicular adenopathies made up of small, hard, mobile, painless lymph nodes. The severe edema of the prepuce made it impossible to uncover the glans, from which oozed thick pus. Palpation of the glans under the prepuce revealed an indurated painful zone the size of a lentil in the region of the frenulum preputii.

Blood examination showed 4,000,000 red cells and 5000 white cells of which 40 per cent were polymorphonuclear neutrophils, 48 per cent lymphocytes, 4 per cent monocytes, 2 per cent plasmocytes, and 5 per cent mononuclear cells.

Three blood cultures proved sterile. The usual serological tests for syphilis and the Nelson test all gave negative results; the Paul-Bunnell reaction, however, was positive.

Local improvement made it possible to uncover on both sides of the frenulum a superficial red, clearly delimited ulceration, the size of a lentil, clean but painful, resting on a larger indurated plaque.

The positive diagnosis was based on the erosive balanoposthitis, the transitory subicterus, the erythematous eruption on the face and trunk, and the fever, asthenia, and adenopathy. The absence of sore throat and of plasmacytosis should be noted.

A series of other cases have been reported, each with preputial ulcerations and positive Paul-Bunnell test reactions. In no case could venereal contamination be proved. The genital lesion, no doubt the portal of entry of the disease, can precede by some two weeks the characteristic alteration in the differential white cell count that suggests determination of the Paul-Bunnell reaction. During this whole prodromal period, diagnosis is impossible.

UROGENITAL DISORDERS IN VARIOUS INFECTIONS BY NONVIRAL AGENTS

INFECTIONS BY AGENTS OF THE PSITTACOSIS-LYMPHOGRANULOMA VENEREUM-TRACHOMA GROUP

The urogenital manifestations of *lymphogranuloma venereum* are discussed in Chapter 52. We shall add here only that the association with epididymitis and even with orchitis was described in 1942.[36]

The agents of the TRIC* group are well known as possible responsible agents in abacterial urethritis. They can be detected in the urogenital system under three different circumstances: in systematic examination of the parents of a newborn infant with inclusion conjunctivitis, as part of the examina-

---

*The term TRIC is applied to the agents of trachoma (TR) and of inclusion conjunctivitis (IC).

tion of patients with ocular infection, and in study of an abacterial urethritis.

Epidemiological investigations have proved that *inclusion conjunctivitis of the newborn* is caused by contamination during birth by an infection of the maternal genital system. As a rule, the maternal infection is asymptomatic or, at the most, is manifested by leukorrhea during pregnancy. It is detected in samples taken at the cervix uteri that reveal inclusion bodies or permit detection of the responsible agent. The infection can exist without obligatorily provoking conjunctivitis in the infant.[23] It is frequently associated with other infestations or infections (trichomoniasis, moniliasis, gonococcal infection) that are probably responsible for any existent clinical signs and symptoms.

The fathers of such infants usually present urethritis with marked functional repercussions, especially dysuria, and mucopurulent discharge; examination reveals inflammation at the urethral meatus with papillary congestion. Examination of samples taken at this level shows cells with inclusions and the agent responsible for the conjunctivitis in the infant.

In the adult *certain ocular syndromes,* inclusion conjunctivitis, punctate keratoconjunctivitis, and even a picture clinically suggestive of trachoma may be associated with an infection of the genital system by an agent of the TRIC group. That the agent of trachoma itself can adopt urogenital localizations does not seem to be demonstrated. It is likely that the agent in all such localizations is that of inclusion conjunctivitis and that in unusually prolonged infections it is capable of creating trachoma-type lesions.[18] The infections of the urogenital pathways associated with these ocular syndromes in adults moreover show the same characteristics found in the parents of newborn infants with conjunctivitis.

These observations have incited systematic search for agents of the TRIC group in subjects with *urethritis.* In the absence of known microbial agents, such research has a particular interest since proof of the etiological role of a TRIC agent would permit a simple and effective treatment with *tetracycline.* Nonetheless the frequency of such infections is still difficult to ascertain. In 22 of 89 cases examined by Dunlop[22] the results of search for a TRIC or inclusion conjunctivitis agent were positive, but the au-

thor, who desired scrupulously to eliminate all possibility of laboratory contamination, proposed to retain only the eight cases in which the isolation was made on first passage. The relationships are still to be exactly determined between these agents and the ocular infections described in the preceding chapters and with syndromes as complex as the Fiessinger-Leroy-Reiter syndrome, in which the urethritis is occasionally associated with agents of the TRIC group.

INFECTION BY MYCOPLASMA

Mycoplasma are fairly frequent in the genital tract in both sexes, and their presence usually occasions no pathological sign. In 1954 Shepard[46] reported study of urethral samples from a patient with nongonococcal urethritis in which he found, in the middle of the larger colonies of *Mycoplasma hominis,* smaller colonies of a mycoplasma that he baptized T strain (T for tiny).

This T strain differs from other mycoplasma not merely by the size of its colonies but also in its staining characteristics and its mode of development on agar.

Since then, systematic search for the T strain in *nongonococcal urethritis* enabled Shepard and numerous other authors to establish the role of this agent in infections of the male genital tract.[47] The urethritis connected with T-strain mycoplasma is a venereal disease with an average incubation period of four weeks (extremes: three and five weeks). Its essential characteristic is urethral discharge, which usually is moderate in abundance, and often mucopurulent, and is associated with dysuria and itching of the urethra. The other associated functional signs—painful erections, inguinal and scrotal pain—are rare. Inguinal adenopathy occurs occasionally, and signs of prostatic involvement (increased volume) are fairly frequent.

The spontaneous evolution of the disease is usually toward chronicity with intermittent bouts of activity. The diagnosis should always be considered in urethritis resistant to penicillin in which gonococci cannot be isolated despite repeated attempts. It can be ascertained, however, only by isolation of the T strain from material obtained by scraping the urethral canal.

Treatment by tetracycline or oxytetracycline in a dose of 500 mg. every six hours for nine days is curative in 80 per cent of cases in the absence of all new infecting contact.

Women carriers of the T strain present no particular sign, but further research is required before the asymptomatic character of the infection in women can be asserted. The T strain is found in the products of urethral or cervical swabbing.

As concerns the other strains of mycoplasma, systematic investigation has revealed them with equal frequency in men with urethritis and in those in apparently excellent health. It is impossible in the present state of research either to affirm or deny with certainty their pathogenic role in the urogenital tract.[8, 15]

Q FEVER

During Q fever a few highly exceptional cases of urogenital manifestations (orchitis[29] and epididymitis[38]) have been reported.

BEHÇET'S SYNDROME

The complexity of Behçet's syndrome is shown by the variety and the number of pathological phenomena described: buccal and genital ulcerations, ocular lesions usually of the iridocyclitis type with hypopyon, more rarely cutaneous, articular, and vascular features. Behçet himself considered the possibility of a viral origin in this disease from the time of his earliest descriptions. The proof, however, has still not been made. In a general review of the subject, Dudgeon[56] noted that the pathogenic organisms isolated belonged to no known microbiological group, that their characteristics, moreover, varied from one author to another, and that their responsibility for the appearance of the disease was in no wise proved.

BIBLIOGRAPHY

1. Andrieu, M., and Guichène, P.: Les orchi-épididymites grippales. Bull. Méd. Paris, *49*:483-486, 1935.
2. Artenstein, M. S., Cadigan, F. C., Jr., and Buescher, E. L.: Clinical and epidemiological features of Coxsackie Group B virus infections. Ann. Intern. Med., *63*:597-603, 1965.
3. Bernd, L. H.: Orchitis as a complication of influenza. Mil. Surgeon, *45*:222, 1919.
4. Bacher. Cited by Morrison and Baird.[39]
5. Blanton, Burham, and Hunter: J.A.M.A., Vol. 72, 1916.
6. Bugbee, H. G.: Infections of genito-urinary tract complicating influenza. J.A.M.A., *73*:1053-1056, 1919.
7. Celers, J.: In: Encyclopédie Médico-Chirurgicale. Maladies Infectieuses. II. 8068 A. 10, 1-10; 8068 A. 30, 1-5. Paris.
8. Chanock, R. M.: Mycoplasma infections of man. New Eng. J. Med., *273*:1199, 1257, 1965.
9. Cheatham, W. J., Weller, T. H., Dolan, T. F., Jr., and Dower, J. C.: Varicella: report of two fatal cases with necropsy, virus isolation, and serologic studies. Amer. J. Path., *32*:1015-1035, 1956.
10. Chiari, H. Cited by Councilman et al.[13]
11. Connolly, N. K.: Mumps orchitis without parotitis in infants. Lancet, *1*:69-70, 1953.
12. Coran, A. G., and Perlmutter, A. D.: Mumps epididymitis without orchitis. New. Eng. J. Med., *272*:735, 1965.
13. Councilman, W. T., Magrath, G. B., and Brinckerhoff, W. R.: Studies on pathology and on etiology of variola and of vaccinia. I. Pathological anatomy and histology of variola. J. Med. Res. 2:12-135, 1904.
14. Craighead, J. E., Mahoney, E. M., Carver, D. H., Naficy, K., and Fremont-Smith, P.: Orchitis due to Coxsackie Virus Group B, type 5. New Eng. J. Med., *267*:498-500, 1962.
15. Csonka, G. W., Williams, R. E. O., and Corse, J.: T-strain mycoplasma in non-gonococcal urethritis. Lancet, *1*:1292-1295, 1966.
16. Curshman, H. Cited by Councilman et al.[13]
17. Dargein, and Germain: Bull. Soc. Méd. Hôp. Paris, May 20, 1929, p. 622.
18. Dawson, C. R., and Schachter, J.: TRIC agent infections of the eye and genital tract. Amer. J. Ophthal., *63*:(Suppl.)1288-1298, 1967.
19. Dixon, C. W.: Smallpox. London J. & A. Churchill, Ltd. 1962, p. 98.
20. Dooley, J. R., and Burkle, J. S.: Three faces of dengue. Arch. Intern. Med., *117*:170-174, 1966.
21. Duboucher. Soc. d'Urologie, Nov. 8, 1920.
22. Dunlop, E. M. C., Freedman, A., Gardland, J. A., Harper, I. A., Jones, B. R., Race, J. W., du Toit, M. S., and Treharne, J. D.: Infection by Bedsoniae and the possibility of spurious isolation. 2. Genital infection, disease of the eye, Reiter's disease. Amer. J. Ophthal., *63*(Suppl.):1073-1081, 1967.
23. Foy, H. M., Wang, S. P., Kenny, G. E., Johnson, W. L. and Grayston, J. T.: Isolation of TRIC agents and mycoplasma from the cervix of pregnant women. Amer. J. Ophthal., *63*(Suppl.): 1053-1056, 1967.
24. Frehse, K.: Med. Klin., Aug. 17, 1935.
25. Fremont-Smith, P.: Orchitis due to Coxsackie Virus Group B, Type 5. New Eng. J. Med., *267*:498-500, 1962.
26. Gellis, S. S., McGuinness, A. C., and Peters, M.: A study of the prevention of mumps orchitis by gamma globulins. Amer. J. Med. Sci., *210*:661-664, 1945.
27. Gerner, K.: Prostatite au cours des oreillons. Pol. Tyg. Lekarski. English summary. 7:1673-1675, 1952.
28. Grégoire, J., Labram, C., Dreyfus, B., Domart, A., and Hazard, J.: Un cas de mononucléose infectieuse avec localisation génitale. Bull. Soc. Méd. Hôp. Paris, *113*:288-290, 1963.
29. Gsell, O.: Klinik und Epidemiologie des Q-

Fiebers. Helv. Med. Acta, *17*:279-300, 1950.

30. Huss. Cited by Morrison and Baird.[39]

31. Jamieson, W. M., and Prinsley, D. M.: Bornholm disease in the tropics. Brit. Med. J., *2*:47-50, 1947.

32. Kocen, R. S., and Critchley, E.: Mumps epididymo-orchitis and its treatment with cortisone. Report of a controlled trial. Brit. Med. J., *2*:20-24, 1961.

33. Lavergne, V. de, and Florentin, P.: Bull. Acad. Méd., 1925, p. 362.

34. Lewis, J. M., and Utz, J. P.: Orchitis, parotitis and meningo-encephalitis due to lymphocytic-choriomeningitis virus. New Eng. J. Med., *265*:776-780, 1961.

35. Mackay-Dick, J. Cited by Riggs and Sanford.[48]

36. Midana, A. Cited by Riggs and Sanford.[48]

37. Mitchell, S. C., and Dempster, G.: The finding of genital lesions in a case of Coxsackie virus infection. Canad. Med. Assoc. J., *72*:117-119, 1955.

38. Moeschlin, S., and Koszewski, B. J.: Komplikationen des Q-fever. Schweiz. Med. Wschr., *80*:929-931, 1950.

39. Morrison, R. J. G., and Baird, J. P.: Orchitis in Bornholm diseases. Brit. Med. J., *1*:198-199, 1952.

40. Norton, R. J.: Use of diethylstilbestrol in orchitis due to mumps. J.A.M.A., *143*:172, 1950.

41. Ormiston, G.: Orchitis as a complication of chicken pox. Brit. Med. J., *1*:1203-1204, 1953.

42. Riggs, S., and Sanford, J. P.: Viral orchitis. New Eng. J. Med., *266*:990-993, 1962.

43. Sabin, A. B.: Dengue. In: Rivers, T. M., and Horsfall, F. L., Jr. (eds.): Viral and Rickettsial Infections of Man. 3rd ed. Philadelphia, J. B. Lippincott Co., 1959, pp. 361-373.

44. Sabrazès, J.: L'orchite de la varicelle. Bull. Acad. Méd. Paris, *98*:122-127, 1927.

45. Savran, J.: Diethylstilbestrol in prevention of orchitis following mumps. Rhode Island. Med. J., *29*:662, 1946.

46. Shepard, M. C.: Recovery of pleuropneumonia-like organisms from Negro men with and without nongonococcal urethritis. Amer. J. Syph., *38*:113-124, 1954.

47. Shepard, M. C., Alexander, C. E., Lunceford, C. D., and Campbell, P. E.: Possible role of T-strain mycoplasma in nongonococcal urethritis. J.A.M.A., *188*:729-735, 1964.

48. Smith, I. M., and Bishir, J. W.: Treatment of mumps orchitis with ACTH and cortisone. New Eng. J. Med., *258*:120-124, 1958.

49. Sulkin, S. E., Burns, K. F., Shelton, D. F., and Wallis, C.: Bat salivary gland virus: infections of man and monkey. Texas Rep. Biol. Med., *20*:113-127, 1962.

50. Tunbridge, R. E., and Gavey, C. J.: Epidemic epididymo-orchitis in Malta. Lancet, *1*:775-779, 1946.

51. Verrier, P., and Burlet, P.: Du syndrome orchite aiguë chez l'adolescent et l'adulte jeune. Lyon Méd., *195*:349-353, 1956.

52. Warin, J. F., Davies, J. B. M., Sanders, F. K., and Vizoso, A. D.: Oxford epidemic of Bornholm disease, 1951. Brit. Med. J., *1*:1345-1351, 1953.

53. Weyrauch, H. M., and Gass, H.: Urogenital complications of dengue fever. J. Urol., *55*:90-93, 1946.

54. Wesselhoeft, C.: Mumps: its glandular and neurologic manifestations. In: Gordon, J. E., et al. (eds.): Virus and Rickettsial Diseases. Cambridge, Harvard University Press, 1943, pp. 309-348.

55. Wesselhoeft, C., and Pearson, C. M.: Orchitis in course of severe chicken pox with pneumonitis followed by testicular atrophy. New Eng. J. Med., *242*:651, 1950.

BEHÇET'S SYNDROME

56. Dudgeon, J. A.: Virological aspects of Behçet's disease. Proc. Roy. Soc. Med., *54*:104-106, 1961.

57. Mortada, A., and Imam, I. Z. E.: Virus aetiology of Behçet's syndrome. Brit. J. Ophthal., *48*:250-259, 1964.

58. Sezer, N.: Further investigations on the virus of Behçet's disease. Amer. J. Ophthal. *41*:41-60, 1956.

PART IX

Involvement of the Eye and Ear During Viral Infections

54

Involvement of the Eyelid, Conjunctiva, Cornea, Sclera, and Anterior Segment*

By R. NATAF AND G. COSCAS

All the membranes, media, and adnexa of the visual organ can be involved directly or indirectly by viruses. For convenience, we shall first consider localized involvements of the eyelid, conjunctiva, cornea, sclera, lacrimal gland, and the anterior portion of the uvea. Certain diseases that provoke ocular syndromes of greater complexity will receive more ample attention: the viral diseases, herpes simplex, and herpes zoster in particular, to which we shall add trachoma and inclusion conjunctivitis although the etiological agents are not viruses but members of the psittacosis-ornithosis-lymphogranuloma venereum group.

LOCALIZED INVOLVEMENTS

THE EYELID AND VIRUSES

Numerous palpebral disorders appear as secondary localizations integrated within the clinical picture of viral disease. Occasionally they can even orient the etiological diagnosis of the viral disease, in cases such as vaccinia, herpes zoster, or herpes simplex.

Palpebral tumors due to viruses will be the essential topic here; the other viral disorders of the eyelids will be described with the symptomatology of the systemic diseases provoked by the virus.

The only viral tumors at present recognized in man show a predilection for the facial skin and the eyelids.

Molluscum Contagiosum. The disease constitutes a clinically and biologically well-defined entity (cf. Chapter 35).

The lesions are usually sufficiently typical in appearance to permit clinical diagnosis. The disease is contagious and inoculable. It often provokes associated conjunctival and corneal disorders. The palpebral localization is among the most frequent, but the disease can involve the skin in a variety of body areas.

The individual lesion characteristic of molluscum contagiosum appears as a small rounded pearl-like tumor that is wider and more spread out in the center than at its pedicle. At the surface the skin is smooth and slightly whitish; it presents a small brown umbilicate depression. On pressure, a grayish-white, greasy-looking matter containing stratum corneum cells and ovoid refringent bodies visible under the microscope oozes from this "umbilicus." As a rule the volume of the tumor is small, rarely exceeding 0.5 to 2 mm. in diameter; it rests on normal-appearing skin. Such tumors are situated on the cutaneous surface of the eyelids, distant from the eyelashes in some instances, but on the palpebral border itself in others.

Usually several small tumors, dispersed or grouped, disseminate over the face. Eberth counted 107 elements on the face of a little girl, 31 of which were on the eyelid.

---

*For figures for this chapter, see color plate.

The local course is benign but protracted. The neoformations may become secondarily infected spontaneously, by scratching, or by eczematization, and may then simulate a malignant tumor. They may also suppurate and discharge their content spontaneously, leaving a scar; even in this case, however, preauricular adenopathy is absent.

Conjunctival complications are frequent, and follicular conjunctivitis often accompanies nodules of molluscum contagiosum situated on the ciliary border.

The cornea, which is more rarely involved, may present different types of keratitis (punctate, marginal, or rosacea) or pseudopannus.

The *diagnosis* of molluscum contagiosum is generally made on the basis of the clinical aspect; it is easily confirmed by biopsy.

Histological examination shows that the tumor is constituted by a genuine invagination in the dermis of piriform epidermic globules with the narrower ends converging toward the center of the tumor. The globules are made up of cells of the malpighian layer that have undergone the double alteration of hyperkeratinization and degeneration and constitute molluscum bodies. These bodies themselves contain the elementary bodies of the causal agent.

The pathogenic agent of molluscum contagiosum is one of the most voluminous of human viruses. It confers no immunity. Its contagiousness and its transmission are well known clinically and experimentally (cf. Chapter 35).

There is no known medical *treatment* of the disease. Only removal of the lesions by surgical means or diathermy seems to be curative. An interesting fact worth emphasis is that ablation of cutaneous tumors distant from the palpebral border suffices to cure the conjunctivitis or keratitis that may result from them.

Warts on the Eyelids. The contagiousness and the frequent auto-inoculation of warts (cf. Chapter 35), as well as the frequency of their palpebral localization, are well-established facts.

Warts, which are characterized by local epithelial hyperplasia, may appear singly or in groups on the eyelid. As in other cutaneous areas, they present different *clinical forms*.

COMMON VERRUCA VULGARIS. This form is characterized by a small grayish or brownish tumor with a nodular or papillary appearance and a prickly surface. It can represent a confluent tumor with an area as large as 1 cm.² to 2 cm.² It is frequent in children but may be seen at all ages.

VERRUCA PLANA. The lesion is smaller than in verruca vulgaris, with a maximum diameter of 1 mm. to 5 mm. It is yellowish and rounded; at the surface small papules are easily visible. Verrucae planae are always multiple; they are most frequent in boys at puberty but occur at all ages.

VERRUCA FILIFORMIS. This type of wart develops in length with a finger-like form and can attain 2 mm. to 10 mm. Its surface becomes keratinized more or less rapidly and produces a so-called horn of the eyelid. This wart has a predilection for the lower eyelid at the limit of the lashes or near the external angle.

CONDYLOMATOMATOUS OR PAPILLOMATOUS VERRUCA. This type is frequent in young adults on the genital organs (venereal warts). It may appear on the eyelids at the limit of the palpebral conjunctiva behind the lashes or on the caruncula. It constitutes a noncorneous red tumefaction with numerous papillomatous digitationes that are prone to hemorrhage and appear raspberry red. These warts are particularly refractory to all treatment, by medical, surgical, or physical agents.

Palpebral warts, whatever their form, like molluscum contagiosum can lead to *true ophthalmological complications:* refractory conjunctivitis, various types of keratitis, and even iridocyclitis.

Histological study of the wart shows a tumor represented by hyperkeratosis englobing papillary hypertrophy with lymphocytic inflammation. It also shows intranuclear and intracytoplasmic inclusions considered to be viral inclusions.

The causal agent is a virus (cf. Chapter 35) represented by a globular body of approximately 50 mμ that can be preserved at low temperature and survive for 30 minutes at 50° C.

THE CONJUNCTIVA AND THE CORNEA AND VIRUSES

Viral conjunctivitis, keratoconjunctivitis, and keratitis are frequent. Moreover, the involvement of the conjunctiva and of the cornea in certain human viral infections can be of first-ranking importance.

Adenoviruses. In the last 15 years or so, it has been shown that adenoviruses are frequently responsible for conjunctivitis and for keratoconjunctivitis.

Whether or not the ocular disorder is part of an "adeno-pharyngo-conjunctival syndrome," the adenoviruses occupy a place of ever-increasing importance in the pathology of viral conjunctivitis and keratoconjunctivitis.

Many cases of follicular or catarrhal conjunctivitis, the viral agent of which was once not definitely known, thus now have an established etiology; at present the number of cases of conjunctivitis and keratoconjunctivitis still "in search of a virus" is small.

The extra-ocular disorders due to adenoviruses are treated in the chapters on the particular type of manifestation they produce, such as acute respiratory disease, and "atypical pneumonia."

We shall consider here the *adeno-pharyngo-conjunctival* syndrome in its classic form, *adenovirus conjunctivitis*, and *epidemic keratoconjunctivitis*.

ADENO - PHARYNGO - CONJUNCTIVAL SYNDROME. This syndrome is characterized by the triad of fever, pharyngitis, and conjunctivitis, with which cervical adenopathy and systemic signs may be associated.

The disorder may take an epidemic, endemic, or sporadic form. Although it was individualized in 1951 by Cockburn and related to APC type 3 (*adenovirus 3*) in 1955 by Bell et al., it seems that this syndrome was described by Beal under the aegis of Morax in 1907. It is now recognized that this adeno-pharyngo-conjunctival fever may be provoked not only by adenovirus type 3, but more or less frequently by types 1 to 7 and type 14. Other adenovirus types may also perhaps be responsible.

The disease occurs in all seasons, but it seems that swimming pools have been the origin of numerous small epidemics involving mainly children and young adults of both sexes. The data on such epidemics suggest that, besides the air-borne transmission generally accepted for all adenoviruses, direct contamination of the eye by Flügge droplets or bathing water can occur. The possible duration of contagiousness is indicated by the length of time during which the virus is present in the pharynx and is thought to be ten days from the onset of the first signs.

After a five- to ten-day *incubation period,* the *course* lasts one or two weeks, or sometimes longer.

The *onset* is abrupt with fever from 38° to 39° C. (100.4° to 102.2° F.), accompanied by more or less acute pharyngitis, cervical adenopathy, fairly intense conjunctivitis, and systemic signs characterized by malaise, muscular and articular aching, and headache.

Conjunctivitis is present in two thirds of cases. It is usually bilateral, acute, and non-purulent, and produces a more or less abundant serous or seromucous discharge associated with hyperplasia of the ocular mucosa.

The conjunctivitis, which is occasionally simply hyperemic and congestive, is usually of the follicular type; the follicles are more pronounced in the lower fornix. The bulbar conjunctiva is usually only slightly involved; the infiltration does not reach the limbus corneae. Photophobia is mild, for the cornea is not always involved, but a superficial punctate keratitis is noted occasionally. Healing almost always is without sequela, unless superinfection occurs.

The adeno-pharyngo-conjunctival syndrome is not always complete: one or several signs may predominate or else be absent. Associated signs may be noted: cough, foamy sputum, thoracic pain, or otitis media, or more rarely nausea, vomiting, and diarrhea.

The etiological diagnosis can be established by the laboratory using serological reactions of complement fixation and neutralization, isolation, and identification of the virus.

Treatment, for the time being, is principally symptomatic; no medication seems to be directly active either on the virus itself or on the pathological process it causes. To avert all secondary infection, disinfection of the respiratory tract and ocular mucosa is, however, recommended.

EPIDEMIC KERATOCONJUNCTIVITIS. Epidemic keratoconjunctivitis constitutes an ophthalmological syndrome that occupies a place of ever-increasing importance in viral ocular pathology. The agent most often recognized at present as the cause of this disease is *adenovirus type 8.* It is possible, however, for other viral agents to be responsible.

The disorder, which is *transmissible and contagious,* occurs at all ages; it can appear in more or less localized epidemics, or in an endemic, or a sporadic form.

It has a certain number of common characteristics: epidemicity or endemicity, a superficial, usually punctate involvement of the cornea, absence of bacterial pathogens, and resistance to treatment.

Epidemics most often occur in collectivities: schools, the armed forces, workshops, and factories. A traumatism often seems to be, if not at the origin of the contamination, at least the factor favoring it, for instance, presence of foreign bodies under the eyelid or on the cornea, irritating smoke, and various microtraumatisms.

Severe epidemics of keratoconjunctivitis have even played a role in national activity. "Shipyard conjunctivitis" in the United States in 1941 and 1943 nearly had infortunate repercussions on the country's maritime construction, in the midst of World War II. In France, the Billancourt epidemic of keratoconjunctivitis in 1948 involved several thousand workers in the automobile industry.

Occasionally even simple ophthalmological measures such as tonometry or instillations of collyrium have provoked small epidemics in patients of dispensaries, hospitals, physicians' offices, and so forth.

All these epidemiological features have posed an important *medico-social problem* in the countries where severe outbreaks of the disease have occurred. Epidemic keratoconjunctivitis is now generally accepted to be a professional disease when outbreaks occur in a work setting.

The *incubation* of the disease is from five to ten days.

Its *onset* is usually abrupt, in the form of follicular conjunctivitis or, simply, intense catarrhal conjunctivitis without perceptible corneal involvement. It is almost always unilateral at the beginning. The other eye is contaminated within a few days, but as a general rule it shows less intense involvement.

The conjunctivitis is characterized by hyperemia and hyperplasia of the ocular mucosa, by numerous follicles and occasionally by suffusions of blood. These signs are more marked at the eyelid and the lower fornix. Lacrimation is intense; photophobia and the sensation of foreign bodies in the eye are marked. The discharge is usually catarrhal; it is rarely seromucous, but it is never purulent.

Periorbital pains are frequent and sharp; they seem to be linked to a sphincteralgic reaction, for when the original miosis is corrected by mydriatic drugs, pain is rapidly relieved.

A preauricular adenopathy is an almost constant feature, with a tumefied, painful pretragal lymph node. This preauricular adenopathy appears fairly early.

More or less marked *systemic signs* may occur from this early phase onward. They consist of moderate fever, dryness of the mouth, irritation of the throat and of the respiratory tract, and headache. Thus a genuine syndrome of adeno-pharyngo-conjunctival fever is often found.

The *keratitis* that is the hallmark in clinical diagnosis appears toward the tenth day. The corneal lesions are constituted by small foci of superficial subepithelial infiltration in the form of thin corneal opacities of variable size and form. Their size ranges from that of the head of a pin to 0.25 mm. in diameter or larger. Their number ranges from a few lesions to several dozens. They are dispersed or grouped, or may follow a crownlike pattern without tendency to confluence; often when they are grouped, they occupy the central area of the cornea and hence produce a severe, but usually transitory, visual impairment.

These foci of corneal infiltration do not always ulcerate. From their initial site in the thickness of the epithelium, they penetrate below it, then penetrate Bowman's membrane and occasionally the superficial layers of the corneal laminae. These corneal lesions may become superinfected in the presence of an erosion; this complication is marked by aggravation of pain and photophobia.

Neovascularization of the cornea does not occur either during the development of the lesions or after it. This feature is, moreover, one of the characteristics of epidemic keratoconjunctivitis.

The *evolution* of the keratoconjunctivitis varies according to the type of epidemic and the type of the causal virus. The disease may last from two weeks to several months, with remissions, outbursts of activity, and recurrences. The evolution of the corneal lesions may be slow, and their definitive disappearance may require weeks, months, or even years after clinical recovery. Healing, however, occurs without appreciable sequelae and with complete return of visual acuity.

The *clinical forms* are numerous and depend on what feature of the disease predominates: the conjunctival lesions or those of the cornea, the degree of tendency toward recurrence, and the form, which may be hemorrhagic, palpebral or conjunctival, or even orbital.

Certain forms of keratoconjunctivitis with an epidemic tendency occasionally appear during systemic diseases of viral origin, such as influenza, measles, or rubella. Rather than true epidemic keratoconjunctivitis, which does not seem to be involved, such cases seem to represent a feature of the systemic disease itself.

The complications and sequelae of epidemic keratoconjunctivitis, the most important of which is the long persistence of the corneal opacities, are almost always transitory. Ulcers are sometimes observed, but they are almost always due to superinfection. Iridic or ciliary impairment may be noted, but in general both are merely inflammatory phenomena.

The *diagnosis* of epidemic keratoconjunctivitis is relatively easy during the phase of full development before onset of any complication, or during an epidemic. At the onset, however, it may be difficult. The diagnosis may be suggested by the clinical characteristics or by microscope examination of smears that show numerous monocytes in the conjunctival discharge.

The etiological diagnosis can be established only by the laboratory: by isolation and culture of the virus (generally in tissue culture), and identification by *group reactions* (complement fixation), and by neutralization tests (revealing *the type* of the causal agent).

The *prognosis* of epidemic conjunctivitis is benign in general, but it should be emphasized that functional recovery is complete only at the end of several months.

The pathology of the disease has been the subject of numerous studies. The corneal subepithelial foci are mainly composed of monocytes. Intranuclear inclusions have been found in the corneal cells of the inoculated rabbit, but such inclusions have hardly been observed in the spontaneous human disease.

The *causal agent* of epidemic keratoconjunctivitis is almost always, if not always, adenovirus type 8. It has been found in numerous epidemics in America, Europe and Asia. Adenovirus 8, which was isolated by Jawetz, Kimura, and Thygeson, presents the characteristics of the group and certain particular characteristics that permitted a type to be individualized (cf. Chapter 44).

No specific *treatment* of epidemic keratoconjunctivitis at present exists. The usual antiseptics and the sulfonamides and antibiotics do not seem to act on the agent itself. However, broad-spectrum antibiotics in topical application (collyrium, oculentum), which act on secondary infections, seem to have a favorable action. Similarly, systemic therapy of various types—antibiotics, sulfonamides, serum therapy, gamma globulins—occasionally seems to improve the results of the topical medication.

OTHER ADENOVIRUS-PROVOKED CONJUNCTIVITIS. Different types of adenoviruses can provoke more ordinary inflammations of the ocular mucosa. The infection most often produces follicular conjunctivitis, or occasionally, simple, acute or subacute, catarrhal conjunctivitis with no defined clinical type. The adenoviruses most often isolated are types 1 to 8 and 14.

CRITERIA OF DIAGNOSIS OF AN ADENOVIRUS INFECTION. The main elements of the diagnosis of adenovirus disorders are summarized as follows:

The *clinical criteria* are their epidemic, often familial, character; a follicular or, particularly, a hyperemic type of conjunctivitis; superficial and punctiform corneal lesions, and systemic signs.

The *laboratory criteria* comprise tissue culture of the virus from ocular, pharyngeal, or other samples, and serological tests (made on a first sample taken within the first five days and a second taken after an evolution of two weeks), in which the complement-fixation reaction determines the *group* and the neutralization test reveals the *type*.

We have considered here only the conjunctival and corneal involvements due to adenoviruses. These viruses are occasionally at the origin of more severe disorders of the eye, in particular iritis, iridocyclitis, and uveitis; we shall return to these infections further on under the appropriate headings.

Other Viruses. CONJUNCTIVITIS IN MOLLUSCUM CONTAGIOSUM. This conjunctivitis is usually of the *follicular type* with predominance of the follicles on the eyelid and the lower fornix.

The *catarrhal type* is less frequent and less characteristic. The hyperemia and hyperplasia are more marked at the same sites as in the follicular type.

The *phlyctenular type* is even rarer; the phlyctenules are multiple not only on the bulbar conjunctiva but also at the sclerocorneal limbus.

The *pseudotumoral form* is the most exceptional. It presents small formations adherent to the conjunctiva but free at the deeper levels. The size of these elements is variable, occasionally reaching the size of a bean; their color is yellowish. Paradoxically, there is no inflammatory reaction of the palpebral mucosa.

Histological examination reinforced by virological study of these neoformations permits their diagnosis.

The *keratoconjunctivitis* due to molluscum contagiosum may present several different clinical forms. The most frequent is superficial punctate keratitis; sometimes corneal ulcers may become superinfected. Another form is marginal pannus-like keratitis; still more rarely, nodular corneolimbic neoformations occur.

Medical treatment is practically ineffectual. Physical and surgical means give better results. Removal of the nodules of molluscum contagiosum, even when they are far from the conjunctiva, leads to healing of the conjunctival and corneal lesions in this disorder.

CONJUNCTIVITIS IN VERRUCA VULGARIS. A wart can provoke a catarrhal type of conjunctivitis or, even more rarely, superficial keratoconjunctivitis. Neither disorder has a distinctive character. Medical treatment is inactive; only exeresis of the wart leads to rapid healing.

CONJUNCTIVITIS IN NEWCASTLE DISEASE. Newcastle disease, a "pseudo-encephalitis fatal in poultry-yard animals," in man is marked by conjunctivitis that is, if not the only manifestation, at least the one most apparent in the human disease. In man, however, a "pneumoconjunctival syndrome" also exists, but the pulmonary involvement is often inconspicuous and unrecognized. Signs or symptoms of encephalitic type are highly exceptional in man and always extremely discreet.

The human disease (distinct from psittacosis and ornithosis) appears mainly in poultry breeders, farmers, and veterinarians, canning and poultry-processing factory laborers, and laboratory workers manipulating the causative virus.

Clinically, Newcastle conjunctivitis presents an acute follicular type of inflammation with preauricular adenopathy.

The *incubation* period is one to two days. The onset, which is often unilateral, is abrupt, with a sensation of a foreign body in the eye, lacrimation, photophobia, and often violent nonlocalized pain of the type involving the sympathetic nervous system.

The ocular mucosa is hyperemic and occasionally dark red; it produces a serous or filamentous discharge that is usually not abundant. Palpebral edema is marked. These signs are often intense, and the patient may present an inflammatory pseudoptosis.

At the acme the bulbar and palpebral conjunctiva take on a venous color that becomes increasingly dark. The tarsal conjunctiva, Douglas' line, and the caruncle are invaded by numerous barely salient, mamillated, red follicles that are more abundant and voluminous in the lower fornix. The picture is occasionally less acute, and the follicles appear pearl gray.

The preauricular adenopathy is a regular feature and is represented by a slightly enlarged, painful lymph node with no tendency toward softening.

The course is relatively short. From the fourth day, and even though the clinical appearance remains unchanged, the intensity of the subjective signs decreases and pain ceases. By the end of the first week the clinical signs begin to improve, and they disappear within a maximum of two weeks to a month.

Systemic signs are discreet, and their presence is irregular. They are weariness, slight fever, sore throat, malaise, and muscular and articular aching.

The *clinical forms* of human conjunctival Newcastle disease do not seem to be numerous. The disorder can, however, appear as a proliferating conjunctivitis with preauricular tumefaction.

The viral origin of the disease was demonstrated in poultry-yard fowl in 1927 by Doyle at Newcastle upon Tyne in England. The first case of human conjunctivitis, however, was reported in only 1943 by Burnet, when three persons in his laboratory were contaminated while working on material infected with Newcastle virus.

The virus is at present identified and cultured with equal facility in the embryonated hen's egg or in tissue culture.

Man can be contaminated by the animal, but the inverse has not yet been demonstrated. Pannarale succeeded in inoculating the disease experimentally and in obtaining interhuman contamination. During recent years Radnót, Nelson, and Postic have shown that Newcastle disease in man is much less rare than previously supposed.

No specific treatment exists, but broad-spectrum antibiotics, applied topically and by the systemic route, avert complications.

THE CONJUNCTIVITIS AND KERATOCON-JUNCTIVITIS OF MEASLES AND RUBELLA mentioned here are limited to those due to the viral diseases themselves. The conjunctiva is a possible portal of entry of measles infection, as it is for numerous other systemic viral diseases. *The conjunctivitis in measles* is benign. It occasionally constitutes the only apparent clinical manifestation (in certain masked forms of measles). Biomicroscopic examination reveals small vesicles; by scrapings from them, Thygeson succeeded in transmitting the disease. A superficial punctate kerato-conjunctivitis occurs in 80 per cent of cases of measles. Except in cases of superinfection, the corneal involvement heals without sequelae. *The ocular symptoms of rubella* are similar to those in measles but generally less intense and more fleeting.

Further on in this chapter, special sections are reserved for the ocular involvements in herpes simplex and herpes zoster, in which the palpebral, conjunctival, corneal, and uveal lesions in these diseases are grouped.

Agents of the Psittacosis-Lymphogranuloma Venereum Group. CONJUNCTIVITIS IN REITER'S DISEASE (FIESSINGER-LEROY-REITER SYNDROME). *Ectodermosis pluri-orificialis,* which is constituted by an *intestinal-conjunctival-urethral-synovial syndrome* comprises conjunctivitis by definition. It is now generally recognized that this syndrome is frequently, if not always, related to an "inclusion body urethritis."

In July, 1916, Feissinger and Leroy noted in members of the French Armed Forces a "urethral-conjunctival-synovial syndrome" in 110 cases of epidemic dysentery. A few months later, Reiter observed in a young German officer a syndrome characterized by the three cardinal signs of arthritis, urethritis, and conjunctivitis, which had followed an episode of diarrhea.

The conjunctivitis that often is the first sign of this disease is mucopurulent, subacute, and bilateral from the onset, without a distinctive character. Pretragal adenopathy is frequent. Iridal and iridal-ciliary complications are exceptional and are found only in the severe, protracted forms of the disease, especially of the recurrent type. The conjunctivitis evolves, as does the disease itself, by bursts of activity that are more or less spaced out during several months or years.

In the etiology of this syndrome the agent most frequently supposed is that of inclusion-body urethritis, which belongs to the psittacosis-lymphogranuloma-trachoma group. Epithelial inclusions with initial bodies and elementary bodies have been found in this disease, frequently in the urethra and the conjunctiva, and less often in the synovial fluid of the articulations involved. Other pathogenic agents can provoke a similar clinical syndrome.

No specific therapy yet exists, but satisfactory results may be obtained by associating topical and systemic use of broad-spectrum antibiotics. This therapy must be repeated periodically and in cycles.

PROLIFERATIVE CONJUNCTIVITIS WITH PREAURICULAR ADENOPATHY. This condition is clinically typified by *Parinaud's conjunctival syndrome,* the etiology of which is highly diverse. In some instances the conjunctivitis represents a localization or a manifestation in the ocular mucosa of certain viral diseases. It can even be the only apparent sign of the disease, as in Newcastle disease. This conjunctival syndrome is more peculiar to lymphogranuloma venereum and cat-scratch disease, of which the first is certainly and the second is perhaps caused by agents of the psittacosis-lymphogranuloma-trachoma group.

In *lymphogranuloma venereum,* conjunctival localization does not seem to be frequent. The involvement is bilateral as a rule. The conjunctiva shows numerous violet-red polypoid formations especially in the fornix, which form a veritable paving. Ulceration does not occur, but the proliferations are covered with a mucofibrinous discharge. Palpebral edema is intense in some cases and may extend as far as the cervicotemporal region.

Preauricular adenopathy is marked. It occurs early: it becomes manifest from the second or the third day. The preauricular tumefaction is mobile and painless; it often evolves toward fistulation. Although usually the lymph node inflammation remains pretragal, it may spread and produce tumefaction of the whole maxillary and cervical region.

The conjunctivo-adenopathic form of the disease is due to contamination of the ocular mucosa by the agent. In such cases no extra-ocular or genital manifestations exist that suggest the diagnosis.

The course drags out over several months. The adenopathy persists a long time, but recovery occurs without conjunctival sequela.

The agent of this disease, *Miyagawanella lymphogranulomatis*, is discussed in Chapter 52. The etiological diagnosis is suggested by the result of the Frei intradermal reaction and confirmed by the laboratory by isolation of the pathogenic agent and the serological reaction.

Conjunctivitis in cat-scratch disease is not rare, since conjunctivo-adenopathic forms of this disease occur in nearly 7 per cent of cases (cf. Chapter 51). The incubation period may last from two weeks to two months; the date of the inoculation may be difficult to determine when the portal of entry was distant from the ocular mucosa. Cases in which the scratch nearest to the eye was noted only on the neck have been reported (Offret).

In clinical practice, the disease is often revealed by an intense palpebral edema.

The palpebral conjunctiva is the one mainly involved. The ocular mucosa, especially in the upper fornix, shows proliferations variable in size but always fairly marked, which are occasionally confluent and even ulcerated. Morax observed genuine phlyctena on the bulbar conjunctiva.

Pretragal adenopathy is always present; it occurs early and may reach the submaxillary and cervical lymph nodes. It can evolve toward softening and even fistulation.

General physical condition is only slightly altered in the conjunctivo-adenopathic form of the disease, which evolves toward recovery in a few weeks.

The etiological diagnosis can be confirmed by the intradermal reaction. Treatment of the disease is based on topical and systemic use of broad-spectrum antibiotics, which shorten the course and permit recovery in about ten days.

The Cornea and Viruses

Viruses in general, and particularly the dermoneurotropic viruses, provoke on the cornea, as they do on the mucosae and the skin, eruptive elements that constitute *viral keratitis*. Such corneal lesions are due in some instances to the direct action of the virus but, in others, to an indirect action consequent to lesions of the trophic and sensory nerves of the cornea.

Viral keratitis occupies a distinct place between infectious inflammatory keratitis and neurotropic keratitis in general. The clinical pictures vary considerably, and it is difficult to study them within the framework of a purely morphological or etiological classification. Different viruses can provoke the same clinical type of keratitis, whereas the same virus can give rise to different-appearing corneal disorders.

Viral keratitis is unilateral as a rule, and only exceptionally bilateral from the onset or successively. Corneal sensitivity is always altered, to a variable degree, ranging from simple hypesthesia to complete anesthesia of the cornea, as in an authentic neuroparalytic keratitis. This alteration of corneal sensitivity has a high value in diagnosis, and in the prognosis, as well. It is often accompanied by subjective hyperesthesia and trigeminal neuralgia.

Viral keratitis also presents certain more or less common characteristics in regard to the circumstances in which the disorder appears. The disease involves young subjects. It often follows an infectious or febrile episode. Reactivation of the disorder is frequent after similar episodes or a local infection, particularly otorhinolaryngeal. An apparently minimal traumatism can set them off; postoperatory viral keratitis is noted occasionally.

The course of viral keratitis often has certain peculiarities. After an acute onset, the disorder becomes torpid, and cicatrization is slow and difficult. Recurrences often occur. Sometimes recurrences have a notably cyclic character, the same eye showing a keratitis clinically identical with that or those that preceded it.

All forms of keratitis—superficial, parenchymatous, or deep-seated—may have a viral etiology.

Superficial keratitis is a disease of young subjects, who show an acute form of corneal involvement. In such cases, the keratitis is usually accompanied by more or less intense signs of inflammation, the picture being that of acute keratoconjunctivitis.

Occasionally the conjunctival element, accompanied by adenopathy, dominates the picture, but neuralgic pain should suggest corneal involvement; systematic biomicroscopic examination reveals it, in a superficial punctate form or that of a more or less well-delimited erosion.

The lesions may be fleeting and discreet, and pass unnoticed. As in the eruptive viral diseases, measles in particular (cf. Chapter 27), superficial viral keratitis may present the appearance of nummular keratitis with large, deeper deposits, the nodules of which may ulcerate and become infected secondarily.

Subepithelial punctate keratitis with a torpid evolution may also be found; it leaves persistent sequelae.

Deep keratitis is most frequently of the *disciformis type*, and the central form is the most characteristic. Certain diffuse forms involving the whole corneal stroma produce a picture of true *parenchymatous interstitial keratitis*. Other sectorial forms, involving a triangular area of the cornea, may suggest an influenzal etiology, for example.

The more or less pure *endothelitides* constitute deep forms limited to the posterior corneal membranes.

Phlyctenular keratoconjunctivitis of limbic form may be caused or, at the least, set off in the young child by intercurrent viral infections: herpes, chickenpox, vaccinia, or measles.

These different types of keratitis have been observed in numerous supposed or proved viral infections: mumps, infectious mononucleosis, aphthosis, and measles, and in many viral diseases with or without an eruptive character. Corneal involvement by the virus of herpes simplex and by that of zoster produce syndromes highly peculiar to each of them.

THE SCLERA AND VIRUSES

Scleritis and episcleritis may be noted during various viral infections. Two clinical types occur.

ANTERIOR SCLERITIS. Usually a papule under the transparent bulbar conjunctiva is apparent. This nodule, which is painful and immobile as a rule, is adherent to the sclera.

POSTERIOR SCLERITIS. The presence of this involvement is announced by orbital pain and, on occasion, by concomitant choroiditis. The scleritis produces inflammation of the posterior segment with edema of

Tenon's capsule. Eyeground examination reveals edema of the whole posterior pole.

The functional signs are more or less discreet; lacrimation occurs; and, in particular, pain is greater in scleritis associated with viral infections than in scleritis of other types.

The scleral nodule or papule of scleritis or of episcleritis is fairly characteristic: it is pink, salient, slightly inflammatory, and surrounded by a zone of more or less apparent congestion. It is fixed and adherent at the scleral level, but the covering conjunctiva remains mobile at its surface.

The scleritis is characterized by diffuse redness in depth accompanied by congestion of Tenon's capsule and by pain. This diffuse injection often contrasts with a white perilimbic circle corresponding to the lymphoid infiltration of the subconjunctival spaces.

The involvement tends to disappear progressively, without sequela. In some cases, however, a bluish gray translucid cicatrix thins away the sclera and can give rise to a scleral ectasia. More rarely, certain cases of scleritis evolve toward scleromalacia and perforation.

Occasionally, the scleral involvements are accompanied by keratitis in the sector corresponding to the area of innervation injured by the scleritis itself.

Episcleritis, scleritis, or sclerokeratitis may be seen in numerous viral infections in man, such as zoster, herpes, chickenpox, mumps, and influenza, as well as in ectodermatosis pluriorificialis.

Treatment should be topical and systemic, symptomatic, and, if possible, causal. The topical therapy varies with the case (in particular, the state of ocular tension) and should be conducted under the direction of an ophthalmologist.

THE LACRIMAL APPARATUS AND VIRUSES

Involvements of the lacrimal apparatus are often observed during regression of systemic viral diseases, those due to adenoviruses, *Myxovirus parainfluenzae*, and rhinoviruses in particular. The lacrimal excretory apparatus, like the secretory apparatus, can be affected. Dacryoadenitis is the most frequent.

ACUTE DACRYOADENITIS. The inflammation occurs during an acute febrile state. It may be unilateral or bilateral, with clinical signs of variable severity. Inflammatory type swelling of the upper eyelid occurs in the external region. The conjunctiva is hyperemic and congested in the external part of the upper fornix. The ocular globe may be deviated downward and inward. In such cases the patient usually complains of diplopia suggesting ocular paralysis.

Lifting up of the choroid, visible by ophthalmoscopy, accompanies dacryoadenitis on occasion. Simultaneously, cutaneous hyperesthesia or hypesthesia may be noted in the malar region.

HYPERACUTE DACRYOADENITIS. Cases of hyperacute dacryoadenitis with a phlegmonous appearance have been reported, but viral acute dacryoadenitis usually heals in a few days.

SUBACUTE OR CHRONIC DACRYOADENITIS. Usually this form represents a residue of an acute attack. Chronic viral dacryoadenitis, however, exists. The inflammation takes on a pseudotumoral appearance, because of obstruction of the small excretory ducts and chronic inflammation of the glandular tissue. Hernia of the palpebral lacrimal gland is disclosed by eversion of the eyelid.

These cases of unilateral or bilateral hypertrophy may also be associated with hypertrophy of the parotid and of the submaxillary glands, thus imitating clinically Mikulicz's disease.

The viral etiology of dacryoadenitis is a possible hypothesis in numerous cases. Only the laboratory can confirm the diagnosis.

THE ANTERIOR UVEA AND VIRUSES

The uvea, a vascular sponge comprising the iris, the ciliary body (anterior uvea), and the choroid (posterior uvea), reacts to all systemic and local infections. The involvement of the uveal tract is not always total and can be limited to either the anterior or the posterior part. In fact, although the inflammatory lesions may predominate in one, the other usually participates in some way, easy to detect or not. We shall consider here only anterior uveitis comprised by iritis and iridocyclitis.

Uveitis occurs in various viral infections in man: herpes, zoster, vaccinia, chickenpox, smallpox, adenovirus infections, influenza, mumps, and measles; it has also been reported during infectious mononucleosis. In these diseases and in primary uveitis direct action of the viral agent has rarely been proved.

Uveitis has no specific symptomatology: the uveal tract seems to respond in an identical, although varied, manner to bacterial and viral infections and to intoxications. Anterior uveitis occurs in young subjects, especially children.

As any uveitis, iridocyclitis can be distinguished by its pattern of development (acute, subacute, or chronic), or by the character of the reaction (serous, fibrinoplastic, hemorrhagic, or purulent), or by its pathological characteristics (nongranular or nodular). The ideal would obviously be an etiological classification, but it is not yet possible.

Iritis and iridocyclitis can often be a manifestation of the viremic phase of a systemic disease, such as influenza, and frequently remain unilateral.

The functional signs are fairly marked: dull, intermittent ocular and periorbital pain accompanied by photophobia and tearing.

The eye becomes red, with conjunctival vasodilatation that predominates around the cornea; the perikeratic injection, of variable intensity, is very different from the diffuse conjunctival hyperemia in conjunctivitis. At the same time the pupil retracts and shows myosis, while the iris remains normal appearing and the cornea intact. An important sign is lack of conjunctival discharge.

Slit-lamp *examination* reveals a typical Tyndall phenomenon of the aqueous humor in the anterior chamber of the eye, which arises from the turbidity and the hyperalbuminosis of the aqueous humor that are fairly characteristic of iridocyclitis. The exudation is manifested, in general, by serofibrinous deposits in the anterior chamber and, especially, on the posterior surface of the cornea on Descemet's membrane. These precipitates are comprised of leukocytes, reticuloendothelial cells, and, on occasion, uveal pigment. They are grayish and usually visible only with the biomicroscope. They can be more or less large or disseminated. Later they may be resorbed, become pigmented, and in large part disappear.

The exudative phenomena are occasionally marked, and flaky exudates are constituted that condense into a small lenticular mass in the pupillary area or occasionally into a hypopyon low in the anterior chamber.

All these inflammatory reactions give rise in time to posterior synechiae, fine irido-crystalline adherences clearly revealed by the irregularity of the pupil on attempt to dilate it. The adherences are fragile at first and may be broken by mydriatics; later these synechiae are firm and definitive. They can lead to deformations and occasionally adhesion: more or less complete "pupillary seclusion."

All the signs can often be seen with the naked eye or a magnifying glass, but bio-microscopic examination reveals them more easily.

Gonioscopy makes it possible to view the iridocorneal angle, by means of a prismat-ic contact lens. It reveals the hyperemia at the base of the iris, the exudates, and oc-casionally fine goniosynechiae that may close off the iridocorneal angle, obstructing the normal pathways of secretion from the aqueous humor and thus causing ocular hy-pertonia.

Puncture of the anterior chamber—useful in both diagnosis and therapy—makes possible biochemical and virological studies of the aqueous humor.

Spontaneously, anterior uveitis (iritis or iridocyclitis) evolves with bursts of activity, which are more or less closely spaced and lasting for several weeks or even several months. They open the door to complica-tions and to severe functional sequelae.

Certain *clinical aspects* deserve indi-vidual mention.

ACUTE SEROUS IRITIS. This form is usually unilateral and occurs mainly in young subjects. Its intensity is variable. As a rule it heals without sequelae in four to six weeks.

HYPERTENSIVE IRIDOCYCLITIS. An in-crease in ocular tension is not rare during iridocyclitis of whatever etiology. This hy-pertonia of the globe can be due to several factors: viscosity of the aqueous humor, exudative block of the iridocorneal angle, closure and blockage of the pupil, and edema of the iridic stroma and of the ciliary body.

Such iridocyclitis raises problems of dif-ferential diagnosis with diverse forms of glaucoma and difficult therapeutic problems, both medical and surgical.

HEMORRHAGIC IRITIS. Particularly in-tense hypervascularization may be compli-cated by hemorrhage of the uveal membrane constituting a hyphema of the anterior cham-ber. Hemorrhages may be recurrent and result in a "hemorrhagic glaucoma."

Subacute and Chronic Uveitis. Subacute uveitis with a protracted chronic course, and which is often recurrent, is fairly frequent. These forms present veritable nodules and granulomas formed by the agglomeration of lymphocytic and plasmocytic elements.

The time of onset is difficult to deter-mine exactly, but the signs are the same, although attenuated, as in acute uveitis. The evolution is slow and progressive; its dura-tion is much longer.

The *complications* as a general rule are the consequence of the inflammatory and exudative reactions. The synechiae may lead to more or less complete pupillary seclusion. Hypertonia and often severe glaucoma may then appear. The inflammatory process may extend to the posterior uvea, which more-over often participates to a variable degree in involvement of the anterior uveal segment. Cataract may be provoked by uveal lesions resulting in malnutrition of the lens and its opacification. In uveitis with a protracted course, all the structures of the ocular globe may become involved and thus result in blindness.

Signs Accompanying Uveitis. Uveitis is sometimes "accompanied" by nonocular signs that should be searched for systemati-cally; in certain cases they suggest a viral etiology and orient the laboratory research.

Meningeal signs are fairly frequent. Even in the absence of clinical signs, system-atic lumbar puncture has revealed menin-geal reactions in apparently isolated uveitis.

Involvement of the optic nerve (uveo-neuraxitis) and *of the auditive nerve* (uveola-byrinthitis) occurs; occasionally, *oculomotor paralyses* are found on the same side as the uveitis. Certain *glandular manifestations* have been reported, such as syndromes of uveoparotitis or association of hypertrophy of the palpebral glands with uveitis.

Cutaneomucosal signs are more sugges-tive of ophthalmic zoster, for example, but are occasionally present in an inconspicuous form in other viral diseases (herpes), or in states such as aphthosis and Vogt-Koya-nagi's syndrome.

Diagnosis. Although clinical diagnosis of a uveitis syndrome is usually easy, the viral etiology of the disease is only rarely proved.

When uveitis occurs during a recognized

viral disease, the possibility of a direct or indirect role of the virus itself easily comes to mind. Often, however, uveitis appears to be a primary disorder. Systematic careful history-taking with a view to disclose an episode of systemic infection, and the detection of the accompanying signs may suggest a viral etiology.

In certain cases the viral etiology could be proved by isolation and identification of the virus in the aqueous humor, cerebrospinal fluid, or blood during the acute phase at the onset of the uveitis. Serological tests can also be useful in diagnosis when the clinical data are sufficiently precise to orient their application.

Treatment. Treatment of iridocyclitis should be both topical and systemic. Topical therapy consists in instillations of collyrium of broad-spectrum antibiotics. Use of mydriatics is indispensable to avert pupillary blockage, but ocular tension should be carefully watched. This treatment requires specialized competence and should be conducted by an ophthalmologist.

Use of corticosteroids should be avoided in the early and the acute phases. Prudent utilization of corticosteroid therapy is, however, permissible under cover of antibiotics in the phase of full installment of the disease and during that of resorption.

COMPLEX OCULAR SYNDROMES

Herpes and the Eye

Herpes is an ectodermoneurotropic viral disease and can involve all the ocular membranes. The most serious ocular involvement is herpetic keratitis.

Herpes of the Eyelids. Herpetic eruption may appear on the cutaneous surface of the eyelids with more or less marked involvement of the free palpebral border. Herpetic blepharitis may thus be noted. The ulcerations of the integuments of the eyelid and its free border may be covered over with false membranes of diphtheroid type. The ciliary bulbi may be destroyed, with consequent definitive loss of the eyelashes. The palpebral eruptions may become superinfected and give rise to a genuine "contagious blepharitic impetigo," especially in children.

The herpetic lesions can also involve the eyebrow region and become superin-

fected, with resultant abscess of the eyebrow.

These palpebral manifestations of herpes may be isolated or associated with other ocular localizations. Preauricular adenopathy is often present, in the form of a small, mobile, barely painful lymph node. In case of secondary infection, however, this preauricular node becomes more voluminous and sensitive.

Herpes of the Conjunctiva. The conjunctiva, like all the other human mucosae, can be involved by herpes. Isolated conjunctival lesions due to herpes are difficult to diagnose. Often the vesiculo-erythematous stage passes unnoticed, and the lesions are observed at their ulcerative stage. The picture noted then is of small ulcerations that are isolated, grouped, or even confluent and covered by a whitish glaze producing fine false membranes, with a few bloody suffusions.

The conjunctivitis in primary herpes infection is often accompanied by an intense follicular reaction that masks the ulcerations. The conjunctival involvement, moreover, is usually much less prominent in the picture than the corneal manifestations.

Herpes and the Uvea. Herpetic iritis and iridocyclitis have the characteristics common to all uveitides, occasionally with a few features peculiar to them.

The uveal tract can doubtless be involved as an isolated manifestation of herpes or in the course of other manifestations of herpes distant from the eye, but during herpetic keratitis, particularly, the cornea seems to become permeable and no longer to resist penetration by the pathogenic agent. The virus has thus been isolated from the aqueous humor of patients with serious keratitis secondarily accompanied by iridocyclitis.

In the course of successive outbursts of herpes, superficial keratitis may occur, then deep keratitis followed by iridocyclitis or global uveitis.

Other Ocular Involvements in Herpes. In the course of herpes, all the ocular membranes—sclera, choroid, and retina—may also be involved. The optic nerve may also be attacked, and likewise the entire oculomotor apparatus of the eye; herpes thus occasions *optic neuritis* and *oculomotor paralysis* of different types.

Herpetic meningitis, encephalitis, meningoencephalitis, and other herpetic disorders can, moreover, lead to neuro-ophthalmological complications or localizations.

Herpes and the Cornea. Corneal attack by herpes is frequent and poses a daily problem to the ophthalmologist. Certain authors even believe that this etiology is to be suspected in the majority of cases of ulcerative keratitis.

Herpes is probably the most widespread human viral disease; recent statistics show that toward age 15 years, 90 per cent of subjects are carriers of the virus in a saprophytic state. Any systemic or localized infection can set off a herpetic keratitis, by a phenomenon of "viral amnestic reaction."

TYPICAL HERPETIC KERATITIS. *Superficial forms* are the most frequent and typical of herpetic involvement of the cornea. *Dendritic* ulcer of the cornea, which is commonest, suggests forthwith the clinical diagnosis of herpes. The subjective signs, which are pronounced, are: sensation of a foreign body in the eye, abundant lacrimation and intense photophobia, and periorbital, supraorbital, and suborbital pain irradiating to the area of the ophthalmic branches of the trigeminal nerve. Often the intensity of the signs of reaction contrasts with the discretion of the organic signs. Examination at this phase reveals a superficial, central or paracentral, corneal erosion that already has a characteristic morphology: ulceration with a distinct linear and arborescent pattern, without underlying infiltration, but more marked at its edges by detachment of the epithelium.

Hypesthesia or anesthesia of the cornea is remarked as a rule.

The mechanisms proposed to explain this anatomical pattern are numerous—for example, edema diffusing into the lymphatic spaces, and dichotomous nervous ramifications. Usually the ulcer is single and unilateral.

The initial stages of this keratitis generally escape detection, and certain authors believe that the erosion is present from the start. However, it may be a consequence of the rupture of epithelial corneal vesicles. This phase of vesicular keratitis is rarely observed owing to its fugacity. It consists of extremely superficial vesicles with a grapelike pattern at the site where the dendritic ulcer later appears.

The course is fairly protracted and is characterized by intermittent bursts of activity that are more or less closely spaced and long lasting. Healing occurs after several weeks and occasionally leaves sequelae "spotting" corneal transparency.

Deep forms are represented especially by disciform keratitis, which is the most frequent and the most characteristic.

Signs of reaction are usually mild, in contrast with those of ulcerous herpetic keratitis, but the patient may complain of periorbital pain. The loss of visual acuity is much greater than in the superficial form. Disciform keratitis appears as interstitial grayish white corneal opacity of disklike form with ill-defined edges situated at the center or paracentrally, while the periphery remains uninvolved and transparent.

Corneal hypesthesia or even anesthesia is marked on the central disk. The zone of corneal opacity is thickened and may be double the normal thickness owing to the infiltration of the corneal stroma by diffuse, especially posterior, edema. Descemet's membrane presents folds and white precipitates evidencing its participation in the process.

The disciform keratitis is torpid appearing and even gives the impression that the lesions are fixed. Although very different from dendritic keratitis, it is also characteristic of the corneal localization of herpes. Its course is generally protracted, and healing occurs slowly after many weeks.

ATYPICAL FORMS OF HERPETIC KERATITIS. The corneal lesions may present different superficial and deep aspects: they represent the atypical forms of herpetic keratitis.

Superficial forms are of two types. *Superficial punctate keratitis* is characterized by numerous small grayish punctiform foci that are very superficial and in variable number, generally in the uncovered corneal area in the region of the palpebral fissure. It most often occurs in young subjects and is frequently accompanied by a vesicular eruption on the eyelid and ciliary border as well as by conjunctivitis of variable intensity.

In general this form occurs in primary infections by herpes and may pose a difficult problem of differential diagnosis with regard to punctate keratoconjunctivitis of other origins. In herpes, however, the disorder is almost always unilateral, and the small ulcerations lie on only discreet underlying foci. Corneal sensitivity is, moreover, always altered.

This form of herpetic punctate keratitis

usually heals in a few days. The ulcerations, however, may spread and become prolonged; they may be stelliform, appear as a striate keratitis, or assume a dendritic type, with all the forms transitional between them.

Marginal herpetic ulcerations represent a localization of herpetic keratitis that is not rare, especially in young children. The corneal erosion is very superficial, without appreciable infiltration, and with irregular detached edges. The surface of the ulcer is hypesthetic, despite neuralgia pain. These ulcers are fleeting but recurrent, a characteristic suggesting a herpetic etiology.

In certain cases the ulcerations extend circularly along the length of the limbus forming erosive *annular ulcers* of the type of Mooren's ulcer. This extension is fortunately extremely rare.

Deep forms show corneal clouding as in disciform keratitis, but the infiltration is not limited to the center; it may occupy the entire corneal surface, thus posing the problem of differential diagnosis of interstitial keratitis. The lesion, however, remains unilateral. Occasionally the opacity occupies only a triangular segment at the base of the limbus and thus constitutes a segmentary keratitis fairly suggestive of its herpetic origin.

In other instances only the deep corneal laminae are involved, and the opacification may occur only in the endothelium, a fact classifying this form as an *endotheliitis* of the Desvignes type. Small, fugacious vesicles may even be seen bulging into the lumen of the anterior chamber.

PATTERNS OF DEVELOPMENT. The distinction between typical and atypical and deep and superficial forms is not absolute, and the types so distinguished can be overlapping.

The line of development of herpetic keratitis of whatever form is hard to schematize, but frequently the inflammation takes a direction toward the subepithelial layers. At the very least, the stroma in its superficial layers is often invaded.

Whereas the lesions of the conjunctiva and of the eyelids heal fairly rapidly without scarring, the corneal lesions become chronic and result in definitive opacities that considerably impair vision. This chronic and recurrent pattern of development can doubtless be explained by the avascularity of the cornea, which hence does not participate in the immune reactions of the rest of the organism.

Herpetic keratitis begins in various ways: occasionally during the regression of another viral or a bacterial infection. In other instances, corneal herpes seems to be provoked by trauma. Such traumatic herpes of the cornea is of special interest because of its relative frequency and of the medicolegal problem it poses.

Neuroparalytic keratitis may follow recurrent bouts of herpetic keratitis. Cerise and Thurel even believe that neuroparalytic keratitis is almost always caused by the herpes simplex virus and that the involvement of the gasserian ganglion plays only a supporting role.

Neuralgic recurrent keratitis is often herpetic, or at least this is a generally accepted hypothesis.

Metaherpetic keratitis is often the consequence of recurrent herpetic keratitis. In this case the ulcers do not have the same superficial character. They are roughly polycyclic with extensive ulcers in a maplike pattern, without separation at the edges. These lesions are accompanied by parenchymatous infiltration. They are tenacious and often serious; neovascularization of the cornea is characteristic. They leave sequelae constituted by corneal leukomas of variable size.

COMPLICATED FORMS. Uveal involvement occurs almost invariably in herpetic keratitis lasting a certain time. Even in superficial herpetic keratitis of two or three weeks' duration, iritis or iridocyclitis of some degree is rarely absent. In certain instances, the uveal involvement in herpetic keratitis can be due to the virus itself.

The "cortisone" forms of herpetic keratitis represent merely the aggravation provoked by corticosteroid therapy applied too early in herpetic keratitis. It seems that in corneal herpes, the topical application of cortisone or its derivatives from the onset of the disorder increases its intensity by diminishing the possibilities of epithelization and cicatrization of the cornea. This action of corticosteroids moreover favors necrosis of the stromal fibers, uveal reactions, and complications due to superinfection. Early application of corticosteroids in herpetic keratitis possibly favors meningeal and meningoencephalitic complications. Further, the corneal leukomas consequent to "cortisone" herpetic keratitis are often more extensive than in herpetic keratitis not treated with corticosteroids.

Superinfection in herpetic keratitis is a

risk in all superficial or deep herpetic keratitis, especially in the recurrent forms. This is particularly true in metaherpetic keratitis. The clinical picture then becomes characteristic of ulceration of microbiotic origin. The total anesthesia of the cornea should attract attention.

Diagnosis of the Ocular Involvement by Herpes. The clinical diagnosis should be suggested by the symptoms of the different manifestations of herpes. The etiological diagnosis is proved by the laboratory (cf. Chapter 34): isolation and identification of herpes virus, and the biological reactions of complement fixation and neutralization.

It is of interest to note that herpes virus was the first human virus to be studied experimentally by inoculation into the rabbit cornea in 1912. This inoculation, which is called Grüter's test, is currently used in ophthalmological practice for the clinical diagnosis of corneal herpes.

Treatment. The topical treatment should always include broad-spectrum antibiotics in oculentum or collyrium to avert all superinfection. Symptomatic, mydriatic, and anti-inflammatory therapy must be added in case of keratitis and uveitis. Ocular pressure must be checked concurrently and frequently.

IDU (5-iodo-2'-deoxyuridine) seems to have an elective activity on the herpes virus by its activity as an antimetabolite. It is applied topically by instillation every hour or every two hours during the day and in gel form during the night. This topical virostatic agent seems to shorten the course but does not prevent recurrences, although they seem to be less intense and shorter when this therapy is used.

Lysozyme and *gamma globulins* by instillation or injection may also be used, as well as various cicatrizing factors.

In herpetic keratitis, abrasion of the lesions, corneal "peeling," and application of antiseptics at this level may be of use. The persistent and obstinate forms, however, present a difficult therapeutic problem: although topical corticosteroid therapy is useful and effective, it carries the risk of serious complications and should not be used except under cover of an extremely strict ophthalmological surveillance.

Systemic treatment consists essentially in medication with a view to reinforcement of the host's defense mechanisms. Corticosteroid therapy by the systemic route is often useful.

Vaccination against herpes, recently introduced, seems to be the hope of the future.

ZOSTER OPHTHALMICUS

The term zoster ophthalmicus applies to the localization of herpes zoster in the nerve trunks of the ocular region and in the cutaneomucosal area innervated by the ophthalmic nerve.

"What characterizes zoster ophthalmicus and gives it a distinct place among the topographical forms of herpes zoster is, on the one hand, the involvement of the eyeball and its adnexa by the direct action on the nerves or its repercussion and, on the other, the oculomotor paralyses" (Brégeat).

Clinical Features. The sensory disturbances are usually more marked in zoster ophthalmicus than in other forms of zoster.

The intensity of pain increases with the patient's age. Pain precedes and accompanies the eruptions and associates neuralgia with pain in the sympathetic system. The neuralgia, which is intermittent, involves the territory of the trigeminal nerve. The pain in the sympathetic system, particularly at the plexuses, may be superficial or deep, but is continuous, with paroxysms of variable duration. The pain often involves an area wider than that governed by the trigeminal and extends to an entire half of the brain. Pain during zoster and after it is particularly intense and hard to bear in some instances.

Anesthesia may be noted; it may be localized at the different points of eruption or may extend to the entire area governed by the involved nerve branch.

The systemic disturbances are those of herpes zoster in general. They are: fever between 38° and 39° C. (100.4° to 102.2° F.), hyperleukocytosis with increase in the polymorphonuclear cells and the neutrophils, and a slight meningeal reaction.

The eruption involves one or both eyelids of the same eye. It does not extend beyond the facial midline and remains localized in the area of the trigeminal branch involved. This eruption goes through the stages usual in zoster. Erythematous patches are followed a few days later by blisters, which are either separate but in clusters, or confluent. On occasion, aberrant vesicles are noted slightly outside the eruptive zone. The elements wither and are covered over by a thin scab that falls between the tenth and the fifteenth day. The healed vesicles leave whitish scars surrounded by a slightly pigmented area that last a variable length of time.

Preauricular adenopathy almost always occurs in zoster ophthalmicus; it appears from the second or the third day of the eruption.

The eyelids show marked edema, as does the conjunctiva, with chemosis, and elements of eruption (only rarely seen at their vesicular stage). Hyperemia and seromucous discharge are fairly marked.

The topography of zoster ophthalmicus is even more characteristic than its morphology. The eruption occurs unilaterally on the dermatomes of the trigeminal nerve with no extension to the other side. The eruption may extend to all the dermatomes innervated by one of several branches. Various topographical distributions are recognizable.

In *frontal zoster* (interior or exterior) the eruption remains localized on the upper eyelid, forehead, and scalp as far as the vertex cranii.

Lacrimal or rather *lacrimotemporal zoster* is characterized by involvement of the upper eyelid, the bulbar conjunctiva, and the integuments of the temporal region.

Nasal zoster may involve only one of the nasociliary branches. In cases of infratrochlear nerve involvement the eruption is localized on the corresponding ala nasi. When zoster involves the anterior ethmoidal nerve, the eruption is characterized by a cluster of vesicles on the tip of the nose. At the same time inflammation of the nasal secretory mucosa may then be noted as well as vesicles on this surface. *The cornea innervated by the infratrochlear nerve can be involved in these forms.*

Most authors agree that zoster ophthalmicus provokes corneal vesicles, followed by ulcerations when the blisters burst. The ulcerations have been observed from the second or third day of the cutaneous eruption. Certain authors believe that the corneal lesions are parenchymatous from the outset and, in their opinion, appear between the fourth and the tenth day of the cutaneous eruption.

The keratitis in zoster is not usually accompanied by deep vascularization, and new-formed blood vessels originating in the limbus ramify at the periphery of the infiltrated cornea. As a rule, fissures occur in the infiltrated corneal areas.

Corneal hypesthesia can exist from the outset. Biomicroscope examination often permits detection of whitish subepithelial or even deep islets, thickening of the corneal nerves, and, on occasion, folds in Descemet's membrane. The primary keratitis in zoster usually heals without sequelae.

Scleral lesions are occasionally associated with those of the cornea and produce a picture of "sclerokeratitis." Such disturbances usually appear late. The scleritis following zoster is characterized by spots that at first are pink and have little vascularization and then appear slate colored; their site is usually at a certain distance from the limbus. This trophic scleritis has a slow course and thins away the ocular covering, with the risk of ectasia and scleromalacia.

Iritis and iridocyclitis in zoster are occasionally isolated, but they are more often associated with the keratitis and constitute an inflammation of the anterior segment. This inflammation often shows a sectorial type of topographical pattern. Systematic biomicroscopic examination of all patients with zona ophthalmica is indispensable.

Iritis, iridocyclitis, and uveitis due to zoster usually have a protracted course but are benign, only rarely leaving synechiae or more severe sequelae. Alteration of ocular pressure is relatively rare. Fairly late-appearing chorioretinal involvement may occur: it usually has a vascular and hemorrhagic character with exudates and, occasionally, venous or arterial thrombosis.

Optic neuritis, pupillary paralysis, and oculomotor paralysis should be searched for systematically. They usually evolve toward recovery, but their duration is highly variable: a few days to several months.

Course. The duration of zoster ophthalmicus is usually the same as that of other forms of zoster, i.e., about two or three weeks. Although the ophthalmic form is benign as a rule, it sometimes leaves functional or sensorial sequelae. The pain subsequent to it is often particularly intense and tenacious.

Diagnosis. Clinical diagnosis is usually easy in view of the unilateral and radicular topography of the erythemovesicular lesions and the pain. Recourse to the laboratory to confirm the etiology is of interest in some cases. Detection of Lipschütz inclusion bodies in smears of the vesicular serosity constitutes an important element in diagnosis; they are also found in chickenpox.

The serological reactions (complement fixation, neutralization tests, or others) are useful (cf. Chapter 30).

Prognosis. In general zoster ophthalmicus is benign. However, the pain subsequent to the ophthalmic form has rather a poor prognosis, owing not only to its intensity and its tenacity but to the paucity of the means available to combat it, particularly in the aged. In certain cases the pain has even led to suicide. The progress of neurosurgery now permits remissions, but the results are not consistent.

Treatment. Antiseptics and antibiotics in collyrium should be applied systematically but with moderation; all medication irritating to the cornea should be avoided.

In presence of a corneal or uveal localization, mydriatic drugs should also be administered, but ocular pressure must be watched. Topical utilization of corticosteroids should be extremely prudent and requires rigorous surveillance.

SYSTEMIC TREATMENT. Broad-spectrum antibiotics seem to have a certain efficacity, although no convincing conclusion can be drawn from the fact. They should, however, be utilized if only to combat secondary bacterial infections. Neurosedatives and analgesics should be associated with all medication directed against infection: aspirin, phenobarbital, tranquilizers, vitamins B_1, B_6, and B_{12}, and so forth.

X-ray therapy and ultraviolet irradiation occasionally lessen pain in zoster.

SURGICAL TREATMENT. In late and persistent pain subsequent to zoster, neurosurgical procedures may be indicated. David, Hécaen, Talairach, and Mounier recommended surgical interventions along the thalamocortical tract, especially in the posterioventral area of the thalamus. Le Beau, Feld, and Bovet advised topectomy. In any event, it seems that neurosurgical techniques may prove particularly useful in therapy of the late algesic phenomena following zoster.

TRACHOMA

Trachoma is a transmissible, specific keratoconjunctivitis, usually with a chronic course. It is characterized by follicles, papillary hyperplasia, and corneal pannus, and later by cicatrization (WHO Expert Committee on Trachoma, Third Report, 1962).

Trachoma is essentially a disease of poverty and of promiscuity, of ignorance, and of childhood.

The disorder, which can be traced back to earliest antiquity, is a worldwide social scourge that involves more than 600 million human beings in numerous regions; it creates some 200 million victims blinded in one or both eyes, or with impaired vision.

The geographical distribution of trachoma covers the greater part of the globe. Only countries with a high living standard are spared. Neither geographical nor racial factors seem to have a sparing action in this disease. On the other hand, the influence of living conditions is too obvious for any specialist in trachoma to consider it to be open to debate. No nation, no climate, and no race is safe against trachoma. With human migrations, the disease appears in regions from which it was previously absent, and it persists there.

Epidemiology. Epidemiological study of trachoma is particularly difficult. The disease is primarily familial: the infant of a mother with trachoma, if he is not infected during birth, contracts the disease in early infancy. Other than, and in addition to, this familial contamination, a large place remains for extrafamilial contamination, at school, in the workshop, in public places, and in assembled groups, for example.

The associated disorders play an important role in the spread of trachoma. Trachoma in itself is thought to be a relatively benign disease if a certain number of factors did not contribute to its aggravation, among which are the lack of elementary hygiene, unsanitary dwellings, overcrowding in conditions of promiscuity, a systemic disease, and other ocular infections.

Trachoma, owing to its involvement of the cornea, reduces the patient's capacities by impairing vision or even producing blindness. This fact makes evident the role played by the disease in the economic, social, and political activity of all the areas where the disease is endemic.

Clinical Studies. Trachoma, even in its pure form and without associated infection, is a chronic and polymorphous disease, without a cyclic course. The evolution is slow and the course punctuated by complications; there is complex overlapping of the different stages until healing finally occurs.

Establishment of an international classification of the different symptoms and stages during the course of trachoma became a necessity. The classification adopted in 1952 by the WHO Expert Committee of Trachoma (Second Report) is the one generally accepted.

TRACHOMA STAGE I. The initial phase of trachoma is marked by only the commonplace symptoms of a prickling sensation, lacrimation, and slight photophobia. The mucosa is occasionally slightly hyperplastic; papillae may be observed at the stage of their onset. Occasionally follicles, which are most easily detected by biomicroscopic examination, are seen from the onset. Even in the initial phase, the first traces of corneal pannus may also be detected; the sign appears early and strongly suggests trachoma (Nataf, 1929)

TRACHOMA STAGE II. The conjunctival mucosa appears rough and granular owing to the follicles and papillae.

Formal distinction between papillae and follicles is possible only under the biomicroscope. The follicle is a barely vascularized, essentially lymphoid element that belongs especially to the symptomatology of trachoma. The papilla, which is essentially vascular and only secondarily lymphoid, is an element commonplace in all conjunctival reactions; its center is marked by a cluster of small capillaries perpendicular to the level of the normal blood vessels.

The follicles of trachoma, when they reach maturity in the chronic stage, resemble "boiled sago" or "frog's spawn." A conjunctival follicle that crumples under slight pressure can not be confounded with any other conjunctival formation.

Frequently at this stage, the naked eye perceives the *corneal pannus,* a "vasculogranular veil." The subjective functional symptoms are intensified with development of this pannus or by secondary infections.

Stage II of trachoma varies in length and has no definite cycle.

TRACHOMA STAGE III. Trachoma ordinarily results in cicatrization by sclerosis on the conjunctiva and the cornea. The length of the precicatricial phase obeys no rule and may appear only after many years. This period is marked by appearance of the characteristic scars while islets of active follicles continue their development. The scars are constituted by extended fibrous ribs and by irregular, starlike, milky white formations the branches of which vary in width and number. These starlike scars are pathognomonic and permit retrospective diagnosis.

TRACHOMA STAGE IV. In this cicatricial or cicatrized stage, the tarsal conjunctiva presents an appearance suggesting the cause. The conjunctiva is streaked by scars in a more or less regular pattern. Most of them converge toward a homogeneous plaque, Arlt's line, situated in the middle third of the tarsal conjunctiva and pathognomonic of trachomatous scarring.

On occasion, conjunctival retraction and atresia of the fornix are noted with narrowing of the palpebral fissure.

PANNUS, KERATITIS, AND CORNEAL LESIONS. Trachomatous pannus is a very early sign of the disease. Trachoma spreads by contiguity and by continuity from the conjunctiva to the cornea and forms a vasculogranular veil over the cornea. In trachoma the pannus usually involves the upper part of the conjunctiva. Infiltration occurs, as well as neovascularization that overlaps the limbus and extends over the cornea, with corneal follicles homologous to the conjunctival follicles. The desquamation of these corneal follicles gives rise to peripheral corneal ulcers that constitute trachomatous keratitis.

PTOSIS, DEFORMATION OF THE TARSUS, AND TRICHIASIS. Trachomatous ptosis corresponds to the increasing heaviness of the upper eyelid. It seems to result from involvement of Müller's muscle (the circular part of the ciliary muscle) and from the tarsal hypertrophy. Frequently a highly peculiar incurvation characterized by arching of the eyelid and an S-shaped deformation of the palpebral border accompanies the tarsal hypertrophy. Trachomatous trichiasis-entropion then arises: it essentially comprises deviation of the eyelashes in the wrong direction, toward the palpebral fissure and the cornea. This development usually occurs late but has been observed in children aged five to ten years.

The trichiasis in trachoma leads to serious corneal lesions such as ulcers and leukomas, to irregular astigmatism and diminished transparency. These complications add to those of trachomatous keratitis itself. The corneal alterations severely impair vision.

COURSE AND CLINICAL FORMS. Trachoma may pursue its chronic course many years or even during an entire lifetime,

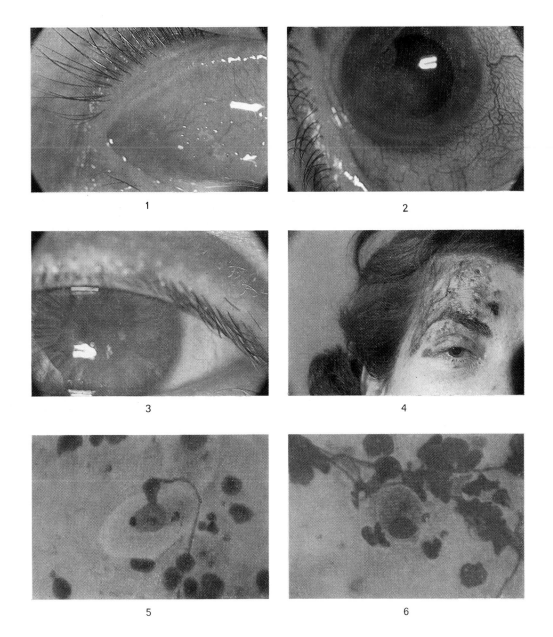

1

2

3

4

5

6

See Chapter 54, page 717.

Figure 54-1. Follicular conjunctivitis. Characteristic hyperemia and hyperplasia of the conjunctiva and follicles visible especially at the angles. (Courtesy of Professor G. Offret.)

Figure 54-2. Herpetic superficial keratitis. Dendritic ulcer of the cornea. Fluorescein staining emphasizes the branches. (Couresty of Professor G. Offret.)

Figure 54-3. Herpetic disciform keratitis. The deep form of herpetic keratitis with interstitial corneal clouding of grayish white tinge with central localization and without vascularization (Courtesy of Professor G. Offret.)

Figure 54-4. Ophthalmic zoster. Frontal eruption with a few elements extending to the lower eyelid, and slight corneal involvement. (Courtesy of Professor G. Offret.)

Figure 54-5. Trachomatous inclusions in an epithelial cell (× 900). Epithelial cell with two inclusions near the nucleus (blue with Giemsa staining). Attentive scrutiny at higher magnification reveals one inclusion full of initial bodies. (Courtesy of the Virological Research Laboratory of the Institute of Ophthalmology, Tunis.)

Figure 54-6. Trachomatous inclusion at a more advanced stage (× 1450). In an epithelial cell, Giemsa's method reveals two blue-stained initial bodies and a multitude of fine elementary bodies distinguished by a violet-red tinge. (Courtesy of the Virological Research Laboratory of the Institute of Ophthalmology, Tunis.)

from the first months after birth to extreme old age. Outbursts of activity may succeed each other in an extremely irregular manner. Trachoma can, however, heal spontaneously, in general after many years.

Certain authors make a distinction between trachoma in the child and trachoma in the adult. But all the various forms and all the complications can occur both in children and in adults.

The division of the clinical forms of trachoma seems rather artificial. Certain forms, however, appear to be more frequent in certain countries than in others. Thus one can describe a florid, a torpid, and a papillary form, diffuse trachoma without follicles, an acute, a mixed, or a unilateral form of trachoma, and even an inapparent form demonstrated both experimentally and clinically (Nataf).

The Etiological Agent of Trachoma.* MORPHOLOGICAL, CHEMICAL AND STAINING CHARACTERISTICS. *"Epithelial inclusions" or Halberstaedter-Prowazek bodies* were discovered and described in 1907. During a mission to Java these pioneers in the study of the disease showed *inclusions in the epithelial cells of the conjunctiva in trachoma*. Since these inclusions seem to be enveloped in a sac (coat or chlamys), Halberstaedter and von Prowazek proposed to classify the agent among the chlamydozoaceae.

After innumerable studies devoted to the subject, the general opinion seems to be that the epithelial inclusion is constituted by an intracellular colony of the pathogenic agent. The etiological agent can thus manifest its presence by *intracytoplasmic inclusions* in the epithelial cells of the conjunctiva or the cornea. These inclusions present different forms at the different stages of their development.

The elementary body, once it has penetrated the cytoplasm, increases in size and becomes basophilic; it is then known as the *initial body*. This phase corresponds to a predominance of deoxyribonucleic acid.

While increasing in size, the inclusion begins to be differentiated into smaller acidophilic elements that reconstitute *elementary bodies*, in which ribonucleic acid gradually replaces deoxyribonucleic acid.

---

*This section was written in collaboration with M. L. Tarizzo.

At the end of the differentiation process, the inclusion is composed essentially of a mass of new elementary bodies capable, in turn, of infecting new cells on liberation by destruction of the host cell or rupture of the cell membrane.

The inclusions are demonstrable by staining smears of corneal scrapings. The techniques most utilized are that of Giemsa (to distinguish the morphological details), iodine staining (to reveal the glycogen in these inclusions), and, especially, immunofluorescence (by which morphological observation can be combined with immunological identification of the agent).

Inclusions are not always found, and the percentage of positive results varies with the stage of the disease, the method of examination, the epidemiological conditions, and according to the authors.

By their morphological characteristics these inclusions are similar to those caused by other microorganisms of the same group as the etiological agent of trachoma.

BIOLOGICAL CHARACTERISTICS. Certain characteristics of the trachoma agent had been studied experimentally even before systematic culture of the agent was achieved. Thygeson and Nataf reviewed the question in 1958.

Systematic culture of the trachoma agent in the yolk sac of the embryonated hen's egg, which has become current in recent years, has made it possible to confirm and to extend knowledge of the facts already known and to open new vistas for study and practical application.

The agent of trachoma is a member of the psittacosis-lymphogranuloma venereum group.

The common characteristics of these agents are their morphology under the light and the electron microscope, their staining characteristics, the simultaneous presence of deoxyribonucleic acid and ribonucleic acid, their sensitivity to certain antibiotics and to sulfonamides, their pattern of replication, and the presence of a group antigen.

Morphology. The morphology of the trachoma agent, cultured in the yolk sac of embryonated hen's eggs, appears *under the light microscope* to be that of a round corpuscle approximately 300 mμ in diameter. Although usually isolated, these bodies may be clustered; they correspond to the elementary bodies seen in the human conjunctiva. Typically, they are red with Machiavello staining, blue when stained by Castañeda's method, and purple with use of Giemsa's method. Typical inclusions may also be found in preparations made by the "imprint" method and in histological sections.

Under the electron microscope these corpuscles have the same typical appearances as the other microorganisms of the same group; a central denser area of somewhat irregular form and a less dense and flattened peripheral area. These characteristics of the elementary body give it a dome-like appearance with a flattened periphery.

Sensitivity to Antibiotics. Sensitivity to antibiotics is variable. The trachoma agent, like all the other agents of the group, is resistant to streptomycin even in high concentration. On the other hand, it is sensitive to the tetracyclines and to erythromycin, as well as to penicillin and, to a less evident degree, to other antibiotics. This sensitivity to antibiotics is linked, in the case of penicillin, to the presence of muramic acid in the corpuscular walls. The sensitivity to sulfonamides of the trachoma agent, like that of the other members of the group, is associated with capacity to metabolize folic acid and its derivatives.

Antigenic Characteristics. The antigenic characteristics of trachoma and their relationships with those of the other agents of the group are now much better known.

Antigens prepared from cultures have enabled demonstration of a *thermostable group antigen*, and that of *complement-fixing antibodies* in a significant percentage of spontaneous clinical cases of trachoma and in practically all cases of the experimental disease.

Other more recent immunological methods, especially application of immunofluorescence to this pathogenic agent, make it possible to perfect even more precise methods of study and diagnosis.

Culture of the Pathogenic Agent of Trachoma in the Embryonated Egg, and Experimental Study of the Pathogenicity of the Agent. Both are possible because the trachoma agent is easily cultured in the yolk sac. Inoculated by this route, the trachoma agent is highly pathogenic for the chick embryo and can kill it in a few days under optimal conditions of development. These conditions are inoculation of the agent into embryonated eggs aged six and eight days, and incubation at 35° C. at approximately 50 per cent relative humidity. The yolk sacs of eggs inoculated with this agent usually show considerable hemorrhage. Histologically, diffuse perivasculitis is noted; petechiae may be found in several organs and tissues of the embryo.

Culture of the trachoma agent in the allantois has also been reported. It was even accomplished on several occasions on the chorioallantoic membrane between 1939 and 1945 at the Pasteur Institute of Tunis, but this culture method could not be perfected at that period, since streptomycin was not yet available.

Small laboratory animals, e.g., mice, guinea pigs, and chickens, are not usually sensitive to the trachoma agent. Some of these animals are utilized for immunological studies, since inoculation of the agent can provoke antibodies in high titer even in absence of clinical evidence of the infection.

Although intraperitoneal, intracerebral, and intravenous inoculation into the mouse of several strains of the trachoma agent shows their lack of pathogenicity for this animal their *toxicity* for the mouse has been demonstrated, as has that of the other agents of this group. Study of this toxin, which is highly labile, has made it possible to differentiate immunologically several strains of trachoma.

Experimental inoculation into man and the monkey of this microorganism cultivated in the egg has confirmed by production of typical forms of the disease that it is really the etiological agent of trachoma. These experimental results make it possible not merely not to specify the etiological role of the pathogenic agent but also to establish the relationships between this agent and the other members of the group and to study the possibility of preventing the disease by immunological means.

Culture of the Trachoma Agent in Tissue Culture. Certain strains adapted to culture in the chick embryo have also been adapted to growth in tissue culture. This method, which presents considerable advantages, has not yet reached the stage of generalized application, and several problems remain to be solved.

Vaccination. Vaccination would seem to be a possibility because of the availability of the pathogenic agent in large quantities and its antigenic characteristics. Several trials have been made in different regions. The results so far obtained would seem to indicate that, although partial and temporary protection has been obtained, vaccination has not emerged from the phase of study and experimentation.

CLASSIFICATION OF THE ETIOLOGICAL AGENT OF TRACHOMA. In 1937 Cuénod and Nataf called attention to similarities and dissimilarities of the trachoma agent in regard to the agents of lymphogranulomatosis venereum and of psittacosis, and to rickettsia. Virological and physicochemical techniques have confirmed and clarified these affinities and differences.

The trachoma agent and the other members of the psittacosis-lymphogranulomatosis venereum-trachoma group cannot be considered to be true viruses according to the definition given by Lwoff: it has been proposed to create for them the Chlamydiaceae family and the genus Chlamydia (cf. Chapter 52).

The trachoma agent and that of inclusion conjunctivitis have proved to be so closely similar that they tend to be grouped under one name: TRIC agents. Some authorities consider that the pathogenic agent is one and the same and that, according to certain conditions (e.g., socioeconomic, climatic) and the pattern of development, it produces trachoma in its classic form in some cases and in others inclusion conjunctivitis, whether it be that of the newborn of genital origin or that of the adult (*vide infra*).

"Trachomatous disease" in its various forms in the newborn as in the adult, although they appear clinically to differ widely, is considered in this hypothesis to form a single entity.

In collaboration with the research team of the Ophthalmology Institute of Tunis we have acquired some recent clinical and experimental data suggesting that although this hypothesis is possible, it is not indisputably demonstrated.

The hypothesis is nonetheless conceivable that if the causal agent belongs to a single genus, it could present different types and strains able to provoke clinical disorders with a range of symptoms extending from trachoma (which could be called classic) in its most varied forms, to inclusion conjunctivitis with its different recognized pathological aspects.

In our view, the facts are insufficiently demonstrated, and wide perspectives lie open for further research by both biologists and clinicians.

Treatment. Sulfonamides by mouth and broad-spectrum antibiotics applied topically have permitted great progress in trachoma therapy. *Improvement of the patient's general physical condition* always plays a highly important role in shortening the course of the disease and in limiting its sequelae.

SULFONAMIDES. A first step forward in therapy of trachoma was made by utilization of sulfonamides by mouth. Among the most generally recommended of these drugs are sulfisoxazole and sulfamethoxypyridazine, for example. Only sulfonamides of low toxicity are permissible. Trachoma is essentially a chronic disease with no defined pattern of development but which is tenacious, subject to outbursts of activity, and to quiescent periods during which it remains contagious. To combat a disease of this type, the medication utilized must have the minimal degree of toxicity but also permit impregnation with an adequate dose over a sufficiently long period to act on the disease process.

ANTIBIOTICS. Topical application of antibiotics is effective in trachoma. Penicillin is weakly active on the trachomatous process; streptomycin has no effect on the trachoma agent. However, broad-spectrum antibiotics have a real activity on the course of the disease; for the moment, those most employed are tetracyclines and erythromycin. Broad-spectrum antibiotics are utilized mainly in an oculentum at 1 per cent to 3 per cent; the second concentration seems to us to be the more effective. The oculentum should be applied several times daily, in any case at least twice a day.

In the active developing phases of trachoma, we advise use of an oculentum containing 3 per cent of Terramycin morning and evening and a collyrium of copper sulfate at noon. We associate with this therapy oral sulfonamides (e.g., sulfamethoxypyridazine) and therapy designed to reinforce the host's general defenses (hormones, vitamins, iron, arsenic, phosphorus).

Recently we have obtained particularly satisfactory and rapid results by association of oxytetracycline (Terramycin), erythromycin, and lysozyme.

Prophylaxis. *All prophylaxis of trachoma* is based on *cleanliness and improvement of living conditions* and of *sanitary organization*.

Betterment of the population's standards

of living and improvement of individual and collective hygiene resulted in disappearance of trachoma in many regions before modern progress in therapy.

The rational, methodical, and complete organization of the fight against ocular diseases and blindness is requisite at both the national and the international level. *In order to be rational, methodical, and complete, the struggle in the involved areas demands a network of centers and of fixed and mobile dispensaries, that covers the whole country in function of its demographic necessities.*

The international prophylaxis of trachoma should be the responsibility of all countries, to assist the unfortunate ones and to safeguard those at present free from endemic trachoma.

Systematic culture of the trachoma agent conjoined with the immunological applications it has already made possible opens new horizons for therapy and prophylaxis.

Trachoma retreats before the advancement of civilization. As of now, eradication of trachoma can be foreseen as the living conditions of man improve.

Inclusion Conjunctivitis

Under this heading we shall discuss inclusion conjunctivitis proper in its two clinical forms: inclusion conjunctivitis of the newborn and follicular conjunctivitis of the adult, of which the most characteristic is "swimming pool conjunctivitis"; and the conjunctivitis observed in cytomegalic inclusion disease.

Inclusion Conjunctivitis. As mentioned earlier, the trachoma agent and that of inclusion conjunctivitis differ so little in their morphological characteristics and in their conditions of intracellular development that they are referred to together as TRIC agents. The pathological and epidemiological characteristics of the second group are greatly dissimilar, however, to those of trachoma.

The agent of inclusion conjunctivitis is a pathogen of the adult genital tract (cf. Chapter 53). It can lead to moderate urethritis in men and to cervicitis in women. The infant is infected during passage through the birth canal and shows a clearly individualized type of conjunctivitis. Transmission of the conjunctivitis from the infant to the adult or

from one adult to another is exceptional. The ocular infections in the adult result mainly from accidental contamination of the eye directly by genital secretions or by the water of unchlorinated swimming pools in which infectious genital secretions subsist.

Inclusion Conjunctivitis of the Newborn. Purulent, nongonococcic, highly contagious conjunctivitis appears in the infant five days to two weeks after birth. It is usually bilateral from the start. Its onset is earlier than that of trachoma, which does not appear in the first weeks of life. It is later than that of gonococcal conjunctivitis, whereas the clinical picture alone is highly similar, with palpebral edema, marked hyperemia and hyperplasia, and abundant purulent discharge. The mucosa becomes granular appearing and, on occasion, even raspberry red. The conjunctiva is extremely fragile and bleeds on the slightest contact.

Corneal complications have been observed in nearly 10 per cent of cases.

Spontaneously, the course of the disease is toward recovery in several months; in the third month persistence of inflammatory lesions of the conjunctiva has been observed. This course is strikingly abbreviated by antibiotics, which cure the disease in ten days, or even less. This characteristic still further differentiates inclusion body conjunctivitis from trachoma, for trachoma heals less rapidly despite treatment with antibiotics and sulfonamides.

Broad-spectrum antibiotics applied topically several times daily by instillation are the most active; their use should be extended a few days after cure to avert relapse. Sulfonamides by the systemic route are occasionally necessary in addition.

Follicular Inclusion Conjunctivitis in the Adult. This acute follicular conjunctivitis appears after eight to ten days' incubation. It is unilateral at first but may involve the other eye after two or three weeks.

The onset is fairly rapid, with photophobia, lacrimation, and mucopurulent discharge. The mucosa is strikingly hyperplastic and becomes dark red, with the color and drupelike surface aspect of a raspberry; papillary and follicular projections occur mainly on the fornix, but the follicles differ considerably from those in trachoma.

Preauricular adenopathy is frequent. The course is uncomplicated. The functional signs regress progressively in three to five weeks, but the appearance of the mucosa remains the same for a fairly long period. The preauricular adenopathy disappears. Healing occurs without sequelae after two or three months, or occasionally longer. Corneal complications are rare; they consist in transitory infiltration of the epithelium or superficial punctate keratitis.

DIAGNOSIS. In the newborn the differential diagnosis principally concerns gonococcal conjunctivitis, but the onset of the gonococcal disease is earlier, i.e., on the second day of life, and can easily be identified by bacteriological examination. In the adult, trachoma is eliminated by the pattern of development: collapse of the infected follicles, pannus formation, and cicatrization are never observed. The characteristic conjunctival follicles predominate at the level of the lower eyelid, whereas in trachoma they are found mainly at the level of the upper eyelid.

Cytomegalic Inclusion Disease (cf. Chapters 23 and 61). The eye can be involved in the generalized forms of the disease, but it is the sole manifestation more often than is yet thought. Cases of keratomalacia, dacryocystitis, dacryoadenitis, scleritis, uveitis, choroiditis, retinitis, neuritis, and cataract have been described. A type of *necrotic conjunctivitis* has been related by certain authors to cytomegalic inclusion disease on the basis of cytomegalic inclusions in the ocular mucosa. *Uveitis* of the newborn and in young subjects are ocular localizations often noted in the more or less complete forms of cytomegalic inclusion disease.

Only the laboratory can confirm the diagnosis. Histopathological examination of the ocular tissues that can be sampled shows typical bird's eye cells due to the cytomegalic inclusions. The same cell formations can be noted in the ocular discharge and from the aqueous humor by puncture of the anterior chamber. The techniques of serodiagnosis (complement-fixation reactions and neutralization tests) are especially useful. Isolation and identification of the virus in tissue culture from an ocular sample may demonstrate its presence in the eye and thus constitute the proof of its direct action on the eye.

At present, treatment does not seem to have any direct effect on the pathologic process of cytomegalic inclusion disease. The benign and masked forms of the disease may, nonetheless, benefit from therapeutic measures that, by their usefulness in combating secondary infections, help the host to fight the infection itself.

BIBLIOGRAPHY

For the literature published before, see Nataf, R., Lépine, P., and Bonamour, G.: Oeil et virus. In: Chapter X, Les embryopathies virales oculaires. Rapport présenté à la Société Française d'Ophtalmologie en 1960. Paris, Masson et Cie.

ADENOVIRUS

1. Dawson, C., et al.: Infections due to adenovirus type 8 in the United States. 1. An outbreak of epidemic keratoconjunctivitis originating in a physician's office. 2. Community-wide infection with adenovirus type 8. New Eng. J. Med., *268*:1031-1034, 1034-1037, 1963.
2. Farkas, E., Jancso, A., and Radnot, M.: Clinical and virologic studies on the first widespread outbreak of epidemic keratoconjunctivitis in Hungary. Amer. J. Ophthal., *60*:78-82, 1965.
3. Hecht, S. D., et al.: Treatment of epidemic keratoconjunctivitis with idoxuridine (IUDR). Arch. Ophthal. (Chicago), *73*:49-54, 1965.
4. Stucchi, C. A.: Particularités cytologiques conjonctivales et éosinophilie avec kératoconjonctivite épidémique (K.C.E.) (étude clinique et microscopique préliminaire). Arch. Ophtal. (Paris), *22*:591-613, 1962.
5. Vass, Z.: Histological findings in epidemic keratoconjunctivitis. Acta Ophthal., *42*:119-121, 1964.

HERPES ZOSTER

6. Radnót, M., and Bajnok, G.: Ophthalmologic correlations of herpes zoster. Szemeszet, *102*:1-4, 1965.

HERPES SIMPLEX

7. Dohlman, C. H., and Zucker, B. B.: Long-term treatment with idoxuridine and steroids. A complication in herpetic keratitis. Arch. Ophthal. (Chicago), *74*:172-174, 1965.
8. Hart, D. R. L., Brightman, V. J. F., Readshaw, G. G., Porter, G. T. J., and Tully, M. G.: Treatment of human herpes simplex keratitis with idoxuridine. A sequential double-blind controlled study. Arch. Ophthal. (Chicago), *73*:623-634, 1965.
9. Hogan, M. J., Kimura, S. J., and Thygeson, P.: Pathology of herpes simplex kerato-iritis. Amer. J. Ophthal., *57*:551-564, 1964.
10. Kaufman, H. E.: Present status of IDU therapy in herpetic keratitis. Eye, Ear, Nose Throat Monthly, *42*:35-37, 1963.
11. Kaufman, H. E., Nesburn, A. B., and Maloney, E. D.: IDU therapy of herpes simplex. Arch. Ophthal. (Chicago), *67*:583-591, 1962.
12. Krwawicz, T.: Application of low temperature in the treatment of herpes simplex keratitis (Polish). Klin. Oczna, *34*:435-439, 1964.
13. Lavrenteva, A. M., and Maevskaya, T. M.: Antigen treatment of herpetic keratitis (Russian). Vestn. Oftal., *3*:29-32, 1963.

14. Liotet, S., and Bonnin, P.: Diagnostic de l'herpès cornéen par immuno-fluorescence. Arch. Ophtal. (Paris), 25:301-304, 1965.

15. Offret, G., Payrau, P., Rudder, J. de, Pouliquen, Y., Faure, J. P., and Cuq, G.: De l'application du vaccin inactivé dans la kératite herpétique. Arch. Ophtal. (Paris), 25:287-300, 1965.

16. Renard, G., and Dhermy, P.: Etude clinique et expérimentale de l'herpès de la cornée et de son traitement par un virusstatique nouveau A.B.O.B. (virustat). Sem. Hôp. Paris, 39:1250-1258, 1963.

17. Rudder, J. de: Le virus de l'herpès. Arch. Ophtal. (Paris), 25:257-286, 1965.

18. Sanna, G., and Serantini, G.: Roentgenterapia indiretta delle cheratiti erpetiche mediante irradiazione dei centri di innervazione trofosensitiva oculare. Ann. Ottal., 90:1-13, 1964.

19. Thomas, C. I., Purnell, E. W., and Rosenthal, M. S.: Treatment of herpetic keratitis with IDU and corticosteroids. Report of 105 cases. Amer. J. Ophthal., 60:204-217, 1965.

20. Vozza, R., and Balducci, D.: The technique of fluorescent antibodies in ophthalmology. A study of herpes simplex and vaccine keratoconjunctivitis and human trachomatous infection. Amer. J. Ophthal., 52:72-77, 1961.

Cytomegalic Inclusions

21. Miklos, G., and Orban, T.: Ophthalmic lesions due to cytomegalic inclusion disease. Ophtalmologica (Basel), 148:98-106, 1964.

22. Miklos, G., and Orban, T.: Ocular changes in cytomegalic inclusion disease. Szemeszet, 101:90-95, 1964.

23. Nataf, R., and Coscas, G.: Manifestations ophtalmologiques et localisations de la maladie des inclusions cytomégaliques. Ann. Oculist. (Paris), 196:7-19, 1963.

Other Viruses

24. Baldwin, B. A.: The presence and properties of Newcastle disease virus in the aqueous humour of chickens. J. Comp. Path., 72:190-197, 1962.

25. Behera, U. C., and Misra, M. C.: Herpes ophthalmicus with varicella. J. Indian Med. Assoc., 38:345-346, 1962.

26. Cairns, J. E.: Varicella of the cornea treated with 5-iodo-2'-deoxyuridine. Brit. J. Ophthal., 48:288-289, 1964.

27. Deduit, Y., and Witmer, R.: The aetiology of uveitis. Results of year of serological studies. Ophthalmologica (Basel), 145:332-340, 1963.

28. Ellis, P. P., and Winograd, L. A.. Ocular vaccinia. A specific treatment. Arch. Ophthal. (Chicago), 68:600-609, 1962.

29. Gould, E. L., Havener, W. H., and Andrew, J. M.: Vaccinia lid infection. Amer. J. Ophthal., 56:830-382, 1963.

30. Jones, B. R., Galbraith, J. E. K., and Al Hussaini, M. K.: Vaccinial keratitis treated with interferon. Lancet, 1:875-879, 1962.

31. Paul, S. D., Ahuja, O., and Shukla, B. R.: Viral uveitis (a review of 11 cases). All India Ophthal. Soc., 12:147-153, 1964.

32. Quere, M. A., and Rey, M.: Les cécités post-rougeoleuses chez l'enfant. In: Enfant en milieu tropical. Dakar et Paris, 1965, No. 23, pp. 3-8.

33. Riffenburgh, R. S.: Ocular manifestations of mumps. Arch. Ophthal. (Chicago), 66:739-743, 1961.

Trachoma and Inclusion Conjunctivitis

34. Al Hussaini, M. K., Jones, B. R., and Dunlop, E. M. C.: Infection of the eye and genital tract by TRIC agent. I. Cytology and isolations. Rev. Int. Trachome, 42:7-13, 1965.

35. Babudieri, B., and Zardi, O.: Isolamento del primo ceppo europeo di virus tracomatose. Boll. Ist. Sieroter Milan., 39:295-297, 1960.

36. Bietti, G. B., Freyche, M. J., and Vozza, R.: La diffusion actuelle du trachome dans le monde. Congrès (19ème) international d'ophtalmologie, New Dehli, 5 décembre, 1962. Rev. Int. Trachome, 39:113-310, 1962.

37. Bernkopf, H.: Trachoma virus. Recent developments. Progr. Med. Virol., 4:119-156, 1962.

38. Bernkopf, H., and Mashiah, P.: The growth cycle of a trachoma agent in FL cell cultures. J. Immun., 88:570-571, 1962.

39. Chang, H. I., Chin, H. Y., and Wang, K. C.: Experimental studies on trachoma vaccine in monkeys. Chin. Med. J. (Peking), 83:755-762, 1964.

40. Collier, L. H.: Experiments with trachoma vaccines. Experimental system using inclusion blennorrhoea virus. Lancet, 1:795-800, 1961.

41. Fujiyama, H.: Culture of trachoma virus in chorioallantoic membrane of developing chick embryo and electron microscopic study thereof (report 2). Rev. Int. Trachome, 40:367-384, 1963.

42. Goto, T., et al.: Antigenic relation of trachoma virus to psittacosis virus. Jap. J. Exp. Med., 31:237-247, 1961.

43. Grayston, J. T., et al.: Field studies of protection from infection by experimental trachoma virus vaccine in preschool-aged children on Taiwan. Proc. Soc. Exp. Biol. Med., 112:589-595, 1963.

44. Hanna, L., et al.: Isolation of viruses from inclusion conjunctivitis in the newborn. Amer. J. Ophthal., 53:774-780, 1962.

45. Harisijades, S., Harisijades, B., and Kuwabarat, T.: Histopathology of the cornea of the chick embryos inoculated with trachoma virus. Acta Med. Iugosl., 17:346-351, 1963.

46. Jones, B. R., Al Hussaini, M. K., and Dunlop, E. M. C.: Infection of the eye and genital tract by TRIC agent. III. Ocular syndromes associated with infection of the genital tract by TRIC agent. Rev. Int. Trachome, 42:21-43, 1965.

47. Kurnosova, L. M., and Lenkevich, M. M.: Mode of action of sulfonamides on trachoma virus. Acta Virol. (Praha), 8:350-358, 1964.

48. Larmande, A., and Longo, A. M.: Les pannus des trachomateux. Rev. Int. Trachome, 37:1-392, 1960.

49. Lassalle, J.: Etude sur cultures cellulaires de l'effet cytolytique des agents du trachome et de la conjonctivite à inclusions. Ann. Inst. Pasteur (Paris), 106:752-761, 1964.

50. Mitsui, Y.: Relation between trachoma and inclusion conjunctivitis. Rev. Int. Trachome, 41:252-261, 1964.

51. Mitsui, Y., et al.: Trachoma and inclusion conjunctivitis agents: adaptation to HeLa cell cultures. Science, 145:715-716, 1964.

52. Nataf, R., Tarizzo, M. L., and Nabli, B.: Etudes sur le trachome. 6. Inoculations expérimentales à l'homme de cultures de virus du trachome et de la conjonctivite à inclusions. Bull. WHO, *29*:95-103, 1963.

53. Roger, A., and Roger, F.: A propos du pouvoir pathogène expérimental et de la culture du virus du trachome. Ann. Inst. Pasteur (Paris), *101*:523-544, 1961.

54. Sédan, J.: Le trachome, fléau infantile. Arch. Franç. Pédiat., *12*:55-65, 1955.

55. T'ang, F. F., et al.: Studies on the etiology of trachoma with special reference to isolation of the virus in chick embryo. Chin. Med. J. (Peking), *75*:429-448, 1957.

56. Tarizzo, M. L., Nataf, R., and Daghfous, T.: Etudes sur le trachome. I. Isolement et culture en série de 12 souches de virus sur oeuf embryonné. 2. Action des antibiotiques sur le virus de trachome cultivé dans les oeufs embryonnés. Bull. WHO, *24*:103-105, 107-113, 1961.

57. Tarizzo, M. L., Nataf, R., Daghfous, T., Nabli, B., and Mitsui, Y.: Etudes sur le trachome. 3. Prés- ence d'anticorps spécifiques déviant le complément dans les sérums trachomateux. 4. Morphologie et réactions tinctoriales du virus cultivé dans le sac vitellin de l'embryon de poulet. 5. Complement-fixation tests in human volunteers. Bull. WHO, *27*:735-749, 1962.

58. Tarizzo, M. L., Nataf, R., and Nabli, B.: Etudes sur le trachome (9ème note). Nouvelles inoculations expérimentales à l'homme des virus du trachome et de la conjonctivite à inclusions. Bull. WHO, *30*:675-691, 1964.

59. Thygeson, P., and Nataf, R.: Les problèmes étiologiques du trachome. Rev. Int. Trachome, *35*:83-175, 1958.

60. Werner, G. H.: Relations immunologiques entre les agents du trachome, de la conjonctivite à inclusions et de la lymphogranulomatose vénérienne. C. R. Acad. Sci. (Paris), *261*:2410-2413, 1963.

61. Werner, G. H.: Recherches expérimentales sur la chimiothérapie du trachome. Ann. Inst. Pasteur (Paris), *100*:93-108, 1961.

55

Choroidoretinitis, Optic Neuritis, and Oculomotor Paralysis

By B. AUVERT

This chapter is intended to specify the different forms taken by viral or presumably viral involvement of the choroid, retina, optic nerve, and oculomotor nerves. The viral etiology of all the clinical pictures described here is not demonstrated—far from it—but it is sufficiently probable to justify their discussion.

CHOROIDITIS

The problems raised by retinochoroiditis have no easy solution. In the first place, the choroid constitutes the posterior uvea, and posterior uveitis is often associated with an- terior uveitis, or iridocyclitis. Second, from the anatomical viewpoint it is sometimes difficult to distinguish between choroidal and retinal lesions, since the uvea and the retina are intimately associated and impairment of one of these membranes almost invariably involves the other. Finally, the papilla is the area of convergence of all the retinal nerve fibers that join to form the optic nerve. A chorioretinal lesion may therefore be complicated by papillitis, optic neuritis, or diffuse neurological manifestations—from which facts arise the terms "uveopapillitis" and "uveomeningitis."

Infection of the choroid sometimes appears as a simple choroiditis. This choroiditis, or posterior uveitis, may be complicated by iridocyclitis, or anterior uveitis, with red eye, and a Tyndall phenomenon, and precipitates seen on slit-lamp examination. Often, however, the reaction of the anterior segment is discreet or absent.

Choroiditis, usually unilateral, manifests itself by decrease in vision and the impression of black spots before the eyes. The degree of lessening of visual acuity depends on that of the turbidity of the vitreous humor and, especially, on the location and size of the retinochoroid lesion. Examination of the fundus oculi, which is hindered by particles floating in the vitreous humor, reveals a blurred papilla, slightly dilated veins, and, above all, a whitish, edematous patch with ill-defined outline on a sector of the retina. After several weeks, scarring occurs. The turbidity of the vitreous humor diminishes, then disappears. The edema surrounding the focus of infection gradually diminishes, and finally a whitish, atrophic patch persists with a surrounding pigmented line. If this scar is situated in a peripheral area it has no functional consequences, but when it is on the macula retinae it causes definitive reduction of visual acuity. New outbursts of inflammation sometimes occur at or around the initial focus of infection.

Jensen's Retinochoroiditis. Infection of the choroid is sometimes accompanied by infection of the retina and produces Jensen's retinochoroiditis.

A young subject presents a sudden visual disorder. Examination reveals a focus of choroiditis situated in contact with, or at a short distance from the papilla. This focus of infection causes a highly characteristic amputation of the visual field. A large scotoma appears contiguous to Mariotte's spot or separated from it (a difference depending on whether the focus is in contact with the papilla) and widens out toward the periphery; it causes an extensive sector of deficiency. This deficit is always greater than the size of the lesion would suggest and, most important, it is permanent. It might result from a vascular lesion of the retina; some authors consider Jensen's retinochoroiditis to be more a retinitis rather than a choroiditis. The scar left by the focus of inflammation appears as a yellowish white spot bordered by a very discreet pigmented line. The juxtapapillary site, the partial amputation of the visual field, and slight or inexistent pigmentary

changes are all signs that permit differentiation between common choroiditis and Jensen's retinochoroiditis.

Uveomeningitis. The group of uveomeningitides is characterized by lesions of the uvea accompanied by meningeal signs. In some instances the meningeal signs predominate, and the uveal signs are so unobtrusive that they have to be searched for; in others the ocular symptoms predominate and the meningeal involvement is reflected only by headaches and alterations of the cerebrospinal fluid and the electroencephalogram. Rouher and Cantat reported 12 cases of uveomeningitis observed in a few years in central France. The ocular disturbances are marked; they are characterized by hypotonia, turbidity of the vitreous humor, and choroidal exudation with bullous protrusion of the retina. The meningoencephalitic disturbances are slight: nausea, signs of diencephalon involvement with disturbances of sleep, thirst, and endocrine modifications, as well as a curious state of euphoria. Spinal puncture shows an increase in the number of cells to between 50 and 500, with predominance of polymorphonuclear leukocytes and an increased protein level. The electroencephalogram shows an arrhythmic tracing without clear localization. Fever is lacking, but blood sedimentation rate is increased. The course is protracted for a year or more.

In the group of uveomeningitides several forms are characterized: Harada's disease, the Vogt-Koyanagi syndrome, and sympathetic ophthalmia.

HARADA'S DISEASE. Harada's disease begins either suddenly by a febrile syndrome, or, on the contrary, progressively. The meningeal signs appear first, with headaches and vomiting. Spinal puncture produces a clear cerebrospinal fluid showing a lymphocytic reaction. The electroencephalogram is abnormal: the tracing is irregular with slow delta and theta dysrhythmia. Then the ocular symptoms appear. With bilateral reduction in visual acuity, examination shows papilledema spreading to the adjacent retina, and haze of the vitreous humor. Several days later, detachment of the retina occurs. This detachment begins in the lower segment and then becomes complete; it is of the exudative type, with wide folds but no tearing. Sometimes the retina appears greenish, or vascular alterations of periarteritis or periphlebitis type occur. Blindness is total, and auditory signs (severe deafness) and cutaneous signs (alopecia) complete the clinical picture. The disease has a protracted course (six months to one year) but a favorable prognosis. The neurological signs disappear, the vitreous humor clears, the folds of detached retina flatten out, and fairly satisfactory visual acuity is recovered. Nevertheless, some sequelae remain apparent in the fundus oculi, e.g., atrophic and pigmentary changes, and vascular modifications. In some cases, a degenerative macular scar results from the severe retinal edema and the slowness with which it regresses, and causes permanent impairment of central visual acuity.

VOGT-KOYANAGI SYNDROME. The Vogt-Koyanagi syndrome can also be included among the uveomeningitides. It affects subjects with a pigmented skin and is a frequent cause of blindness in South America and the Far East, whereas it is exceptional in France, for example. The disease is characterized by the extent of the ocular signs, especially prominent in the anterior uvea, where iridocyclitis with precipitates and thick synechiae are noted. When examination of the posterior segment is possible, the vitreous humor appears hazy, and large exudative patches of retinochoroiditis are noted with bullous protrusion of the retina. The meningoencephalitic syndrome is represented only by occasional headaches and modifications of the cerebrospinal fluid. The syndrome includes disorders of hearing and cutaneous symptoms: alopecia, poliosis, and vitiligo. The gravity of the Vogt-Koyanagi syndrome results from the ocular lesions, in particular development of cataract behind an iris that is blocked by thick synechiae. Surgical treatment is extremely difficult, and usually the extent of the lesions of the posterior segment renders functional improvement illusory.

SYMPATHETIC OPHTHALMIA. The Harada and the Vogt-Koyanagi syndrome represent uveomeningitides with a probable viral etiology. They have sometimes been related to sympathetic ophthalmia, a uveomeningitis that occurs under particular circumstances. After accidental or surgical perforation of the eye, or more rarely, during the development of an intraocular tumor, bilateral uveitis can occur, affecting the wounded ("exciting") eye and the healthy eye (rendered "excited"). This uveitis, of an anterior or a posterior type, is accompanied by mild meningeal signs, and auditory and skin disorders. Although it was frequent in the past and the fear of every ophthalmologist who treated perforating ocular wounds, sympathetic ophthalmia is rarer at present. It usually develops as a posterior uveitis of the Harada type and responds relatively well to treatment with corticosteroids. The pathogenesis of sympathetic ophthalmia remains a mystery. Sympathetic ophthalmia occurs in perforating wounds with iridal debris. It does not occur in perforating wounds with microbial superinfection, hypopyon, or panophthalmitis.

PART PLAYED BY VIRUSES IN THE ETIOLOGY OF CHOROIDITIS. Choroiditis may arise from a great variety of causes. The uvea is an extremely sensitive tissue, ready to react to microbial, parasitic or viral agressions, whether they occur in the region of the choroid itself or in any other part of the body. Choroiditis occurs during recognized viral disease. Despite intensive etiological investigations, the origin of a certain number of cases of retinochoroiditis is still unknown. It can be hoped that discovery of new viruses will help to clarify this mysterious ophthalmological problem.

Jensen's retinochoroiditis was long considered to be an atypical form of ocular tuberculosis. Today it is thought to be a syndrome provoked by causes as varied as tuberculosis, syphilis, multiple sclerosis, parasitoses (toxoplasmosis, in particular), and certain viral diseases. Jensen's choroiditis has been observed during the regression of viral and microbial sore throat, and after influenza.

The viral origin of uveomeningitides remains to be proved. A certain number of cases seem to be due to rickettsial or neo-rickettsial disease. In others a viral origin is likely. Various arguments have been advanced in favor of a viral origin.

Clinical Arguments. Uveomeningitis affects young subjects; it frequently begins suddenly by a systemic influenza-like syndrome and can occur in small epidemics. It can be a complication of a known viral disease (mumps, influenza, herpes zoster). Sympathetic ophthalmia can be a complication of herpes of the cornea. Serious lesions of the choroid and retina, or a uveopapillitis may be found in cases of cytomegalic inclusion disease.

Laboratory Arguments. In such cases

before recent years no virus had ever been isolated from the aqueous humor,* blood, or spinal fluid. It is impossible to perform a biopsy of the choroid, which would permit a direct search for virus. However, cells containing inclusions have been found in the aqueous humor of a patient with sympathetic ophthalmia and in the subretinal fluid of a patient with Harada's disease, and certain uveomeningitides have been transmitted to animals.

Is sympathetic ophthalmia due to a virus, introduced by the traumatism, that reaches the meningeal spaces via the optic nerve of the wounded eye and, from there, the healthy eye via the other optic nerve? Is it an allergic reaction, a particular sensitivity of the eye to the traumatized uveal pigment? Is it a coincidence, i.e., a viral uveomeningitis bearing no direct relationship to the ocular wound?

The doubtful pathogenesis explains the fact that the treatment of viral retinochoroiditis and uveomeningitis is nonspecific. Treatment is based on use of corticosteroids and broad-spectrum antibiotics; high doses are necessary because of the low intraocular penetration.

RETINITIS

Involvement of the retina may be secondary to that of the choroid, but it can be primary. Certain vascular disorders of the retina can be of viral origin.

Localized retinal periphlebitis is discovered by routine examination of the fundus oculi. In the course of influenza or infectious mononucleosis a small whitish coating of a retinal vein with a few hemorrhages may be discovered.

In other instances, a subject, who is young and apparently in good health, has a sudden visual disturbance in one eye. Examination shows typical *venous thrombosis,* affecting the trunk of the central vein of the retina or one of its branches. Upstream from the thrombosis, the vein is severely dilated and shows diffuse hemorrhagic suffusions. These retinal venous thromboses occurring in young subjects without diabetes or any vascular disorder suggest the possibility of a

rickettsial, a neorickettsial, or a viral disease. Similar venous thrombosis may occur during a known viral disease such as mumps or influenza. The prognosis in such cases of venous thrombosis is favorable. Even if the thrombosis involves the trunk of the central vein, recovery of sight can be hoped for; usually the complications of the hemorrhagic glaucoma type do not occur as in older subjects with arteriosclerosis.

The vascular involvement of the retina during a virus disease sometimes manifests itself by the appearance of small whitish spots or nodules. This phenomenon was once called Roth's septic retinitis and considered to be due to a microbial embolus in the small retinal arterioles. In the course of certain virus diseases *nodules dysoriques** are observed that seem to be due to small foci of retinal endotheliitis.

In some cases, severe macular edema is the principal manifestation of viral involvement of the retina. This picture is presented by *central exudative retinitis* (retinitis stellata) and by unilateral, pseudoalbuminuric retinitis. This macular edema can result from a vascular disturbance from subjacent choroiditis, or from spread of papillary edema to the retina.

Can certain viruses cause *massive destruction of the retina?* In a case of neonatal herpes with fever and meningoencephalitic reaction, examination of the fundus oculi showed hemorrhages and exudates. Death occurred three months after onset of the disease. Histopathological examination of the eye revealed diffuse lesions of the retina and optic nerve with necrosis and glial alterations; the choroid remained intact (Cogan).

A transitory *spasm* or definitive obliteration of *the central artery of the retina* in some instances complicates the course of a viral disease. The clinical picture of *pigmentary pseudoretinitis of viral origin* is highly individual: this rare, but very serious,

---

*Herpes simplex virus was isolated from the anterior chamber of a woman with bilateral severe panuveitis.[16]

*Nodules on the retina or near the papilla, in the form of nacreous spots, brilliantly white as compared to cotton wool, two or three in number, not exceeding ten, in cases of severe alteration of general physical condition in infections, intoxications, and collagenoses. The course of these nodules is parallel with that of the associated disease. Histological examination reveals hypertrophy of the nerve fibers and of the eyeball, with cytoid bodies corresponding to varicose degeneration of the nerve fibers. (Translator's note)

syndrome occurs after rubella, vaccinia, or encephalitis, but more often during regression of measles complicated by encephalitis or sometimes during that of even common measles.

About a week after onset of the illness, blindness suddenly occurs; the pupils are dilated and do not react to light. Examination of the fundus oculi reveals bilateral occlusion of the central artery of the retina with filiform vessels and retinal edema on which the cherry red color of the macula clearly distinguished it. Total blindness persists for several weeks and then regresses: the child is able to see sufficiently to guide himself, the photomotor reflex reappears, and the retinal edema disappears, but the vessels remain narrow and the optic disc becomes atrophied. The period of recuperation is protracted, and recovery is incomplete. Not only does visual acuity not return to normal but, still more serious, a secondary deterioration occurs in the following years, evolving as a pigmentary retinitis with hemeralopia, concentric shrinkage of the visual field, and peripheral pigmentation of the retina.

The pathogenesis of viral pigmentary pseudoretinitis is much debated. Is vascular spasm in the retina involved? Is the cause a direct or an indirect action of the virus on retinal metabolism? Or could the disease be attributed to variations of allergy related to the viral disease? Does viral pigmentary pseudoretinitis occur in predisposed subjects? Does the viral disease set off a latent hereditary degenerative retinitis pigmentosa, or is there a genetic predisposition to this retinal manifestation in the course of viral infection? Franceschetti, Babel, and Amman considered the problem of heredity with regard to the following case. In a child born of consanguineous parents, viral retinitis developed at 3 years of age; at age 20 the patient had typical retinitis pigmentosa, and it was subsequently discovered that two of his cousins, a girl and a boy, also had retinitis pigmentosa.

Several studies have been made on changes of the electroretinogram during viral pigmentary retinitis. In some cases, the electroretinogram is completely extinguished as in true hereditary retinitis pigmentosa. In other cases, it is only altered, but the changes become more pronounced with the clinical aggravation of the disease.

OPTIC NEURITIS

Viral infection of the optic nerve manifests itself in various ways. The optic nerve may be involved only along the macular fasciculus (producing axial or retrobulbar optic neuritis), or it may be involved through its entire thickness (producing transverse optic neuritis). The orbital course of the optic nerve is the most frequently involved, but the nerve may also be affected at the optic disk (producing papillitis), at the optic canal (yielding acute optic neuritis of the canal), or along its intracranial course. Involvement may be unilateral or bilateral.

Signs and symptoms of retrobular neuritis are occasionally discreet. A young patient complains of periocular pain, and moderate loss of visual acuity in one eye follows. The fundus oculi appears normal, but examination of the visual field reveals a small central scotoma. The disease regresses rapidly toward recovery.

In some cases, the picture is more alarming: visual impairment is severe. The central scotoma is large and may attain 20° to 30°, leaving only peripheral vision. The prognosis, however, is favorable. The scotoma regresses, and central vision is recovered, but the temporal segment of the optic disk often appears pale.

In *transverse optic neuritis,* blindness is complete. The fundus oculi appears normal, or the optic disk is congested, with a blurred outline. Functional recuperation is more or less complete, but optic atrophy almost always occurs subsequently. Parallelism between vision and the appearance of the fundus oculi is not obligatory; an appearance of total optical atrophy may coexist with scarcely modified visual acuity.

Acute papillitis causes a severe loss of visual acuity, and the fundus oculi presents severe alterations. The papillary edema is marked and extends into the retina. The veins are dilated, and peripapillary hemorrhages are noted. The papillary edema regresses gradually, but optic atrophy is the sequela of papillitis.

Sometimes, the reduction of the visual field during viral infection of the optic nerve does not take the form compatible with a central scotoma. When the deficit is in a sector or a quadrant of the visual field, compression of the edematous optic nerve in an unexpanding bony canal is to be considered.

On occasion, visual acuity is not modified, but systematic eyeground examination reveals *papillary hyperemia,* or even marked *papilledema.* This picture reflects a reaction of the fundus oculi to intracranial hypertension, and not optic neuritis.

Involvement of the optic nerve may be associated with uveitis (*uveopapillitis*), or with encephalitic, myelitic or meningeal involvement. These neuropapillitides associate a unilateral or a bilateral papillitis with an unobtrusive meningeal or encephalitic reaction, which is detected by spinal puncture and the electroencephalogram.

Devic's disease, or *acute neuromyelitis optica,* constitutes an individualized clinical entity because of the association of a bilateral optic neuritis with a myelitic syndrome. This disease, which affects young subjects, begins by a sudden bilateral drop in visual acuity, preceded by ocular pain and systemic signs and symptoms. The eyeground may be normal or show papilledema. The myelitis generally occurs after the ocular symptoms in the form of a flaccid paralysis with sphincteral disorders. The prognosis is highly variable: death may be rapid as a result of secondary complications, or recovery may occur with neurological and ocular sequelae, the neurological sequelae being the more pronounced.

In isolated retrobulbar neuritis in a young patient, the first diagnosis that should come to mind is *multiple sclerosis:* it is well known that this disease frequently begins with optic neuritis. The likelihood of an acute viral disease should, nonetheless, be considered on the basis of the clinical data: when a young subject, after a short bout of fever, shows a discreet optic neuritis that rapidly regresses.

Often, however, viral optic neuritis does not appear in isolation but is a complication of a known viral disease. Optic neuritis due to ophthalmic herpes zoster is rare, despite the frequent meningeal reaction that accompanies this disease: it is unilateral, on the same side as the eruption, and is masked by the palpebral edema and keratitis. Sometimes it is detected only at the stage of sequelae. Optic neuritis can complicate influenza, chickenpox, infectious mononucleosis, choriomeningitis, and measles, but is most frequent in mumps.

Mumps optic neuritis often takes the form of papillitis. It occurs during the acute phase of the disease, at the same time as parotitis, but it may develop later, during convalescence. If parotitis has been only slight, it may be difficult to relate the papillitis to its real cause. The time of appearance may have a certain importance in prognosis. Early papillitis, developing with parotitis, regresses in ten days to two weeks, whereas papillitis occurring later is thought often to lead to optical atrophy.

Neuropapillitis, which associates meningeal and encephalitic symptoms with optic neuritis, has sometimes been attributed to known viruses: those of mumps, lymphocytic choriomeningitis, Coxsackie infections, influenza, and various encephalitides.

Although acute neuromyelitis optica, or Devic's disease, is generally considered to be a demyelinating disease of the nervous system closely related to encephalitis periaxialis, it has been described as a complication of measles, or in association with a systemic infectious syndrome suggesting the possibility of a viral etiology.

Even the *mechanism* of viral involvement of the optic nerve is unknown. Various processes have been suggested: among them, proliferation of a virus in the region of the optic nerve itself, an allergic reaction of the optic nerve during a viral infection, or a mechanical edematous reaction resulting from intracranial hypertension. In certain cases involvement of the optic nerve occurring during influenza seemed to be the consequence of sinusitis complicating the influenza.

The inflammatory process sometimes occurs first in the sheaths of the optic nerve and then gains the fasciculi themselves.

The lesions of the optic nerve associated with uveitis or meningoencephalitis also give rise to pathogenic problems as yet unsolved. Is the involvement of the optic nerve ascending, i.e., from the uvea toward the encephalon, or descending, i.e., from the encephalon toward the uvea, or does it simultaneously involve the uvea, the optic nerve, and the encephalon?

OCULOMOTOR PARALYSIS

Viral disease may compromise the extrinsic or the intrinsic motility of the eye. The nerve most often affected is the sixth cranial, with resultant paralysis of abduction and homonymous, horizontal diplopia. Involvement of the fourth cranial nerve causes vertical diplopia increased in downward vision; it thus hinders walking and reading. Involvement of the third cranial nerve is rarely total; it causes ptosis, limitation of adduction, and hence of raising and of lowering the eyes, mydriasis, and paralysis of accommodation. Usually the lesion is only partial and is reflected by ptosis alone, or by an isolated lesion of an oculomotor muscle (rectus oculi medialis, superior rectus, inferior rectus, or inferior obliquus), by paralysis of accommodation, or mydriasis.

Functional paralyses affecting convergence and accommodation are also seen.

Oculomotor paralyses of viral origin occur in young patients. After an influenza-like episode, diplopia develops suddenly. This diplopia is due to oculomotor paralysis, but it may be mild. Paralytic strabismus is barely apparent, decreased motility is not obvious and the paralysis of the muscle is usually discovered only by special tests (study of diplopia with red glass, Lancaster examination or the Hess Lees coordimeter). Within a few days or weeks, everything usually returns to normal. However, in the young child whose binocular vision is still fragile, or who has a unilateral ametropia, this oculomotor paralysis results in strabismus. Paralysis of one oculomotor muscle causes contraction of the antagonistic muscle, and this contracture persists even when the paralysis has disappeared. Consequent to oculomuscular paralysis, *concomitant strabismus* that thereafter progresses on its own thus occurs in children. When the child is seen at this stage, initial oculomotor paralysis has disappeared. Paralysis of the fourth nerve due to virus infection is thought to be relatively frequent and to explain why so many cases of concomitant strabismus in children include a vertical factor. Another possible consequence of viral oculomotor paralysis in children is ocular torticollis; to compensate for diplopia, the child adopts a head tilt that persists even after disappearance of oculomotor paralysis.

Although isolated oculomotor involvement of viral origin is possible, the involvement frequently appears as the complication of a known virus disease. All the neurotropic viral infections can result in oculomotor paralysis; they appear, for example, in herpes, all viral encephalitis, and the brain stem forms of *poliomyelitis*. An isolated paralysis of the inferior oblique muscle of the eye has been described during infection by Coxsackie B5 virus.

In ophthalmic herpes zoster, involvement of the third cranial nerve, which is fairly frequent, is hard to detect. Ptosis is masked by palpebral edema, diplopia goes unnoticed, and atropine-induced mydriasis masks paralytic mydriasis. In the stages of sequelae, when a mydriasis is discovered, sometimes with dissociation of pupillary reflexes resembling an Argyll-Robertson sign, it is not always clear whether the pathology is the consequence of paralysis of the third nerve or of iridic atrophy following iridocyclitis due to zoster.

In chickenpox, a pupillary syndrome, resembling Adie's syndrome, can suddenly appear and be definitive. In *mumps encephalitis,* transitory paralysis of accommodation functions has been observed either alone, or in conjunction with pupillary disturbances. Other viral diseases, such as measles and vaccinia, and infectious mononucleosis may become complicated by oculomotor paralysis.

The pathogenic mechanism of viral infection of the oculomotor system most often remains unknown. The lesion seems to be situated on the nerve trunk itself or in the oculomotor nucleus, or it appears to be supranuclear. If in some cases, impairment of the oculomotor system is primary, in others it is the consequence of viral meningoencephalitis.

To relate an isolated case of oculomotor paralysis to a viral etiology is often difficult. However, with regard to oculomotor paralysis, the possibility of this etiology should be considered; probably certain disorders of binocular vision in the child are the consequence of an unrecognized oculomotor virus infection.

BIBLIOGRAPHY

An extensive bibliography can be found in the report of Nataf, Lépine, and Bonamour, 1960. We cite only works published since that date.

1. Birge, H. L.: Ocular virology and mycology. Amer. J. Med. Sci. *246*:239-244, 1963.
2. Blancard, P., Guillaumat, L., Sorato, M., and Brunell, J. C.: Deux cas d'uvéoméningite avec décollement de la rétine. Bull. Soc. Ophtal. Franç., *63*:427-433, 1963.

3. Bonamour, G., and Bonnet, M.: Rétinite grave post-morbilleuse. Bull. Soc. Ophtal. Franç., *65*:517, 1965.

4. Bonnet, J. L., and Istre, M.: Neuromyélite optique et rougeole. Bull. Soc. Ophtal. Franç., *64*:135-137, 1964.

5. Bouzas, A.: Les signes ophtalmoscopiques dans la poliomyélite antérieure. Bull. Soc. Ophtal., Franç., *75*:366-379, 1962.

6. Cogan, D. G.: Herpes simplex retinopathy in an infant. Arch. Ophthal. (Chicago), *72*:641-645, 1964.

7. Collier, M.: Problèmes étio-pathogéniques posés par la choriorétinite juxta-papillaire, type Jensen. Bull. Soc. Ophtal. Franç., *63*:44-53, 1963.

8. Ferrero, N.: Contribution à l'étude des névrites optiques de l'enfant. Thèse, Paris, A.G.E.M.P., 1962.

9. Franceschetti, A., Babel, J., and Amman, F.: La pseudo-rétinopathie pigmentaire post-morbilleuse est-elle une manifestation aiguë d'une hérédo-dégénérescence familiale? Bull. Soc. Franç. Ophtal., *77*:549-557, 1964.

10. Kissel, P., et al.: Paralysie des VI et VII nerfs craniens au cours d'une méningo-encéphalite à virus Coxsackie B5. Rev. Otoneuroophtal., *36*:195, 1964.

11. Martenet, A. C.: Neuro-rétinite grave post-morbilleuse. Ophthalmologica (Basel), *145*:384-391, 1963.

12. Morrison, F. D.: Transient accommodative paresis complicating mumps. With preservation of pupillary constriction for near vision. Arch. Ophthal. (Chicago), *73*:86, 1965.

13. Nataf, R., and Coscas, G.: Manifestations et localisations ophtalmologiques de la "maladie des inclusions cytomégaliques." Ann. Oculist. (Paris), *1*:7-20, 1963.

14. Nataf, R., Lépine, P., and Bonamour, G.: Oeil et virus. In: Chapter X, Les embryopathies virales

oculaires. Rapport présenté à la Société Française d' Ophtalmologie en 1960. Paris, Masson et Cie.

15. Offret, G., and Campinchi, R.: Traitement des uvéo-papillites. Année Thér. Clin., *15*:173-188, 1964.

16. Pavan-Langston, D., and Brockhurst, R. J.: Herpes simplex panuveitis. Arch. Ophthal. (Chicago), *81*:783-787, 1969.

17. Paufique, L., Audibert, J., Dorne, and Bonnet-Gehin, M.: Uvéite avec atteinte choriorétinienne d'origine ourlienne. Bull. Soc. Ophtal. Franç., *63*:226-228, 1963.

18. Pemberton, J. W.: Optic atrophy in herpes zoster ophthalmicus. Amer. J. Ophthal., *58*:852-854, 1964.

19. Puscariu, E.: L'hérédité des syndromes hérédo-familiaux. La rétinite pigmentaire d'origine médicamenteuse et après des maladies à virus. Arch. Ophtal. (Paris), *22*:253-258, 1962.

20. Riffenburgh, R. S.: Ocular manifestations of mumps. Arch. Ophthal. (Chicago), *66*:739-743, 1961.

21. Rogers, J. W.: Internal ophthalmoplegia following chickenpox. Arch. Ophthal. (Chicago), *71*:617-618, 1964.

22. Rouher, F., and Cantat, M. A.: Aspect clinique d'une épidémie d'uvéo-méningite. Ann. Oculist. (Paris), *194*:577-588, 1961.

23. Royer, J.: Manifestations rétiniennes des maladies à virus. J. Méd. Lyon, *40*:675-681, 1959.

24. Schlaegel, T. F., and Morris, W. R.: Virus-like inclusion bodies in subretinal fluid in uveo-encephalitis. Amer. J. Ophthal., *58*:940-945, 1964.

25. Thieffry, S., et al.: Etude clinique, virologique et sérologique systématique de 473 cas d'affections du système nerveux par les entérovirus. In: VII Symposium de la Poliomyélite, Paris, Masson et Cie., p. 185.

56

Ocular Lesions of Viral Embryopathies

By B. AUVERT AND G. COSCAS

Among virus infections occurring during intrauterine life only those in the first months of gestation affect a nondifferentiated organ and are capable of producing a congenital malformation. Multiple malforma-

tions are observed that differ greatly from the chronological viewpoint.

Viral infection of the mother during pregnancy can have a serious effect on the development of the fetal eye. Two anomalies are particularly frequent: congenital cataract and pigmentary pseudoretinitis.

CATARACT

Congenital cataract alone represents nine tenths of ocular viral embryopathies. It occurs in 40 to 50 per cent of cases of embryopathies of viral origin. For this reason, when a newborn infant has a cataract, the first reaction of the ophthalmologist is to inquire whether the mother had rubella during the first three months of pregnancy.

Although the cataract can be unilateral, it is most often bilateral. It may be unequally developed, i.e., more marked in one eye than in the other. No specific feature differentiates it from other congenital cataracts. It may be total, or a central cataract involving only the embryonic nucleus. It is sometimes incomplete at birth and subsequently becomes complete. On the other hand, it may be complete at birth and later regress, with resultant shrunken or membranous cataract.

Congenital cataract of viral origin raises therapeutic problems. A unilateral rubella cataract should not be treated surgically until much later, for aesthetic reasons. A bilateral central cataract, which permits the infant to make certain visual acquisitions, can be relieved surgically much later than complete bilateral cataract. The latter should be handled surgically early enough to aid the child's psychomotor development; however, the frequent association with cardiopathy complicates the problem of anesthesia. Difficulties arise in surgery, for the eyeball is abnormally small (microphthalmia), the pupil dilates poorly, the anterior chamber is narrow, and discission of a dense nucleus is difficult. Subsequently, the cortex is badly resorbed. Repeated discissions are necessary.

The functional results are often disappointing because of associated retinal lesions and mental retardation. Even when the cataract is diagnosed and operated on in early childhood in patients with normal psychomotor development, the congenital cataract causes profound and lasting amblyopia; the child begins to see clearly only when he is able to wear corrective spectacles at age three to four years. Even then vision is not good, because of inability to accommodate and lack of perception of the relief of objects and their depth. Recent attempts to adapt scleral or corneal contact lenses seem promising, but these lenses present difficult practical problems in such cases.

Numerous histological studies have been made of lesions of the crystalline lens caused by rubella virus. It seems that the primary fibers derived from the posterior epithelium of the lens are the first to be impaired and that impairment of the secondary fibers originating from the equator lentis follows.

Before rubella cataract is diagnosed, it is necessary to eliminate the possibility of congenital cataracts of other etiologies and of neonatal cataracts that appear within the first few days or weeks after birth. *Hereditary cataracts* are frequent; their diagnosis is facilitated by the fact that there are other cases in the family. Cataracts resulting from galactosemia, or the Lowe-Bickel-Mac-Lachlan-Terry syndrome,* are rarer. The other embryopathies likely to cause cataracts should be taken into consideration (e.g., those of toxic origin, or due to drugs, or to radiation).

PIGMENTARY PSEUDORETINITIS

The most frequent complication of viral embryopathy, after cataract, is pigmentary pseudoretinitis. It may occur alone, but it can also be associated with cataract, as is revealed by examination in unilateral cataract or after surgery when the cataract is bilateral.

An abnormal pigmentation covers the posterior pole of the retina and considerably overlaps the macular region; it appears as small, more or less darkly pigmented patches, of irregular outline, but that differ clearly from the osteoblast-like deposits of a true retinitis pigmentosa. This pigmentary rearrangement often coexists with small yellowish white degenerative lacunae, from which arises the "salt-and-pepper" appearance of the posterior pole. The color of the papilla is normal, and the retinal vessels are not narrowed.

A histological study showed that the lesions involved the choroid and pigmentary epithelium, whereas the sensory retina remained intact. These facts explain why the electroretinogram is either normal or subnormal.

---

*A syndrome that comprises aminoaciduria, congenital nuclear cataract, glaucoma, hypotrophy of weight and height, and bone disorders (Translator's note)

The effect of these lesions on visual acuity is difficult to ascertain, since they are often associated with cataracts, nystagmus, deafness, and mental retardation. However, these lesions in themselves seem to be compatible with relatively satisfactory vision. Moreover, they are static and do not progress as in true retinitis pigmentosa.

Differential diagnosis concerns hereditary retinitis pigmentosa. The parents are usually consanguineous, and eyeground examination reveals a pale pupilla, narrowed vessels, and peripheral osteoblast-like pigmentation. The electroretinogram is extinguished or severely altered in the hereditary disease, which is progressive. Hemeralopia is accompanied by an annular scotoma and, later, by a concentric diminution of the visual field, resulting in blindness. However, consanguinity is not always found. Atypical forms of retinitis pigmentosa, in which the pigmentation occurs centrally rather than peripherally, can be observed. In both cases, deafness and mental retardation are often associated with the abnormal retinal pigmentation. The association of retinitis pigmentosa with deafness is frequent. In institutions for the deaf, routine ophthalmological examination often reveals pseudoretinitis and, consequently, deafness can be ascribed to maternal rubella.

Congenital pseudoretinitis pigmentosa due to rubella rarely poses a problem of differentiation from acquired viral pseudoretinitis pigmentosa (cf. Chapter 55), which appears as a complication of measles, for example, in childhood.

OTHER OCULAR MALFORMATIONS

Rubella infection during pregnancy can result in numerous other ocular malformations.

Microphthalmia with Microcornea. The condition may occur alone or with cataract and pigmentary pseudoretinitis.

Buphthalmos. Buphthalmos, related to a malformation of the anterior chamber angle, has been described. Maternal rubella is, however, rarely the cause of infantile glaucoma.

Corneal Opacities. Such opacities are possible after maternal rubella. Posterior embryotoxon has been reported; it represents a congenital opacity of the posterior layers of the cornea.

Lesions of the Iris. After maternal rubella, atrophy of the stroma iriditis, heterochromia, and persistence of the pupillary membrane have all been described. Atrophy of the dilator iridis might be responsible for the myosis that often accompanies rubella cataract.

Lesions of the Crystalline Lens. Apart from cataract, other malformations of the crystalline lens are observed: abnormal position (ectopia), deformation of the anterior or the posterior surface (anterior or posterior lenticonus), or absence of the lens (aphakia).

Strabismus. The occurrence of strabismus is illustrated by a case reported by Paufique. A child, aged 7 years, whose mother had had rubella during the second month of gestation showed a posterior embryotoxon, vestiges of pupillary membrane, poor pupillary dilation, and degenerative abnormalities of the retina with peripapillary degeneration. Visual acuity was 6/20, but alternant convergent strabismus was associated with musculotendinous abnormalities and cardiac malformation.

Nystagmus. If the ocular lesions allow a certain degree of vision, nystagmus often aggravates visual deficiency.

Complex Lesions. Maternal rubella frequently produces complex ocular lesions in the fetus that result in the blindness.

Wolter et al. studied an eyeball removed for esthetic reasons from a girl whose mother had had rubella during the first trimester of pregnancy. The microphthalmic eyeball measured 17 mm.; the white, opaque cornea could not be distinguished from the sclera. The anterior chamber, lens, iris, and ciliary body were absent, and the eyeball was filled only with vitreous humor. The retina was thin, with several folds and peripheral cavities. On the whole, the retina and optic nerve showed a relatively satisfactory development that contrasted with the severe anomalies of the anterior segment.

When the ocular lesions are highly complex, a diagnosis of viral embryopathy may be difficult. The possibility of fetal iridochoroiditis or of chromosomal anomaly enter into the debate.

RESPONSIBLE VIRUSES

Although rubella virus is generally recognized as responsible for most ocular embryopathies of viral origin, other viruses have been accused, especially those of mumps, measles, and influenza, as well as cytomegalovirus. The action of these viruses on the embryo is not proved. The question is discussed in Chapter 61 on prenatal viral infection.

BIBLIOGRAPHY

1. Francois, J.: Les cataractes congénitales. In: Chapter XV, Embryopathie d'origine infectieuse. Rapport présenté à la Société Française d'Ophtalmologie en 1959. Paris, Masson et Cie.
2. Holowach, J., Thurston, D. L., and Becker, B.: Congenital defects in infants following mumps during pregnancy. A review of the literature and a report of chorioretinitis due to fetal infection. J. Pediat., 50:689-694, 1957.
3. Nataf, R., Lépine, P., and Bonamour, G.: Oeil et virus. In: Chapter X, Les embryopathies virales oculaires. Rapport présenté à la Société Française d'Ophtalmologie en 1960. Paris, Masson et Cie. (This chapter contains a good bibliography.)
4. Paufique, L., Ravault, P., Lequin, M., and Sourdille, P.: Malformations oculaires multiples et embryopathie rubéoleuse. Bull. Soc. Ophtal. Franç., 65:535-537, 1965.
5. Thomas, C., Cordier, J., and Rény, A.: Embryopathie oculaire et rubéole pré-conceptionnelle. Bull. Soc. Franç. Ophtal. 77:334-340, 1964.
6. Wolter, J. R., Hall, R. C., and Mason, G. L.: Unilateral primary congenital aphakia. Amer. J. Ophthal. 58:1011-1016, 1964.

57

Involvement of the Ear and of the Vestibular-Labyrinthine Tracts in Viral Infections

By M. AUBRY AND P. PIALOUX

Pathological involvement of the ear by viral infection has been known for years. Deafness in mumps and the cochleovestibular participation in zoster of the head are well characterized clinically, as are the aural consequences of maternal rubella for the future infant. On the other hand, in sudden deafness by selective involvement of the inner ear, a whole group of disorders exists in which a viral etiology may be suspected but is difficult to affirm. Viral involvement of the middle ear certainly exists, but this etiology is difficult to identify, and hence its frequency cannot be exactly specified.

We shall consider in this chapter first the middle ear, then the inner ear, and in the last section the cases in which a nerve lesion, or perhaps involvement of the nucleus of the auditory nerve, is considered probable.

VIRAL LESIONS OF THE MIDDLE EAR

Viral involvement of the middle ear is theoretically probable. Simple serous otitis media, catarrhal inflammation also involving the eustachian tube and the tympanum, and suppurative otitis media all frequently follow coryza, rhinopharyngitis, or sore throat. The preponderance of viruses is recognized in the etiology of many cases of inflammation of the nasal fossae, of the pharynx, and of the tonsils. This inflammatory condition is attended first by dryness, and the mucosa appears dark red; then it is the site of an abundant clear nonpurulent discharge. The sense of smell and the conjunctiva may be affected in addition. In practice, the viral origin of the ear involvement is hard to ascertain: on the one hand, identification of the virus is difficult and is rarely attempted; on the other, secondary infection by common bacteria almost always, if not always, occurs. Probably in the large majority of cases in which suppuration appears, it is due to microbial superinfection.

Tubotympanal Catarrh and Serous Otitis. When the cause is not simply mechanical (obstruction of the eustachian tube) but inflammatory, the viral origin that is still unproved is, nonetheless, probable. The reason for this likelihood is the viral etiology of the coryza or of the rhinopharyngeal infection, especially when the tubotympanal inflammation and the primary infection of the nasal fossae or of the rhinopharynx are concomitant and microbial superinfection has not had time to occur. Moreover, in such cases, the fluid aspirated on myringotomy is bacteriologically sterile, a fact that may constitute indirect proof of nonmicrobial contamination.

Suppurative Otitis Media. A viral origin in such cases is also extremely difficult to identify. Several studies have been made. Grönroos et al. investigated 322 cases of otitis media but were unable to isolate a virus in any of them. Laxdal et al. also failed in this respect in 18 patients, but in two they found positive serological reactions. Yochie isolated a virus in four of ten subjects with otitis media; two showed antibodies. In nine of ten children, Berglund et al. identified a virus in the auricular effusion and in the pharynx. Halstead et al. investigated 106 cases in children but managed to isolate a virus from the auricular fluid in only one, although they found a virus in the pharynx in ten; results of serological tests were positive in 15.

More recently Tilles et al. attempted to identify a virus in 90 children with auricular effusion. They isolated a virus in only two: adenovirus type 3 in one and Coxsackie B4 in the other. In 73 of the 90 children, the serological reactions were tested; they gave positive results in 19. After this brief glimpse of the problem, the great difficulty for the time being of ascertaining precisely the viral origin of acute suppurative otitis media seems evident.

In the rare cases in which viral involvement, or at least a viral association, has been proved, the clinical picture of acute suppurative otitis media seems impossible to differentiate from other forms. The systemic and functional signs are identical. Otoscopic examination also shows the same picture, with a red bulging eardrum. The course does not present any etiologically specific characteristic. One case complicated by mastoiditis was reported by Van Dishoeck, but to draw any conclusion from a single case is really difficult.

Other Forms of Otitis Media. Several types deserve especial mention.

MYRINGITIS. The inflammation of the tympanum is often attended by blister formation. Serous effusion may or may not be present. The condition often appears during influenza. It does not usually evolve toward suppuration. This form does not generally necessitate paracentesis, although occasionally simple evacuation of the serous effusion by aspiration is required. Merifield and Miller found no positive serological result in the 23 cases of this type investigated, despite utilization of numerous different antigens. Rifkind et al., however, produced otitis of this type in 12 of a series of 27 adult volunteers inoculated with *Mycoplasma pneumoniae*. Sobeslavsky et al. isolated and identified this same microorganism in one case both in the auricular effusion and in the pharynx. Many authors tend, moreover, to consider that this clinical form of otitis is very probably of viral origin or due to a mycoplasma; the probable role of *Mycoplasma pneumoniae* is particularly emphasized even though the probable role of this agent is difficult to determine exactly.

HYPERACUTE FORM. The otitis is characterized by intense pain often associated with cerebromeningeal signs; general physical condition is altered rapidly, and fever is high. This form of otitis media with sanguinolent effusion is exceptional today. It was complicated within a few hours by myringitis, and by mastoid and meningeal signs. This particular form has been attributed to viruses but also to certain streptococci and pneumococci.

OTHER FORMS OF POSSIBLE VIRAL ORIGIN. In some forms occurring during measles or influenza, viral etiology is probable, but the proof has almost never been made. The serosanguinolent effusion with functional involvement of the inner ear is, however, accepted as a valuable element in the diagnosis.

Therapy of Viral Lesions of the Middle Ear. The forms described do not present any particular indications different from those in the other clinical forms. If signs of inner ear involvement appear, the antibiotic treatment should be reinforced to combat the secondary bacterial superinfection.

VIRAL INVOLVEMENT OF THE INNER EAR

These forms are much more interesting from the virological standpoint. The exact diagnosis is not, however, always made. In certain cases it is made only because of the clinical context: mumps, rubella, influenza, or viral pneumopathy. In other cases the virus can be identified in samples from the nasopharynx, the blood, or the cerebrospinal fluid; antibodies against the virus can be determined. When a precise clinical context is absent, the physician searches in the patient's history for precedent rhinopharyngitis, periods of malaise, asthenia, and predominantly posterior headache. Aside from the diseases already mentioned, upper respiratory infection seems to be among the most frequently discovered elements in the history of inner ear infection. We shall discuss the epidemiology, then the pathology, clinical aspects, diagnosis, and treatment of the disorder. In the section on clinical features we shall go into the involvement of the labyrinth in known viral diseases such as mumps and rubella and also discuss the group of disorders marked by sudden deafness, the viral origin of which is possible.

EPIDEMIOLOGY AND PATHOGENESIS

The disease seems to arise from the propagation of a virus present first in the upper or lower respiratory tract. When an attempt has been made to pinpoint the viral etiology, a virus has been isolated a certain number of times at one level or another in the respiratory system. In general, the most frequent point of departure would seem to be rhinopharyngitis, tracheobronchitis, or viral pneumopathy.

No precise knowledge at present exists in otorhinolaryngology as regards contagion during the propagation of a virus toward the labyrinth. Contagion does not seem to be frequent, however. In a family with several children, mumps as a rule spreads to all of them and in a few cases to one of the adults. It is rare, on the other hand, for several to present an auricular complication; the complication appears in only one person. Van Dishoeck, however, reported the following case. During the regression of a viral pneumopathy, a mother presented sudden irreversible deafness. Her son living with her also had pneumopathy and deafness, but in him the deafness regressed. This case report is not conclusive, because the origin in the labyrinth of the son's deafness cannot be affirmed for want of an audiogram.

The date of the appearance of the auricular involvement in regard to the course of the viral disease is not always easy to ascertain. During mumps, the ear complication usually occurs a few days after the appearance of parotid tumefaction. It seems to be related to the severity of the clinical syndrome and especially to that of the meningeal reaction. These data cannot, however, be considered absolute. In the course of viral respiratory disease, involvement of the ear seems to appear more frequently during the regression of the illness.

It is difficult to be precise as to the nature of viruses with a specificity for the cochleovestibular system, with the exception of those of measles, mumps, rubella, and herpes zoster, and to a lesser degree, chickenpox and smallpox. Influenza viruses must also be mentioned. Earlier in this chapter we emphasized the probable role of adenoviruses, influenza type A, and Coxsackie B4, as well as *Mycoplasma pneumoniae*. Van Dishoeck called attention to Columbia SK virus,* as well as Coxsackie viruses. In reality, it seems difficult to be affirmative in the matter at the present time.

The propagation of viruses to the inner ear and the acoustic nerve seems to occur by three pathways: directly from the middle ear, by the meninges and the cerebrospinal fluid, and by the blood.

The first hypothesis seems to be valid in measles and chickenpox especially when, in presence of otitis media, an involvement of the inner ear, labyrinthitis, occurs secondarily, even when the otitis interna is nonsuppurative. In such cases propagation via the blood cannot be excluded in view of the arterial connection between the two organs.

In the course of mumps and of all viral infections leading to meningeal involvement,

---

*Encephalomyocarditis virus, pathogenic in rodents, pigs, monkeys, and rarely in man; it belongs, like Coxsackie viruses, to the picornavirus group.

the cerebrospinal fluid is considered to be the vehicle. This pathway seems likely and its plausibility is reinforced by a certain number of histopathological data.

Work in the United States tends to demonstrate that the blood route plays a preponderant role. Lindsay considers, on the basis of a histopathological research, that propagation via the blood is the most plausible mechanism.

Until recent years, a certain number of factors were suggested: edema in the labyrinth of allergic origin, vascular spasm, sunstroke, a chill, or psychological shock. Probably these elements exist, but they tend increasingly to be considered as factors that set off a latent viral infection.

PATHOLOGY

Study of the pathology is the only scientific basis on which one can found an attempt to understand the pathogenesis of viral involvement of the labyrinth and the acoustic nerve.

In cases of involvement by the meningeal route, Nager made a study in 1907 that is still valid because of its precision and because the results have since been confirmed. The perilabyrinthine spaces showed a generalized fibrous reaction with bony neoformation in spots. Degenerative lesions were found in the nerve elements, the psalterial cord, and Corti's organ. The cochlear canal was obliterated.

Among authors of recent work, Schuknecht et al. studied four cases of sudden deafness, and Lindsay reported four: one in measles, one in rubella, and two in mumps. A certain reserve is, nonetheless, legitimate, for most of these histological studies were made long after the occurrence of deafness. As Lindsay himself emphasized, reactions of cicatricial type can alter the specific appearance. In one of his cases, however, the examination was made fairly early at the "subacute stage."

Lindsay found that, in function of the case, the lesions can be limited to the cochlea, or involve only the cochlea and the sacculus. They can involve the cochlea, sacculus, utricle, and semicircular canals. The initial inflammatory reaction develops in the blood vessels. Secondary alteration appears in the endolymph. Progressive degeneration of the sensory cells, the sustaining cells, and the nerve elements follows the initial lesions.

In the case of rubella he studied, Lindsay found that the degenerative lesions were limited to the structures of the cochlear canal and to those of the sacculus. In the two cases of mumps, the involvement was confined to the cochlear canal and its content, with, however, discrete degenerative lesions of the spiral ganglion.

Schuknecht et al. made their histological studies in four cases of sudden deafness long after its advent, but their conclusion nonetheless seems worth mention. As concerns Corti's organ, they found several degrees. These were: disappearance of the ciliated cells with intact sustaining cells; disappearance of the hair cells and collapse of the supporting structures; atrophy of all of Corti's organ, and, lastly, disappearance of the organ. In one case these authors also noted disappearance of the sensorial cells of the saccular macula. They found different degrees of degeneration of the cells of the spiral ganglion and observed that the severity of this degeneration was proportional to that of the alteration of the supporting cells in Corti's organ.

They concluded that the degeneration is secondary to the alteration of the supporting structures. Schuknecht et al. also found involvement of the tectorial membrane. In all four cases, the stria vascularis was involved, although to different degrees. However, an important fact, all these lesions differed clearly from those seen in cases of vascular obstruction, i.e., those in deafness of vascular origin.

CLINICAL FEATURES

A characteristic common to all auricular involvement of viral origin is its gravity from the functional standpoint because of the difficulty and the slightness of effect of treatment.

During *mumps,* tinnitus may be the first symptom of the labyrinthine complication. It is barely marked in the child, who does not always pay attention to it. The tinnitus nonetheless seems to increase progressively; within a few hours hearing loss and vertigo appear. The degree of hearing impairment rapidly increases in 24 or 48 hours, or occasionally in three or four days, and then becomes stable. The degree of loss varies with the subject. It may attain total deafness, although absolute loss of hearing is infrequent. The impairment presents all the characteristics of an endocochlear lesion: perceptive deafness and phenomenon of recruitment. Air conduction and bone conduction are both involved, in the low frequencies less than the high frequencies. In the days following, some recuperation may occur, but it is never complete, and it is inversely proportional to the severity of the earlier deafness. In the great majority of cases, unilateral impairment of hearing occurs. In the rare cases in which the involvement is bilateral, it is distinctly asymmetrical. Vertigo and disturbances in balance are usually slight except at the onset, when severe vertigo of the whirling type with repeated vomiting occasionally occurs. The vertigo and vomiting may, moreover, be related to a meningeal syndrome. The syndrome of vertigo disappears in the following days in children. In the adult the disequilibrium may persist longer. At this point vestibular hypoactivity is revealed by testing. This hypoactivity seems fairly rare in children.

Hearing loss consequent to *rubella* is always bilateral and asymmetrical, and is always severe. The impairment is of the perceptive type with recruitment. The audiometric curves may assume any type, showing loss in high frequencies, in all frequencies, in a U-shaped curve, or involvement in the low frequencies. Associated vestibular involvement is fairly common, but not a regular occurrence. Usually it is manifested by bilateral, asymmetrical hypoactivity without severe functional disturbances. In rubella the consequences of the auricular lesions are particularly serious, for the child is born deaf. All the problems of auditory education arise and are often difficult to solve.

In *sudden deafness,* the hearing impairment is often preceded by phenomena such as buzzing and tinnitus of variable degree. As soon as the hearing loss begins, these phenomena are regularly present and are usually acute. The impairment develops within a few hours or two or three days as a rule. Occasionally it occurs with the suddenness of the drop of a curtain over the acoustic duct. Several cases have been reported in which it occurred during a telephone conversation. The intensity of the deafness varies. It is usually fairly marked, of the order of 50 to 60 decibels of loss, but it may be complete. Impairment is of the perceptive type with recruitment. The audiometric curves

vary in form: usually they are steep, occasionally horizontal, or with predominances in the low frequencies. Recuperation is not common. When it occurs, it is rarely complete and always progressive. It may occur quickly, in five to ten days, but more often is fairly slow, over a period of months. Burton et al. reported a case in which hearing improvement was detected only after nine months. In this case viral origin was proved. Fairly often sudden deafness is accompanied by vertigo, at least at the onset. The attack of whirling vertigo, of variable intensity, at the onset is followed by slight phenomena of positional type vertigo, or by instability in walking. These disturbances usually dsisappear progressively with sole sequel of more or less marked vestibular hypoactivity. They may persist, however, especially in persons past middle age. In a few cases episodic attacks of slight vertigo over several weeks may be the earliest sign of the endolabyrinthine involvement. We have seen two cases of the type, the viral origin of which was strongly suspected.

DIAGNOSIS

Diagnosis is easy in a precise clinical context such as measles, mumps, or rubella, known or probable, in the first two months of pregnancy. Mumps can present clinical forms leaving uncertainty. In a family, all the children but one present mumps in a regular and manifest order. One is apparently not infected. He presented only a vague earache, headache, or isolated rise in temperature. He is usually thought to have escaped mumps. Hearing impairment is noted only days or months later. The same may be true of an adult in the same family who had had "parotitis" in childhood or adolescence. Careful questioning at the time when deafness appears reveals in the history a degree of asthenia or vague pains at the nape of the neck during a mumps epidemic.

In presence of sudden deafness, viral origin is extremely difficult to ascertain; isolation of a virus from the blood or the cerebrospinal fluid and probative determination of antibodies are often difficult at the stage when deafness is detected. Only the first result establishes the evidence. A certain suspicion arises when a virus is found in the nasopharynx. Likewise, knowledge of recent influenza, rhinopharyngitis, or bronchopulmonary illness is an argument as to the probability of a viral etiology.

TREATMENT

Viral deafness presents considerable problems. Practically, no effective therapy exists. Antibiotics are useful only against secondary infection. Corticosteroid therapy is of questionable usefulness and is considered dangerous in viral infections such as varicella, herpes, and others. Some antiviral-type drugs such as ABOB (see p. 43) can, however, be tried, although their efficacy is highly questionable. Prescription of vitamins seems desirable, especially all the group B vitamins. Some authors recommend vasodilators in view of the similarity to sudden deafness of purely vascular origin. The histological lesions that Lindsay and Schuknecht et al. found in the stria vascularis do not seem to indicate such therapy. Moreover, treatment with vasodilators cannot be undertaken until the time when the lesions are already established, and, in consequence, they are ineffective. Therapy seems, hence, to belong to the realm of the future.

NEURAL INVOLVEMENT

In this last section we shall consider cephalitic zoster and isolated vestibular involvements (sometimes called neuraxitis or neuronitis).

HERPES ZOSTER

In zoster oticus, but also in other forms of cephalic zoster and even that of the superficial cervical plexus, cochleovestibular involvement may appear. It is most frequently related to zoster oticus. According to statistics compiled by Ramsay Hunt, this complication occurs in one case in three.

The site of the lesions is essentially the geniculate ganglion and Scarpa's and Corti's ganglion. A nuclear involvement, however, appears probable. Lhermitte and Nicolas published a histopathological study of a case in which they found lesions of the cerebral trunk. A similar case was reported by Wohlwill. We ourselves observed a patient who, on the fifteenth day of the eruption of zoster, presented a central vestibular syndrome characterized by multiple nystagmus and severe bilateral hypoactivity of the labyrinthine reactions with normal hearing. The lesions therefore seem to be of a ganglioradicular type; they may also involve the nuclear bulbopontine area.

Clinical Features. Zoster oticus is marked by the triad: earache, eruption of zoster, and facial paralysis. Earache is the first symptom; the eruption appears toward the fourth or the fifth day, and the facial paralysis follows.

If cochleovestibular involvement occurs, it is contemporaneous with the eruption or appears, as a rule, within the 48 hours following its appearance. In certain cases, the two are dissociated; in such cases, the auricular vestibule seems to be the organ most readily involved.

The involvement manifests itself abruptly by a severe crisis of whirling vertigo that lasts two or three hours and is repeated during two or three days at variable intervals. During these intervals, a subvertiginous state persists. More rarely, the phenomena of vertigo are milder. Objectively, the vertigo is manifested by spontaneous nystagmus of the horizontal rotary type. The intensity varies. Vestibular hypoactivity is more usually shown by testing, but hyperactivity is found occasionally. Later, recuperation occurs, but is fairly slow.

Tinnitus and hearing loss attend the crises of vertigo. Impairment of hearing develops progressively. It is of the perceptive type without recruitment, i.e., of retrocochlear type. The audiometric curve is usually normal up to the 1000 frequency. Beyond this point, it falls sharply. Occasionally, however, the impairment is parallel for all frequencies. We have observed two cases of this type. The prognosis of the hearing impairment is not excellent: recuperation occasionally does not occur, and when it does, is always slow and often incomplete. Recuperation seems to be related to the severity of the original hearing impairment.

ISOLATED UNILATERAL VESTIBULAR NEURITIS

The disease is still called neuronitis vestibularis (Dix and Hallpike) or neuropathia vestibularis (Stenger). Ruttin distinguished it as an entity in 1909 and attributed it to inflammation, without examination by spinal puncture.

The cause is ill known. No alteration of the cerebrospinal fluid has been found. Most authors consider vascular or angioneurotic disturbances to be probable. Others have proposed the hypothesis of allergy or of focal infection. In 1949 Winther described a vestibular neuraxitis. Aschan described a vestibular nucleoreticular syndrome arising from involvement of the central nuclei.

Dix and Hallpike believed that cause of neuronitis vestibularis is vascular but may also have an inflammatory cause without its being possible, clinically, to distinguish these two forms.

Podrebersek considers that the origin may be viral and hence necessitates serological examination. To date no precise information has been reported in this regard. The cases reported by Dalsgaard and Nielson seem to give some support to the hypothesis of a viral origin, for they reported a small epidemic. The viral hypothesis seems to be supported by the report of muscular and articular aches and pains and febrile influenza-like state preceding or accompanying the attacks of vertigo.

Clinical Features. Posterior cephalgia is often a premonitory sign; then a sudden crisis of vertigo appears in association with sudden unilateral loss of vestibular function. As a predisposing cause, cold has been accused, in circumstances of work or travel, supposedly more frequently in men aged 30 to 40 years.

The vestibular syndrome is characterized by severe true vertigo that may appear in the middle of the night and is occasionally accompanied by diplopia. This state of vertigo may continue several weeks. The accompanying nystagmus is typical of vestibular destruction (hence noted on the uninvolved side); complete loss of vestibular function or marked hypoactivity are found as a rule. In rare instances, examination shows hyperactivity. The vertigo is accompanied by fairly marked neurovegetative signs. On the other hand, signs of cochlear origin are absent, and the cerebrospinal fluid is normal. The prognosis is favorable, despite frequent persistence of some degree of vestibular hypoactivity.

Diagnosis. The disorder requires differentiation from a sudden attack of vertigo in Ménière's syndrome, but the absence of cochlear signs suffices to eliminate Ménière's syndrome. Positional nystagmus is also easy to eliminate in view of the absence of cochlear signs; in this disorder, vertigo occurs in only certain head positions.

Treatment. Sudation, corticosteroids, and vasodilators have been recommended without a conclusion as to the proper treatment. A focal disorder should be searched for (Mündnich, Pfaltz).

BIBLIOGRAPHY

1. Aubry, M., and Pialoux, P.: Maladies de l'oreille interne et oto-neurologie. Paris, Editions Masson, 1957.
2. Berglund, B., Salmivalli, A., Toivanen, P., and Wickstrom, J.: Isolation of respiratory syncytial virus from middle ear exudates of infants. Arch. Dis. Child., *41*:554, 1966.
3. Coffey, J. D., Jr.: Otitis media in the practice of pediatrics: bacteriological and clinical observations. Pediatrics, *38*:25-32, 1966.
4. Feingold, M., et al.: Acute otitis media in children. Bacteriological findings in middle ear fluid obtained by needle aspiration. Amer. J. Dis. Child., *111*:361-365, 1966.
5. Fishman, L. Z., Lennette, E. H., and Dannenberg, T. B.: Indolent, or so-called serous otitis media, including combined allergy and virus studies. Arch. Otolaryng., *72*:25-30, 1960.
6. Foy, H. M., Grayston, J. T., Kenny, G. E., Alexander, E. R., and McMahon, R.: Epidemiology of Mycoplasma pneumoniae infection in families. J.A.M.A., *197*:859-866, 1966.
7. Grönroos, J. A., Kortekangas, A. E., Ojala, L., and Vuori, M.: Aetiology of acute middle ear infection. Acta Otolaryng. (Stockholm), *58*:149-158, 1964.
8. Halstead, C., Lepow, M. L., and Wolinsky, E.: Personal communication from M. L. Lepow, January 16, 1967.
9. Lahikainen, E. A.: Clinicobacteriologic studies on acute otitis media: aspiration of tympanum as diagnostic and therapeutic method. Acta Otolaryng. (Stockholm), Suppl. 107, pp. 1-82, 1953.
10. Laxdal, O. E., Blake, R. M., Cartmill, T., and Robertson, H. E.: Etiology of acute otitis media of infants and children. Canad. Med. Assoc. J., *94*:159-163, 1966.
11. Leading article. Mycoplasmas. Lancet, *2*:248, 1967.
12. Lindsay J. R.: Viral labyrinthitis – histopathologic characteristics. Acta Otolaryng. (Stockholm), *63*:2-3, 1967.
13. Merifield, D. O., and Miller, G. S.: Etiology and clinical course of bullous myringitis. Arch. Otolaryng. *84*:487-489, 1966.
14. Mortimer, E. A., Jr., and Watterson, R. L., Jr.: Bacteriologic investigation of otitis media in infancy. Pediatrics, *17*:359-369, 1956.
15. Nelson, W. E.: Textbook of Pediatrics. Philadelphia, W. B. Saunders Co., 1964, p. 819.
16. Nielsen, J. C.: Studies of the Aetiology of Acute Otitis Media. Copenhagen, Munksgaard, 1945.
17. Pfaltz, C. R.: Differentialdiagnostische Probleme bei Vestibularisstörungen. HNO, *8*:217, 1960.
18. Rifkind, D., Chanock, R., Kravetz, H., Johnson, K., and Knight, V.: Ear involvement (myringitis) and primary atypical pneumonia following inoculation of volunteers with Eaton agent. Amer. Rev. Resp. Dis., *85*:479-489, 1962.
19. Sever, J. L.: Application of microtechnique to viral serological investigations. J. Immun., *88*:320-329, 1962.

20. Siirala, U., Tarpila, S., and Halonen, P.: Inhibitory effect of sterile otitis media exudates on the cytopathogenicity of herpes simplex poliomyelitis and adenoviruses in HeLa cells. Acta Otolaryng. (Stockholm), *53*:230-236, 1961.

21. Sobeslavsky, L., Syucek, L., Bruckova, M., and Abrahamovic, M.: Etiological role of Mycoplasma pneumoniae in otitis media in children. Pediatrics, *35*:652-657, 1965.

22. Spigland, I., et al.: Virus watch program: continuing surveillance of viral infection in metropolitan New York families. II. Laboratory methods and preliminary report on infections revealed by virus isolation. Amer. J. Epidemiol., *83*:413-435, 1966.

23. Stenger, M. M.: HNO, Vol. 3, Part 3, 1928.

24. United States Department of Health, Education, and Welfare, Public Health Service. Diagnostic Complement Fixation Method (L.C.E.). Laboratory Branch Training Manual. Atlanta, Georgia, Communicable Disease Center, 1962.

25. Van Dishoeck, H. A. E.: Viral infection in two cases of sudden perceptive deafness. Acta Otolaryng. (Stockholm), Suppl. 183, pp. 30-33, 1963.

26. Vogel, J., and Shelokof, A.: Adsorption-hemagglutination test for influenza virus in monkey kidney tissue culture. Science, *126*:358, 1957.

27. Yochie, C.: On isolation of influenza virus from middle ear exudates of infants. Arch. Dis. Child., *41*:554, 1966.

PART X

Viral Infections in Relation to Other Conditions

58

Acute Febrile Syndromes

By C. HANNOUN

INTRODUCTION

The first symptoms of attack of the human organism by an infectious agent are almost always the same, whatever the agent may be. With a few rare exceptions, all virus diseases begin with a "prodromic" phase during which the signs and symptoms are considered to be "undifferentiated," but systemic. Often this initial phase or *acute febrile syndrome* is considered preliminary; hence the term prodromic phase (from the Greek word for forerunning) or *premonitory symptoms*. Whatever may be the virus disease, it is now clear that this febrile state is, in fact, *one of the stages of infection*. Though the infection is not yet specifically identifiable at this stage, an irreversible process has already begun, the character of which will become more specific in the hours and days that follow.

ISOLATED ACUTE FEBRILE SYNDROMES

Such syndromes are characterized by sudden appearance of a clinical picture that may be more or less dramatic, but is always complex. The predominant features are hyperthermia with chills and malaise. Frequent additional components are frontal headache, ocular pains with photophobia, muscular and/or articular pain, slight stiffness of the neck and back, and anorexia. Occasional components are vomiting, abdominal discomfort, a red throat, abundant sweating, and congestion of the face and conjunctiva.

These symptoms are of moderate intensity at the outset. None of them predomi-

nates sufficiently to guide the clinical diagnosis in any well marked direction. *It is important to bear in mind that this clinical picture can represent, or at least mark the beginning of, almost any virus disease, including those diseases that have other, specific symptoms later on.*

This clinical picture can appear and develop with variable degrees of intensity. At one extreme, all the symptoms that compose the picture can be so discrete that they are overlooked completely. This is the case in *inapparent primary viral infection*. When they are mild, they represent a slightly apparent primary infection that usually escapes the physician's observation, for the malaise rapidly disappears and the patient notices it only slightly, and, in any event, does not consult a physician. When the symptoms are more marked, a *typical acute febrile syndrome* is observed with all or part of the classic picture. In this case, the physician is often consulted and must make a diagnosis and decide a therapy. Diagnosis at this time is still difficult. In addition to the clinical data, an ensemble of external factors must be considered, such as living conditions, general epidemiological context, and age and previous history of the subject.

When the infection is in fact viral, two main possibilities then exist. Either the course will be degressive and clear up definitively, with recovery at this point, or else, perhaps after several days of remission or even apparent recovery, new signs and symptoms will develop more or less rapidly and create a new picture. In this second phase of the disease, it may be easier to make a specific diagnosis. This diagnosis often is

761

made in vague general terms such as "viral pneumopathy," or "viral encephalitis." Laboratory tests are necessary to determine the exact etiology, even though definition of the cause is not always of great importance in the decision as to treatment. The patient also may be examined only during the second phase of the disease, the initial febrile syndrome having passed unnoticed.

Thus the course of most virus diseases can be schematically divided into several phases. The first lies *between* the infecting contact with the virus and the onset of signs and symptoms. This is the *incubation phase,* during which the virus begins to invade the organism. This phase could be called the silent invasion phase. The second is the prodromic period, during which symptoms and signs appear suddenly in a single system or involve the entire organism. The first symptoms are subjective (malaise, fatigue); then objective signs appear (hyperthermia, congestion). This phase is now generally called an acute febrile syndrome; it is the one discussed in this chapter.

The third phase, which does not necessarily occur in all diseases or even in every case of a single disease, is that during which the *characteristic symptoms* appear. These symptoms occasionally permit diagnosis, as in measles or poliomyelitis, or at least help to direct the diagnosis, toward respiratory viral disease, for example.

It is thus important, when a patient is seen in the second phase of disease, to try to determine whether signs and symptoms represent the whole disease, as in an "influenza-like" syndrome, or a "dengue-like fever," or whether the disease will probably develop toward a more specific clinical picture.

Although, as mentioned earlier, the picture noted during the febrile phase is common and nonspecific, it nonetheless corresponds to specific phenomena of the viral infection and represents tendencies, intensification of which may later lead to more specific symptoms. For example, in its classic form dengue provokes a few hemorrhagic phenomena that may pass for a somewhat uncharacteristic manifestation of the disease. However, this symptom is marked in the "hemorrhagic fever" form of the disease caused by the same virus and occupies the foreground. It is useful to examine individually each of the principal phenomena during "undifferentiated" febrile states, especially the systemic disturbances, viremia, fever, tendency to hemorrhage, exanthem, inflammatory reaction, and leukopenia.

SYSTEMIC DISORDERS

An ensemble of subjective systemic symptoms precedes or accompanies the appearance of precise objective signs. At first, with a vague sensation of malaise and fatigue, the patient feels limp, loses appetite, and has diffuse unsystematized pain in bones, joints, and muscles. These disturbances are the prelude to various other pathological phenomena, of which they are the first subjective manifestation.

During this time, the virus is multiplying and invading a tissue, a system, or the whole organism. The disorders reflect: *viral multiplication* in certain susceptible cells the physiological functions of which are then disturbed; the presence of viruses in the blood (viremia) owing to the *toxicity* proper to certain viruses; the presence in tissues and the blood of *degradation products* from the involved or destroyed cells, and the appearance of a degree of *vascular and circulatory disturbance.*

This undifferentiated syndrome may be followed secondarily by more specific disorders or lesions of one or another organ system that progressively yield the clinical picture specific to the infection.

VIREMIA

Invasion by virus via the blood occurs in most viral infections that involve tissues and organs far from the portal of entry. This invasion via the circulation occurs by the intermediary of the lymphatic system, by active or passive transport of the virus by circulating cells (leukocytes), by spread of the infection from vascular epithelium, or by direct transport by the blood plasma. Viremia begins during the incubation phase and persists for a variable length of time during the acute phase of the disease. Sometimes it occurs in several stages: *primary viremia* during which, from its entrance point, the virus invades susceptible organs (lymphatic system, spleen) where it actively multiplies and from which sites a more abundant *secondary viremia* arises. The virus then totally invades the organism. The prodromic acute febrile syndrome appears, not at the time when the virus enters the organism, but during one or even both of these phases of viremia. During them, the concentration of virus in the blood may reach a high level. Since viremia is an early phenomenon, the attempt to isolate the virus must often be made soon after the first signs. Several examples have been reported of isolation of arboviruses from blood samples taken one or two days before the appearance of symptoms. The level of viremia decreases as soon as circulating antibodies appear, although virus isolation is not necessarily impossible, owing to the weak avidity of the earliest antibodies.

FEBRILE STATE

Fever occurs during most viral diseases and is often the first measurable objective sign. Impairment of thermoregulatory mechanisms indicates important organic dysfunction, the causes and consequences of which are essential in the complex process of infection. Various series of experiments have been performed in an attempt to understand how this impairment occurs, especially during viral infections. One elementary and easily demonstrated fact is the pyrogenic effect proper to certain preparations of viruses. After earlier studies had elucidated certain aspects of the pyrogenic effect of bacterial toxins, in 1949 Wagner, Bennett, and Le Quire[86] studied the effect of injection into rabbits of purified influenza virus. Although little or no viral multiplication occurs in this animal, such injection provokes marked rise in temperature after a brief latent period. This period is about one hour, which is distinctly longer than that produced by bacterial pyrogens and hence indicates a difference in the mode of action. The effect of viruses is indirect. A pyrogenic substance different from the virus itself appears in the sera of inoculated rabbits. When this substance is injected into a new series of rabbits, it elicits an immediate rise in temperature and has effects similar to those produced in polymorphonuclear leukocytes by contact with bacterial endotoxins (Atkins and Huang[6]). In 1964 King observed the same phenomenon with use of Coxsackie B1 virus.

A similar pyrogenic substance was obtained by Atkins et al.[5] in 1964: after incubation of purified parainfluenza virus with rabbit leukocytes, the cells produced a substance capable of eliciting an immediate pyrogenic effect. Nonstimulated leukocytes or mononuclear cells from various sources, such as lymph nodes and spleen, did not produce a pyrogenic substance. The cells responsible for production of this factor are probably the polymorphonuclear leukocytes. Injection of either a virus or a virus-induced pyrogenic substance, moreover, simultaneously produces lymphocytopenia, a fact that suggests cell damage. The rise in temperature produced by injection of the pyrogenic substance is diphasic. The first phase corresponds to direct stimulation of the thermoregulatory centers, the second probably to a new liberation of the pyrogen. Rabbits subjected to a first injection of the virus or the pyrogen are rendered tolerant as concerns a second injection of the virus but respond to a second injection of the pyrogenic substance by hyperthermia due to direct action as in the first phase of the diphasic response. The mechanism hence appears to be complex and is explained by an action of the virus on the sensitive cells that are probably altered and liberate products acting on the thermoregulatory centers.

Hyperthermia is a reaction that may play a favorable role in the development of the infection. A. Lwoff and M. Lwoff in work published in 1959 and 1960 demonstrated that systemic rise in temperature or a rise localized at an inflammatory focus can inhibit or even totally block viral development and thus limit the infection. The degree of inhibition depends on the temperature attained and the sensitivity of the virus in question. Numerous observations of the favorable effects of hyperthermia in several virus infections of man and of animals have been published, among them those of A. Lwoff (1959) on myxoma, herpes, Coxsackie viruses, and poliomyelitis. At least one mechanism is known: the thermoresistance of viruses in certain phases of development is related to their virulence. The most sensitive strains are inhibited when temperature rises and are hence of low virulence, whereas thermoresistant strains are more virulent, since they are not affected by this mechanism. A. Lwoff considered that hyperthermia is one of the important nonspecific factors that determine the development of a viral infection and the outcome in the infected subject.

TENDENCY TO HEMORRHAGE

In a certain number of acute febrile syndromes, signs indicate a tendency to hemorrhage, among them, *lowered platelet count* and *capillary fragility*. A few cutaneous manifestations may be found, and more or less abundant hemorrhage occur.

This tendency is variable. With certain viruses the intensity of these phenomena varies from one epidemic and from one geographic region to another. Dengue, a disease that always causes a certain degree of thrombocytopenia,[52] under certain conditions provokes hemorrhagic fevers that sometimes have been taken for a totally different disease.

The physiopathology of these phenomena has not been clearly elucidated, but many hypotheses have been proposed. According to certain authors, the virus acts directly on the platelets: the virus can incorporate itself into the platelet or become affixed to it. In the case of the influenza virus, this phenomenon has been demonstrated,[36] as well as that of platelet agglutination.[50] These interactions modify the platelets, which liberate sialic acid, and the virus-platelet complex is then probably eliminated by the reticuloendothelial system. Other authors have proposed an allergic mechanism to explain the same phenomena. In this hypothesis the virus renders the subject's platelets antigenic; production of antiplatelet antibodies is hence supposed, with resultant thrombocytopenia.[44]

Another explanation concerns the direct action of the virus on the bone marrow, in which, according to Nelson and Bierman,[52] dengue virus causes marked aplasia of all elements. In certain cases they found no megakaryocytes. Aplasia could obviously explain not only the reduction in platelet count but also that of the granulocytes; in general, leukocyte count is much more reduced by viral infection than that of the lymphoid cells. In the case of dengue, from the seventh day on, the bone marrow resumes its activity and even becomes hyperplastic; young cells of all types become extremely abundant. The bone marrow returns to normal only toward the twelfth day of disease. Moreover, thrombocytopenia is accompanied by decreased activity of factors V and VII + X and decrease of prothrombin.

According to Halstead,[28] the mechanism of shock during acute hemorrhagic infections begins by virus-produced lesions in the capillary system. The intensity of this generalized impairment varies from one virus to another. When it is marked, it has severe conse-

quences. In hemorrhagic fever syndromes, for example, capillary lesions result in modification of vascular permeability. Fluids, including proteins, leak into the intracellular spaces. This phenomenon, coupled with dehydration due to hemoconcentration and decrease in blood volume, overloads the heart and causes a degree of hypoxia. Hypoxia and other ensuing factors of toxicity result in acidosis and hyponatremia. Progressive hepatic alterations, revealed by increase in transaminase level and decrease in clotting factors, are accompanied by thrombocytopenia. These disorders initiate a cyclic aggravation of the syndrome: they increase the endothelial lesions, the effects of which become more marked, and these effects in turn accelerate the disease process. Without treatment, this accelerated course ends in a state of shock characteristic of hemorrhagic fevers, for example. In the case of the less pathogenic viruses, however, the disease process may not reach such an extreme; it may even go no further than the stage of "tendency to hemorrhage."

EXANTHEMAS

Exanthemas associated with virus diseases usually have distinctive characteristics familiar to clinicians. In many cases, the date of onset of these cutaneous signs, and their appearance, extent, and course make possible a quasi-certain clinical diagnosis. However, during the first phase of an acute febrile syndrome, all of these elements are not always evident, and diagnosis may be difficult. Cutaneous manifestations of viral infections are discussed in Chapters 27 and 28. We shall consider here only the preliminary aspects of viral exanthemas, but shall include those in viral infections not specifically considered to be eruptive.

Skin damage during viral infection obviously is the direct or indirect consequence of intracellular viral reproduction and its primary pathogenic effect on sensitive cells. The lesions are local and centered around clusters of cells infected or even destroyed by the virus. The most typical lesions seem to consist of foci of infection in the capillary endothelium. These lesions originate from virus particles that attached themselves, during viremia, to cells of the vascular walls, infected them and then, by dissemination from cell to cell, induce a focus of infection. After each cycle of cellular infection the virus is shed into the blood, and comes into direct contact with neighboring cells. Thus two phenomena occur together: viral dissemination, which can be massive and increase the titer of viremia, and a necrotic, microfocus of infection.

INFLAMMATORY REACTION

The alteration of infected cells that degenerate and are finally lysed elicits secondarily an inflammatory response probably related to diffusion of certain by-products of the cellular degeneration. The nature of these by-products conditions the forms taken by the inflammatory process and may give a clinically specific character to the lesions produced by a particular virus.

Inflammation is not limited to cutaneous lesions. Usually, around superficial or deep foci of viral multiplication, an ordinary type of inflammatory response appears that is in no way specific as concerns any particular virus. Early-appearing and persistent edema is often noted, especially in viral upper respiratory tract infections and encephalitis.

The cellular characteristics of the response to inflammation in viral infection differ greatly from those of the response in bacterial diseases. The typical initial response is mononucleosis that consists of mobilization and afflux of macrophages, plasmocytes, and lymphocytes. However, at least transitory polymorphonuclear infiltration occurs occasionally and certain infections are not attended by cellular infiltration.

LEUKOPENIA

Leukopenia is a fairly general characteristic of viral infection in its acute phase. The number of leukocytes often decreases to 3000 per cu. mm. Since polymorphonuclear leukocytes are more affected than lymphocytes, the result is a shift to moderate lymphocytosis. Secondary polynucleosis often occurs after this phase.

The mechanism of these reactions has been only partially elucidated. As in the case of megakaryocytes, the germinal line of polymorphonuclear cells seems to be affected by the viral invasion. This phenomenon could represent a direct or an indirect effect of the virus on the myelocytes, since the bone marrow appears aplastic while the activity of the lymphatic system is normal or even, perhaps as a reaction, intensified. On the other hand, when this effect of the virus disappears the bone marrow becomes hyperactive, and numerous polymorphonuclear leukocytes reappear in the blood.

It should, however, be mentioned that experiments with influenza virus in rabbits showed an opposite reaction: rabbits present leukopenia with relative hypergranulocytosis; the number of lymphocytes is specifically lowered.[32]

LABORATORY DIAGNOSIS

To determine the specific etiology of an acute febrile syndrome, in addition to consideration of the clinical facts it is sometimes useful to request virological laboratory investigation; the results make it possible to incriminate or eliminate a particular virus. The cases in which the laboratory can provide useful information are, however, limited by a certain number of factors.

The acute febrile syndrome is transitory and after a few hours or days evolves either toward a more specific picture or toward spontaneous recovery. In the first instance, clinical diagnosis becomes easier, if not evident, and the requested investigation risks proving useless. In the second instance, diagnosis has only an epidemiological or purely informative interest.

Biological procedures in virology are difficult and slow. The earliest serological reactions (those of complement fixation) begin to be of interest only after the fifth or sixth day of disease. Under the best conditions, isolation and identification of a virus require at least a week. The results hence arrive long after the acute phase of the disease. Even if no diagnosis has yet been made, the results of therapy, in particular, are already evident. However, the use of rapid new tests, by immunofluorescence for example, will doubtless accelerate diagnosis when they have been sufficiently perfected technically to enter routine practice.

Too many different viruses produce the same picture for the clinician or even the biologist to be able to decide easily during an acute febrile syndrome what specific tests should be made. One solution would be to perform a battery of serological tests or to try to isolate the virus by all known techniques. Even though this *modus operandi* is feasible in some particularly well equipped institutions, it is obviously too complex technically and too expensive to be used routinely. A selection, a preliminary choice must therefore be made to permit decision as to the gamut of tests to be requested. This choice in itself is difficult, for the usefulness of the techniques selected largely depends on it. Several guide points should be applied. In the *clinical context* the predominant symptoms provide a matter from which the physician can make certain presumptions concerning a likely etiology. Also to be taken into consideration are factors concerning the patient: age, general health, socioeconomic context, history, and vaccinations. The *epidemiological context,* during an epidemic, for example, facilitates rapid presumptive diagnosis for which biological confirmation is then requested from the laboratory. The *geographical location* or the *season of the year* makes certain etiologies likely or unlikely. Taken as a whole, these elements are valuable when isolation of the virus is attempted as well as in proper direction of merely serological diagnosis.

ISOLATION OF VIRUSES

The choice of the organic matter from which to attempt isolation of a virus depends on the type of virus to be sought; i.e., it depends on the presumptions made previously.

For a certain number of viral diseases in which the febrile phase of invasion is regularly or possibly accompanied by viremia, this material is blood or serum. In particular, blood is always used for arboviruses, for they produce viremia that sometimes attains an extremely high titer. At this phase, the virus can easily be isolated by inoculation of whole blood, serum, or blood cell suspensions into the brains of mice 1 to 3 days old. One of the difficulties here is to choose when to make the sample. It must correspond to the period of viremia, which sometimes is brief. The other difficulty is the fragility of the virus; the time between drawing the blood and inoculating it must be short. Samples should be sent "express" by the most rapid means possible with precise indications to avoid hesitations or delays after delivery. To insure favorable conditions of transport, samples should be packed in ice or Dry Ice.

The chances of isolating the virus are a function of these various factors. The virus can also be isolated from the blood in infections by Coxsackie viruses, and in measles and rubella (cf. Chapters 3, 22, and 27).

Especially in search for the viruses of *influenza, poliomyelitis,* and *Coxsackie* and *adenovirus* infections, the *pharyngeal* mucus is sampled by sterile swab. The specimens are placed in a tube containing a small quantity of appropriate medium containing antibiotics (see the chapter concerning each of these viruses). The samples are then inoculated into chick embryos or tissue cultures. Here again, delivery to the laboratory must be made by the most rapid means available.

Feces or rectal swabs can be used for isolation of *enteroviruses* (polioviruses, Coxsackie and ECHO viruses) and for that of adenoviruses in cultures of various cell types (KB, HeLa, monkey kidney, human diploid, thyroid, or amniotic cells).

The appearance of signs of nervous system involvement sometimes suggests the utility of lumbar puncture; the *cerebrospinal fluid* serves not only for cytological and biochemical tests, but also for virus isolation.

When the laboratory isolates a virus from these specimens, it performs several passages and then identifies it. Because of the time required, the clinician is frequently informed that a virus has been found, that it probably belongs to such and such a group, and that complete identification is under way.

SEROLOGICAL TESTS

Serological examinations are theoretically easier to carry out, since the period during which specimens should be taken is less strictly limited. However, as for all serological tests in viral diseases and perhaps even more specifically in acute febrile syndromes that are often caused by the commonest viruses, the immunological status of the patient *before* the onset of disease, or at the beginning, is extremely important. Establishing the existence of even a relatively high level of antibodies for influenza or poliomyelitis on the fifteenth day of an acute febrile syndrome is of little diagnostic value if the level before the onset of this disease is unknown. In most cases, serological confirmation can be made only by comparing the level before the onset (that is to say, in practice, the level in the serum taken at the earliest possible moment after the onset of symptoms but before the beginning of immunological response) with the serum level later on (10 to 30 days later). This is especially true for antibodies that persist long after an infection (hemagglutination-inhibiting antibodies), or even longer (neutralizing antibodies). In the case of complement-fixing antibodies, the fact that in some viral infections they disappear rapidly makes possible a presumptive diagnosis of a specific infection, even from one specimen, if the antibody titer is sufficiently high.

The major drawback to these techniques is that the results come in much too late to be of practical interest as concerns the patient himself. The interest is of a general, collective, epidemiological nature, particularly if, during this time, other cases are declared in the same group or region. More or less specific means of prophylaxis can then be considered (quarantine, vaccination, disinfection).

In the cases of acute febrile syndromes, tests are most often made for influenza, adenovirus and Coxsackie virus infections, ornithosis, and Q fever (see the corresponding chapters). The technical details are found in specialized manuals.

INTERPRETATION OF RESULTS

Correct interpretation of results is more difficult than for other diagnostic procedures. Isolation of virus from a patient does not prove that this agent is the cause of the disease. The frequent isolation of certain viruses from "normal" subjects is only one of the reasons for prudence in interpreting results. In particular, it must be ascertained that specific antibodies actually appeared or that their level significantly increased. Taken together, isolation of a virus and the appearance of the corresponding antibodies indicates contact with the virus or active infection by it. The conclusion that this infection is the cause of the observed disease obligatorily rests on other evidence, such as results excluding all other etiologies.

ETIOLOGY OF ACUTE FEBRILE SYNDROMES

Acute febrile syndromes can be induced by almost any of the known viruses. The diseases caused by certain viruses in their typical form are discussed in other chapters in this book. Here we shall mention only the preliminary stages of some of these diseases: stages taking the form of a more or less transitory acute febrile syndrome that usually evolves toward a more typical form of disease. However, in many cases, these diseases occur in an attenuated, "abortive," or "atypical" form limited to the acute febrile syndrome; the fact appears clearly in the results of attempted isolation of viruses by certain large laboratories specialized in diagnostic virology. For example, Coxsackie virus is isolated from patients of whom more than 10 per cent show only an undifferentiated febrile syndrome.

Many strains of poliovirus, adenovirus, and influenza virus have been isolated from patients with a similar syndrome. As concerns Q fever (a rickettsial disease) 26 per cent of the strains are isolated in such "atypical" febrile conditions. Arboviruses, many of which are responsible for undifferentiated fevers, will be discussed in some detail.

POLIOMYELITIS VIRUS

The poliomyelitis virus enters the body via the respiratory and digestive tracts. It is present in the throat and intestine one to two weeks before the appearance of paralytic symptoms both in the chimpanzee under experimental conditions and in man during the disease or after vaccination with attenuated living virus. Later, the virus moves into the lymphatic system and the circulating blood, still during a preliminary phase of the disease. This secondary viremia is concomitant with minor illness.[34] Dissemination of the virus launches a third phase of multiplication, and the amount of virus present in the body increases greatly. These various stages of infection are part of the so-called presymptomatic or prodromic phase. This phase in fact corresponds to systemic infection or invasion of the organism and is evidenced by minor nonspecific symptoms comparable to those brought on by less pathogenic viruses. By analogy with what is known about the pathways of dissemination of exanthema-producing viruses and arboviruses, involvement of the central nervous system can be attributed to the movement of the blood-borne virus toward the neural cells. Other mechanisms are certainly involved, such as the propagation of poliovirus from cell to cell within the central or peripheral nervous system (Bodian, 1949).

The minor illness can be more or less apparent; it can, moreover, either represent the only form of infection or be followed by a typical form of the disease. According to the estimate made by Paul in 1955,[55] 90 to 95 per cent of the infections are entirely inapparent, 4 to 5 per cent are abortive, i.e., go no further than the minor illness, and 1 to 2 per cent develop into clinically apparent poliomyelitis. A few cases of poliomyelitis may not have been preceded by the minor illness. Chronologically, the slight illness theoretically occurs three to seven days after contact with the virus; the neural phase begins from the tenth day forward.

Only the first phase is discussed in this chapter. This minor illness (Paul, 1932) rapidly follows the appearance of virus in the throat and feces and coincides with viremia. The symptoms are: moderate rise in temperature, headache, and vomiting. They last only 24 to 48 hours, and can very well go unnoticed in benign forms or not require a physician. The first signs of the neural phase of the disease begin three to four days after remission of the phase of systemic infection.

Etiological diagnosis of the minor illness in its abortive form can be made only by the laboratory. The attempt to isolate the virus at the beginning of disease is made from the throat and the feces; the search is also made for complement-fixing or neutralizing antibodies.

COXSACKIE VIRUSES

Approximately half the type A and all type B Coxsackie viruses can cause an "undifferentiated febrile disease." This form of disease may be a step in a progression toward other manifestations or represent, in itself, the complete clinical picture of the disease.

Usual symptoms are fever, at the beginning (or after a latent period), general malaise, anorexia, nausea, and abdominal pain. Later symptoms are headache, vertigo, vomiting, more or less marked stiffness of the neck and back, myalgia, and myocarditis (see Chapters 20 and 36). Here again, if infection is expressed only as a febrile syndrome, diagnosis can be made only from laboratory test results.

As for other related viruses, diagnosis of *infection* does not necessarily give the etiology of the *disease* since these viruses are frequently found in healthy subjects. A consideration of the *clinical* and the *epidemiological* context is indispensible.

ECHO VIRUSES

Echo virus is especially known for the small, limited and localized epidemics of in-

fectious or meningeal syndromes that it causes. However, it can also manifest itself among young children within an epidemic focus as an acute febrile disorder, with discreet maculopapular rashes in a large proportion of patients. The types best known as a cause of this type of disease are Echo viruses 2, 4, 6, 9, 11, 14, 16, and 18. From one type to another, the course of the disease they cause differs: in length of the febrile period, in chronological appearance of fever and rash, and in the localization and aspect of rash.

Search for the virus is made in feces, in cerebrospinal fluid if signs of meningitis are present, and in specimens from the throat, but the epidemiological data are of great interest for the diagnosis, as soon as the etiology of the first cases can be determined.

REOVIRUSES

The role of reoviruses in human disease has not been clearly established. These viruses have, on occasion, been isolated from children during febrile diseases, but also during many other diseases, as well as from healthy subjects. Diagnosis is made by isolating the virus in tissue culture, then identifying it by hemagglutination-inhibition techniques. Hemagglutination-inhibiting antibodies develop in infected patients and persist for at least a year. Normal subjects often have antibodies, so that testing of a pair of sera is required to demonstrate a sharp rise in the antibody titer.

INFLUENZA VIRUSES

In the first stages of influenza before the respiratory symptoms appear, the clinical picture is that of an acute febrile syndrome. The term influenza-like syndrome refers to this picture. The problem of etiological diagnosis of syndromes so called is the topic here. A certain ambiguity is evident even in the terms, since the words "flu" or "influenza" do not mean the same thing to the clinician and to the virologist. For the clinician, the influenza syndrome is the whole group of symptoms described in the preceding pages. To the virologist, it is a disease provoked by the influenza virus. This ambiguity presents evident difficulty when the laboratory receives specimens for "the diagnosis of flu." To the clinician, this obviously does not mean only "search for influenza virus," and the virologist must then put into operation a series of procedures to identify the agent in question and ascertain whether it is really an influenza virus, or an adenovirus, a Coxsackie virus, or even an arbovirus. The difficulty lies in the choice of the procedures to be undertaken as concerns the specimen. This is why it is useful to stress again the importance of sending, with the specimen, precise observations including (besides the essential clinical information and indication of the exact date of onset) information concerning the epidemiological context: the existence of other cases in the surrounding area, contact with other sick persons, and also information as to the patient's habitation, presence of animals, abundance of arthropods, and the like. This information facilitates the virologist's work and his choice of techniques or of the specific serological reactions to be used.

In regard to the influenza virus itself, isolation is performed by inoculating chick embryos or tissue cultures. Serological procedures offer the choice between group diagnosis by complement-fixation or type identification by hemagglutination-inhibition (Hirst reaction).

These tests are indispensable, particularly in all acute febrile diseases of sudden onset that last three to four days, occur in groups, present no additional symptoms representative of other recognized infections, and occur from December to May.

PARAINFLUENZA VIRUSES AND RESPIRATORY SYNCYTIAL VIRUS

A certain number of other respiratory viruses cause bouts of fever, especially in children. Other symptoms are often present, such as cough, rhinitis, and a red throat, as well as signs of laryngeal or bronchopulmonary localization of infection with subcrepitus detected by auscultation. This evident respiratory localization can facilitate diagnosis by at least limiting the choice of tests to be requested from the laboratory. The four types of parainfluenza virus could be responsible for these disorders, but especially types 1 and 3, and also respiratory syncytial virus.

Laboratory diagnosis is made by attempt to isolate the parainfluenza or respiratory syncytial virus in tissue culture (from pharyngeal specimens) or by corresponding serological tests.

MEASLES VIRUS

The prodromic phase of measles, before the eruption that permits easy identification of the disease, marks the end of the incubation period and represents a short intermediate phase. Besides the fever, this phase is characterized by respiratory symptoms and the injected ocular conjunctiva. The appearance of the characteristic enanthem precedes that of the rash, which spreads over the whole body and is followed by a drop in the fever.

Apart from leukopenia, which excludes a diagnosis of bacterial infection, the results of laboratory tests are of no great practical value.

RUBELLA VIRUS

The prodromic phase of rubella is sometimes asymptomatic. Usually, it is expressed by general malaise, slight rise in temperature, headaches, irritation of the conjunctiva, and sore throat. Lymphadenopathies, especially of the cervical nodes, may occur several days before the rash. Differential diagnosis during this phase is sometimes difficult, for other viral exanthematous diseases, due to Echo viruses and arboviruses, can have the same aspect (including that of the rash). Diagnosis of rubella is hence sometimes false. Present techniques of isolation and serological methods permit verification of the etiologies of these diseases. Noneruptive febrile forms of rubella are brought to light by systematic studies of persons in contact with evident rubella. The virus is usually isolated from the throat, but may be found in the blood, feces, and urine.

EXANTHEMA SUBITUM

The rash appears after three to four days of fever and is accompanied by one or more common symptoms such as suboccipital and postauricular adenopathies. Leukopenia with an increase of lymphocytes occurs during this phase. Rash seems often not to appear under normal conditions, and it does not appear in experimental attempts to transmit the disease to man or to the monkey. In such cases, an acute febrile syndrome is the only expression of the disease.

ADENOVIRUSES

The first symptoms of adenovirus infections are often systemic. They consist in gradual rise in temperature with chills, headache, malaise, and anorexia. Specific localized symptoms, such as pharyngitis or conjunctivitis, usually appear a little later. The acute febrile syndrome lasts from two to five days and disappears slowly. In a number of experimentally induced infections in man, the disease was limited to this febrile phase. In most cases, biological confirmation is necessary for diagnosis. The virus is easily isolated from specimens of feces or from the pharynx or the conjunctiva. Complement-fixing antibodies for the group antigen appear as early as the seventh day of disease.

ORNITHOSIS-PSITTACOSIS

Although the agents of this disease are no longer considered to be viruses, ornithosis-psittacosis must be mentioned. The severity of infections produced by agents of this group vary greatly. Many cases undoubtedly go unnoticed, and a certain number appear only as a minor "flu-like" episode. In Paris between 1954 and 1959, of 442 patients infected by the ornithosis agent as diagnosed by complement fixation, 281 (53.5 per cent) had typical pulmonary localization of infection, but 23 (5.2 per cent) had "flu-like" syndromes, and 42 (9.6 per cent) had only febrile syndromes, which did or did not recur.

Q FEVER

Q fever is an acute disease caused by a rickettsia that has various complications. Its initial phase is an acute febrile syndrome, that is to say, a complex and fairly severe combination of intense frontal headache, general malaise, anorexia, myalgia, and chills. The fever fluctuates and can last more than two weeks; it rarely lasts less than ten days.

That Q fever is considered to be a disease of the respiratory system probably stems from the fact that it is commonly transmitted by air. When the agent is airborne, it produces pneumonia. The disease is, however, systemic, with the rickettsia in the blood. Pneumonia, if it occurs, is only one of the expressions of the disease.

The diagnosis is, in part, epidemiological (contact with animals, for example, is taken into account) and in part biological

(*Coxiella burnetii* is isolated from the blood, or agglutinating or complement-fixing antibodies are demonstrated).

HUMAN INFECTIONS DUE TO ARBOVIRUSES

Arboviruses are characterized by their mode of transmission from vertebrate to vertebrate by certain hematophagic arthropods in which the virus can multiply. Infection of the arthropod occurs while the insect feeds on the blood of a viremic vertebrate. Inoculation of the virus to healthy vertebrates is then accomplished by injection of virus-containing saliva during the vector's feeding on a new host.

This group of viruses is defined by an ensemble of biochemical criteria: ribonucleic acid content, and sensitivity to ether and to deoxycholate. The term arbovirus derives from the mode of transmission: *ar*thropod-*bo*rne-virus.

This important and constantly increasing group of some 200 different viruses is divided into a certain number of serologically defined subgroups by hemagglutination-inhibition reactions (Casals, 1957). The types A, B, and C (and others not designated by letters) assemble viruses with few common clinical properties: the agents of equine encephalitis and Chikungunya virus are in group A; tick-borne encephalitis and dengue are in group B. However, these viruses have in common the fundamental properties of arboviruses and are serologically related.

Few groups of viruses show as great a variety of clinical manifestations as arboviruses. The first virus identified as responsible for a human disease, that of yellow fever, belongs to this group. It was identified by Reed and Carrol in 1902, a time when even the nature of viruses was not yet well defined. The agents of various forms of encephalitis also belong to this group; their characteristics appear in other chapters of this book. St. Louis, Murray Valley, and Japanese encephalitis are transmitted by mosquitoes; the group of tick-borne encephalitis (the forms of Central Europe and the Far Orient, louping ill, and others) are arboviruses. Many arboviruses are responsible for acute febrile diseases accompanied by some more or less regular symptoms or other signs. A great variety of terms are applied to them, such as: "pseudo-influenza," "summer influenza," "three day fever," "swamp fever," and "dengue-like fever syndromes." Epidemiological studies have shown that for each clinical case of these diseases, whatever the form, a certain number of inapparent infections occur, often in the proportion of 100 to 1000 for one clinical case.

One of the most striking features of the diseases caused is the regularity of systemic febrile infection. This fever syndrome constitutes the main picture of the first phase of these infections, and is sometimes the only one. We shall review the facts known about the viruses of this group in this chapter, since acute febrile syndromes occur whenever arbovirus infection is clinically apparent. In many countries, research on this subject is only beginning, and these viruses are certainly more widespread than is generally believed. No region is free of them, although they are especially abundant in the tropics. They have been reported on numerous occasions even in arctic regions.

The basic epidemiological characteristics of this group consist of active transmission by arthropod vectors (most frequently mosquitoes and ticks), and their wide pathogenic range, which permits them to infect species belonging to wide classes: Arachnida, insects, reptiles, birds, and mammals. We shall discuss particularly the viruses not covered in other chapters of this book as concerns the pathogenic characteristics peculiar to them.

ARBOVIRUS OF GROUP A

Chikungunya. CLINICAL FEATURES. A dengue-like disease was observed in Tanganyika in 1952. Its incubation period is from three to 12 days and begins suddenly with *severe articular pains* accompanied by *high fever*. In the local language, the name of the disease means "bent over" because of the joint pains and of the posture they often force the patient to assume. The pain is localized especially in the limbs and spinal column. The disease is often biphasic: a two-day remission is followed by reappearance of the fever with, most frequently, a maculo-papular rash on the trunk and limbs. Sometimes after recovery, which occurs about ten days later, recurrences of articular pain are noted, but without lasting sequelae. The Chikungunya virus is also involved in "hemorrhagic fever" syndromes in Asia, but

some of its clinical features differ from those of dengue and are usually less severe.

THE VIRUS. Chikungunya virus has been isolated from patients' blood during the acute phase of the disease (Ross, 1956; Hammon et al., 1960) and from mosquitoes. It kills intraperitoneally inoculated newborn mice, but not adult mice. It multiplies in tissue culture in HeLa cells, duck kidney, monkey kidney, and chick embryo fibroblasts and causes plaque formation. In the brain of baby mice and in tissue culture, it produces a hemagglutinin active on goose red blood cells at pH 6.2, a property useful for the detection of antibodies by hemagglutination inhibition. The virus is inactivated by ether and deoxycholate.

LABORATORY DIAGNOSIS. The virus can be isolated by inoculation of the material to be studied into the brains of mice 1 to 4 days old. The sensitivity of the virus to deoxycholate is tested first. It is identified by complement fixation and hemagglutination inhibition techniques with use of reference sera. The material to use for isolation studies is blood, taken during the acute phase of the disease and sent to the laboratory without delay. The serological tests are those used for other arboviruses: complement fixation, hemagglutination inhibition, and seroneutralization in the mouse or in tissue culture.

Diagnosis requires comparison of the titer of complement-fixing antibodies at the onset of disease and several days after it. The antigenic relationships between this virus and the O'nyong-nyong virus sometimes make the results difficult to interpret.

EPIDEMIOLOGY. Chikungunya virus causes widespread epidemics, like that in Tanganyika in 1952. Sometimes nearly half the population is stricken. The disease has been found in Central and East Africa, as well as in Asia, Thailand, India, and Cambodia. In Africa, the known vectors are mainly *Aedes aegypti* and *Aedes africanus*, but other species of mosquitoes have been found to be virus carriers, for example, the genera *Culex* and *Mansonia*. The life cycle of the virus is unknown. Only chimpanzees have been found to have antibodies; they could hence be considered to be possible intermediate hosts.

O'nyong-nyong Virus. CLINICAL FEATURES. A disease strikingly similar to that provoked by Chikungunya virus appeared in Uganda in 1959. At the onset it presents the picture of an acute febrile syndrome, but violent pain in all limb joints rapidly appears. After a few days, a morbilliform pruritic rash appears and lasts four to seven days; it is accompanied by adenopathy, especially in the cervical area. The local name for the disease means "joint-breaker."

THE VIRUS. Although this disease is similar to that provoked by Chikungunya virus, O'nyong-nyong virus has characteristics that justify the distinction made between the two agents, despite their close serological relationship. The O'nyong-nyong virus is sometimes pathogenic for newborn mice, but adaptation of the virus to this animal is laborious. During the first passages, mice show no distinct pathological signs other than retarded growth and tendency to development of areas of alopecia. By intracerebral passages from animal to animal, Haddow et al. (1960) obtained a mouse-adapted virus. Later, the same virus was easily isolated in adapted mice from the patients' blood and from mosquitoes, usually of the genus *Anopheles*. The biological properties of O'nyong-nyong virus are similar to those of Chikungunya virus.

EPIDEMIOLOGY. In 1959 an epidemic exploded that spread from Uganda south, across Tanganyika and Nyasaland; it even reached Rhodesia. Serological investigations have indicated that the virus is widespread in all of East Africa, except in regions at high altitude. The number of cases observed between 1959 and 1962 was estimated at 2,000,000. This number represents a high percentage of the total population, but no deaths were attributed to the disease. The O'nyong-nyong virus was the first arbovirus for which the vector role of *Anopheles* was thoroughly established. No hosts other than *Anopheles* and man are known.

Mayaro Virus. CLINICAL FEATURES. Mayaro virus was isolated from the blood of patients with fever in Trinidad (Anderson et al., 1957), in Brazil, and in Bolivia (Uruma strain[67]). A benign febrile syndrome lasting two to six days is accompanied by headache and sometimes by moderate icterus. The disease was apparently more severe in Bolivia.

THE VIRUS. Isolation is made by intraperitoneal or intracerebral inoculation into suckling mice; so introduced, the virus is lethal. The adult mouse is not usually susceptible. The virus is also pathogenic for young hamsters and chick embryos. It multiplies in tissue culture (in HeLa cells, in kidney cells of duck, mouse, and hamster, and in chick embryo fibroblasts). The size of

the virus was estimated to be between 17 and 21 mμ by Schmidt et al.[67]

EPIDEMIOLOGY. The virus was isolated from the mosquito *Mansonia venezueliensis*. It can be transmitted experimentally by *Aedes aegypti* and *Anopheles quadrimaculatus*. The viral cycle is unknown, but the percentage of serologically positive subjects is higher among men than among women, a fact suggesting that contamination probably occurs in the forest.[22]

Sindbis Virus. CLINICAL FEATURES. This virus can induce a benign febrile disease with headache and muscular pain. In one case, a rash with vesicular elements was noted, and the virus was isolated from the vesicles.

THE VIRUS. Sindbis virus was isolated from mosquitoes in Egypt by Taylor et al.[79] Its chemical composition and morphology have been studied particularly,[51, 58] since it multiplies easily and abundantly in the brain of suckling mice and in tissue culture. These characteristics constitute a model system often used in basic research in virology. Sindbis virus is nonpathogenic for the adult mouse. It reproduces in vitro in a large variety of cells and produces well marked plaques on chick embryo cells.

EPIDEMIOLOGY. The virus is not dangerous to man. Only six cases of Sindbis virus infection have been reported so far; all were benign. The geographical distribution of the virus is wide. It extends in Africa from Egypt to South Africa, and has been found in Malaysia, India, the Philippines, and Australia. Serologically positive subjects are often found in the regions involved. The virus has been isolated from several species of *Culex* (*univittatus, tritaeniorhynchus*, and others) and from birds. The presumed cycle is from bird to mosquito (or other arthropod) to bird, with man as a possible but relatively rare host.

Equine Encephalitis Viruses. These viruses, which also belong to the group A arboviruses and are pathogenic in man, are discussed in Chapter 11. They are distinguished according to the distribution of types that differ in their serological properties: Eastern equine encephalitis virus (EEE), Western equine encephalitis (WEE), and Venezuela equine encephalitis (VEE).

GROUP B ARBOVIRUSES

West Nile Virus. CLINICAL FEATURES. The clinical form of the disease varies according to the patient's age. Although children, younger adults, and older adults present the same symptoms, the difference in their intensity results in a considerable difference in the clinical picture. After the first isolation of the virus in Egypt from patients with "slight fever without an etiology or other notable clinical signs" (Smithburn et al.[71]), large epidemics were carefully studied by Israeli workers.[10, 26, 45] Moreover, in 1951 Southam and Moore inoculated West Nile virus into patients with cancer, in a therapeutic trial. Their observations revealed the clinical picture of this disease in aged adults after inoculation with large amounts of the virus. These circumstances differed considerably from natural conditions, but the description is valuable, nonetheless.

In children, the main sign is fever of sudden onset, often accompanied by chills. Temperature rises as high as 39° or 39.5° C. (102.2° to 103.1° F.); on occasion it reaches 40° C. (104° F.). The incubation period that follows an infecting contact seems to be from two to three days. The fever lasts one to four days. In some cases, a second rise in temperature occurs toward the sixth or seventh day, after a remission of one or two days. *Exanthem* then appears, with a frequency inversely proportional to age: it occurs in 90 per cent of patients aged less than 2 years but in only 25 per cent of those aged 6 to 11 years. The eruption is constituted by discreet rounded slightly pink maculae with slightly salient papules 2 to 4 mm. in diameter. The exanthem appears during the febrile phase and sometimes persists afterward. It remains discreet and nonpruritic; it may be overlooked, since it is short lasting (one to four days) and inconspicuous. It is usually localized on the trunk and limbs; the face is sometimes also involved. Headache, on the other hand, seems rather infrequent and not severe in young children, in so far as this symptom can be determined in view of their age. Vomiting is frequent in children (it occurs in approximately half the cases). *Abdominal pain,* diarrhea, and anorexia occur occasionally. Lymph node enlargement is relatively infrequent in children. Blood count shows leukopenia with relative lymphocytosis during the acute phase. Recovery is rapid and complete, without asthenia or after-effects.

In young adults, fever is also a prominant symptom, although nearly afebrile cases have been reported, for example, in six

of the 37 cases reported by Bernkopf et al.[10] The onset is sudden, and the febrile period usually lasts three to five days. It is accompanied by violent chills reminiscent of those in malaria, and by attacks of vertigo. The face is congested and the conjunctiva red. Exanthem is a more irregular symptom. Although it is reported in only 14 per cent of cases in the adult, this relative infrequency may be due to difficulty of detection; the eruption appears more clearly immediately after a hot shower. Headache is much more frequent and severe in the adult; it is reported in 78 per cent of adults but in only 37 per cent of children; pain in the ocular muscles is sometimes noted. Vomiting is much rarer, as are abdominal signs. In the adult, on the other hand, marked adenopathy of the submaxillary and occipital nodes is seen. These enlargements vary in size from that of a pea to a cherry, and by their extent and size sometimes suggest Hodgkin's disease. Recovery is spontaneous and rapid, but convalescence is long. The patient often remains asthenic for several weeks and occasionally presents short recurrences with hyperthermia. The lymph node reaction regresses only progressively over a period sometimes as long as two to three months. One case complicated by myocarditis was reported by Albagali and Chaimoff.[1]

In adults past middle age (after age 50) most authors have noted a less prominent febrile syndrome and less adenopathy and exanthem, whereas the predominance of meningoencephalitic signs and symptoms is marked. Among 49 patients with disease due to West Nile virus, Spigland et al.[77] reported a more or less typical febrile syndrome in 33, in 12 severe meningoencephalitis with recovery, and in four fulminating fatal encephalitis confirmed by histopathological examinations. Appearance of complement-fixing antibodies was retarded and attained only a low level. In a similar age group, Pruzanski and Altman[60] reported seven cases of encephalitis with high fever, convulsions, and meningeal and pyramidal signs; in six recovery occurred in one to two weeks, with no after-effects. Among the patients in Southam and Moore's study reported in 1951, a certain number had encephalitis, which was severe in a few.

In summary, the typical clinical forms of West Nile disease are an acute benign febrile disease among children, and a more severe febrile disease in adults, accompanied either by adenopathies or by exanthem or by both, and, in adults aged over 50, a disease with less typical systemic signs but a definite tendency to localize or to produce complications in the central nervous system.

THE VIRUS. The structure of the West Nile virus is relatively well known. It is formed of spherical particles with an estimated diameter of 35 mμ by the electron microscope and 20 to 30 mμ by ultrafiltration. It contains several antigenic constituents demonstrable by hemagglutination and by complement fixation (Smith and Holt, 1961). The virus contains ribonucleic acid that can be separated from the viral envelope without losing its capacity to replicate (hence its infectivity). It is pathogenic for suckling mice, adult mice, and hamsters inoculated intracerebrally, and for the baby mouse inoculated intraperitoneally. The virus induces inapparent infections in a number of animal species, a fact important in studies of its epidemiological pattern. West Nile virus multiplies and is cytopathogenic in tissue culture (for example, in HeLa, KB, and hamster kidney cells). It induces plaque formation in cultures of chick embryo cells and of duck kidney cells under agar. It also multiplies in chick embryos.

DIAGNOSIS. Although various clinical forms of the disease have been fairly well defined, the picture is not sufficiently characteristic to permit accurate diagnosis except during a declared epidemic. The first elements that help to guide the etiological diagnosis of a febrile disease toward West Nile fever concern not only the patient, but extrinsic factors, such as the season, the abundance of mosquitoes, and previous knowledge of the presence of West Nile virus in the area. Specific diagnosis can be made by *isolation* of the virus from the patient's *blood*. The virus is present one to two days before onset of the first symptoms and remains present until the fourth or fifth day. It is relatively easy to isolate by inoculation into newborn mice. In this instance, isolation of the virus can be considered to be a practical means of diagnosis if the following essential precautions are observed: the specimen must be taken early under sterile conditions, and without addition of coagulants or preservatives; it must be delivered rapidly to the laboratory with precise accompanying information. Serological tests are performed under the usual conditions: complement-fixation and hemagglutination-inhibition tests are

made on two samples taken two weeks apart.

EPIDEMIOLOGY. The virus has a wide geographical distribution, for it has been isolated in Africa (Uganda, Egypt, Ethiopia, the Congo, and South Africa[65]), in Asia (Israel, India, and Western Pakistan) (cf. Barnett, 1964, and Work et al., 1964), and in Europe.[31] Specific antibodies have been found in even more remote areas (as far as the Philippines). Some viruses described under other names are either identical with West Nile virus or closely related to it, for example the Astrakhan virus described by Chumakov, according to Kunz[38] and "Israel turkey disease" virus. Whatever the country, West Nile virus provokes disease of variable gravity in man, and varies in its extension in the area involved. It seems, however, to manifest its activity according to two main patterns. One pattern is exemplified in Egypt where the virus goes almost unnoticed; children are involved and present only a benign febrile illness, after which they are immune. The second pattern is exemplified in Israel. There, an epidemic develops, especially in the communities, and involves members of all age groups, most of whom are not native to the region. This distinction is important and should be borne in mind in studies of the epidemiological characteristics of the virus. Cases of West Nile virus infection usually occur during a limited period of the year, i.e., from May to October, except in the tropics, where cases are sometimes seen during the winter months. These periods correspond to those of maximum prevalence of mosquitoes.

Serological studies have shown that, wherever the virus is present, the number of persons infected is far greater than the number of cases of clinically apparent disease. In Egypt, the number of subjects with antibodies increases in the first year of life; it reaches 70 per cent at age 4 years, and 80 per cent by the end of adolescence (Melnick et al., 1951; Taylor et al., 1956). The adult population thus has a high level of immunity; the fact demonstrates the endemicity of the virus. Severe clinical forms of the disease are unknown. In Israel, in the nonimmune adult population, the disease can take a serious epidemic form and involve many individuals. One of the first epidemics studied produced clinically apparent disease in 60 per cent of the population. In southern France and in Corsica, the situation seems intermediate between these extremes. From one area to another, 20 to 50 per cent of the adult population has antibodies probably acquired from an unnoticed infection contracted in childhood. In this instance, the virus is also endemic, but at a lower level than in Egypt.

Search for antibodies in other animal species reveals the wide distribution of West Nile virus. In endemic regions, immunization occurs among horses, sheep, Bovidae, various species of birds such as crows and pigeons, rodents, and so forth. In most cases, these animals were probably infected without showing pathological signs. The sensitivity of birds, for example, has never been demonstrated even though they show viremia after natural or experimental inoculation of the virus. Moreover, in young birds this viremia is often protracted and of so high a titer that birds in endemic regions can be considered important members of the reservoir species. The virus was isolated once in Egypt from the brain of a horse with fatal encephalitis[66] and once in France from the spinal cord of a foal with fatal encephalomyelitis.[54] The role of the horse is not, however, limited to that of "susceptible host," since recent experiments show that, after experimental inoculation of the virus by peripheral injection, the foal can have a sufficiently high titer of viremia to permit initiation of a new cycle of infection of mosquitoes.

The known vectors differ with the region: in Egypt *Culex antennatus* and *C. univittatus,* in Israel *C. modestus* and *C. univittatus,* in India *C. vishnui,* and in France *C. modestus.* Numerous other species of *Culex, Aedes* and *Mansonia* are able to transmit the virus under experimental conditions, but their role in nature has not been clearly established. However, the virus has been isolated from *Argas reflexus hermanii,* a tick living in pigeon houses, and a possible vector of the virus.

The life cycle of the virus could, therefore, be schematically and temporarily outlined as a continuous circulation from one vertebrate to another by the intermediate of mosquitoes of the genus *Culex.* Birds, with their intense protracted viremia, are undoubtedly hosts of prime importance, and the horses may well play a role in disseminating the virus. Rodents are perhaps also implicated in the cycle. Man, however, does not appear to play any part except that of susceptible host. The species of *Culex* incriminated are precisely the ones prevalent around the various animal species, and they feed on birds, horses, rodents, and man. This picture does not satisfactorily explain the way by which the virus overwinters, but several points are currently being investigated by numerous workers. One is the role of ticks, which can transmit certain arboviruses via the ovary to their progeny. Another is the role of hibernating mosquitoes, which possibly remain carriers of virus during their quiescent period and initiate a new cycle of viral activity as soon as warm weather returns. The role of hibernating vertebrates (rodents, bats) or of reptiles as reservoirs of the virus is under study, as is the possibility of an annual reintroduction of virus by migratory animals either by a prolonged viremia or by the infected parasites they transport.

Cases of West Nile virus infections in laboratory workers have resulted from accidental contamination. In these cases, it would seem that the virus penetrates through small skin lesions or by exposure to aerosols, or to projections without the precise tegumentary portal of entry being known. Such cases suggest the possibility of airborne transmission of the virus, a hypothesis corroborated by the results of experimental infection of animals by aerosols of the virus.[53]

Ilheus Virus. CLINICAL FEATURES. In some cases of acute febrile disease, occasionally with symptoms of moderate involvement of the nervous system, Ilheus virus was isolated in Brazil[16] and in Trinidad.[76] Inoculations of this virus into patients with cancer during therapeutic trials by Southam and Moore produced the same clinical disease.

THE VIRUS. Ilheus, which also belongs to group B, is closely related to but distinct from West Nile virus and from that of St. Louis encephalitis. Its isolation was reported in 1947 by Laemmert and Hughes, from mosquitoes captured in the Brazilian forest; later it was isolated from birds, as well, in other South American countries and in the Caribbean Islands. The virus is pathogenic for mice inoculated intracerebrally and for various tissue culture systems.

EPIDEMIOLOGY. The epidemiological cycle of this virus is ill known. The virus might have a natural avian reservoir and use Culicidae of the genus *Psorophora* as its principal vector.

Dengue Virus. CLINICAL FEATURES. Dengue is a disease familiar to clinicians in the countries where it is prevalent. In endemic areas it involves mostly children. When epidemics appear, they involve a great many people of all ages. Because the disease is well known, it tends to be confounded with clinically similar or identical syndromes due to other viruses. Where dengue is present, clinicians tend to call "dengue" whatever resembles it, especially certain other arbovirus infections. The expression dengue-like fevers hence arises similarly to the term influenza-like fevers.

In its typical form, dengue is an acute benign disease characterized by fever, headache, prostration, hemorrhagic eruption, and leukopenia with relative lymphocytosis. After four to eight days' incubation, the disease begins with a period of *general malaise* or *sudden fever*. The temperature is high and persists for some days, with or without remission; its curve is sometimes diphasic. Pulse rate may at first rise proportionally to the temperature, but if so it becomes dissociated during the disease, and bradycardia persists at least until convalescence. At the beginning of the acute phase, headache is severe and accompanied by a wide variety of painful phenomena, especially pain in muscles, joints, and the back. During the acute and the later stages, the patient is anorexic and extremely weak, or even prostrate. Convalescence lasts several weeks. Lymph node reactions are usual, but always of moderate intensity. Adenopathy occurs in various sites and is sometimes generalized. The eruption seems to occur in two stages, which are not, however, always observed in the same case. First, erythema appears in patches on various parts of the body along with a punctiform rash on the elbows and knees. Then, toward the third or the fifth day, a maculopapular rash appears on the trunk, limbs, and face. The rash is scarlatiniform in some cases. Even in this typical benign form of the disease, the classic descriptions note tendency to hemorrhages. They often mention epistaxis, hematemesis, and intestinal or cutaneous hemorrhages. The tourniquet test is frequently positive. It was proposed as an important aid in early diagnosis after an epidemic in Greece in 1927 to 1928.

Another form of true dengue recognized in 1954 and known as hemorrhagic fever is seen in children. It is characterized by sudden onset of an acute febrile syndrome that is unexpectedly complicated a few days later by extremely serious shock. Severe signs of hemorrhage appear simultaneously. The prognosis is often poor (cf. Chapter 47).

THE VIRUS. Dengue virus has been known since the work of Ashburn and Craig in 1907 but was studied especially by Sabin (1945 to 1952). The virus measures 17 to 24 mμ, contains ribonucleic acid, and causes hemagglutination of goose red cells. At least four types of dengue virus (and perhaps six) are known. Types 1 and 2 (Hawaii and New Guinea) were described by Sabin, and then types 3 and 4 were discovered in 1961 by Hammon in the Philippines during an epidemic of hemorrhagic fever. No relationship exists between serological type and pathogenicity, since hemorrhagic fever can be due to any of the four types. Hammon proposed prototype strains 5 and 6, which may be variants of types 2 and 1, respectively.

Other than man, the species that contract the disease after subcutaneous inoculation are few: even monkeys do not manifest disease. The mouse inoculated intracerebrally is the best animal to use in study. For isolation of the virus, newborn mice are used, but blind passages are often required to adapt the virus to this animal. Dengue virus seems particularly difficult to isolate, at least during certain epidemics. The non-adapted virus does not multiply in chick embryos. Among other laboratory animals, only the newborn hamster is utilizable to obtain viral propagation. Mouse-adapted strains cause lesions in tissue culture under only special conditions that must be rigorously observed. These strains produce, for example, slow cytopathogenic effects in hamster kidney cells[35] and in certain strains of HeLa cells;[12] they induce plaque formation under methylcellulose gel overlays in KB cells.

LABORATORY DIAGNOSIS. The clinical picture is never rigorously specific, and biological diagnosis runs into serious difficulties. Isolation of dengue virus presents the difficulties already mentioned. During some epidemics such as that in the Caribbean Islands in 1963, millions of people were attacked. Clinical and epidemiological data strongly suggested dengue. Serological tests were positive for group B arboviruses and for various types of dengue virus, in particular. The virus was rarely isolated, despite numerous attempts by various laboratories using specimens taken under optimum conditions. During other epidemics and under similar working conditions, numerous strains were isolated. Technical problems apparently remain to be solved, or the virus is not identical in different epidemics. In any event, isolation of the virus, which is the best method of biological diagnosis, cannot always be easily achieved.

In addition, dengue viruses, which are themselves serologically similar, are related to other Group B arboviruses. These serological relationships are so close that cross-reactions are frequent and intense; they sometimes exceed the homotypic response in studies of experimentally induced infections. During a primary infection, this relationship complicates matters. But when dengue follows infection by another group B virus, serological diagnosis becomes impossible. Serological reactions are then positive for all viruses of group B, including, for example, yellow fever, so that the member responsible for the current infection cannot be distinguished. This response is so characteristic that it permits detection of patients undergoing a secondary response with relation to group B, but it gives no further detail. Frequently, in the same region several type B arboviruses are active simultaneously: two different types of dengue, or dengue and Japanese B encephalitis, or dengue and Ilheus virus, and so forth. Moreover, the different reactions utilizable are not always evaluated similarly by different authors. According to some investigators, complement fixation is the more specific reaction, whereas others consider passive hemagglutination to be preferable (Lim and Phoon, 1962). In dengue, hemagglutination-inhibiting antibodies persist so long that retrospective study of the 1927 epidemic in Greece permitted identification of dengue virus as its cause some 30 years later (Theiler et al., 1960; Pavlatos and Smith, 1964).

EPIDEMIOLOGY. Man alone seems to be susceptible to dengue viruses. Inoculation of monkeys results in only an inapparent infection with no febrile phase but with viremia, followed by appearance of circulating antibodies. Other animal species are not susceptible and do not seem to be naturally infected. The principal vector is *Aedes aegypti*; the role

of other species of *Aedes (albopictus, scutellaris, polynesiensis)* is probably minor in comparison. The cycle of transmission of dengue as we know it is from man to *Aedes aegypti* to man. It thus differs from that of sylvan yellow fever, in which man is an intermediate host in a cycle passing essentially from mosquito to monkey to mosquito. The cycle, however, resembles that in urban yellow fever.

Many observations and arguments confirm the ways in which this cycle occurs. First, the geographic distribution of the disease corresponds to that of *Aedes aegypti*: tropical America, the Caribbean Islands, Egypt, the Middle East, western and equatorial Africa, India, Southeast Asia, Australia, and the Pacific Islands. In Europe, dengue has occurred episodically in Portugal and in the whole Mediterranean region except France, it seems. In Greece, the 1927 to 1928 epidemic was part of a pandemic that involved all western Mediterranean countries. Dengue seems to be contained within the northern and southern parallels of 40° latitude, i.e., close to the 20° C. isothermic line. These limits are hence wider than those of yellow fever, although both diseases are carried by the same vector.

Epidemics of dengue are not deadly, for the disease is rarely fatal. Their diffusion among the populations they strike is, however, extraordinary. Endemic zones are well known; in them, infections unnoticed or barely remarked in childhood probably immunize the population. But when a new adult population moves into such areas, the situation changes: susceptible adults are then exposed to a virus with an apparently high diffusion potential. In the Philippines from 1905 to 1924 the difference in proportion of cases of dengue among American and native soldiers was striking: on the average, 95 per 1000 in the Americans, but 17 per 1000 in the Philippine group. The autochthones were thus five times less susceptible to dengue than outsiders. This situation has occurred in many other countries of Southeast Asia, such as Vietnam and Malaysia. The endemic zones include, besides this area of Asia, the coasts of central Africa, India, and some countries of the Middle East.

Dengue takes an epidemic or even a pandemic form when the virus enters a region that has not been contaminated for some years, where the population is hence susceptible and *Aedes aegypti* abounds. An example was the 1927 to 1928 epidemic in Greece. The virus was probably introduced by travelers from Alexandria in the autumn of 1927. A limited epidemic arose, and 20,000 cases occurred before winter. But the season was already too advanced for the *A. aegypti* to be active enough and able to infect many more people. In April, a few cases occurred when the mosquitoes reappeared; then, during the pullulation of *Aedes* in July, one of the most overwhelming outbreaks ever known burst forth. In Athens an estimated 90 per cent of the inhabitants were stricken within a few weeks; among the remaining 10 per cent, many persons had contracted the disease in the autumn of the preceding year.

From Athens, the epidemic rapidly spread to the Ionian Islands, to Thessaly, to Macedonia, to Epirus, to Peloponnesus and to the islands in the Aegean Sea, but did not reach neighboring countries. An epidemic of comparable scope had been observed in the same region in 1889 but spread to Asia Minor, Palestine, and Egypt.

How the virus survived the winter is uncertain. One current hypothesis concerns the possibility that some *Aedes* infected during the autumn wintered in a tunnel then under construction in Athens. The mosquitoes could have found shelter there. The first cases that appeared at the end of the following spring occurred in this section of town, and the epidemic spread from this primary focus. Infected mosquitoes remain carriers of the virus (hence potential vectors) throughout their lives, which have been as long as 200 days under experimental conditions. The chance that such a preservation mechanism can function depends on the number of viremic human beings. Widespread epidemics such as those of dengue, with only one susceptible vertebrate host, have a self-regulatory mechanism. After such a massive invasion, almost the entire population is immune, viremic individuals disappear, and the virus is no longer carried by the vector, as the infected arthropods have disappeared.

Serological surveys permit study of these phenomena, even retrospectively. The agent (dengue type 1) in the Greek epidemic was identified long afterwards, since neutralizing or hemagglutination-inhibiting antibodies subsist a long time.

Such research is possible only where a single group B arbovirus is present, for cross-reactions otherwise make the results uninterpretable. A serologically related virus, however, does not confer substantial cross-immunity. A convalescent from dengue is immunized against the homologous virus and apparently against a closely related type, but only the homologous immunity lasts. Infection by type 1 dengue virus has been reported in patients who had been infected by type 2 dengue virus 10 years earlier.[21] In endemic areas, serological testing shows a high percentage of adults immune to all the group B viruses present, a fact ascertained especially in Vietnam and the Caribbean islands. Hence in these countries, only young children and foreigners are attacked. As concerns young children, the illness is usually slight, and this first involvement protects them thereafter. However, since 1954, the hemorrhagic form has occurred frequently in children, especially in Asia. This clinical form of the disease was not unknown previously. Even during the epidemic in Greece, clinicians often had noted "a tendency toward the hemorrhagic type that may take the form of menorrhagia, hematuria, and hemorrhagic eruption, or bleeding of the nose or gums" (Epidemiological Report of League of Nations, 1928). However, this form has become much more apparent in recent years, and its dramatic aspect, with a spectacular hemorrhagic-shock syndrome, has drawn particular attention to it.

Other Group B African Arboviruses: Uganda S, Spondweni, Wesselsbron, and Zika. These four viruses were isolated from the blood of febrile children or adults in various regions of Africa. They do not apparently represent agents of great importance to man, but perhaps have a greater responsibility in disease than is at present suspected. Moreover, they are antigenically related to other more dangerous viruses: yellow fever, dengue, and West Nile. Their presence can make the interpretation of serological results much more difficult in areas where several Group B viruses are present.

Uganda S virus, which was isolated by Dick and Haddow[18] from *Aedes* mosquitoes, exists in East and South Africa. *Spondweni virus* was discovered in South Africa by Kokernot et al. in 1955 in a group of *Taeniorhynchus uniformis;* it is also present in Nigeria. *Wesselsbron virus* differs in that it provokes abortions in ewes, an effect experimentally reproduced in guinea pigs and rabbits.[87] A certain number of human diseases due to Wesselsbron virus have been recognized, whether contracted naturally or in the laboratory. The virus seems to invade the whole body, including the spleen and liver; some degree of splenomegaly and hepatomegaly sometimes occurs in man. The virus is found in South Africa, Rhodesia, and Portuguese East Africa.

Zika virus was isolated in 1947 by Dick et al. (report published in 1952)[19] from monkeys experimentally exposed to mosquitoes in the Zika forest (Uganda). The virus was later frequently found in *Aedes africanus*. Although antibodies against this virus are frequently found in man, few cases of disease are recorded. Simpson[69] described the disease in himself. The onset was sudden, with slight frontal headache the first day. On the second day, a discreet macropapular rash appeared on the face, trunk, and arms that spread rapidly; fever and malaise set in the same day. Hyperthermia lasted only a few hours, and the rash alone persisted for four days; all other symptoms disappeared rapidly. This benign illness resembles those induced by other arboviruses but is not accompanied by adenopathy or notable articular pain.

GROUP C ARBOVIRUSES

Nine arboviruses are classified in Group C (Causey et al., 1961). Eight of them were isolated from the blood of human beings. The patients were mostly forest workers or laboratory technicians.[25] The disease appears as a systemic syndrome including fever, intense headache, and muscular pain. On occasion, a few signs of nervous system involvement are noted: bouts of vertigo, photophobia, and prostration. The disease is sometimes diphasic. It is always benign, but is followed by protracted asthenia.

These viruses (Apeu, Caraparu, Itaqui, Madrid, Marituba, Murutucu, Oriboca, Ossa, and Nepuyo) all originate from Belém in Brazil, Trinidad, or Panama. Despite this apparently restricted geographical distribution, antibodies have been found in man in Puerto Rico, Africa, and the U.S.S.R.

These viruses are pathogenic for suckling and adult mice. In the baby mouse, the virus is found in especially large quantity in the blood and liver; the brain is less rich in virus. Mouse serum is used in preparation of hemagglutination antigens; their titer is often low. Group C viruses have been isolated

from rodents and certain species of mosquitoes.

ARBOVIRUSES OF OTHER GROUPS

The Bunyamwera Group. Among the 16 known types of viruses of the Bunyamwera group, only four are considered to be responsible for human diseases. *Bunyamwera virus* itself was discovered in 1964 in Uganda by Smithburn et al. They isolated it from a few cases of febrile disease, some due to laboratory contamination, in Uganda, South Africa, and Nigeria. The symptoms were fever, headache, and other pain. In one case an eruption was noted; abdominal pain occurred in several other cases. Recovery always took place without after-effects. However, in four of Southam and Moore's patients experimentally inoculated with Bunyamwera virus, serious nonfatal encephalitis developed.

Ilesha virus, a member of the group, produced the same type of disease in Nigeria as *Germistan* virus in South Africa. *Guaroa virus,* another member of the Bunyamwera group, was isolated from man in several instances during febrile diseases, but also from numerous normal subjects; 44 per cent of the inhabitants of the village in which the virus was isolated had antibodies.

Bwamba Virus. Bwamba fever, observed in 1937 in Uganda,[73] is caused by a virus that, with *Pongola virus*, constitutes a distinct serological group. The disease is similar to others described in this chapter. It often seems to be inapparent: epidemiological investigation shows a high percentage of immune subjects in East Africa and South Africa. Antibodies are also found in wild monkeys.

Colorado Tick Fever. CLINICAL FEATURES. The main symptoms of this disease,[85] which is frequent in the Rocky Mountain area especially, are fever, chills, headache, and lumbar pain. Onset is sudden, four or five days after the tick bite. *Fever* rises rapidly as high as 39.5° C. (103.1° F.) and lasts two to three days. It disappears for one or two days, but often rises again and lasts at least one or two days. *Leukopenia* is a regular sign. In children, *neurological symptoms* are frequent. They are a meningeal syndrome with a lymphocytic reaction, somnolence sometimes bordering on coma, mental confusion, delirium, and agitation.

Severe *hemorrhagic signs* are also seen in children: nasal, buccal, and digestive tract hemorrhages occur and may even necessitate blood transfusion because of the severity of anemia. Generalized macular eruption, morbilliform rash of the early type, or petechial eruption around the mouth has been reported in certain cases. The clinical picture may be alarming, but fatal cases are rare.

THE VIRUS. The first isolations were made by inoculation into hamsters of blood from patients in the febrile period. The animals presented only leukopenia. This leukopenia was reproduced by serial passage. After several series passages in hamsters, and demonstration that the agent traverses Seitz and collodion filters, Florio et al. reproduced the disease in man.[24] The virus proved pathogenic for mice inoculated intraperitoneally or intracerebrally. The isolation technique used is intraperitoneal inoculation of blood into mice 3 to 4 days old. With this technique, Eklund et al. isolated 552 strains of virus between 1948 and 1959. The virus does not produce a hemagglutinin.

LABORATORY DIAGNOSIS. In contrast to most other arboviruses, Colorado tick fever virus is remarkably stable, especially in whole blood, and isolation does not pose the same problems of preservation. Moreover, the period of viremia is long. Isolation is achieved regularly during the first eight days of disease, but the virus has been isolated from blood specimens taken up to the seventeenth day. Diagnosis by isolation of the virus is recommended in this instance; it can be confirmed later by the usual serological tests of complement fixation (these antibodies appear after a four week interval) or neutralization.

EPIDEMIOLOGY. The virus is localized in the Rocky Mountain area and all the western states (Colorado, Idaho, Nevada, Montana, Wyoming, Utah, South Dakota, California, and Washington). The disease occurs from March to August with a sharp *peak in May and June*. The virus was first isolated from the tick *Dermacentor andersoni*, particularly in the mountainous regions where the vector seems to be most heavily infected. The virus accompanies the tick from one stage to another: the infected larvae pass the infection to the nymphs and to the adult ticks that transmit the virus, but transovarial transmission in the tick has not been demonstrated. The virus has been isolated from numerous species of rodents on which the tick larvae feed: squirrels, porcupines, and mice, for example. The ecological cycle of the virus seems to be established. The infected nymphs preserve the virus during the winter, then bite rodents on which larvae become infected; the larvae, which remain infected, develop during the summer, and in turn pass the following winter in the form of nymphs.

Phlebotomus Fever Viruses (Three-Day Fever, Pappataci Fever, Pym Fever, Pick Fever, Sandfly Fever).

CLINICAL FEATURES. Pym, in 1804, and Burnett, in 1816, described a febrile disease lasting three days and occurring in the European and African basin of the Mediterranean. This disease was particularly frequent on the island of Malta, where the English military surgeons called it "summer fever." During the movement of British troops toward the Crimea in 1855 and 1865, many cases were observed. The role of *Phlebotomus papatasii* in the disease was suspected as early as 1905 by Taussig, but the first important studies of the disease were those published in 1909 by Doerr, Franz, and Taussig. From that time on, "sandfly fever" was observed in numerous regions.

The *incubation period* varies from three to seven days. The first symptoms are malaise, lassitude, and generalized pain. *Onset* is sudden, with chills and headache; the pain becomes localized gradually; the conjunctiva are injected, and the face becomes so red that it suggests an erythematous rash, which can last several days after the febrile phase, and then suddenly disappears (Castellani, 1917). The skin is hot and dry, despite temporary bouts of abundant sweating. At the onset the temperature rises rapidly, attaining 39° to 40° C. (102.2° to 104° F.) in 24 hours. Pulse rate is not accelerated or increases only slightly; true bradycardia with 50 to 60 pulsations per minute occurs on occasion. Ocular movements are painful; muscular, bone, and joint pains are frequent. The patient either cannot sleep or remains prostrate. Abdominal pains are common, and anorexia is the rule. In the course of the disease, the throat becomes red, and sometimes a dry cough appears, as well as enanthem of a peculiar type, with small, rounded, hyperemic spots, on the hard palate.

The acute febrile phase lasts three days as a general rule (in 80 per cent of cases), but occasionally lasts as long as nine days. At the time when fever drops, the other symptoms disappear, but the patient remains weak, and convalescence is slow. A more or less prolonged recurrence sometimes occurs immediately after the disappearance of fever. During the febrile phase, moderate leukopenia (4000 leukocytes) is usual, with relative lymphocytosis.

Differential diagnosis is based on the following elements: sudden onset of fever, lasting three days with no rubelliform rash; severe, generalized pains; absence of splenomegaly; and persistent erythema on the face and neck.

THE VIRUS. Two serologically different types of virus were isolated by Sabin in 1955 from specimens taken almost ten years earlier from soldiers of the American Expeditionary Corps during the Italian campaign, in Sicily and in Naples. The two types of virus are named for the places where they were found. After a sometimes difficult adaptation, these viruses are pathogenic for suckling and adult mice inoculated intracerebrally. Complement-fixing and hemagglutinating antigens are prepared from infected mouse brain. The Naples type virus is related to various other viruses isolated in the Americas: *Icoraci, Bujaru, Anhaga,* and *Candiru* in Brazil,[16] *Itaporanga* also isolated in Brazil, and *Chagres* in Panama.[57] The viruses have been isolated several times in Iran and Pakistan.[9] *Candiru* and *Chagres* viruses were isolated from febrile patients. The *Naples* and *Sicily* types of phlebotomus fever are serologically unrelated, but one of the viruses isolated in Iran (I 58 type) reacts with both antigens and probably represents an intermediate type.

These viruses multiply with cytopathogenic effects in various tissue culture systems (primary cultures of human or mouse kidney, HeLa cells).

EPIDEMIOLOGY. The disease occurs in the Mediterranean basin (littorals and islands), but also farther east, in Iran, southern Russia, and Central Asia. Its distribution corresponds to the hot, dry climates in which *P. papatasii* thrives. Several reports mention clinical cases of the disease without laboratory confirmation, but some of them probably have another etiology, since the other arboviruses can produce a three-day fever. No hosts other than man are known, nor is it known how the virus survives the winter.

Oropouche Virus. CLINICAL FEATURES. An epidemic disease was first observed in Trinidad (Anderson et al., 1955), and then in Belém, Brazil in 1961.[83] It consists of a febrile illness (sometimes with a temperature of 40° C. (104° F.), accompanied by malaise, headache, generalized muscular and articular pain, and injection of the conjunctiva. The disease, which is always benign, lasts from two to seven days, and has no after-effects. Leukopenia is a regular sign during the acute phase.

THE VIRUS. Isolation is made from the serum of febrile patients. The virus is pathogenic for suckling and adult mice inoculated intracerebrally. Intraperitoneal inoculation is without effect except in newborn mice. The virus kills guinea pigs on intracerebral injection, is pathogenic for the hamster, and can be cultured in chick embryos. Experimental inoculation into monkeys demonstrated the possibility of inducing viremia and antibody production in this animal, which shows no disease.

The virus multiplies in various species of mosquitoes inoculated parenterally.

Complement-fixing (but not hemagglutinating) antigens can be prepared from the brains of infected mice. *Oropouche virus* is serologically related to *Simbu* virus, which was isolated in Africa.

EPIDEMIOLOGY. The studies undertaken after isolation of this virus demonstrated antibodies in a small proportion of the inhabitants of the region in which Oropouche virus was originally found and in a third of the monkeys examined. The virus was isolated from mosquitoes of the genus *Mansonia* in Trinidad, and from the species *Aedes serratus* in Brazil. During the Belém epidemic in which 7000 cases were recorded, numerous strains of virus were isolated, and serological tests showed that inapparent infections were frequent.

Rift Valley Fever Virus. CLINICAL FEATURES. Rift Valley fever (or enzootic hepatitis) is essentially a disease of domestic animals. It attacks calves and young lambs, and causes abortion in mares, ewes, and cows. The disease is transmissible to man by contact with infected animals or laboratory contamination. It is fairly severe, but not fatal. The first symptoms appear suddenly after a four to six day incubation period. They are fever, general malaise, nausea, and vomiting. The course of the disease is often diphasic, with remission of one to two days. Other usual symptoms are headache, muscular pains, vertigo, and sensations of discomfort in the liver area. Hemorrhages are seen on occasion. Convalescence is long: asthenia lasts several weeks. Ocular complications have been reported (disturbed vision with retinal involvement). After a short period of leukocytosis, leukopenia appears and is prolonged beyond the acute phase.

THE VIRUS. Morphological studies by electron microscopy have shown that the virus consists in spherical particles 60 to 75 mμ in diameter according to Levitt et al.[40] or 90 mμ according to McGavran and Easterday.[43] The virus is sensitive to ether, a general characteristic of arboviruses that indicates the presence of a lipidic envelope.

Rift Valley fever virus is highly pathogenic under natural and experimental conditions for young lambs, in which the infection is rapidly fatal. Adult sheep are less susceptible. In calves the disease is usually fatal. The pig is not susceptible. Monkeys and rodents in nature show a period of viremia followed by immunization. The virus is highly pathogenic for laboratory rodents (mice, hamsters, rats), in which it causes serious hepatic lesions with foci of necrosis and petechial hemorrhages. The virus reaches a high titer in the serum of inoculated mice; after treatment with acetone and ether the serum is used in preparation of hemagglutinating antigens.[49] The virus multiplies readily in the chick embryo and in various types of tissue culture, for example, fibroblasts of various origin and hamster kidney cells.

DIAGNOSIS. Where the disease is enzootic and when contact with sick animals is known, presumptive clinical diagnosis is easy. It is confirmed by isolating the virus; the patient's serum is inoculated into mice or tissue cultures. Easterday and Jaeger[23] perfected a technique applying immunofluorescence to inoculated tissue cultures. The method permits diagnosis in 24 hours, according to the authors.

Diagnosis may also be facilitated by search for antibodies of the complement-fixing, neutralizing, or hemagglutination-inhibiting types. Since this virus has no serological relationship with other viruses, the immunological reactions are more easily interpreted.

EPIDEMIOLOGY. This disease, named after an area of Kenya, is seen especially in South Africa where it causes severe losses in cattle herds and numerous cases of the disease in man. Antibodies are prevalent in the inhabitants of regions where the animal disease is widespread. The enzootic areas are localized in the forested areas where the cycle includes passage by mosquito. The virus has been isolated from various species of mosquitoes of the genera *Eretmapodites* in Uganda, and *Aedes* and *Culex* in South Africa.

The disease is a characteristic anthropozoonosis since both animals and man are infected in the areas where the virus is present. Probably, in addition to the transmission typical of arboviruses, this virus is capable of infecting directly persons handling animals or meat, for the disease is frequent among professional breeders, veterinarians, and butchers. The virus is stable in aerosols, and could enter the human organism by the respiratory tract.[48]

An attenuated live vaccine is used for animals. In man, trials with an inactivated vaccine prepared in monkey kidney cells suggest that it produces a good antibody response in man without dangerous side effects.[61]

Viruses of the California Complex. CLINICAL FEATURES. Of the viruses in this group, only two seem to cause human disease: the *California encephalitis virus* and *Tahyna virus*.

The California virus was first isolated in 1943 by Hammon and Reeves from mosquitoes. Later it was isolated on several occasions in the same region from mosquitoes and ticks, and from the blood of a hare in Montana. Serological studies then showed that several patients convalescent from encephalitis in California had antibodies against this virus. It was hence called *California encephalitis virus*. More than 20 years later, Thompson et al.,[84] during examination of specimens of brain from earlier cases of encephalitis, isolated the same virus from the brain of a child aged 4 years who had died from meningoencephalitis in 1960 in Wisconsin. Serological investigation revealed antibodies in the persons who had been close to the child and hence the existence of inapparent or scarcely apparent infections.

Tahyna virus, which was isolated in Czechoslovakia,[8] is serologically related closely to the California encephalitis virus. It has been isolated from mosquitoes but not as yet directly from human patients. It has been found in pools of "normal" human plasma in Yugoslavia.[41] However, studies by Bardos et al. (1964) of patients hospitalized for various infections revealed that antibody production against Tahyna virus was occurring in many of these patients. Whereas of 121 patients without an infectious febrile syndrome only one showed a serological conversion, 20 of the 99 patients in the febrile group in whom antibodies had appeared showed neither characteristic signs nor complications; 13 of the 111 in the febrile group had complications, usually pulmonary. Although serological evidence constitutes only indirect and not formal proof, it seems certain that the Tahyna virus is an etiological agent in certain human febrile diseases.

THE VIRUSES. Members of this group are easily adapted to suckling and adult mice inoculated intracerebrally. They can be cultured in various types of tissue culture, for example, chick embryo, hamster kidney, and HeLa cells. They form plaques under agar in cultures of chick embryo cells.[47]

The virus isolated by inoculation into mice is highly neurotropic. The titer of virus in the blood and spleen remains low. However, strains not adapted to the nervous system can be obtained by passages with use of the parenteral route. The virus thus obtained reaches a high titer in the blood, spleen, lung, and muscle of the mouse during the phase of invasion. The virus multiplies secondarily in the brain. This nonadapted virus is less pathogenic for primary cultures of hamster kidney cells.

Inoculation of Tahyna virus into foals provokes viremia lasting three to five days at a titer that may reach 1.5 log DL_{50} per 0.03 ml. In piglets, the viremia is of similar duration, but occasionally of even higher titer. Neither the foal nor the piglet shows any pathological sign during experimental infection.

In the hedgehog viremia also follows inoculation of the virus; if the animal goes into hibernation after inoculation of the virus, the time of appearance of the viremia is delayed by the duration of hibernation. Thus, when the hedgehog awakes from hibernation after completion of the incubation period, it shows a high titer of viremia that can last as long as ten days.

EPIDEMIOLOGY. As regards the California encephalitis virus, studies made in Wisconsin after isolation of the virus showed that in certain professional categories such as forest rangers, a high percentage (34 per cent) were immune; of veterinarians in this state, 11 per cent had protective antibodies, as did 9 per cent of young campers in the

region. Serological conversions were observed during the summer of 1963. The regions where the virus seems to be active are wooded hills separated by valleys through which flow small streams that join the Mississippi. Subjects found already to have antibodies, like those in whom they developed during the summer, had not had notable infections. Only a bout of simple undifferentiated fever was occasionally remembered. Hence this virus, which is capable of provoking encephalitis, as often causes mild or inapparent infections.

The situation is similar for Tahyna virus in Europe. Antibodies have been found in human sera in Czechoslovakia, Austria, Hungary, Albania, Finland, Italy, and southern France. The percentages of subjects with antibodies are often high, especially when the seroneutralization reaction is used; in the normal population, they often exceed 50 per cent. Moreover, research in animals has shown that pigs, wild rodents, rabbits, and horses frequently had antibodies. For example, 16 of 88 pigs examined by Bardos and Adamcova[7] in Slovakia had antibodies; 46 of 47 horses in the Camargue region of southern France had neutralizing antibodies. The Tahyna virus has been isolated from mosquitoes or from human plasma in Czechoslovakia, Yugoslavia, Austria, and France.[30] The mosquitoes from which the virus has been isolated and which are hence involved in the transmission cycle of the virus are *Aedes vexans* in Czechoslovakia and Austria, and *Aedes caspius* in Czechoslovakia and France. Studies of the possible transmission of the virus by *Aedes vexans*[17] showed that when the virus titer is sufficiently high in the donor's blood, 80 to 90 per cent of the mosquitoes can become vectors. The blood level of virus required to infect mosquitoes has to be at least 1.5 to 1.8 log DL_{50} per 0.03 ml.

Serological and virological studies on experimentally induced infections show that several species of domestic and wild animals are reservoirs or possible intermediary and amplifying hosts: horse, pig, and hedgehog.

Quaranfil Virus. THE VIRUS. In Egypt, Taylor et al.[80] isolated on two occasions between 1952 and 1954 strains of *Quaranfil virus* from the blood of children with ordinary febrile diseases. This virus had been isolated on numerous other occasions in this area from the ticks *Argas arboreus* and *Argas hermanni*. It has also been isolated from the blood of young egrets (*Bubulcus ibis ibis*) in the same region.

The virus has all the characteristics of other arboviruses, but does not produce a hemagglutinin. It is pathogenic for suckling mice on intracerebral or intraperitoneal inoculation, for adult mice on intracerebral inoculation, and for chick embryos, chickens, pigeons, and hamsters.

Chenuda virus, closely related to Quaranfil virus, has never been isolated from man and is much less pathogenic for laboratory animals (it is pathogenic only for suckling mice). Its manner of propagation in ticks, but not in mosquitoes, creates a relationship between Chenuda virus and Colorado tick fever virus.

EPIDEMIOLOGY. A large proportion of the inhabitants of the region where Quaranfil virus was isolated have neutralizing antibodies against it from an early age. These antibodies are also prevalent in pigeons and egrets, but not in chickens, ducks, geese, or crows. Similar viruses have been isolated in South Africa. The epidemiological cycle implicates ticks (*Argas*), which are habitual parasites of birds living in pigeon houses or under the bark of the trees in which the egrets nest. The virus is probably fairly widespread, but these ticks rarely bite man. The virus has never been found in other common species of ticks. Moreover, infections are rare, and children may be more exposed to them if they climb trees or come in contact with the ticks in pigeon houses. The main life cycle of the virus seems to be through bird-tick-bird transmission; man seems to be only an accidental host.

OTHER ARBOVIRUSES

Two viruses of the *Guama* group have been isolated from man. The patients were foresters in the Belém region in Brazil (Causey et al., 1961). The patients presented a syndrome with hyperthermia (38.5° C.; 101.3° F.), headache, muscular and articular pains, and, on occasion, bouts of nausea and vertigo. The characteristics of the virus are those of arboviruses, but only two cases of disease are known to have been caused by *Guama* virus and four by *Catu* virus, a similar but not identical agent.

The *Semunya* (or *Nakiwogo*) virus originates in East Africa. It was isolated on five occasions from patients with acute febrile syndromes. *Piry* virus (Belém, Brazil) was isolated in four cases.

PROPHYLAXIS AND THERAPY OF DISEASE DUE TO ARBOVIRUSES

The arboviruses responsible for only acute benign febrile syndromes have not been closely studied from the viewpoint of vaccines. The only vaccines against an arbovirus currently available for use in man are those for protection against yellow fever. The other vaccines utilizable, but still in only the experimental stages, are those against tick-borne encephalitis and Rift Valley fever. As concerns several other arboviruses, in general those responsible for the most serious diseases, research is under way to obtain either concentrated potent but safe inactivated vaccines or noninactivated greatly attenuated live vaccines. These studies are being carried out on equine encephalitis (Western equine and Venezuelan equine encephalitis), Japanese encephalitis, and dengue. Price et al.[59] proposed successive immunization for group B viruses with yellow fever vaccine, an attenuated West Nile vaccine, and attenuated Langat vaccine. The Langat virus belongs to the subgroup of tick-borne encephalitis. In the monkey, this three-stage vaccination elicited a high titer of antibodies against all group B viruses and protected the animals against inoculation of several of the challenge viruses used.

Another general prophylactic method used in the fight against arboviruses is the attempt to eradicate their vectors. Mass campaigns to eradicate mosquitoes can be undertaken to rid a limited area of Culicidae. The best results, however, are obtained by use of laborious techniques of detection of the mosquitoes' breeding places and individual treatment of these sites. These methods cannot be applied to extensive swamps and forests; they are applicable only to cities and to limited areas. Individual protection can always be attempted by spraying insecticides inside houses, placing mosquito screens on windows and doors and mosquito nets over beds, use of insect repellents on exposed parts of the body, and wearing boots in tick-infested areas.

The treatment of febrile syndromes caused by arboviruses, like that of other such syndromes caused by other viruses, is only symptomatic.

BIBLIOGRAPHY

1. Albagali, C., and Chaimoff, R.: A case of West Nile fever myocarditis. Harefuah, *57*:275-276, 1959.

2. Anderson, C. R., Aitken, T. H. G., Downs, W. G., and Spence, L.: The isolation of St. Louis virus from Trinidad mosquitoes. Amer. J. Trop. Med., 6:688-692, 1957.

3. Anderson, C. R., and Wattley, G. H.: The isolation of yellow fever virus from human liver obtained at autopsy. Trans. Roy. Soc. Trop. Med. Hyg., 49:580-581, 1955.

4. Ashburn, P. M., and Craig, C. F.: J. Infect. Dis., 4:440-475, 1907.

5. Atkins, E., Cronin, M., and Isacson, P.: Endogenous pyrogen release from rabbit blood cells incubated *in vitro* with parainfluenza virus. Science, 146:1469, 1964.

6. Atkins, E., and Huang, W. C.: Studies on the pathogenesis of fever with influenza viruses. II. Effects of endogenous pyrogen in normal and virus-tolerant recipients. J. Exp. Med., 107:403, 1958.

7. Bardos, V., and Adamcova, J.: J. Vet. Cas., 9:349, 1960.

8. Bardos, V., and Danielova, V.: The Tahyna virus. A virus isolated from mosquitoes in Czechoslovakia, J. Hyg. Epidem. (Praha), 3:264-276, 1959.

9. Barnett, H. C., and Suyemoto, W.: Field studies on sandfly fever and kala-azar in Pakistan, in Iran, in Baltistan (Little Tibet), Kashmir. Trans. N.Y. Acad. Sci., 23:609-617, 1961.

10. Bernkopf, H., Levine, S., and Nerson, R.: Isolation of West Nile virus in Israel. J. Infect. Dis., 93:207-218, 1953.

11. Bodian, D.: Differentiation of types of polyomyelitis viruses. I. Reinfection experiments in monkeys (second attacks). Amer. J. Hyg., 49:200-224, 1949.

12. Buckley, S.: Serial propagation of types 1, 2, 3 and 4 dengue virus in HeLa cells with concomitant cytopathic effect. Nature, 192:778-779, 1961.

13. Casals, J.: The arthropod-borne group of animal viruses, Trans. N.Y. Acad. Sci., 19:219-235, 1957.

14. Casals, J., and Clarke, D. H.: In: Horsfall, F. L., Jr., and Tamm, I. (eds.): Viral and Rickettsial Infections of Man. 4th ed. Philadelphia, J. B. Lippincott, 1965, pp. 583-598.

15. Castellani: J. Trop. Med., Aug. 15, 1917.

16. Causey, O. R., Causey, C. E., Maroja, O. M., and Macedo, D. G.: The isolation of arthropod-borne viruses including members of two hitherto undescribed serological groups in the Amazon region of Brazil. Amer. J. Trop. Med., 10:227-249, 1961.

17. Danielova, V.: Quantitative relationships of Tahyna virus and the mosquito Aedes vexans. Acta Virol. (Praha), 10:62-65, 1966.

18. Dick, G. W. A., and Haddow, A. J.: (Praha), Uganda S virus. A hitherto unrecorded virus isolated from mosquitoes in Uganda. I. Isolation and pathogenicity. Trans. Roy. Soc. Trop. Med. Hyg., 46:600-618, 1952.

19. Dick, G. W. A., Kitchen, S. F., and Haddow, A. J.: Zika virus. Isolations and serological specificity. Trans. Roy. Soc. Trop. Med. Hyg., 46:509-520, 1952.

20. Doerr, R., Franz, K., and Taussig, S.: Das Pappatacifieber. Leipzig, Deuticke. 1909.

21. Doherty, R. L., and Carley, J. G.: Studies of arthropod-borne virus infections in Queensland. J. Exp. Biol. Med., 38:427, 1960.

22. Downs, W. G., and Anderson, C. R.: Distribution of immunity to Mayaro virus infection in the West Indies. W. Indian Med. J., 7:190-195, 1958.

23. Easterday, B. C., and Jaeger, R. F.: The detection of Rift Valley fever virus by a tissue culture fluorescein labelled antibody method. J. Infect. Dis., 112:1-6, 1963.

24. Florio, L., Stewart, M. O., and Mugrage, E. R.: The experimental transmission of Colorado tick fever. J. Exp. Med., 80:165-188, 1946.

25. Gibbs, C. J., Jr., Bruckner, E. A., and Schenker, S.: A case of Apeu virus infection. Amer. J. Trop. Med., 113:108-113, 1964.

26. Goldblum, N., Sterk, V. V., and Paderski, B.: West Nile fever. The clinical features of the disease and the isolation of West Nile virus from the blood of nine human cases. Amer. J. Hyg., 59:89-103, 1954.

27. Haddow, A. J., Davies, C. W., and Walker, A. J.: O'nyong-nyong fever: an epidemic virus disease in East Africa. I. Introduction. Trans. Roy. Soc. Trop. Med. Hyg., 54:517-522, 1960.

28. Halstead, S. B.: Mosquito-borne hemorrhagic fevers of South and Southeast Asia. Bull. WHO, 1965.

29. Hammon, W. McD., Rudnick, A., and Sather, G. E.: Viruses associated with epidemic hemorrhagic fevers of the Philippines and Thailand. Science, 131:1102-1103, 1960.

30. Hannoun, C., Panthier, R., and Corniou, B.: Isolation of Tahyna virus in the South of France, Acta Virol. (Praha), 10:362-364, 1966.

31. Hannoun, C., Panthier, R., Mouchet, J., and Eouzan, J. P.: Isolement en France du virus West Nile à partir de malades et du vecteur *Culex Modestus Ficalli*. C. R. Acad. Sci. (Paris), 259:4170, 1964.

32. Harris, S., and Henle, W.: Lymphocytopenia in rabbits following intravenous injection of influenzal virus. J. Immun., 59:9-20, 1948.

33. Horsfall, F. L., and Tamm, I.: Viral and Rickettsial Infections of Man. 4th ed. Philadelphia, J. B. Lippincott, 1965.

34. Horstmann, D. M., McCollum, R. W., and Mascola, A. D.: Viremia in human poliomyelitis. J. Exp. Med., 99:355-369, 1954.

35. Hotta, S., Oyama, A., Yamada, T., and Awai, T.: Cultivation of mouse-passaged dengue viruses in human and animal tissue cultures. Jap. J. Microbiol., 5:77-88, 1961.

36. Jerushalmy, Z., Kohn, A., and Devries, A.: Interaction of myxoviruses with human blood platelets in vitro. Proc. Soc. Exp. Biol. Med., 106:462, 1961.

37. Kokernot, R. H., Heymann, C. S., Muspratt, J., and Wolstenholme, B.: Studies on arthropod-borne viruses of Tongaland. V. Isolation of Bunyamwera and Rift Valley fever viruses from mosquitoes. S. Afr. J. Med. Sci., 22:77-80, 1957.

38. Kunz, C.: Immunological relationship between Astrakhan and West Nile viruses. Arch. Ges. Virusforsch., 5:674-675, 1965.

39. Lépine, P.: Techniques de laboratoire en virologie humaine. Paris, Masson et Cie, 1964.

40. Levitt, J., Naude, W. du T., and Polson, A.: Purification and electron microscopy of pantropic Rift Valley fever virus. Virology, 20:530-533, 1963.

41. Likar, M., and Casals, J.: Isolation from man in Slovenia of a virus belonging to the California complex of arthropod-borne viruses. Nature, *197*:1131, 1963.

42. Lwoff, A., and Lwoff, M.: Sur les facteurs du developpement viral et leur rôle dans l'évolution de l'infection. Ann. Inst. Pasteur (Paris), *98*:173-203, 1960.

43. McGavran, M. H., and Easterday, B. C.: Rift Valley fever virus hepatitis. Light and electron microscopy studies in the mouse. Amer. J. Path., *42*:587-607, 1963.

44. Magnusson, J. H.: Acute thrombocytopenic purpura following rubella. Acta Med. Scandinav., *126*:40, 1946.

45. Marberg, K., Goldblum, N., Sterk, V. V., Jasinska-Klingberg, W., and Klingberg, A. M.: The natural history of West Nile fever. I. Clinical observations during an epidemic in Israel. Amer. J. Hyg, *64*:259-269, 1956.

46. Mayerova, A., and Mayer, V.: Improved plaque assay of Tahyna virus (complex of California encephalitis). Acta Virol. (Praha), *8*:95, 1964.

47. Melnick, J. L., Paul, J. R., Riordan, J. T., Barnett, J. H., Goldblum, N., and Zabin, E.: Isolation from human sera in Egypt of a virus apparently identical to West Nile virus. Proc. Soc. Exp. Biol., *77*:661, 1951.

48. Miller, W. S., Demchak, P., Rosenberger, C. R., Dominik, J. W., and Bradshaw, J. C.: Stability and infectivity of airborne yellow fever and Rift Valley fever viruses. Amer. J. Hyg., *77*:114-121, 1963.

49. Mims, C. A., and Mason, P. J.: Rift Valley fever virus in mice. V. The properties of haemagglutinin present in infective serum. Brit. J. Exp. Path., *37*:423-433, 1956.

50. Motulsky, A. B.: Platelet agglutination by influenza virus. Clin. Res. Proc. pp. 1-100, 1953 (abstract).

51. Mussgay, M., and Rott, R.: Studies on the structure of a haemagglutinin component of a group A arbovirus (Sindbis). Virology, *17*:202-204, 1964.

52. Nelson, E. R., and Bierman, H. R.: Dengue fever: a thrombocytopenic disease? J.A.M.A., *190*:99-103, 1964.

53. Nir, Y. D.: Airborne West Nile virus infection. Amer. J. Trop. Med. *8*:537, 1959.

54. Panthier, R., Hannoun, C., Oudar, J., Beytout, D., Corniou, B., Joubert, L., Guillon, J. C., and Mouchet, J.: Isolement du virus West Nile chez un cheval de Camargue atteint d'encéphalomyélite. C.R. Acad. Sci. (Paris), *202*: 1308, 1966.

55. Paul, J. R.: Epidemiology of Poliomyelitis. WHO Monogr. Ser., *9*:29, 1955.

56. Pavlatos, M., and Smith, C. E. G.: Antibodies to arthropod-borne viruses in Greece. Trans. Roy. Soc. Trop. Med. Hyg., *58*:422, 1964.

57. Peraltra, P. H., Shelokov, A., and Brody, J. A.: Chagres virus: A new human isolate from Panama. Amer. J. Trop. Med., *14*:146-151, 1965.

58. Pfefferkorn, E. R., and Clifford, R. L.: The origin of the protein of Sindbis virus. Virology, *23*:217-223, 1964.

59. Price, W. H., Parks, J., Ganaway, J., Lee, R., and O'Leary, W.: A sequential immunization procedure against certain group B arboviruses. Amer. J. Trop. Med., *12*:624-638, 1963.

60. Pruzanski, W., and Altman, R.: Encephalitis due to West Nile fever virus. World Neurol., *3*:524, 1962.

61. Randall, R., Binn, L. N., and Harrisson, V. R.: Rift Valley fever virus vaccine. Amer. J. Trop. Med., *12*:11-15, 1963.

62. Reed and Carrol: Amer. Med. J., p. 301, 1902.

63. Ross, R. W.: The Newala epidemic. III. The virus: isolation, pathogenic properties and relationship to the epidemic. J. Hyg., *54*:177-191, 1956.

64. Sabin, A. B.: The dengue group of viruses and its family relationships. Bact. Rev. *14*:225-232, 1950.

65. Schmidt, J. R.: West Nile fever. E. Afr. Med. J., *42*:207-212, 1965.

66. Schmidt, J. R., and El Mansoury, H. K.: Natural and experimental infection of Egyptian equines with West Nile virus. Ann. Trop. Med. Parasit., *57*:415-427, 1963.

67. Schmidt, J. R., Gadjusek, D. C., Schaeffer, M., and Gorrie, R. H.: Epidemic jungle fever among Okinawan colonists in the Bolivian rain forest. II. Isolation and characterization of Uruma virus, a newly recognized human pathogen. Amer. J. Trop. Med., *8*:479-487, 1959.

68. Schulze, I. T., and Schlesinger, R. W.: Plaque assay of dengue and other group B arthropod-borne viruses under methyl cellulose overlay media. Virology, *19*:40-48, 1963.

69. Simpson, D. I. H.: Zika virus infection in man. Trans. Roy. Soc. Trop. Med. Hyg., *58*:335, 1964.

70. Smith, C. E. G., and Holt, D.: Chromatography of arthropod-borne viruses on calcium phosphate columns. Bull. WHO, *24*:749-759, 1961.

71. Smithburn, K. C., Hughes, T. P., Burke, A. W., and Paul, J. H.: Neurotropic virus isolated from blood of nature of Uganda. Amer. J. Trop. Med., *20*:471-492, 1940.

72. Smithburn, K. C., Mahaffy, A. F., and Haddow, A. J.: A neurotropic virus isolated from Aedes mosquitoes caught in the Semliki forest. Amer. J. Trop. Med., *26*:189-208, 1946.

73. Smithburn, K. C., Mahaffy, A. F., and Paul, J. H.: Bwamba fever and its causative virus. Amer. J. Trop. Med., *21*:75-90, 1941.

74. Sohier, R.: Diagnostic des maladies à virus. Paris, Editions Médicales Flammarion, 1964.

75. Southam, C. M., and Moore, A. E.: West Nile Ilheus and Bunyawera virus infections in man. Amer. J. Trop. Med., *31*:724-741, 1951.

76. Spence, L., Anderson, C. R., and Downs, W. G.: Isolation of Ilheus virus from human beings in Trinidad. Tr. Roy. Soc. Trop. Med. Hyg., *56*:504-509, 1962.

76a. Spence, L., Downs, W. G., and Boyd, C.: Isolation of St. Louis encephalitis virus from the blood of a child in Trinidad. W. Indian Med. J., *8*:195-198, 1959.

77. Spigland, I., Jasinska-Klingberg, W., Hofshi, E., and Goldblum, N.: Clinical and laboratory observations in an outbreak of West Nile fever in Israel. Harefuah, *54*:275-281 [English Summary].

78. Taussig, S.: Die Hundskrankheit (Endemischer Magenkatarrh) in der Herzegovina. Wien Klin. Wschr., *18*:129-136, 163-169, 1905.

79. Taylor, R. M., Hurlbut, H. S., Work, T. H., Kingston, J. R., and Frothingham, T. E.: Sindbis virus:

A newly recognized arthropod-transmitted virus. Amer. J. Trop. Med., *4*:844-862, 1955.

80. Taylor, R. M., Hurlbut, H. S., Work, T. H., Kingston, J. R., and Hoogstraal, H.: Arboviruses isolated from Argas in Egypt: Quaranfil, Chenuda and Nyamanini. Amer. J. Trop. Med., *15*:76-86, 1966.

81. Taylor, R. M., Work, T. H., Hurlbut, H. S., and Rizk, F.: A study of the ecology of West Nile virus in Egypt. Amer. J. Trop. Med., *5*:579-620, 1956.

82. Theiler, M., Casals, J., and Moutousses, C.: Etiology on the 1927-1928 epidemic of dengue in Greece. Proc. Soc. Exp. Biol. Med., *103*:244-246, 1960.

83. Theiler, M., and Downs, W. G.: Oropouche: the story of a new virus. Yale Sci. Magazine, *37*:6, 1963.

84. Thompson, W. H., Kalfayan, B., and Anslow, R. O.: Isolation of California encephalitis group virus from a fatal human illness. Amer. J. Epidem., *81*:245-253, 1964.

85. Topping, N. H., Cullyford, J. S., and Davis, G. E.: Colorado tick fever. Public Health Rep., *55*: 2224-2237, 1940.

86. Wagner, R. R., Bennett, I. L., Jr., and Le Quire, V. S.: The production of fever by influenzal viruses. I. Factors influencing the febrile response to single injections of virus. J. Exp. Med., *90*: 321, 1949.

87. Weiss, K. E., Haig, D. A., and Alexander, R. A.: Wesselsbron virus: a virus not previously described associated with abortion in domestic animal. Onderstepoort J. Vet. Res., *27*:183-195, 1956.

59

Sudden Death and Viruses

By J. COUVREUR

Sudden death is especially frequent in young children. "Crib death" with no apparent cause usually remains an enigma both for the attending physician and for the histopathologist. Its frequency, although estimated differently by different authors, is nonetheless considerable in pediatrics from the end of the newborn period to age 2 years. Stowens[16] found that unexplained sudden death represented 4 per cent of the total deaths in pediatric practice and 16 per cent of the deaths before age 6 months in which autopsy was performed. Coe[7] reported that 10 per cent of deaths of infants aged from 5 days to 1 year were sudden and unexpected; the majority (85 per cent) of them occurred before age 6 months. In recent years the hypotheses most often proposed to explain these phenomena are: hypogammaglobulinemia, a massive visceroviseral reflex, bronchial aspiration of milk with hypersensitivity, and viral infection. Although none of these hypotheses has been fully verified, a certain number of observations draw attention to each of them. Since Adams[1] proposed the viral hypothesis in 1943, numerous investigations have been made in an attempt to verify it.[2, 7, 9, 11, 13, 14, 17]

The arguments in favor of the viral origin of sudden, unexplained death are of three types: epidemiological and clinical, histopathological, and virological. In most cases, they suggest respiratory infection.

Clinical and Epidemiological Data. The sudden unexplained death of young children is clearly more frequent in the winter months. Arey and Sotos[3] noted that 85 to 114 cases of sudden death in children occurred between September and April. Banks,[4] Jacobsen, and Carpenter and Shaddick[5] found a striking increase in January, February, and March. All the authors concerned with sudden, unexplained death agree on this point.

Thorough and detailed analysis of the minor signs and symptoms of the children during the two weeks preceding death has revealed deviations from normal in almost all cases.[9] The disturbances were associated in their large majority with benign-appearing upper respiratory infection.[7, 11] In 50 per cent of cases the children's parents had consulted a physician before the child's death.[5] When inquiry was made among the persons in the child's surroundings, it revealed the frequency of respiratory infections. Coe[7] found such infection in either the child or the persons in contact with him in a total of nearly 53 per cent of cases. Adelson and Kinney[2] found manifestations of respiratory infection in the human surroundings in 54 per cent of cases.

The age of maximum frequency of sudden death (1 to 6 months), it should be emphasized, is situated precisely at a period when the infant is especially susceptible to this type of infection. The increased frequency of sudden death both in children and in adults during the severe pandemics of influenza of 1919 to 1920 and of 1957[15] is also to be noted.

Anatomical and Histopathological Data. The arguments in favor of respiratory infection are weighty.[1, 2, 11, 12, 18] Adelson and Kinney[2] studied 126 cases, in 74 (58 per cent) of which they found proof of laryngitis (necrotizing in 11), tracheitis in 37, bronchitis or bronchiolitis in 19, pneumonia with purulent bronchitis in 24, and interstitial pneumonia in four. Histological signs of respiratory tract inflammation existed in a total of 106 cases. In 47 of 52 cases Gruenwald and Jacob[12] found a mononuclear cell pneumopathy, the infectious or viral origin of which they affirmed unhesitantly. Werne and Garrow[18] found signs of respiratory tract infection in 30 of 50 cases. None of these authors seems, however, to have found histological signs suggesting any specific viral etiology. Although Adelson and Kinney[2] found four cases of interstitial pneumonia, they did not find giant cell pneumonia and rarely remarked an element suggesting viral infection, such as inclusion cells.

The Virological Hypothesis. In contrast with the frequency of the anatomical signs of respiratory infection, the paucity of results of bacteriological investigations must be emphasized. Staphylococci in pure culture were isolated by Werne and Garrow[18] in 11 of 31 cases. Adelson and Kinney,[2] whose search gave negative results in 95 of the 120 cases so investigated, however, rejected the determining role of bacterial invasion in any of their cases.

It would hence seem logical to try to explain the facts observed by a *viral infection.* During the incubation period of such infections viruses can multiply massively in the organism. For death to occur in a highly susceptible subject during massive viremia before any symptom appears seems a possibility. In ectromelia of the mouse, it has been demonstrated[10] that certain animals die during the incubation period of the experimental disease, during which the virus abounds in the liver and the spleen and has already produced necrotic phenomena.

After Bowden and French, a certain number of other authors have made systematic attempts to isolate viruses in the blood and viscera of subjects who died suddenly. Among them, Adelson and Kinney[2] failed to isolate any virus in 120 cases; it must be added that, at the time, they utilized only methods of inoculation into mice. Four groups of research studies have obtained more encouraging results since 1961.

Gold et al.[11] used tissue culture and animal inoculations in study of samples of blood, stools, lymph nodes, lung, spleen, heart, and cerebrospinal fluid, of pharyngeal and laryngeal secretions, and of brain and spinal cord from 48 children. They isolated 12 strains of viruses, five of them from the pharynx and the stools and seven from the cerebrospinal axis (25 per cent of cases). Coxsackie A4 virus was found in eight cases (in six from the neuraxis), Coxsackie A8 in two cases in the stools, and poliomyelitis type 3 in the cerebrospinal axis in one case in which a Coxsackie A4 virus was isolated from the stools as well. On the other hand, Valdes Dapena and Hummeler,[17] who studied 109 cases and attempted to isolate a virus in each of them from eight organ fragments by inoculation into the adult and the newborn mouse, the embryonated egg, HeLa and monkey kidney cells, isolated only one virus, a Coxsackie B, in the lung of an infant with no histological signs of pneumopathy but epiglottitis and tracheitis.

Moore et al.[14] analyzed 45 specimens of different organs from children; they isolated one or several viruses in seven of the ten cases studied: Echo 7 in the stools in three, in the liver, the lung, or the brain in two; Echo 22 in the stools in one, and poliomyelitis type 1 both in the stools and the liver in one case.

Holy and Vanecek[13] isolated viruses from 11 of 254 infants who had died at age 3 months to 29 months: Echo 26 (one case); Echo 12 (one case) in the bronchial secretions; a Coxsackie virus (two cases); an unidentified enterovirus (four cases); adenovirus type 6 in the trachea, myocardium, and intestines (one case); and an unidentified adenovirus (two cases). In all these cases histopathological study revealed signs of inflammation of the respiratory tract: rhinitis, pharyngitis, bronchiolitis, tracheobronchitis, or interstitial pneumonia.

Such are the observed facts. What remains to be discussed is the relationship between the demonstration of a virus in the viscera and sudden death. The hypothesis of absence of any etiological relationship is defendable. A certain disproportion is manifest between the low frequency of virus isolation and the quality of the techniques utilized that should permit demonstration of most of the known enteroviruses. Autopsy samples can be contaminated. The wide diffusion of viruses in the population makes it possible to consider the presence of the agents isolated as a matter of chance. The facts can also be emphasized that few were isolated in the neuraxis and that they were evidenced only after passage in the newborn mouse. Moreover, Gold et al.[11] noted that no histological alteration was detected in the brain or the spinal cord in the cases in which a virus was isolated. However, the Coxsackie A viruses could act in the nursling infant as in the mouse and multiply in the brain without producing lesions detectable at present. It has, moreover, been demonstrated that enteroviruses can be detected in the cerebral tissue before histological alterations appear (Melnick and Goldman). To accept the responsibility of these viruses in the death, the possibilities to be considered are biochemical disturbances leading to functional involvement of the nerve cells or of lesions so localized that they could have escaped detection in the histological investigations (Gold et al.).

The elements of conjecture give the measure of present uncertainty in regard to the role of viruses in sudden unexplained death in pediatrics. The intervention of viruses seems possible. Even in the cases with demonstrated presence of a virus, it is, however, difficult to explain the so frequent contrast between the discreteness, if not the absence, of lesions provoked by it and the dramatic course. The intervention of other factors inherent to the host, in particular, may be considered.

BIBLIOGRAPHY

1. Adams, J. M.: Sudden death in infants due to pneumonia. J. Pediat., *23*:189, 1943.
2. Adelson, L., and Kinney, E. R.: Sudden and unexpected death in infancy. Pediatrics, *17*:663, 1956.
3. Arey, J. P., and Sotos, J.: Unexpected death in early life. J. Pediat., *49*:523, 1956.
3a. Balduzzi, P. C., and Greendyke, R. M.: Sudden unexpected death in infancy and viral infection. Pediatrics, *38*:201, 1968.
4. Banks, A. L.: An enquiry into sudden death in infancy. Monthly Bull. Minist. Health, *17*:182, 1958.
4a. Bricout, F., Regnard, J., Huraux, J.-M., Fontaine, J.-L., Guy-Grand, D., and Boccon-Gibod, L.: Recherches de virus au cours des autopsies. Un virus peut-il être rendu réellement responsable dans certains cas de mort subite dans l'enfance? Arch. Franç. Pédiat., *26*:669, 1969.
5. Carpenter, R. G., and Shaddick, C. W.: Role of infection, suffocation and bottle-feeding in cot deaths. An analysis of some factors in the histories of 110 cases and their controls. Brit. J. Prev. Soc. Med., *19*:1, 1965.
6. Cochard, A. M., Le Tan Vinh, and Lelong, M.: Le placenta dans la cytomégalie congénitale. Etude anatomoclinique de 3 observations personnelles. Arch. Franç Pédiat., *20*:35, 1963.
7. Coe, J. I., and Hartman, E. E.: Sudden unexpected death in infancy. J. Pediat., *56*:786, 1960.
8. Collins, J. D., and Piper, P. G.: Sudden unexpected death in infancy. A disease of theories. Wisconsin Med. J., *60*:571, 1961.
9. Emery, J. L., and Crowley, E. M.: Clinical histories of infants reported to coroner as cases of sudden unexpected deaths. Brit. Med. J., *2*:1518, 1956.
10. Fenner, F.: Pathogenesis of acute exanthems: interpretation based on experimental investigation with mouse-pox (infectious ectromelia of mice). Lancet, *2*:915, 1948.
11. Gold, E., et al.: Viral infection. A possible cause of sudden unexpected deaths in infants. New Eng. J. Med., *264*:53, 1961.
12. Gruenwald, P., and Jacob, M.: Mononuclear pneumonia in sudden death or rapidly fatal illness in infants. J. Pediat., *39*:650, 1951.
13. Holy, J., and Vanecek, K.: Die Virusinfektion und der plötzliche Tod der Säuglinge und Kleinkinder. Zbl. Bakt., *192*:183, 1964.
14. Moore, M. L., et al.: Sudden unexpected death in infancy. Isolations of ECHO type 7 virus. Proc. Soc. Exp. Biol. Med., *116*:231, 1964.
15. Neilson, D. B.: Sudden death due to fulminating influenza. Brit. Med. J., *1*:420, 1958.
16. Stowens, D.: Sudden unexpected death. A major problem in infancy and early childhood. A.M.A. Arch. Path., *61*:341, 1956.
17. Valdes Dapena, M. A., and Hummeler, K.: Sudden and unexpected death in infants. 2. Viral infections as causative factors. J. Pediat., *63*:398, 1963.
18. Werne, J., and Garrow, I.: Sudden apparently unexplained death during infancy. Amer. J. Path., *29*:633, 1953.

60

Prenatal, Transnatal, and Postnatal Viral Diseases and Malformations

INTRODUCTION
by R. Debré

The chapters that follow are devoted to the viral diseases that affect the child before birth, during it, or immediately after his arrival in the world. It is obvious that, to the first category, is linked the problem of congenital malformations of viral origin. To the second belong accidents of direct contamination during childbirth, the child being infected on contact with the genital pathways. To the third category is related the behavior peculiar to the newborn with regard to a viral contamination; it is different from that observed in the older child.

Naturally, the neonatal period must first be defined: in conformity with the generally accepted conventions, this period will be considered to extend up to the end of the fourth week; the early neonatal period, that which concerns the first week of life, will be distinguished, as will the late neonatal period that covers the three weeks following.

It is sometimes extremely difficult to know when and how the child was contaminated. Sometimes the viral infection of the neonatal period stems from a transplacental involvement consecutive to a viremia in the pregnant woman (rubella is the typical example of this first category, doubtless by far the most frequent). Sometimes the contamination is connected, not with a hematogenous and transplacentary

infection, but with a step-by-step infection by contiguity starting from an endometrial infection that, in its turn, can either infect the fetus by the blood pathway, or infect it by the intermediary of the amniotic fluid, itself contaminated across the membrane (this pathway seems to be without decisive proof and very rare for viral diseases). Sometimes the infection is due to contamination during childbirth itself (some neonatal herpes infections seem certainly to be linked to the genital herpes of the mother). Sometimes it is consecutive to an infection occurring shortly before birth (certain viral epidemic respiratory infections seem to enter into this framework).

New research work should be pursued in order to study more closely the transmission of viral infections at the prenatal, transnatal, and neonatal period. Table 60-1, which is that of Gillot and Bodin[1] slightly modified, gives an idea of the pathways that are considered to be generally followed in the neonatal viroses.

The links between the viroses and the host cells are so intimate and the importance of cellular metabolism is so fundamental that one understands the entire singularity of the problem set up by the relationships between the viruses and an embryonic tissue in course of rapid development. The speed of growth and the forces brought into play in the formation and the complex construction of a new being can not fail to play a role in the host-virus relationships in the embryonic,

Table 60-1   *Microorganisms Responsible for Neonatal Infection and Their Pathways*

MICROORGANISMS*	TRANSMISSION		
	Antenatal Intrauterine Transplacental Infection	Transnatal During Delivery	Postnatal Exogenous Infection after Delivery
VIRUSES			
Adenoviruses	+ ?		+
Coxsackie viruses	+ ?		+
Echo viruses	+ ?		+
Influenza viruses	?		+
Viral hepatitis	+ ?		
Herpes simplex	+	+ + +	+
Cytomegaloviruses	+ + +		+
Myxoviruses parainfluenzae. R.S. viruses			+
Mumps	+ ?		
Poliomyelitis	+ + +	+	+
Measles	+ ?		+
Rubella	+ + +		
Vaccinia	+		+
Varicella-herpes zoster	+		+
Smallpox-alastrim	+		+
TRIC AGENT†			
Inclusion conjunctivitis		+ + +	

*Transmission: + ? = very questionable; + ? = possible but not proved; + = demonstrated; + + + = usual.
†Group including the agents of trachoma and inclusion conjunctivitis.

fetal, and neonatal period. Few glimmers of light illuminate this domain. It is necessary, however, to recall the interest that is attached to certain experimental infections in the newborn animal: the particular sensitivity of the baby mouse to infections with Coxsackie virus, for example. Moreover, the cultures of rubella virus on human embryonic tissues, in revealing chromosome breakages, show that, in the course of cellular division, the daughter cells inheriting the damaged chromosomes are not viable, so that, at each division, a more or less elevated proportion of cells disappears, which explains the low birth weight and the disturbances of cellular differentiation (cf. Chapter 61).

The study of the means of defense of the developing organism against viral aggression brings up numerous problems as yet insufficiently studied. They are the role of the cutaneous covering, with the peculiar structure of the skin at birth; the role of the mucosae in connection with the transnatal and postnatal penetration of germs from the exterior world, the capacities, different and varying according to the stages of development, of the cellular defenses (phagocytosis), tissular defenses (inflammation), and general defenses (fever). The variations in the phenomenon of tolerance, of allergy, and of interferon production can only be mentioned here in order to show their interest in the understanding of viral antenatal, transnatal, and postnatal infections. The protective antibodies have been studied more thoroughly, and the knowledge acquired in this domain is more important to the clinician.

Three main types of immunoglobulins, IgA, IgM, IgC, are distinguished. The last two are detectable in the fetus from the eighteenth to the twentieth week on, and progressively increase. It is thought that the level in the cord blood is comparable to that in the maternal blood. The M immunoglobulins present in the 20 week old fetus represent, at birth, less than 10 per cent of the values in the adult. As to the A immunoglobulins, they seem to be detectable in the circulation only after 20 days of extrauterine life.

It does not seem open to doubt that the greatest quantity of immunoglobulins present in the fetus and the newborn are of maternal origin. It is, however, an acquired fact that a part of the fetal immunoglobulins are elaborated by the fetus itself.

The maternal antibodies in man are transmitted by the placenta, and it does not seem possible to envisage antenatal digestive absorption of the antibodies in the amniotic sac—in our species—or their postnatal absorption from colostrum. The antibodies transmitted are the maternal IgG antibodies, the only ones able to traverse the placenta. They protect the child during intrauterine life and up to approximately the sixth month after birth (of course, *when* the mother possesses them). The fact does not in the least contradict that, from as early as fetal life, the infant is able to synthesize immunoglobulins, although antibodies of maternal origin may have some inhibitory action on antibody formation by the child. This capacity of the newborn, even premature, to form antibodies should be borne in mind. It will be considered in connection with early vaccinations (cf. Chapter 63).

In short, if, in certain cases—as in measles and poliomyelitis—the IgG antibodies protect the fetus and the newborn, for a certain time, against the infection, in other cases this protection is lacking. The fetus or the child synthesizes IgM antibodies before synthesizing appreciable quantities of IgG antibodies like the adult.

BIBLIOGRAPHY

1. Gillot, F., and Bodin, G.: Etiologie et voies de l'infection néonatale. In XXI Congrès de l'Association des pédiatres de langue française. Paris, Expansion Scientifique Française, 1967, Vol. 3, pp. 71-137.

PRENATAL VIRUS INFECTIONS
by J. A. DUDGEON

During intrauterine life the embryo or fetus,* which at conception has a reasonable expectation of being normal, may be subjected to a number of external or environmental influences capable of affecting its subsequent growth and development. Environmental agents, such as toxic substances or infections, are in the main transmitted to the fetus via the placenta and not via genetic pathways. They are impor-

---

*Terminology is discussed on page 793.

tant because in many instances the fetus can be protected by some appropriate measure, e.g., chemotherapy, immunization, avoiding exposure, or withholding toxic substances during pregnancy. The effect of environmental agents on the fetus may become manifest in several different ways. Such agents may lead to fetal death, to stillbirth, or to a malformation. Depending on the stage of pregnancy at which the insult occurs, and on other circumstances, the fetus may escape without any adverse effect.

At one time infections in pregnancy were regarded as the principal cause of congenital malformations. If syphilis or any febrile disorder preceded the birth of a child with a deformity, it was assumed that the deformity was due to the maternal infection. The concept that infection was the cause of malformations fell into disrepute when it became clear that the incidence of congenital malformations remained unaltered despite the decline in the incidence of syphilis and other infectious diseases, a process that has been accelerated by general public health measures and by the advent of chemotherapy. Virus infections are of special interest in this context. It has been known for many years that certain virus infections in pregnancy—measles, mumps, and smallpox—might cause fetal death or stillbirth, while in others transplacental infection might result, with clinical evidence of the maternal infection in the fetus or infant at birth. The discovery by Gregg in 1941 that rubella in early pregnancy was often followed by the birth of infants with congenital deformities raised the possibility that other viruses might also have a teratogenic action. In Table 60-2 are listed the more important virus diseases of man which have from time to time been associated with reports of fetal damage or which constitute a potential hazard to the fetus if they should occur in pregnancy. Many of these infections are essentially diseases of childhood, and others can be prevented by immunization, so that the actual risk of primary infection in pregnancy is not very great, as most individuals will already have experienced infection by the time of child-bearing age. However, with the changing pattern in the natural history of disease some individuals will undoubtedly escape infection in childhood and may therefore be exposed for the first time in pregnancy.

Extensive studies to adduce the effect of

Table 60-2. *Virus Diseases in Pregnancy That Are Potential Causes of Fetal Infection*

Rubella	Hepatitis
Measles	Smallpox
Varicella	Vaccinia
Mumps	Herpes simplex
Poliomyelitis	Zoster
Coxsackie virus infections	Cytomegalic inclusion disease
Echo virus infections	Influenza

virus infections on the fetus have confirmed the fact that certain of these infections may be followed by abortion or stillbirth (in many instances the risk appears to have been exaggerated). No conclusive evidence has yet been produced, however, that these viruses, except for rubella and cytomegalovirus, can cause congenital malformations. That malformations may follow infections such as measles and mumps there is no doubt, but as they cannot be distinguished from coincidental associations their causative role cannot be assumed.

For many years the association between rubella in pregnancy and congenital malformations depended on statistical evidence. Little was known about the virus or about the way in which defects were produced. Moreover, undue emphasis was placed on one aspect of fetal damage—malformations. With the isolation of the rubella virus in 1962 and the development of laboratory procedures, much new knowledge has been gained about the pathogenesis of rubella and about possible mechanisms of fetal damage. Malformations following maternal rubella now seem to be but one aspect of the overall picture of fetal damage. Maternal rubella may lead to abortion, stillbirth, death in infancy, major and minor malformations, a chronic virus infection with and without malformation, subclinical infection—and also to an uninfected and undamaged infant. Much has still to be learned about this important problem and in particular why one virus can deform some fetuses and not others, and why other viruses with a basically similar pathogenesis have no such action. In this chapter on prenatal virus infections the effect of rubella virus on the fetus will be discussed first, and then congenital cytomegalovirus infections will be described. Finally, against the background knowledge gained from the study of these two viruses, the ef-

fect of other human viruses on the fetus will be considered.

A comment on terminology would appear to be relevant at this point. The usually accepted definition of the term congenital malformation is an abnormality of structure present at birth and attributable to faulty development during the period of organogenesis. Most rubella malformations fall into this category, but strictly speaking those caused by cytomegalovirus do not, as in this condition the anomalies present are in most instances caused by secondary destruction of formed organs. The same holds for structural changes found in congenital syphilis and toxoplasmosis. It is doubtful whether much is to be gained by too strict adherence to the precise definition of the term congenital malformation. In this chapter it is proposed to consider the effect of fetal damage in the widest sense and to consider any adverse effect in fetal development attributable to virus infection. The term defect rather than malformation will be used to denote structural anomalies present at birth irrespective of the stage in development at which they have occurred, because the word defect has a somewhat broader meaning.

The period of prenatal life with which this chapter is concerned extends from the time of conception to the time of birth. This will therefore include the stage of the developing ovum, the embryo (second to eighth week), and the fetus (the third lunar month). It would be impossible within the context of this chapter to adhere to the precise use of terms used in developmental anatomy. The term "fetus" will therefore be used to denote the developing human organism at the stage of embryo as well as that of the fetus.

CONGENITAL RUBELLA

HISTORY OF CONGENITAL RUBELLA

In 1941 Gregg[14] recorded a series of cataracts in 78 newborn infants which he had observed in Sydney, Australia. Many infants had bilateral cataracts and three-quarters had congenital heart disease. According to Gregg,[14] "many of the infants were of small size, ill-nourished and difficult to feed." In 68 of the first 78 cases Gregg obtained a history from the mothers that rubella had occurred in early pregnancy, most frequently in the first and second months. Further cases were described in which the outstanding anomalies were cataracts, cardiac disease, deafness, and mental retardation. Swan et al.,[37] from South Australia, collected data on 120 cases of rubella in pregnancy followed by congenital malformations in 101 cases. In nearly all cases maternal rubella had occurred in the first trimester. The most frequent malformations encountered were microcephaly (62 per cent), cardiac disease (52 per cent), deaf-mutism and deafness (48 per cent), cataract (18 per cent), and mental deficiency (5 per cent). These defects occurred singly or in combination. This retrospective survey[37] revealed instances of many other defects, for example, strabismus, cryptorchidism, inguinal hernia, hydrocele, spina bifida, spastic diplegia, high-arched palate, mongolism, speech defect, pyloric stenosis, buphthalmos, hypospadias, optic atrophy, failure of closure of the choroidal fissure of the eye, obliteration of the bile ducts, and talipes equinovarus. Although no connection has been established between rubella and many of these defects, there are some (buphthalmos and strabismus) which may be causally related, and in the light of recent work on rubella the possibility remains that other defects may be caused by this virus.

In an analysis of 558 cases of congenital malformations from all parts of the world, Swan[36] found that in 519 cases (93 per cent) the mother had contracted rubella in the first four months of pregnancy, and he concluded that the risk of congenital malformations following rubella in the first, second, and third trimesters was 98 per cent, 81 per cent, and 72 per cent, respectively.

MORBIDITY AND MORTALITY FOLLOWING RUBELLA IN PREGNANCY

These early studies clearly demonstrated the close association between rubella in early pregnancy and congenital defects, but for several reasons they overestimated the risk. The enquiries were made retrospectively; they depended on the mothers' memory, and often opinion, of an illness in pregnancy, and they did not take into consideration the number of normal children that were born following maternal rubella. A more accurate assessment of the risk has been obtained in recent years by prospective studies, i.e., by observing, in the first instance, the attack of rubella in pregnant women and subsequently examining the offspring. Estimates of risk obtained in this way indicate that the incidence of fetal damage is much lower and is in the region of 25 to 30 per cent following rubella in early pregnancy. Even the prospective studies have differed markedly from each other, depending on methods used in the survey and in particular on the age at which medical examinations were undertaken and on the criteria used for accepting congenital defects as due to rubella. Many such surveys have been carried out, and special reference will be made to two surveys carried out between 1950 and 1952 in which the outcome of rubella in pregnancy was studied in a large group of women and in which matched controls were also studied. These are the surveys carried out in Sweden by Lundström[19] in 1951 and the British survey carried out under the auspices of the Ministry of Health in 1950-1952 and reported by Manson et al.[20]

Statistical studies show that for the fetus exposed to intrauterine rubella the critical period is the first 16 weeks of pregnancy, after which the risk of fetal damage declines sharply. During this time the period of greatest risk is the first four weeks, and during each successive four-week period the incidence declines to the sixteenth week. Thereafter the risk is slight.

Spontaneous Abortions. The incidence of spontaneous abortions in 13 prospective studies from different parts of the world summarized by Lundström[19] varied from nil to 36 per cent, with a mean incidence of 14 per cent. In the study carried out in Great Britain the incidence of spontaneous abortions was 5 per cent following first trimester rubella, compared with 2.4 per cent in the controls.

Stillbirths and Deaths of Liveborn Infants. The incidence of stillbirths in 295 cases of maternal rubella from the same 13 studies plus one other was 7.5 per cent, but again there was wide variation in some series.

In Table 60-3 are shown the figures for abortions, stillbirths, livebirths, deaths under two years of age, and defects, obtained in the British survey of 1950-1952.[20] The overall effect on the fetus is noticeably

Table 60-3. *Effect of Maternal Rubella in Pregnancy*

	PER CENT INCIDENCE OF EFFECTS OF FETAL DAMAGE						
Time of Maternal Rubella	*Abortions*	*Stillbirths*	*Liveborn Infants*	*Major Defects in Liveborn Infants*	*Death under 2 yr.*	*Alive at 2 yr.*	*Major Defects at 2 yr.*
Rubella up to 12 wk.	5.0	4.5	90.5	15.8	6.9	83.6	13.0
Controls	2.4	2.4	95.2	2.3	2.4	92.8	1.5
Rubella at 13 wk. and over	0.3	3.0	96.7	2.2	2.7	94.0	1.1
Controls	0.5	2.6	96.9	2.3	2.6	96.3	1.5

Details abstracted from Manson et al.[20]

higher following rubella in the first trimester than after the thirteenth week or in the control group.

Incidence of Congenital Malformations. The incidence of congenital defects after rubella in several prospective studies is shown in Table 60-4. It can be seen that there is considerable variation in the incidence of defects obtained from these studies. The reasons for this are not clear. To some extent it may be due to small numbers in the study groups, to local epidemiological conditions, and to methods of assessment. In column 1 of Table 60-4 are shown the results obtained from 15 prospective studies summarized by Lundström.[19] Four of these are shown separately in column 2, since, according to Bradford-Hill and his associates,[5] the methods of conducting the surveys were very similar. The details in column 3 (also included in column 1), from Lamy and Séror's investigation in France in 1953-1954,[17] are shown separately because of the extremely high incidence of defects. Again, the reasons for this are not clear. The figures from the Swedish (column 4) and British (column 5) surveys are shown with those of the controls. It is clear from these figures that the risk of fetal damage is greater following maternal rubella in the first 12 weeks of

Table 60-4. *Incidence of Congenital Malformations Following Rubella in Pregnancy. Data from Several Prospective Studies*

	SUMMARY OF 15 STUDIES, 1946-1961, QUOTED BY LUNDSTROM[19]		BRADFORD-HILL ET AL.[5] 1949-1954, SUMMARY FROM 4 STUDIES		LAMY AND SÉROR[17] FRANCE, 1953-1954		LUNDSTRÖM[19] SWEDEN, 1951		MANSON ET AL.[20] GREAT BRITAIN, 1950-1952	
	Rubella	*Controls*	*Rubella*	*Controls*	*Rubella*	*Controls*	*Rubella*	*Controls*	*Rubella*	*Controls*
Number of cases of rubella in pregnancy	Not stated	None	104	None	48	57	1146	712	578	5717
Number of liveborn infants	1231		Not recorded		42	559	1121	698	547	5655
Number with major malformations	96*		17†		23*	0	51*	5	37‡	128
Per cent incidence of malformations										
0- 4 wk.	33.0		50.0		100		11.0		15.6	
5- 8 wk.	25.0		25.0		63.0		11.0		19.7	
9-12 wk.	9.0		17.0		40.0		8.0		13.0	
13-16 wk.	4.0		11.0		75.0 (13-20 wk.)		1.4		4.2	
17 wk. or later	1.0		6.0 (17-24 wk.)				0.5		2.2	
1st trimester	20.0		30.6		66.6		10.0	0.7	15.6	2.3
Total pregnancy	8.0		16.4		50.0	0	6.6	0.7	6.4	2.3

*Rubella syndrome type defects of the heart, eye, and hearing only.
†11 infants born following maternal rubella in first 8 weeks had rubella syndrome defects. Of 3 infants following rubella in the 3rd month, 2 had CDH, 1 had harelip and cleft palate. Of 3 infants born following rubella in 4th to 6th month, 2 had CDH and 1 anencephaly.
‡These figures include all major defects. Corrected figure for rubella syndrome defects is 25 (13.6% 0-12 wk., 4.2% total pregnancy). See Table 25 in Manson et al.[20]

pregnancy than in any other period, but, taking malformations separately, the risk continues up to the sixteenth week and is proportionately greater in the first than in the second and third months of pregnancy. The age at which medical examinations are carried out is important in assessing the incidence of fetal damage. In the studies referred to in Table 60-4 most of the examinations were carried out at birth or soon after and were repeated at one to three years of age. In the British survey further examinations at three and seven years* revealed a considerable increase in the number of hearing defects from 6.0 per cent to 12 per cent following rubella in the first 16 weeks. No other major defects such as cataracts or congenital heart disease were encountered. In a final assessment at 8 to 11 years Sheridan[33] found that a further 16 per cent of children in the original survey had minor defects such as unilateral hearing loss, squints, and defective vision. In a preliminary assessment of the effect of rubella on 6000 pregnancies during the United States rubella epidemic of 1964, Sever and his associates have recorded the incidence of abnormalities detected during the *perinatal period* (first 28 days) as 10 per cent.[31] Many defects caused by rubella, such as heart disease and deafness, are not obvious in the very young infant, and it is probable that this number will be increased on subsequent examinations.

Taken as a whole, the overall effect of rubella in the first 12 weeks of pregnancy, with fetal damage by abortion, stillbirth, death in infancy, and major congenital malformations detectable by the age of one to three years, is approximately 25 to 35 per cent.

CLINICAL MANIFESTATIONS OF CONGENITAL RUBELLA

The classic defects following maternal rubella in early pregnancy are those involving the eye, the heart, and the hearing organs. These defects, which may occur singly or in combination, have been referred to as the "rubella syndrome." In addition to this triad of sequelae, affected children are often underweight and may have microcephaly. Following the 1964-1965 rubella epidemic in the United States many infants

*See Table 42 in the report by Manson et al.[20]

were born with congenital rubella defects; some of them showed the classic symptoms of the "rubella syndrome," while others had defects which either had not previously been recognized or had not been recorded as a specific manifestation of congenital rubella. These included neonatal purpura and thrombocytopenia, hepatosplenomegaly, jaundice, hepatitis, anemia, pneumonitis, myocardial damage, central nervous system involvement, and osseous lesions.[27] In addition, many infants were found to have multiple abnormalities, including those of the classical type, while in others the only manifestation of intrauterine infection was an inapparent illness with persistence of virus in the absence of any gross defects at birth.[29] Many infants also exposed to maternal rubella at the most susceptible stage in intrauterine life were born without obvious stigmata. These new manifestations which commonly appeared in the newborn have been referred to as "the expanded rubella syndrome" or acute disseminated congenital rubella. In this chapter they will be considered together under the heading of congenital rubella.

Cardiac Malformations

INCIDENCE. Congenital heart disease (CHD) is one of the commonest manifestations of congenital rubella. Its incidence following rubella during the first trimester is 7.0 per cent; and in children with congenital rubella it is 50 to 60 per cent.

TYPE OF DEFECT. Cardiac defects are usually of the acyanotic or potentially cyanotic type. A patent ductus arteriosus (PDA) is the most common. Next in order of frequency are interatrial defects (ASD) and interventricular septal defects (VSD) and Fallot's tetralogy. In the past the assessment of a cardiac defect depended on a clinical diagnosis. Now, with improved methods of diagnosis, it is possible to reach a more definitive diagnosis in a greater number of cases of cardiac disease. Out of 58 patients with congenital heart disease following maternal rubella seen at the Hospital for Sick Children, Great Ormond Street, London, 34 had PDA and a further six had a patent ductus with some other defect. In 60 per cent some other rubella defect was also present.

A high incidence of cardiac defects (60 to 70 per cent) was encountered among cases of congenital rubella following the United States epidemic. Patent ductus arteriosus was the most frequent type of cardiac lesion, but a number of cases of coarctation of the pulmonary artery and its branches were also encountered.

Eye Defects. The most important and frequent eye defects encountered are cataracts. Approximately 70 per cent of cataracts are bilateral, and they are commonly associated with other rubella defects.

INCIDENCE. The incidence of cataracts following rubella during the first trimester is 5.5 per cent; and in infants with congenital rubella it is 40 per cent.

TYPE OF CATARACT. Three types of cataracts have been described. The most frequent are subtotal and appear as dense white opacities, often with a pearly center surrounded by a zone of less dense opaque material and an outer peripheral zone of clear cortex. In other cataracts the contrast between the central and intermediate zones is less pronounced. A membranous type of cataract may also be found. Cataracts may not appear for some weeks after birth. Those present at birth may increase in size during the early weeks of life.

OTHER EYE DEFECTS. Cataracts are frequently associated with microphthalmia. Pigmentary changes in the retina are also common, being most apparent in eyes without cataracts. The retinal lesions, which have been described as "rubella retinitis" and "pseudoretinitis pigmentosa," appear as pepper and salt changes and result from a lack of pigment formation and not from an inflammatory reaction such as occurs in cytomegalic inclusion disease and in toxoplasmosis. Other eye conditions seen less commonly are glaucoma and corneal opacities and clouding of the cornea without increase in ocular tension. Congenital glaucoma may be the only manifestation of congenital rubella, but it is more often associated with other rubella defects such as heart disease and purpura. As with cataracts, glaucoma may not become obvious for several months. A transient clouding of the cornea may also occur, but without any corneal enlargement or increase in tension. This usually subsides without surgical treatment being necessary. Coloboma and failure of closure of the choroidal fissure have been reported.

Hearing Defects

INCIDENCE. The incidence of hearing defects following rubella in the first trimester is 6.5 per cent at age one to three years, but 22 per cent when reassessed at five to seven years. The incidence of deafness in infants with congenital rubella is 50 per cent.

TYPE OF HEARING DEFECT. The defect is a form of congenital perceptive deafness due to maldevelopment or degenerative changes in the cochlea and organ of Corti. The vestibular apparatus is unaffected. The loss of hearing has been described as deaf-mutism, but the loss of hearing is not absolute and the term "profound childhood deafness" for the severe forms of deafness is preferable to deaf-mutism. The failure to speak is caused not by any pathological lesion of the speech apparatus but by damage to the inner ear; this can frequently be remedied by proper training. Marked variation in the degree of hearing loss is encountered in rubella. It may be so severe as to be suspected in the first few months of life, particularly if other rubella defects are present, or it may not be suspected until later when there may be evidence of delayed or defective speech. In approximately 30 per cent of cases deafness is unilateral and in 70 per cent it is bilateral; these latter cases are commonly associated with speech defects. Asymmetry is often found. Even in the most severe cases of deafness loss of hearing is not absolute. Early recognition of hearing defects is of the utmost importance so that appropriate training and education can be arranged. Deafness should always be suspected in patients with known history of maternal rubella and with other rubella defects. In rubella deafness the pattern of the audiogram is characteristically flat, with the greater hearing loss in the higher frequencies. Deafness can be assumed if the audiogram shows a hearing loss of 20 decibels or more in two adjacent frequencies or of 30 decibels in a single frequency. Follow-up studies with audiometric examination have shown that the incidence of deafness following first trimester rubella may be as high as 20 to 30 per cent when assessed at five to seven years of age compared with six per cent at two years.[3, 16]

Following the 1964-1965 rubella epidemic in the United States many infants were born with rubella defects of an unusual kind in addition to the classic rubella syndrome defects. Many of these defects were multiple and of an acute nature and were recognizable in the neonatal period.[27] The incidence of these manifestations from several reported series is shown in Table 60-5.

Dysmaturity. Intrauterine growth retardation is common. In most instances immaturity (birth weight less than 2500 gm.) is associated with a normal or near normal ges-

Table 60-5. *Predominant Clinical Features in Five Studies on Congenital Rubella, 1964-1965*

SIGNS AND SYMPTOMS	RUDOLPH ET AL. HOUSTON	COOPER ET AL. NEW YORK	PLOTKIN ET AL. PHILADELPHIA	LINDQUIST ET AL. PHILADELPHIA	HORSTMANN ET AL. NEW HAVEN
Birth weight ≦ 2500 gm.	80%	60%	57%	50%	50%
Purpura	80%	70%			50%
Thrombocytopenia	80%	86%	43%	20%	50%
Hepatomegaly	80%	72%	33%	20%	55%
Splenomegaly	70%	69%			
Cardiac defects	70%	67%	67%	75%	86%
Eye defects	45%	45%	76%	60%	66%
Full fontanelle	45%	Not recorded	24%	25%	Not recorded
X-ray changes in long bones	60%	22%	33%	50%	Not recorded

Rudolph et al., J.A.M.A., *191*:843, 1965.
Cooper et al., Amer. J. Dis. Child., *110*:416, 1965.
Plotkin et al., J. Pediat., *67*:182, 1965.
Lindquist et al., Brit. Med. J., *2*:1401, 1965.
Horstmann et al., Amer. J. Dis. Child., *110*:408, 1965.

tational age. The incidence of malformations is higher in infants with low birth weights. Lundström[19] found that the mean length of infants with defects at birth was 47.8 cm.; in those exposed to maternal rubella but without defects it was 50 cm., and in the controls, 51.0 cm. Sixty-six per cent of infants with defects had a length of 41 to 49 cm. compared with 18 per cent of short length in the controls. At follow-up at one to three years 27 per cent of the infants with defects were found to be subnormal in size, 47 per cent had a subnormal head circumference, and 36 per cent had delayed functional development.

In the British series the proportion of premature births (between the twenty-ninth and thirty-sixth weeks of gestation) was 4.7 per cent in the rubella group as a whole and 4.4 per cent in the controls, but the figure was higher when rubella had occurred in the first 12 weeks. There was also a greater risk of a lower birth weight in the rubella group; in first trimester cases 17 per cent had birth weights less than 5.5 lb. compared with 4.3 per cent in the control group.

It can be seen from Table 60-5 that 50 to 80 per cent of infants born following the United States rubella epidemic of 1964-1965 had birth weights of 2500 gm. or less. In the series reported by Cooper and associates[9] 60 per cent of infants fell below the tenth percentile and 90 per cent below the fiftieth percentile levels. The mean birth weight with a normal gestational age was 2270 gm.

Neonatal Purpura and Thrombocytope- nia. Purpuric lesions appear as red-purplish macules approximately 3 to 6 mm. in diameter on the face, trunk, and arms. In some cases a generalized eruption develops involving the whole trunk, palms, and soles of the feet. The rash may consist of a few skin petechiae or a large blotchy mass of coalescing purpuric lesions. Purpura usually develops within 48 hours of birth and starts to fade within seven to ten days. A few cases have been observed of purpura developing several months after birth. In most cases of neonatal purpura the platelet count ranges from 60,000 to 100,000 per cubic millimeter. Marrow specimens may reveal a paucity of megakaryocytes. Both platelets and megakaryocytes usually return to normal within six to eight weeks.

Hepatomegaly and Splenomegaly. An enlarged liver and spleen are commonly found soon after birth, but this may not develop or be noticed until the second or third month of life. The organs are usually firm and may extend to 3 to 4 cm. below the costal margin; occasionally the enlargement is confined to one organ.

Hepatitis and Jaundice. Hepatomegaly may be associated with jaundice. Usually this appears during the first 48 hours of life and is associated with high levels of direct-reacting bilirubin. Hepatitis without jaundice may also occur; the transaminase levels may be elevated for several weeks before returning to normal. Liver biopsies reveal changes similar to those seen in giant cell hepatitis or any focal areas of damaged cells.

Bone Changes. Radiological changes can be found in the long bones.[28] These consist of an alteration in the trabecular pattern of the metaphyses, being most evident in the distal end of the femur and the proximal end of the tibia. Linear areas of translucency can be seen, and the zones of calcification are clearly defined. These bone changes are seen more often in the neonatal period than in older children with the rubella syndrome. Periosteal reactions are not seen. In the skull a widening of the anterior fontanelle may be present.

Central Nervous System Changes. A persistently full anterior fontanelle with raised cerebrospinal fluid pressure may be present. There may also be an increase in the protein content and a pleocytosis. Convulsions and seizures may occur, and abnormal electroencephalographic recordings in some cases suggest that encephalopathy may be present.

Other Manifestations. Cases of congenital rubella have been described with a maculopapular rash and enlarged cervical, occipital, and postauricular nodes similar to childhood or adult rubella. Hemolytic anemia, myocardial damage, interstitial pneumonitis, and splenic fibrosis have also been described.

PATHOLOGY OF CONGENITAL RUBELLA

Ocular Lesions. The lesions are mainly confined to the lens and retina. Macroscopically the whole eye, including the lens, may be small. Lens opacities are caused by necrosis of cells in the central nuclear portion and to a lesser extent in the cortical zone. The nucleus may undergo complete necrosis and appear as an amorphous mass. Lens fibers comprising the cortical zone, particularly those in the equatorial region, may become degenerate and separated by vacuoles from the unaffected segment. In the retina focal areas can be found in which there is a lack of pigment epithelium due to an interference with normal development of pigment epithelium.

The Ear. The general anatomical configuration of the middle ear, auditory ossicles and inner ear is normal. The main pathological lesion in rubella is the lack of differentiation of primitive cells to form the organ of Corti. In other cases, in which the

organ of Corti may have reached maturation, hemorrhages may be found in the cochlea and stria vascularis. Inflammatory changes with granulation tissue and degenerating cells may be found in differentiated organs of Corti and in the basilar membrane, causing adhesions to the delicate tectorial membrane.

Heart. In patent ductus arteriosus the lumen is often larger and thinner than normal with some loss of fibers in the internal elastic lamina. Connective tissue may be found replacing muscle at the margin of septal defects. Varying degrees of myocardial damage have been described. There may be a few fragmented muscle fibers or complete disruption of normal myocardial architecture with extensive vacuolization and gross nuclear changes. There is little or no inflammatory response.

Other Organs. In the *brain,* necrosis of paraventricular white matter has been described with calcification around the capillaries of the white matter, corpus striatum, and some cortical areas.[18] No perivascular cuffing was found. In the *lung,* there may be an interstitial pneumonitis and thickening of the alveolar septa due to fibrosis, and, in the *spleen,* marked fibrosis in a neonate has been described, suggesting that the inflammatory process was of long standing. In the *liver* there may be swelling of parenchymal cells and fusion to form multinucleate cells with infiltration of mononuclear cells in the portal tract and foci of hepatic necrosis.

Placenta. The changes are mainly in the decidual cells. Vesiculation occurs with balloon degeneration, and varying cytoplasmic inclusion bodies can be found. Necrosis is not a marked feature, and only a minimal inflammatory reaction with lymphocytes is seen. The chorionic villi and endometrial glands appear normal.

EPIDEMIOLOGY OF CONGENITAL RUBELLA

The epidemiology of rubella in children and adults is discussed in Chapter 27. The following points are of special significance to the context of congenital rubella.

Epidemicity. Rubella has a worldwide distribution; therefore congenital rubella may occur in all parts of the world. Epidemics occur with less regularity than with measles, usually every five to six years, with major epidemics every nine to ten years.

Infectiousness. Rubella is on the whole less infectious than measles but subclinical infection occurs more often in rubella than in measles. The disease is uncommon in preschool children and has its highest incidence in older children and adolescents. Rubella can be highly infectious under conditions of close contact, as, for example, in a family or household, and in schools and institutions. Under these circumstances the infection rate may be close to 100 per cent. The ratio of subclinical to overt infection may range from 1:1 in institutions to 6:1 in service recruit establishments. Subclinical infection may lead to fetal infection and to congenital defects.

Immune Status and Fetal Infection. A close correlation exists between susceptibility to rubella and the absence of circulating antibody at the onset of infection. Conversely, the development of resistance is accompanied by the appearance of antibody. Approximately 15 to 25 per cent of adults of both sexes may reach adult life without being infected with rubella. The proportion of women of child-bearing age without rubella antibody is approximately 15 to 20 per cent,[11, 32] but it may be higher in nonwhite populations. The incidence of fetal abnormalities is closely related to the incidence of primary infections, clinical or subclinical, in women during the first 16 weeks of pregnancy. The period of birth of infants with defects (autumn-winter) tends to correspond with the seasonal incidence of rubella (spring-summer).

PATHOGENESIS OF CONGENITAL RUBELLA

The main features of the pathogenesis of congenital rubella (see Fig. 60-1) can be con-

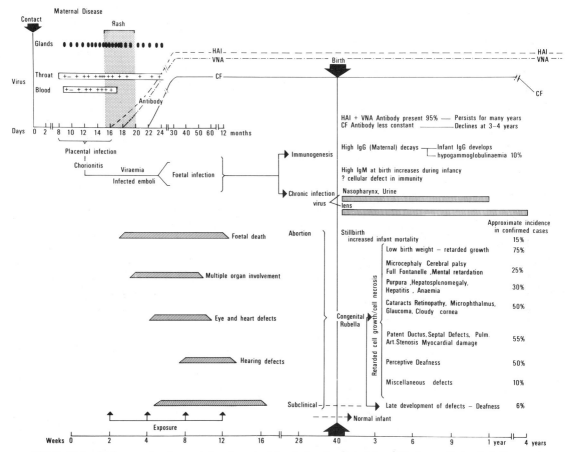

Figure 60-1. Pathogenesis of prenatal and postnatal rubella. Reprinted from Dudgeon, J. A., Rubella vaccines. Brit. Med. Bull., *25*:159, 1969; reproduced by kind permission of the Editors of the British Medical Bulletin.

sidered under four main headings. Further details on the pathogenesis of the disease in adults, with which fetal infection is closely linked, can be found in Chapter 27.

Maternal-Placental-Fetal Infection. In maternal rubella the incubation period between the time of exposure and onset of rash is approximately 14 to 16 days. Virus may be present in the nasopharynx and in the blood for up to seven days before the appearance of the rash and in the nasopharynx for up to 21 days after the rash. Viremia, on the other hand, seldom persists after the rash has appeared, and by this time virus will probably have reached the fetus. Whether viremia is as prolonged in subclinical as in clinical infections is not known, but the extent of fetal damage may be equally severe following both types of infection. The next stage is infection of the placenta. Virus has been recovered from the placenta and from membranes from aborted material following maternal infection in the first 12 to 16 weeks of pregnancy,[2] and histological evidence of placental involvement has also been demonstrated.

Fetal Infection. Virus can be recovered from the fetus and from isolated organs and tissues of the fetus following maternal rubella in the early weeks of pregnancy.[2] It persists in fetal tissues for long periods, having been recovered from fetuses of gestational age varying from 12 to 23 weeks.

Postnatal Infection. Fetal infection may become chronic and persist after birth.[15] Virus can readily be recovered from the nasopharynx and from the urine and also from cataractous material. The number of infants excreting virus may be as high as 60 per cent in the first month of life, 30 per cent at six months, and 7 per cent at 10 months.[10] Virus excretion has not been detected over the age of two years. Both nasopharyngeal secretions and urine constitute a source of infection, and cases of rubella have been reported in nurses and doctors caring for infants with the rubella syndrome. Virus has been recovered from 14 per cent of newborn infants without observable defects at birth.[29] Such cases need careful observation for late development of defects, particularly deafness. In fatal cases virus has been recovered from nearly every organ in the body: liver, brain, spinal cord, spinal fluid, heart muscle, cataractous tissue, lymph gland, spleen, thymus, adrenal, kidney, and bone. Quantitative estimations of virus show high concentrations of virus in certain organs, particularly the lymphoreticular tissue, thymus, kidney, and cataractous tissue.

Immunogenesis. The presence of rubella neutralizing antibody in infants with congenital rubella has been demonstrated by Dudgeon and associates[11, 12, 26] and by Weller and his associates.[38] In most cases the antibody titer in infants with rubella is equal to or greater than that in the mother. It persists at a high level throughout the first year of life and probably indefinitely. Approximately 90 per cent of infants and children aged six months to five years with rubella defects following intrauterine rubella in the first trimester have significantly raised levels of rubella antibody compared with their normal cohorts. Five to 10 per cent of children born with rubella defects and following a history of maternal rubella are found to be without antibody. Serological evidence of subclinical infection of the fetus has been demonstrated by Butler and his associates.[8] It is probable that antibody is produced either by the fetus late in intrauterine life or soon after birth, and the initial response is predominantly IgM. This view is confirmed by the finding that high levels of IgM (19S) globulin have been demonstrated in sera from infants with congenital rubella aged three weeks to six months.[34] As the macroglobulins do not normally pass across the placenta, it seems likely that the IgM in infants with congenital rubella is fetal in origin. In fetal sera the levels of rubella neutralizing antibody in specimens collected from the twelfth to sixteenth week are considerably lower than in the mother. This antibody is predominantly IgG (7S) globulin and is presumably maternal in origin. At birth large amounts of IgG and IgM antibody are present. The level of IgG declines during the first few months of life and subsequently rises again toward the end of the first year of life, and during this time the high level of IgM is maintained.[1, 4] A few cases of congenital acquired hypogammaglobulinemia have been reported.[34] Thus fetal infection with rubella does not lead to immunological tolerance in the accepted sense of the term. The fetus appears to be able to tolerate the viral antigen, as shown by the persistence of virus for many months, but this does not prevent the production of neutralizing antibody. It seems probable that some defect in the cellular immune mechanism is responsible for the persistence of virus in the presence of antibody in congenital rubella. A similar series of events occurs in cytomegalic inclusion disease.

Pathogenesis at the Cellular Level. The abnormalities in congenital rubella are of two main types. First, there are malformations or changes which are essentially due to retardation of growth of developing organs, and, second, there are secondary changes due to destruction of formed organs. Both can be correlated with the multiplication of virus in the tissues. Rubella-infected infants are characteristically subnormal in size in relation to normal gestational age. The small size of certain organs such as the pancreas and adrenals appears to be due to a subnormal number of morphologically normal cells.[22] A possible explanation for this is provided by observations on the growth of rubella virus in cell culture, in which the main effect is the arrest of mitotic activity.[24] The arrest of mitosis may therefore lead either to a defect or to a limitation in growth of a normal organ, depending on the stage in gestation at which infection is initiated. This is the predominant effect of rubella virus on the fetus, but secondary destruction of formed tissues and organs can occur, as for example in infants with hepatitis, myocardial damage, pneumonitis, and splenic fibrosis.

Pathogenesis of Congenital Rubella: A Synthesis. The sequence of events is summarized in Figure 60-1. Although the duration of viremia probably varies from case to case, it is probable that the fetus is infected at or soon after the appearance of the maternal rash. The capacity of the virus to infect and invade the fetus is closely related to gestational age, but other factors such as duration of viremia, prophylactic use of gamma globulin, or resistance of the host may affect the outcome of maternal-fetal infection. Most cases of fetal infection leading to fetal death or malformations have followed rubella in the first 16 weeks of pregnancy. Thereafter the risk appears to be slight. As a general rule, multiple defects are related to early infection (in the first eight weeks), whereas single organ defects tend to occur with later infection. Eye lesions occur with greatest frequency after infection at the sixth to eighth week, cardiac lesions between the

ninth and tenth weeks, and hearing defects from the eighth to twelfth week, but throughout this period there is marked variation in the type of response. Both subclinically infected and unaffected infants may be born after fetal infection throughout this period of maximum susceptibility.

DIAGNOSIS OF CONGENITAL RUBELLA

The following methods can be used to establish the diagnosis of congenital rubella in the laboratory (details will be found in Chapter 27): (1) isolation of virus; (2) serological methods to detect rubella antibody; and (3) immunoglobulin estimations.

Virus Isolation. Rubella virus can be isolated in primary African green monkey kidney culture (AGMK) using the interference technique with Echo 11 virus or Coxsackie A 9 as the challenge agent. Specimens should be inoculated into four AGMK culture tubes and incubated at 35° C. for seven to ten days, after which time two culture tubes are challenged with 1000 tissue culture doses ($TCID_{50}$) Echo 11 virus. If no interference is detectable after primary inoculation, at least one further passage should be made.

An alternative technique is to inoculate specimens into cell cultures prepared from a continuous line of rabbit kidney cultures, the RK 13 cell line. Inoculated cultures should be observed for the presence of cytopathic changes, which in the case of rubella appear as focal areas of degeneration in seven to ten days. In most cases a second passage is necessary before typical cytopathic changes appear. Both methods are equally sensitive. Any agent showing interference or cytopathic change should be identified by a neutralization with a specific rubella antiserum. The cytopathic changes in RK 13 cells produced by rubella virus from a case of congenital rubella are shown in Figure 60-2.

Serology

NEUTRALIZATION TEST. Antibody can be measured by the interference-inhibition test in AGMK cultures, or by the cytopathic-inhibition test in RK 13 cells. Both methods are reliable and yield results which are comparable.

COMPLEMENT-FIXATION TEST. Complement-fixing antibody can be titrated by

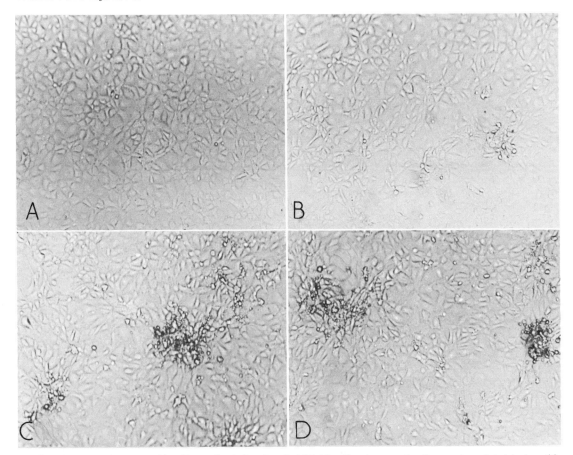

Figure 60-2. The cytopathic effects of rubella virus in RK 13 cells: *A*, control culture uninoculated (cytopathic inhibition with rubella antiserum is similar); *B*, six days after inoculation with nasopharyngeal swab; *C*, after passage with material shown in *B*; *D*, after inoculation with cataractous tissue from cases of congenital rubella.

means of a microtechnique with cell-associated antigens prepared in RK 13 cells or AGMK cultures[30] or in a chronically infected line of LLC MK2 cells.[35]

Complement-fixing antibody in congenital rubella does not parallel neutralizing antibody. In some cases it is present in high titer at birth and persists throughout the first year of life. In others a rising titer can be demonstrated at about three months of age. Unlike neutralizing antibody, complement-fixing antibody tends to decline between the second and third years of life.

FLUORESCENT ANTIGEN-ANTIBODY TEST. A fluorescent antigen-antibody test has also been described[7] but does not appear to have any advantage over the neutralization test in the study of congenital rubella.

Immunoglobulin Estimation. This can be detected by the gel-diffusion precipitation technique. The IgM levels are usually found to be grossly elevated in infants with congenital rubella,[34] and this provides additional confirmatory evidence of infection acquired before or very shortly after birth.

PROPHYLAXIS OF RUBELLA

The prophylaxis of virus infections is largely dependent on immunization, either by active or passive means, both of which are mediated through specific circulating antibody. On theoretical grounds, therefore, it should be possible to prevent maternal rubella, and hence infection of the fetus, either by passive immunization with gamma globulin or by active immunization with a vaccine. At present only limited experience is available with the use of rubella vaccines, and the results of prophylaxis with gamma globulin are in the main contradictory.[13, 19]

Passive Immunization with Gamma

Globulin. In measles and hepatitis gamma globulin is administered with the object of modifying or preventing symptomatic disease. In rubella in pregnancy gamma globulin is administered with the intention of suppressing the viremia. This is difficult to achieve on account of the peculiarities of the natural history of rubella. The prophylactic value of gamma globulin in rubella has been studied experimentally by Green and his associates.[13] Gamma globulin was administered in a dosage of 0.15 ml. per pound of body weight to groups of individuals who were then exposed to rubella in such a way as to simulate infection by either brief contact or prolonged exposure. Of 33 subjects given gamma globulin, 18 (55 per cent) developed clinical rubella and 9 (27 per cent) subclinical infection, a total of 27 (82 per cent) infected. In the controls the corresponding figures were 21 (57 per cent) with clinical rubella and 13 (35 per cent) with subclinical rubella, a total of 34 (92 per cent) infected. Gamma globulin did not prevent viremia, but appeared to reduce its duration. However, subjects with antibody, even at low levels, were protected. In a study in Alaska it was found that commercial gamma globulin (0.25 ml. per pound) prevented rubella infection in 56 per cent of the male subjects under investigation and also suppressed symptoms, but not infection, in a third of the remainder. In this study the gamma globulin was administered during the incubation period and in many cases before exposure.[6] The results of trials of gamma globulin in preventing rubella in pregnancy are extremely variable. A significant degree of protection has been recorded with commercial gamma globulin and with convalescent rubella gamma globulin.[19] Protection has also been recorded by McDonald with 750 and 1500 mg. of pooled gamma globulin.[22] In the 1964 epidemic in the United States, Cooper and his associates[9] found little evidence that gamma globulin prevented maternal rubella, whereas other observers did.[29, 31]

There are a number of possible explanations for these discrepancies in the efficacy of gamma globulin in rubella. They could be due to differences in (1) antibody titer between batches of gamma globulin, (2) the time of administration and dosage, and (3) time, degree, and length of contact before the gamma globulin was administered. This last point is of special importance in view of the fact that patients with rubella (and this applies to subclinical infections as well) may be infectious for a week before the onset of the rash. The timing of first contact may therefore be difficult to ascertain.

Despite these variable results and until such time as a rubella vaccine for active immunization can be developed, gamma globulin is the only method of prophylaxis available. Although gamma globulin may not prevent maternal rubella it may reduce the risk of serious malformations. The dosage recommended for pregnant women in the first 16 weeks of pregnancy is 1500 mg. (approximately 0.2 ml. per pound).

Active Immunization. The use of cell culture techniques has opened up the way to the development of a vaccine against rubella as it has in other virus diseases. Currently research is directed toward both an inactivated and an attenuated vaccine, but difficulties have been encountered with both types of vaccine. The potency of an inactivated vaccine depends initially on the amount of viral antigen present. Production of rubella virus in high titer presents certain problems, and the antigenicity may be lost by inactivation procedures. Preliminary experiments to induce active immunity with culture fluids containing live virus have encountered an obstacle in that the vaccinees developed a transmissible infection.[25] Recently the development of a live attenuated rubella vaccine has been reported which produces an active infection, does not appear to be contagious, and produces an immune response in 94 per cent of susceptible children.[21]

Since these initial trials[21] in 1966 rapid progress has been made and several attenuated rubella vaccines have been developed by serial passage of the virus in different cell culture systems. The details of three such vaccines are shown in Table 60-6. These vaccines have now been administered to many thousands of susceptible individuals.[38a, b] Very few reactions have been observed except for some cases of joint involvement in adult females; reactions in children have been few and very mild. A high proportion of vaccines excreted virus in the nasopharynx, but no evidence of communicability has been demonstrated. Of special importance is the fact that the seroconversion rates in susceptible vaccinated individuals has been close on 100

Table 60-6. *Details of Three Attenuated Rubella Vaccines*

VACCINE STRAIN AND DESIGNATION	CELL SUBSTRATE	PASSAGE DETAILS
Cendehill vaccine Cendehill 51/2	Primary rabbit kidney	51st passage
Duck embryo vaccine HPV/77:DE5	Duck embryo tissue culture	HPV/77 + duck embryo 5
Diploid vaccine RA27/3	Human diploid fibroblast (WI-38)	Seed virus in 25th passage; two additional passages in WI-38 in United Kingdom

per cent and antibody appears to be well maintained. Two of the vaccines mentioned in Table 60-6, Cendehill and duck embryo have now been licensed for general use in certain countries. The current problem is to decide how best they can be used. This will to a large extent depend on the epidemiological background created by rubella in each country, but it is important to stress that although the vaccine strains have been attenuated their effect on the human fetus is not known. Rubella vaccines should not, therefore, be given to anyone who could be pregnant. There are two alternative approaches to rubella immunization: (1) mass immunization of young children of both sexes with the object or eradication of rubella as a disease, or (2) selective immunization of prepubertal girls. The pros and cons of each approach have been discussed by Dudgeon in two recent reviews.[38c, d]

CYTOMEGALIC INCLUSION DISEASE

This disease has been variously described as salivary gland inclusion disease, inclusion disease, and generalized cytomegalic inclusion disease. Originally recognized many years ago as a pathological entity on account of bizarre inclusion-bearing cells found in autopsy material, it was not until 1952 that the disease was recognized during life with the discovery by Fetterman[39] that intranuclear inclusions in epithelial cells could be found in urinary

sediments. In 1956 the causative virus was isolated in tissue culture.[43, 45] The inclusions in cytomegalic inclusion disease are essentially similar in appearance to those that are found in the salivary glands of many normal animals. They are caused by the salivary gland viruses (SGV), a group of distinct species-specific viruses which are widely distributed throughout the animal kingdom. The human strain which shares a common antigen with one of the simian strains is referred to as cytomegalovirus (CMV).

CLINICAL MANIFESTATIONS

Four main types of infection with cytomegalovirus may occur:

1. An asymptomatic infection with localized infection. Infants may excrete virus at birth. This is probably the most common form of infection.

2. Mental retardation, microcephaly, and convulsions, often with a delayed onset.

3. A neurological disease with low birth weight, microcephaly, chorioretinitis, occasionally cerebral calcification, and motor disabilities.

4. A generalized infection with low birth weight, hepatosplenomegaly, jaundice, and hepatitis. Neurological deficits may develop later. This is the most severe form of the disease, but the least common.

Only this last form of cytomegalic inclusion disease will be considered in this chapter.

The fulminating form of the disease usually presents at or soon after birth.[44] The main clinical features are a low birth weight

(2500 to 3000 gm.), prematurity, microcephaly, jaundice, and petechiae. The liver and spleen are frequently enlarged. There is usually an early onset of lethargy, difficulty in feeding, convulsions, and respiratory distress. Jaundice may persist for several weeks, but the petechiae usually disappear in a few days. Both the liver and spleen may remain enlarged and firm for several months. Neurological sequelae in infants who survive are common and represent the most serious aspect of infection with this virus.[40, 44] Microcephaly, mental retardation, paralysis, and spasticity are frequently encountered. The spinal fluid may show an increase in the protein content and a pleocytosis. Choroidoretinitis and cerebral calcification occur in about 25 per cent of cases. Malformation of the brain has been reported, pointing to developmental arrest during gestation.[42]

EPIDEMIOLOGY

Cytomegalovirus infections have been identified in many parts of the world. The presence of neutralizing and complement-fixing antibodies in the absence of clinical disease indicates that infection is both widespread and usually subclinical.[42] Approximately 50 to 60 per cent of adults may have antibody to cytomegalovirus. Antibody to cytomegalovirus can be demonstrated in human gamma globulin. Clinical disease in those over the age of one year is uncommon.

The majority of severe generalized infections develop in the newborn period and in most instances within two to three days of birth. These presumably result from intrauterine infection. In about 15 per cent of reported cases symptoms have appeared between the fourth and eighth week, and in these cases infection could have been contracted postnatally. The incubation period is not known. Infants with cytomegalic inclusion disease harbor virus in the nasopharynx and urine for many months after birth[45] and can presumably spread infection in the same way as do infants with congenital rubella. In the general population virus is probably spread from asymptomatic carriers via nasopharyngeal secretions and urine.

PATHOLOGY

The characteristic large epithelial cells with both intranuclear and intracytoplasmic inclusion bodies may be found in 10 per cent of all infant autopsies. Inclusion-bearing cells may be found throughout the body and particularly in the salivary glands, kidney, liver, adrenals, pancreas, gastrointestinal tract, spleen, and thymus. In the brain there may be extensive necrotizing granulomatous

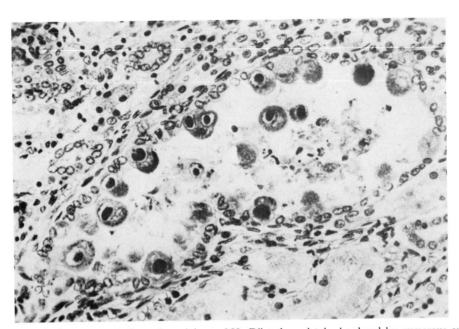

Figure 60-3. Kidney, hematoxylin-eosin staining × 350. Dilated renal tube bordered by numerous cytomegalic cells some of which have fallen into the tubular lumen and are ready to be eliminated in the flow of urine. (Photomicrograph by Le Tan Vinh.)

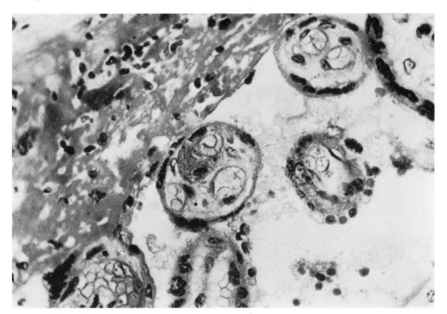

Figure 60-4. Placenta, hematoxylin-eosin staining × 450. In the center is a well distinguished cytomegalic inclusion cell in the mesenchymal axis of a chorionic villus. At lower right, hyaline membrane with numerous leukocytes. (Photomicrograph by Le Tan Vinh.)

PATHOGENESIS

lesions with calcification and choroidoretinitis. In the liver, focal areas of necrosis with multinucleate giant cell formation may be found.

PATHOGENESIS

Little is known about the pathogenesis of congenital cytomegalovirus infections, as the disease in the mother is invariably asymptomatic, but it is presumed that the fetus is infected following a primary infection with viremia in the mother. It is possible that infection could follow reactivation of latent virus.

In the newborn the virus can be recovered from the urine, the nasopharynx, and also the liver.[45] Virus may persist in the urine for six months to four years and in the liver for three months. Antibody can be demonstrated in the presence of virus excretion. Whether cytomegalovirus infection results in abortion or stillbirth is not known, but it would be surprising if it did not. Very rarely malformations of the brain have been reported in congenital cytomegalovirus infection, but most of the congenital abnormalities are the result of destruction of formed organs and not of defects in organogenesis. A summary of the facts concerning

the pathogenesis of congenital rubella and cytomegalovirus is shown in Table 60-7.

DIAGNOSIS

Characteristic cytomegalic cells with inclusions may be found in urinary sediments or in autopsy material from the kidney and other viscera. When present they are of considerable diagnostic value, but experience is required in detecting them in urine specimens. Of greater value is the isolation of the causative virus from the nasopharynx and urine by inoculation of cell cultures of human fibroblasts. Serological tests are also useful. The finding of a persistent high titer of neutralizing antibody to cytomegalovirus in the first few months of life is strongly suggestive of congenital cytomegalovirus infection. The complement-fixation test is of less value in the first year of life.[44] Complement-fixing antibody, presumably maternal in origin, may be found in the first weeks of life; it then disappears and may reappear during the second year of life. The IgM levels are usually elevated in congenital cytomegalovirus infection, with near normal levels of IgA.[41] IgA has been reported as elevated in congenital cytomegalovirus infection in the newborn.[41] A raised IgM value in the first

Table 60-7. *Summary of the Effects of Rubella and Cytomegalovirus on the Fetus*

FETAL INFECTION	FETAL DEATH	FETAL MALFORMATIONS/ABNORMALITIES
Rubella		
Invasion and multiplication of virus in fetal organs	Increase in	*Dysmaturity*
	Abortions	Low birth weight, subnormal height, and retarded development
Isolation of virus from fetus and newborn	Stillbirths	*Malformations* of eye, heart, ear, and other organs due to defects during organogenesis
Chronic virus infection, with persistence of virus and antibody after birth	Deaths in infancy	*Abnormalities* of liver, lung, myocardium, etc., due to secondary destruction
Cytomegalovirus		
Same as above	Abortions and stillbirths not known	Low birth weight and retarded development
	Mortality rate in infancy increased	Rarely malformation of brain
		Abnormalities with destruction of tissue in many organs

year of life is a useful additional diagnostic finding.

PROPHYLAXIS AND TREATMENT

There is no form of specific treatment or prophylaxis.

THE EFFECT OF OTHER VIRUSES ON THE FETUS

The other viruses which present a potential hazard to the fetus if infection should occur in pregnancy have been listed in Table 60-2. These comprise the viruses responsible for the acute viral exanthems, the acute epidemic infections, a virus used in a live vaccine (vaccinia), and a number of others. With few exceptions primary infection with these viruses is associated with viremia. Thus, from the theoretical point of view, virus can reach the fetus by transplacental infection. In the case of influenza, viremia has never been convincingly demonstrated, but the accompanying toxemia could explain the damage to the fetus that sometimes occurs.

The overall effect of these viruses on the fetus is summarized in Table 60-8. Evidence of fetal infection in certain instances follows from reports of rashes and pock marks in fetuses and the newborn following infection with measles, varicella, smallpox, vaccinia, and herpes. Similarly, signs and symptoms of the maternal illness appearing within a few days of birth in cases of poliomyelitis or Coxsackie B indicates that fetal infection can occur if allowance is made for the known incubation period of these diseases. There is also clear-cut evidence of an increase in fetal deaths following measles, mumps, smallpox, vaccinia, poliomyelitis, and influenza, but in some instances, to be discussed, the risk appears to have been exaggerated. On the other hand, clear-cut evidence that these viruses can cause congenital malformations is lacking, but this aspect of the problem requires more detailed study.

Measles. Measles in early pregnancy can result in an increased number of abortions, but the British Survey[57]* showed that

---

*See Table G in Manson et al.[57]

Table 60-8. Effect on Fetus of Other Virus Infections in Pregnancy

Virus Disease	Fetal Infection	Fetal Death	Fetal Malformation/ Abnormalities
Measles	+	+	−
Varicella	+	−	−
Mumps	?	+	?
Smallpox	+	+	−
Vaccinia	+	+	−
Hepatitis	?	−	?
Poliomyelitis	+	+	−
Coxsackie A	−	−	−
Coxsackie B	+	?	?
Echo	−	−	−
Herpes simplex	+	−	−
Zoster	?	−	−
Influenza	−	+	?

the risk was less serious than was generally supposed. Similar findings were reported by Bradford-Hill and associates.[47] In the British survey the incidence of malformed infants following measles in the first trimester was 7 per cent compared with 2.3 per cent in the controls, but these consisted of many different defects with little consistent pattern. At least one patient had a rubella-like defect (cardiac lesion and eye defect), so there could have been a mistake in the diagnosis of the maternal illness. This has been reported before.[46] No association between measles and congenital malformation was reported by Bradford-Hill et al.[47]

Varicella. Varicella in the newborn is not uncommon. A fatal disseminated infection with visceral necrosis may also occur. Herpes zoster in the newborn may follow maternal varicella late in pregnancy.

Variola. The risk of spontaneous abortion is considerably increased following variola in pregnancy. This risk can be eliminated by vaccination *prior* to pregnancy.

Vaccinia Virus. Administration of vaccinia virus during pregnancy may lead to an increase in abortions, and a few cases of fetal vaccinia have been reported with extensive cutaneous and visceral lesions following primary vaccination in pregnancy.[54, 56, 58] The appearance of the lesions and reports of virus isolation from the aborted fetuses indicate that vaccinia virus can persist for several weeks in the fetus.

Other Live Viral Vaccines. There is no indication that other live human virus vac-

cines, yellow fever vaccine or oral poliovaccine, have produced any adverse effect on the fetus, although on general principles their administration in pregnancy is considered inadvisable Fetal damage can also follow the use of certain live animal virus vaccines, such as hog cholera vaccine and blue tongue virus of sheep.

Mumps. Mumps in early pregnancy is commonly supposed to cause an increase in abortions, but the findings in the British survey (Table G in the article cited)[57] did not support this view. A high incidence of defects following mumps in the first trimester has been reported from Finland,[62] a finding that has not since been confirmed. Recent studies[59] have indicated that children with endocardial fibroelastosis show a marked hypersensitivity skin reaction to mumps virus antigen. It has been postulated that the skin reaction results from fetal infection with resulting immunological deficiency, whereby the fetus or infant is rendered incapable of forming antibody but can produce a delayed-type hypersensitivity reaction. Further reports on the association between mumps virus and fibroelastosis are conflicting.[51, 60]

Poliomyelitis. Poliomyelitis is associated with an increase in abortions and stillbirths, and the general effect on the fetus is poor. In the British survey only 55.6 per cent of infants were alive at two years following poliomyelitis in the first trimester, compared with 91.2 per cent in the controls.

There is no indication that any of the Echo viruses in sporadic or epidemic form cause fetal damage. Extensive studies following Echo 9 epidemics in the United States[52] and in Scotland[55] failed to reveal any evidence of an increase in malformations.

Coxsackie B virus infection can cause a disseminated infection in the newborn, and cases of endocardial fibroelastosis and cardiac defects have been attributed to fetal damage with Coxsackie B strains.[50] This report needs further investigation.

Hepatitis. The effect of hepatitis on the fetus is not known. Reports[49] that a "virus" has been isolated from cases of neonatal hepatitis and biliary atresia have not yet been confirmed. Similar pathological changes can be found in the liver in cases of congenital rubella and cytomegalovirus with neonatal hepatitis.

Influenza. Influenza may lead to an increase in abortions and stillbirths. No such effects were observed following epidemic influenza in Britain in 1950-1951,[57] but an increase in deaths of liveborn infants under two years of age was noted following maternal influenza between the twelfth and twenty-eighth weeks. An increase in malformations of the central nervous system was reported from Dublin in 1951 following the Asian influenza pandemic,[48] but there was no evidence of such malformations following the epidemic in the United States.[61]

Herpes Simplex. On rare occasions herpes simplex may produce a disseminated infection in the newborn. In most cases infection was probably acquired at or shortly after birth, but transplacental infection can occur. Fetal defects have not been observed.

BIBLIOGRAPHY

Rubella

1. Alford, C. A.: Studies on antibody in congenital rubella infections. Amer. J. Dis. Child., *110*:455, 1965.
2. Alford, C. A., Neva, F. A., and Weller, T. H.: Virologic and serologic studies on human products of conception after maternal rubella. New Eng. J. Med., *271*:1276, 1964.
3. Barr, B., and Lundström. R.: Deafness following maternal rubella. Acta Otolaryng., *53*:413, 1961.
4. Bellanti, J. A., Artenstein, M. S., Olson, L. C., Buescher, E. L., Luhrs, C. E., and Milstead, K. L.: Congenital rubella. Amer. J. Dis. Child., *110*:464, 1965.
5. Bradford-Hill, A., Doll, R., Galloway, T. M., and Hughes, J. P. W.: Virus diseases in pregnancy and congenital defects. Brit. J. Prev. Soc.. Med., *12*:1, 1958.
6. Brody, J. A., Sever, J. L., and Schiff, G. M.: Prevention of rubella by gamma globulin during an epidemic in Alaska. New Eng. J. Med., *272*:127, 1965.
7. Brown, G. G., Maassab, H. F., Veronelli, J. A., and Francis, T.: Detection of rubella antibodies in human serum by the indirect fluorescent antibody technique. Arch. Ges. Virusforsch., *16*:459, 1965.
8. Butler, N. R., Dudgeon, J. A., Peckham, C. S., Hayes, K., and Wybar, K.: Persistance of rubella antibody with and without embryopathy. Brit. Med. J., *2*:1027, 1965.
9. Cooper, L. Z., Green, R. H., Krugman, S., Giles, J. P., and Mirick, G. S.: Neonatal thrombocytopenic purpura and other manifestations of rubella contracted in Utero. Amer. J. Dis. Child., *110*:416, 1965.
10. Cooper, L. Z., and Krugman, S.: Diagnosis and management: congenital rubella. Pediatrics, *37*:335, 1966.
11. Dudgeon, J. A.: Serological studies on the rubella syndrome. Presented at the Seminar on Measles and Rubella, Paris. Arch. Ges. Virusforsch., *16*:501, 1965.
12. Dudgeon, J. A., Butler, N. R., and Plotkin, S. A.: Further serological studies on the rubella syndrome. Brit. Med. J., *2*:155, 1964.
13. Green, R. H., Balsamo, M. R., Giles, J. P., Krugman, S., and Mirick, G. S.: Studies on the natural history and prevention of rubella. Amer. J. Dis. Child., *110*:348, 1965.
14. Gregg, N. M.: Congenital cataract following German measles in the mother. Trans. Ophth. Soc. Aust., *3*:35, 1941.
15. Horstmann, D. M., Banatvala, J. E., Riordan, J. T., Payne, M. C., Whittemore, R., Opton, E. M., and Florey, C. V.: Maternal rubella and the rubella syndrome in infants. Amer. J. Dis. Child., *110*:408, 1965.
16. Jackson, A. D. M., and Fisch, L.: Deafness following maternal rubella. Lancet, *2*:1241, 1958.
17. Lamy, M., and Séror, M. E.: La rubeole de la femme enceinte. Arch. Ges. Virusforsch., *16*:377, 1965.
18. Lindquist, J. M., Plotkin, S. A., Shaw, L., Gilden, R. V., and Williams, M. L.: Congenital rubella syndrome as a systemic infection. Brit. Med., J., *2*:1401, 1965.
19. Lundström, R.: Rubella during pregnancy. Acta Paediat. (Uppsala), Suppl. No. 133, 1962.
20. Manson, M. M., Logan, W. P. D., and Loy, R. M.: Rubella and other virus infections in pregnancy. Reports on Publ. Hlth. & Med. Subj., H.M.S.O., London, No. 101, 1960.
21. Meyer, H. M., Jr., Parkman, P. D., and Panos, T. C.: Attenuated rubella virus. II. Production of an experimental live virus vaccine and clinical trial. New Eng. J. Med., *275*:575, 1966.
22. McDonald, J. C.: Gamma globulin for prevention of rubella in pregnancy. Brit. Med. J., *2*:416, 1963.
23. Naeye, R. L., and Blanc, W.: Pathogenesis of congenital rubella. J.A.M.A., *194*:1277, 1965.
24. Plotkin, S. A., Boué, A., and Boué, J. G.: The in vitro growth of rubella viruses in human embryo cells. Amer. J. Epidem., *81*:71, 1965.

25. Plotkin, S. A., Cornfeld, D., and Ingalls, T. H.: Studies on immunization with living rubella virus. Amer. J. Dis. Child., *110*:381, 1966.

26. Plotkin, S. A., Dudgeon, J. A., and Ramsay, A. M.: Laboratory studies on rubella and the rubella syndrome. Brit. Med. J., *2*:1296, 1963.

27. Rubella Symposium. Amer. J. Dis. Child., *110*:345-478, 1965.

28. Rudolph, A. J., Singleton, E. B., Rosenberg, H. S., Singer, D. B., and Phillips, C. A.: Osseous manifestations of the congenital rubella syndrome. Amer. J. Dis. Child., *110*:428, 1965.

29. Schiff, G. M., Sutherland, J. M., Light, I. L., and Bloom, J. E.: Studies on congenital rubella. Amer. J. Dis. Child., *110*:441, 1965.

30. Sever, J. L., Huebner, R. J., Castellano, G. A., Sarma, P. S., Fabivy, A., Schiff, G. M., and Cusumano, C. L.: Rubella complement fixation test. Science, *148*:385, 1965.

31. Sever, J. L., Nelson, K. B., and Gilkeson, M. R.: Rubella epidemic, 1964: Effect on 6,000 pregnancies. Amer. J. Dis. Child., *110*:395, 1965.

32. Sever, J. L., Schiff, G. M., Bell, J. A., Kapikian, A. Z., Huebner, R. J., and Traub, R. G.: Frequency of rubella antibody. Pediatrics, *35*:996, 1965.

33. Sheridan, M. D.: Final report of a prospective study of children whose mothers had rubella in early pregnancy. Brit. Med. J., *2*:536, 1964.

34. Soothill, J. F., Hayes, K., and Dudgeon, J. A.: The immunoglobulins in congenital rubella. Lancet, *1*:1385, 1966.

35. Stern, H.: Rubella virus complement fixation test. Nature, *208*:200, 1965.

36. Swan, C.: Rubella in pregnancy as an aetiological factor in congenital malformation, stillbirth, miscarriage and abortion. J. Obstet. Gynaec. Brit. Emp., *56*:341, 591, 1949.

37. Swan, C., Tostevin, A. L., Moore, B., Mayo, H., and Black, G. H. B.: Congenital defects in infants following infectious diseases in pregnancy. Med. J. Aust., *2*:201, 1943.

38. Weller, T. H., Alford, C. A., and Neva, F. A.: Retrospective diagnosis by serologic means of congenitally acquired rubella infections. New Eng. J. Med., *270*:1039, 1964.

38a. Proceedings of the 23rd Symposium on Microbiological Standardisation, Rubella Vaccines, London, November 1968. Karger, Basel, 1969.

38b. International Conference on Rubella Immunization. Amer. J. Dis. Child., *118*:155-410, 1969.

38c. Dudgeon, J. A.: Rubella vaccines. Brit. Med. Bull., *25*:159, 1969.

38d. Dudgeon, J. A.: Immunization against rubella. Nature, *223*:674, 1969.

CYTOMEGALOVIRUS

39. Fetterman, G. H.: New laboratory aid in clinical diagnosis of inclusion disease of infancy. Amer. J. Clin. Path., *22*:424, 1952.

40. Hanshaw, J. B.: Congenital and acquired cytomegaloviruses infection. Pediat. Clin. North Amer., *13*:279, 1966.

41. McCracken, G. H., Jr., and Shinefield, H. R.: Immunoglobulin concentrations in newborn infants with congenital cytomegalic inclusion disease. Pediatrics, *36*:933, 1965.

42. Rowe, W. P.: Adenovirus and salivary gland virus infection in children. *In*: Rose, H. M. (ed.): Viral infections of infancy and childhood. Hoe-

ber, Division of Harper & Row, New York, 1960.

43. Smith, M. G.: Propagation in tissue culture of a cytopathogenic virus from human salivary gland virus (SGV). Proc. Soc. Exp. Biol. Med., *92*:424, 1956.

44. Weller, T. H., and Hanshaw, J. B.: Virologic and clinical observations on cytomegalic inclusion disease. New Eng. J. Med., *266*:1233, 1962.

45. Weller, T. H., Macaulay, J. C., Craig, J. M., and Wirth, P.: Isolation of intranuclear inclusion producing agents from infants with illnesses resembling cytomegalic inclusion disease. Proc. Soc. Exp. Biol. Med., *94*:4, 1957.

OTHER VIRUSES

46. Albaugh, C. H.: Congenital anomalies following maternal rubella in early weeks of pregnancy. J.A.M.A., *129*:719, 1945.

47. Bradford-Hill, A., Doll, R., Galloway, T. M., and Hughes, J. P. W.: Virus diseases in pregnancy and congenital defects. Brit. J. Prev. Soc. Med., *12*:1, 1958.

48. Coffey, V. P., and Jessop, W. J. E.: Maternal influenza and congenital deformities. Lancet, *2*:935, 1959.

49. Cole, R. A., Danks, D. M., and Campbell, P. E.: Hepatitis virus in neonatal liver disease. Lancet, *1*:1368, 1965.

50. Fruhling, L., Korn, R., Lavillaureix, J., Surjus, A., and Foussereau, S.: La myo-endocardite chronique fibro-elastique du nouveau-né et du nourrisson. Ann. Anat. Path., *7*:227, 1962.

51. Gersony, W. M., Katz, S. L., and Nadas, A. S.: Endocardial fibroelastosis and the mumps virus. Pediatrics, *37*:430, 1966.

52. Green, D. M., Reid, S. M., and Rhaney, K.: Generalized vaccinia in the human fetus. Lancet, *1*:1296, 1966.

53. Kleinman, H., Ramras, D. G., Cooney, M. K., and Boyd, L.: Echo 9 virus infection and congenital abnormalities. A negative result. Pediatrics, *29*:261, 1962.

54. Landsman, J. B., Grist, N. R., and Ross, C. A. C.: Echo 9 virus infection and congenital malformations. Brit. J. Prev. Soc. Med., *18*:152, 1964.

55. Lynch, F. W.: Dermatologic conditions of the fetus with particular references to variola and vaccinia. Arch. Dermat. Syph., *26*:997, 1932.

56. MacArthur, P.: Congenital vaccinia and vaccinia gravidarum. Lancet, *2*:1104, 1952.

57. Manson, M. M., Logan, W. P. D., and Loy, R. M.: Rubella and other virus infections in pregnancy. Reports on Publ. Hlth. & Med. Subj., H.M.S.O., London, No. 101, 1960.

58. McDonald, A. M., and MacArthur, P.: Foetal vaccinia. Arch. Dis. Child., *28*:311, 1953.

59. Noren, G. B., Adams, P., and Anderson, R. C.: Positive skin reactivity to mumps virus antigen in endocardial fibroelastosis. J. Pediat., *62*:604, 1963.

60. Shone, J. D., Armas, S. M., Manning, J. A., and Keith, J. D.: Mumps antigen skin test in endocardial fibroelastosis. Pediatrics, *37*:423, 1966.

61. Walker, W. M., and McKeen, A. P.: Asian influenza in pregnancy relationship to foetal abnormalities. Obstet. Gynaec., *13*:394, 1959.

62. Ylinen, O., and Jarvienen, P. A.: Parotitis during pregnancy. Acta Obst. Gynaec. Scand., *32*:121, 1953.

NEONATAL VIRAL INFECTIONS

by R. Debré, A. Rossier, Le Tan Vinh, and D. Alagille

Elsewhere in this book different authors have traced the physiognomy of the newborn contaminated in utero by rubella, by cytomegalic inclusion disease, and by herpes, and, as concerns herpes especially, the picture produced in the newborn by infection contracted during birth or shortly after it. Here we shall review some of the viral infections contracted during the last days of pregnancy or the first few days after birth.

NEONATAL MEASLES

The contrast between measles and rubella is striking. It seems to arise from the greater pathogenicity of measles virus for the embryo. Whereas measles in the mother apparently kills the embryo, rubella virus can vegetate in the child-to-be until birth and after it. Rubella thus often causes the syndromes compatible with life that are described in the preceding section. In cases of prenatal contamination by measles virus, spontaneous abortions and stillbirths predominate. Malformations attributed to measles are rare, and their etiology is debatable.

For centuries physicians have studied the effects of measles on the infant when the mother is infected close to term, at the time of delivery, or immediately after it. In such cases it is often extremely difficult to determine exactly whether the contamination was prenatal, or occurred during birth or immediately after it.[1-5] In any event, the newborn present a characteristic disease during the first days of life. The eruption varies in intensity. On occasion, the rash is typical, dense, and of relatively long duration; it may be extremely sparse and fleeting. The greatly attenuated character of the rash in some cases makes probable the existence of congenital measles without exanthem. Koplik's spots are present as a rule, and sometimes the elements of the exanthem are even especially abundant. Since the rash may be fleeting and the oculonasal catarrh extremely mild, detection of Koplik's spots is particularly valuable. The rash may appear in both mother and child at the time of delivery. More often, the time of delivery coincides with that of development of the eruption in the mother. The child is born without manifestations of measles, which sometimes appear the day after birth or within the following days. As a rule, the rash appears during the first week of life or even the second week. Under certain conditions, when the incubation period is spontaneously long or has been prolonged by injection of gamma globulins at birth, the eruption develops during the third week, i.e., in the late postnatal period.

Congenital measles is serious. The prognosis is not, however, invariably fatal, as has been said: it varies with certain features of the disease process. For example, developed measles with the signs characteristic of the disease seems to be less serious than the other forms of congenital measles, in which death occurs without appearance of the signs typical of the infection.

Theopold[7] studied a case of measles in a newborn infant in whom the rash appeared 11 days after that in the mother. He emphasized the low titer of neutralizing antibodies in the infant, which decreased further even 18 weeks after measles, while the titer in the mother remained high.

The best means to protect the newborn against measles is to prevent measles in the pregnant woman. All pregnant women without a history of measles who have come into contact with the disease should be tested for neutralizing antibodies against measles. In absence of proof of these antibodies, the expectant mother should receive a preventive injection of gamma globulins in suitable dosage. Another precaution indicated to prevent or attenuate congenital measles is systematic injection of gamma globulin as soon after birth as possible in all infants born to mothers with measles when the baby has no sign of the disease at birth.

NEONATAL CHICKENPOX

Varicella may manifest itself in the newborn either at birth or some days later. In 1964 Pearson[10] reviewed 33 cases from the literature, with onset during the first ten days of life, of which ten were fatal. The early forms, in which the eruption is present at birth or appears before age five days, seem to be less serious.

Neonatal varicella results from infection of the mother before delivery or from contamination of the infant just after birth. In fatal cases the virus can be isolated not only from the skin but from other organs such as the lung and the liver. Ehrlich et al.[7a] isolated the virus at autopsy from the skin and the lung. Varicella had erupted in the mother two days before delivery; the disease had appeared in the infant on the sixth day of life and terminated fatally on the twelfth. In 1963 Garcia[9] described acidophilic intranuclear inclusions in the decidual cells of the placenta in a case of fetal varicella.

According to a report by Manson et al., chickenpox during pregnancy seems not to be responsible for congenital malformations (cf. bibliography to the preceding chapter).

NEONATAL POLIOMYELITIS

As mentioned earlier in this book, poliomyelitis during pregnancy may cause abortions or stillbirths, but not malformations, it seems.

Neonatal poliomyelitis is exceptional. Since the first case reported in 1941 by Aycock[11] a few other cases have been reported. In 1950 Mouton et al.[15] found 10 cases by review of the literature. In 1953 Rocco[16] discovered 50. Two years later Bates[12] reported 58 cases in infants less than one month old. Among them 15 became apparent during the first five days of life, 30 between age five days and fifteen days, and 13 in the second two weeks after birth. In 1962 Soulié[20] reported five more cases in the newborn of which two occurred in premature infants; in one of these cases, hospital contamination seemed probable. Smallpeice and Ounsted[19] reported a small epidemic of three cases in a hospital. Sims Roberts and Thomson[18] observed four cases, three of them fatal, that occurred in close succession in a small lying-in hospital; all were due to poliovirus type 3.

The infant born of a mother with acute poliomyelitis may seem normal and even show a rise in antibody level corresponding to inapparent poliomyelitis.[17] In other cases, however, marked hypotonia with flaccid paralysis of one or more limbs appears within a few days, as a rule before the fifth day of life. The course is not always fatal, but death may ensue.

The virus has been isolated from the meconium and the placenta, and in fatal cases from the child's nervous system. It is found in the mother's stools, a fact suggesting the possibility of contamination during birth. In the mother and child, antibody level rises significantly as regards the causative type of poliovirus. Histopathological study of the child's nervous system has revealed alterations typical of poliomyelitis.[13]

When antibodies are absent from the mother's blood, their presence in that of a newborn infant is proof that the child was contaminated after birth: five days is accepted as the minimum length of the incubation period, and antibodies appear from the eighth day of the disease.

NEONATAL HEPATITIS

Viral hepatitis in the newborn may be evidenced by hyperacute, acute, or subacute icterus. When other clinical signs are associated with the icterus and the case history reveals certain data in addition, they sometimes raise a suspicion as to the nature of the virus responsible. Only virological and serological studies, however, can ascertain the precise etiology. Stokes et al.[27] affirmed as far back as 1951 that viral hepatitis should be considered to be one etiological element in icterus of the newborn; decisive progress has, moreover, been made since then in knowledge of viral hepatitis, for example, that due to herpes, cytomegalic inclusion disease, and rubella. Nonetheless, data sufficiently precise to incriminate one particular virus rather than another are wanting in most cases.

As a rule the history of the pregnancy fails to contribute any exact element of information to the diagnosis. For the mother to have presented icterogenic hepatitis in the last months of pregnancy or previously is exceptional. Occasionally, several siblings also presented neonatal hepatitis; here a question arises as to the possible presence and permanence of viremia in the mother.

The importance of the problem is emphasized by the frequency of viral hepatitis in the newborn period. In a statistical study[21] of 347 cases of nonhemolytic, nonphysiological neonatal icterus, hepatitis accounted for 170 cases (48.99 per cent). The cases in which a virus was clearly determined, however, were rare: rubella hepatitis in three (0.86 per cent), cytomegalic inclusion disease in four (1.15 per cent), and herpetic hepatitis in two (0.58 per cent).

Three main forms of icterogenic viral hepatitis are distinguished in the newborn.

THE COMMON FORM

In the most usual form, icterus appears in a premature newborn infant or one of low birth weight (47.6 per cent); sex is often male (68.2 per cent). This icterus may appear at birth during, the first days of life, or after a free interval of a few weeks. Occasionally it succeeds "simple" neonatal icterus, and an icterus-free interval of variable duration occurs. Its intensity is inconstant. It is accompanied by dark, bile-pigment-containing urine and by pale stools decolorized to a variable degree. Frequently (but not always) the picture appears during regression of a digestive upset comprised of vomiting, diarrhea, and systemic disturbances (fever, dehydration, and weight loss). The liver is moderately increased in volume, as is the spleen as well, in many cases.

Diagnosis. BIOLOGICAL STUDY. Tests reveal direct- and indirect-reacting blood bilirubin, i.e., mixed hyperbilirubinemia. The humoral signs of biliary retention are clear: blood cholesterol and blood lipids may reach extremely high levels. The signs of hepatocellular involvement are present but are often moderate and short lived. Usually signs of inflammation are lacking. Results of flocculation tests are always negative in the neonatal period. Only increase in the levels of alpha-1-globulins and, especially, of alpha-2-globulins is usual; this increase is a feature of most neonatal infections. Hematological disturbances are frequent, in particular, normochromic anemia with secondary increase in circulating reticulocytes, and thrombocytopenia in some cases.

HISTOPATHOLOGICAL STUDY. Needle biopsy of the liver yields elements important in *histological diagnosis*. Schematically, they consist in: a mesenchymatous reaction almost always associating inflammatory infiltration with erythrogranulocytic infiltration of the porta hepatis; cellular impairment, including clarification of the cytoplasm, anisocytosis, and nuclear alterations that may go as far as pyknosis; intralobular and intracellular retention of pigment in the porta hepatis without obstruction of the biliary ducts by bile; and a more or less active process of regeneration sometimes represented by binucleated or multinucleated cellular formations.

The Course. The prognosis of the common form is variable. In roughly half the cases, icterus disappears in a few days or weeks. The stagnation of the infant's weight gives place to renewal of weight increase. Recovery can be obtained as is shown both by a healthy clinical appearance and a return to normal of the results of biological tests.

Complications. The most frequent complications arise from bacterial or pyogenic superinfection, with various localizations: pulmonary, urinary, osseous, and so forth. The vulnerability to infection of infants with such hepatic disease is particularly great. On the other hand, a subacute cirrhogenic course appears in only rare cases (3.5 per cent). The difficult problem posed by these common forms of icterogenic viral hepatitis is that of *sequelae.* Neurological sequelae occur and are feared especially because manifestations appear in the acute phase in 31 per cent of cases of such hepatitis in the newborn. Osseous sequelae are frequent: they take the form of osteomalacic rickets with multiple fractures. They can usually be averted by parenteral administration of vitamin D in high dosage and supplementary calcium intake. Dental sequelae, such as chlorodentia and hypoplasia of the enamel are, in contrast, relatively rare (2.3 per cent of cases).

FATAL HYPERACUTE FORMS

Rapid death is not exceptional in neonatal hepatitis. Death may be due to the intensity of the viral infectious syndrome, to dehydration, or to bacterial superinfections, particularly by *Escherichia coli.* Alarming signs may appear at the onset (in 2.88 per cent of cases). In such cases jaundice remains moderate, but diffuse hemorrhages and serious disturbances of the nervous system occur; death ensues in a few days.

The diagnosis is sometimes made only retrospectively on the basis of the *histological findings* in infants whose clinical history had not suggested viral hepatitis. In the hyperacute forms, histological examination reveals the disappearance by autolysis of almost all the parenchymatous cells and their replacement by granulation tissue and collagen fibers. The undestroyed islets of hepatic cells are isolated, without vascular or biliary connection. In such cases hematopoietic foci are always extremely numerous.

CHOLESTATIC FORMS

From the onset or later, icterogenic viral hepatitis in the newborn often (in 30 per cent of cases) assumes the characteristics of retention jaundice, evidenced by clay-colored stools over a long period. Despite the disappearance of digestive and systemic signs, the jaundice drags on, often after several variations, and takes on an aspect closely resembling that of genuine malformation of the bile ducts. Jaundice progressively deepens, and hepatomegaly develops little by little.

Diagnosis. The *biological signs* of bile retention are patent, whereas the initial signs of hepatocellular involvement fairly rapidly disappear. If the hepatitis at the onset is known directly or significant elements can be detected by questioning, diagnosis is relatively easy. At the onset, however, the digestive and infectious signs may have been slight or absent, with the result that the child is first examined when the picture is identical with that in malformation of the extrahepatic bile ducts. To resolve the frequent and difficult problem of differential diagnosis in such cases, the procedure usually followed is either *needle biopsy* for histological examination or *surgical exploration.*

The histological picture is important, since bile plugs in the biliary ducts of the porta hepatis are pathognomonic of true malformation of the extrahepatic bile ducts. However, not all sections of the bile ducts in the porta hepatis are obstructed by such plugs, and analytical study of the portal spaces, which is easy in autopsy specimens, is often difficult and unrewarding on small fragments of liver parenchyma obtained by aspiration biopsy. Moreover, the histological picture of "biliary angiomatosis" of the porta hepatis suggests extrahepatic blockade only in the advanced cases in which biliary cirrhosis is already marked.

The Course. In neonatal hepatitis, the course of cholestasis may be reversible within a few weeks; its regression is sometimes hastened by choleretic medication. In such cases, the stools recover their normal color, jaundice regresses gradually but finally disappears, and the child recovers. This favorable process occurs in most cases of treated neonatal cholestatic hepatitis. At present, surgical exploration is required in only a minority of cases. Some years ago the main purpose of such operations was diagnostic— to distinguish between cholestatic hepatitis of other causes and true malformations of the extrahepatic biliary ducts. Today surgical exploration presents a therapeutic interest inasmuch as the absence of extrahepatic biliary ducts in most cases may result from viral hepatitis. Congenital absence of these ducts due to true agenesis seems relatively rare. In most cases their absence seems to be secondary to inflammatory involvement of biliary ducts formed normally in the embryonic period. The inflammatory process apparently results in *biliary atresia during antenatal life or after birth.* This concept is supported by observation of elements of different types. One of them is the frequency of normal-colored stools during the first days or weeks of life in children in whom, at the time of surgical exploration, no biliary duct is permeable. Another is the frequency with which the histological picture strongly suggests hepatitis in infants in whom autopsy or surgical examination reveals an anomaly of the extrahepatic biliary ducts. Furthermore, repermeabilization of the extrahepatic ducts sometimes occurs paradoxically after they had been considered impermeable during surgical exploration. Moreover, some siblings present true neonatal hepatitis and others an anomaly of the extrahepatic biliary duct, or partial absence of intrahepatic biliary tracts.

The recent knowledge that neonatal viral hepatitis may provoke atresia of the intrahepatic and extrahepatic ducts is the reason for the present policy of never deferring surgical exploration in a young infant with retention jaundice. The operation presents a real therapeutic interest, since in certain cases the preoperative instrumental maneuvers result in recuperation of extrahepatic biliary ducts in the process of atresia but still in a phase in which the obstruction is not definitive and irreversible.

Doubtless certain congenital and familial cirrhoses[24] of which the etiology remains obscure are related to the group of cholestatic cirrhosis.

Treatment. The principal arm available at present is corticosteroid therapy in relatively high dosage (2 mg. per. kg. of body weight) administered for several weeks or even several months in the hope of arresting the inflammatory process and of averting fibrosis. Treatment with suitable antibiotics, management of coagulation disorders, use of sorbitol, arginine, and sodium dehydrocholate, and medical drainage by duodenal intubation or surgical drainage in cases of pseudomalformation are indicated in association with corticosteroid therapy.

NEONATAL COXSACKIE VIRUS INFECTIONS

Coxsackie virus infections can be serious in the newborn, whereas they are much more benign past early infancy.

COXSACKIE A VIRUSES

The role of Coxsackie A viruses is still not well established. A certain number of isolated case reports suggest that prenatal contamination is possible, perhaps with embryopathy or fetopathy. In a case reported by Makower et al.[47] a Coxsackie A virus was isolated from the meconium of a newborn who died of bronchopneumopathy at age four days and had multiple malformations. Gold et al.[37] incriminated Coxsackie A viruses as a cause of sudden death in nursling infants. These authors isolated Coxsackie A 4 or A 8 in 18 cases, but the age was not stated exactly ("less than 16 months old" was used universally in their study of sudden death in children). Coxsackie A viruses seem to produce sporadic cases of meningitis.[39]

Other disorders may be related to Coxsackie A viruses. Wright et al.[67] reported a case in which "herpetiform" lesions of the lingual mucosa had been noted as early as the third day of life along with intestinal and cardiac disturbances. Death occurred at age seven weeks; Coxsackie A 16 virus was isolated from the heart and the intestines. According to these authors "herpetiform" mucosal lesions may suggest this type of virus. Such lesions in association with a vesicular exanthem of the hands and feet constitute the hand, foot, and mouth syndrome, of which Cherry and Jahn[31] observed two cases at age six weeks. Marie et al.[48] related neonatal ulcerohemorrhagic enterocolitis to Coxsackie A 9 virus.

COXSACKIE B VIRUSES

The type B viruses take a sporadic or, especially, an epidemic form. South African investigators were the first to relate epidemics of neonatal myocarditis due to Coxsackie B viruses in maternity hospitals. Montgomery et al.[50] in 1955 reported three cases, one of them fatal, in which Coxsackie B 4 virus was isolated; Javett et al.[40] reported ten cases with one death that occurred in 1955. In the Netherlands the following year Van Creveld and de Jager[63] and Verlinde and Van Tongeren[65] published five fatal cases of myocarditis in the newborn with isolation of Coxsackie B 4 virus from the myocardium. An epidemic of pleurodynia and lymphocytic meningitis raged in the country during the same period, it should be noted.

After these early reports numerous others succeeded them. Suckling and Vogelpoel[60] in Capetown reported an epidemic in 1957 in a maternity hospital; nine cases occurred with four deaths; Coxsackie B 3 was isolated. In 1959 Vanek et al.[64] from Czechoslovakia reported five cases with one death, in which Coxsackie B 3 was also isolated. From Budapest, Lukacs and Romhanyi[46] reported in 1960 their observations, made during an epidemic of Bornholm disease, of an epidemic in a maternity hospital in which 17 newborn infants were involved, with one death. In this instance, in which Coxsackie B 3 was again isolated, the disease presented encephalomeningeal, rather than cardiac, symptoms. In Germany, Schenck et al.[56] reported in 1964 an epidemic striking seven newborn babies and one young infant grouped in a hospital service. Coxsackie B 3 was isolated. The disease took the form of meningoencephalitis with myocarditis; it was fatal in three of the newborn infants. In the United States, Brightman et al.[29] observed an epidemic in three units of a maternity hospital among three full-term newborns and 14 premature infants. The signs were of mild lymphocytic meningitis without myocarditis, and all the children recovered.

Sporadic cases were reported during the same period. These forms were severe and always fatal. Some cases were of encephalomyocarditis due to Coxsackie B 4; others took the form of a generalized infection.[33, 43, 55, 62] In France, Bach et al.[28] reported two cases of myocarditis due to Coxsackie B 3 in newborn twins, one of whom died on the ninth day and the other on the thirteenth. They made a study of the subject in general. Most cases, they found, occur in an epidemic situation. In the same region where an epidemic of "summer grippe," "pleurodynia," or "aseptic meningitis" is raging, the same virus is isolated from sick adults and from involved newborn children. For example, in the small epidemic in the newborn reported by Schenck et al.,[56] a member of the personnel in the same hospital had meningitis with pleurodynia. The infants are all very young. In their review, Bach et al. classified the 61 cases in which age was known as follows: age less than seven days, 38 cases; age 8 to 14 days, 13 cases; age 15 to 21 days, seven cases, and age more than 21 days, three cases.

The disease is particularly frequent in summer and autumn. The source of contamination is usually the mother, occasionally the father or a sibling, or a nurse. The adults in question have a nonlocalized febrile illness or on occasion febrile illness with muscular aching or a meningeal reaction;[46] they are sometimes healthy carriers with a high blood titer of antibodies.[28]

The Pathways of Contamination. The infant seems usually to be contaminated after birth; the incubation period is short—two to four days, and as a rule the onset in the newborn is at the end of four to six days. The transplacentary route is also possible. It has been proved in different cases. In the one reported by Delaney and Fukunaga,[33] a Coxsackie B 4 virus was isolated before delivery from the mother, who had meningoencephalitis. Makower et al.[47] isolated a Coxsackie A 4 from the first meconium. The same route was found by Kibrick[44] in two infants: the mother of one of them had a febrile respiratory disease a few days before delivery by cesarean section and the infant was immediately placed in isolation. The other infant, who was born to a mother who had presented pleurodynia a week before delivery, showed first symptoms a few hours after birth. The isolation by Brightman et al.[29] of a Coxsackie B 5 virus from the placenta of a premature infant who presented an inapparent infection proves the reality of contagion *in utero*. Prenatal contamination is, however, the exception. It was proved in only five of the 54 cases reviewed by Katz and Kilbrick.[41]

Clinical Features. Coxsackie virus infections occur in the newborn under two quite different epidemiological circumstances: in sporadic forms, which are invariably fatal; and in epidemic forms, in which recovery occurs in more than half the cases. The commonest clinical picture is that of meningoencephalo-myocarditis, but other manifestations are observed.

The onset is usually between the third and the eighth day of life. The first disturbances are characterized by feeding difficulties and/or a slight spike of fever, or occasionally coryza, or a beginning of diarrhea. The case reported by McLean et al.,[49] in which the child was born with a papular rash (that lasted four days), represents a rarity.

In most cases this initial period is followed by an interval of apparent recovery lasting two to seven days. The second phase attracts more notice, for it is characterized by marked deterioration of general physical condition, vomiting, refusal to drink, and inconstant fever; sometimes eruption (fleeting rash or purpura) occurs. Anemia may be noted, occasionally with leukocytosis and polynucleosis.[28] Three types of disorder may occur, alone or in association: signs of cardiac, nervous system, and hepatic involvement.

CARDIAC SIGNS. Almost all cases of neonatal myocarditis due to Coxsackie viruses are caused by type B (with the exception of a case reported by Hosier and Newton,[39] who found a Coxsackie A 9 virus in the feces of a newborn infant with fatal myocarditis).

The cardiac involvement is evidenced by respiratory distress, with cyanosis, pallor, dyspnea, and inspiratory retraction, by severe tachycardia sometimes exceeding 200 beats per minute, by muffled heart sounds, and by increase in heart volume ascertained in x-ray films, by edema of the lower extremities, and by hepatomegaly. Disturbances of the electrocardiogram may occur; they consist in low voltage, alteration of the ST segment, flattening of the T waves, and perturbed rhythm. None of the different signs is specific, however, and their variability has been emphasized.[61]

Electrocardiographic signs usually appear some 24 hours later than the clinical signs or, occasionally, even later. Sometimes, however, they exist in absence of any clinical signs of the myocarditis, or the electrocardiogram may be normal in the presence of clinically evident signs of myocarditis. The electrocardiographic signs regress slowly and may persist several weeks, or even months.

The gravity of the cardiac forms arises from the complete unpredictability of their course. Numerous authors have observed sudden unexpected collapse resulting in death within a few hours, as in the second case reported by Bach et al., or even sudden unexpected death.[28]

NEUROLOGICAL SIGNS. Although frequent, nervous system signs are not always in the foreground of the clinical picture. They may be limited to somnolence, slight convulsive movements, and loss of the earliest reflexes. In other instances, the neurological signs are predominant and distinguish a meningoencephalitic form. In such cases the fever is accompanied by meningeal signs, tension of the fontanel, disturbances in tonus, and ocular signs (strabismus, nystagmus). The cerebrospinal fluid is usually altered and shows lymphocytic pleocytosis and an increased albumin level. The electroencephalogram also presents the changes typically associated with meningoencephalitis.[28]

HEPATIC SIGNS. Icterus is often reported. During the first days, it is not always easy to distinguish from physiological jaundice. When it is associated with an enlarged hard liver or with splenomegaly in the midst of a picture of a severe illness, it suggests neonatal hepatitis. It may predominate and be associated with edema, a hemorrhagic syndrome, coagulation disorders, and severe alteration of hepatic functions shown by considerable fall in level of esterified cholesterol and a considerable increase in that of transaminases.[28, 44]

On the sixth day the newborn infant observed by Rawls et al.[54] presented somnolence with jaundice, purpura, and an enlarged liver, and died on the tenth day. The lesions consisted in necrosis of the liver without lesions of the encephalon or the myocardium. The cerebrospinal fluid and the tissues sampled (liver, kidney, and spleen) permitted isolation of Coxsackie A 23 (now classified as Echo 9).

Diarrhea is often mentioned in Coxsackie B infections; it is occasionally intense and prolonged. Koch[45] asserted the presence of pancreatitis on the basis of a high level of amylasuria. The blood count shows no characteristic feature. Sussman et al.[62] reported a leukocytosis with 21,900 white cells of which 72 per cent were polymorphonuclear. Coxsackie virus infection might account for a certain number of cases of sudden death in early infancy (cf. Chapter 59).

The Course. The disease is often rapidly fatal in two to four days, particularly in the sporadic cases. Death is due to aggravation of the encephalitic signs and to hyperthermia, to progressive heart failure, or, more often, to sudden collapse or irreversible apnea. In other cases the course is protracted and may end in recovery. Most of the forms with recovery, however, have been detected during epidemics in which the coincidence of fatal forms permitted their identification. A fairly recent review by Patois[53] reported 38 cases of recovery in 65 epidemic cases, whereas 34 sporadic cases were all fatal except one.

Pathology. Autopsy shows that the disease is generalized, with plurivisceral involvement in which the myocardial alterations predominate.

MYOCARDIAL LESIONS. The cardiac muscle is pale. Petechiae and foci of necrosis under the epicardium are frequent findings.

Microscopic examination shows that the lesions, which are occasionally diffuse, are often localized in the left ventricle. They consist in zones of necrosis with fragmentation of the fibers and loss of the double striation. The associated lesions are infiltration of mononuclear cells localized near the blood vessels, and interfascicular edema in limited patches. Endocardial and pericardial participation is of variable degree and occurs irregularly.

LESIONS OF THE CENTRAL NERVOUS SYSTEM. Meningeal congestion, meningeal petechiae,[51] and thickening of the arachnoid in the fissure of Sylvius[63] are found.

Microscopic examination reveals mononuclear and lymphocytic infiltrates especially in the spinal cord and brain stem; perivascular lesions in the cortex and bulb; inflammatory lesions of the brain, especially of the mesencephalon, with particular involvement of the olivary nuclei and the basilar region. Degeneration of the ganglionic cells of the anterior horn of the spinal cord has also been described.[34] This degeneration, however, also selectively involves the perivascular cells of the white matter, a fact differentiating the lesions from those of poliomyelitis.

HEPATIC LESIONS. Fatty degeneration, necrotic and inflammatory foci, and even necrosis extending to almost the entire parenchyma have been described.[28, 62]

OTHER LESIONS. Mononuclear infiltration of the small intestine, inflammatory reactions of the lung or the kidney, and necrotic foci have been reported in a few cases. Spleen, bone marrow, lymph nodes, thymus, and muscles may be the seat of inflammatory or necrotic foci. The lungs may show hemorrhagic foci and, occasionally, lesions of interstitial pneumonia.

Virology. ISOLATION OF COXSACKIE VIRUSES. The virus may be isolated from pharyngeal swabs or, especially, stool specimens, from cerebrospinal fluid, or from the blood.

In newborn infants, Coxsackie A viruses have not often been incriminated. Aside from the case of myocarditis due to Coxsackie A 9 reported by Hosier and Newton,[39] Marie et al.[48] reported one case and Wright et al.[67] another of infection due to Coxsackie A viruses (type 9 and type 16), and it should be noted that the symptoms were exclusively intestinal in the first and predominantly intestinal in the second.

Nearly always Coxsackie B 3, B 4, and B 5 are isolated in the epidemic forms and types B 2, B 3, B 4, and B 5 in the sporadic forms.

In fatal cases, numerous investigators have isolated the virus from the myocardium, brain, and other organs: in particular, the kidney, spleen, lymph nodes, lungs, pancreas, and intestines. The affinity of Coxsackie B viruses for the myocardium is remarkable. It is almost always isolated from the myocardium in fatal cases, and its titer may be as much as 1000 times higher than in the other organs.[30]

This fact leads to consideration of the possible relationship between Coxsackie viruses and subendocardial fibroelastosis. Schneegans et al.[57] studied 20 cases of fibroelastosis and, from autopsy specimens, isolated a Coxsackie virus 14 times, in 13 of them a Coxsackie B 3 virus. They remarked that the frequency of fibroelastosis increased during Coxsackie virus epidemics, and histological examination revealed inflammatory signs evidencing a process of interstitial myocarditis. They concluded that fibroelastosis could occur if myocardial inflammation was sufficiently prolonged. When the viral infection occurs after formation of the embryonic heart, the late action of maternal antibodies might permit a protracted inflammatory reaction of the myocardium leading to fibroelastosis. Nevertheless, the absence of serological control reactions makes these results difficult to interpret.

Other authors—Noren et al.[52] in 1963, Sellers et al.[58] in 1964, Vosburgh et al.[66] in 1965, and Shone et al.[59] in 1966—found that children with fibroelastosis had a positive skin reaction to a solution of mumps antigen* injected intradermally, whereas the reaction was negative in the control groups. According to Shone et al., however, the patients show no rise in the corresponding serum antibodies. Gersony, Katz, and Nadas[36] undertook similar research and found no correlation between fibroelastosis and these skin tests. No certain conclusion can be drawn at present.

Neutralizing Antibodies. Most authors have studied the neutralizing antibodies, which appear rapidly and have already reached their peak level by the fifteenth day of the disease. Lukacs and Romhanyi[46] found them in seven of 15 newborn infants with Coxsackie infection and in ten of 12 mothers. The presence of these antibodies and the concomitant rise of titer in the mothers constitute an essential proof of the congenital nature of the infection.[44] Their increase in the newborn indicates that not only transmitted antibodies but also antibodies elaborated by the child himself are involved, as was observed by

Koch et al.[45] in four newborn babies with lymphocytic meningitis due to Coxsackie B 5. Neutralizing antibodies may be absent in such cases, however. The possible hypotheses are that either the maternal antibodies were not transmitted, or the infant was unable to produce them. Owing to the rapidity of death in numerous cases, study of this question has usually been impossible.

Treatment. Therapy is symptomatic. Use of corticosteroids can be considered. Although they may have an unfavorable effect under experimental conditions, in numerous instances they seem to have benefited patients. Antibiotics should be associated. Most especially, intensive treatment should be undertaken with digitalin in high dosage over a long period. Because of these conditions, Digilanid or digoxin is often preferred to digitalin.

Attentive prophylaxis should be instituted in maternity hospitals or departments when an epidemic of pleurodynia or other infection due to Coxsackie viruses is suspected. Every febrile parturient recently exposed to an infection, and her child, as well, should be rigorously isolated. Every possible measure should be undertaken to detect larvate forms in the medical and nursing staff. In certain instances, it is indispensable to close a maternity hospital or department infected by a Coxsackie virus.

VIRAL INFECTIONS OF THE RESPIRATORY TRACT IN THE NEONATAL PERIOD

Although numerous studies have been published as regards nurslings and young children, they unfortunately contain little precise information concerning the neonatal period.

Etiology and Epidemiology

Cases are rarely isolated; they usually appear as small epidemics in lying-in hospitals or centers for premature infants. One of the first authors to touch on this problem was Adams[68] in 1948. He mentioned epidemics of "common" respiratory infections in young children and, in a certain number of cases, discovered cells with cytoplasmic inclusions in pharyngeal specimens. He suspected, although without the proof, the role of a virus in these "primary pneumonias." The question remained in suspense until 1953, when Sano

---

*Prepared from the allantoic fluid of embryonated hens' eggs.

et al.[93, 94] reported the same facts in an epidemic in Sendai, Japan, involving 17 newborn infants. The authors were enabled to prove the viral origin of this "inclusion body pneumonia" by Kuroya et al.,[90] who isolated a virus similar to that of influenza but with certain distinguishing characteristics. The virus was later denominated parainfluenza 1, type Sendai, in the myxovirus group. Other Japanese investigators, Matsuyama et al.[91] described in 1957 an epidemic of fatal pneumopathies due to the same virus in three young nursling infants. Other parainfluenza type 1 epidemics were described by Chanock et al.[77] in 1959, by Beem et al.[71] in 1962, and by other authors. Parainfluenza 3 was isolated in other epidemics, especially in premature infants.[72] More rarely influenza viruses A and B were noted in the very young child (Chanock et al.,[77, 78] Beem et al.,[71] and Gaburro[86]).

Respiratory syncytial virus (RSV) was isolated by Chanock et al.[79] in 1957 in two cases of acute pneumopathy in children. This virus was identified with the chimpanzee coryza agent (CCA), a virus discovered by Morris (1956). It has been the object of numerous publications. It seems to be responsible for the majority of respiratory infections in early infancy and has been found in epidemics of capillary bronchitis or bronchoalveolitis by Chanock et al.,[77] Chany et al.,[82] Beem et al.,[71] Breton et al.,[74] Sandiford and Spencer,[92] Hilleman,[88] Gernez-Rieux et al.,[87] Adams et al.,[69] Berkovich,[72] Fandre et al.,[85] and Sterner et al.[96] The reports by the last two groups of investigators concerned premature infants.

Additional etiological agents were discovered in isolated cases or in epidemics of respiratory infections (nasopharyngeal or pulmonary). Adenoviruses were incriminated by Hilleman,[88] Chany,[80] and Beem et al.[71] Echo viruses were found by Butterfield et al.,[75] and Berkovich.[72] Coxsackie B viruses were isolated in respiratory infections in children by Seringe et al.,[95] and Gaburro.[86] Infectious mononucleosis was also indicated by Gaburro.[86]

Positive serological reactions in the newborn are particularly valuable in diagnosis because certain studies have emphasized the rarity of natural antibodies acquired during the first weeks of life. Hornsleth and Volkert,[89] for instance, showed the fact in regard to respiratory syncytial virus. To be demonstrative, a rise in antibody level must be detected in serum samples taken within a two-week interval, as usual. This rise, however, is inversely proportionate to age. In an epidemic of respiratory syncytial virus infections (Randall strain) Beem et al.[70] detected an increase in four of 11 nursling infants, whereas it occurred in ten of 17 older children.

In an epidemic studied by Berkovich[72] in 14 premature children aged 11 to 184 days, 12 nurslings elaborated neutralizing and complement-fixing antibodies for respiratory syncytial virus, and in eight of them the level quadrupled at least, during the illness. In the nurslings involved, the author found a rash associated with a rise of $1/4$ to $1/3$ in antibodies against measles. Questions hence arise concerning the possible role of measles in certain pneumopathies in infancy and the association of measles with another viral disease.

NEONATAL DIARRHEA AND VIRAL INFECTIONS

In various epidemics, the role of viral infections in intestinal disorders of the newborn has been suspected. In most instances this role remained open to question, since no decisive proof was made of a pathogenic relationship between the disorder and the viruses isolated (Echo, Coxsackie, and adenovirus of different types). We teach that a normal bacterial flora exists from the second or third day of life, but that no "viral flora" is normally present in the first days or weeks of infancy. Intestinal viruses in the newborn should be considered pathological, as Sabin et al.[112] demonstrated on isolation of an Echo virus in rectal samples from seven of 58 infants born at home. Eichenwald and Kotsevalov[99] studied 4000 young nursling infants under nursery conditions by systematic . stool sampling, with regularly negative results.

It is evident, however, that the presence of a virus in the stools does not prove its pathogenic role and that neutralizing antibodies can be transmitted by the mother. In general, maternal antibodies protect the newborn child. When they are insufficiently protective, a secondary rise in their level is evidence of acquired infection. Such a rise during epidemics due to Echo 18 in 12 premature infants and older nurslings was found by Eichenwald et al.,[98] and in epidemics of neonatal diarrhea associated with Echo 9, adenoviruses, and Coxsackie viruses.

TREATMENT

A proper technique of rehydration and of reanimation should be applied immediately in viral diarrhea of the newborn. Cardiorespiratory analeptics and corticosteroid therapy are indicated in some cases, in addition. The essential in neonatal viral infections is their prophylaxis. In hospital maternity departments and lying-in hospitals, centers for premature children, and nurseries for young nursling infants, preventive measures should be rigorously applied. They consist in close check of the adults for viral infections, measures of eviction, and closure of contaminated services.

BIBLIOGRAPHY

Neonatal Measles

1. Debré, R., et al.: La rougeole congénitale. Le nourrisson, *13*:249, 1925.
2. Debré, R., and Joannon, P.: La rougeole. Epidémiologie. Immunologie. Prophylaxie. Préface du Pr. Léon Bernard. Paris, Masson et Cie, 1926.
3. Debré, R.: Some remarks to the problem of inborn measles. Česk. Pediat., *22*:391-395, 1967.
4. Dyer, J.: Measles complicating pregnancy. Southern Med. J., *33*:601, 1940.
5. Kugel, R. B.: Measles in a newborn premature infant. Amer. J. Dis. Child., *93*:306, 1957.
6. Smith, J.: Delivery: The mother suffering from prodromata of measles; the disease developed in both mother and child on the succeeding day. Amer. J. Med. Sci., *59*:282, 1870.
7. Theopold, W.: Maserninfektion bei einem Neugeborenen. Arch. Kinderheilk., *166*:174-177, 1962.

Neonatal Chickenpox

7a. Ehrlich, R. M., et al.: Neonatal varicella. A case report with isolation of the virus. J. Pediat., *53*:139, 1958.
8. Freud, P.: Congenital varicella. A.M.A. J. Dis. Child., *96*:730, 1958.
9. Garcia, A. G. P.: Fetal infection in chickenpox and alastrim, with histopathologic study of the placenta. Pediatrics, *32*:895, 1963.
10. Pearson, H. E.: Parturition varicella-zoster. Obstet. Gynec., *23*:21, 1964.

Neonatal Poliomyelitis

11. Aycock, W. L.: The frequency of poliomyelitis in pregnancy. New Eng. J. Med., *225*:405, 1941.
12. Bates, T.: Poliomyelitis in pregnancy, fetus and and newborn. Amer. J. Dis. Child., *90*:189-195, 1955.
13. Elliott, G. B., and MacAllister, J. E.: Fetal poliomyelitis. Amer. J. Obstet. Gynec., *72*:896, 1956.
14. Lycke, E., and Nilsson, L. R.: Poliomyelitis in a newborn due to intrauterine infection. Acta Paediat., *51*:661, 1962.
15. Mouton, C. M., Smillie, J. G., and Bower, A. G.: Report of ten cases of poliomyelitis in infants under six months of age. J. Pediat., *36*:482, 1950.

16. Rocco, L.: Considerazioni so un caso di poliomielite in un immaturo de due mesi. Lattante, *24*:7, 1953.
17. Shelokov, A., and Habel, K.: Subclinical poliomyelitis in a newborn infant due to intrauterine infection. J.A.M.A., *160*:465-466, 1956.
18. Sims Roberts, J. T. C., and Thomson, D.: Poliomyelitis in infancy, especially in the neonatal period. Monthly Bull. Minist. Health, *12*:152-163, 1953.
19. Smallpeice, V., and Ounsted, C.: Cerebral poliomyelitis in early infancy. J. Neurol. Neurosurg. Psychiat., *15*:13, 1952.
20. Soulié, J. E. C. M.: A propos de cinq observations de poliomyélite chez des enfants nouveau-nés. Paris, Dactylographie médicale, 1962. Thèse, Paris, Faculté de Médecine, 1962, No. 166.

Neonatal Hepatitis

21. Alagille, D.: Les ictères du nouveau-né. Päd. Fortbild., *15*:43-56, 1965.
22. Aterman, K.: Neonatal hepatitis and its relation to viral hepatitis of mother. Amer. J. Dis. Child., *105*:395-416, 1963.
23. Chaptal, J., et al.: Les ictères par hépatite infectieuse du nouveau-né et du nourrisson. Rapport au 17ème Congrès de l' Association des Pédiatres de Langue Française, 1959, Vol. 3, p. 111.
24. Debré, R., and Lamy, M.: La cirrhose hépatique congénitale et familiale. Ann. Med., *47*:48-87, 1946.
25. Dible, J. H., et al.: Foetal and neo-natal hepatitis and its sequelae. J. Path. Bact., *67*:195, 1954.
26. Gellis, S., et al.: Prolonged obstructive jaundice in infancy. IV. Neo-natal hepatitis. Amer. J. Dis. Child., *88*:285, 1954.
27. Stokes, J., Jr., Wolman, I. J., Blanchard, M. C., and Farquhar, J. D.: Viral hepatitis in the newborn: clinical features, epidemiology and pathology. Amer. J. Dis. Child., *82*:213-216, 1951.

Neonatal Coxsackie Virus Infections

28. Bach, C., Seringe, P., and Bocquet, L.: L'infection à virus Coxsackie B du nouveau-né. I. Etude clinique et anatomique. Sem. Hôp. Paris, *37*:2883-2892, 1961.
29. Brightman, V., Scott, T., Westphal, M., and Boggs, T.: An outbreak of Coxsackie B 5 virus infection in a newborn nursery. J. Pediat., *69*:179-192, 1966.
30. Carré, M., Virat, J., and Maurin, J.: L'infection à virus Coxsackie B du nouveau-né. A propos de deux cas familiaux. II. Etude virologique. Sem. Hôp. Paris, *37*:2892-2895, 1961.
31. Cherry, J., and Jahn, C.: Hand, foot and mouth syndrome. Pediatrics, *37*:637-643, 1966.
32. Couvreur, J.: Les infections à virus Coxsackie. Arch. Ges. Virusforsch., *13*:104-127, 1963.
33. Delaney, T. B., and Fukunaga, F.: Myocarditis in a newborn infant with encephalomeningitis due to Coxsackie virus group B, type 4. New Eng. J. Med., *259*:234-236, 1958.
34. Fechner, R., Smith, M., and Middelkamp, J.: Coxsackie B virus infection of the new-born. Amer. J. Path., *42*:493, 1963.
35. Gear, J.: Coxsackie virus infections of the newborn. Progr. Med. Virol., *7*:106, 1958.

36. Gersony, W., Katz, S., Nadas, A.: Endocardial fibroelastosis and the mumps virus. Pediatrics, *37*:430-434, 1966.

37. Gold, E., Carver, D., et al.: Viral infection: possible cause of sudden unexpected death in infants. New Eng. J. Med., *264*:53-60, 1961.

38. Grenier, B.: Les myocardites aiguës primitives de l'enfant et les virus Coxsackie. Paris, Masson et Cie, 1958.

39. Hosier, D., and Newton, W.: Serious Coxsackie infection in infants and children. A.M.A. J. Dis. Child., *96*:251-267, 1958.

40. Javett, S., Heymann, S., et al.: Myocarditis in the newborn infant. J. Pediat., *48*:1, 1956.

41. Katz, S. L., and Kibrick, S.: Nonbacterial infections of the newborn. Pediat. Clin. N. Amer., *8*:493, 1961.

42. Kibrick, S., and Benirschke, K.: Acute aseptic myocarditis and meningo-encephalitis in the newborn child infected with Coxsackie virus group B type 3. New Eng. J. Med., *255*:883, 1965.

43. Kibrick, S., and Benirschke, K.: Severe generalized disease in the newborn due to Coxsackie virus group B. A.M.A. J. Dis. Child., *96*:498, 1958; Pediatrics, *22*:857, 1958.

44. Kibrick, S.: The role of Coxsackie and ECHO viruses in human disease. Med. Clin. N. Amer., *43*:1291-1308, 1959.

45. Koch, F., Enders-Ruckle, G., and Wokittel, E.: Coxsackie B 5 infektionen mit signifikanter Antikörperentwicklung bei Neugeborenen. Arch. Kinderheilk, *165*:245-258, 1965.

46. Lukacs, V., and Romhanyi, J.: Über eine meningoencephalo-myocarditis Epidemie bei Neugeborenen während der Epidemic von Bornholmischer Krankheit in Ungarn in Yare 1958. Ann. Paediat. (Basel), *194*:89, 1960.

47. Makower, H., et al.: On transplacental infection with Coxsackie virus. Texas Rep. Biol. Med., *16*:346-354, 1958.

48. Marie, J., et al.: Entérocolite ulcéro-hémorragique du nouveau-né avec présence dans l'intestin du virus Coxsackie A 9. Sem. Hôp. Paris, *40*:275-282, 1964.

49. McLean, D., et al.: Coxsackie B 5 virus as a cause of neonatal encephalitis and myocarditis. Canad. Med. Assoc. J., *85*:1046, 1961.

50. Montgomery, J., Gear, J., Prinsloo, F., Kahn, M., and Kirsch, Z.: Myocarditis of the newborn. S. Afr. Med. J., *29*:608-612, 1955.

51. Moossy, J., and Geer, J.: Encephalomyelitis, myocarditis and adrenal cortical necrosis in Coxsackie B3 virus infection. Distribution of the central nervous system lesions. A.M.A. Arch. Path., *70*:614-622, 1960.

52. Noren, G., Adams, P., and Anderson, R.: Positive skin reactivity to mumps virus antigen in endocardial fibroelastosis. J. Pediat., *62*:604-606, 1963.

53. Patois, B.: Considérations sur la myocardite à coxsackie, à propos de 3 observations. Thèse, Paris, 1965, No. 222

54. Rawls, W., Shorter, R., and Herrmann, E.: Fatal neonatal illness associated with ECHO 9 (Coxsackie A 23) virus. Pediatrics, *33*:278-280, 1964.

55. Schaeffer, R., Rohrs, K., and Vivell, O.: Encephalomyokarditis Syndrom beim Neugeborenen infolge Infektion mit Coxsackie-virus vom Typ B 4. Münch. Med. Wschr., *101*:740-744, 1959.

56. Schenck, W., Vivell, O., et al.: Eine Epidemie durch Coxsackie virus Typ B 5 auf einer Neugeborenen- und Säuglingssation. Arch. Kinderheilk, *170*:41, 1964.

57. Schneegans, E., Frühling, L., et al.: Etude anatomo-clinique et étiologique de 20 cas de myoendocardite chronique fibro-élastique de nourrisson. Arch. Franç. Pédiat., *20*:645, 1963.

58. Sellers, F. J., Keith, J. D., and Manning, J. A.: The diagnosis of primary endocardial fibroelastosis. Circulation, *29*:49, 1964.

59. Shone, J., Munoz Armas, S., Manning, J., and Keith, J.: The mumps antigen skin test in endocardial fibroelastosis. Pediatrics, *37*:423-429, 1966.

60. Suckling, P., and Vogelpoel, L.: Coxsackie myocarditis of the newborn. Med. Proc. (Johannesb.), *4*:372-389, 1958.

61. Surjus, A.: Les maladies à virus Coxsackie en Alsace. Etude générale, fréquence et gravité au cours des années 1956 à 1961. Thèse, Strasbourg, 1962, No. 20.

62. Sussman, M., Strauss, L., and Hodes, H.: Fatal Coxsackie group B virus infection in the newborn. A.M.A. J. Dis. Child., *97*:483, 1959.

63. Van Creveld, S., and de Jager, H.: Myocarditis in newborns caused by Coxsackie virus. Clinical and pathological data. Ann. Paediat. (Basel), *187*:100; 1956.

64. Vanek, J., Lukes, J., Potuznik, V., Polednikova, I., and Vilim, N.: Myocarditis and encephalitis in newborn infants, caused by Coxsackie B virus. J. Hyg. Epidem. (Praha), *3*:283, 1959.

65. Verlinde, J., and Van Tongeren, M.: Myocarditis in newborns due to Group B Coxsackie virus. Ann. paediat. (Basel), *187*:113, 1956.

66. Vosburgh, J., Diehl, A., Liu, C., Lauer, R., and Fabiyi, A.: Relationship of mumps to endocardial fibroelastosis. Amer. J. Dis. Child., *109*:69, 1965.

67. Wright, H., et al.: Fatal infection in an infant associated with Coxsackie virus group A, type 16. New. Eng. J. Med., *268*:1041-1044, 1963.

VIRAL INFECTIONS OF THE RESPIRATORY TRACT IN THE NEONATAL PERIOD

68. Adams, J.: Common respiratory tract infections in childhood. J. Pediat., *33*:499, 1948.

69. Adams, M. O., et al.: R. S. virus infections in the North West of England. Arch. Ges. Virusforsch., *13*:268-271, 1963.

70. Beem, M., Wright, F., et al.: Association of the chimpanzee coryza agent with acute respiratory disease in children. New Eng. J. Med., *263*:523-530, 1960.

71. Beem, M., Wright, F., et al.: Observations on the etiology of acute bronchiolitis in infants. J. Pediat. *61*:864-869, 1962.

72. Berkovich, S.: Acute respiratory illness in the premature nursery associated with respiratory syncytial virus infections. Pediatrics, *34*:753-760, 1964.

73. Breton, A., Gaudier, B., Ponte, C., and Samaille, J.: Les bronchopneumopathies à virus de l'enfant. Etude épidémiologique, clinique et paraclinique. Critique des méthodes de diagnostic. In:18ème Congrès Association des Pédiatres de Langue Française, Genève, 1961, pp. 64-169.

74. Breton, A., Samaille, J., Gaudier, B., Lefebvre, G.,

and Ponte, C.: Isolement de virus syncytial au cours de manifestations respiratoires bénignes épidémiques chez des prématurés. Arch. Franç. Pédiat., *18*:459-467, 1961.

75. Butterfield, J., et al.: Cystic emphysema in premature infants. A report of an outbreak with the isolation of type 19 ECHO virus in one case. New Eng. J. Med., *268*:18-21, 1963.

76. Chanock, R., et al.: Newly recognized myxoviruses from children with respiratory disease. New Eng. J. Med., *258*:207-213, 1958.

77. Chanock, R., et al.: Association of hemadsorption viruses with respiratory illness in childhood. J.A.M.A., *169*:548-553, 1959.

78. Chanock, R., et al.: Association of hemadsorption viruses (parainfluenza) and other viruses in children with and without respiratory disease. Pediatrics, *26*:243, 1960.

79. Chanock, R., et al.: Respiratory syncytial virus. J.A.M.A., *176*:647-653, 1961.

80. Chany, C.: Infections à adénovirus chez l'enfant. Arch. Ges. Virusforsch., *13*:294-301, 1963.

81. Chany, C., Robbe-Fossat, F., and Couvreur, J.: Enquête sérologique sur le rôle épidémiologique du myxovirus para-influenzae type 3, Souche EA 102. Bull. Acad. Nat. Méd. (Paris), *143*:106-110, 1959.

82. Chany, C., Daniel, P., Robbe-Fossat, F., Vialatte, J., Lépine, P., and Lelong, M.: Isolement et étude d'un virus syncytial non identifié associé à des affections respiratoires aiguës du nourrisson. Ann. Inst. Pasteur (Paris), *95*:721-731, 1958.

83. Chany, C., Lépine, P., Lelong, M., Le Tan Vinh, and Virat, J.: Severe and fatal pneumonia in infants and young children associated with adenovirus infections. Amer. J. Hyg., *67*:367-378, 1958.

84. Couvreur, J., Cook, C., Chany, C., Gerbeaux, J.: Une épidémie d'exanthème à virus ECHO 16. Arch. Ges. Virusforsch., *13*:215-232, 1963.

85. Fandre, M., Dropsy, G., Coffin, R., et al.: Epidémie de bronchiolite aiguë du nourrisson. Isolement d'un virus R.S. Arch. Franç. Pédiat., *21*:1189-1195, 1964.

86. Gaburro, D.: Le pneumopatie da virus (e da rickettsie) nell'immaturo. Minerva Pediat., *8*:345-351, 1956.

87. Gernez-Rieux, C., Breton, A., et al.: Isolement du virus R. S. (C.C.A. de Morris) au cours d'une épidémie de manifestations respiratoires bénignes chez des prématurés. Arch. Ges. Virusforsch., *13*:265-267, 1963.

88. Hilleman, M.: Respiratory syncytial virus. Amer. Rev. Resp. Dis., *88*:181-189, 1963.

89. Hornsleth, A., and Volkert, M.: The incidence of complement-fixing antibodies to the respiratory syncytial virus (0-19 years). Acta Path. Microbiol. Scand., *62*:421-431, 1964.

90. Kuroya, M., Ishida, N., and Shiratori, T.: Newborn virus pneumonitis (type Sendai). Isolation of a new virus with hemangglutinin activity. Yokohama Med. Bull., *4*:217-233, 1953.

91. Matsuyama, T., Marak, et al.: The isolation of a virus from an epidemic of fatal suckling pneumonitis. Gunma. J. Med. Sci., *6*:1, 1957.

92. Sandiford, B., and Spencer, B.: Respiratory syncytial virus in epidemic bronchiolitis. Brit. Med. J., *309*:881-882, 1962.

93. Sano, T., Niitsu, I., and Nakagawa, I.: Newborn virus pneumonitis, type Sendai. Yokohama Med. Bull., *4*:199-216, 1953.

94. Sano, T., Niitsu, I., Nakagawa, I., and Ando, T.: Newborn virus pneumonitis (type Sendai). I. The clinical observations. II. The isolation of a new virus. III. Pathological study. Tohoku J. Exp. Med., *58*:56-82, 1953.

95. Seringe, P., Bach, C., Virat, J., Carré, M., et al.: L'exploration virologique dans les infections respiratoires d'un service de pédiatrie parisien. Sem. Hôp. Paris, *37*:2895-2898, 1961.

96. Sterner, G., Wolontis, S., Bloth, B., and Dehevesy, G.: Respiratory syncytial virus. Acta Paediat. Scand., *55*:273-279, 1966.

NEONATAL DIARRHEA AND VIRAL INFECTIONS

97. Berkovich, S., and Kibrick, S.: Echo 11 outbreak in newborn infants and mothers. Pediatrics, *33*:534-540, 1964.

98. Eichenwald, H. F., Ababio, A., Arky, A. M., and Hartman, A. P.: Epidemic diarrhea in premature and older infants caused by ECHO virus type 18. J.A.M.A., *166*:1563-1566, 1958.

99. Eichenwald, H., and Kotsevalov, O.: Immunologic responses of premature and full-term infants to infection with certain viruses. Pediatrics, *25*:828-839, 1960.

100. Galbraith, N.: A survey of enteroviruses and adenoviruses in the feces of normal children aged 0-4 years. J. Hyg. (Lond.), *63*:441-455, 1965.

101. Jordan, W., et al.: Acquisition of type-specific antibodies in the first 5 years of life. New Eng. J. Med., *258*:1041-1044, 1958.

102. Kibrick, S., et al.: Clinical associations of enteric viruses. Ann. N.Y. Acad. Sci., *67*:311-325, 1957.

103. Lenner, L. de: Le problème étiologique de la diarrhée épidémique des nouveau-nés. Arch. Franç Pédiat., *5*:324-329, 1948.

104. Light, J., and Hodes, H.: Studies on epidemic diarrhea of the newborn infant: Isolation of a filtrable agent causing diarrhea in calves. Amer. J. Public Health, *33*:1451, 1943.

105. Marie, J., Hennequet, A., Bonissol, C., Watchi, J., Cayroche, P., and Eschwege, F.: Entérocolite ulcérohémorragique du nouveau-né avec présence dans l'intestin du virus Coxsackie A 9. Sem. Hôp. Paris, *40*:275-282, 1964.

106. Moscovici, C., and Maisel, J.: Intestinal viruses of newborn and older prematures. Amer. J. Dis. Child., *102*:771, 1961.

107. Ramos-Alvarez, M., and Sabin, A. B.: Intestinal viral flora of healthy children demonstrable by monkey kidney tissue culture. Amer. J. Public Health, *46*:295, 1956.

108. Ramos-Alvarez, M.: Cytopathogenic enteric-viruses associated with undifferentiated diarrheal syndromes in early childhood. Ann. N.Y. Acad. Sci., *67*:326-331, 1957.

109. Ramos-Alvarez, M., and Sabin, A. B.: Enteropathogenic viruses and bacteria. Role in summer diarrheal diseases of infancy and early childhood. J.A.M.A., *167*:147, 1958.

110. Ramos-Alvarez, M., and Olarte, J.: Diarrheal diseases of children. Amer. J. Dis. Child., *107*:218, 1964.

111. Rossier, A., Sarrut, S., and Delplanque, J.: Entero-

colite ulcéro-nécrotique du prématuré. Sem. Hôp. Paris, *35*:2428, 1959.

112. Sabin, A. B., Ramos-Alvarez, M., et al.: Live orally given poliovirus vaccine: effects of rapid mass immunization on population under conditions of massive enteric infection with other viruses. J.A.M.A., *173*:1521-1526, 1960.

113. Samaille, J., Maurin, J., Lépine, P., Dubois, O., and Carré, M.: Isolement du virus ECHO 14 au cours d'une épidémie de crèches de gastro-entérite. Ann. Inst. Pasteur (Paris), *99*:2, 1960.

114. Yow, M., Melnick, J., Blattner, R., and Rasmussen, L.: Enteroviruses in infantile diarrhea. Amer. J. Hyg., *77*:283, 1963.

61

Viruses and Chromosomes

By A. BOUÉ AND J. G. BOUÉ

For the physician, a virus is a pathogenic microorganism which, as a free-living agent, infects an individual and, in infecting him, produces pathological changes.

But, if we consider the same phenomena from the viewpoint of cellular biology, we may then think of a virus as "a nucleic acid, capable of introducing itself into a cell, which possesses the necessary information for its precise replication and, at times, that necessary for the synthesis and assembly of protective elements (components of virions and of infectious virus particles); these components enable the virus to remain temporarily in the external environment and to pass to a new host cell, the virion only being a means of transport for genetic information" (Berkaloff[1]).

Inside the cell, the presence and replication of a virus, whether in complete or in incomplete form, does not always result in damage (e.g., cell death, inclusion bodies, or giant cells) and we must study the consequences of the prolonged presence of a virus in a host cell and in its descendants, where the passage of viral genome to daughter cells at the time of cell division may, in some cases, form the only method of transmission. In such circumstances, virus represents a superimposed nucleic acid and it will be of value to trace the fate of the genetic capital of the cell and its expression; a possible approach to the study of these events is afforded by cytogenetic observations.

In 1962, W. Nichols[24] produced evidence of chromosomal breaks in white blood cells taken from children during the course of measles. These early observations led to numerous studies, in particular of cells cultivated in vitro. Of especial interest is the work carried out in human diploid cell lines; through the experience acquired during the past few years in human cytogenetics, it is possible, in some instances, to establish correlations between a chromosomal change induced in a human cell in vitro and a similar change observed in pathological conditions in man.

In all these investigations, varying types of chromosomal change have been observed (Table 61-1).

At first, *an inhibition of cellular division*, shown by a very marked diminution or even a complete absence of metaphases, occurs following virus infection. This has been induced experimentally in some human embryo cells by infection with rubella virus[2, 3] and this mitotic inhibition has since been observed in leukocyte cultures taken during the acute phase of infective hepatitis[17] and also in congenital rubella during the first months of life.[19, 26]

Chromosomal breakages comprise the most commonly observed lesions; their significance is assessed by estimating the percentage of metaphases which show one or more true breaks in one or two chromatids.

Table 61-1. *Chromosomal Modifications Observed in Human Cells After Viral Infection*

TYPE OF MODIFICATION	CELL SYSTEM STUDIED		VIRAL INFECTION (NATURAL OR EXPERIMENTAL)
Inhibition of cell division	In vivo		Congenital rubella (first months of life), infectious hepatitis
	In vitro	Diploid cells	Rubella virus
Breaks	In vivo		Measles, chickenpox, infectious hepatitis, rubella, congenital rubella (age 1 year), vaccination against yellow fever
	In vitro	Leukocytes Diploid cells	Measles virus, Rous sarcoma virus, rubella virus, adenoviruses
Chromosomal pulverizations	In vitro	Diploid cells	Measles virus, herpes simplex virus, chickenpox virus, parainfluenza viruses
Modifications of the number of the chromosomes	In vitro	Diploid cells	SV 40, Rous sarcoma virus

It is important to know the localization of these breaks, which may affect the chromosomes randomly or, on the contrary, may have sites of predilection; for example, chromosomes 1 and 17 are damaged after infection with adenovirus 12.[31] We should also note whether the breaks are associated with chromosomal morphological changes such as dicentric chromosomes, rearrangements, or ring chromosomes. Observation of an increase in chromosome breaks must always be made with considerable care; indeed, both in vivo and in vitro, there is a low percentage of cells (about 5 per cent) in which breaks are found normally and it is only by comparison with control cells that any appraisal of this phenomenon may be made.

Chromosomal changes may be more marked, for example, the appearances of *chromosomal pulverization* which are observed in vitro following the inoculation of certain cytopathogenic viruses, in particular the myxoviruses;[5, 22, 23] it is difficult in this case to dissociate such lesions from the group of phenomena which end in the death of the cell.

Finally, associated or not with morphological lesions, we may observe *alterations in the number of chromosomes*, arising during the development of human cells which are chronically infected, whether with infectious virus or some subviral element.

But, whatever the nature and degree of the chromosomal changes which follow the entry of a virus into a cell, it is essential to know whether this cell may give rise to viable daughter cells and what will be the characteristics of the chromosomes typical of the cell population arising from the mother cell.

Whether *the lesions produced in this way are stable or, on the contrary, continue to progress*, we may visualize the intervention of a factor of viral origin into two regions of pathology: teratogenesis and oncogenesis.

In some cases, chromosomal anomalies are seen in a cellular population maintained in vitro without any morphological changes in the cells. Such a situation is found in infections of human diploid cells with rubella virus. Although no cytopathic effect is observed in spite of viral replication, an action of this virus on the mechanism of cellular division has been demonstrated.

In diploid cells derived from kidney, hypophysis, and lung, infection with rubella virus leads to inhibition of cellular division, shown by diminution, then complete absence of mitoses after the initial passages of cultures. As against this, virus infection of cell cultures derived from skin, muscle, and pharyngeal mucosa, and under the same experimental conditions, does not inhibit cellular division and these cultures may be maintained in a state of chronic infection for months. Cytogenetic examination of these chronically infected diploid cell lines shows an increase

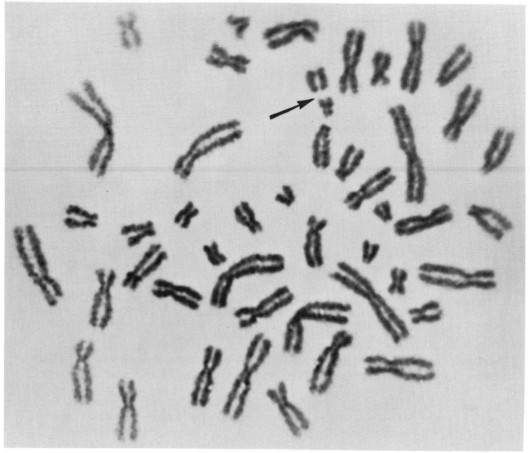

Figure 61-1. Metaphase of a human diploid cell chronically infected in vitro by rubella virus and presenting a break in the two chromatids of a D chromosome. Such a lesion is probably lethal for the daughter cells.

in the percentage of chromosomal breaks, which remains at 20 to 25 per cent during the whole life of the culture, control diploid lines always having lower levels of about 10 per cent.[3, 5] If these chronically infected cell cultures progress toward the stage of senescence without any sign of transformation being observed, nevertheless, their span of life is shortened when compared with control diploid cell lines.

These experimental facts have been confirmed by observations made during the course of congenital rubella. A high proportion of chromosomal breaks has been observed in cell cultures established from embryos taken at "therapeutic" abortions carried out because of maternal rubella, but only in those cases where virus was demonstrable.[8] Cell lines have been established from tissue taken at autopsy from neonates who died from congenital rubella; these cell lines grow sluggishly and their life span is shorter than

those of normal diploid cells.[27] Cultures of leukocytes taken from children affected by congenital rubella have shown, during the first months of life, an inhibition of cellular division,[19, 26] then as the age of one year approaches, a significant increase in the proportion of chromosomal breaks is found.[25]

Experimental data, confirmed by these clinical observations, allow us to put forward a hypothesis of the pathogenesis of defects in embryonic development.

Inhibition of cellular division and, above all, its selective nature are thus reconciled to the selective action of the virus in the localization of defects in the embryo. We do not think that it is possible to draw too close a parallel between in vivo and in vitro observations as regards different tissues; cells in the course of adaptation to an in vitro existence are subject to phenomena of dedifferentiation, as yet too little understood to enable us to attempt such a comparison. But we can see in the diverse effects of viral action on cellular division an experimental model of the selective character of this action which may well be determined by cellular differentiation.

Such facts agree well with the anatomical findings of Tondury[30] which demonstrate that this "endosymbiosis" of virus and host cell may not have any overt effect until particular stages of cellular differentiation are reached.

Inhibition of cellular division does not lead to the immediate destruction of the cell, which may survive without morphological change. During organogenesis, the cells thus attacked, but incapable of dividing, may remain in situ and hinder their own replacement by the healthy cells which should be supplanting them.

An increase in percentage of chromosomal breaks influences the growth of the entire cellular population. When a chromosomal break is produced during the course of a single cell division, the daughter cell which incorporates the damaged chromosome will not be viable (the two daughter cells, if there have been breaks in two chromatids). There is, therefore, at each reduplication of the whole cell population, a proportion of cells which is not viable: this leads to diminution in the growth rhythm and may explain the low birth weight which is one of the most constant features of congenital rubella; the anatomical studies of Naeye and Blanc[21] on neonates who have died from congenital rubella have shown a diminution in weight of certain organs and especially a decrease in the cellular density, disclosing a growth retardation in the cell population.

The lesions observed in congenital rubella may therefore be explained by an action of the virus upon cellular division, whether this inhibitory action prevents specifically the

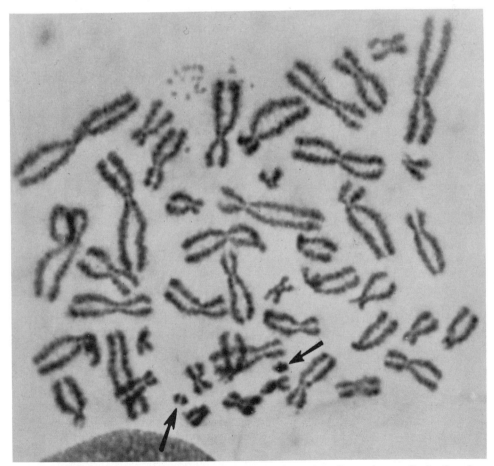

Figure 61-2.   Metaphase plate from a primary spleen culture of an embryo from a therapeutic abortion after maternal rubella. Note a break of the two chromatids of a G chromosome. The distal acentric fragment represents a small loss of genetic material; such a cell may give a viable pathologic clone.

development of particular cells, or whether it is an action on the chromosomal structure resulting in a diminution of growth rhythm in the majority of cellular tissues and, by the same token, the whole embryo.

In other cases, chromosomal anomalies are observed in *a cell population where significant morphological transformation appears*. This is what is seen in infection of human diploid cells by oncogenic viruses. Most studies have been made with a DNA virus, SV40,[11, 28] but more recently we have been able to study the evolution of chromosomal changes after infection with an RNA virus (Rous sarcoma).[7] If one tries to analyze the successive events which occur in these experiments, at first the normal cycle of viral replication is modified and, in place of the production of a complete virion — a virus in its infective form — an abortive cycle of viral replication takes place in which only antigens, and not the complete infective particle, are synthesized. This modification of the viral cycle may follow a period when the cycle is normal (with SV40[10, 11]) or may be established from the onset (Rous sarcoma). Morphological transformations seem, in general, to precede chromosomal changes (at least in those cases detectable by the techniques in use at present). These chromosomal changes are, in the first place, chromosomal breaks in a large proportion which may be accompanied by abnormal chromosomes (dicentrics, ring chromosomes[20]). Then changes in the number of chromosomes appear. These differ according to the virus studied. With SV40, it is, above all, progress toward subdiploidy and subtetraploidy, with loss of chromosomes in group G especially and also in group D. With Rous sarcoma, it is an evolution toward trisomies and double trisomies, found mainly in group C.

We must observe that chromosomes of group D and G, acrocentric chromosomes with satellites, are involved in the formation of the nucleolus, that SV40 is a DNA virus present in the nucleus and that infected cells show early lesions in the nucleolus; it is thus possible to visualize viral mediation here at the time of cellular division. Compared with this, Rous sarcoma is an RNA virus; the chromosomal changes observed with this virus are the result of nondisjunction, for monosomic C cells may be observed at the time when trisomic C cells appear: we may suppose that the action of the virus occurs at the time of metaphase and anaphase, when there is no longer any nuclear membrane, during the formation of the spindle.

Up to now, only two viruses have been studied in human cell cultures and, in the case of Rous sarcoma in particular, the amount of experience is, as yet, limited. The chromosomal changes observed during these experiments represent different types of response by living human cells to the action of oncogenic viruses without allowing us to attribute any specificity to these lesions.

When we compare the results of these experiments with observations made in human cancers, we can see some resemblances. In a statistical study of chromosomal changes observed in human tumors, Levan[15] has shown that these do not occur at random; in cell populations obtained from these human tumors, group C chromosomes tended to be in excess, while, on the contrary, group D and G chromosomes have tended to be deficient in number. We found the changes observed in vitro in human cells infected with Rous sarcoma on one hand and with SV40 on the other.

Other observations agree in general with these findings; in the evolution of cell lines derived from Burkitt tumors, trisomy C, then double trisomies C have been observed.[12] The phenomenon of duplication of the supernumerary chromosome has been observed by J. Lejeune in the karyotypic evolution of human tumors, but it could be nondisjunctive phenomena as with Rous sarcoma virus: a cell of 47 chromosomes gives rise to two complementary cells of 46 and 48 chromosomes.

May we consider the role of viruses in other chromosomal anomalies, in particular in the chromosomal abnormalities observed in man? Such a hypothesis has already been put forward by a number of workers; we know that the chromosomal abnormalities recognized in man and, in particular, the 21-trisomy responsible for Down's syndrome, do not arise by chance and that there exist variations in time and space in the frequency of these abnormalities. In Australia, Stoller and Collman[29] have been able to show a significant correlation between the incidence of cases of infective hepatitis and the frequency of children with "trisomy-21" who were born nine months later. Observations on spontaneous abortions have shown that chromosomal abnormalities occur in 40 per cent of cases;[6] the influence of maternal age is found in the trisomies of the acrocentric chromosomes (D and G), an observation already made in living children with this abnormality, the role of maternal age is not observed in the other trisomies or in the monosomies affecting the X chromosome.

We have just seen that oncogenic viruses may, in vitro, alter the chromosomal complement. In such cases, the chromosomal alterations do not remain stable but continue to evolve. MacPherson[16] has shown in cloned BHK 21 cells (hamster-derived), which had been transformed by Rous sarcoma virus, that a reversion could be seen and that some cells, having lost their viral genome, reverted to a normal morphology.

Following the manifestation of a chromosomal change, may a similar phenomenon occur, which leads to the stability of the chromosomal change?

Up to now, it has proved to be impossible to induce chromosomal aberrations with other, nononcogenic, viruses.

Many factors remain to be discovered in the mechanism of formation of chromosomal abnormalities and there is no doubt that the genetic inheritance of the cell influences the frequency or scarcity of such changes in each cell population. The variations in time and space of the frequencies with which such abnormalities occur remain, however, to be explained and it seems likely that external factors play a part, among which viruses represent serious candidates, for we have seen that, in vitro, they may produce analogous abnormalities.

BIBLIOGRAPHY

1. Berkaloff, A., Bourguet, J., Favard, P., and Guinnebault, M.: Biologie et Physiologie cellulaire. Paris, Hermann, 1967, p. 301.
2. Boué, A., Plotkin, S. A., and Boué, J. G.: Action inhibitrice du virus de la rubéole sur la multiplication de différentes cellules embryonnaires humaines cultivées in vitro. C. R. Acad. Sci. (Paris), 259:489, 1964.
3. Boué, A., Plotkin, S. A., and Boué, J. G.: Action du virus de la rubéole sur différents systèmes de cultures de cellules embryonnaires humaines. Arch. Ges. Virusforsch., 16:443, 1965.
4. Boué, A., and Boué, J. G.: Effects of rubella infection on division of human cells. Am. J. Dis. Children, 118:45-48, 1969.
5. Boué, J. G., Boué, A., Moorhead, P. S., and Plotkin, S. A.: Altérations chromosomiques induites par le virus de la rubéole dans les cellules embryonnaires diploïdes humaines cultivées in vitro. C. R. Acad. Sci. (Paris), 259:687, 1964.
6. Boué, J. G., Boué, A., and Lazar, P.: Altérations chromosomiques induites par le virus de la rubéole et par le virus de la rougeole dans les cellules

diploïdes humaines cultivées in vitro. Path. Biol. (Paris), 15:997, 1967.
7. Boué, J. G., Boué, A., and Lazar, P.: Les aberrations chromosomiques dans les avortements. Ann. Génét. (Paris), 10:179, 1967.
8. Boué, J. G., Boué, A., Montagnier, L., and Vigier, P.: Evolution chromosomique d'un clone de cellules humaines transformés par le virus du sarcome de Rous, C. R. Acad. Sci. (Paris), 266, serie D:178, 1968.
9. Evans, H. J.: The nucleolus, virus infection, and trisomy in man. Nature, 214:361, 1967.
10. Girardi, A. J., Jensen, F. C., and Koprowski, H.: SV 40 induced transformation of human diploid cells, crisis and recovery. J. Cell. Comp. Physiol., 65:69-81, 1965.
11. Girardi, A. J., Weinstein, D., and Moorhead, P. S.: SV 40 transformation of human diploid cells: parallel studies of viral and karyological parameters. Ann. Med. Exp. Fenn., 44:242, 1966.
12. Henle, W., Diehel, V., Kohn, G., Zur Hausen, H., and Henle, G.: Herpes-type virus and chromosome marker in normal leukocytes after growth with irradiated Burkitt cells. Science, 157:1064, 1967.
13. Koprowski, H., Ponten, J. A., Jensen, F., Moorhead, P., and Saksela, E.: Transformation of cultures of human tissue infected with simian virus SV 40. J. Cell. Comp. Physiol., 59:281, 1962.
14. Lejeune, J.: In Le concept d'évolution caryotypique. Les chromosomes humains. Paris, Gauthier-Villars, 1965, p. 210.
15. Levan, A.: Nonrandom representation of chromosome types in human tumor stemlines. Hereditas (Lund), 55:28, 1966.
15a. Levan, A.: Some current problems of cancer cytogenetics. Hereditas (Lund), 57:343, 1967.
16. MacPherson, I.: Recent advances in the study of viral oncogenesis. Brit. Med. Bull., 23:144, 1967.
17. Mella, B., and Lang, D. J.: Leucocyte mitosis: suppression in vitro associated with acute infectious hepatitis. Science, 155:80, 1967.
18. Montagnier, L., Vigier, P., Boué, J., and Boué, A.: Transformation en milieu gelifié d'une souche diploïde de cellules humaines par le virus de Rous. C. R. Acad. Sci. (Paris), 265, serie D, 2161-2164, 1967.
19. Montgomery, J. R., South, M. A., Rawls, W. E., Melnick, J. L., Olson, G. B., Dent, P. B., and Good, R. A.: Viral inhibition of lymphocyte response to phytohemagglutinin. Science, 157:1068, 1967.
20. Moorhead, P. S., and Saksela, E.: The sequence of chromosome aberrations during SV 40 transformation of a human diploid cell strain. Hereditas (Lund), 52:271-284, 1965.
21. Naeye, R. L., and Blanc, W.: Pathogenesis of congenital rubella. J.A.M.A., 194:169, 1965.
22. Nichols, W. W., Levan, A., Aula, P., and Norrby, E.: Extreme chromosome breakage induced by measles virus in different in vitro systems. Preliminary communication. Hereditas (Lund), 51:380-382, 1964.
23. Nichols, W. W., Levan, A., Aula, P., and Norrby, E.: Chromosome damage associated with the measles virus in vitro. Hereditas (Lund), 54:101, 1965.
24. Nichols, W. W., Levan, A., Hall, B., and Ostengren, G.: Measles associated chromosome breakage. Hereditas (Lund), 48:367, 1962.
25. Nusbacher, J., Hirschhorn, K., and Cooper, L. Z.:

Chromosomal studies on congenital rubella. New Eng. J. Med., *276*:1409, 1967.

26. Olson, G. B., South, M. A., and Good, R. A.: Phytohaemagglutinin unresponsiveness of lymphocytes from babies with congenital rubella. Nature, *214*:695, 1967.

27. Rawls, W. E., and Melnick, J. L.: Rubella virus carrier cultures derived from congenitally infected infants. J. Exp. Med., *123*:795, 1966.

28. Shein, H. M., and Enders, J. F.: Transformation induced by simian virus 40 in human renal cell cultures. I. Morphology and growth characteristics. Proc. Nat. Acad. Sci. U.S.A., *48*:1164-1172, 1962.

29. Stoller, A., and Collman, R. D.: Incidence of infective hepatitis followed by Down's syndrome nine months later. Lancet, *2*:1221, 1965.

30. Tondury, G., and Smith, D. W.: Fetal rubella pathology. J. Pediat., *68*:867, 1966.

31. Zur Hausen, H.: Virus-cell genome interactions. I. Induction of specific chromosomal aberrations by adenovirus type 12 in human embryonic kidney cells. J. Virol., *1*:1174, 1967.

62

Tumor Viruses

By SVEN GARD

The first successful experimental transmission of a neoplastic condition which is on record seems to be the production of warts in man after inoculation of material derived from juvenile verrucae as reported in 1894 by Variot.[15] Thirteen years later Ciuffo[3] repeated the experiment with filtered, cell-free extracts. These observations seem not to have attracted the attention they actually deserved.

The same was true of the report in 1908 by Ellerman and Bang[5] that fowl myeloblastosis could be transferred to healthy birds by passage of cell-free plasma. The reason for the general lack of interest in this discovery was no doubt the fact that leukemia at this time was considered to represent not a neoplastic but rather a special type of inflammatory reaction.

When, however, Peyton Rous,[10] after first having established the transplantability of a certain spontaneous chicken sarcoma, in 1911 described the successful serial transfer of this neoplasm by intramuscular inoculation of cell-free tumor filtrates, the scientific world sat up and took notice. At first high hopes were attached to this discovery; the solution to the problem of the cause of cancer seemed to be within easy reach.

Innumerable attempts to reproduce Rous' results with other tumors in other species of animals were made but were consistently unsuccessful. Hope faded rapidly, and the question of the true nature of the Rous sarcoma was raised: neoplasm or hyperplasia? This discussion is not yet entirely ended.

Slowly, however, evidence of viruses as causative agents of true neoplastic conditions accumulated. In 1933 Shope[11] could show that papillomas which occur spontaneously in wild cottontail rabbits and which not seldom develop into cancer could be passed with cell-free extracts to cottontail as well as to domesticated rabbits. Bittner,[1] who for several years had studied mammary cancer of mice, in 1936 felt justified to conclude that a milk-borne factor which might be a virus played a decisive role in the genesis of the tumors. In 1951 Gross[7] described the cell-free transfer of lymphatic leukemia to low-leukemia strains of mice.

Since then the development has begun to run at a faster rate, thanks in large measure to the introduction into virology of tissue culture as an invaluable routine procedure. With the discovery in 1957 of the polyoma virus of mice (Stewart et al.[12]), in 1960 of the SV40 (Sweet and Hilleman[13]), and in 1962 of the oncogenic capacity of adenoviruses (Trentin et al.[14]), the stage was set for today's dramatic, world-wide activity in the tumor virus field.

Terminology. Tissue culture is one of the most important tools in the study of tumor-inducing viruses, and consequently many of the terms used to describe the properties and behavior of such agents refer to tissue culture studies. Since this technique is now being used for many different purposes and in various branches of science, it is not surprising that a certain terminological confusion has ensued, the same term sometimes being used in different connotations and different terms being used to describe the same phenomenon. To bring some order into the field of nomenclature, the American Tissue Culture Association has made certain recommendations which will be followed in this review.

ONCOGENIC VIRUSES; GENERAL PROPERTIES

The term *oncogenic* is used only in reference to a tumor-inducing agent; a cell having the capacity of producing a tumor is described as *tumorigenic*.

The number of known oncogenic viruses now is considerable. A summary of the present status of knowledge is presented in Table 62-1. In this list all of the four main groups of DNA viruses are represented and two of the seven RNA groups.

Table 62-1. *Viruses of Known Oncogenic Capacity*

GROUP	TYPE	HOST
DNA-viruses		
Poxvirus	molluscum contagiosum	man
	Yabe	monkey
	fibroma	rabbit, deer
Herpesvirus	bovine rhinotracheitis	cattle
	Lucké	frog
Adenovirus	8 human	
	6 simian	hamster, mouse
	1 bovine	
	1 avian	
Papovavirus	papilloma subgroup	man, several species of mammals
	polyoma	mouse and other rodents
	SV40	hamster
RNA-viruses		
Paramyxovirus	—	
Rhabdovirus	—	
Myxovirus	—	
Leukosis virus	fowl leukosis, several immunological types	chicken and other birds
	Rous sarcoma	birds, several mammals
	murine leukosis, several immunological types	mouse, rat
	Bittner	mouse
	cat leukemia	cat
Reovirus	wound tumor	plants
Arbovirus	—	—
Picornavirus	—	—

Whether or not a pattern can be distinguished here is at present uncertain, since sufficiently detailed information on the fine structure of all viruses involved is not yet available. It may be significant that no viruses belonging to groups with a proved helically symmetrical structure (paramyxoviruses, rhabdoviruses, and myxoviruses) have as yet been found to be oncogenic. It may likewise be more than a coincidence that the picornavirus group is not represented. Picornaviruses seem to be the only animal viruses which cause a true lysis of the host cell and which, like bacteriophages, are released in a distinct "burst."

One group of viruses was not included in Table 62-1, the picodnaviruses. This comprises the very small (20 to 22 mμ) single-stranded DNA viruses: the adenosatellite viruses, the rat viruses K and X14, and Toolan's hamster virus H. Knowledge about the properties of these viruses is still incomplete. Some of them seem to have quite remarkable biological effects; to what extent they might participate in tumor formation must at present be left an open question.

Since the human adenoviruses fall into three distinct groups as regards oncogenicity—highly and moderately oncogenic and nononcogenic—attempts have been made to relate these characteristics to chemical composition and other definable structural properties. Green and co-workers determined DNA content, base ratio, and homology of the first 28 immunological types of human adenoviruses and found a pattern of a certain consistency. Thus the highly oncogenic types 12 and 18 had significantly lower DNA and guanine + cytosine contents than the other types. Structural homology between the DNA's of the two types was estimated at 79 per cent, whereas homology tests with either one of them versus those of types 2, 4, or 7 yielded values in the range of 9 to 26 per cent. Comparisons between moderately oncogenic and nononcogenic types gave less clear-cut results.

When trying to evaluate these observations one must keep in mind that, at the time, the existence of adenosatellite viruses was not yet recognized. Many adenovirus strains have since been found to be sometimes heavily contaminated by satellite virus. The DNA content of these small viruses is significantly higher than that of adenovirus, and the presence of such contaminants could, therefore, greatly affect the result of quantitative determinations. It is, therefore, desirable that the above-mentioned observations be confirmed with the use of material known to be free from contaminants.

Biologically, oncogenic viruses display hardly any distinctive characteristics apart from the capacity to cause transformation of the host cell. Their behavior in vitro varies considerably from one type to another. Some leukosis viruses have not yet been grown in cell cultures. The molluscum contagiosum agent produces cytopathic lesions on primary inoculation, but has not been maintained in passages. Some strains of Rous sarcoma virus (RSV) are defective and cannot produce mature virions in the absence of a helper virus. In some adenovirus-cell systems simultaneous infection with two genetically distinct viruses seems to be a requirement for multiplication.

As regards in vitro cytopathic effects, leukosis viruses as a rule multiply without producing any demonstrable changes in cell morphology or viability—apart from occasional transformations. Most other oncogenic viruses produce cytopathic effects of essentially the same character as those found in cells infected with nononcogenic types belonging to the same group. The interaction between virus and host cell varies considerably, however. Host and viral factors are in this respect of equal importance. SV40 may be mentioned as an example. It multiplies abundantly in primary rhesus or cynomolgus kidney cells without any apparent or only insignificant cytopathic effects, whereas infected cercopithecus kidney cells undergo a characteristic vacuolation and eventual total destruction.

In summary, observations so far made have not provided much information on the structural or genetic basis for the oncogenic capacity of a certain virus. No simple tests have as yet been devised by which oncogenic and nononcogenic viruses might be distinguished.

TRANSFORMATION

In the present context the term transformation will be used to imply a *hereditary* change of a cell. In turn this, of course, means that a transformed cell has retained its viability and reproductive capacity; degenerative changes ultimately leading to cell death are not included.

Transformation may express itself in several ways. Some of the changes observed may be objectively recorded and measured, while others are less well defined. Some are demonstrable in vitro, others only in vivo.

Growth Characteristics. Normal tissue cells cultivated in vitro are characterized by sensitivity to contact inhibition, by a moderate growth rate, and by a finite lifetime. Physical contact with another cell inhibits both motility and mitotic activity. Normal cells, therefore, do not ordinarily form multilayered cultures. Occasionally, however, fibroblasts in a monolayer culture produce a sheet of extracellular fibers on which a second monolayer of cells may grow out. Normal cells seem incapable of growing indefinitely in vitro. After a certain number of successive divisions (for human fibroblasts 50 ± 10) the cells go into senescence; mitotic activity is retarded and becomes irregular, and eventually the cells die.

Changes in growth characteristics are regular manifestations of virus-induced transformation. Insensitivity to contact inhibition is practically always observed. Multilayered growth can be measured in terms of number of cell nuclei per unit of culture surface area. Increased growth rate is a common feature, and not seldom the transformed cells have acquired the capacity of unlimited growth.

Morphology. Transformation is often associated with morphological changes which, coupled with multilayered growth, make colonies of transformed cells, appearing in a monolayer culture, stand out as distinct pocks. Transformed fibroblasts are shorter, more plump than the normal cells, irregularly arranged, and carry a thick coat of a mucopolysaccharide. Cells of other origin often assume rounded or polygonal shapes.

Chromosomal abnormalities may appear. Whereas normal animal cells are diploid with a normal chromosome idiogram, transformation is often followed by, in the initial stage, tetraploidy which later, in connection with other mitotic irregularities, may develop into aneuploidy and heteroploidy.

Morphological changes cannot readily be classified or quantitated.

Immunological Characteristics. Immunological changes as part of the transformation phenomena are of great theoretical interest and presumably of a considerable practical importance.

Antigenic properties of transformed cells have been studied with the aid of complement fixation, immunofluorescence, cytotoxicity, and transplantation reaction techniques. It is not always clear to what extent the various methods indicate identical or distinct antigens.

Virus-transformed cells seem invariably to have acquired antigens not found in normal cells. The use of immunofluorescence on acetone-fixed or sectioned cells has demonstrated the existence of both intranuclear and cytoplasmic antigens, and application of the same technique on living cells has shown the presence of specific surface antigens as well.

Immunofluorescence is relatively insensitive; unless the density of specific antigenic sites is sufficiently high no visible reaction will take place. A thinly spread antigen could therefore escape detection even if the total antigenic mass were large, while a locally concentrated small amount of antigen can be spotted. Complement fixation, on the other hand, using cell extracts as reagents, would preferably indicate antigens present in large quantities but would naturally give no information about their distribution or localization. Thus, even though in principle the two reactions should indicate the same antigenic specificities, each might add some information that the other cannot.

Cytotoxicity and transplantation (graft rejection) reactions presumably involve only antigenic sites on the cell surface. The cytotoxic effect is mediated by antibodies and is complement dependent. It is measured variously by direct microscopy of cultured cells, with the aid of vital staining, or by the leakage of isotope from prelabeled cells. The principal mechanism in graft rejection most probably is cell-associated immunity.

Circulating antibodies play a somewhat ambiguous role in this connection. Sometimes they seem to act in synergism with, sometimes in antagonism to, the cell-bound factor. The explanation probably is to be found in the distribution of antigenic sites on the cell surface. An antibody-mediated cytotoxic effect requires a certain density of reactive sites. If this density falls below a critical level the cell will be "antibody-resistant," presumably because it is capable of counteracting the scattered lytic attacks on the cell membrane by reparative processes. At the same time the antibody-covered antigenic sites seem to be inaccessible to the sensitized lymphocytes which are responsible for the true graft rejection reaction. The smaller the number of reactive sites on the surface of a transformed cell, the greater will be the chance that they all become blocked by antibodies and consequently protected from cell-associated immunoreactions. This antagonistic antibody effect is known under the name of *enhancement,* which refers to the enhancing effect on the capacity for survival of a graft.

The cytotoxic effect of antibodies is readily assayable in vitro, whereas attempts to establish in vitro procedures for demonstration and measurement of cell-associated immunity have not been unequivocally successful. At present, therefore, we have to rely upon animal experiments for the latter test. This means that only tumorigenic cells can be examined by this method. Since transformed cells seem to retain most of their normal isoantigens, it follows that availability of syngeneic animals is another requirement; non-tumor-specific isoimmune rejection in allogeneic recipients would completely obscure any tumor-specific reactions.

Specific antigens demonstrable with the above-mentioned methods were first found in polyomavirus-induced tumors. The relevant antigens were apparently present in the cell membrane, and they were shown to differ from any antigens found in the virion of the inducing virus. These tumor-specific antigens were thus nonviral but still virus specific in the sense that all tumors induced by the same virus carried the same antigenic specificity irrespective of the nature of the tissue in which they originated or the species of animal in which they developed. The same seems to be true of all cells transformed by the naked DNA viruses of the papovavirus and adenovirus groups.

Leukosis virus-induced transformation presents a somewhat different picture. In most cases the surface antigen of the transformed cell is indistinguishable from that of the inducing virion. This is not surprising, since the virus envelope is derived from the cell surface. However, a cell transformed by a defective and nonreproducing Rous sarcoma virus (RSV) does not carry any surface antigen that is demonstrably both virus specific and tumor specific. This fact is as yet unexplained.

As regards terminology, the definitions are neither very distinct nor very rational. Three terms are in general use. Intranuclear antigens demonstrable by means of immunofluorescence in papovavirus- and adenovirus-transformed cells are usually referred to as neoantigens. Antigens detectable in a complement-fixation test are called tumor or T-antigens. Finally, antigens responsible for graft rejection are labeled tumor-specific transplantation or TST-antigens. Obviously the first two as well as the last two categories might well overlap.

Cell Physiology and Biochemistry. In addition to such transformation-associated changes as were already discussed, various shifts in the metabolic pattern of transformed cells have been described. The significance of such alterations is not always clear.

The possible causal relationship between immunologic abnormalities and leukemia is attracting increasing interest. Such autoimmunologic manifestations as hemolytic anemia are not infrequent in cases of human leukemia. Changes in immunologic responsiveness in leukosis virus-infected mice demonstrable before the onset of leukemia have been reported. Of particular interest is the recent observation that a certain mouse line, NZB/BL, is highly prone to develop autoimmune disease followed some time later by leukemia. This line has been shown to carry a leukosis virus.

The question in this case is whether a hereditary predisposition for an immunological anomaly paves the way for neoplastic transformation or whether the functional abnormality of the lymphatic system marks an early step in a progressive, virus-induced transformation process. In line with the latter alternative it has also been suggested that lymphomatosis might represent an abnormally violent manifestation of cell-associated immunity to transformed cells of a nonlymphocyte nature. At present a discussion of these phenomena would of necessity be mainly conjectural, but obviously the problem is well worth further study.

Tumorigenicity. As indicated in the introduction, the nature of the tumors induced by viruses has been, and in some quarters still is, under discussion. The question raised has been whether the growths should be classified as simple hyperplasia or as true neoplasms. There can now be little doubt that virus-induced tumors may eventually develop true neoplastic properties. The point is whether this is attributable to the virus alone or whether a contribution by additional factors is needed.

There is probably no simple answer to these questions. In some typical virus infections, such as vaccinia, hypertrophy of infected cells and hyperplasia are a characteristic of the initial stage, followed later by degeneration and disintegration. In molluscum contagiosum the tumor character is more pronounced; the incubation period is considerably longer, between 15 and 50 days; the course is protracted over several months; the wart-like growths produce no reaction in surrounding tissue and eventually disappear, presumably by a process of slow degeneration.

Still another picture is presented by, for instance, the Shope papilloma of rabbits and the mammary cancer of mice. In domesticated rabbits virus-induced papillomas undergo regression, leaving behind a solid immunity; they cannot be propagated serially in these animals. In wild cottontails, on the other hand, they continue to grow, sometimes to an enormous size, and they often develop into malignant carcinomas. In Bittner virus-carrying mice "hyperplastic nodules" are almost always to be found in the mammary glands. Cancer may develop, always starting in such nodules, but practically only in females of certain breeds and after one or more pregnancies.

Finally, some tumors, such as those induced by polyomavirus, display clear-cut neoplastic characteristics right from their first appearance.

Presence or absence of tumorigenic capacity cannot be determined on the basis of any in vitro criteria. Most but not all tumorigenic cells possess a majority of the features of transformation mentioned earlier. On the other hand, cells that appear thoroughly transformed in vitro may lack the capacity of forming tumors in vivo. There are as yet no clues to these obviously important problems.

MECHANISMS OF TRANSFORMATION

Growth Control. Morphology, physiology, and other properties of tumor cells and their relations to surrounding tissue show at least as much variation as do the corresponding characteristics of normal cells. The only feature they have in common is partial or complete insensitivity to the mechanisms regulating cell growth in the macroorganism. A thorough knowledge of the various factors controlling development, growth, and interrelationships of cells, tissues, and organs would thus seem to be an imperative requirement for a real understanding of the nature of neoplasia. Unfortunately, our knowledge in this area is still pitifully inadequate.

In principle, growth control might be imposed upon the cell in three different ways.

1. By direct action of inhibitors or activators of a hormonal nature. Such agents apparently act selectively, which might be explained by differences in composition and permeability of the membranes of the various cells.

2. Indirectly by agents—chemical, physical, or even mechanical—acting upon the cell membrane. This would imply the presence on the cell surface of specific receptors capable of triggering certain feedback mechanisms. Contact inhibition might belong in this category.

3. By induction or repression of gene activity. This is a mechanism of presumably primary importance in the ontogenic differentiation processes. Every cell in the macroorganism, as a descendant of one and the same fertilized ovum, has the same karyotype and should have the same complement of the estimated number of well over 2 million genes. The regularity of ontogenesis excludes a differentiation by mutational processes, leaving as the most probable alternative a selective repression of gene activity. In a differentiated cell presumably only a minor fraction of the genes are functioning at any given time, although the whole genome most probably retains the potential of activity. Consequently, differentiation is not the result of a change in or addition of genetic material but of a partial repression of the potentialities of a genetically omnipotent cell. Thus, there should be a wide margin for inductive or repressive influences.

Virus Replication. The amount of genetic material in a virion is small compared to that of the cell, ranging from two or three genes in the dwarf RNA phages to an estimated number of 400 in the largest members of the poxvirus group. The middle-sized viruses, among which most of the tumor viruses are to be found, contain on the order of 40 to 50 genes. A certain number of genes are needed to code for the various structural proteins entering into the coat of the virion. Others code for specific enzymes necessary for the synthesis of the virus nucleic acid. The thousands of enzymes mediating the fundamental metabolic processes which furnish energy and basic building blocks have to be provided by the cell, as are the ribosomes, principal tools for protein synthesis. It has to be expected that DNA and RNA virus replication follow slightly different paths.

DNA Viruses. Like that of the DNA phages the animal DNA virus genome seems to contain two operons coupled in a switch mechanism. After penetration and decoating of the virion the virus genome is released and the first operon is activated while the second one seems to stay inactive. Messenger RNA is produced and so-called early proteins are synthesized. These seem to represent mainly enzymes, such as specific DNA polymerase, thymidyl kinase, and others needed for synthesis of virus DNA.

In most cases cell DNA activity is blocked, leading to complete inhibition of synthesis of cell DNA, RNA, and protein. This effect is probably mediated by a virus protein which in some cases might be preformed as a component of the virion (e.g., in bacteriophage and poxvirus); in other cases it is probably synthesized together with the early proteins or possibly at a still later stage.

When the sufficient amount and number of virus-specific enzymes have been produced, synthesis of virus DNA is initiated. By a mechanism not yet identified, this seems to switch off the first and switch on the second operon. Synthesis of early proteins ceases, and the supply of such proteins accumulated during the first phase is gradually depleted. At the time of virus maturation and release early proteins are usually no longer demonstrable.

Shortly after initiation of DNA synthesis, structural proteins, immunologically identifiable with components of the mature virion, begin to appear and increase continuously in quantity. Finally mature virions are formed and active virus is released. In most systems, however, the major part of the virus remains cell associated.

At the time when cell-DNA activity is blocked the cell contains a supply of enzymes sufficient for maintenance, at least

temporarily, of a basal metabolism at an undiminished rate. Since the content of enzymes is no longer replenished by active synthesis, the supply is gradually exhausted. Sooner or later some essential enzyme gives out completely, bringing metabolism to a halt. When this happens, virus synthesis stops because of lack of building blocks and energy, and the cell slowly deteriorates. The cell does not undergo a true lysis.

Synthesis of poxviruses in its entirety is located in the cytoplasm. As regards other DNA viruses, the early protein is apparently formed in the nucleus and so is presumably the virus DNA. The structural proteins, on the other hand, seem to be produced in the cytoplasm. They are later transferred to the nucleus, where maturation takes place. This transport seems to be mediated by a specific protein coded for by the virus genome.

If formation of virus DNA is inhibited by means of 5-fluorodeoxyuridine (FUDR), the above-mentioned switch mechanism is not triggered. Early proteins are continuously synthesized, but no DNA or structural proteins are produced. Early proteins may appear extracellularly, which in a regular cytocidal reproduction cycle they do not do.

RNA Viruses. Most viruses in this category contain single-stranded RNA. After decoating, the virus RNA seems capable of functioning directly as a messenger-RNA, which, in contradistinction to cellular m-RNA, appears to be completely stable. As an indication hereof it forms polysomes of an unusual size containing 40 or more ribosomes. No distinct separation of early and late phases of synthesis are observed; virus-associated enzymes, RNA, and structural proteins appear in close succession and are continuously produced through the whole cycle of replication.

Synthesis of nucleic acid, both DNA and RNA, generally requires a template consisting of two complementary strands. Synthesis of virus RNA seems to conform to this pattern. The first phase in RNA replication thus is the formation of double-stranded RNA. Consequently, the infected cell will contain three categories of virus RNA: (1) one part functioning as m-RNA in the synthesis of enzymes and structural proteins, (2) the double-stranded replicating form, and (3) a pool of newly synthesized single-stranded, virus-precursor RNA.

Several RNA virus groups are completely independent of any DNA activity, and in fact they themselves block the cell DNA, causing cessation of synthesis of cell DNA, RNA, and protein. However, the members of three groups, myxoviruses, reoviruses, and fowl leukosis viruses, do not go into replication in cells whose DNA is blocked by actinomycin D. This does not necessarily imply that host-directed enzyme formation is required for virus synthesis. A more likely explanation is that an inducible cell enzyme is needed for decoating and release of virus nucleic acid.

However, fowl leukosis viruses differ from other RNA viruses so far studied inasmuch as they seem to require a continued cell DNA activity throughout the replication cycle. Thus, if actinomycin D is added to an infected culture at any time within the first 48 hours, virus replication will not start, and if it is added to a culture already producing mature virus, virus synthesis will be interrupted. The explanation for these facts is still obscure. It has been suggested that a virus-directed synthesis of DNA might be the first step in the replication process and that this DNA rather than double-stranded RNA serves as the template in virus RNA formation.

The site of RNA virus synthesis, as far as it is demonstrable with the aid of immunofluorescence, in most cases is in the cytoplasm of the host cell. However, the internal protein and presumably the nucleic acid of influenza viruses are synthesized in the nucleus. As regards fowl leukosis viruses, viral antigens are not regularly found intranuclearly, although the nucleus seems to participate somehow in virus replication as indicated by the constant, considerable enlargement of the nucleoli.

Maturation. It should be recalled that enveloped viruses undergo the last step in the maturation process right at the surface of the cell. The viral nucleocapsid seems to push the cell membrane outward, and the extrusion thus formed is then detached from the cell. The envelope of the virion is thus derived from the cell membrane. By means of isotope labeling it has been shown that the lipids of the envelope are preformed cell structures, whereas the protein parts, the "spikes," are coded for in the virus genome.

Transformation. Rous sarcoma virus seems to transform every infected cell. In most other systems transformation is a rare event, involving only 1 per cent or even as little as 10^{-6} of the infected cells. Some viruses, like polyomavirus, may transform any type of cell; others, like fowl myeloblastoma virus, display a strictly specific transforming activity, although they are capable of infecting and multiplying in many types of cells. Leukosis virus-transformed cells in most cases continue to produce and release virus, whereas in other systems the transformed cells neither release nor produce any virus.

In a description of the phenomenology of transformation, RNA and DNA viruses are best considered separately. Among the former, the fowl leukosis viruses, and particularly the RSV, have been most extensively studied. Leukosis viruses in general do not inhibit host cell metabolism; they do not produce cytopathic changes and do not affect the viability of the host cell. Infected cells thus grow and divide while continuously producing and releasing virus, although at a very moderate rate when compared to most other cell-virus systems.

As already mentioned, the RSV seems to cause transformation in practically 100 per cent of infected cells. Fibroblasts are the main target, but transformation of epithelial cells is also known to occur. At least some strains of RSV have been found to be genetically defective, unable to induce synthesis of mature virions without the aid of a helper virus. This fact offers special opportunities for studies of the basic mechanisms of tumor induction.

The virion of a defective RSV is apparently made up of an RSV genome in a helper virus envelope. The external protein, responsible for serological specificity of the virion and host cell affinity, is thus provided by the helper virus. To what extent the internal structural proteins are coded for in the RSV genome is not yet clear.

A cell singly infected with RSV is readily transformed, but it does not produce or release any virus (nonproducers). Transformed cells grow faster than normal cells and are tumorigenic. They usually show characteristic morphological changes, typical of the infecting strain of virus. However, fetal calf serum incorporated in the tissue culture medium suppresses morphological changes without apparently affecting other properties of the infected cells.

Nonproducing cells are reported not to have undergone any immunological changes. Immunofluorescence tests do not detect any virus-specific intracellular or membrane antigens, and the cells do not induce cell-associated transplantation immunity in chickens. In this respect, however, the issue is not clear. The nonproducing tumors that can be induced in mammals by certain strains of RSV seem to possess specific transplantation antigens. In the search for an explanation for this apparent discrepancy the possibility of enhancement as a complicating factor ought to be investigated. It may be a question of the concentration of a presumptive surface antigen. The sensitivity of the tests thus far applied did not permit detection of antigen concentrations below 15 per cent of those found in virus-producing cells.

It has been convincingly shown that contact inhibition, as regards cell migration as well as mitotic activity, is triggered from the cell surface. Although a loss of sensitivity to such inhibition could be explained by a block in essential intracellular feedback mechanisms, the most logical place to look for the cause of such a loss would be the cell surface itself. Surface alterations as manifested by immunological changes seem to be a characteristic of all other tumorigenic cells examined, and a divergent behavior of RSV-induced chicken cells should not be acknowledged unless proved beyond reasonable doubt. This situation seems not to prevail.

On the other hand, appearance of a new antigen in the cell membrane is per se not sufficient to cause transformation or tumorigenicity. Several of the RSV helper viruses (Rous-associated viruses, RAV1, RAV2, and so forth), which in the absence of RSV multiply and cause immunological transformation of infected cells, do not induce morphological changes or tumorigenicity. It might be of special interest that avian myeloblastosis virus, oncogenic in its own right but only in myeloid cells, multiplies in fibroblasts and serves as a Rous helper virus.

To what extent the RSV genome is defective is not known. Apart from what in this writer's opinion is the likely possibility that singly infected transformed cells produce a specific surface protein, no synthesis of early or structural proteins, detectable by immunological methods, seems to be induced. Neither is there any direct evidence of any synthesis of virus RNA. Since, however, the amount of virus RNA at any given time remains very small even in producing cells, the failure to find it in nonproducing cells cannot be assigned too much weight.

As already mentioned, the dependence of virus synthesis as well as transformation on an intact cell DNA activity has actuated the assumption of an integration of the virus code, if not the virus RNA itself, into the cell genome. The hereditary character of transformation undoubtedly serves to support this hypothesis. The probability that an independently replicating cytoplasmic unit would get lost in a series of successive cell divisions would seem to be considerable.

Some of the DNA viruses seem to present a somewhat stronger case for the integration hypothesis. In the first place, the theoretical conditions are more favorable; the virus DNA penetrates into the cell nucleus and a direct integration without a preceding transcription of the genetic code would be technically possible. Furthermore, some kind of repressor mechanism, reminiscent of that of the bacteriophages, seems to regulate the activity of the two operons apparently contained in the virus genome (cf. p. 836).

The hereditary character of transformation might, as in the case of RSV, be considered circumstantial evidence of integration. As shown by immunofluorescence, early proteins (neoantigens) are continuously being synthesized by transformed cells, but apparently no virus DNA or structural proteins and no mature virus is produced. These facts taken together indicate that the virus-directed regulation of the activity of the various parts of the virus genome is paralyzed, which in turn points toward the existence of a special "replicator" gene with the double function of initiating DNA replication and synthesis of structural proteins and switching of the "early" operon. This would be a mechanism analogous to the one supposed to regulate the activity of temperate phages and such nonviral episomes as the fertility factor of certain bacteria.

Direct evidence of integration is not yet available. Attempts by means of DNA homology tests to detect the presence of virus DNA in the cell genome have not yielded conclusive results. Actually, this technique is hardly sensitive enough for this purpose. It has not been possible unequivocally to induce virus multiplication in transformed cells by agents known to induce prophages. A repressor mechanism of the type responsible for the "immunity" of lysogenic bacteria seems not to operate in the animal virus systems. A virus-transformed, nonproducing cell might thus be susceptible to superinfection with the same virus. However, resistance to superinfection varies considerably from one transformed cell line to another. The possibility that varying numbers of integrated virus genomes might account for differences in resistance should be kept in mind.

A constant feature of DNA virus transformation is the appearance of a virus-specific transplantation antigen. The naked papovaviruses and adenoviruses which undergo complete maturation in the interior of the cell do not incorporate any cell membrane constituents into the virion. It is therefore not surprising that the TST-antigen in these cases is distinct from the viral antigens. Whether the TST-antigen is formed also in a cytocidal cycle of infection is not known, although it would seem plausible that this be the case.

An interesting phenomenon is the so-called "hybridization" between SV40 and various adenovirus types. A cell doubly infected with SV40 and the weakly oncogenic adenovirus type 7 might produce highly oncogenic virions with the immunologic and other in vitro characteristics of the adenovirus but producing tumors carrying the SV40-specific TST-antigen. These "hybrids" are defective, incapable by themselves of inducing formation of any mature virus but doing so in coinfections with adeno helper viruses. The virions thus produced carry the immunological characteristics of the helper. Presumably these "hybrids" may be regarded as "incomplete" viruses, containing only the "early" operon of the SV40 in an adenovirus coat.

In an attempt to sum up and sort out the relevant facts on which a general hypothesis of the mechanism of oncogenesis could be based, one might proceed as follows:

1. Formation of a specific cell surface antigen seems to be of essential importance, as this signals a change in the structure of the surface proteins which might account for loss of sensitivity to contact inhibition and acquisition of invasive activity. This may be a necessary prerequisite for tumorigenic transformation but it obviously is not a sufficient explanation of the mechanism.

2. The cytocidal effect of the virus must be blocked. Leukosis viruses do not inhibit cell DNA activity and seem not to cause cytopathic changes. This, however, is true of SV40, polyomaviruses, and adenoviruses. Members of the last-mentioned group produce a "cytotoxic" factor capable of blocking DNA, RNA, and protein synthesis. The toxin has been identified with the structural penton protein which most probably is coded for in the second operon and therefore probably is not to be found in the early protein fraction. Repression of the hypothetical replicator gene should then inhibit both virus replication and cytopathic activity.

3. Transformation may thus be regarded as a consequence of a defense reaction of the cell against virus infection. At least three different mechanisms for control of virus activity are conceivable: (a) the virus itself might be defective, e.g., RSV and SV40-adenovirus hybrids; (b) induction of interferon-like substances, which might inhibit specific sectors of the virus activity; (c) integration, by which process the cell DNA replicator gene would assume control of and synchronize virus DNA replication. Interferon production is sometimes but not regularly observed. RSV-transformed nonproducing cells remain fully susceptible to superinfection by RAV; infection with helper virus, on the other hand, induces resistance against RSV. In this case interference as a controlling factor can apparently be ruled out.

4. If integration served no other function than to block the cytocidal effects of the virus while permitting the virus-directed synthesis of the essential cell surface components, it could not be accepted as an unconditional explanation of oncogenesis. Fibroblasts infected with avian myeloblastosis virus show no cytopathic changes and they carry the virus-specific surface antigen; yet they are not tumorigenic. Transformation takes place only if the same virus enters a myeloid cell. If, therefore, integration is essential, it must also be assumed to permit expression of some virus gene which normally remains inactive, or alternatively affect some part of the cell genome by induction or repression.

5. It would seem that the many problems concerning the mechanisms of viral oncogenesis still unresolved might be fruitfully attacked with such techniques of experimental cytogenetics as hybridization of normal and transformed cells in vitro.

VIRUSES AND HUMAN CANCER

The discovery of oncogenic properties of such common and widespread human pathogens as the adenoviruses and the relative ease with which transformation of human tissue can be achieved in vitro with certain viruses have, of course, encouraged comprehensive projects of screening human tumors and tumor patients' sera for immunological indications of a possible etiological importance of known oncogenic viruses. So far all attempts in this direction seem to have yielded negative results.

In one field of human tumor research more promising results have been obtained, however. In 1957 Dmochowski described electron microscopy of material derived from a case of human leukemia and the detection in such preparations of virus-like particles. These studies have gradually been extended, in vitro culture of leukemic cells has been introduced, and immunological studies have been initiated.

With a remarkably high frequency virus-like particles of the "C" type, characteristic of fowl and mouse leukosis viruses, have been observed in fresh leukemic material as well as in cultured cells. Formation of such particles through the process of "budding" from the cell surface is likewise relatively frequently observed. Of immunological methods tested, immunofluorescence has shown a certain promise. When applied as membrane fluorescence on living cells this technique has yielded preliminary results which suggest a certain pattern with respect to reactivity of cells of different origin as well as to prevalence of antibodies in sera from various categories of human donors. Thus, there seems to be a significant difference between leukemic and normal white blood cells. Leukemic sera have almost always been found to react with positive cells; a large proportion of close contacts to leukemic patients have given positive serologic reactions, whereas healthy young adults without such contact have given largely negative reactions.

A study of Burkitt's African lymphoma has led to another type of so far rather puzzling observations. In a large proportion of cell strains derived from cases of this disease, intracellular virus-like particles have been found. These particles, which appear both in the nucleus and in the cytoplasm, when isolated and purified show an architec-ture of distinct icosahedral symmetry of the type found in the capsid of members of the herpesvirus group. They seem to differ from these viruses by their consistently smaller size, by about 20 per cent, and by their immunological specificity. Only a minor fraction of the cells carry such particles at any one time, and maturation and release of virus from the cells have not yet been observed. Coincidentally with the appearance of particles the cells acquire the capacity of staining intranuclearly and cytoplasmatically in the immunofluorescence tests with a high proportion of human sera.

Recently, strong circumstantial evidence has been presented to show that the herpesvirus-like particles are indeed the etiological agent of mononucleosis. Their causal relationship to Burkitt's lymphoma must therefore at present remain in doubt.

Since animal experiments have shown that an effective immunoprophylaxis against virus-induced leukemia is, indeed, a definite possibility, we can at least hope for a breakthrough in the field of human leukemia research in the not too distant future.

BIBLIOGRAPHY

1. Bittner, J. J.: Some possible effects of nursing on the mammary gland tumor incidence in mice. Science, *84*:162, 1936.
2. Burkitt, D.: A tumor syndrome affecting children in tropical Africa. Postgrad. Med. J., *38*:71, 1962.
3. Ciuffo, G.: Investo positivo confiltrate di verruca vulgare. Giornale Italiano della Malattie Veneree, *42*:12, 1907.
4. Dmochowski, L., Grey, C. E., Sykes, J. A., Shullenberger, C. C., and Howe, C. D.: Studies on human leukemia. Proc. Soc. Exp. Biol. Med., *101*:686, 1959.
5. Ellerman, V., and Bang, O.: Experimentelle Leukämi bei Hühmen. Zbl. Bakt. Abt. I. Orig., *46*:595, 1908.
6. Epstein, M. A., Achong, B. G., and Barr, Y. M.: Virus particles in cultured lymphoblasts from Burkitt's lymphoma. Lancet, *1*:702, 1964.
7. Gross, L.: "Spontaneous" leukemia developing in C3H mice following inoculation in infancy, with AK-leukemic extracts, or AK embryos. Proc. Soc. Exp. Biol. Med., *76*:27, 1951.
8. Lacy, S., Sr., and Green, M.: Adenovirus multiplication: Genetic relatedness of tumorigenic human adenovirus type 7, 12, and 18. Science, *150*:1296, 1965.
9. Piña, M., and Green, M.: Biochemical studies on adenovirus multiplication. IX. Chemical and base composition analysis of 28 human adenoviruses. Proc. Nat. Acad. Sci. USA, *54*:547, 1965.
10. Rous, P.: A sarcoma of the fowl transmissible by

an agent separable from the tumor cells. J. Exp. Med., *13*:397, 1911.

11. Shope, R. E.: Infectious papillomatosis of rabbits. J. Exp. Med., *58*:607, 1933.

12. Stewart, S. E., Eddy, B. E., Gochenour, A. M., Bargese, N. G., and Grubbs, G. E.: The induction of neoplasms with a substance released from mouse tumors by tissue culture. Virology, *3*:380, 1957.

13. Sweet, B. H., and Hilleman, M. R.: The vacuolating virus, SV40. Proc. Soc. Exp. Biol. Med., *105*:420, 1960.

14. Trentin, J. J., Yabe, Y., and Taylor, G.: The quest for human cancer viruses. Science, *137*:835, 1962.

15. Variot, G.: Un cas d'inoculation expérimentale des verrues de l'enfant à l'homme. J. Clin. Therap. Infant, *2*:529, 1894.

REVIEWS

16. Burdette, W. J. (ed.): Viruses Inducing Cancer. University of Utah Press, Salt Lake City, Utah, 1966.

17. Gross, L.: Oncogenic Viruses. Pergamon Press, New York, 1961.

18. Vogt, P. K.: Avian tumor viruses. *In*; Smith, K. M., and Lauffer, M. A. (eds.): Advances in Virus Research. Academic Press, New York, 1965.

63

Vaccinations Against Viral Diseases: Their Place in the Vaccination Calendar

By R. MANDE

The near absolute lack of specific therapy for viral infections makes prevention all the more important. Measures of general hygiene, moreover, have almost no effect against the viruses most widespread in developed countries. Vaccination, which induces preventively and artificially the immunity normally elicited by the infection, is hence the ideal method of defense against viral diseases.

The first two effective vaccines known were those against smallpox and rabies, i.e., viral diseases; the fact is particularly remarkable. However, after the discovery of vaccination against rabies, almost a century passed without much further progress in control of viral diseases. The possibility of growing viruses in tissue cultures (Enders) suddenly changed this situation. It provided a basis for preparation of new vaccines from which we can reasonably hope to obtain the extreme rarification of some of the most widespread viral diseases.

Three live vaccines are already in current use: those against smallpox, poliomyelitis, and measles. Vaccines against influenza and other respiratory diseases exist. A vaccine against German measles and one against mumps will soon be generally available. In short, the number of vaccinations, which is already high, is certain to increase further. The size of the arsenal makes it necessary to decide at what ages vaccines begin to be effective, the order in which they should be administered, and the possibilities of associating viral vaccines with each other and with bacterial or antitoxic vaccines. Formulation of what, by common agreement, has been called for some years a vaccination calendar has become particularly important for the vaccines to be administered during the first years of life, and especially during the first months.

The fact is that no ideal "calendar" can be established that is valid for all countries or for any country over a long period. The calendar must be adapted to the epidemiological situation in each particular country. It should be modified, within that country, in function of variations in the particular epidemiological situation and in function of the quality of the vaccinal antigens available.

RECEPTIVITY OF CHILDREN TO VIRAL INFECTIONS

Before an ideal order can be defined, two factors must be ascertained. One is the age at which the child begins to be exposed to the different infections he can be protected against. The other is the age at which the capacity to produce immunizing antibodies is on hand to respond to the different antigenic stimuli.

The receptivity of an infant to infectious diseases varies considerably with the phases of his physiological development. Pediatricians recognized long ago that the European newborn ordinarily have a substantial degree of resistance against diphtheria, poliomyelitis, and measles. These diseases are almost never seen before age three months and are exceptional before age six months. Although mumps and varicella are not common in the first three months of life, they are much more frequent. Whooping cough, on the other hand, is not a rarity during even the first weeks of life.

The infant hence seems to be born more or less completely immune to some of the commoner viral diseases. This immunity is ephemeral. Even when it was total during the first three or six months, it disappears during the second semester of life and gives way to the well known susceptibility of children to these same viral infections. Passive immunity is transmitted from mother to child. Its duration is equivalent to the time the child's organism takes to eliminate maternal gamma globulins. Such passive immunity is in no way automatic and exists only if maternal immunoglobulins had developed after either patent or inapparent infection, or vaccination. In a population in which measles, for example, is a rare disease, children born to mothers who had never been in contact with measles virus may be victims during the first weeks of life of an occasional epidemic of measles.

The receptivity of small children to poliomyelitis is a good illustration of the role of maternal antibodies. In 1960 to 1961, the question was studied[22] in 75 unvaccinated expectant mothers in the Paris area. The titer of neutralizing antibodies was less than or equal to $\frac{1}{64}$ in 43 for type I, in 32 for type II, and in 50 for type III. The antibodies enter the child's circulatory system at the titer they had reached in the mother, but their level decreases rapidly. Their average half-life is estimated to be 30 to 45 days; i.e., every 30 to 45 days the titer decreases by 50 per cent. The hypothesis was hence that 50 to 60 per cent of the children born to the 75 expectant mothers would no longer be protected against types I and III after age three months. Antibody determination in 25 of these children showed the truth of the prediction.

These data applied to the epidemiology of the disease in general suggest that a certain number of children are receptive to poliomyelitis as early as the third month of life. Study of the age distribution of cases of the disease in France during the 1957 epidemic revealed 198 (4 per cent of all cases) in children aged less than one year. Only 5 per cent were noted before age three months, but 22 per cent occurred between age three and six months. Poliomyelitis may hence be contracted during the first semester of life, and this fact spotlights the importance of beginning immunization as early as possible.

However effective the child's passive immunity may be at birth, it lasts only a few months. This early immunity is therefore not a valid argument against early vaccination. On the contrary, the temptation is to take advantage of the period in which an infant is covered by a certain immunity inherited from the mother to undertake active immunization by vaccines. Two fundamental questions arise, however. The first is whether antibody-producing capacity exists during the first months of life. The second is whether the presence of maternal antibodies in the child hinders an active immunitary response. In function of the country and the epoch, different answers to these two questions have given rise to different policies in regard to vaccination during the first months of life.

ANTIBODY-PRODUCING CAPACITY IN THE CHILD

The premise held for years was that the antibody-forming system is not fully developed at birth and matures progressively, as do many other systems and apparatuses. The date at which this system was assumed to be functionally complete has been set diversely, and perhaps a little arbitrarily. For example, in the 1940's, French law fixed the age for diphtheria and tetanus vaccination at age 18 months because of the supposed inaptitude of the child's organism to react sooner to antigenic stimuli by the vaccines in question. In fact, a great deal of recent work shows the necessity to revise this traditional position.

The normal fetus synthesizes little gamma globulin. As early as the tenth or twelfth week of intrauterine life, the child-to-be begins to receive via the placenta the principal proteins in adult blood. Among them, gamma globulins rank high. They can be detected in fetal blood at the third or fourth month. They increase progressively, and reach a level at term approximately equal to the maternal level. They comprise, among other elements, antibodies against viruses. These antibodies are transmitted individually and in variable proportions. The level of some is lower than in the mother; the levels in mother and child are sometimes identical, or the infant may have a level higher than the mother's. The mechanism of this active selection is ill known. It has received attention especially since fractionation of gamma globulins. γG globulins (sedimentation constant, 7S) traverse the placenta best; the reason seems to be linked more closely to their structure than to their low molecular weight. The γG globulins, as indicated elsewhere in this book, are the main constituent of the antibodies neutralizing viruses. The γA and γM globulins do not traverse the placenta.

After birth, the level of passively acquired γG globulins falls; their half-life is estimated at about four weeks. The newborn organism begins progressively to elaborate its own immunoglobulins in response to aggression by various infectious agents or even to vaccinal stimuli. γM globulins appear first, then γA globulins, and lastly γG globulins; the third group gradually becomes the major fraction of the immunoglobulins. Although the fetus is not ordinarily able to synthesize gamma globulins, apparently even in utero γM globulins are elaborated in response to infection (rubella, for example). Synthesis of γA and γG globulins is possible only later on, toward the second or third month after birth. The level of immunoglobulins produced in infants rises progressively and can attain the one found in adults only toward the end of the first year. An infant's antibody-forming capacity is therefore certainly less than that of adults. The traditional cautious attitude hostile to early vaccination takes account of this aspect of the problem.

What is important is that *the capacity exists*, however imperfect it may be. Over the past 15 years, numerous studies, inspired especially by a desire to protect infants as early as possible against whooping cough, have demonstrated that this capacity is real and is effective. The names of Sako, and of di Sant'agnese,[11-14] with those of their co-workers are attached to this research. Sako et al.[30] first showed that good production of agglutinins against whooping cough could be obtained by vaccination as early as the sixth week of life. Later, Goerke et al.[16] made the same discovery as concerns diphtheria and tetanus toxoids in infants who received the first injection of vaccine at age six weeks.

From all these studies, which have been repeated and the results of which have been confirmed by many authors, it is clear that as early as the sixth to the eighth week a baby reacts to the antigenic stimulus of a vaccine by an immune response. In short, he can be vaccinated.

The infant's immunological immaturity is evidenced until the third or fourth month by a weak, or sometimes an undetectable response to the first injection of a vaccine. This fact is evident in the work of Martin du Pan and Zourbas,[24] who studied the results of associated diphtheria-tetanus-pertussis vaccines in infants of various ages from birth to 16 months. Four weeks after the first injection, no agglutinin was detectable, or the titer had not increased from that in the cord blood of infants who received the initial injection during the first days of life. The titer increased slightly in infants vaccinated at age one month, and it reached $1/160$ in those more than six months old at the time of the first injection. From this study, however, as from that of Ungar[32] a supplementary conclusion emerges: although the first antigenic stimulus by a vaccine during the first weeks of life does not elicit a measurable rise in antibody level, it is not without effect.

In another study by Zourbas,[38] 82 per cent of the children who had received a first injection of whooping cough vaccine at age one month had an agglutinin level equal to or greater than $1/320$ after the third injection (i.e., during the fourth month of life). This level is generally considered to reflect good clinical protection. The work of Vahlquist and Nordbring[34] showed that some antibody production can be obtained even in premature infants, although the reaction is weaker and, especially, slower to appear than in full-term newborn infants.

It therefore certainly seems that the principle of efficacy of vaccination as early as the first months of life should be accepted, and that henceforth public health programs should be directed toward early vaccination. However, emphasis should be placed on the almost unanimous opinion of investigators that the level of antibodies obtained by vaccination during the first months drops during the second semester of life and that a booster injection given between age 12 and 18 months is indispensable.

THE INHIBITORY EFFECT OF ANTIBODIES OF MATERNAL ORIGIN

The second problem mentioned earlier (vide supra) is that of the possible inhibitory role of passive antibodies of maternal origin on active antibody formation in the infant. This inhibitory effect certainly exists, but it varies according to the quality of the vaccinal antigens. When the vaccine has strong antigenic potency, as is generally the case for toxoids, formation of active antibodies is barely affected.

Comparative dosage of antibodies in the cord blood with those in the blood of infants vaccinated during the first weeks of life is an elegant method of measuring the inhibitory effect of maternal antibodies on active immunization of the child. Goerke et al.[16] made a study of this type bearing on the possibility of immunization during the first weeks of life with diphtheria toxoid. The study was based on 42 cases. Only nine of the 42 samples revealed antitoxin either in the mother's blood or in the cord blood. In seven, antitoxin level reached 0.01 U. per cm.[3]; in 12, 0.1 U.; and in two, 1 U. per cm.[3] In 22 of the children, Goerke et al. were able to measure the antitoxin level one month after toxoid vaccination made during the first weeks of life. In 18 the level was higher than in that of the cord blood, in one it was the same, and in three it was lower. Bousfield[3] reported that in practically all children vaccinated before age six months, the Schick reaction remained negative several

years after the vaccination. Both these studies demonstrated that antitoxins of maternal origin do not notably hinder active production of antitoxins after vaccination. The same conclusion was reached in studies made by Ramon, Lelong, Richou and Rossier, Barr, Glenny and Butler, and Vahlquist.

These conclusions do not, however, hold for all vaccinal antigens. In vaccination against smallpox, poliomyelitis, and measles, maternal antibodies certainly inhibit development of active immunity in the infant.

Smallpox Vaccine. All observers agree that smallpox vaccination does not take at present during the first weeks of life as often as it did years ago, at least in countries where the vaccination is a routine practice. The fact has been established in most European countries and in North America. It has led to postponement of smallpox vaccination, once practiced shortly after birth, until the beginning of, or during the second semester or even the second year of life.

Poliomyelitis Vaccines. In vaccination against poliomyelitis, the influence of maternal antibodies is more or less clear in function of whether inactivated or live vaccines are used.

INACTIVATED VACCINE. The results of different studies with inactivated vaccines are dissimilar. Batson et al.[2] found that inactivated vaccine elicited a good immune response as early as the first months. Brown and Kendrick[5] noted an inhibitory effect of maternal antibodies on development of active antibodies. Their study, made in 1958, concerned 48 infants. An important fact is that most of the mothers had been vaccinated against poliomyelitis during their pregnancy or within the preceding two years. At the time of the first injection of vaccine between the second and fourth month of life, a high proportion of the children had detectable serum antibodies. Among the others, 18 lacked antibodies for type I, 10 for type II, and 22 for type III. The vaccination consisted in three injections at one-month intervals. Antibody determination after the end of the primary vaccination showed a low level of acquired antibodies in subjects who had had detectable antibodies before the first injection. When antibodies had been undetectable in the original test, seven of the 18 children negative for type I, nine of the 10 negative for type II, and eighteen of the 22 negative for type III acquired an acceptable level. In contrast, among the subjects who had had antibodies, only five of 30 were apparently vaccinated against type I, eight of 38 for type II, and seven of 26 for type III. The increases occurred in the subjects with the lowest levels before vaccination. When antibody titers had been high originally, they decreased or even disappeared several weeks after the third injection in some instances.

These results are particularly significant because in 1954, when the inactivated poliomyelitis vaccine had not yet entered widely into practice, Brown and Smith[7] had noted, on the contrary, a good serological response in children aged 2 to 4 months.

Comparison of the results of these two studies made at several years' interval, one before and the other after widespread use of the vaccine, shows that ability to produce antibodies against poliomyelitis exists in fact as early as the first months but that it can be more or less completely inhibited by transmitted maternal antibodies, in high titer especially.

In a more recent study Brown et al.[6] observed that development of antibodies against poliomyelitis, which is poor when an inactivated vaccine is first injected in the third month and followed up by monthly injections, is greatly enhanced when the vaccine is injected at two-month intervals. This improvement of the immune response has two explanations. When the injections are separated by two months, the last is made at age seven to eight months, i.e., at a time when immunological maturity has greatly progressed; moreover, the second and third injections occur when the level of transmitted maternal antibodies, however high it was at birth, is practically nil. One of these mechanisms or both may enter into play. The first results of the investigation concerning the rhythm of vaccinations pursued at present by the International Children's Center (Paris) also show that the response to injections of inactivated poliomyelitis vaccine initiated at age three months and continued at the rate of one injection per month is much less satisfactory than when such vaccination is begun after age six months. All these data show clearly that, at least with the current preparations of inactivated vaccine, vaccination begun in the third month of life does not give as good results as when it is begun after the sixth month.

LIVE SABIN VACCINE. The results with live Sabin vaccine are different. As early as the first weeks of life, multiplication of the vaccinal virus is detected in the intestine.[29]

This multiplication is directly influenced by the titer of maternal antibodies, and fecal excretion of the virus is inversely proportional in amount and length to the titer of maternal antibodies.[28] This implantation and multiplication of the vaccinal strain occurs in the newborn without simultaneous and automatic production of antibodies. Antibodies were detected in only 35 to 50 per cent of cases (in function of the virus type introduced).

Antibody-forming capacity rapidly improves. At age three months, the immune response to the live vaccine is entirely satisfactory and comparable to that in older children. Debré, Celers, and Drouhet[10] obtained measurable antibody levels in 90 per cent of 21 children for type I, and 100 per cent for types II and III by administering monovalent vaccines as early as the third month of life. The first results of the study by the International Children's Center on the rhythm of vaccinations showed that, in 75 children who received the first dose of trivalent Sabin vaccine at age three months and later received two further doses at six-week intervals, antibody level at age nine months was satisfactory.

Measles Vaccines. Theoretically, there is every reason to believe that the presence in infants of maternal antibodies against measles at a level sufficient to insure satisfactory immunity for the first six months of life should exert a certain interference with the production of active antibodies by vaccination during this period. With regard to the live vaccine, this inhibitory action is apparent until the sixth, or even the eighth month of life.

As concerns the inactivated vaccine, Brown[4] noted that the presence of maternal antibodies had less marked but evident inhibitory effect in children who received a first injection of the vaccine at age three months. This inhibition was inversely proportional to the titer of maternal antibodies. If the primary injection was given at age five months, a time when the level of passive antibodies has greatly diminished, the results were much better. Antibody formation occurred in 60 per cent of cases, whereas the proportion was only 28 per cent in the children who received the first injection at age three months. These considerable differences in response to the primary vaccination did not, however, reappear when a booster dose was given at age 18 months. In general, response to the booster was excellent and similar in the two groups, whether inactivated or live vaccine had been used.[18, 19] These two facts unfortunately present only theoretical interest, since the inactivated vaccine has been at least temporarily abandoned because of the reactions it causes in certain subjects on subsequent natural infection by measles or even on injection of an attenuated vaccine.

Age hence strongly influences development of antibodies when primary vaccination with an attenuated vaccine is undertaken during the first months of life. Beyond this period, Satgé et al.[31] showed that the rate of conversion (from absence to presence of antibodies) and average antibody titer are practically the same between ages eight months and one year, between ages one and two years, and past age two years. The desirable moment for vaccination with attenuated live vaccine seems to be situated before the end of the first year of life.

AGE FOR PRIMARY VACCINATIONS VERSUS MATERNAL ANTIBODIES

Presence of maternal antibodies can strongly inhibit the efficacy of vaccination against smallpox, against poliomyelitis with inactivated virus, and against measles when vaccination is undertaken during the first months of life. This fact suggests postponement of smallpox vaccination until after age six months and the advice that vaccination against poliomyelitis with inactivated virus and against measles be undertaken only during the second semester of life. On the other hand, use of Sabin live vaccine of either the monovalent or the trivalent type elicits an excellent antibody response as early as the third month of life, and vaccination can be achieved at that time. Moreover, the inhibitory effect of maternal antibodies in the child obviously varies with the antigenic potency of the vaccine. Better results could doubtless be obtained in smallpox vaccination and in poliomyelitis vaccination with inactivated virus by preparation and use of more potent vaccines.

COMBINED VACCINES

The difficulty of evaluating the efficacy of an isolated vaccine is relatively slight as compared with the problems in determining that of combined vaccines. Vaccines against viruses are already utilized in a combined form in certain instances and will shortly be utilized in others. Triple diphtheria-tetanus-poliomyelitis vaccine and a quadruple diphtheria-pertussis-tetanus-poliomyelitis (DTPP) vaccine both exist. The immune responses obtained with these different preparations are not all equally well known. The responses are also notably influenced by the age at which vaccination is begun and the intervals between injections.

In the triple diphtheria-tetanus-poliomyelitis vaccine, the poliomyelitis component yields the same results as when the inactivated poliomyelitis vaccine is used separately; the response shows neither interference between the antigens nor enhancement. The problem of the quadruple vaccine, the one of most interest to mothers, physicians, and health administrators, is much more complex and still not completely solved. To read the immunization programs adopted in certain countries might well give the impression that all the difficulties have been eliminated and that the quadruple vaccine has definitely proved its efficacy. Unfortunately, this impression does not always fit the facts.

In recent years, a great number of studies over a period of some years have emphasized the difficulty of obtaining a stable vaccine preparation that contains both pertussis and poliomyelitis antigens mixed with toxoids. Pertussis vaccine is generally considered an excellent adjuvant to diphtheria and tetanus toxoids. It does not play the same role with respect to inactivated poliomyelitis vaccine; prolonged contact between these two antigens is apparently deleterious to both of them. For this reason the quadruple vaccine has not so far been used in certain countries, among them France. Quadruple vaccination can be achieved either by injecting the triple diphtheria-tetanus-pertussis vaccine into one site and the poliomyelitis vaccine into another, or by using a two-stage syringe that makes possible successive injection of the triple vaccine and the poliomyelitis vaccine without a change in site.

Preparations of quadruple vaccine are utilized in numerous countries, particularly in the United States. Agreement is, however, far from unanimous as to their efficacy, especially in young children. For example, Barrett et al.[1a] reported the results of a controlled study made with one of the commercial vaccines most widely used in the United States. The conclusions were that, to obtain satisfactory immunization initiated at age three months, a series of four injections, rather than the usual three, was required and that the booster injection should be made six months after the end of the primary vaccination. Brown et al.[6] made a systematic study of the immunization possibilities of another quadruple vaccine used in the United States. By varying the time of the initial injection and the intervals between the various injections, they established nine trial schedules of immunization. The efficacy of the pertussis antigen in their mixture proved to be below the optimum. The most notable results were that the diphtheria and tetanus toxoids consistently elicited satisfactory reactions even when immunization was begun at age three months, whereas production of pertussis agglutinins and poliomyelitis antibodies was always poorer when the vaccination was begun at age three months than at six months. In the same series of experiments, they noted that production of agglutinins and of poliomyelitis antibodies was much more satisfactory when the interval between injections was two months instead of one. These investigators explained this difference not as a direct consequence of spacing out the injections, but by the fact that when the interval between the injections is two months, the vaccination initiated at age three months is completed at age seven months. The child hence receives the last two injections at a time when antibody-producing capacity has improved and the level of passive maternal antibodies that could inhibit elaboration of active antibodies is practically nil. Despite some years' intensive utilization of this quadruple vaccine during the first months of life, agreement that the vaccine completely fulfills its purpose is less than complete.

The difficulties inherent in a certain incompatibility between the pertussis vaccine and the inactivated poliomyelitis vaccine mixed in the same ampule may well disappear because of the increasingly widespread use of live poliomyelitis vaccine. A child can easily receive at the same time a triple diphtheria-tetanus-pertussis (DTP) vaccine by injection and poliomyelitis vaccine by mouth. This method affords proper development of the different antibodies, provided the antigens are good. A study on the rhythm of vaccinations by the International Children's Center showed that immune responses to trivalent Sabin vaccine administered orally at the same time as the triple DTP vaccine by injection are completely satisfactory: of 75 children, 97 per cent acquired antibodies for types II and III poliovirus and 90 per cent for type I.

Combination of inactivated measles vaccine with inactivated poliomyelitis, studied by Brown[4] and by Warren et al.,[35] showed that mixture of these two antigens did not modify the rate of appearance of the respective antibodies. The fact has its interest even though inactivated measles vaccine is no longer used.

SPACING OF INJECTIONS

Response to vaccines varies essentially in function of the reactive capacity in children and of the quality of the vaccinal antigens, but it is also influenced by the rhythm of administration of vaccines. An interval of less than three weeks between two injections is universally accepted to be insufficient: it does not permit the second dose to produce an adequate antigenic stimulus. Studies that permit specification of the optimal interval between doses are few indeed, however, as are those that reveal whether the interval between the first two injections should be the same as between the second and the third. Most countries have adopted an average interval of one month between each of the three injections. For this reason most studies on vaccination against various pathogens during recent years have utilized the same interval. The opinion is general that, on the average, it permits good production of antibodies. The possibility nonetheless exists that this rhythm should be varied in function of different periods in life, as the results of the study by Brown et al.[6] mentioned earlier strongly suggest.

The fact likewise seems well established that, whereas the interval between the first dose of a vaccine and the second must not be too long (not over a maximum of eight weeks), the interval between the second dose and the third can be much longer. Thus in the United States and many other countries, the interval between the second and third injection of inactivated poliomyelitis vaccine was fixed at six months.

On this precise subject of the optimal interval between injections of a vaccine, the programs adopted arise mainly from a heavy dose of empiricism. Many points need to be specifically elucidated that can be thoroughly studied in only large-scale investigations by use of different schedules of immunization and of control groups. Such study, which necessitates a large number of blood samples from very small children, is difficult to carry out. At present the International Children's

Center is investigating the intervals for vaccinations during the first year of life. The data collected during this study will provide a degree of precision that has so far been lacking.

BOOSTER INJECTIONS

Inactivated Virus Vaccines. Whatever the age at which vaccination was begun and the intervals between injections, one fact is certain and of fundamental importance: during the year that follows the primary vaccination, a booster injection must be given. The idea should be anchored firmly that all vaccination is incomplete, and therefore has every chance of being at least partially ineffective, unless it includes a booster. The current tendency, remarked earlier as regards the work of Barrett et al., is to advance the date of booster injection after a primary vaccination initiated at age three months. The booster consistently elicits a manifest increase in antibody level. Usually the immunity so obtained lasts several years. It does not, however, last a lifetime. Boosters at five-year intervals are indicated until age 21 years.

Attenuated Live Virus Vaccines. The approach to the problem is somewhat different with attenuated live virus vaccines. The need for boosters depends not only on the antigenic potency of the vaccine used, but on the immunological and epidemiological characteristics of the infection it creates, and of the one that it helps to combat when the two infections are not identical as, for example, vaccinia and smallpox.

SMALLPOX VACCINATION. Revaccination is practiced in many countries every five or ten years until age 21 years. Further revaccination is practiced during an epidemic or before a trip into an endemic area.

ORAL VACCINATION AGAINST POLIOMYELITIS. With attenuated live virus vaccine, the utility of a booster during the year that follows the three doses of trivalent vaccine given at correct intervals is debated. The immunity conferred by effective primary vaccination persists at least four years. If this immunity is sufficiently high, it can hinder a revaccination practiced too close to the primary series. Nonetheless, in absence of systematic verification of the titer of neutralizing antibodies against poliomyelitis in each individual, which is difficult, this first booster dose should be given. It enhances the low levels of antibodies that occur in some subjects and completes the vaccination when one

of the three poliovirus types has not taken effect previously. Later on, the trivalent oral vaccine must be taken every five years until age 21 years. Supplementary vaccination is required during epidemic periods or on travel in endemic areas.

HYPERATTENUATED MEASLES VACCINE. How the immunity to measles conferred by hyperattenuated live vaccine evolves is not yet known thoroughly enough for a rhythm of booster injections to be established. Antibodies seem to persist at an effective level for several years. There is hence no reason to give a booster dose during the first year following the primary vaccination.

SIDE EFFECTS

The child's reaction to vaccines, and the incidents or accidents to which vaccination gives rise at different times in life, are factors to be taken into consideration before setting up a vaccination schedule.

Poliomyelitis Vaccine. Whether live attenuated virus or an inactivated vaccine is utilized, vaccination against poliomyelitis is always well tolerated at whatever age.

Hyperattenuated Measles Vaccine. The vaccination always elicits a substantially similar type of reaction. However, more numerous febrile and systemic reactions have been seen among young children who live in collective conditions than in those of the same age (one to four years) who live in families.[22] These incidents seem to be due to the greater diffusion in institutions and the like of other acute viral infections that become manifest after vaccination among children in this type of environment. If the phenomenon is not accidental, it should lead to vaccination of children living under such circumstances by small groups rather than to change in the age for vaccination.

Smallpox Vaccination. In vaccination against smallpox the question of age in relation to side effects is of particular importance. The generally accepted view until fairly recently was that postvaccinial encephalitis was extremely rare or never occurred during the first year of life and was exceptional before age eighteen months. Practically all cases were thought to follow late vaccinations, i.e., involved children vaccinated for the first time after age two. This traditional idea has been contested in Great Britain, where study of administrative documents collected between 1951 and 1957 showed that the percentage of encephalitis was clearly higher during the first year of life than between age one and two years. According to the figures cited by Conybeare,[8] the incidence of diseases of the central nervous system before age one was 1.46 per 100,000 vaccinations, whereas it was 0.33 per 100,000 between age one year and age two.

These data were behind the flexible attitude adopted during a symposium on vaccination held in London in 1959. The symposium indicated simply that the initial smallpox vaccination should be effectuated during the first five years of life. Parish,[24] who was secretary of this meeting, however, estimated that the majority of English physicians continued to vaccinate against smallpox between age five months and six months. This age is currently recommended in most countries. For the moment, there is no decisive evidence that vaccination at other times is less dangerous. Nothing is, in fact, more difficult than to affirm a posteriori the legitimacy of a diagnosis of vaccinial encephalitis. Moreover, conclusions drawn from observations in this matter in Great Britain cannot be transposed per se to all countries. Smallpox vaccination is not compulsory in Great Britain; it is practiced less systematically than in many other European countries. For example, the better protection of French children against encephalitis during the first year of life may arise from the fact that most of them inherit partial immunity from their mothers, who have been vaccinated.

The English figures in this matter show that epidemiological data are changeable and should be frequently revised. Investigations in the United States[24a, 24b] confirmed that postvaccinal encephalitis occurred more often in the second semester of life.[1] For the moment similar data have not been reported elsewhere. The wiser policy hence seems to be to continue to vaccinate against smallpox, at least in countries where the entire population is generally vaccinated, between age six months and seven. At this age the child has lost maternal antibody protection but still seems to be well enough protected against the cerebral complications of the vaccination.

EPIDEMIOLOGY AND SANITATION

THE BASIC CONCEPTS

The points discussed earlier make it possible to establish a vaccination calendar

in consideration of the child's capacity for immunization and the antigenic potency of different viral vaccines, utilized separately or in combination. The fundamentals also compromise not only the epidemiology of viral diseases in different countries, but the country's budgetary possibilities, and the equipment of its health services. The epidemiological pattern creates imperatives. Poliomyelitis represents a danger from the end of the first year of life in all children. The same is not true of measles, for instance. Whereas measles is a serious and a frequent disease in infancy south of the Sahara in Africa, it occurs at a later period and is usually benign in Europe, for example. The place to be reserved for poliomyelitis vaccination ought to be similar, within the limits of feasibility, whatever the country, but in Africa vaccination against measles demands a priority. In western Europe and North America, whooping cough represents the most serious danger today during the first months of life. The fact accounts for the pediatrician's desire to vaccinate against whooping cough at the earliest age possible, by a single vaccine or one associated with toxoids, in conjunction with live poliomyelitis vaccine or not.

In certain cases the epidemiological patterns of a disease may influence less imperatively the age for vaccination than the fact that the dangerous consequences of the disease occur only at certain times in life. Rubella is a characteristic example. The possibility of vaccination against rubella doubtless will soon be available everywhere, but it is useless to incorporate immunization against this disease early in the vaccination calendar. Rubella is so consistently benign in children that its prevention during childhood is not an objective: the disease confers solid lifelong immunity, whereas vaccination has not been proved to confer as durable an immunity or as solid a defense. Moreover, rubella presents no danger to boys. It therefore seems desirable during the early years of study at least, to confine systematic vaccination against rubella to girls at puberty.

The possibilities of practical application obviously play a considerable role in the programming of an ideal vaccination calendar in general. It would be utopic to imagine that the same program is applicable to countries presenting widely different conditions. It seems more reasonable to propose two models of a vaccination calendar, one adapted to well equipped countries, the other to the developing countries with inadequate health services.

Vaccinations against viral diseases, it should be remembered, are part of the general program into which other vaccinations by toxoids and microbian vaccines must be integrated. The possibility of administering several vaccines at once should receive hospitable consideration everywhere, but especially in ill equipped countries.

The place to be reserved for vaccinations against bacterial diseases is subject to the same variations. Vaccination against tuberculosis is a good example. In many countries, tuberculosis continues to be a serious menace as early as the first months of life. In such countries BCG should be administered as soon as possible after birth. In other countries with a much lower morbidity rate for tuberculosis, vaccination can well be postponed until the age when the child enters school (Denmark) or leaves school (Norway and Great Britain). In countries where smallpox is still endemic, the same imperatives govern smallpox vaccination. Association of BCG with smallpox vaccination has long been hoped for by many developing countries. The studies of Balthazar, Machoun, Sabeti and Siadat, and that of Huang in Formosa for W.H.O. have shown that this association is not dangerous and that the two vaccines produce their usual effects.

IDEAL ORDER

Schedules Applicable in Countries with Adequate Public Health Facilities. The schedule in Table 63-1 represents the ideal order in general currently desirable, but it supposes the availability of good antigens and a good medicosocial infrastructure.

BCG can be given at birth or during the first weeks of life if the morbidity rate of tuberculosis is high. If not, it should be put off until after the end of the first series of vaccinations, until schooling starts, or until the end of schooling, in function of the prevalence of tuberculosis in the population under consideration. Between ages three and five months, injection of diphtheria-pertussis-tetanus vaccine (preferably adsorbed) is advisable and effective. Three doses of live trivalent poliomyelitis vaccine can be given during the same period at six-week intervals. Smallpox vaccination has its place in the program toward the sixth month. Between ages seven and nine months, if the child has not

Table 63-1. *Proposed Schedule for Countries or Regions with Adequate Public Health Facilities*

AGE	IMMUNIZATION
First days of life	BCG vaccination
3 4 months 5	Triple vaccination: diphtheria-tetanus-pertussis vaccine + three oral doses of trivalent live poliomyelitis vaccine at six-week intervals
6 to 7 months	Smallpox vaccination
8 9 months 10	Poliomyelitis vaccination with inactivated virus if live vaccine not utilized earlier Hyperattenuated live measles vaccine in the tenth month
11 to 12 months	BCG if not received at birth
15 months to 2 years	*One year after the initial vaccination:* Booster injection of diphtheria-tetanus-pertussis vaccine Another oral dose of live attenuated trivalent poliomyelitis vaccine *or* Booster injection of inactivated poliomyelitis vaccine
6 years	BCG if not received earlier Booster injection of diphtheria-tetanus-inactivated poliomyelitis vaccine *or* Diphtheria-tetanus-pertussis + another dose of live trivalent poliomyelitis vaccine
10 years	Smallpox revaccination
11 years	Diphtheria-tetanus-inactivated poliomyelitis vaccine booster *or* Diphtheria-tetanus booster + live trivalent poliomyelitis vaccine
16 years	Booster injection of tetanus-inactivated poliomyelitis vaccine *or* Tetanus booster + another dose of live trivalent poliomyelitis vaccine
21 years	As at age 16 years, boosters

been vaccinated earlier against poliomyelitis, three doses of oral vaccine or three injections of inactivated vaccine yield excellent protection. Administration of hyperattenuated live vaccine against measles is absolutely required toward age ten months in countries where measles is a serious hazard. Whatever the country, it is also indicated for children with bronchopulmonary malformations, asthma, mucoviscidosis, or any other cause of respiratory tract fragility. Adherence to this schedule means that, before the end of the first year of life, the child has received all the principal vaccines.

These primary vaccinations, however, are never sufficient. They must always be complemented, or rather completed, by a booster injection during the second year of life. Between age 15 months and two years, the child should receive an injection of triple diphtheria-tetanus-pertussis vaccine and a dose of trivalent Sabin vaccine, or an injection of the triple DTP vaccine with inactivated poliomyelitis vaccine conjointly.

At age six and eleven years, another booster of triple vaccine associated with another dose of trivalent Sabin vaccine or a booster dose of quadruple vaccine is indicated. At age sixteen years, the diphtheria toxoid component in vaccination is abandoned in certain countries, whereas in others it is not. In accord with national practice, diphtheria and tetanus toxoids in combination, or tetanus toxoid alone, is injected. Inactivated poliomyelitis vaccine can be associated with either preparation. If trivalent Sabin vaccine is preferred, a booster dose of oral vaccine is indicated. Although smallpox revaccination is required every three years by international regulations within certain countries, France among them, it is recommended only at age 10 and 20 years.

IDEAL ORDER AND REALITY: GUIDE TO PRACTICE AND COMPROMISE

Programs in Developing Countries. *In ill equipped countries, such a program obviously cannot be executed. The schedule represented in Table 63-2 was proposed during a W.H.O. Experts' meeting in 1966.*[41] It differs from the first only by greater intervals between the injections, by decrease in the number of injections of diphtheria-tetanus-pertussis associated vaccine, reduced from three to two, and by the limitation of the number of booster injections.

Such a program is still, in fact, beyond the possibilities of many poorly equipped countries. In some of them it is applied to children in large centers of population where a mother-and-child welfare organization operates. In rural areas, however, the density of health service personnel is much too low to permit regular application of even a simplified program of this type. Naturally, to

Table 63-2. *Proposed Schedule for Countries with Inadequate Public Health Facilities*

AGE	IMMUNIZATION
0-1 month	BCG vaccination
3 to 6 months	Simultaneous administration of smallpox vaccine and first dose of alum-adsorbed diphtheria-pertussis-tetanus (DPT) triple vaccine Second dose of DPT triple vaccine, one to three months after first dose First dose of oral poliomyelitis vaccine
6 to 12 months	Second dose of oral poliomyelitis vaccine Live, hyperattenuated measles vaccine
5 to 6 years	Booster dose of diphtheria-tetanus vaccine Simultaneous smallpox vaccination

adhere as closely as possible to the schedule is manifestly desirable. When, as is often the case, vaccinations can be administered only by itinerant teams, the schedule inevitably is governed primarily by the possibility to displace the team under the given circumstances and not by the age of the child. Thus the various immunizations recommended in Table 63-2 during the first semester of life may be delayed by circumstance until age three years or even six, according to the sector. In such situations, the great desirability of *associated vaccinations* is evident. Simultaneous vaccination with BCG and smallpox vaccine, combined vaccine against yellow fever and smallpox (used currently in French-speaking West Africa), and the more recent formula associating vaccines against yellow fever, smallpox, and measles have been studied in countries with this type of problem.

In many of these countries, the *hierarchy of dangers* often differs from that in Europe and in North America. The result is a change in order of vaccinations. In Africa south of the Sahara, vaccination against smallpox and measles usually requires a priority over that against diphtheria and tetanus.

In insufficiently equipped countries, as elsewhere, primary vaccination does not always confer lasting immunity. *Periodic booster injections* must be given; usually they are possible only during itinerant campaigns by polyvalent teams.

Another aspect of immunization programs must be taken seriously into account in countries where regular, for example annual, vaccination is impossible. Part of the population remains unvaccinated and constitutes a permanent reservoir of pathogenic viruses. In countries where vaccinations can be administered regularly every year to all children, progressive disappearance of the virus reservoir is a highly important epidemiological fact that makes a significant contribution to the total effect of vaccination.

Another difficulty arises in tropical countries, most of which are inadequately equipped. It concerns vaccination against poliomyelitis, in particular. Infections by other enteroviruses are extremely frequent, and they interfere with the implantation of live vaccine strains in the subject to be vaccinated.

In such countries, where the public health infrastructure is ill proportioned to need, execution of coherent programs of immunization is handicapped by numerous difficulties. Such programs nonetheless constitute one of the least debatable of priorities. It is hence desirable that the authorities responsible for public health fully understand the importance of this priority and that they find possibilities of assistance from international organizations.

Special Cases

The vaccination calendars in which the program is established in function of public health equipment, and of the epidemiological and immunological situation generally prevalent in each country or group of countries sometimes need to be supplemented by so-called exceptional vaccination. The indications may be of a purely individual character, or are collective. Examples are the particular sensitivity of certain patients to an infectious disease, and unusual epidemiological circumstances, as when a virus suddenly spreads into a region ordinarily free of it, or when travel brings people into areas where the endemic viruses are different from those in their country of origin.

During the wait for instauration of more extensive prophylaxis of viral respiratory diseases,[15, 20, 36] vaccination against influenza is especially opportune in certain categories of patients. The vaccine should be capable of reinforcing previously acquired immunity and of eliciting antibodies specific for the strain prevalent at the time of vaccination (cf. Chapter 39). It is formally indicated for certain subjects with chronic diseases: cardiopathy, mucoviscidosis, chronic pulmonary diseases, and respiratory insufficiency of neurological or muscular origin.

We mentioned earlier the problem of vaccination against rubella. Vaccination against mumps could be recommended for young men assembled in conditions of collective living, for example, in military personnel known to be receptive to mumps (cf. Chapter 23).

In face of the threat of a smallpox epidemic, the imperative indication for smallpox vaccination (cf. Chapter 31) comes to every physician's mind, as does the necessity to revaccinate any person planning a trip into an endemic area. This revaccination against smallpox should be associated with a booster against poliomyelitis and, for travelers to tropical Africa and South America, with yellow fever vaccination.

Aside from the immunoprophylactic treatment given after rabies infection, which prevents the disease when the incubation period is long enough, systematic vaccination of high-risk groups is under consideration in certain countries, including the United States (cf. Chapter 10).

THE PRESENT AND THE FUTURE

The different types of calendar proposed or considered here can represent only *a guideline as to desirable policies of immunization in a given country or group of countries, valid for a certain epoch, and with certain types of vaccines.* Discoveries and improvements rapidly follow one another in this field in our time, and calendars, it must be admitted, are soon out-of-date. Nonetheless, the idea that a certain preferential order must be respected retains its validity. Many fundamental points still need to be more exactly determined. Attempts to define immunization policy should be based in the future on more precise knowledge of the child's ability to acquire immunity in function of the age at which vaccination is begun, the nature of the antigens and their various associations, the order in which they are administered, and the interval between different vaccinations. Elucidation of these problems is the aim of study that is being pursued by the International Children's Center.

BIBLIOGRAPHY

1. American Academy of Pediatrics. Report on the Control of Infectious Diseases, 1966.

1a. Barrett, C. D., et al.: Multiple antigen immunization of infants against poliomyelitis, diphtheria, pertussis and tetanus. Pediatrics, *30*:720-736, 1962.

2. Batson, R., et al.: Response of the young infant to poliomyelitis vaccine given separately and combined with other antigens. Pediatrics, *21*:1-7, 1958.

3. Bousfield, G.: Combined immunization against diphtheria and whooping-cough in infants aged 2-5 months. Brit. Med. J., *2*:1216, 1957.

4. Brown, G. C.: Immunologic response of infants to combined inactivated measles-poliomyelitis vaccine. Arch. Ges. Virusforsch., *16*:353-357, 1965.

5. Brown, G. C., and Kendrick, P. L.: Réponse sérologique des nourrissons vaccinés simultanément contre la diphtérie, le tétanos, la coqueluche et la poliomyélite en fonction de la présence d'anticorps spécifiques d'origine maternelle. In: Calendrier des vaccinations. Paris, Masson et Cie, 1960, pp. 131-143.

6. Brown, G. C., et al.: Responses of infants to D.T.P.-P. vaccine used in nine injection schedules. Public Health Rep., *79*:585-602, 1964.

7. Brown, G. C., and Smith, D. C.: Serologic response of infants and preschool children to poliomyelitis vaccine. J.A.M.A., *161*:399-403, 1950.

8. Conybeare, E. T.: Illness attributed to smallpox vaccination during 1951-1960. 1. Illnesses reported as "generalized vaccinia." 2. Illnesses reported as affecting the central nervous system. Monthly Bull. Minist. Health, *23*:126-133, 150-159, 1964.

9. Debré, R.: Vaccinations. In: Journées de Pédiatrie. Paris, Lanord, 1958, pp. 227-237.

10. Debré, R., Celers, J., and Drouhet, V.: Vaccination antipoliomyélitique par voie orale avec le vaccin à virus atténués (souches Sabin) à partir de l'âge de 3 mois. C. R. Acad. Sci. (Paris), *254*:195-199, 1963.

11. di Sant'agnese, P. A.: Combined immunization against diphtheria, tetanus and pertussis in newborn infants; production of antibodies in early infancy. Pediatrics, *3*:20-33, 1949.

12. di Sant'agnese, P. A.: Combined immunization against diphtheria, tetanus and pertussis in newborn infants; duration of antibody levels; antibody titers after booster dose; effect of passive immunity to diphtheria on active immunization with diphtheria toxoid. Pediatrics, *3*:181-194, 1949.

13. di Sant'agnese, P. A.: Combined immunization against diphtheria, tetanus and pertussis in newborn infants; relationship of age to antibody formation. Pediatrics, *3*:333-343, 1949.

14. di Sant'agnese, P. A.: Simultaneous immunization of newborn against D.T.P. Amer. J. Public Health, *40*:674-680, 1950.

15. Fulginiti, V. A., Amer, J., Eller, J. J., Joyner, J. W., and Askin, P.: Parainfluenza virus immunization. IV. Simultaneous immunization with parainfluenza types 1, 2 and 3 aqueous vaccines. Amer. J. Dis. Child., *114*:26-28, 1967.

16. Goerke, L. S., et al.: Neo-natal responses to D.T.P. vaccines. Public Health Rep., *73*:511-518, 1958.

17. Janeway, C. A.: The immunological system of the child. I. Development of immunity in the child. II. Immunological deficiency states. Arch. Dis. Child., *41*:358-374, 1966.

18. Karelitz, S., Schluederberg, A., et al.: Killed measles vaccine prior to seven months of age followed by attenuated live virus vaccine at nine months. Arch. Ges. Virusforsch., *16*:343-346, 1965.

19. Krugman, S.: Measles immunization: combined vaccinations. Arch. Ges. Virusforsch., *16*:339-342, 1965.

20. Leagus, M. B., Weibel, R. E., Mascoli, C. C., Stokes, J., Jr., and Hilleman, M. R.: Respiratory virus vaccines. VI. Serologic responses to heptavalent vaccine among young children in families. Amer. Rev. Resp. Dis., *95*:838-844, 1957.

21. Mande, R.: Données fondamentales pour l'établissement d'un calendrier des vaccinations chez l'enfant. Rev. Immun. (Paris), *21B*:225-264, 1960.

22. Mande, R., Jammet, M. L., Celers, J., and Boué, A.: A propos de la vaccination contre la rougeole. Résultats des premiers essais de vaccination antimorbilleuse en France avec le vaccin à virus vivant hyperatténué (souche Schwarz). Ann. Pédiat. (Paris), *1*:66-73, 1967.

23. Mayer, M., Raimbault, G., Morali-Daninos, A., Ducas, P., Celers, J., Drouhet, V., and Boué, A.: Transmission de l'immunité spontanée antipoliomyélitique de la mère à l'enfant. Sa durée et son incidence sur l'immunisation vaccinale. Presse Méd., *19*:961-962, 1963.

24. Martin du Pan, R., and Zourbas, J.: La vaccination anticoquelucheuse chez le nourrisson. Praxis, *46*: 24-30, 1957.

24a. Neff, J. M., Lane, J. M., Pert, J. H., Moore, H., Millar, J. D., and Henderson, D. A.: Complications of smallpox vaccination. I. National survey in the United States. New Eng. J. Med., *276*:125-132, 1967.

24b. Neff, J. M., Levine, R. H., Lane, J. M., Ager, E. A., Moore, H., Rosenstein, B. J., Millar, J. D., and Henderson, D. A.: Complications of smallpox vaccination in the United States 1963. 2. Results obtained by four statewide surveys. Pediatrics, *39*:916-923, 1967.

25. Parish, H. J.: Calendrier des vaccinations en Grande-Bretagne. In: Calendrier des vaccinations. Paris, Masson et Cie, 1960, pp. 305-310.

26. Preston, N. W.: Effectiveness of pertussis vaccine. Brit. Med. J., *2*:11-13, 1965.

27. Ramon, G., Lelong, M., Richou, E., and Rossier, A.: La vaccination antidiphtérique réalisée dans différentes conditions chez l'enfant et en particulier chez le nourrisson de moins de 1 an, ses résultats. Rev. Immun. (Paris), *14*:1-8, 1950.

28. Sabin, A. B., et al.: Live, orally given poliovirus vaccine. Effects of rapid mass immunization on population under conditions of massive enteric infection with other viruses. J.A.M.A., *173*:1521-1526, 1960.

29. Sabin, A. B., et al.: Effect of oral poliovirus vaccine in newborn children. 1. Excretion of virus after ingestion of large doses of type 1 or of mixture of all 3 types, in relation to level of placentally transmitted antibody. 2. Intestinal resistance and antibody response at 6 months in children fed type 1 vaccine at birth. Pediatrics, *31*:623-640, 641-650, 1963.

30. Sako, W., et al.: Early immunization against pertussis with alum-precipitated vaccine. J.A.M.A., *127*:379, 1945.

31. Satgé, P., Baylet, R., et al.: Possibilités d'utilisation du vaccin rougeoleux inactivé en association. Arch. Ges. Virusforsch., *16*:358-365, 1965.

32. Ungar, J.: Réponse sérologique à la vaccination anti-

coquelucheuse chez les enfants. La coqueluche. Séminaire du Centre International de l'Enfance. Paris, Masson et Cie, 1959, pp. 65-79.

33. Vahlquist, B.: Vaccination systématique des nourrissons avec un vaccin associé. Etude sérologique et clinique. La coqueluche. Séminaire du Centre International de l'Enfance. Paris, Masson et Cie, 1959, pp. 168-182.

34. Vahlquist, B., and Nordbring, F.: Studies on diphtheria. The effect of diphtheria immunization of newborn prematures. Acta Paediat., *41*:53-56, 1952.

35. Warren, J., Feldman, H. A., et al.: The response of children to combined measles-poliomyelitis vaccine. J.A.M.A., *186*:533-536, 1963.

36. Weibel, R. E., Stokes, J., Jr., Mascoli, C. C., Leagus, M. B., Woodhous, A. F., Tytell, A. C., Vella, P. P., and Hilleman, M. R.: Respiratory virus vaccines. VII. Field evaluation of respiratory syncytial, parainfluenza 1, 2, 3 and Mycoplasma pneumoniae vaccines, 1965 to 1966. Amer. Rev. Resp. Dis., *96*:724-739, 1967.

37. Winter, P. A.: Combined immunization against poliomyelitis, diphtheria, whooping cough, tetanus and smallpox. S. Afr. Med. J., *19*:513-515, 1963.

38. Zourbas, J.: Etude immunologique et épidémiologique des nourrissons immunisés à l'aide de différents vaccins anticoquelucheux simples ou associés. La coqueluche. Séminaire du Centre International de l'Enfance. Paris, Masson et Cie, 1959, pp. 124-167.

39. Séminaire sur le Calendrier des Vaccinations organisé par le Centre International de l'Enfance. Rev. Immun. (Paris), vol. 24, no. 1-2, 1960.

40. Conférence sur la lutte contre les maladies infectieuses par les programmes de vaccination. World Health Organization, Rabat, 23-31 Oct., 1959.

41. Symposium de l'OMS sur les maladies à virus, Moscou. WHO Chron., *20*:494-500, 1966.

Index

Numbers in *italics* refer to illustrations; (t) refers to tables.